America's Best Hospitals

America's Best Hospitals

The Editors of *U.S.News & World Report*

With the National Opinion Research Center at the University of Chicago

JOHN WILEY & SONS, INC.

New York / Chichester / Brisbane / Toronto / Singapore

Library of Congress Cataloging in Publication Data:
America's Best Hospitals/U.S.News & World Report—0–471–12614–4

Printed in the United States of America

10 9 8 7 6 5 4 3 2 1

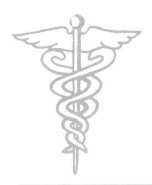

Contributors

Editor: Avery Comarow

Writers: Susan Brink, Doug Podolsky, Rita Rubin

Research: Elizabeth Mueller Gross

Production: Karen S. Chevalier, Stephanie Sisle, Janie S. Price, Mark O. Emerson, Lowell Vitangcol, Kathleen Phillips

Coordinator: Katherine T. Beddingfield

Rankings design: Sarah Shaw

Rankings methodology: Craig Hill and Krishna Winfrey at the National Opinion Research Center

ACKNOWLEDGMENTS

"How in God's name is anybody supposed to know what hospital to go to?" *U.S.News & World Report* Editor-in-Chief Mortimer B. Zuckerman asked one day in 1988. It was a provocative question without an answer—then. The one-of-a-kind rankings his question inspired have now appeared in the magazine annually for six years. The latest version forms the foundation of this book—which you would not now be reading had it not been for Executive Editor Peter Bernstein's encouragement and advice. In addition, Co-editors Michael Ruby and Merrill McLoughlin were unfailingly supportive. Kathryn Bushkin and Gail Lione at *U.S. News* carefully maneuvered the project around numerous black holes.

The good thinkers at the National Opinion Research Center (NORC) at the University of Chicago have been invaluable partners since 1991. NORC Senior Analyst Craig Hill and his former colleague, Analyst Barbara Rudolph, coached by Senior Vice-President Norman Bradburn, created the ground-breaking methodology behind the *U.S. News* rankings. Analyst Krishna Winfrey joined the NORC team for the latest rankings and quickly became indispensable. NORC has indefatigably refined the methodology every year to make the rankings even more credible.

To Susan Barry, the John Wiley & Sons editor who envisioned a book in the *U.S. News* rankings and made others see it, too, heartfelt thanks. Thanks go as well to Myles Thompson, Erika Pendleton, Janice Weisner, and Jody Siegartel at John Wiley for their patience and inspiration.

An immeasurable debt is owed the hundreds of readers who have called and written over the years to keep us on course. You have let us know how you or someone you love turned to the rankings in time of need. You have entrusted us with stories both tragic and inspiring. And you have suggested, always with astonishing deference, countless ways in which the rankings might be improved. Over and over, you have shown us the importance of Mort Zuckerman's question.

—AVERY COMAROW, EDITOR
America's Best Hospitals

||...||..||.||.||.||.||.||..|..||.|||.||.|.|.|||..||.|||..||.||.| ********************************** 3-DIGIT 078

NANCY T REILLY
RR 1 BX
GREAT MEADOWS   NJ   07838-9801   12

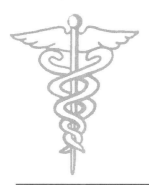

Preface

On a warm spring evening in 1983, I found myself on my back in a hospital bed, facing a decision I was ill equipped and far from willing to make. A dye had been squirted a few hours before through my heart's coronary arteries that made blockages easy to see in X rays—blockages that had been wrapping my chest in an excruciating hug several mornings a week. The results had come back. I needed coronary artery bypass surgery, said my doctor. I could have the surgery done anywhere I wanted.

The local newspaper had reported a few years before that the large teaching hospital in which I was a temporary resident had less than a sterling reputation for heart surgery. About five percent of bypass patients died, a rate four or five times higher than the acceptable benchmark. But I trusted my doctor. "What would you do?" I asked him. "What would you say if your wife or father or daughter were in this bed?"

"I would tell them to come here," he answered unhesitatingly. "A new chief of cardiac surgery was hired recently, and he has recruited a fine young surgeon to work with him."

The young surgeon came to my room to discuss the surgery, obviously exhausted—I learned later that he had performed three major operations that day. He radiated a quiet confidence that inspired faith, but first I had a question: Had he ever lost a patient whose age and medical profile were similar to mine?

Never, he answered, squarely meeting my eyes and calming my apprehension. And today, more than 12 years later, I am quite literally living evidence that my faith in Dr. Nevin Katz was not misplaced. His needle-point on my heart returned me to an entirely normal life, and then some—a marriage now in its 27th year, children on the verge of adulthood, newfound physical discipline that allowed me to finish three marathons.

This personal tale has two messages. The first and most important is: Ask questions, many questions, when your life and health are on the line. And do not forget to ask: "Doctor, how have you done with patients like me?"

The other message is that a guide to the nation's hospitals would have kept me anchored and given me perspective, had a publication of this type existed back then. In 1990, such a guide became available. *America's Best Hospitals*, a special issue published annually ever since by *U.S.News & World Report*, is aimed at patients like the one in that hospital bed on that warm spring evening—frightened and looking for credible information.

This book grew out of the *U.S. News* project. If it falls to you to consult it, my hope is that it blunts your fears and contributes in a small way to the renewed health of you or someone you love.

—AVERY COMAROW, EDITOR
America's Best Hospitals

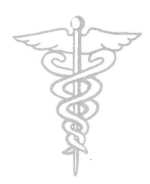

Contents

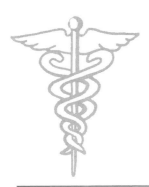

Introduction

America's hospitals are in a Darwinian struggle to survive. They are merging, consolidating, downsizing, forging alliances, diversifying—anything to avoid going the way of the dinosaur. Even the elite among the nation's 1,631 tertiary-care hospitals, universally respected for the kind of cutting-edge, high-technology care that brings royalty, sheiks, and movie stars to their doors, face the woes of empty beds and budget shortfalls.

A massive shift to managed care is largely responsible for this struggle because of a new emphasis on cost control. The change has been wrenching, with shorter hospital stays and fewer choices for patients and greater numbers of empty beds for hospitals. In 1994, the country's hospitals filled only about 60 percent of their available beds, down from 69 percent 10 years earlier.

To make up for the loss of acute-care patients, hospitals have branched out. In 1985, only 54 percent of hospitals offered outpatient services like ambulatory-care centers and outpatient surgery centers. By 1992, the latest year about which information is available, 89 percent of hospitals had such services. In 1983, 24 percent of surgeries in community hospitals were outpatient procedures; by 1993, 55 percent of all surgeries were. Rather than watch patients slip away into other settings, hospitals are setting up birthing centers, outpatient surgery centers, and home health-delivery organizations.

The institutional giants that once competed in major cities are uniting to achieve economies of scale and to avoid duplicating services and technologies. Massachusetts General Hospital and Brigham and Women's Hospital in Boston, for instance, are now affiliated. In St. Louis, Barnes Hospital, Children's Hospital and Jewish Hospital, acute-care teaching hospitals a block apart, became one and soon after brought in Christian Health Services, a suburban network of hospitals. In a blockbuster merger of for-profit hospitals, Columbia Health Care Corporation bought the Hospital Corporation of America, creating a system of 192 hospitals under one corporate roof.

FREE SPENDING? NO MORE

The belt-tightening of the 1990s is a far cry from the free-spending ways sparked by Medicare's passage in 1965. Cost-based reimbursement assured that when a physician or hospital submitted a bill, the government program would pay a set percentage of it, no matter what the procedures or how long the care took. Hospitals could count on a steady income with few questions asked. Teaching hospitals blossomed, with high-ticket items like organ transplants and assorted cardiac procedures augmented by a growing arsenal of high-technology instruments.

Then came the 1980s and a move to slow down escalating health care costs. Medicare switched to diagnosis related groups, or DRGs, to compute payment. The government would pay a fixed sum for a specific diagnosis—and no more. If the hospital could perform the service for less, it could keep the change. But if a patient's care cost more, the hospital would eat the loss. At the same time, the private insurance sector began marching toward capitated payment. Every year, physician groups, managed-care plans, and hospitals would receive a total sum based on the number of patients expected to come through the door over the course of the year and the services they would need. If doctors and hospitals could serve their patient load for less than the annual sum of the capitated payments, all would prosper. If not, they would run a loss.

Payment incentives were abruptly thrown into reverse. Doctors and hospitals felt pressured to shorten hospital stays and perform fewer tests and procedures. Yet medical ethics, the Hippocratic Oath, and even the bottom line still encourage the traditional goal of high-quality, uncomplicated care. A patient diagnosed and treated early and successfully is a lower-cost patient than one whose disease has been allowed to progress. And complications caused by inadequate care are costly.

YARDSTICKS WANTED

To help inform all medical consumers, from individuals to the employers who provide health coverage and the insurers who pay for it, experts have been pressing for yardsticks that measure hospital quality. They are coming—slowly. The Joint Commission on Accreditation of Healthcare Organizations (JCAHO), the major accrediting body for hospitals, nursing homes, and mental-health, ambulatory-care, and long-term care facilities, has begun releasing information from its surveys; information on nearly a quarter of hospitals is available. Checking out a hospital or two doesn't come cheap, however. A four-page performance report for one hospital, with accompanying explanation, costs $30. In a few years, the JCAHO plans to be able to tell consumers how well patients actually fare in various procedures—the percentage of patients who survive quadruple bypass surgery or deliver vaginally after having a cesarean section, for example.

The National Committee for Quality Assurance, which accredits health maintenance organizations

(HMOs), has conducted a pilot study of 21 HMOs, using standardized measures of performance. But the committee had to manually gather much of the information they needed, because it was unavailable in any computer files.

In such a volatile climate, the annual rankings of America's hospitals that have appeared in *U.S. News* for six years are a friend to health consumers. They are still the only comprehensive effort to identify the best hospitals in objective fashion—and the guide you are now reading represents a significant advance.

The first *U.S. News* venture into ranking hospitals was 1990, when 400 leading doctors in 12 specialties from AIDS to urology were asked to recommend the ten best institutions in their specialty. Their responses became the basis for reputational rankings. In 1991, *U.S. News* joined forces with the National Opinion Research Center, a respected social science research arm of the University of Chicago. Four specialties were added in the 1992 rankings.

The rankings became far more sophisticated in 1993, when death rates for hospitals in 12 specialties were combined with various categories of hard data, such as the ratio of registered nurses to beds. Four specialties—ophthalmology, pediatrics, psychiatry, and rehabilitation—continue to be ranked on reputation alone. Mortality is irrelevant, since deaths rarely are a consequence of care in departments of ophthalmology, pediatrics, psychiatry, or rehabilitation.

Now *America's Best Hospitals* takes another step. Thanks to the expansiveness afforded by publication in book form, this edition assesses the quality of every one of the 1,631 hospitals in the country with a tie to a medical school or heavy emphasis on modern medical technology—so-called tertiary-care hospitals. We wanted to provide a national perspective and bring the results close to home. So the top 50 hospitals in each of 12 specialties are ranked nationally—but you will also find all of the tertiary-care hospitals ranked state by state, again in each of 12 specialties. Hospitals located in the 10 largest U.S. metropolitan areas get a separate set of rankings in the 12 specialties.

Anyone who needs the best care available needs it *now*, not next month or next year. Those are the consumers for whom this book is intended. Use it well. And may your good health, or the health of someone you love, be restored.

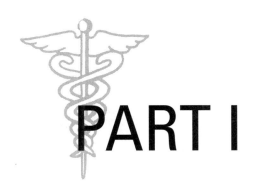

PART I

YOU, THE PATIENT

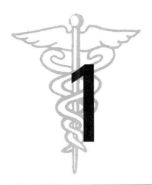

When a Top Hospital Can Make a Difference

Hospitals traffic in miracles so routinely that we rarely think about them. Sprawling urban giant and six-bed rural clinic alike serve up fresh new babies and thump stilled hearts back to life with ho-hum matter-of-factness. It is no more than what Americans have come to expect.

Yet some miracles demand skills that not all hospitals can supply. General hospitals and nonspecialized clinics, lumped together in the vocabulary of health professionals as primary-care facilities, meet the day-to-day medical needs of their local communities in fine fashion. But they wouldn't be your first choice if you needed a heart transplant or an experimental cancer treatment. Nor should they be.

If you or someone close to you is seriously ill or has a condition that puzzles doctors you have consulted, you will want to think about seeking care at one of the nation's 1,631 tertiary-care centers. These major medical centers, such as Johns Hopkins Hospital in Baltimore and Massachusetts General Hospital in Boston, conduct advanced clinical research and tend to attract the best and brightest doctors. Most are teaching hospitals that train the nation's physicians or are affiliated with a teaching hospital. Most are large, with hundreds of beds.

Because of their research and training mission and their size, these medical centers confront illnesses and perform procedures every day that doctors in community hospitals may encounter only a few times a year. That is vital to excellence. Like the old joke about the lost tourist in New York City who asked how to get to Carnegie Hall and was told "Practice, practice, practice," countless studies show that in general, the more often an operation or other medical procedure is performed, the better the outcome is likely to be. At major centers, the surgeon, anesthesiologist, technicians, and nurses who make up the surgical teams have joined hands on hundreds or even thousands of difficult operations and mesh like an elite ballet company.

EQUAL AT THE TOP?

Your search for the best care shouldn't cease once you've found a top hospital in the specialty you require. Even leading centers have differing degrees of expertise in treating specific maladies. Many hospitals excel at neurological care, for instance, but only a handful—including Massachusetts General Hospital and the Mayo Clinic—are on the forefront of treating brain aneurysms, in which arteries balloon and can suddenly burst, causing symptoms similar to those of a stroke. And because cancer is really many different diseases, even large hospitals often have expertise in diagnosing and treating only a few types of cancer.

Many patients in need of expert attention travel long distances to get it. Typically, 10 to 20 percent of patients come from outside the region or state—and in some highly specialized areas of medicine, the figure is higher. An amazing 67 percent of the patients who are seen at the neurology department at the Mayo Clinic in Rochester, Minnesota, one of the country's top neurology centers, hail from out of state.

WHO DECIDES?

The choice of hospital is rarely up to the patient alone, of course. As a practical matter, where you live, your income, and your health coverage narrow the selection. Health maintenance organizations and other managed-care plans typically handle requests to go outside the system case by case, and patients often must pay part of the cost—sometimes all of it.

When to seek out a top medical center does not become an automatic decision at some well-defined point. The balance tips at some point because of the nature and severity of the problem or its treatment. A look at various problems suggests where the tipping point might appear.

AIDS

Ideally, every HIV-infected patient could live near a top-rated AIDS hospital. But moving away from family and friends to find such care generally isn't necessary, and the loss of familiar surroundings and emotional support at home can wipe out some of the advantages of state-of-the-art care. Moreover, outpatient care has become the rule. Most patients both prefer to stay at home and run less of a risk from hospital-based infections. And since most treatments use drugs and not technology against HIV infection, AIDS, and the opportunistic diseases that the weakened immune system cannot fight effectively, local hospitals can serve patients well as long as the staffers have experience. Still, medical centers that serve as hubs for research and training are the places to go for the most up-to-date care and experimental treatments.

Arthritis

For someone with severe arthritic flare-ups, which can damage the lungs or other organs, a top rheumatology staff is an obvious resource. Or perhaps a joint has deteriorated to the point that replacement is recommended. A rheumatology department with access to up-to-date radiological equipment—such as the latest in diagnostic arthroscopy, which lets doctors peer directly into diseased tissue—can be consulted to verify the need for a new joint. Ernest Brahn, assistant professor of rheumatology at UCLA medical center, notes that surgeons at

community hospitals who perform hip and knee replacements may not always know the latest techniques to hasten recovery and make the recuperative period more comfortable, such as the use of screws and plates rather than body casts.

Cancer

The usual reaction to a diagnosis of cancer is to head for the nearest major medical center, first for a second opinion and then for treatment. That's not a bad response. Cancer is too deadly and unpredictable—and the array of available treatments too vast—to entrust care to less than the best. Renowned hospitals deliver up-to-date care that includes clinical trials of new drugs and experimental therapies. Their doctors tend to be leaders in their fields. And they provide much-needed emotional support through well-established programs.

That said, it is no longer always necessary to bypass your local hospital. Increasing numbers of community hospitals deliver state-of-the-art cancer treatment, thanks in part to a nationwide computer network called PDQ, for Physicians Data Query. This reference service gives doctors (cancer patients can access it, too) detailed information on current therapies and how well they are working in which types of patients. For many cancer patients, where to go will depend on whether they can enter a clinical trial. If so, they may have to travel to a center in another city. If not, a local hospital may be the best choice.

Ear, Nose, and Throat

Top hospitals are the choice for relatively rare conditions such as tumors of the acoustic nerve, which few otolaryngologists, as ear, nose, and throat specialists are called, ever see if they practice outside major centers. They also treat deafness and complicated cancers of the throat and larynx. Brian McCabe, a professor in the department of otolaryngology at the University of Iowa Hospitals and Clinics, says that anyone seeking care for, say, throat or sinus cancer, which may involve reconstructive surgery, should be sure the department has not only diagnosticians, surgeons, oncologists, and high-technology radiation therapists but also speech pathologists and specialists in the construction of prostheses—artificial facial replacements. "When we can't reconstruct a part of a face, we can make a prosthesis that would not be discernible as artificial from across a room," McCabe says.

Much of the work of otolaryngologists still deals with common conditions such as sinus and ear infections, which can be treated at small hospitals. Most local doctors and hospitals perform enough bread-and-butter otolaryngology procedures—removing tonsils, repairing deviated septums, excising small internal tumors of the head and neck—to stay sharp.

Eye Problems

Ophthalmology is largely technology driven, and it is the big centers that have the most sophisticated equipment—like laser beams and ocular ultrasound equipment, important in treating tumors. Same-day surgery is now the rule for most eye operations. You have to pack a bag only for involved procedures, such as reconnecting a detached retina or removing a tumor.

Gastroenterology

Community hospitals' gastroenterology departments can handle such routine problems as heartburn, ulcers, and gallstones. Liver transplants, of course, are best done at major medical centers. But patients would also be well advised to seek out a center renowned for difficult diagnostic problems, even prosaic-sounding symptoms like chronic nausea or abdominal pain. At community hospitals, such complaints often lead to barium enema tests that show little. But at top centers, they might trigger complex electrical and pressure measurements of the stomach and intestinal tract that might point up a need for specific treatment. Top centers are also the only places that offer special stents, or tubes, that keep blocked pancreatic or bile ducts open.

Gynecology

Diseases like endometriosis, ectopic pregnancy, uterine bleeding, and fibroid tumors may suggest a medical center with a strong reputation in gynecology. Confusing diagnoses, rare complications, or failure to respond to treatment also merit such referrals. As Charles Hammond, chairman of the obstetrics and gynecology department at Duke University, says: "A doctor at a community hospital may see one placental tumor in a lifetime, but a top center may have half a dozen cases at any one time."

Most such centers also offer obstetric services, although they are reserved mainly for difficult and high-risk pregnancies. Some hospitals offer the most sophisticated technology available for overcoming infertility. Based purely on logic, the decision to travel to a major institution is defensible if a couple's problem is particularly hard to treat. But because of the need for many return visits, most people may be better off at an in vitro fertilization clinic close to home.

The majority of obstetric and gynecological problems, in fact, can be treated locally. It is true that community hospitals are geared to routine care, but they can open doors to a nearby network of larger, more sophisticated hospitals, where specialists can treat early-stage cancers and care for high-risk mothers or low-birthweight newborns.

The Heart

From angina, or chest pain, to clogged coronary arteries, most community hospitals can safely and skillfully perform routine diagnostic tests, such as angiography and coronary bypass surgery. Still, you need to apply the practice-makes-perfect yardstick: The hospital you choose should perform the procedure you need at least once or twice a day, or 300 to 500 times per year. Patients who need a repeat bypass, or who are on their second or third angioplasty to clear out clogged arteries, may benefit from a trip to a renowned hospital where physicians face especially complex cases weekly.

A top medical center would be a resource for a heart patient who has an unusual or complex problem involving congenital heart disease, valve problems, or a rhythm disorder. Heart conditions complicated by serious lung problems also call for special attention at a major center.

Mental Illness

Because of improved drugs, cost-cutting pressure from insurers, and greater understanding of emotional disorders, hospitalization for mental illness is rarer, and stays are shorter, than was the case a few years ago. Most community hospitals with psychiatric units can provide adequate care when severe depression or alcohol- or drug-related problems strike. But mending the mind takes a human touch. The best medical centers increasingly emphasize a proper balance between drugs and psychotherapy. Steven Mirin, psychiatrist in chief at McLean Hospital in Belmont, Massachusetts, advises looking for a continuum of care that extends beyond the patient's hospital stay. His checklist of questions includes: Are there day and evening programs for expatient or outpatient psychotherapy provided by the same people who treated the patient in the hospital? Is partial hospitalization available—nights only, for example, if that makes sense? When patients are discharged, Mirin says, they should get more than a phone number. They should feel that the medical center will be there for them when and if they need it.

Muscular and Neurological Problems

Only at major centers—and not even at all of those—can individuals find comprehensive care and treatment of muscle and central nervous system problems, from parkinsonism and multiple sclerosis to Alzheimer's disease, epilepsy, stroke, and spinal-cord injuries. Lewis Rowland, chief of neurology at Columbia Presbyterian Medical Center in New York City, notes that his department has many superspecialists—in movement disorders, neuromuscular diseases, and dementia-related problems, just to name three areas. "The amount of knowledge available is so huge," he says, "that physicians have to focus if they're going to be on the front lines." Superspecialists can best diagnose such conditions early. That's important, because those types of disorders are best managed early on.

Old Age

Aging patients often suffer from an assortment of chronic illnesses, such as diabetes, heart disease, and arthritis. Patients who worry that their care is not well coordinated should look for geriatrics programs at large centers that offer comprehensive assessments. Robert Butler, chief of geriatrics at Mount Sinai Medical Center in New York City, notes that diseases affect older people differently than they affect other patients. A heart attack, for instance, may cause confusion rather than chest pain. "Because we have the expertise to provide the primary care for all of our patients' medical problems, there is better coordination," he says.

That may mean calling in an endocrinologist, who treats diseases marked by overproduction or underproduction of hormones. These conditions include osteoporosis, menstrual irregularities, and rare conditions such as hormone-producing tumors. Henry Kronenberg, head of the endocrinology unit at Massachusetts General Hospital, says that intellectual rigor—knowing which tests should be done and which treatments are indicated—is the key and is much more important than the presence of high technology. And access to surgeons with a complete understanding of endocrinology is a feature offered almost exclusively by big academic or clinical centers.

Pediatric Illnesses

For children who need routine hospital care, convenience is paramount. Why bring a child to a strange city and disrupt family and work routines needlessly? Besides, doctors in pediatric units of general hospitals have the expertise to repair a hernia, remove an inflamed appendix, and treat most other childhood illnesses. But children who are very sick or who have rare disorders like glycogen storage disease, a treatable metabolic problem, belong in specialized children's hospitals. There's nothing exotic about most of the technology used in these hospitals to diagnose illness, but experts can better interpret test results. A large, hazy shadow on an X ray of an adult lung, for example, often means lung cancer. In babies, it may signal sequestered lobe, a rare lung disorder curable by surgery. And surgery is done with children in mind. Operating room staffs know how to cater to a newborn's special needs, from transfusions to anesthesia. Finally, children's hospitals maintain support groups that educate parents and help prop up entire families enduring difficult times.

Urology

Kidney stones, routine bladder infections, and an enlarged prostate may receive perfectly adequate care at a community hospital. But for major problems with the kidneys, bladder, or prostate, it's time to seek care at a major medical center. Top centers, of course, are best equipped for kidney transplants, treating severe bladder problems resulting from complex nerve abnormalities, and prostate cancer. Treatment of the latter calls for a top center because the risk of impotence and incontinence is relatively high when less than the latest techniques are used. Major centers are first to perfect techniques such as nerve-sparing prostate surgery, which dramatically reduces the chances of side effects such as impotence and incontinence. In such cases, a top hospital can truly make a difference.

FOR MORE HELP

- **American Academy of Orthopaedic Surgeons,** P.O. Box 618, Park Ridge, IL 60068. Free information is available by sending a stamped, self-addressed envelope.
- **The American Foundation for Urologic Disease.** Patient information on urologic diseases can be obtained by calling (800) 242-2383; information on prostate cancer support groups is available by calling (800) 828-7866.
- **American Thyroid Association,** (800) 542-6687. The association offers pamphlets and referrals to board-certified endocrinologists.
- *Gut Reactions,* **by W. Grant Thompson, M.D.** (New York: Plenum Press, 1989, $22.95). This publication is a lay-language discussion of digestive disorders.

- **National Association of Psychiatric Health Systems,** (202) 393-6700. The association provides a list of facilities in your area and special programs offered, such as centers that treat alcoholism.
- **National Council on Independent Living,** (518) 274-1979. The council offers support to patients following rehabilitation.
- **National Eye Institute,** Bldg. 31, Room 6A-32, 31 Center Drive MSC2510, Bethesda, MD 20892. The institute offers basic information and lists of clinical trials.

- **The National Multiple Sclerosis Society,** (800) 344-4867. Alzheimer's Association, (312) 335-8700.
- **National Women's Health Network,** (202) 347-1140. Packets on health issues of concern to women are available for a $7.50 donation.
- **Neurology self-help groups.** ALS Association, (818) 340-7500. Parkinson Support Groups of America, (301) 937-1545.
- **Self-Help for Hard of Hearing People,** (301) 657-2248. For a $20 annual membership fee, this organization provides information and referrals.

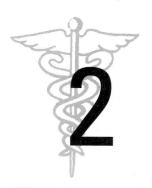

2

How to Get Admitted to a Top Center

I n what many people now remember fondly as the golden age of health care (in reality only a few years ago), most people's health insurance at least covered catastrophic care. Consumers may have had to open their wallets for well-baby visits and routine checkups, but when they got seriously ill, they could pick any hospital in the country and had to worry only about how to pay to get there.

Now health plans cover routine care, and most provide preventive services as well, strategies that health insurance companies have found make both medical and economic sense. But the health plan, not the consumer, chooses the hospital. At the beginning of 1994, some 100 million Americans were enrolled in some form of managed care. It usually takes the form of a health maintenance organization (HMO) or a preferred-provider organization, which offers health care through a network of contracted providers, most of which offer unlimited primary-care visits for no charge or with a low copayment.

But when it comes to old-fashioned catastrophic care—hospital care—managed care can seem like an unyielding obstacle instead of a comforting bulwark. Patients and their families can spend time and energy doing battle with the system's bureaucracy rather than fighting illness. Even people with traditional fee-for-service health plans are sometimes offered the incentive of a lower deductible if they choose a hospital recommended by their plan.

So when a seriously ill patient is well-informed—and adamant—about going to a specific institution outside the plan, the battle for coverage can rival the struggle against the disease itself. Armed with a list of the best hospitals in America, however, and a conviction that a particular hospital can make a difference, patients and their advocates can often push their insurance plans to do the right thing.

You do not have to gird for battle with the health plan right away. Most top-notch hospitals can help people get in (that is their business, after all). When you have digested this guide, talked with your doctor, done your homework, and decided on a specific hospital, contact the hospital's physician referral service. To get into any hospital, a patient must go through a doctor who has admitting privileges. That means you have to find a doctor at the hospital who believes you will benefit by being admitted. The referral service will help you select a doctor and schedule an initial appointment. The service also will brief you on costs and help you make arrangements for a place to stay if you're coming from out of town.

The first appointment—but not travel or lodging—often will be covered by your health plan, as a second opinion. In addition to medical matters, you need to discuss with the physician how much he or she will be your advocate in fighting for insurance coverage if necessary.

It may not be easy. But veterans of the admitting wars—patients, doctors, hospital administrators—have valuable tips to share. Their key advice, backed up by their personal perspective, should go a long way toward getting you in the door and the cost covered.

ADVICE FROM VETERANS OF THE ADMITTING WAR

1. "Game" the System—but Be Careful

If the hospital you want is outside your health plan's network of providers, and if the time is right, consider changing health plans. Most large employers have an annual open-enrollment period during which employees can change health insurance plans with no waiting period for coverage and without having to disclose preexisting conditions. But be very careful to check the new plan's fine print, making sure there are no waiting periods or exclusions for preexisting conditions. And make sure the treating physician agrees that the procedure can wait until the next open-enrollment period with no danger that the condition will worsen.

Personal Perspective

Say you've got intermittent esotropia, a condition in which the eye muscles cause the eyes to cross occasionally. Some people live with it, but it can become too annoying, or too severe, to ignore. "For most patients, nothing will be harmed if they have to wait a couple of months," says David Guyton, an ophthalmologist at the Wilmer Eye Institute at Johns Hopkins Hospital.

Many ophthalmologists clip and suture the eye muscles to correct the problem. But at some major eye centers, including the Massachusetts Eye and Ear Infirmary and the Wilmer Eye Institute, surgeons have advanced the standard procedure by using adjustable sutures. They leave the suture ends exposed outside the eye. Then, when the patient's patches come off, the surgeon uses the suture ends to finely adjust the muscle length. Wilmer ophthalmologists have cut the reoperation rate in half, from 20 to 10 percent, by using adjustable sutures. A patient whose plan will not approve the procedure at a specialized eye center might want to wait for open-enrollment time and switch to a fee-for-service plan that allows maximum choice of physician and institution.

2. Be Prepared to Prove that Experience Pays Off

As was noted in Chapter 1, the more procedures physicians or institutions do, the fewer the complications and deaths. As a rule, volume equals skill. Coronary bypass surgery, by now fairly routine, is a good example. The American Heart Association and the American College of Cardiology advise picking a hospital that does at least 200 to 300 open-heart operations a year and a surgeon who does at least 100. Any surgeon should be able to provide such figures. Alternatively, many local and state health departments collect volume data on hospitals.

Personal Perspective

Jonathan Miller is 27, a resident of Concord, Massachusetts. A fringe benefit that comes with living in a Boston suburb is the certainty that you are at the center of the medical universe. Bostonians like to call the city a "medical mecca," with three medical schools in town and a fourth in Worcester, a stone's throw to the west. Boston's teaching hospitals draw patients from around the world. And that was Miller's problem.

"There was a feeling that if an operation can't be done in Boston, why not?" says Miller. But the operation he needed was *not* done in Boston, and Miller was left to prove its value to highly sophisticated health plan bureaucrats.

Miller has a condition called avascular necrosis, a degenerative bone disease that gradually kills the hip bones of young adults. It strikes patients at an average age of 34. Normally, surgeons replace the hip with an artificial hip joint, a kind of surgery generally helpful for elderly adults whose hips are lost to osteoarthritis or other disease. But the artificial hip, surgically supported by implanted bone from a cadaver, fractures more easily than living bone does. Although the surgery can serve older patients well, becuase they are relatively sedentary, it is less successful with younger, more active patients— who need working hips far longer than elderly patients do. Artificial hips last an average of 20 years; younger avascular necrosis patients therefore face two or three replacement hips during the course of their lives.

James Urbaniak, chief of orthopedic surgery at Duke University Medical Center, developed a procedure in 1979 to get around the replacement problem. He explains: "We remove the dead bone and replace it with a bone graft from the patient's own fibula [the thinner of two long bones of the lower leg], along with the blood vessels," says Urbaniak. He removes the diseased portions of the hip bone and builds a new bone around what is left with the graft from the fibula. Then he hooks up the graft's blood vessels to the blood that serves the remaining live bone in the old hip. "The bone stays alive and stimulates other new bone to form," says Urbaniak, who has now done the procedure more than 600 times, on patients from all but a few states. He has taught a handful of other surgeons the procedure. One was in

Boston—but that surgeon, to whom Miller was referred by his health plan, had not done the procedure since training with Urbaniak.

"He decided I was a good candidate for this procedure," says Miller. "But I would have been his first patient, and that's something that I didn't want to be. He didn't want it, either."

The surgeon urged Miller to go to North Carolina to meet Urbaniak. The health insurer balked at coverage—and would not tell Miller whether the surgery at Duke would be covered—right up to the Friday morning Miller arrived in North Carolina in preparation for a Monday morning operation. The last word he had before heading for a round of presurgical exams, X rays, and laboratory tests was that the plan considered the $25,000 operation experimental, even though Miller would be patient number 580 for Urbaniak. But Miller's family didn't give up. Even as his son was preparing for surgery, Miller's father worked the phone, hounding health plan administrators. Finally, on Friday afternoon, coverage was approved.

Miller later had the other hip replaced at Duke as well—and approval, by comparison, went smoothly. Now an old hand at paperwork battles, Miller offers this advice: "Get your paperwork in right away and then follow up. Get the name of who it goes to and make sure everything is moving along. Know as much as you can about the chain of command that the paperwork goes through. You don't want to be in a situation where you're going through a six-hour operation, you'll be on crutches for six months, and you don't know if the paperwork is taken care of."

3. Become a Dogged Researcher by Tracking down Relevant Studies and Numbers

Get statistics that are as tailor-made to your condition as possible. The less common the disease or procedure, the fewer the institutions that will have had significant experience with it—and the more an individual will likely benefit from finding the hospital with the most experience. It may take a surgeon 10 years or longer—performing a new procedure, training other surgeons, and gathering follow-up data on patients—to get to the point of publishing results in a peer-reviewed journal. Insurance companies look to such journals when making payment decisions, but some doctors can make convincing arguments about a procedure's benefits long before they're able to publish. Ask your doctor if anyone at the hospital of choice is doing research on your condition, using patients from that institution.

Personal Perspective

Dr. John Cameron, chief of surgery at Johns Hopkins Hospital, was frequently called on to rally his staff, his expertise, and even his charm to help desperately ill patients get what they and he felt to be the best care possible for pancreatic cancer. He and colleagues at Hopkins had developed a complex surgical procedure called the Whipple procedure that they report results in a five-year survival rate of 26 percent—remarkably high considering that this form of cancer has a one-year mortality rate in excess of 90 percent. The procedure involves removing part of the pancreas along with all of the duodenum (the upper portion of the small intestine), the gallbladder, and sometimes part of the stomach. Other Maryland hospitals do the procedure, but much less often.

To help get patients needing the procedure into Johns Hopkins, Cameron would write letters on their behalf. He would call medical directors of managed-care plans. Armed with numbers, he would make a sterling case for Hopkins's expertise, often adding that outcomes there were so superior that it would be unconscionable to send a patient anywhere else in the region for the risky surgery.

After much correspondence and cajoling, even managed-care organizations that did not have a relationship with Hopkins usually came around. But some didn't. And occasionally someone would get miffed. "Sometimes a medical director would call our president and say that we were using unfair pressure," says Cameron.

Cameron concluded that he had to make an unshakable case for the surgery. So he and Toby Gordon, vice-president for planning and marketing, authored a study. Published in January 1995 in *Annals of Surgery*, it examined all 501 cases of pancreatic cancer in Maryland from the years 1988 to mid-1993 in which the Whipple procedure was used. Hopkins performed 54 percent of the procedures, with the others parceled out among 38 hospitals. The in-hospital death rate at Hopkins was 2.2 percent; the average rate at the other hospitals was 13.5 percent. Moreover, the cost of the procedure at Hopkins was $26,204, compared to an average $31,659 elsewhere. "All of a sudden, we didn't have any problem getting patients in our hospital," says Cameron. He adds somewhat cynically: "It wasn't the outcomes. It was the lower cost."

4. Keep an Open Mind about the Hospital Recommended by Your Health Plan

Managed-care plans try to control costs not only by holding down expensive tests and procedures but also by minimizing costly complications. They have often done considerable research to find the institutions that have the most experience and the best outcomes.

Personal Perspective

In 1988, Prudential Insurance Company created a program that steers patients to "institutes of quality"—hospitals that seem to offer the best chance for successful results in such high-technology medical areas as organ transplant and rehabilitation services. Those hospitals are available to patients whose serious medical problems, in the opinion of the HMO, can be better addressed by hospitals outside the usual network. The health insurer judges each hospital by reviewing the professional literature and by conducting on-site inspections and personal interviews. Other health plans call such hospitals "centers of excellence." "These are blue-ribbon institutions with very good outcomes," says William Roper, Prudential's senior vice-president and chief medical officer. For liver transplants, for example, Prudential's list includes seven institutions: Cedars Sinai Medical Center in Los Angeles; Children's Hospital in Boston; Emory University Hospital in Atlanta; Massachusetts General Hospital in Boston; Mayo Clinic in Rochester, Minnesota; University of California at San Francisco Medical Center; and the University of Chicago Medical Center.

The plan refers patients to the nearest facility and pays for travel expenses for the patient and a companion. In some cases, the companion's meals and lodging expenses are covered as well.

Patients appreciate the higher standards that Prudential applies to the hospitals that make the list. Or most patients do. Roper spoke with one physician who worked for Prudential who said his patient, who needed a new liver, wanted the transplant done at his local hospital rather than at one of Prudential's "institutes of quality." Why? "He found out he would be the very first transplant patient at his local hospital," says Roper. That kind of honor, he notes, a patient is better off doing without.

5. Play "Let's Make a Deal"

See if the hospital you have in mind will settle for the reimbursement rates that your health insurer pays its member hospitals. The negotiating is done between hospital administrators and health plan medical directors, so suggest it to your plan's director.

Personal Perspective

To attract more managed-care patients, Children's Hospital in Los Angeles has changed the way it charges insurers by setting a flat fee for a given procedure or operation. The "case rate," as the fee is called, can be adjusted—for out-of-town patients, say, who may return home to get follow-up care. A patient needing a bone marrow transplant, for example, could be charged a lower case rate if a managed-care plan wanted to take on some of the preoperative and postoperative care and the long-term follow-up care. "Preoperative care, scans, blood work—we won't repeat any of it. And we'll cut the cost accordingly," says Bart Wald, a pediatric oncologist who left clinical medicine to market Children's services. And if the managed-care plan also took on the typical 100 days of follow-up care included in the normal case rate, the hospital would make an appropriate downward adjustment.

6. Freedom of Choice Is Available if You're Willing to Pay

You may have a strong preference for a hospital, but your insurance plan may have an equally good case to make for choosing another institution. Your preference may be important enough to you that you'll shell out.

Personal Perspective

Mark Feierberg of Highland Park, a suburb of Chicago, knew he would eventually need a heart valve replaced because blood leaked through even when the valve was closed. The deformity, known technically as mitral valve prolapse (and informally as floppy valve syndrome), does not always require treatment. In Feierberg's case, after 15 years of living with the condition, tests showed that the leakage had increased to the point where his heart might fail if the valve were not replaced. His doctors at Rush-Presbyterian Medical Center and Northwestern University Hospital in Chicago agreed that he would need the surgery within about six months. A surgeon at the Cleveland Clinic was known for his expertise in the procedure, both doctors told him. Feierberg used his six months to determine which institutions and doctors were most familiar with the procedure he needed.

Everything pointed to Cleveland Clinic, an institution known for excellent cardiac care. He found out that surgeons there do the procedure he'd need at about the rate of two a day. But he was covered by a Blue Cross/Blue Shield preferred provider organization (PPO) with strong financial incentives to keep patients within a Chicago-area network of providers. He would pay $1,000 out of pocket if he stayed within the network. The PPO would permit him to go to Cleveland, but he went there believing he would have to pay $4,000 of the expense. In November 1994, Feierberg had valve replacement surgery—at the Cleveland Clinic. "I only have one heart," he says. "If there were any complications, I wanted to be where they had seen it all before." The total bill was $36,000. Feierberg says that if he had been forced to pay the entire bill himself, he probably would have stayed in Illinois and within his provider network.

7. Persistence Pays—So Does the Threat of a Lawsuit

If your insurer won't cover a hospitalization or procedure, pull out all the stops. Write and call insurance company officials. Have your spouse or friends make calls. Make your insurance company wish you'd go away. Nag. Nag. Nag. Call it follow-up, call it hounding, call it harassment, but keep calling. And if they don't respond the way you believe they should, hire a lawyer.

Personal Perspective

Doris Dunkleburger's metastatic breast cancer was diagnosed in November of 1992. Her insurer, Empire Blue Cross/Blue Shield, declined to pay the $190,000 cost of the recommended treatment—high-dose chemotherapy followed by a bone marrow transplant—arguing that it was considered experimental. If the Clifton Park, N.Y., kindergarten teacher and Jay, her engineer husband, had to come up with the money themselves, they could not have done it, and Doris would have died. Doctors at Memorial Sloan-Kettering, a prominent cancer center in New York City, encouraged her to have the procedure and worry about bills later, since the procedure was her only hope.

Doris could not do that. "I told Jay, 'I'm not going without insurance. I'm not leaving you with a legacy of bills,'" she says. Jay, of course, was urging her to go anyway and hang the cost, but she would have none of it. So she and Jay plunged into research. He called and wrote Empire's vice-president for medical policy and research, who continued to insist that the procedure was experimental. Jay got the names of the company's board members and wrote to them. The Dunkleburgers had always been active in church, school, and scouting in Clifton Park, a community of 35,000, creating a ready-made base for networking their appeals. Friends of theirs who were also friends of Empire's board members hand delivered letters of appeal. The business manager at Doris's school kept up a two-month-long bombardment of Empire with missives and calls. Sloan-Kettering itself jumped in, probing the insurance company for specific reasons why they were denying coverage. "We're tena-

cious," says Janice Levy, director of the hospital's patient representative department. "We research the medical journals to provide evidence on why these patients are good candidates. Usually, the insurance companies at least take a second look."

But finally, the risk of further delay was too great to wait much longer, and Jay contacted a legal aid society, which helped them find Carla Hogan, an Albany, N.Y., attorney willing to take the case *pro bono*. She filed a complaint on Dunkleburger's behalf—and within a week Empire agreed to pay.

Enlisting a lawyer tends to lead to that outcome. A study in the February 17, 1994, issue of the *New England Journal of Medicine* by researchers at the Duke University Bone Marrow Transplant Program examined insurance company decisions on coverage of bone marrow transplants for the treatment of breast cancer. The process, they concluded, is "arbitrary and capricious." They also found that of 39 women whose insurance companies had first refused and then agreed to cover the procedure, 19 had hired an attorney.

The study shortly followed news of a 38-year-old California woman whose family successfully sued Health Net, her HMO. Nelene Fox died in April 1993. Her HMO had denied coverage of the same long-shot, last-hope procedure Dunkleburger was to have. Fox's friends and family rallied, with bake sales, car washes, Bingo games, and personal loans, so that she could eventually have the procedure and pay for it herself—but not until eight months after her doctor first recommended it. Her lawyers argued after her death that by then it was already too late. The procedure would have cost the HMO $212,000. The jury awarded $89 million in punitive and compensatory damages.

Doris Dunkleburger's treatment was concluded in May 1993, by all appearances successfully. She walks two miles a day, teaches 26 kindergartners, sings in the church choir, and does volunteer work. She is grateful beyond words for her life—yet she still would not have agreed to the procedure without insurance coverage. "The love that [Jay] had for me in insisting that I go anyway was the same love I had for him in saying I wouldn't leave him destitute," she says. "If I had died, he would still have to live."

8. Look for Savings by Checking out Free or Low-Cost Transportation or Lodging

The hospital's physician referral service or social services department may be able to arrange for discount plane fares and housing for patients and family members.

Personal Perspective

The three months that Doris Dunkleburger spent in treatment at Memorial Sloan-Kettering coincided with the opening of a new Ronald McDonald House in New York City. During those months, the temporary housing meant for families of seriously ill children had vacancies among its 86 beds—so they allowed Jay Dunkleburger to live there for $20 a night and Doris to stay there the two days a week when she could leave the hospital, even though as an adult patient she was technically ineligible.

9. Check Your Policy for Catch-22s

The fine print may give your plan ammunition to drop you.

Personal Perspective

Robert Abbas thought that health coverage for his then 19-year-old daughter, Bethany, was secure. She had always been a healthy child and was doing well at Cedarville College in Cedarville, Ohio, the college where her father teaches, when she was diagnosed with leukemia. Treatment at Miami Valley Hospital in Dayton was going well when the Abbas family was notified that Bethany was being dropped from coverage. To continue coverage on her father's insurance plan beyond the age of 18, Bethany had to maintain her status as a full-time student—which was impossible because she was in a hospital, being treated for leukemia. "That was scary," says Abbas. "It's the kind of thing you don't need when your daughter is in the hospital."

Bethany's cancer is in remission, but the chemotherapy damaged her hips, requiring the same hip-replacement surgery that Jonathan Miller had at Duke University Hospital. Her father's health plan, like Miller's, at first suggested the surgery was experimental and agreed to cover only 60 percent of the cost, instead of the 90 percent Abbas hoped for. But when Abbas hired an attorney, the plan capitulated.

During recovery from leukemia and two hip replacements, including physical therapy to relearn to walk, Bethany, now 21, has managed to remain a full-time student, mostly through independent study, in order to retain insurance coverage. It helps that she goes to a school where her father teaches and where many of her professors have known her since childhood.

FOR MORE HELP

- **American Cancer Society's Guestroom Program**, (800) 227-2345. This program helps cancer patients and their families away from home arrange for free or reduced-rate hotel and motel accommodations.
- **Air Care Alliance**, Manassas, VA, (800) 296-1217. This group helps patients connect with airlines that offer discounts to patients and their families who need to travel for medical treatment. The group also locates volunteer pilots who donate their time and aircraft to help people get to the medical care they need.
- **Family Inn**, 70 Sewall Avenue, Brookline, MA 02146, (617) 566-3430. Jamie Fiske was the country's youngest-ever liver-transplant patient in November 1982. In gratitude, her parents created the Family Inn, which provides housing in the Boston suburb at $10 a night for families of people awaiting organ transplants. A second facility is scheduled to open in Chicago in early 1996, and a third in Palo Alto, Calif., is in the early planning stages. Jamie is now 13.
- *Health Pages*, 135 Fifth Avenue, 7th Floor, New York, NY 10010, (212) 505-0103. These are regional guides, currently covering Atlanta, Boston/Worcester, Cincinnati/Columbus/Dayton, Pittsburgh, and St. Louis, that describe services, backgrounds, and prices charged by participating doctors and hospitals.
- *The HMO Health Care Companion: A Consumer's Guide to Managed-Care Networks,* by Alan G. Raymond (HarperPerennial, 1994, $10). This paperback guide, by the vice-president for public affairs at the Harvard Community Health Plan in Cambridge, Mass., includes chapters on how to receive the best care for specific health problems like asthma, heart disease, diabetes, and cancer and what to do if you are dissatisfied with your plan or want to appeal a coverage decision.
- **Ronald McDonald House**, Chicago (312) 836-7384. The Ronald McDonald House provides free or low-cost temporary housing for families of seriously ill children.
- *Through the Patient's Eyes: Understanding and Promoting Patient-Centered Care,* edited by Margaret Gerteis, Susan Edgman-Levitan, Jennifer Daley, and Thomas L. Delbanco (Jossey-Bass, 1993, $29.95). This is a compilation of various surveys of patient satisfaction by the former Picker/Commonwealth Program for Patient-Centered Care, now called the Picker Institute. It is an overview of what patients actually experience when they go to hospitals, and it explores models of care that can make the experience more humane.

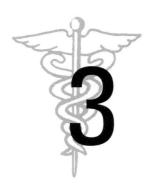

The Local Alternative

Tucked into the foothills of the Allegheny Mountains in central Pennsylvania, Altoona boasts the world's oldest wooden roller coaster and a theater where Sarah Bernhardt and W.C. Fields once performed. Its streets are safe, its housing affordable. And on top of all that, Altoona happens to be home to a hospital with one of the lowest death rates from coronary bypass surgery in the state.

As competition for patients intensifies, large urban teaching hospitals are having to look over their shoulders at upstart community hospitals that provide the same or better care at a lower price. From New York to California, hospital "report cards" based on death rates and other data are drawing attention to hospitals little known outside their immediate areas.

Although there is an ongoing debate about how best to assess hospital quality, most of the parties involved would agree that large tertiary-care centers don't have a lock on it. "I think we can give care that's at least as good as any academic medical center," notes Eric Sundel, a pediatrician on staff at Bryn Mawr Hospital, a community hospital just outside Philadelphia.

Take cardiac bypass surgery. Many hospitals that do not appear at the top of this guide's national rankings in cardiology perform the operation competently, and Altoona Hospital is one of them. In fact, its record on bypass surgery offers a prime example of the quality and value available beyond the walls of high-profile urban medical centers.

ALTOONA'S STORY

The 1995 edition of *A Consumer Guide to Coronary Artery Bypass Graft Surgery,* published by the Pennsylvania Health Care Cost Containment Council, a state agency, tells the story of Altoona Hospital. Of 41 medical centers in Pennsylvania that performed the operation in 1993—the latest year for which data were available—the 354-bed hospital was one of only three whose death rates were lower than expected, considering the kinds of patients each hospital treated. Only three of Altoona Hospital's 462 bypass patients died; the expected number of deaths—taking into account the age, gender, and medical condition of the hospital's bypass patients—ranged from four to 14, according to the report.

And Altoona Hospital is a bargain. The other two hospitals with exemplary bypass surgery death rates, Temple University Hospital of Philadelphia and Allegheny General Hospital in Pittsburgh, are major urban teaching centers whose average charges are considerably higher than those at Altoona Hospital. Temple's average charge for bypass surgery was $85,310—the fifth highest in the state—while Allegheny General's was $55,879. But Altoona's average charge was only $37,895, the 10th lowest in Pennsylvania. Smack dab in the middle between Pittsburgh and Harrisburg, Altoona Hospital, which has residents only in family practice, attracts patients from eight rural counties, says spokesman Rick Reeves.

Not surprisingly, many hospitals that don't score as well on such report cards question the methods used. "We must again raise concerns over the use of charges to measure cost of services," Paul Boehringer, executive director of Temple University Hospital, wrote in response to the 1995 edition of the Pennsylvania heart bypass guide. "We appreciate that the availability of charges makes them a likely means of measurement; however, charges are simply not a meaningful indicator of cost."

Boehringer's pique is understandable. Academic medical centers tend to be costlier, because training doctors and caring for large numbers of uninsured patients is an expensive proposition. Their administrators argue that few patients actually pay the average charge, which is much higher than the discounted price offered to big employers or the amount that Medicare or Medicaid reimburses. Average charges "give a misleading and inaccurate picture of what hospitals actually receive in payment for CABG [coronary artery bypass graft] surgery or any procedure," Samuel Steinberg, chief executive officer of The Graduate Hospital, a Philadelphia teaching hospital, wrote in response to the 1995 bypass surgery guide.

In every one of the four annual guides that have been published so far, Steinberg's institution has topped the state chart with the highest average charge for bypass surgery. Its 1993 average charge, as reported in the 1995 guide, was $103,000—nearly four times the state's lowest average charge for bypass surgery: $26,000 at Robert Packer Hospital in Sayre.

Joe Martin, spokesman for the Cost Containment Council, has heard the arguments before. "Charges are the only information that's available to us at the moment," he says. "We know that they're not exactly the same as payments. We don't think payments are going to provide any more consistent information, because you have so many different payment schemes in some areas."

A DEBATE OVER DEATH RATES

Publishing mortality rates is just as controversial as publishing charges. Academic medical centers argue that they tend to attract riskier cases that inflate their death rates. In determining death rates, however, the Cost Containment Council does weigh the condition of the patients when they were admitted to the hospital. The range of expected deaths reported in the guide is adjusted according to their degree of illness. An example from the guide: "A patient with congestive heart failure who had a previous coronary bypass operation will have a higher risk of dying in the hospital than a patient with no significant risk factors." Patients who are women or who need kidney dialysis also face an increased chance of death from bypass surgery.

Hospitals argue that the system used to adjust death rates still needs more fine-tuning. In a letter to the Cost Containment Council, Robert Costello, director of public relations for Mercy Hospital in Scranton, expressed concern that his institution's bypass patients actually were sicker than the state analysts had classified them, so the expected number of deaths should have been higher.

And plain bad luck is one component that just cannot be factored into analyses of death rates, says Steinberg, whose hospital's death rate fell right in the middle of its expected range, according to the Cost Containment Council's report. "We continue to believe that numerous interrelated and complex factors, including random chance, can affect outcomes on a year-to-year basis with no proven correlation to hospital quality or the competence of the surgeons performing the procedure," Steinberg commented in his letter to the council. One factor hospitals have repeatedly suggested should be added to the severity-of-illness criteria is whether patients were transferred from another institution that had turned them down for being too sick.

Despite this ongoing debate, Martin credits the annual bypass surgery reports with helping to reduce death rates and the growth in charges in the state. "Certainly there have been a lot of pressures on hospitals in terms of managed care and just a general outcry about the cost of health care," says Martin, "but I think it's fair to say that we've contributed to that pressure."

The statewide death rate for coronary bypass surgery in Pennsylvania fell from 3.9 percent in 1990 to 2.9 percent in 1993. That's a drop of more than one fourth. And although the average charge for a coronary bypass operation in the state rose by nearly 10 percent from 1990 to 1991, it increased only 4.6 percent from 1992 to 1993. "Many of our council members feel a lot of the reason is because the hospitals have to face the local newspaper headlines when this comes out," says Martin.

Pennsylvania hospitals might not agree with Martin's assessment, but at least one New York hospital acknowledges that publicity about its poor performance spurred it to make drastic changes in its heart bypass program. In 1989, the first year for which the New York State Health Department published hospitals' bypass death rates, Winthrop-University Hospital on Long Island looked terrible. Of the 30 hospitals approved to perform the operation in the state, it ranked number 29, with an adjusted mortality rate of 9.56 percent—about twice the statewide average that year.

So the hospital recruited surgeon William Scott from Yale-New Haven Hospital to overhaul its department of thoracic and cardiovascular surgery. Scott hired specialists in vital areas—cardiac anesthesia, nursing, administration, and intensive care. The 591-bed hospital began requiring that surgeons perform at least 100 open-heart operations to keep their privileges. "All of these changes have resulted in dramatic improvement in the quality of patient care," Scott said at the June 1995 press conference held by the New York State Health Department to release its analysis of 1993 death rates.

The numbers back him up. According to the state's bypass surgery report, Winthrop, which performed 534 of the operations in 1993, had an adjusted death rate of just 1.69 percent—the second best in the state—compared to the statewide average of 2.56 percent. As in Pennsylvania, adjusted death rates take into account how sick patients are and other factors that might affect survival, so they're different from the actual death rates.

New York's annual bypass surgery reports also seem to have had a similarly favorable effect on the statewide average death rate. "It really is designed as a quality-improvement tool," says Frances Tarlton, a health department spokeswoman. In 1991, the adjusted death rate was 3.38, according to the health department. The success of the heart bypass reports has led the department to begin working on similar analyses of balloon angioplasty and infant mortality.

GETTING THE TOTAL PICTURE

However they are determined, though, death rates do not give a total picture of how well a hospital performs a procedure like heart bypass surgery. Simply surviving surgery does not guarantee a lack of complications, let alone a normal life. That is one reason Iowa does not include mortality rates in its hospital report cards, says Pierce Wilson, a management analyst with the state health department. Iowa has published hospital-specific data about length of stay, complication rates, and number of procedures for heart bypass operations as well as for the 25 most common Medicare diagnostic related groups, or DRGs.

Death is just one of several possible complications of disk surgery considered by the California Hospital Outcomes Project. The project's first report—which assessed hospitals' success in treating disk surgery and heart attack patients—appeared in December 1993. (A second, expanded report—scheduled for release in late 1995—also assesses hospitals' competence in performing vaginal deliveries and cesarean sections.) Other complications for disk surgery include an unplanned second operation before discharge and postoperative infections, according to the first edition of the California report.

"These complications were chosen by reviewing the medical literature and consulting with expert advisors, such as orthopedic surgeons and neurosurgeons," the report states. "Although some complications are more serious than others, all of the chosen complications are associated with longer hospital stays and higher costs." Unusually long hospital stays were considered separately as another outcome of disk surgery.

The problem, acknowledges the Outcomes Project, is that no one yet knows the genuine usefulness of such an analysis for picking a good hospital in which to have disk surgery. It's unclear whether disk surgery patients who stay in the hospital for a long time or who experience complications do worse in the long run. In addition, hospitals may report complications inconsistently, according to the Outcomes Project. Finally, the California project considered only deaths in the hospital within 30 days of admission in evaluating hospitals' success in treating heart attack patients. As with bypass surgery, mortality rates alone don't provide any information about the health status of patients who survived.

The project's reports do not list hospitals' specific death or complication rates. The first report noted only whether a hospital performed significantly better than expected; the second report will also cite hospitals for performing significantly worse than expected. "As more years of data become available, one will be more confident of results for hospitals and more confident in the ability to distinguish among them," according to the first report. "Therefore, this first report should be viewed as a baseline against which to view future reports. As such, it probably will be more useful to health care providers than to purchasers or consumers; however, it can certainly be used to stimulate discussions among these communities."

Providers, purchasers, and consumers of health care are all taking advantage of the Missouri Department of Health "show me" philosophy. The health department issues annual regional "buyer's guides" for outpatient care at hospitals or ambulatory surgical centers. Procedures covered in the ambulatory care guides range from CAT scans to cataract removals. The guides list facilities' charges for the procedures and whether they perform many or relatively few.

In addition, the state health department each year publishes regional buyer's guides for a particular type of hospital care. The first such set of booklets, on obstetrical services, includes hospital-specific information on charges, patient satisfaction levels, cesarean section rates, ultrasound use, and number of very low birth-weight babies. The second special buyer's guide, scheduled for publication in late 1995 or early 1996, will focus on emergency services. "When choosing a provider, you should weigh all of the quality and cost indicators," the obstetrical guide cautions. "No one indicator alone is a direct measure of a provider's quality of care."

Although consumers do often have to pay deductibles and copayments, the main purchasers of health care are employers. So it's not surprising that the driving force behind the publication of health care report cards is the business community. Employers hope that such information will help them get the most for their money and foster greater cost and quality consciousness among workers.

In several cities around the country, employers have hooked up with *Health Pages*, a magazine that publishes data about local hospitals, doctors, and health plans in a readable format. The magazines comes out two to four times a year, depending on the market, and feature articles about various health topics as well as cost and quality data. "It's on the newsstands and we work with the American Association of Retired Persons and other organizations, but it's still the large employers who buy the magazine and make it feasible for us to do it," says Publisher and Editor Martin Schneider. Those employers include Bank One, based in Columbus, Ohio; US West in Denver; and McDonnell Douglas in St. Louis. "Here in St. Louis," says Jim Proffitt, director of health and welfare benefits at McDonnell Douglas, "we have never had anything in English that people can actually read."

FOR MORE HELP

Hospital report cards—sometimes available for doctors and health plans as well—are available for a variety of states, regions, and cities. You can get copies by writing to the following addresses. Unless noted, the reports are free.

- Atlanta, Boston, Cincinnati, Columbus, Colorado, Dayton, Fort Lauderdale, Los Angeles, Miami, Phoenix, Pittsburgh, St. Louis, South Florida, Tucson, West Palm Beach: *Health Pages*, 135 5th Avenue, 7th Floor, New York, NY 10010; $3.95 plus $2.50 shipping and handling.
- California: *Study Overview and Results Summary* of the California Hospital Outcomes Project, OSHPD Data Users Support Group, 818 K Street, Room 500, Sacramento, CA 95814.
- Iowa: **Iowa Health Data Commission**, 601 Locust St., Suite 330, Des Moines, IO 50309-3774.
- Missouri: *Buyer's Guides* for obstetrical services, ambulatory care, and, as of late 1995, emergency services are available for $3 each from the Missouri Department of Health, P.O. Box 570, Jefferson City, MO 65102.
- New York: *Cardiac Report,* Box 2000, Albany, NY 12220.
- Pennsylvania: *Consumer Guide to Coronary Artery Bypass Surgery*, and *The Hospital Effectiveness Report* (hospital-specific information—including average charges and lengths of stay—for 59 common diagnoses), Pennsylvania Health Care Cost Containment Council, Suite 400, 225 Market St., Harrisburg, PA 17101.

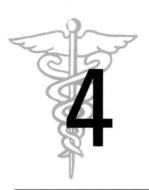

4

What to Expect When You Go

That no one looks forward to going into the hospital, except perhaps for the birth of a baby, is a platitude among platitudes. The language and surroundings are unfamiliar, the required garb too revealing, the food no threat even to a mediocre restaurant. And with care increasingly being provided on an outpatient basis, the kinds of patients admitted to a hospital these days are more likely than in years past to be dealing with serious ailments.

These factors combine to make even assertive, thick-skinned individuals feel vulnerable. But if you are one of the more than 30 million hospital admissions this year in the United States, you can take steps that not only will make you feel more in control but also will ensure that your stay is as pleasant—and as conducive to your recovery—as possible.

If you're being admitted for an elective procedure, you have the luxury of time to prepare for your hospital stay. Knowing what to expect can greatly lessen your anxiety, so it's important to ask your doctor questions, even if you think he or she already might have answered them. "The more you know, the more power you have and the better you can handle it," notes Anita Woodward, director of customer relations at Fairview General Hospital in suburban Cleveland and president of the National Society for Patient Representation and Consumer Affairs, an arm of the American Hospital Association.

"Director of customer relations" is a relatively new title at a hospital and is a bit hard to take for some old-timers—for it represents a sea change in the way health care providers regard patients. "It reminds us in a subtle way that these are people with choices and rights who can choose to go elsewhere if their needs and rights aren't met," says Woodward. True, the growth of HMOs and other forms of managed care has restricted patients' choice of doctors and hospitals. But if patients are dissatisfied enough, they can pressure their employers to switch health plans, says Woodward. "Now, all of a sudden, the provider is at risk not just of losing you, but of losing 5,000 employees of your company."

YOU, THE CUSTOMER

Still, even people who spend hours reading consumer magazines and grilling salesmen before buying a car or a computer tend to become trusting sheep in the hands of their health care providers, says Edward Bradley, a surgeon and author of *A Patient's Guide to Surgery* (Consumer Reports Books, 1994, $16.95). "This is a *service* industry," stresses Bradley. "Patients have a right to know what is being provided, and they have a right to have input into that."

Bradley, vice-chairman of the surgery department at the State University of New York at Buffalo, thinks patients are too reluctant to question their doctors. "On any given day, I could visit with Mrs. Jones and tell her we were going to schedule a cranial removal, and Mrs.

Jones would say, 'Yes, doctor,' " says Bradley. Mrs. Jones's absence of curiosity would mean waking up from the anesthesia to find she had lost her skull.

Understandably, the mind tends to shut down when a doctor first talks about a need for hospitalization. Once the shock has worn off and your brain has kicked back into gear, you should jot down all of those questions you forgot to ask, as well as what you recall of your doctor's comments, for a follow-up session. You may feel more comfortable bringing a friend or relative to act as a second set of ears at a subsequent meeting with the doctor.

Key points to go over with your doctor include the nature of any tests you will encounter and, if you're having surgery, what tests you can expect afterward. All patients undergo a battery of medical tests, often before they are admitted as well as while they're hospitalized. Make sure you understand the purpose of the tests and determine that they're absolutely necessary. That might require putting your doctor on the spot and doing a little homework, such as looking up the tests in a book that describes medical procedures in lay terms; a good one is the *Mayo Clinic Family Health Book* (Morrow, 1990, $40). Excessive medical tests are a major contributor to health care costs, and no procedure is totally free from risk. Even a routine test can backfire if done incompetently. Drawing blood can be done painlessly in 30 seconds—or it can take half an hour of agonizing poking, leaving bruises, raising your blood pressure, and even inducing a heart attack. (Hint: Ask that blood be drawn by a phlebotomist or at least by a staff member who knows how to do it right.)

SURGERY QUESTIONS

If you face surgery, ask how long it will last and whether you will go back to a regular patient room afterward. Sometimes patients are kept in the recovery area or placed in the intensive care unit so they can be closely monitored after an operation. Your surgeon can explain about the array of tubes you might find extending from your body after surgery. While you are anesthetized, a Foley catheter may be inserted into your bladder to drain urine. (If you are a male, here is a tip to minimize discomfort: Ask beforehand for lubricated tubing.) A nasogastric tube will be threaded through your nose and into your stomach if you have abdominal surgery. After such surgery, it can take several days for your digestive tract to resume functioning normally, and during that period, the nasogastric tube keeps your stomach empty so you won't regurgitate.

Don't be afraid to ask your doctor about pain—how much you can expect afterward and how it will be con-

trolled. Request patient-controlled analgesia if possible. Many hospitals now have pumps that allow patients to push a button to administer an intravenous dose of painkiller. Research shows that patients who use these pumps actually require less painkiller and feel more comfortable than those who must depend on their doctor or nurse to regulate their analgesia. Your doctor should be able to estimate how long you'll be in the hospital and how soon you'll be able to return to work and resume your other normal daily activities.

Ask to speak with the anesthesiologist with whom your surgeon will be working. Many patients never meet the anesthesiologist until they're wheeled into the operating room, by which time they've usually been given medication to take the edge off their anxiety that leaves their thinking too foggy for intelligent conversation. A thorough, presurgery explanation of anesthesia's administration and effects—especially general anesthesia, which represents the ultimate loss of control—can provide reassurance. If you have sensitive skin, you may also want to pass on a request, since your eyes may be taped shut during surgery: Ask for hypoallergenic tape, which will peel off later without taking your skin with it.

FAMILIARIZATION TOUR

If you are lucky, your hospital has a formal preadmission program. Such programs provide patients with the opportunity to visit the hospital a week or so before admission, to talk with a nurse and other staff members who might be caring for them. Even if your hospital lacks a formal program, you can still ask to talk with a nurse before you are admitted.

Getting an estimate of the total cost of your stay, let alone your share, can be tricky. The doctors involved in your case should be able to give you a rough idea of their charges, and you can call the hospital business office to find out at least what its room rates are. A private room can make your hospital stay more tolerable. Although insurance plans usually cover only a semiprivate room, the cost difference may be small enough that you will want to pay out of pocket for the added privacy.

In most cases, you will actually enter the hospital the day of surgery, perhaps as early as 5:30 A.M. With one eye always on costs, health plans rarely pay these days for an overnight stay before surgery. And that's not so bad. A good night's sleep can be far more elusive in the hospital than at home.

Do not bring jewelry or other valuables. Hospitals are public places, and when you're in surgery or recovery or simply asleep in your room, you could be a target of theft. In addition, you should check with the hospital before you bring a razor, hair dryer, or other plug-in appliance. (Be forewarned: You might not be allowed to take a shower or wash your hair for several days, depending on the nature of your surgery.) Do be sure to pack your health insurance card, slippers, a robe, sleepwear, toiletries, and just enough money to buy the daily paper or inexpensive items from the hospital gift shop. It may turn out to be helpful to bring a written list of all your medications and medical complaints and a description of your medical history.

Once installed in your room, you may be taken aback by some of the reading material you receive. In 1990, Congress enacted a law requiring hospitals to inform all adult patients upon admission about their rights to make decisions about their medical care, including a right to formulate an "advance directive," better known as a living will. This is not the best time to start thinking about the person to designate to make decisions about your care should you become incapacitated or whether your doctors should take heroic measures to keep you alive. Do it beforehand, when you are at home and have your wits—and your family—about you. But remember to make your wishes known to your family and your doctor.

A BILL OF RIGHTS

You are also likely to receive your hospital's version of "A Patient's Bill of Rights," adopted in 1973 and revised in 1992 by the American Hospital Association. It will include the right to make decisions about care and the right to know hospital policies related to patient care, such as the availability of resources for resolving disputes.

The Joint Commission on Accreditation of Health Care Organizations—the accrediting body, as you will recall—stipulates that every hospital must have a mechanism in place to deal with patients' grievances. This is a relatively recent idea for an industry that used to assume its customers were satisfied simply if the operation was a success. Most patients are hardly equipped to assess the finer points of their clinical care, of course. "What you *can* evaluate is, 'Did they treat me like a human being, or did they treat me like a liver? Was the place clean? Was the food good?' " says Woodward of Fairview General.

More than half of U.S. hospitals have staff members such as Woodward who function as patient advocates. "We tend to be the generalists who can respond to any questions, concerns, or unmet needs the patients might have," says Donna Davison-Smith, patient representative

director for Glens Falls Hospital in Glens Falls, New York. If you have a problem, you should contact a patient representative while you are still in the hospital, not after you go home, advises Mindy Raymond, an executive director of patient services at Boca Raton Community Hospital in Florida. Often, patients mistakenly suffer through whatever is bothering them because they figure they'll be discharged in a few days, says Raymond. "It's unfortunate that one bad experience can really affect their whole perception of their hospital stay," she laments.

Cultivate assertiveness. It is a quality that can prove valuable in a hospitalized patient to minimize the chance of errors—and hospitals make a lot of them. "If someone is coming into your room with a treatment, ask them about the treatment. What is it? What is it for?" urges Bradley, the surgeon. "One doesn't have to be completely passive." If your condition might interfere with your ability to monitor your care or make decisions, ask a friend or relative to accompany you to the hospital to serve as your representative.

Just as patients have to take the initiative and ask questions, health care providers should be willing to supply information. Not all are. "Part of the fault lies with the provider side," says Alexandra Gekas, executive director of the National Society of Patient Representation and Consumer Affairs. "We don't give enough information voluntarily." A patient may wait all day for a scheduled test that never happens, and no one explains that two emergency cases bumped the patient to the next day. "The nurse might think it's none of the patient's business," says Gekas.

That kind of paternalistic attitude is becoming rarer as hospitals compete for business. Glens Falls Hospital, whose logo includes the phrase "Responding to You," invites former patients back to the hospital to provide feedback in focus groups. One focus group of patients who had all undergone surgery around the same time complained that they had been rushed through and had not had enough time to ask questions. The hospital looked into the problem, and now patients are invited to ask questions when they come in for tests a few days before surgery.

Before leaving the hospital, you should receive a written explanation of how to take care of yourself at home. The explanation should include information about restrictions on activity or diet, medications, and wound care. Your doctor and a nurse should be available to answer any of your questions. Even once you are home, don't be afraid to ask questions. The informed patient, the patient who plays an active role in his or her care, is likely to recover more quickly.

ADVICE FROM A COMBAT VETERAN

Susan Rogers has valuable lessons to teach about ways in which families and friends can make a hospital stay as tolerable as possible—and even brighten the medical outcome. The Dover, Massachusetts woman's insights are born not of professional expertise but of personal tragedy. In the summer of 1994, Rogers's baby daughter, Emily, contracted a virus that led to meningitis, encephalitis, and seizures. Emily spent most of that August and September in Boston Children's Hospital. After a brief return home, Emily was readmitted to the hospital's intensive care unit. Recurring seizures caused brain damage, and she eventually could no longer move or even swallow. By the time Emily died in January of 1995, 70 days into her second hospital admission, she had been under the care of 63 different doctors and 55 nurses.

"My footprints are still in the hallways from pacing," Rogers said several months after her nine-month-old daughter's death. She feels driven to share what she learned during those long hours and days. And her advice applies to patients of all ages and conditions, not just to seriously ill babies or children.

Little things, for instance, can make a sterile hospital room more pleasant. A scented pillow can help cut through antiseptic hospital smells. A favorite sweater, book, or photo can help familiarize strange surroundings. Rogers made tapes so that Emily could hear her parents and Louisa, her three-year-old sister, even when they couldn't be with her. Rogers posted notes reminding hospital staff that Emily liked to listen to the tapes. For an adult patient, a sign could be posted to inform staff members that the patient likes to get the paper every morning or to sleep with socks on at night—"just something you would point out if you were sitting there," says Rogers.

Even Louisa got involved. "Everyone thinks 'don't bring the other kids in,'" says Rogers. "Bring them. Otherwise, you're doing a real number on them. We had a house rule: Whenever Louisa wanted to go in, she went in." Not being able to see and touch her little sister would have been more traumatic than anything she encountered in the hospital, Rogers says. No matter how many wires and tubes came between them, Louisa would step up on a stool at Emily's side and help bathe her or simply hold her hand. When Louisa wasn't at the hospital, she frequently would talk to Emily over the phone.

Rogers's common-sense tips can make life easier for friends and family as well. For example, if you park in the hospital's garage, "mark your parking tickets with the number or designation of the floor on which you parked your car," she suggests. "You never know what your state of mind may be at the end of the day." If a short cord makes it difficult to hand the hospital room phone to the patient or visitors, buy a longer one at Radio Shack and bring it in. Take advantage of friends' offers to cook, run errands, or perform other tasks, especially if a family member will be hospitalized for a long time.

Perhaps the most important lesson Rogers learned is that the responsibility for optimal medical care cannot rest solely on the professionals. "When you check your kid in or you check your mom in, you've got to check in, too," she says. "You just can't assume that everything that's being done is right." Before Emily's illness, Rogers had taken for granted, as many do, that doctors alone possess the ability to make sick people better and that they do so unerringly. But "doctors don't know your child or your husband or your sister the way you do," Rogers notes. "I can count at least 10 times I saved Emily's life. I could look at her and say, 'There's something wrong here.'"

To support her observations, Rogers could turn to the daily journal she kept about Emily's condition and care. The journal was particularly helpful to doctors and nurses new to her case. Emily's medical chart was as thick as three New York City phone books, so Rogers's notes came in handy when time was at a premium. On more than one occasion, she would tell doctors or nurses, "Look, let me cut your paperwork in half here. This is what we did a month ago." Such efforts, Rogers is convinced, helped keep her tiny daughter fighting for life longer than anyone had expected.

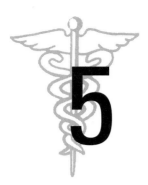

5

The Nursing Factor

After the surgeon peels off the latex gloves; after the radiologist, pathologist, and anesthesiologist go home; after the last visitor says goodbye; the hospital ward is left to the patients—alone and frightened—and to the nurses. Cost-saving alternatives like outpatient surgery, home health aides, and ambulatory-care centers tend to keep sick people at home. So the patients left in hospital beds when nearly everyone else has gone home are *very* sick. They are people who truly need nursing care, and need it around the clock.

It is in that dependent, vulnerable state that most people first begin to understand good and bad nursing. "You push a button and nobody comes. You've got tubes and restraints, and you can't get up, and you need a bed pan, and nobody comes. Or you're lying there in searing pain and nobody comes," says Ralph Seeley, 45, a Tacoma attorney with chordoma, a rare form of cancer of the spinal column.

He had been a patient in other hospitals before cancer struck. But since his diagnosis nine years ago, he's gotten all his care at the University of Washington Medical Center in Seattle, a hospital recently singled out by the American Nurses Credentialing Center for excellence in nursing. He discovered the difference high-quality bedside care can make. "It's hard to quantify. One of the problems in dealing with cancer is that you go through long phases where you don't feel any pleasure. When you're on chemotherapy, you never smile. You can't get past how *bad* you feel," he says. "The nurses at the University of Washington always come through the door looking like they're glad to see you. In some intangible way, it very much helps your psychological well-being, knowing you can push the button and ask for help and someone will come through the door with a smile."

The importance of a good nursing staff goes beyond a quick response and a smile, however. The way nurses monitor their patients can spell the difference between speedy recovery and relapse—even between life and death. In *U.S. News* surveys, physicians repeatedly rank the quality of nursing care second only to the quality of the medical staff as the chief predictor of overall patient care in a hospital. Nursing care is considered more important than state-of-the-art technology, than research capability, than the quality of teaching in hospitals affiliated with medical schools. Geriatricians, who treat the elderly, consider nurses more important even than the quality of a hospital's doctors.

LIVES SAVED

The surveys are right in emphasizing nursing care. Studies confirm what nurses and doctors have long believed: Good nursing can save lives. The most comprehensive study to date, which appeared in August 1994 in the nursing journal *Medical Care*, showed that hospitals judged as having excellent nursing care had fewer deaths among Medicare patients than did a comparison group of other hospitals. Researchers looked at mortality rates among Medicare patients at 39 hospitals chosen by nurses surveyed to determine institutions that provide high-quality nursing care. Mortality rates at recommended hospitals were then compared with mortality rates at 195 other hospitals similar to the nurse-chosen hospitals in size, organizational structure, and other measures. Good nursing saved five lives for every 1,000 Medicare patients, says Linda Aiken, the study's lead author and director of the Center for Health Services and Policy Research at the University of Pennsylvania School of Nursing.

The nurse-chosen hospitals, dubbed "magnet hospitals," were identified during the nursing shortages of the 1980s, when the American Academy of Nursing identified hospitals with excellent nursing reputations and an ability to attract and keep nurses when many hospitals were experiencing high turnover. These hospitals were practically immune from nursing shortages, even as many hospitals were dangling sign-up bonuses, free parking spots, and health club memberships. The academy then sent nursing experts to the nominated hospitals and came up with 41 that were "magnets" to nurses. Reevaluated in 1986 and 1989, the magnet hospitals—now reduced to 39 for various reasons having nothing to do with quality—have become known as nursing's gold standard of excellence.

POWERFUL MAGNETS

The magnet hospitals are not the only hospitals that boast excellent nursing care, of course. The American Nurses Credentialing Center now has a program that allow hospitals to apply for magnet status. So far, 49 hospitals have done so. But the program is relatively new; only the University of Washington Medical Center and Hackensack Medical Center in New Jersey have completed the lengthy review process and met the new standards. Magnet status means that in those hospitals nurses feel respected, not overworked, and believe that doctors and administrators support them in organizing and delivering excellent nursing care. The assumption is that what's good for nurses is good for patients, too. Aiken's study is the first to back up that assumption with figures.

Other studies have shown a link between relative numbers of registered nurses (RNs) and patient outcomes—which is why you will see it included as a factor in the rankings in this guide. A 1989 study in the *New England Journal of Medicine* examined various characteristics of 3,100 hospitals, among them the relationship between the percentage of nurses on staff who are registered and the hospital's death rates. The researchers found that when hospitals were ranked according to their RNs as a percentage of total nurses, the hospitals in the top quarter had six fewer deaths per 1,000 patients than did those in the bottom quarter. A review of various studies, reported in 1993 in *Nursing Economics*, found that the higher the overall nurse staffing, the lower a hospital's mortality rate.

Although the sheer quantity of nurses seems related to the quality of care, no accepted standard exists for the perfect ratio of nurses to patients or for the best mix of RNs, licensed practical nurses (LPNs), and unlicensed nursing aides. Nationwide, 28 percent of RNs come from two-year associate's degree programs and 30 percent from four-year bachelor's degree programs. Another 34 percent are trained in three-year hospital-based training programs, 3 percent are trained in a foreign country, and about 8 percent have a master's degree or higher. "This hospital has 95 percent or more at the bachelor's degree or master's level. That's very high," says Joyce Clifford, vice-president for nursing and nurse in chief at Beth Israel Hospital in Boston, a hospital long recognized for excellent and innovative nursing.

Nationally, the mix of RNs to LPNs, whose post-high school training is a 12- to 14-month course focusing on basic nursing care, is 85 percent RNs to 15 percent LPNs, according to figures from the American Hospital Association (AHA). Smaller hospitals, with fewer than 25 beds, average about 70 percent to 30 percent, while hospitals with more than 500 beds average about 90 percent to 10 percent, according to the AHA. Hospitals also have unlicensed aides who traditionally have done chores such as making beds. But as hospitals seek to cut costs, the aides have received more responsibility for direct care.

To a bed-bound patient, uniformed care givers look pretty much the same, whether RNs or housekeeping staff. But bedside observations made by a trained observer can alter an outcome or save a life. Many unlicensed staffers, for example, are perfectly capable of taking a temperature or measuring blood pressure. But a sudden change in blood pressure, coupled with a rise in temperature, sounds warning bells for a trained nurse that may not alarm a staffer with less training. Add clammy skin and a change in respiratory rate, and the patient could be slipping into septic shock—a potentially fatal infection that demands an immediate response. "A nurse would know what that array of symptoms could mean, run through the preliminary diagnoses, and quickly inform the physician," says Diane Soules, associate administrator for patient care services at the University of Washington Medical Center.

For a quick response, those at the bedside must be links in a strict chain of command that leads to a licensed, accountable nurse. But as hospitals seek to cut costs, more of them are retraining nonmedical staffers in medical services that give them more contact with patients—not always with a solidly accountable chain of command. In at least one state, the trend has resulted in a consumer warning.

Indiana Attorney General Pamela Carter received enough complaints through the state's Consumer Protection Agency to hold a press conference in March 1995, warning consumers that unlicensed and untrained hospital staff were in over their heads in providing medical services and performing medical procedures at some Indiana hospitals. The reports to her office included some indicating that staff trained only in basic first aid were performing emergency room procedures such as stapling head wounds. Carter suggested that consumers ask staff members for their titles and training before accepting treatment—though that may be less than totally practical if you're bleeding all over the emergency room. The state is investigating the complaints. Naomi Patchin, executive director of the Indiana State Nurses Association, says, "Indiana is not unique, except that we have an attorney general who is willing to speak up."

The American Nurses Association (ANA) also suggests that patients ask bedside care givers for their title. The ANA says hospitalized patients should expect a visit every hour by an RN, no matter how many visits they get from aides or housekeeping staff.

Unlicensed staffers are increasingly undergoing what the industry calls cross-training. A housekeeper might deliver a tray, give a bath, hand out medicine, and handle other nonmedical tasks traditionally done by nurses. Since most state nurse licensing boards hold the nurse responsible for care delivered by a delegated staff member, the cross-trained staffer should be able to let patients know the name of the nurse who ordered the bath, the medications, or other care.

A BLOOD-DRAWING SECRETARY

The background and training of staffers trained on the job does not always inspire confidence. Patchin recalls a recent employment ad placed by a large, urban hospital that read: "Unit secretary. Secretarial skills required. Do phlebotomy [draw blood], make medical rounds, and give medications." Consumers would do well to ask anyone who approaches the bed for their credentials.

The ANA suggests as a minimum an overall ratio of one RN to every five patients on a typical hospital medical-surgical floor. For intensive-care units, the ANA's guideline is one to two. But those numbers are not accepted industrywide. Even some nurses worry that any accepted minimum standard will quickly become the industry maximum. "The floor too often becomes the ceiling. That's what has happened in nursing homes," says Janet Heinrich, director of the American Academy of Nursing, an elite group of nurses selected from ANA membership for their leadership in nursing research, practice, or teaching. But Arthur Levin, director of the Center for Medical Consumers in New York, a non-profit consumer advocacy group, believes patients have a right to know the staffing required for good care. "You can't always make judgments on ratios, but there have to be minimum standards below which you know you can't go," says Levin. Given the lack of an agreed-upon standard, consumers can ask the level of nurse staffing and how the hospital came to consider that level adequate. "Our staff runs five or six patients per nurse as a high average. I've been in hospitals that talked about 15 patients per nurse," says Beth Israel's Clifford. Staffing information should be available through the department of nursing services or perhaps through the public relations department.

Determining the nature of a particular hospital's nursing care ahead of time takes digging. Physicians are an obvious source, since they rely on accurate observations of the hospital's nurses to make a quick diagnosis or an over-the-phone modification in treatment. Ask your doctor if he or she does rounds with nurses or holds meetings that include nurses in discussions of patient care—indicators of a good, working team effort between doctors and nurses. Nurses themselves can provide invaluable inside information. "If you know a nurse, ask him or her what he or she thinks of a hospital's nursing staff," says Heinrich.

Aiken, Clifford, and other nursing professionals are adamant about not hiring a private-duty nurse, who comes from an agency and is paid at an hourly rate. A hospital should be expected to provide a level of nursing attention that should make a private-duty nurse unnecessary. "It's a very bad sign to be encouraged to bring your own nurse. If you should ever feel you have to bring your own nurse, you shouldn't go to that hospital. A private nurse would never be able to communicate with the rest of the staff, with the doctors, or know the technology available the way a staff nurse would," says Aiken.

On the other hand, bringing a spouse, a family member, or a trusted friend may be vital. "I think the one single thing that a consumer can do is to take an advocate along—a family member, or a friend, who will be responsible for observing care, asking questions. You almost need someone there 24 hours a day," says Sandra Gainer, an RN and West Virginia state coordinator for the National Center for Patients' Rights.

Having an advocate is especially important for patients with new limitations—from a stroke, for example—that call for strong nursing care. An articulate family member can speak out if a bedridden patient is not regularly repositioned to prevent painful bedsores and serious infections. A patient advocate can make sure the recovering stroke patient is fed slowly, to reduce the risk of choking. And stroke patients need rehabilitation efforts, such as range-of-motion exercises to keep blood freely circulating, reducing the chances of life-threatening blood clots.

Patients know what they like and, when asked, can provide some of the best consumer guidelines of all. Most hospitals at least pay lip service to patient satisfaction surveys, and a growing number are using standardized, objective measures of satisfaction like one developed by the Picker Institute, formerly called the Picker/ Commonwealth Program for Patient-Centered Care. The Picker survey has so far asked more than 6,000 hospital patients from 62 hospitals about their experiences. Surveyers found that patients wanted from nurses good physical care, relief from discomfort, and personal attention. Some 28 percent of patients surveyed said their nurses sometimes seemed too busy to take care of them, and 5 percent reported having to wait more than 15 minutes to have a call button answered. Most hospitals use such surveys internally as a way of knowing where changes are needed, not to provide information to consumers. But patients can ask if the hospital surveys patients, and, if they do, what changes have resulted.

Many hospitals assign one nurse to be responsible for a patient's care from preadmission through discharge. That nurse is with the patient through a normal eight-hour shift but is still responsible for a written care plan telling nurses on other shifts what needs to be done, when, and how. "Patients don't feel that they have to repeat things over and over," says Clifford. Patients or their families can ask which nurse will be primarily responsible for care and how the care is kept consistent across shifts.

Ruthann Goularte, 44, is a liver transplant patient who spent a two-month stretch in the University of Washington Medical Center waiting for a suitable donor organ. She has sclerosing cholangitis, a degenerative disease that eventually closed her bile ducts, making a transplant the one option that could save her life. Her long hospital wait gave her plenty of opportunity to reflect on the importance of nursing care. "I think the consistency made a difference, having a few nurses that saw me regularly," says Goularte.

Following surgery, Goularte's trust in her nurses paid off during painful and frightening times. "One nurse that came in would immediately make me relax simply by the way she talked to me. She'd say, 'Ruthann, it's going to be okay.' Somehow, it would register and I could relax," says Goularte.

Consistency of care led to trusting talks and soothing voices. "This sounds odd," says Goularte, who owns a housewares store in Olympia, Washington. "But as a person in retail, I felt like they treated me like a customer—like someone they cared enough about to try to please," she says. Of course, nurses are not merchants who peddle cutlery, cars, or computer chips. They peddle nothing—but they provide a component of hospital care that can make all the difference.

FOR MORE HELP

- **The American Nurses Credentialing Center**, 600 Maryland Avenue S.W., Suite 100 West, Washington DC 20024, (800) 284-2378. The center can tell consumers which hospitals have applied for "magnet" status, a rigorous quality standard indicating excellent nursing.

- **Picker Institute**, 1295 Boylston Street, Suite 100, Boston, MA 02215, (617) 667-2388. Formerly called the Picker/Commonwealth Program for Patient-Centered Care, the institute uses state-of-the-art surveys to find out what patients do and don't want during their hospital stays—including what satisfies them about nursing care.

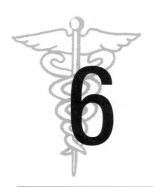

6

Going Home Quicker, Sicker, and Poorer

Congratulations, says the doctor—you can leave the hospital and go home. That's almost always welcome news, though these days patients are getting sprung from medical centers sicker, quicker, and poorer than ever before. Fortunately, patients can take steps to ease their recuperation at home and prevent shock from the hospital bill.

Avoiding headaches over charges requires a good deal of bedside chutzpah during hospitalization. Patients can ask doctors before they perform diagnostic procedures or treatments, for instance, to accept the insurance payment and waive the rest of the usual fee. Some physicians will go along with this request, especially if the charges would impose an undue burden. And patients should try to keep track of which doctors they saw as well as the tests, services, and procedures they received while hospitalized or should have someone do it for them. Knowing how much time they've spent in the operating and recovery rooms, for example, is particularly important, since at $300 to $500 an hour, operating-room charges can be extremely steep. Keeping track of such matters will be of immeasurable help when it finally comes time to review the bills.

First, of course, patients need to recuperate, and that may call for planning. People with family members or friends who can help care for them while they recover at home may require only a group conversation with their doctors or nurses. But those who will need professional help should speak with a social worker or other

"discharge planner" early during their stay, rather than when they're on their way out the door. Such hospital staff members can help arrange for the care patients may need at home, including physical therapy, medical treatments, nursing services, meals on wheels, and other assistance. Some patients may be surprised at the thought of a bedside visit with a social worker during their hospitalization. But social workers are responsible for assessing patients' more complicated posthospitalization needs and their ability to deal with their aftercare. They help involve patients and their families in making decisions about such needs, and they coordinate the plans with doctors, nurses, physical therapists, and other care givers.

GETTING PERSONAL

In fact, in hospitals that do a good job coordinating care, patients should expect a social worker to come calling during the first couple of days of a hospital stay. After all, patients and their families need sufficient time to make decisions and to adapt to their situation. But before patients divulge personal details about their needs or their ability to pay for services that may be necessary at home, they should make certain they really are talking to a hospital social worker and not a "case manager" or "cost reducer" from the hospital's billing office, says Jim Brennan, a senior staff associate for health and mental

26

services at the National Association of Social Workers, an umbrella organization. He says he has received reports of patients fooled by visits with hospital billing office staff whose intentions are to cut costs by *limiting* aftercare services to patients instead of setting it up. And patients at high risk for postdischarge difficulties because they are frail, live alone, or require a high level of care at home should receive a follow-up assessment from a social worker within a week of discharge.

HOME HELP

Patients may require visits at home from a skilled nurse to set up infusion therapy or to ensure that pills are taken as directed. Social workers can help patients handle logistical problems, such as getting to and from their doctor's office for follow-up visits and tests, by arranging for transportation services such as those offered by the American Cancer Society for patients receiving chemotherapy. Social workers can help put patients in touch with financial assistance programs, other community agencies, and information and referral services as well as provide emotional support and counseling. On the other hand, "chore workers" may be all that are needed—volunteers or unskilled employees of home health agencies who handle shopping and cleaning. Typically, such service agencies are community based or affiliated with hospitals.

"To social workers, the key is creating options for very concrete problems," says Brennan. For example, at the Mayo Clinic in Rochester, Minnesota, where two-thirds of neurology patients are from out of state, social workers even help coordinate patients' aftercare needs back home. "Typically, we'll help locate providers of home care services in the patient's community that can meet the patient's needs," says Michael O'Brien, director of medical social services at Mayo. "We'll even work with third-party payers and family members to see if types of services the patient requires are covered. And if not, we'll see if there are alternatives. Perhaps there's an agency that's subsidized by the United Way or agencies that provide services on a sliding scale or charity." O'Brien will also help coordinate Mayo doctors' orders for follow-up tests, treatments, and checkups with hometown doctors. Usually there's no need: Mayo physicians and hometown doctors communicate directly about follow-up care, and out-of-town patients are sent home with copies of doctors' orders, O'Brien says.

For people over age 65 and others who qualify for Medicare, the federal program generally covers most home health care if services are ordered by a physician and if the home health agency is certified. Many supplemental insurance policies also offer home health care as a covered benefit, and virtually all HMOs offer home care as part of their program, says the American Hospital Association. Of course, patients can also order home health services themselves, without a doctor. But if they do, they'll probably have to pay the bills out of their own pocket. Keep in mind, also, that homemaker and housekeeper services normally are not covered.

Home health agencies charge either an hourly rate for their services or a by-the-visit fee. Medicare pays on a per-visit basis. But patients with private insurance should ask the home health agency to accept their insurance company's payment as payment in full, advises the American Hospital Association (AHA). And patients should be aware of the fine print in home care contracts. What may seem like a lower hourly rate may really end up costing more than paying by the visit. That is because some home health agencies charge a minimum number of hours each day and days per week, says the AHA. And medical supplies and equipment are almost always extra. Even if a home health agency advertises that it will accept insurance, this does not mean that your insurance company will necessarily cover the particular agency.

HALVING THE BILL

Nursing care at home costs about half what it does at nursing homes, according to the AHA. What's more, studies comparing hospital care to home care costs show dramatic differences, according to a report by the National Association for Home Care, a trade group. For example, caring for a low-birth-weight baby typically costs $26,190 per month in a hospital. But for well-selected infants who can be sent home early, the cost is only $330 per month when family members—aided by periodic visits from a nurse—provide the 24-hour watch. And caring for a ventilator-dependent adult may cost $21,570 per month in a hospital, but minus room and nursing charges, only $7,050 per month at home when home care attendants help out.

But despite assurances of discounted care, consumers are well-advised to enter into agreements only after doing some sleuthing, particularly in the burgeoning and virtually unregulated field of intravenous drug and nutrition services known as home infusion therapy. Federal investigators have investigated dozens of reports involving kickbacks from home infusion companies to physicians for referrals as well as false Medicare claims. With only a handful of states now licensing home infusion services, more insurers are probing bills for padding and negotiating discounts. Consumers can further protect themselves from overcharges and other problems with a bit of common sense:

- *Check your coverage.* Many patients run up huge home care tabs only to have the insurer refuse payment or to find they have exhausted their policy's lifetime limit. Some insurers still insist on a hospital stay before approving home care. To avoid billing problems, find out if your infusion service is among your insurer's approved providers and ask about limits to coverage; some insurers, for instance, will pay for only up to eight weeks of antibiotic infusion.
- *Get an independent second opinion.* "A second opinion is always useful," says Michael Mangano, principal deputy inspector general at the U.S. Department of Health and Human Services (HHS). The trick is to ensure an *independent* second opinion. Roughly half the states forbid physicians from referring patients to home care or other companies in which they have a financial stake. The local health department can tell you if the state has banned physician self-referral. Otherwise, the only way to ferret out any business ties is to ask the doctor.
- *Haggle with suppliers.* You do not have to be a hospital or health insurer to bargain down the price of in-home care. "Call several services and ask how much it will cost," suggests Laurie Bodenheimer, home care manager at Blue Cross and Blue Shield of the National Capital Area, based in Washington, D.C. You may not get the 50 percent discounts many health organizations have negotiated, but most infusion firms will reduce their rates upon learning another local outfit will do the job for less. Or ask your insurer to do the bargaining. Experts also advise asking whether generic drugs are available.
- *Scrutinize supplies.* A company's first delivery may provide more gauze, syringes, and other commodities than the patient can use in a month—all of which inflate the tab and are unreturnable. Alerting the infusion company to hold up on restocking should alleviate the excess. Care givers should also examine medications; even the most reliable service can deliver the wrong goods.
- *Watch for swindles.* If a company tries peddling medical equipment or services directly to you as a patient, chances are you are being scammed. Most insurers require a prescription or physician's referral for reimbursement. And so does the government. "Any time you hear the words, 'Medicare will pay, and it won't cost you

a thing,' that should be a red flag," a program analyst in the inspector general's office of HHS told *U.S. News.*

The lack of national or state licensing standards has prompted a growing number of home infusion companies to seek industry accreditation from the Joint Commission on Accreditation of Healthcare Organizations (JCAHO), the group that also accredits hospitals. Besides accrediting companies that provide home medical equipment, the JCAHO accredits organizations that provide any of the following:

- Nursing services; medical social work; and physical, speech, and occupational therapy
- Personal care, including bathing and household maintenance
- Pharmaceutical services, including monitoring patients' clinical status and their medication regimen
- Respiratory services, including monitoring vital signs and administering therapeutic treatments

The JCAHO now releases reports on home care organizations that have passed the commission's accreditation process, including those that have passed with special commendation. The special category was created in 1991 to recognize exemplary performance in selected health care organizations. To earn and maintain accreditation, home care organizations must pass an on-site survey at least every three years during which they are scored on 400 standards of performance. Reports are available for organizations surveyed after January 1, 1994. Each performance report costs $30 and includes the organization's overall evaluation score compared with those of similar organizations surveyed; the organization's performance in areas such as infection control and patients' assessments; and recommendations for improvement.

Eventually, recuperating patients must deal with their hospital bill. Typically, it's a whopper—and if their fee-for-service plan is also typical, they will owe 20 percent, up to a maximum of $1,500 or so. Patients also have to pay all physician charges that exceed their insurer's notion of "reasonable and customary." A hospital bill for a five-day stay can easily run to 10 pages of single-spaced entries. Large hospitals have thousands of separate numerical codes for procedures, medication, and other charges, to say nothing of the medical jargon used to describe them. And keeping track of every poke, prod, and prescription drug a patient has been given during a long hospital stay is simply impossible.

But patients can help minimize billing errors, cut down on excessive charges, and get relief from overcharges. Simply fulfilling an insurance company's requirements for precertification before a hospital stay or operation can help patients sort out major costs and head off problems. Before contacting an insurer, ask doctors for the medical name and billing codes of the major procedures that were performed, as well as the fees. A hospital's billing office can explain what these procedures typically cost and can provide the hospital's daily room rate, operating-room charges, and recovery-room charges. The insurance company will then determine if the charges are within the "customary and reasonable" amounts covered by the policy. If not, patients should discuss them with their doctors, who may be willing to reduce the fee. It's often a good idea for patients to jot down the codes and fees for later reference.

Billing mistakes usually occur when numerical codes are confused. The code for a specific test may differ from another by no more than a single digit in a four- to eight-digit code, but inadvertently swapping the codes may increase the cost by $100 or more. Many hospitals also automatically bill for equipment or services typically associated with a procedure whether you get them or not.

That is why patients should ask for an itemized bill as well as the standard "summary." When you get it, first double-check the obvious, such as the number of days you were hospitalized and the charges for time in the recovery and operating rooms. Detecting errors in medication, services, tests, and physician visits will be harder, but it will help that you tried to keep track while in the hospital. You should watch for medication charges that shoot up dramatically in a single day or charges for a procedure you cannot remember. An excess of miscellaneous charges may also signal a problem.

Hospital bills are rife with errors and overcharges, a government audit suggests. And deciphering abbreviations and diagnostic codes is both a necessity and a nightmare. Bills are so confusing that services have sprung up to help patients sort through them. (The National Association of Claims Assistance Professionals, a referral group, can provide help and is listed among the resources below.) Typically, such firms have registered nurses and people with insurance backgrounds check bills for obvious goofs, such as three casts for one broken leg, as well as for lesser sins, such as too many antibiotics. Patients get a plain-language explanation or report that flags unusual charges. Some firms will confront the hospital with discrepancies. If not, patients can ask the hospital's billing supervisor or audit nurse to check the suspect charges and respond within 30 days with a corrected bill. A call to the hospital administrator's office can some-

times cut through lingering red tape that threatens to tie patients, and their savings, in knots.

Unhappy patients can ask for a "utilization review" from their health insurer—an in-depth accounting of their hospital stay—and can ask the hospital to formally audit the charges. That can take weeks or months. Also, the JCAHO requires that every hospital have a formal mechanism for dealing with patients' complaints—including billing disputes. Your doctor also may help you plead your case. But if your insurance company and hospital ultimately agree that the charges were correct and legitimate, you will have little choice but to pay up or hire a lawyer, always an expensive proposition. In that case, you may be better off just to get on with your recovery.

FOR MORE HELP

- *Better Health Care for Less,* by Neil Shulman and Letitia Sweitzer (Hippocrene, 1993, $14.95). This publication offers a section on hospital stays with 33 money-saving tips, from avoiding unnecessary tests to exploring outpatient options.
- *Extended Health Care at Home,* by Evelyn Baulch (Celestial Arts, 1988, $9.95). This publication provides information on caring for patients at home, including advice on how to prepare and where to seek help and burnout advice for care givers.
- **The Joint Commission on Accreditation of Healthcare Organizations,** One Renaissance Blvd., Oakbrook Terrace, IL 60181, (708) 916-5754. This not-for-profit accrediting organization reports whether home care agencies meet requirements for personnel, safety, and infection control procedures. Inquiries about home infusion companies should specify the name of the local branch, since many infusion companies are part of conglomerates. For a self-addressed, stamped envelope, the commission will provide a free list of questions to ask when choosing a home care firm, such as whether a provider offers 24-hour telephone service.
- **National Association of Social Workers,** 750 First Street, N.E., Suite 700, Washington D.C. 20002, (202) 408-8600. This association provides information on standards and credentials of social workers who serve as hospital discharge planners.
- *Take This Book to the Hospital With You,* by Charles Inlander and Ed Weiner (People's Medical Society, 1993, $14.95). This book makes it easier to log tests, medications, and charges.

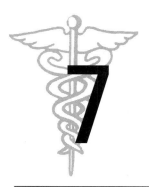

Alternatives to Hospitalization

Not everyone needs the high-octane care offered by a top hospital. For that matter, not everyone needs to check into a hospital at all. Over 2,500 procedures, from cataract surgery to mastectomies, are being done on an outpatient basis at same-day surgical centers. More patients who need minor surgery and routine diagnostic tests are getting them at their doctors' offices. Patients with minor pains and sprains are bypassing hospital emergency rooms for less hectic walk-in care at "emergicenters." And patients who do need to go to a hospital are finding that they no longer must trek very far for access to resources of some major hospitals—now they can visit their satellite clinics.

In an astonishing display of medical efficiency, nudged by financial pressures, most operations no longer call for an overnight stay. About 55 percent of surgeries are now done on an outpatient basis. More than 90 percent of hospitals either have outpatient departments where same-day surgeries are done or are affiliated with free-standing "surgicenters." Outpatient surgery costs less since no hospital stay is necessary. Surgicenters, of course, don't carry the huge overhead that hospitals do. From the patient's perspective, a huge plus is that recuperating at home limits exposure to infection; incorrect treatments; and the inherent risk of drugs, X rays, and false lab tests. Besides, it's more pleasant. Patients indeed seem pleased. In a survey by the Department of Health and Human Services, 98 percent of Medicare patients who had surgery at ambulatory

centers rated them good or excellent, as did 94 percent of those who went to outpatient departments.

Same-day surgery is no longer just for patients needing an abscess drained or a bunion excised. Outpatient surgical centers are doing far more complex procedures in specialties from gastroenterology and gynecology to neurology and plastic surgery. Much of the credit goes to new combinations of anesthesia drugs that limit nausea and pain, such as scopolamine patches. The other major factor is the blossoming use of "keyhole" surgery done through small incisions. The surgeon manipulates instruments, a light, and a fiber optic link to a video monitor through tiny tubes. Even coronary bypass surgery might be done that way before too long, allowing the patient to go home the same day.

OUTPATIENT MASTECTOMIES?

At Johns Hopkins Hospital in Baltimore, doctors are beginning to do outpatient hysterectomies, mastectomies, and even cleft palate procedures. By May 1995, 28 women had undergone breast cancer surgery as outpatients. Other hospitals are developing similar capabilities. So far, Hopkins's doctors have found that although about 80 percent of mastectomy patients qualify for same-day mastectomies—they do not have chronic medical problems, and someone is at home who can help them recuperate— almost all initially decline. Most are worried about the procedure and want to be hospitalized in case of complications or pain afterwards. Those who have taken the same-day option have done so only after thoughtful discussions with their doctor, social worker, occupational therapist, and a nurse. Even then, most don't finally agree to give up a hospital room until they wake up in the recovery room. Traditionally, inpatient costs are about $4,500; an outpatient mastectomy can cost $1,500 to $2,500. Hopkins is also among the first centers to do same-day vaginal hysterectomies, eliminating the traditional three- to five-day hospital stay. Such outpatient hysterectomies cost about $1,750 compared to $5,000 when done as an inpatient procedure. After same-day surgery, the patient is evaluated for several hours and sent home. That night, a nurse stops by to give medication and to show the patient how to change dressings and avoid infection.

Patients who have same-day surgery are largely on their own after the operation, making the quality of the surgery center paramount. Fortunately, patients can check up on centers near them. Hospital outpatient departments and other ambulatory-surgery centers that do not accept Medicare reimbursement are automatically suspect. The federal Health Care Financing Administration (HCFA), which oversees the Medicare system, halts payments to centers that it judges inadequate in some way. Your state health department can tell you whether Medicare privileges are suspended or if the outpatient center is on probation.

Although freestanding ambulatory-care centers that receive Medicare reimbursement are all federally certified and must pass state licensure reviews, only about 20 to 30 percent have passed additional quality reviews by private agencies. About 450 are currently accredited by the nonprofit Accreditation Association for Ambulatory Health Care (AAAHC), and 350 by the Joint Commission on Accreditation of Healthcare Organizations (JCAHO). In their definition of ambulatory-care centers, both groups include emergency-care centers, community-health centers, ambulatory-surgery centers and even some types of group practices. Both send inspectors—by appointment—for announced periodic checkups. The AAAHC's reviews are tailored to the type, size, and range of services offered; reviewers are specialists in the type of care given.

The JCAHO suggests that patients begin by asking their doctor or insurer to recommend several ambulatory care organizations. A visit to several, armed with pointed questions for the manager, should leave you confident of your choice. Some possible questions are:

- *How often is the procedure performed and what is the facility's success rate?* (Answers, of course, should show that the facility is experienced and adept, performing the procedure once or twice a day.)
- *What is the specific training of the physician who will be performing the procedure?* (Physicians should be certified by the appropriate medical specialty board. To verify a physician's certification, call the American Board of Medical Specialties at 800-776-2378.)
- *Is the center affiliated with an area hospital, and if so what is the transfer arrangement in case of emergency?* (Surgicenter affiliation with a full-service hospital is a major plus; patients can be rushed there if complications arise.)
- *Does the center have a 24-hour phone number to call in the event of complications?* (Walk out of any center that does not have one. As for others, ask if a nurse or doctor will answer the phone and what the procedure is for dealing with after-hour emergencies.)
- *Has the center passed muster with an accrediting organization, such as the JCAHO?* (JCAHO accreditation means the organization has met national health and safety standards. Information is available on individual ambulatory-care centers by calling the JCAHO at (708) 916-5800. For $30, the commission will send a report that includes the accreditation decision and overall evaluation and performance scores, as well as specific recommendations in areas that come up short in some way.)

SURGERY IN THE DOCTOR'S OFFICE

Many low-level procedures can be performed in an office setting just as safely and far more cheaply than in either hospitals or surgicenters. Examination and biopsy of a gastric ulcer with a tube called an endoscope cost $548, on average, instead of the $1,100 charged at a surgicenter and somewhat more in a hospital, according to data reported in July 1993 in the *Journal of Family Practice.*

Doctors would love to do more procedures in their offices. To keep down the unnecessary use of expensive medical facilities, Medicare reimburses at a higher rate if certain procedures are done in an office setting rather than in hospitals or surgicenters; patients' out-of-pocket copayments are lower, too. In 1994, the HCFA published a list of 550 codes for procedures the agency would like to see done in offices more often. That was 120 more than in 1992, when the first list was published. And where HCFA's Medicare program leads, private insurers usually follow.

But patients need to know what should—and should not—be done in a doctor's office. "Anything involving general anesthesia should be reserved for hospitals, though not necessarily an overnight stay," says Richard Schilsky, director of the Cancer Research Center at the University of Chicago. A hospital is also the safest setting for patients with bleeding disorders, serious lung disease, or abnormal heart rhythms.

Even excising a bunion may be dangerous for patients who have diabetes or hypertension that is not under firm control, says Glenn Gastwirth, deputy executive director of the American Podiatric Medical Association. And many experts advise making sure that doctors who plan to operate in their offices have privileges to perform the same procedures in a hospital.

"DOC-IN-A-BOX"

Emergency-care clinics have come to be known as "urgi-centers" or "doc-in-the-boxes" (because they sometimes are found in strip malls alongside fast-food restaurants) can be good bets for relatively minor emergency cases. Charles Inlander, head of the People's Medical Society, a consumer-advocacy group in Allentown, Pennsylvania, suggests scouting out local emergency-care clinics for future use in a non-life-threatening situation—say, a severely sprained ankle. The wait will be shorter than at a hospital emergency room and your visit cheaper.

Homey birthing centers, usually staffed by midwives, became an alternative to the bright lights and metallic feel of big hospitals' labor-and-delivery rooms many years ago, and their popularity continues. A good clinic will not accept high-risk patients and will whisk you to a hospital if your labor goes awry. Some hospitals have fought back by offering their own birthing centers, which combine an unthreateningly low-technology environment with the security of an operating room a gurney ride away in case of emergency. Nonhospital birthing centers are about one third cheaper than those in hospitals. In an uncomplicated pregnancy, the choice of venue is mostly a matter of personal preference. A study of birthing centers several years ago showed the same rate of infant death for labors begun in birthing centers and those begun in hospitals. It is worth noting, however, that one of six women who started out in a birthing center wound up delivering their babies in a hospital because of various complications. More than half the states license these centers. Check with the local health department to see if the one you have in mind is licensed.

Surgical patients who do need hospitalization may be able to receive treatment from some of the best hospitals in the country without traveling vast distances, by visiting their satellite clinics. Treatment at the vaunted Mayo Clinic, Cleveland Clinic, or M.D. Anderson Cancer Center, for instance, no longer requires a trek to Minnesota or Ohio or Texas. Chasing shifting demographics, all three institutions have opened up shop in the Sun Belt, in well-off cities near plenty of potential patients. Mayo launched its first satellite clinic in Jacksonville, Florida, in 1986 and established a second in Scottsdale, Arizona, a year later. The Cleveland Clinic has since opened a Fort Lauderdale facility. And M.D. Anderson joined with a local hospital to open the Orlando Cancer Center.

All have thrived. Mayo says its surveys show that patients at its two new locales are as satisfied with the care they receive as are patients at its Rochester, Minnesota, center. And all the satellites have added doctors and office space since opening; the Mayo centers, for example, have gone from a couple of dozen physicians to more than 120 doctors in each new site. That's peanuts compared with roughly 1,000 in Minnesota but plenty to permit the open consultation between doctors that is the main advantage of clinic-style medicine.

Patients who live nearby like the convenience. For many terminal cancer patients, for instance, it would be tough to fly to M.D. Anderson in Houston or to drive several hours to a university center every three months to have specialists perform a delicate procedure to slow the growth of a liver tumor. One patient, for instance, now makes a 30-minute trip to Orlando instead. "Cancer disrupts your life," he told *U.S.News & World Report.* "Travel would disrupt it so much more." He and others praise the doctors' and nurses' skills, thorough history taking and the feeling that the doctors—who work on salary rather than for fees—don't see them as cash cows.

The clinics have gone to great lengths to reproduce the ambiance of their home bases, right down to the fish tanks gracing the waiting rooms of M.D. Anderson's Houston and Orlando centers. Every month, an M.D. Anderson physician comes to Florida for a week to meet with Orlando confreres, and all Orlando doctors spend at least one week a year in Houston. Ninety percent of the physicians at the Jacksonville Mayo Clinic took at least part of their training in Minnesota, and a third of the doctors staffing the Cleveland Clinic's Fort Lauderdale outpost moved down from Ohio. All three home bases maintain satellite linkups so doctors can send X rays and other data back and forth for consultation. And patients can enroll in most of the research protocols offered back home.

A few big-ticket items are absent. Mayo, for example, has a gamma knife—a multimillion-dollar gamma-ray generator that can destroy diseased tissue deep within the brain without surgery—only in Minnesota. The Cleveland Clinic satellite in Fort Lauderdale sends cancer patients to a local facility for radiation therapy. Orlando Cancer Center doctors still consider sending patients with very rare conditions back to Houston. On the other hand, some procedures are available only in Orlando, such as experimental radioactive implants for brain tumors.

Satellite clinics aside, some hospitals are offering patient-friendlier alternatives in-house. The ninth through 13th floors of New York University Medical Center's Arnold and Marie Schwartz Health Care Center have the air of a Manhattan hotel, what with Impressionist prints on the walls and Chinese takeout menus piled near the elevator. Moreover, the rooms can be locked, the twin beds are framed in oak, and the windows offer breathtaking views of the Hudson and East rivers.

Can this be a hospital? The usual blood pressure monitors and oxygen-tank hookups lining the wall are missing; so are the bright lights and the nursing station at the end of the hall. Only the extra-wide halls and doors and the emergency-call pull chain in the bathroom are standard hospital issue.

The patients, on the other hand, are no different from those on the floors below. Many are recovering from surgery or are scheduled for an operation, high-dose chemotherapy, or an invasive procedure like cardiac catheterization. But their care is different. They and their doctors have opted for the cooperative approach, in which a relative or friend stays with the patient in the 104-patient Cooperative Care Center night and day. After instruction, the "care partner" dispenses oral medications, brings the patient to examining rooms and the cafeteria, and watches for symptoms such as rapid breathing that call for a nurse or doctor from the 14th floor.

The patient-empowerment movement of recent years has given the idea a boost. Medical Center Hospital of Vermont has a 10-bed unit, Rhode Island Hospital has a 74-bed version, and other hospitals have incorporated bits and pieces of cooperative care. And seven hospitals in California, New York, and Oregon have units designed by Program Planetree, a San Francisco consumer-health group, in which health care workers teach patients about

their ailments and patients have far more than the usual autonomy. As at NYU, there's no dress code, visitors can come anytime, and no one bursts in at 6 A.M. to draw blood without a good reason. The point is to enlist the patient in the medical team. Patients spend hours talking with hospital staff about their illness, treatment, and recovery and have access to their medical records.

A recent Johns Hopkins-NYU evaluation showed that the lack of close nursing supervision does not hurt. Cooperative-care patients needed no extra care after discharge, and they had easier transitions from hospital to home because they knew more about their illness and medications. Insurers readily pay for NYU's cooperative care—which costs about a third less than a normal hospital room—and Planetree's, which costs the same.

Any patient can borrow from cooperative-style care. While in the hospital, you can set up a formal appointment with your attending physician to plan your at-home care. You can ask that a friend or relative be present for all discussions with your doctors and nurses. You can talk to the nurses about wearing your own clothes or ordering food in and can ask your doctor to limit nocturnal visits from the nursing staff. Inlander of the People's Medical Society suggests that you think of yourself not as an inmate but as a paying customer, with the right to be as comfortable as you can. That's not easy when you're really sick, but it can make you feel at least a little better.

FOR MORE HELP

- *Helping You Choose Quality Ambulatory Care* (Joint Commission on Accreditation of Healthcare Organizations, 708-916-5800). A free pamphlet lists questions to ask before choosing ambulatory-care services. Callers can also check whether an ambulatory care center is accredited; a full report costs $30.
- *Questions and Answers about the Accreditation Association for Ambulatory Health Care, Inc.,* (708-676-9610). A free pamphlet explains the accreditation process and how it relates to patient care. The AAAHC will also send a free list of accredited organizations.

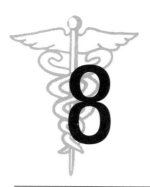

8

Health Reform in Spite of Itself

Health care reform is dead; long live health care reform. President Clinton's failure to muster congressional support in 1994 notwithstanding, the delivery of health care is undergoing a major revolution.

The economics of health care delivery once meant that a patient plus a hospital bed automatically equaled profits all around. Now a patient who stays too long in a hospital, or who requires complex technological care, is likely to represent an economic liability to the hospital and to the patient's physician. Medicine used to reward specialists handsomely for focusing on the heart, the bones, the skin, the brain. Now it is internists and other primary-care providers who have the best shot at job security, with health maintenance organizations (HMOs) and other managed-care plans scrambling to hire them.

The switch in emphasis from more to less and from specialized care to primary care can be laid at the doorstep of managed care, which got under way in 1945 in California with Kaiser Permanente, the first HMO. Managed-care plans provide virtually all of an individual's health care needs, typically short of dental, for a set fee. The lack of variation in the fee over the course of a year, and the cradle-to-grave coverage of health needs, has made managed care very popular indeed with consumers. Kaiser Permanente now has 6.7 million members in 16 states and the District of Columbia, and some 100 million Americans are enrolled in some form of managed-care plan, according to the Health Insurance Association of America.

The move to care paid for in advance through negotiated fees creates an incentive for insurers to provide the least care that will yield the best result—because, of course, poor outcomes and complications from inadequate care also can be costly to the insurer. It means, too, that care provided by primary-care physicians is valued for its low-cost efficiency, and referrals to higher-cost specialists can become liabilities to the insurer if the same quality can be achieved at a cheaper price.

WANT FREE CHOICE? IT'LL COST YOU

The ongoing revolution to convert the public to managed care has shoved aside the short-lived effort led by President Clinton and First Lady Hillary Rodham Clinton to provide affordable, universal health care in some form. The failure of the Clinton plan, says Uwe Reinhardt, professor of political economy at Princeton University, means a three-tiered medical system is in the works. Reinhardt sees managed care, the largest tier, reserved for the middle class. Traditional fee-for-service plans, which permit consumers to pick their doctors and hospitals out of the *Yellow Pages* if they so desire, will become more and more expensive, their sky-high premiums eventually restricting their use to the wealthy. And public hospitals and clinics, together with low-cost

Medicaid managed-care plans being developed by a growing number of states, will provide care to the uninsured and poor.

For now, managed care is at center stage. It comes in four basic flavors: HMOs, physician provider organizations (PPOs), exclusive provider organizations (EPOs) and point-of-service plans (POS).

Health maintenance organizations provide health services to their patients from womb to tomb. Doctors are paid a salary as HMO employees or receive a set fee, called a capitated payment, to care for each patient's needs. In either case, the insurer makes a profit on an individual when the patient needs few medical services and loses money if the patient's medical needs are costly. The financial incentives for providers are exactly reversed from those for fee-for-service care, where physicians make more money if they order more tests and perform more procedures.

About 51 percent of HMOs are federally qualified, a necessary step for organizations that want to offer care to Medicare recipients. Most others adhere to the federal guidelines in most respects. The guidelines call for providing 10 basic benefits:

- Physician services and referrals
- Hospitalization
- Preventive care (including well child care, prenatal care, routine health exams, eye and ear exams for children under 18, immunizations, and infertility services)
- Emergency treatment inside and outside the HMO's service area
- Diagnostic tests and services, such as pap smear tests for cervical cancer
- Rehabilitation services for conditions like hip replacement surgery or, when appropriate, for relatively minor conditions like tennis elbow
- Up to two months of physical, occupational, and speech therapy
- 20 outpatient mental health visits
- Drug and alcohol treatment
- Home health care

Although most HMOs have these benefits in common, significant differences exist from one HMO to the next. "Staff model" HMOs, such as Kaiser Permanente and the Harvard Community Health Plan, hire physicians and pay them a salary. All care—routine care from a general internist, complex care from a specialist, laboratory tests, and pharmacy needs—can often be delivered from the same clinic location. Another kind of HMO is an independent practice association, or IPA, such as U.S. Healthcare. An IPA contracts with individual physicians in private practice to provide services to plan members, again at a prepaid rate per patient. Physicians maintain their own offices and can still see nonplan patients. A primary-care provider in an IPA can refer patients in the plan only to specialists who are also in the plan. Most patients in any form of HMO pay $5 or less per office visit.

Phsician provider organizations are more flexible than HMOs. Consumers are free to choose any doctor, although the PPO tries to control costs by directing patients to providers with proven records of cost-effective care delivery. If a consumer wants to choose a less efficient doctor, he or she will pay more out of pocket.

Exclusive provider organizations are a version of PPOs in which consumers who stray from the recommended physicians pay the entire cost of care out of pocket. And a *POS* is a hybrid of all of the above, giving consumers a list of doctors to visit and charging a low fee for their services, but adding the option of choosing an out-of-plan provider at any time and for any reason. POS plans carry either a high premium, a high deductible, or a higher copayment for choosing an out-of-plan provider.

Managed-care enrollees include 3 million Medicare recipients. That is still only a small percentage of all seniors but represents a whopping 16 percent jump from 1993 to 1994 and is expected to skyrocket by the year 2000. "We don't want to use the word 'coerce,' but we will make it very attractive for Medicare recipients to want to move to a managed-care system," Republican Senator Bob Packwood of Oregon predicted at the 1995 annual meeting of Group Health Association of America, (GHAA), the largest trade group that represents HMOs. The appeal will come, as for those under the age of 65, from the lower copayments and out-of-pocket costs offered by managed care.

THE GATEKEEPER

In any managed-care plan, a patient's "gatekeeper," or primary-care physician, is the foundation. That doctor—a general internist, family practice physician or pediatrician, and in some cases an obstetrician/gynecologist—steers each patient through whatever medical maze lies ahead. Consumers uncomfortable with letting one doctor determine their health care services might want to forget about managed care—if they can afford a fee-for-service plan. The primary-care physician in a managed-care organization provides all routine care to each patient and refers patients to specialists only if the problem is severe.

"Routine" and "severe" are defined through internal reviews that tend to be unavailable to consumers. The plan's administrators look over the primary-care doctors' pattern of referrals, lab tests, and drugs and compare each doctor to all others. About half of HMOs use such records to adjust physician compensation, rewarding doctors with bonuses for holding down costs. Only about 20 percent of HMOs peg doctors' pay to reports of members' satisfaction. An HMO that does might be worth a look.

Utilization reviews—internal reviews of how an HMO's doctors order tests, prescribe drugs, and refer to specialists—have become a way of life at virtually every health plan. For example, a child with a persistent ear infection may not respond to a low-cost antibiotic, so a physician might prescribe a higher-cost alternative. That might be enough to trigger a call from a utilization review staffer—sometimes a doctor or nurse, but not always—questioning the use of the pricier medication.

Critics deride reviewers as "health care police" because they step in and reach conclusions after the fact. Some state medical boards are taking steps to hold HMO medical directors responsible when a utilization reviews inappropriately denies coverage. And in Minnesota, a law has been introduced to require that anyone performing utilization reviews be a physician licensed in the state.

Although most HMOs provide prescription drugs free or at low cost, some 86 percent of HMOs surveyed by the GHAA control prescription costs by using drug formularies, or lists of approved drugs. The lists, usually developed by committees that include physicians, administrators, pharmacists, and sometimes consumers, are often simply guidelines for doctors, encouraging them to use lower-cost drugs over similar higher-cost drugs. But a few HMOs have what are called "closed formularies" and will cover only prescriptions on the list. Consumers can ask their managed-care physician if he or she is prescribing the most appropriate drug available or simply the most appropriate drug available through the formulary.

HOW CONSUMERS FEEL ABOUT MANAGED CARE

Surveys show that consumers are still sorting out their feelings about managed-care plans. People choose plans like HMOs primarily because premiums are lower and they like the range of services offered. They also appreci-

ate that once they sign on, there's almost no paperwork involved in receiving care. But they are struggling to get used to the gatekeeper concept, which many believe limits their choices, and are often frustrated at having to wait longer than they want to for information and appointments. A report published in the May 25, 1994, *Journal of the American Medical Association*, for example, found that 30 percent of HMO patients said they had trouble reaching a doctor with a question, while only 20 percent of fee-for-service patients said it was a problem. And 37 percent of HMO members thought it was hard to get an appointment right away, while 18 percent of fee-for-service patients thought they waited too long for an appointment.

What now remains of federal government efforts to reform the health care delivery system is vastly scaled down from the heady days of President Clinton's Health Security Act. That 1,342-page tome called for coverage for everyone, emphasized preventive care, and would have created a complex system involving groups of insurance plans in an attempt to offer at least some degree of choice to consumers.

Instead, experts predict that Congress will tackle a mere handful of noncontroversial items in the next year or two. "Modest insurance reform will pass," predicted Packwood at the annual GHAA meeting. That includes such things as limiting insurers' ability to exclude people because of preexisting conditions. Someone recovering from cancer, say, should be able to shop around and switch insurance plans and still be covered for cancer. "That doesn't mean they'll have to sell it to you at the same price," says Robert Blendon, chairman of the department of health policy and management at the Harvard School of Public Health. But the higher premiums of those with preexisting conditions, or older people at higher risk for disease, will at least be capped—perhaps at 150 percent of the average premium. Malpractice reform, also considered a modest insurance reform, would limit jury awards to patients injured by negligence, mistakes, and incompetence, presumably lowering the cost of malpractice insurance. As further disincentive to file lawsuits, the loser in a malpractice case would pay court costs under a proposal by Texas Senator Phil Gramm.

On the other side of the aisle, Representative Richard Gephardt, a Missouri Democrat, also predicts a move toward laws guaranteeing that insurance benefits will be portable, so people won't be forced to remain with an employer solely out of fear of losing coverage if they move or change jobs. "I think people will begin to have confidence that, no matter what, they'll have health insurance coverage," he says.

Another proposed way out of the quagmire is to establish tax-free medical savings accounts, nicknamed "medisave" or "medical IRAs"—not to be confused with existing arrangements at many companies that allow employees to set aside pretax dollars to pay for out-of-pocket medical expenses. Medisave accounts would go hand in hand with reduced health insurance coverage and are a cornerstone of many Republican health reform plans, including that of Senator Gramm. The money in a medisave account would cover the cost of routine and preventive care.

Medisave accounts would be an option for employees willing to gamble on coverage that carried a high deductible and paid for high-ticket care like surgery but not for lower-cost care like annual checkups or new eyeglasses. Since employers would pay a lower premium on the high-deductible policy, employers might be required to put some of their savings into the medisave accounts. Employees might also contribute their own money in pretax dollars. As noncritical medical needs like a sore throat or a pulled muscle arose during the year, the employee could draw from the account to cover medical expenses, with no tax penalty. If the money contributed by the employer ran out before the deductible was met, however, the employee would have to pay out of pocket until the deductible was met and catastrophic coverage would kick in.

The gamble is that by keeping medical expenses low, an employee could end up with an annual bonus consisting of any unused medical savings. But an unexpected illness could wipe out the account—and then some. Supporters say it would give consumers strong incentives to shop around for efficient health care and would discourage them from overspending on unnecessary care. But critics say medical savings accounts could discourage people from using preventive medical care, perhaps delaying diagnosis of diseases like breast cancer which have better survival odds when caught early.

So far, the federal changes proposed are small, especially when compared with President Clinton's Health Security Act. But still on the back burner, and destined to remain simmering, says Vermont's Governor Howard Dean, is the single-payer plan—a proposal for national health insurance covering everyone. The government would collect premiums in the form of a payroll tax that would be used to pay providers. Medical care would be provided free to all Americans, who would choose their own doctors. As of summer 1995, a single-payer plan proposed by Representative Jim McDermott, Democrat from Washington, had 90 sponsors—and not a prayer of a chance. But if small changes don't soon make people feel more comfortable about such important considerations as the cost and portability of insurance, Dean says, the single-payer plan just may make a surprising comeback.

The pace of change in the states, once considered percolating laboratories of reform ideas, has slowed, according to researchers at the George Washington University Intergovernmental Health Policy Project. In Massachusetts, for example, the state's 1988 Health Security Act, authored by then-presidential candidate Michael Dukakis, was put on hold for a third time, postponing the start date to January 1996. Its main provision, that employers provide health insurance for all employees or pay a fine that helps pay to cover uninsured Bay Staters—a concept called "play or pay"—was originally to start on January 1992.

In Minnesota, a move is under way to repeal or delay a reform that would set fees for physicians who remain in the fee-for-service setting. Oregon's controversial Medicaid reform, establishing a prioritized list of illnesses that will be covered only as deep into the list as state money lasts each year, is still on track. The state's plan to require employers to provide health insurance or pay a fine, with the money subsidizing universal health care, however, is off the table.

For a while, then, Americans will continue to watch the rise and fall and rise again of federal health care reform ideas, along with the charge and retreat of state health care reform plans. But the real shake-up for consumers is here and now, right in their own doctors' offices.

FOR MORE HELP

- *Radical Surgery: What's Next for America's Health Care*, by Joseph A. Califano, Jr. (Times Books, 1994, $25). The Secretary of Health, Education and Welfare from 1977 to 1979 tells consumers what a changing health care delivery system means to them.
- **The Kaiser Family Foundation** offers publications on health policy topics, including *The New American Electorate and Health Reform* and *What Shapes Lawmakers' Views: A Survey of Members of Congress and Key Staff on Health Care Reform*. For a complete list of publications or to order single copies, call (800) 656-4533.

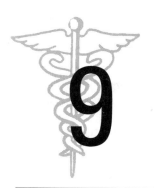

What to Do When Emergency Strikes

The key to getting the best care in an emergency is no different than in a less stressful moment: You have to take charge. That calls for advance planning so that when illness or injury strikes, you can move with calm certainty into take-charge mode.

Every potential emergency room candidate—which means everyone—can benefit by scouting out the best emergency room or ambulance service. For anyone with a history of stroke, heart disease, asthma, or falls, however, as well as for those with young children at home, the exercise is no less than crucial. Yet very few people make even rudimentary contingency plans, such as asking their physician what to do should chest pains strike. Studies show that 92 out of 100 people with heart attack symptoms call a neighbor first—or their spouse, which is even worse. In several studies, investigators have found that three to four hours may be lost while mates worry about what to do.

Phoning your physician for help, while understandable, can delay getting to a hospital, according to a study of stroke victims in several cities. By the time doctors returned their calls, told them to go to the hospital, and they arrived, an average of 10 hours had elapsed from their initial symptoms. The delay is not all the physicians' fault; most patients took nearly six hours to actually get to the hospital, says study author William Barsan, who is in charge of emergency medicine at the University of Michigan Medical Center.

Calling a pediatrician or racing a child to the doctor's office instead of dialing 911 during an emergency is similarly risky. Only 43 percent of the pediatricians recently surveyed by Johns Hopkins Medical School said they had all the equipment and drugs on a list of commonly used emergency equipment in their offices. Children need smaller oxygen masks, for example, and using adult-size blood pressure cuffs on a child, which many hospitals still do, often results in inaccurate readings. Because children have smaller lungs and airways, they require plastic airway tubes less than half as wide as those made for adults. (Any pediatrician, however, should have the basic equipment to perform cardiopulmonary resuscitation and to restore breathing and should have epinephrine, a heart stimulant, on hand for an emergency that occurs in the office.)

DON'T CALL THE ER

A direct call to an emergency room might seem logical but can elicit bad advice. Investigators at the University of Pittsburgh School of Medicine anonymously telephoned 61 emergency departments and said that their five-week-old baby had symptoms that should have been recognized as signs of meningitis, a swift and deadly infection. Only 32 advised bringing the baby in immediately. In a previous study, the Pittsburgh team called 46 emergency departments and said a parent was having heart attack symptoms. Only four emergency departments suggested calling 911. A majority of the others told the caller to drive the parent in; others suggested taking antacids or borrowing someone's nitroglycerin tablets.

Despite anecdotal reports of horrendous waits, the best advice is still to call 911 or the emergency number listed in the phone book. A recent *U.S.News & World Report* survey of the state and local emergency medical service (EMS) in eight cities and 12 suburbs found that reported response times generally met the deadline for starting cardiopulmonary resuscitation, or CPR, and for reviving a heart with a shock from a defibrillator.

CLOCKING THE RESPONSE

But not all emergency services are equally prompt, and digging out the average response time can take determination. The first stop should be the EMS division of the local fire department. If officials say they don't track response times, ask for the number of the EMS state office—it is usually part of the state department of health. The best indicator of performance is "standard response time"—how long it takes an ambulance to respond in 90 percent of the calls—but many offices are not this exact. Residents of cities where the standard response time exceeds nine minutes may want to look into private or volunteer ambulance services. The Hatzoloh ambulance service, which covers most of New York City, boasted response times of two and a half to four minutes in 1992, compared with the city's 911-dispatched median arrival time of about nine minutes. Run by a small group of Orthodox Jews, Hatzoloh—Hebrew for rescue—is one of the largest U.S. volunteer ambulance services.

Volunteer services, however, often suffer from a lack of funds for training and equipment. The percentage of paramedics on staff (the higher the better) and the presence of defibrillators are keys to good service. Parents might ask whether rescuers are trained for pediatric emergencies. According to national surveys, one urban crew in seven lacks such training. Advanced courses for critical-care technicians and paramedics devote no more than 10 of the 200 to 1,000 hours of training to children. In New Jersey, for example, the state department of health concedes that only one in 20 paramedics is certified in advanced pediatric life support. Emergency medical technicians (EMTs) are even more in the dark; only two of the 110-hours of training EMTs get is spent on the prehospital emergency care of infants and children.

Emergency crews refer to the window during which a seriously ill or injured adult must be treated the "golden hour." For children, they call it the "platinum half-hour." The younger the child, the smaller the margin for error. Unless rescuers must spend time freeing an accident victim, an average on-scene time of 20 minutes or more usually means inefficient care and needless delay. That information can be gleaned from listings on ambulance run sheets, which reputable companies should make available.

The next chore is to get the patient to the best emergency room. Normally, ambulance crews consult by radio with emergency-department physicians from different hospitals who serve on a rotating basis. Using standardized severity-of-illness guidelines and patient-destination policies approved by the local EMS agency, the crew and the doctor decide where the patient should go. Rescuers should determine, for instance, whether the patient suffers from any chronic conditions such as cirrhosis, bleeding problems, or diabetes. All can increase the risk of death in an injury victim. Many cities and suburbs have devised hospital referral lists that distinguish among emergency rooms adequate for setting fractures, for treating seriously sick children, and for dealing with full-fledged trauma. The information is sometimes available from state or local EMS coordinators and local hospital associations—but not always in writing, since the explanations can be highly technical.

All of the guidelines notwithstanding, critics charge that gravely ill and injured children too often are taken to the wrong place. Usually, they are rushed to the nearest hospital—even though a pediatrician may not be on duty, the nursing staff has no special training in pediatrics, equipment designed for children is not available, and critical specialists such as neurosurgeons are not present. In a large percentage of these cases, the child must be transferred to another hospital. The delay, which can last several hours, can prove fatal. Surprisingly, kids in many of the nation's nicest communities are most at risk. Sick children whose middle-class parents instinctively take them to modern community hospitals in safe, tree-lined neighborhoods may be less likely to receive optimal care than inner-city kids who live closer to teaching hospitals with advanced pediatric services. The startling fact is that unless critically ill children are taken to a sophisticated children's hospital or one especially geared for pediatric emergencies, the treatment they will receive is dicey at best.

How many children suffer as a result of these systemic problems is impossible to know. Most medical personnel, especially doctors, refuse to talk openly about specific cases that go awry. This code of silence is partly fueled by a fear that speaking up could lead to malpractice suits and loss of patient referrals—or even their jobs.

It also stems from a reluctance to alienate colleagues and other key medical players whose cooperation is needed to improve the system. Reformers face another obstacle: Most Americans, including many pediatricians, do not know the extent of the problem. Rightly proud of medical technology's dazzling progress, many find it impossible to believe that a system that can coax a one-pound premature baby to robust health cannot adequately treat children who become gravely ill.

When key players and institutions cooperate, improvement can be striking. It was once common for rescue squads to pick up a critically ill or injured child and race to the nearest hospital, a process known as "scoop and run." Today paramedics and emergency medical technicians are much more likely to deliver children to hospitals with intravenous lines and ventilators already in place. But there are only a few strong communitywide systems—two pioneering examples are in Maryland and Los Angeles—for treating desperately ill children.

Partly in response, the American Board of Medical Specialties not long ago approved a subspecialty in pediatric emergency medicine, which may lessen the rivalries between pediatricians and emergency physicians and could make the field more attractive to the next generation of doctors. The goal is to have 1,000 board-certified pediatric emergency doctors in the United States by the year 2000. That is not a large number, considering the need, but supporters of the subspecialty hope these new doctors will have a ripple effect, inspiring many communities to deal with this problem.

Other experts in both pediatrics and emergency medicine argue that more reforms are needed—including greater access to equipment designed for children; 24-hour staffing by pediatricians and other doctors and nurses with pediatric training in hospital and wards that treat children; more training of emergency rescue personnel; and better coordination between them and hospitals to get sick children to the right place quickly.

ADULT EMERGENCIES

Emergency treatment for adults is more straightforward. The medical crew is generally supposed to assess the severity of the problem and make tracks for the closest appropriate facility. Unhappy patients can transfer to another hospital once their condition has stabilized. But if the move is not for medical reasons, you will likely bear the cost. If your doctor has told you to go to a particular hospital in case of, say, a stroke or a fall, you should expect to be taken where you want to go, as long as you can speak up for yourself. But anyone in immediate danger of losing life or limb will undoubtedly be sped to the nearest hospital, then transferred when it's safer.

To pick the overall best emergency room in your area for adults, you'll need to write each hospital's quality-assurance representative or emergency room chief. You should pose the following questions:

- *What is the proportion of part-time or moonlighting doctors to full-time emergency physicians?* The answer should indicate a low ratio. David Sklar, president of the Society for Academic Emergency Medicine, goes so far as to say that there should be *no* moonlighting doctors in an ER. "Those doctors are trying to earn a little extra money during their residencies in, say, neurology or radiology or anesthesiology . . . and not only aren't they qualified, they potentially could be dangerous," he says.

- *Are most of the physicians fully certified in emergency medicine?* Those doctors completed a residency training program in emergency medicine and passed a two-part examination by the American Board of Emergency Medicine. Doctors who may not have taken a residency program, but who are career emergency physicians or who have passed the certification exam by drawing on years of experience in ERs, are fine, too. Realistically, however, only about half of the nation's 25,000 emergency-room doctors would meet Sklar's standards, according to a September 1994 report by a panel of health experts chaired by the president of the National Board of Medical Examiners.

- *What proportion of patients make an unplanned return visit for the same problem within 72 hours?* Look for a number in the range of 2 to 3 percent, Sklar says. But remember that emergency physicians often see someone in different phases of an illness as it progresses. In appendicitis, for instance, the initial nausea and abdominal pain could mean nothing at all; many patients are sent home only to return 12 to 24 hours later with an obviously inflamed appendix. "But a good emergency physician," Sklar says, "will educate the patient on the initial visit that the symptoms may progress and that if they do the patients should come back."

- *How often does a discrepancy between an emergency room doctor's reading of X-ray reports and a radiologist's interpretations require a patient to return to see a specialist?* Significant errors should happen no more than 1 percent to 2 percent of the time, says Sklar. Often, a radiologist who has little information on the patient's complaints will flag anything in an X ray that's unusual or suggestive and will call the patient back for X rays, MRIs, or CT scans that might be unnecessary. On the other hand, an emergency physician may miss a fracture that the radiologist will pick up the next day—in time for treatment.

Additional questions will help determine the quality of care that your community's emergency facilities deliver to children:

- *What percent of the EMTs are trained in advanced pediatric life support?* An ideal system would provide such training to all EMTs, all of whom would also have child-size resuscitation equipment to stabilize a child.
- *Does the system in your town allow EMTs or paramedics to bypass the nearest hospital in favor of the nearest facility that might be better for a given illness or injury?* The system should also have communication links permitting rescue crews to talk to hospital-based pediatric specialists before and while a child is on the way.
- *Which of your nearest hospitals has an organized team of doctors, nurses, and respiratory specialists with pediatric training on duty 24 hours a day?* Since most community hospitals do not have in-house pediatricians, it is crucial for the emergency room staff to be able to stabilize your child until a pediatrician arrives. Surgeons should also be available quickly, especially to place an IV line properly.
- *Which is the closest regional pediatric critical-care center?* Any local hospital with an emergency room should be able to answer this.
- *Is a mobile intensive-care unit (ICU) available to move a child from a community hospital to a regional pediatric critical-care center?* Such transport systems exist in most places for neonatal patients, but they are not as widely available for older children.
- *Will a child in serious condition be placed in an ICU especially designed and staffed for children or in the regular adult ICU?* Nurses in adult ICUs, for example, may be unfamiliar with the special needs of children and how to assess their condition.

Once you identify the best emergency room, use it strictly for emergencies. In a typical ER, 60 percent to 80 percent of those waiting for a doctor need only stitches or have simple problems that a neighborhood "doc in the box" clinic could handle—a fact that explains the average two-hour emergency room wait for non-life-threatening conditions. Such emergency-care clinics can be good bets for relatively minor emergency cases. Charles Inlander of the People's Medical Society suggests that you scout them out for use when someone is hurt but in no special danger—with a twisted knee, say. The wait will be shorter and your visit cheaper. These centers, essentially doctors' offices, require no private accreditation. Look at a facility's waiting room to see if it seems well organized, or find people who have tried it. And considering how easy it is to end up at the wrong ER, prospective patients need to know where to go for back pain as opposed to chest pain. In the midst of an actual emergency, most victims make poor shoppers.

FOR MORE HELP

- *First Aid Handbook* (National Safety Council). This $10.95 illustrated manual shows the steps to take for most injuries, and sudden illnesses. Although information is useful for treating all age groups, the book stresses actions to take in adult injuries.
- *A Parents Guide to Child Safety* (National Safety Council, 1121 Spring Lake Drive, Itasca, IL 60143). This $5 book covers safety tips exclusively for children from infancy through 12 years of age, including helpful information on child-proofing homes, sports injuries, and safety around pets.
- *What You Should Know About Emergency Care* (Emergency Brochure, ACEP, 1111 19th Street, N.W., Suite 650, Washington DC 20036). This free pamphlet developed by the American College of Emergency Physicians covers such things as warning signs of a medical emergency and what to say when calling 911 for help. Send a self-addressed, stamped envelope.

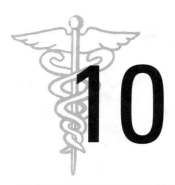

10

The Quest to Measure Quality

When it comes to health care, quality, like most of life's intangibles, is in the eye of the beholder. To employers, quality might mean lower costs—the size of an employee's medical bill and how quickly the employee returns to work. To a pediatrician at a health maintenance organization (HMO), it might be the percentage of children in his or her HMO who are properly immunized. And to a patient, quality might simply translate as less pain—or simply how long it takes to see a doctor. "The way a consumer defines quality of care is pretty straightforward: Do I feel better? Can I do what I want to do with my life?" says Ann Mond Johnson, senior vice-president of the Sachs Group of Evanston, Illinois, a strategic planning and marketing information company that conducts annual surveys of health plan members to see how satisfied they are.

These disparate agendas have not discouraged accrediting organizations, state legislatures, employer coalitions, consumer groups, and health care providers themselves from trying to develop report cards that rate the performance of doctors, hospitals, and health plans. Such efforts could backfire, warn policy experts. Although the report cards could help consumers make better choices and could spur improvements, health care providers might try to inflate their grades by accepting only patients they think will do well, rejecting the very old or sick. And, like students who get their test questions in advance, health care providers might focus all

their energies on only those areas in which they know they will be graded.

The possibility that grades or numbers could be manipulated or misunderstood led the federal government in 1995 to stop compiling hospital-by-hospital mortality rates. (The mortality rates that appear in this guide were compiled by a private firm for *U.S. News & World Report.*) It is true that mortality rates for some hospitals, especially those in inner cities, suffer because a disproportionate share of their patients are poor and uninsured and thus more likely to suffer complications. But published mortality rates adjust for the case mix— the age of patients and the severity of their illness. Hospitals with relatively low mortality rates also tend to do best in the reputational surveys conducted for the *U.S. News* annual hospital rankings, validating the use of death data. Many of those high-ranking hospitals are located in the inner city.

THE BEST EVERYDAY CARE

Although the *U.S. News* rankings are intended to help consumers identify the best hospitals for diagnosing or treating the most complex and serious illnesses, more resources are emerging that help locate high-quality sources of routine care. Laws in at least 39 states require various healthcare providers to supply such information as charges, length of stay, mortality rates for certain procedures, and other measurable data to state agencies or independent commissions. Some states publish this information for consumers. California, Missouri, New York, Pennsylvania, and Wisconsin have pioneered such efforts.

Other states collect similar data but release it only to those who provide or pay for care—namely hospitals, doctors, and employers. "This report card business has sort of gotten out of hand," says Pete Bailey of South Carolina's Office of Research and Statistics, part of the state's Budget and Control Board. "We believe the public will have difficulty understanding them and using them appropriately." Bailey's office has released information to consumers about individual hospitals' services and lengths of stay and charges for certain ailments and procedures. But data related to how well patients do who have those ailments or undergo those procedures are not available to consumers. "We believe we should make this information available to providers," Bailey says. "If they know how they compare and where they're out of line, they will get in line. You relieve the public of a very difficult effort of trying to figure out what in the world does all this mean."

Another option, of course, is to figure out a way to convert this information into a format that doesn't require a doctorate in statistics. Such efforts are in their infancy, but as the demand increases, many health policy experts predict, the quality of available information will improve. In late 1994, the Joint Commission on Accreditation of Healthcare Organizations (JCAHO) began releasing its accreditation reports for individual hospitals, nursing homes, and ambulatory-care clinics. But JCAHO accredits institutions on a three-year cycle, so reports will not become available for all 11,000 institutions it reviews—including 80 percent of U.S. hospitals—until the end of 1996. Each report includes an overall score and individual scores in such areas as ensuring proper medication use and checking nurses' qualifications. How a center compares with similar institutions is also shown. But the reports don't rate individual medical specialties.

Checking out JCAHO's opinion of a community's entire roster of medical centers doesn't come cheap, at $30 for each four-page report. That might be one reason why only about 450 reports were ordered during the first six months the JCAHO made them available. For now, the reports relate the ways in which a facility does or does not meet JCAHO accreditation standards. Most experts think of those standards—on physician licensing and infection-control programs, for example—as proxies for quality rather than direct measures. In a few years, JCAHO plans to be able to tell consumers how well patients actually fare at individual hospitals in specific procedures. For instance, a report might include the percentage of patients who survive quadruple-bypass surgery, or who can deliver vaginally after having had a cesarean section previously.

The biggest demand for the JCAHO reports has come from hospitals themselves and from health plans, says John Laing, a JCAHO vice-president. "Hospitals want to know how somebody down the street is doing," says Laing, while some for-profit hospital chains are using the reports as a management tool. Laing says HMOs and other health plans want the information to help them make decisions about which hospitals they should incorporate into their networks of healthcare providers.

WHICH HMO?

For more and more Americans, the main health care decision is not which hospital, but which health plan. The growth of managed care means that more people are finding their choice of hospitals limited except in unusual circumstances to those in their health plan's network. Many health experts believe that it is managed-care plans that need evaluating, since for many people their plan dictates the quality of their care. Some HMOs, such as U.S. Healthcare in the Northeast—which mainly serves the Northeast, have conducted in-house quality surveys for their members, but the resulting data cannot be used to compare different plans. However, such information can help plan members pick their primary-care doctors, as well as assist the plans themselves in pinpointing trouble spots.

The biggest nationwide assessment of health plans is conducted by the U.S. Office of Personnel Management, which hopes to set an example for the private sector. It is a survey of members' satisfaction, not a report that measures performance. In 1994, the office randomly surveyed federal employees in 261 HMOs and fee-for-service plans throughout the country (203 other plans available to federal workers were not included because they chose not to participate, had too few federal workers as members or as survey respondents, or were not offered as choices in 1994). Some 90,000 people responded to the survey, which asked the plan members to rate the accessibility and quality of care in their plans, the availability of doctors they wanted to see, the range of covered services, and customer service. The eight-page report issued by the Office of Personnel Management in October 1994 broke the plans down by state and presented overall satisfaction ratings for each, as well as ratings for the individual components of satisfaction. Information in the report would also be useful to nonfederal workers trying to pick a health plan. Differences among the plans in the 1994 report are far from striking, however. Fewer than a handful have overall satisfaction ratings below 70 percent; most fall in the 80 percent to 95 percent range. In Georgia for example, Aetna and PruCare of Atlanta scored an overall satisfaction rating of 85 percent, while Kaiser-Permanente of Atlanta scored 88 percent. Office of Personnel Management officials expect the survey will be conducted annually. The Center for the Study of Services, which devised and conducted the survey for the government, sells a minutely detailed report about the findings, including information on costs.

THE MOVE TO ACCREDIT

One of the other leaders in assessing HMOs, as in assessing hospitals, is an accrediting organization. In 1994, the Washington, D.C.-based National Committee for Quality Assurance (NCQA) began making public the status of HMOs that seek accreditation. Since then, the NCQA has updated the list monthly. When selecting health plans, many employers place great value on NCQA accreditation, so an increasing number of HMOs are seeking that seal of approval. JCAHO, too, is getting into the HMO-accrediting business but had accredited only nine plans by mid-1995. In comparison, the NCQA's accreditation status list by that time included 168 HMOs. Of those HMOs, a third had received a full three-year accreditation, 40 percent a one-year accreditation, and 14 percent provisional accreditation. Another 12 percent were denied accreditation, while 1 percent are appealing the NCQA's original decision. In addition, 17 HMOs were awaiting the results of their first review, and 118 had reviews scheduled. After a team of doctors and managed-care experts conducts on-site and off-site evaluations, a committee of physicians analyzes the findings. Accreditation is based on how the plan's performance holds its own against 50 NCQA standards. The yardsticks fall into six categories: quality improvement, physician credentials, members' rights and responsibilities, preventive health services, utilization management (whether the plan is reasonable and consistent in deciding the services appropriate to an individual's needs), and medical record keeping.

As with JCAHO accreditation of hospitals, meeting the standards does not necessarily mean that an HMO provides satisfactory care. A written disclaimer from the NCQA states: "Accreditation status is not a guarantee of the quality of care that any individual patient will receive or that any individual physician or other provider delivers."

To fill the quality-information gap, the NCQA, along with health plans and employers, developed 28 standardized measures of performance that it calls the Health Plan Employer Data and Information Set— HEDIS for short. HEDIS measures such factors as physician turnover, cesarean-section rates, and the percentage of adults who have their cholesterol levels checked. Twenty-one plans that serve nearly 10 million members around the country participated in a year-long pilot study of a core set of 28 HEDIS measures, which was published in February 1995. In addition to the HEDIS measures, the NCQA conducted a telephone survey of plan members to assess their satisfaction with their plans. The survey asked enrollees such questions as whether they would recommend their health plan to others. The NCQA hopes to be able to apply HEDIS to all accredited plans within a few years.

Consumers, of course, want to know about health plans in their community. The NCQA's project was a good start, "but not very helpful for consumers unless it's produced at the local level," says Martin Schneider, publisher and editor of a group of city and regional consumer magazines called *Health Pages* and a member of the steering committee for the pilot HEDIS project. The NCQA agreed. So in the summer of 1995, it used HEDIS to evaluate managed-care plans in a handful of cities, enabling employers in those areas to compare all of the plans in their markets. NCQA will be widely disseminating the findings from that research. Some HMOs have used the HEDIS standards to develop their own report cards. But employers and consumers should keep in mind that—unlike the NCQA's evaluations—such data are not audited by an outside organization, so their accuracy cannot be assured.

Schneider, whose magazines feature data about local doctors, hospitals, and some HMOs as well as articles about personal health, has a surefire way to ensure that HMOs don't exaggerate their performance records: "We tell the plans we will publish their unaudited information one time and one time only." Thereafter, *Health Pages* will print only data audited by a credible authority, and those data will be published along with the previous unaudited information. "If they want to go up one year by lying, they're going to look really bad the next," says Schneider. "That seems to send a message." In St. Louis, the city's HMO association is now auditing information that its members submit to *Health Pages*, and an employer coalition in California hired an outside firm to do the job with its local plans.

So far, *Health Pages* magazines have reported on health care providers in nine different cities or regions, including some of those participating in the local HEDIS project. The cities covered by the magazine, which is available on newsstands and distributed by companies to their employees, range from Dayton to Los Angeles. All of *Health Pages'* 1995 fall editions feature plan-specific information about local HMOs.

Everyone trying to develop consumer-friendly report cards for health care is grappling with the problem suggested by South Carolina's Pete Bailey: When is enough enough? Overwhelm consumers with details, and they're likely to miss the forest for the trees. Provide too little information, and consumers might not get a complete picture. In focus groups, the NCQA found that consumers tend to think most about hands-on characteristics like accessibility of care and bedside manner when defining health plan quality. But that is not true in every city. Ann Mond Johnson of the Sachs Group observes that people in cities where health care is largely provided by HMOs, such as Sacramento or San Francisco, tend to cite the importance of the quality of physicians. "How they're judging that, I can't tell," she adds.

Recognizing the push to assess health plans, *U.S. News* asked the National Opinion Research Center at the University of Chicago to survey doctors about how they would rank 31 possible indicators of HMO quality. Of the seven indicators placed at the top by the physicians, four had to do with preventive medicine: a high rate of childhood immunizations; aggressive preventive-medicine efforts, such as writing or calling to remind patients to schedule checkups; a high mammography rate, and a heavy dose of prenatal services.

A comparable survey of consumers would probably yield far different results. "There seems to be a big gap right now between what the experts think is important and what the consumers think is important," says Alan Raymond, vice-president for public affairs at the Harvard Community Health Plan in Boston and author of *The HMO Health Care Companion.*

For its 1994 annual report, the Harvard plan surveyed 750 U.S. adults about the factors they used to choose their health coverage. Asked to compare three standardized measures of quality, half the respondents put "success rates for various medical procedures" at the top. Only a quarter named childhood immunization

rates, and only a quarter cited screening for cancer or heart disease. In fact, more than half of the respondents based their choice on a plan's reputation with friends and neighbors. Although those involved in developing report cards deserve an A for effort, they may have a tough time changing consumers' ingrained decision-making habits.

FOR MORE HELP

- **Health Insurance Guide for Federal Employees,** a detailed report of the federal government's annual survey of federal workers about their health plans, can be ordered by writing the Center for the Study of Services, 733 15th Street, N.W., Suite 820, Washington DC 20005. It costs $8.50 plus $1.50 shipping and handling.
- **"How Members Rated Their Health Plans"** is an eight-page report from the U.S. Office of Personnel Management (OPM) that rates 90,000 federal government workers' satisfaction with 261 health plans throughout the country. Most of the plans count non-government workers among their members as well. To get a copy of the free report, write to OPM, Box 707, 1900 E Street, N.W., Washington DC 20415.
- **The Joint Commission on Accreditation of Healthcare Organizations** has reports available on each hospital it has reviewed. Because hospitals are reviewed only once every three years, reports on every institution checked out by the JCAHO will not be available until the end of 1996. The four-page reports, which cost $30 each, can be ordered by calling (708) 916-5800.
- **The National Committee for Quality Assurance,** the main accrediting body for HMOs, updates its list of plans' accreditation status every month. To get a free copy, write to the NCQA at 2000 L Street, N.W., Suite 500, Washington DC 20036.
- **The Ultimate HMO Handbook,** by Rhys Jones, and, **The HMO Health Care Companion** by Alan Raymond, explain how to use HMOs. Jones's book costs $7.95 and can be ordered from TTM Health Publishing, 1070 Neilson Street, Albany, CA 94706, (510) 524-4200. Raymond's book, published by HarperPerennial, costs $10 and is available in book-stores.

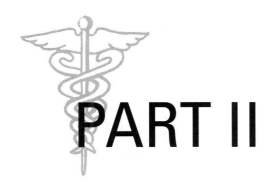

PART II

THE RANKINGS

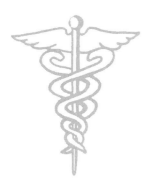

How to Interpret the Rankings

For six years, *U.S.News & World Report* has assessed the quality of care at major medical centers throughout the nation, publishing the results for the top hospitals in the pages of the magazine. This book goes much further. It includes scores for every one of the nation's tertiary-care centers—something no government agency and no research group has done before. It includes national rankings based on objective data and does so specialty by specialty.

The hospitals named had to meet at least one of the following requirements: membership in the elite Council of Teaching Hospitals, affiliation with a medical school, or a score of at least 10 on an index of medical technology. Each hospital also had to satisfy certain specialty-specific standards. Cardiology departments, for example, had to admit a minimum of 824 Medicare patients during the previous year, and the hospital must operate a cardiac catheterization lab or, alternatively, offer open-heart surgery, angioplasty, or cardiac rehabilitation services.

The scores and rankings drew upon a mathematical model developed for *U.S. News* by Senior Analyst Craig Hill and Analyst Barbara Rudolph of the National Opinion Research Center (NORC), a widely respected social-science research group at the University of Chicago. This year's work was aided by Analyst Krishna Winfrey. For 12 of the 16 specialties—from AIDS to urology—each hospital received a *U.S. News* Index score. The Index sums up three dimensions of quality,

each weighted equally: *reputation* of a specialized department among a national cross-section of board-certified specialists; *mortality rate*, the rate of patient deaths from the date of admission to discharge; and other *objective indicators* that vary by specialty, such as the ratio of cardiologists to beds.

The rankings for four specialties—ophthalmology, pediatrics, psychiatry, and rehabilitation—are based solely on reputation. For those specialties, mortality is irrelevant, since deaths rarely occur as a result of care at a hospital's ophthalmology, pediatrics, psychiatry, or rehabilitation departments.

All reputational results are based on annual surveys of a geographic cross-section of 150 board-certified specialists in each of the 16 specialities—2,400 doctors in all. The physicians were asked to nominate the top five hospitals in their specialty, without considering location or expense. Results of three such surveys, conducted in 1993, 1994 and 1995, were pooled and averaged.

Another of the trio of quality indicators, the specialty-specific death rate, is based on pooled mortality figures for 1992 and 1993, the two most recent years with complete data. Pooling data smooths out blips in the death rate that may not be related to the quality of care provided by a hospital. Mortality figures used by NORC were calculated by MEDSTAT Group Inc., an Ann Arbor, Michigan-based healthcare information-management firm, using a collection of data called MEDPARS that was obtained from the federal Health Care Financing

Administration. MEDSTAT applied a clinical measure of disease severity that is commonly used by the health care industry when analyzing death rates.

Of the 12 objectively rated specialties, mortality rates for seven are specialty specific, based on illness and procedure classifications called diagnosis related groups, or DRGs, for medical and surgical procedures reimbursed by Medicare. Diagnosis related groups could not be used for AIDS, geriatrics, gynecology, otolaryngology, or rheumatology, mainly because relatively few patients are admitted to hospitals for DRG procedures in those specialties.

The third factor in the *U.S. News* ratings comes from a specialty-specific combination of nine quality indicators ranging from the number of geriatric services to the ratio of registered nurses to beds. (You'll find a glossary of the indicators below.)

The national rankings on the following pages show the top 50 hospitals across the nation in each of the 12 objectively ranked specialties. (The state-by-state and metropolitan-area listings call out hospitals in the top 100 institutions nationally, even though the national rankings only show the top 50.) For the four reputationally ranked specialties, state-by-state and metropolitan-area rankings are not included because they would not be statistically valid. The national rankings for these four specialties show the hospitals that were named by at least 3 percent of the physicians surveyed.

In the state-by-state and metropolitan-area rankings, the hospitals are grouped into four levels, or tiers. The number of hospitals in each tier varies somewhat by specialty. All of the hospitals in Tier Four have a *U.S. News* Index score at or below the mean for the specialty. Tier Three hospitals have higher scores—up to one standard deviation above the mean, in the jargon of statistics. Tier Two hospitals score up to two standard deviations above the mean. And Tier One hospitals score higher than two standard deviations above the mean.

Here's how to put that into perspective. If a statistician plotted all of the hospital scores as a graph, they would form a bell-shaped curve; about 95 percent of all of the hospitals would fall within a range from two standard deviations above the mean to two standard deviations below it. That 95 percent would include the hospitals in Tiers Two, Three and Four. Tier One consists of the relatively few hospitals with scores at the very top within each specialty. Given the high standards for Tier One, it should not be surprising that some states, especially if they are thinly populated, lack a single Tier One hospital.

Since scores are especially critical at the top of the rankings, the hospitals in Tier One are listed in the order

of their *U.S. News* Index score. Hospitals in Tiers Two, Three, and Four are listed alphabetically, because minor score differences at those levels are not meaningful.

To assess the quality of a hospital across different specialties, you should look at the tiers in which the hospital appears and not at its *U.S. News* Index scores, which cannot be directly compared across specialties. A score of 80 in AIDS, for example, does not mean the same as a score of 80 in cancer. But knowing that a hospital is in Tier One both for AIDS and cancer indicates top care in both specialties.

The rankings highlight real differences in the quality of care dispensed by the nation's tertiary-care centers. There are relatively few outstanding hospitals. There are a large number of hospitals that provide good care. And there are relatively few hospitals where care is merely adequate. This does not imply that care delivered at the "best" hospitals will be free of problems, even in the specialty for which a hospital is cited—nor does it suggest that care is invariably iffy at hospitals with low scores. Still, with the overwhelming majority of tertiary-care hospitals falling below the top tier, it is clear that patients need all the help they can get finding the best care possible when serious illness strikes.

WHAT THE TERMS MEAN

- *Rank* is based on the *U.S. News* Index.
- The *U.S. News* Index is an all-inclusive measure of a hospital's quality of care. One third is based on *reputational score*; one third on *mortality rate*; and one third on other objective measures, which vary by specialty. The top-ranked hospital in each specialty is assigned a score of 100.
- *Reputational score* is the average percentage of board-certified doctors surveyed in 1993, 1994, and 1995 who named the hospital.
- *Mortality rate* is the ratio of actual to expected deaths from the date of admission to the date of discharge. Unless noted otherwise, the mortality rate is specialty specific. Lower is better.
- *COTH member* indicates membership in the elite Council of Teaching Hospitals. About 77 percent of the 1,631 medical centers analyzed this year are members.
- *Interns and residents to beds* is the ratio of doctors in training to beds. Higher is better, indicating commitment to teaching and research.
- *R.N.s to beds* is the ratio of full-time registered nurses to beds. Higher is better. The ratio in any eight-hour shift will be about one third of the figure shown.

- *Board-certified specialists to beds* is a ratio that reflects the number of staff specialists relative to a hospital's size. Higher is better. A board-certified specialist must complete three to seven years of training beyond residency and pass qualifying exams.
- *Procedures to beds* is the ratio of surgical and nonsurgical procedures to beds. It is specialty-specific unless noted otherwise. Higher is better—quality usually improves with volume.
- *Technology score* is related to high-tech services, such as sophisticated imaging devices, available on premises in a specialty. The highest possible score ranged from 5 in orthopedics and rheumatology to 26 for ophthalmology.

- *Discharge planning* indicates availability of a staffed social work department and patient-representative services.
- *Service mix* indicates availability of such outpatient and community services as specialized AIDS care, substance abuse programs, genetic counseling, home health services, and fertility counseling.
- *Geriatric services* are comprehensive geriatric assessment, Alzheimer's diagnostics assessment services, geriatric acute care, geriatric clinics, adult day care, respite care, emergency response for the elderly, senior membership services, and patient-representative services.

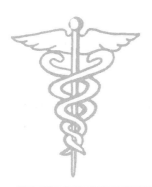

The 16 Specialties, from AIDS to Urology

For 12 of the 16 specialties in which the nation's hospitals were judged for this book, the ranking of a particular hospital is based on its score—its U.S. News Index. (Rankings for the other four specialties are explained below.) The Index, in turn, is made up of three parts, each weighted equally: reputation, mortality rate, and a number of categories ranging from technology to the ratio of physicians to beds.

For the four remaining specialties, rankings are based solely on reputation. But what about the specialties themselves? What do doctors who specialize in endocrinology or gastroenterology do? You'll find out here.

THE 12 OBJECTIVELY RANKED SPECIALTIES

AIDS

At hospitals that excel in treating people infected with HIV (human immunodeficiency virus) or suffering from active AIDS, doctors mingle healing and research, moving from one drug combination to another to battle the infections that develop as the body's immune system deteriorates. Some success has been registered against one type of mycobacterial infection, which causes fever, night sweats, chills, weight loss, and weakness: *Pneumocystis carinii* pneumonia, a deadly respira-

tory infection, and toxoplasmosis, an infection of the nervous system. The next step is to find a way to ward off cytomegalovirus infection, which in the most severe adult cases causes fever and inflames the liver and lungs. Top hospitals are far more than glorified pharmacies, however. They have comprehensive outpatient programs to enable patients to live at home and come to the hospital only when necessary. These hospitals also maintain pediatric intensive care units for the youngest sufferers. Social workers and patient representatives are much in evidence, to help cope with paperwork, family problems, and home care from nursing to meals.

Cancer

Cancer is not a single disease but many with a common element: cells grow unchecked and may spread throughout the body. In the latest developments, cancer researchers are zeroing in on what regulates this out-of-control proliferation. The findings have led to trials of experimental therapies that target the process. Doctors at top hospitals constantly test and fine-tune the mix of surgery, chemotherapy, and radiation used to fight most forms of cancer. The ability to deliver megavoltage radiation therapy, an especially high-powered form of radiation treatment, and to perform stereotactic radiosurgery, in which a computer permits precise positioning of surgical tools, are two examples of the high technology that has become a hallmark of the best cancer care. Approaches to treatment for many common and lethal cancers vary from specialist to specialist and hospital to hospital. Where you are treated for cancer, and by whom, can make a greater difference than for any other disease.

Cardiology

Cardiologists diagnose and treat heart and circulatory disorders ranging from arrhythmia, or abnormal heartbeat, to congestive heart failure. Cardiac surgeons specialize in heart operations such as coronary bypass, which can now be done safely and skillfully at many community hospitals, especially those that perform at least 300 to 500 a year. Cardiologists in major medical centers have expertise in treating unusual or especially complicated cases—for example, those involving congenital heart disease, valve problems, and serious rhythm disorders. And they are more apt to be up on the very latest research. Cardiac rehabilitation facilities that help patients along the road to recovery are as much a mark of top care as is the latest in high-technology imaging equipment and intensive-care facilities.

Endocrinology

Endocrinologists diagnose and treat patients who have problems involving the hormone-secreting endocrine glands. Overproduction or underproduction of those hormones affects rate of growth, metabolism, and sexual development. At top hospitals, clinical endocrinologists are consultants to virtually every other department, meeting with other specialists to discuss such disorders as diabetes, osteoporosis, menstrual irregularities, thyroid disorders, infertility, high cholesterol, and hormone-producing tumors. And at top centers, endocrinologists' armamentarium includes such advanced technology as radioisotope facilities, which employ radiation both for diagnosis and therapeutic purposes.

Gastroenterology

For a specialty, gastroenterology is strikingly broad. Its practitioners treat digestive disorders from routine heartburn, diarrhea, and intestinal pain to ulcers, gallbladder problems, liver disease, and cancer. People who require a liver transplant, of course, are well-advised to go to a major medical center, as are patients with difficult diagnostic problems. Gastroenterologists at top hospitals often become subspecialists—in diseases of the liver and gallbladder, for example. Most have become adept within the last several years at using endoscopes—light- and tool-tipped flexible tubes enabling doctors to peer into the esophagus, stomach, and intestinal tract and snip off bits of suspect tissue for examination. Endoscopic ultrasound—organ scans painted with sound waves generated from inside the body—has boosted cancer-screening effectiveness, and drugs that suppress the immune system have turned liver transplants into reliable lifesavers when cirrhosis has ravaged the organ.

Geriatrics

Geriatrics is a relatively new specialty, with fewer than 800 board-certified geriatricians in the entire country. That older patients are different from younger ones is a reality that these specialists confront every day. The efficiency of the kidneys and lungs, for example, drops off with age. A minor infection in a 20-year-old thus can become life-threatening in an 80-year-old. Because medications pass through older bodies at a more leisurely rate, the risk of overdose is greater; geriatricians must keep that in mind when they prescribe. Drugs, illness,and a move to a hospital can create disorientation that can be confused with dementia, and top geriatrics hospitals provide specialists who know the difference. They also coordinate care for age-related ailments from atherosclerosis to osteoporosis. The hospitals that appear in the rankings offer specialty services as well, such as Alzheimer's diagnostic assessment, adult day care services, psychiatric education, and hospice care.

Gynecology

Gynecology, usually twinned with obstetrics, provides counseling on contraception, prenatal care during pregnancy, routine deliveries, cesarean sections, treatment for sexually transmitted diseases, and counseling to keep STDs at bay. Leading ob/gyn centers also shepherd women through high-risk pregnancies and generally have neonatal intensive-care units at the ready for fragile or early-term newborns. Increasingly, infertility experts within the specialty are providing hope for couples who once would have remained childless through a growing list of treatment options that include artificial insemination and in vitro fertilization. Top centers can provide state-of-the-art genetics counseling. The hospitals listed here provide diagnostic mammograms to screen for breast cancer. They are equipped to handle the most difficult deliveries and most incorporate neonatal intensive-care centers for immediate, high-technology care of very sick newborns.

Neurology

Neurology covers the nervous system and its disorders, such as Parkinson's disease, multiple sclerosis, and various forms of dementia including Alzheimer's disease. Neurologists have an understanding of the brain, spinal cord, and nerves. Only a handful of years ago, few disorders of the nervous system could be effectively treated. Now, new treatments are being developed, including drug treatments like Tacrine for patients with Alzheimer's disease or Betaseron for multiple sclerosis. Many leading hospitals have dedicated centers for such disorders as Lou Gehrig's disease, epilepsy, stroke, and spinal cord injuries to deal with the explosion of knowledge. In brain and spinal cord disorders, experts rely heavily on imaging technologies like CT scanners and magnetic resonance imaging, and leading centers have available neuroradiologists who specialize in imaging of the nervous system. Access to such sophisticated technology and the presence of experts who can put it to good use has much to do with a hospital's ranking.

Orthopedics

Orthopedics is the branch of surgery that deals with bones, joints, and muscles. The specialty serves children born with skeletal disorders like spina bifida, injured athletes of all ages, and seniors crippled by diseases like osteoporosis. Orthopedics offers surgery or rehabilitation to help people keep moving, and leading centers take on complex cases like delicate spine or hand surgery or total replacement of the hip or knee joints. Such procedures require intensive rehabilitation for full recovery, and top centers have physical therapists on staff. Since the odds of surgical success improve with the experience of the surgical team, the hospitals listed here must do at least 283 orthopedic surgical procedures annually to be considered. Some orthopedic procedures take less of a toll than in years past, thanks to new technology like the arthroscope—a tube that enables the physician to look inside a joint and perform delicate surgery, such as the removal of damaged cartilage, with no more than one or two small incisions.

Otolaryngology

Otolaryngologists deal with the ear, nose, and throat. Relatively uncomplicated problems include infected tonsils and sinuses and deviated septums. But leading centers can take on head and neck cancers, deafness, and reconstructive facial surgery. Recent breakthroughs in this field include cochlear implants—tiny devices wired

to the inner ear that can help some deaf people hear again. The implants are constantly being improved, and top centers are up on the improvements. Speech pathologists can be key players in the recovery of patients undergoing throat or ear surgery. Radiologists in otolaryngology departments are likely to be practiced at using imaging technology that zeros in on the inner ear or the vocal cords as opposed to scanning the entire head. Specialists in this field say a good hospitals should have a wide range of imaging technology available. The hospitals listed have seen at least 3,500 cases annually, considered a minimum for high-quality outcomes.

Rheumatology

Rheumatologists diagnose and treat diseases of the muscles, bones, joints, and connective tissue. These ailments are major causes of chronic pain and physical handicaps. Some rheumatic diseases, such as rheumatoid arthritis, are autoimmune disorders in which the patient's own immune system attacks normal tissue. Other rheumatic ailments, such as Lyme disease, are triggered by an infection. Diagnosing rheumatic diseases depends mainly on a thorough medical history and examination. Leading rheumatology hospitals are equipped with a variety of imaging devices enabling doctors to peer into patients' bodies. Although gout can be controlled with medication and Lyme disease treated with antibiotics, there are no specific treatments for most chronic rheumatic ailments. Orthopedic surgeons as well as rheumatologists are often involved in caring for patients with these diseases, and physical and occupational therapists help patients minimize disability and adjust to any impairment.

Urology

Urologists treat disorders of the urinary tract in men and women and reproductive problems in men. Such ailments range from annoying bladder infections to life-threatening kidney cancer. Urinalysis is probably the best tip-off to these diseases. The presence of glucose, blood, nitrogen, or excessive amounts of protein in urine can be symptoms of a variety of problems linked to the urinary tract. Urologists also focus on the prostate, a gland that often enlarges with age and is one of the main cancer sites in men. How aggressively prostate cancer should be treated is not always clear. In ranking urology centers, one of the factors taken into account was whether a hospital has such sophisticated technology as a lithotripter to crush kidney stones or special radiation machines to treat prostate cancer.

REPUTATION-RANKED SPECIALTIES

For these specialties, reputation alone determines rank. This is because mortality rates are either unavailable (in the case of pediatrics) or irrelevant (virtually no one dies as a result of care at a hospital's ophthalmology, psychiatric or rehabilitation departments). A hospital's reputational score comes from the same three years' worth of surveys that supplied reputational scores for the other 12 specialties. Other information (such as technology score) is included because many doctors consider it relevant, but it plays no role in the rankings.

Ophthalmology

Ophthalmologists treat diseases of the eye, most of the time on an outpatient basis—which is why many top hospitals maintain separate eye clinics. In Americans older than 65, age-related macular degeneration—marked by a slow or sudden but painless loss of central vision—is the leading cause of irreversible blindness. In younger people, AIDS and diabetes are major contributors to vision problems. About one in four AIDS patients will develop inflammation of the retina from cytomegalovirus infection. And in one study, about three quarters of patients with diabetes developed diabetic retinopathy—a noninflammatory disease of the retina—over a 10-year period. Less debilitating, near-sightedness affects about one in four Americans. A growing number of them are undergoing surgery called radial keratotomy. A recent study found that the procedure corrected patients' vision to at least 20/25 in all but a tiny fraction of cases. However, 10 years after the operation, a number of patients had become farsighted. A good ophthalmology department will be aware of seeming breakthroughs—and on top of their drawbacks.

Pediatrics

Most pediatricians are primary-care providers who try to keep their patients well by preventing diseases or at least diagnosing and treating them early. The doctors who spend much of their time in the top pediatrics hospitals are subspecialists. Their patients range from the fetus under the perinatologist's care to the teenager seen by the adolescent-medicine specialist. Other pediatric subspecialists focus on certain parts of the body, such as the nervous, cardiovascular, or genitourinary systems, or on certain types of diseases, such as cancer or infections. Pediatricians recognize that child health involves the interplay of several components, including behavioral, sociological, economic, and political factors. Thus, the large dose of practical and emotional support for patients and their families that high-ranking hospitals supply is as important as the medical care they dispense. Perhaps no better example of this interaction is HIV infection, an increasingly common problem in children's hospitals and wards.

Psychiatry

Recent studies suggest that psychiatric disorders may be more common than previously thought. To complicate matters, these disorders tend to concentrate in certain people who may suffer from three or more at the same time. Understandably, an individual with multiple psychiatric disorders usually is harder to diagnose and treat than is someone with only a single ailment—and is less likely to do well, besides. Researchers are still trying to unravel the causes of mental illness. Increasingly, they are finding evidence of biological factors behind major disorders like schizophrenia. Techniques such as magnetic resonance imaging have revealed differences between the brains of people with schizophrenia and those without it. Psychiatrists also are involved in caring for people with other types of illnesses whose depression or dementia could lengthen their hospital stay. Compared to top medical centers in other specialties, the best psychiatric hospitals offer low-technology care that combines medication and talk therapy.

Rehabilitation

The growth of rehabilitation services available for patients recovering from injuries or disabling illnesses has led to a dramatic increase in the number of doctors in this specialty. By the end of 1994, some 4,600 physicians were certified as specialists in physical medicine and rehabilitation—more than double the number of such doctors just a decade earlier. These specialists, called physiatrists, traditionally have treated patients with stroke, brain injury, amputation, and spinal cord injury. Some physiatrists subspecialize in treating children, athletes, or victims of spinal cord injuries. Increasingly, physiatrists also are called upon to work with organ transplant or cancer patients who have become debilitated after being hospitalized for long periods. Other members of the rehabilitation team at top hospitals include physical, speech, and occupational therapists; psychologists; and social workers and nurses who continue to work with patients after they've been discharged. As a general rule, the earlier rehabilitation starts, the shorter the hospital stay and the lower the rate of complications and deaths.

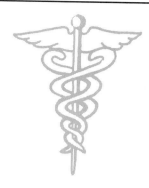

The *U.S. News* Honor Roll

The hospitals named here belong to an elite group: All scored high in the *U.S. News* national rankings—and did so in at least three specialties. Such all-around competence suggests unusually high performance. To make the *U.S. News* honor roll, a hospital had to rank among the top 10 hospitals in at least three specialties and score 10 or more points. (A number 1 ranking in a specialty earned 10 points, a number 2 ranking nine points and so on, down to 1 point for a number 10 ranking.)

1. Johns Hopkins Hospital, Baltimore
    (119 points in 15 specialties)
2. Mayo Clinic, Rochester, Minn.
    (107 points in 14 specialties)
3. Massachusetts General Hospital, Boston
    (75 points in 10 specialties)
4. UCLA Medical Center
    (65 points in 12 specialties)
5. Duke University Medical Center, Durham, N.C.
    (42 points in 9 specialties)
6. Cleveland Clinic
    (40 points in 8 specialties)
7. University of California San Francisco Medical Center
    (30 points in 6 specialties)
8. Brigham & Women's Hospital, Boston
    (22 points in 5 specialties)
9. University of Texas M.D. Anderson Cancer Center, Houston
    (21 points in 4 specialties)
10. University of Washington Medical Center, Seattle
    (19 points in 6 specialties)
11. Barnes Hospital, St. Louis
    (19 points in 5 specialties)
12. Memorial Sloan-Kettering Cancer Center, New York
    (15 points in 3 specialties)
13. Stanford University Medical Center, Stanford, Calif.
    (15 points in 3 specialties)
14. New York University Medical Center, New York
    (14 points in 4 specialties)
15. University of Iowa Hospitals and Clinics, Iowa City
    (14 points in 3 specialties)
16. University of Michigan Medical Center, Ann Arbor
    (13 points in 3 specialties)
17. New York Hospital—Cornell Medical Center, New York
    (11 points in 3 specialties)
18. University of Chicago Hospitals
    (10 points in 4 specialties)

AIDS

Rank	Hospital	U.S. News index	Reputational score	Hospitalwide mortality rate	COTH member	Interns and residents to beds	Technology score (of 11)	Discharge planning (of 2)	R.N.'s to beds	Board-certified internists to beds
1	San Francisco General Hospital Medical Center	100.0	59.1%	0.95	No	1.19	8	2	1.52	0.011
2	Johns Hopkins Hospital, Baltimore	66.1	31.2%	0.97	Yes	0.73	11	2	1.43	0.084
3	Massachusetts General Hospital, Boston	62.3	26.8%	0.88	Yes	1.00	11	2	1.14	0.085
4	University of California, San Francisco Medical Center	55.0	19.4%	0.89	Yes	1.03	10	2	1.82	0.435
5	UCLA Medical Center, Los Angeles	54.2	19.7%	0.66	Yes	1.52	11	2	1.20	0.023
6	University of Miami, Jackson Memorial Hospital	42.8	15.4%	1.12	Yes	0.85	8	2	1.39	0.046
7	Memorial Sloan-Kettering Cancer Center, New York	41.4	12.6%	0.91	Yes	0.38	7	2	1.37	0.074
8	New York University Medical Center	39.5	9.7%	0.98	Yes	1.30	8	2	1.15	0.360
9	New York Hospital-Cornell Medical Center	37.9	10.9%	1.07	Yes	0.79	10	2	1.00	0.113
10	University of Washington Medical Center, Seattle	35.6	4.3%	0.84	Yes	1.05	8	2	2.06	0.440
11	Stanford University Hospital, Stanford, Calif.	35.4	6.1%	0.90	Yes	1.34	9	2	0.86	0.147
12	Beth Israel Hospital, Boston	35.2	4.4%	0.85	Yes	0.57	8	2	1.93	0.590
13	New England Deaconess Hospital, Boston	35.2	7.2%	0.99	Yes	1.08	9	2	1.33	0.089
14	Duke University Medical Center, Durham, N.C.	34.5	5.0%	0.90	Yes	0.91	10	2	1.61	0.081
15	UCSD Medical Center, San Diego	33.6	2.8%	0.75	Yes	1.65	8	2	2.17	0.049
16	Columbia-Presbyterian Medical Center, New York	33.0	8.3%	1.25	Yes	0.85	11	2	1.05	0.111
17	Northwestern Memorial Hospital, Chicago	32.7	6.4%	0.99	Yes	0.43	9	2	1.03	0.134
18	Rush-Presbyterian-St. Luke's Medical Center, Chicago	32.3	2.9%	0.81	Yes	1.05	10	2	1.24	0.224
19	Mount Sinai Medical Center, New York	31.6	4.9%	1.09	Yes	0.99	9	2	1.50	0.253
20	University Hospital, Portland, Ore.	31.1	0.3%	0.80	Yes	1.54	9	2	2.31	0.164
21	Boston City Hospital	31.0	1.8%	0.75	No	1.64	7	2	1.37	0.545
22	Barnes Hospital, St. Louis	30.8	4.0%	0.98	Yes	0.89	9	2	0.82	0.273
23	Montefiore Medical Center, Bronx, N.Y.	30.3	6.2%	1.19	Yes	0.53	10	2	1.28	0.095
24	Henry Ford Hospital, Detroit	30.2	1.3%	0.96	Yes	1.34	10	2	1.50	0.301
25	Cleveland Clinic	30.1	1.2%	0.87	Yes	1.22	10	2	1.47	0.015
26	Brigham and Women's Hospital, Boston	30.0	2.1%	0.91	Yes	1.49	8	2	0.79	0.179
27	Hospital of the University of Pennsylvania, Philadelphia	30.0	2.0%	0.97	Yes	1.72	9	2	1.33	0.007
28	Los Angeles County-USC Medical Center	29.8	1.9%	0.88	Yes	1.21	9	1	1.30	0.052
29	Cook County Hospital, Chicago	29.5	1.3%	0.55	Yes	1.00	9	2	1.43	0.073
30	University of Chicago Hospitals	29.5	0.2%	0.80	Yes	1.64	9	2	1.38	0.074
31	New England Medical Center, Boston	29.3	1.0%	0.86	Yes	1.07	8	2	1.66	0.086
32	University of Illinois Hospital and Clinics, Chicago	29.3	0.0%	0.83	Yes	1.29	9	2	1.95	0.056
33	University of Maryland Medical System, Baltimore	29.1	1.4%	0.98	Yes	0.96	9	2	1.67	0.281
34	University of California, Davis Medical Center	28.8	0.0%	1.01	Yes	1.54	9	2	2.81	0.032
35	Georgetown University Hospital, Washington, D.C.	28.8	1.6%	0.97	Yes	0.92	9	2	1.59	0.140
36	Los Angeles County-Harbor-UCLA Medical Center	28.7	1.6%	0.91	No	1.53	8	2	1.33	0.148
37	University of Michigan Medical Center, Ann Arbor	28.6	1.8%	0.98	Yes	1.00	10	2	1.29	0.086
38	Yale-New Haven Hospital, New Haven, Conn.	28.6	2.6%	1.06	Yes	1.12	10	2	1.23	0.094
39	Vanderbilt University Hospital and Clinic, Nashville	28.5	1.5%	1.01	Yes	1.21	10	2	1.29	0.171
40	Thomas Jefferson University Hospital, Philadelphia	28.3	0.5%	0.85	Yes	0.96	9	2	1.44	0.042
41	University of Texas, M.D. Anderson Cancer Ctr., Houston	28.2	0.4%	0.38	Yes	0.70	8	2	1.88	0.083
42	University Hospital, Denver	28.1	1.1%	0.89	Yes	0.76	9	2	1.05	0.044
43	Mayo Clinic, Rochester, Minn.	28.0	2.7%	0.72	Yes	0.24	7	2	0.77	0.060
44	University of North Carolina Hospitals, Chapel Hill	27.8	2.4%	1.23	Yes	1.41	9	2	1.71	0.246
45	University of Wisconsin Hospital and Clinics, Madison	27.7	0.4%	0.95	Yes	1.30	10	2	1.24	0.037
46	University of Minnesota Hospital and Clinic, Minneapolis	27.6	1.3%	0.81	Yes	0.59	8	2	0.86	0.133
47	University Hospitals of Cleveland	27.6	0.3%	1.07	Yes	1.60	11	2	1.73	0.080
48	University Hospitals, Oklahoma City	27.5	0.0%	0.98	Yes	1.60	9	2	1.56	0.040
49	Boston University Medical Center-University Hospital	27.4	0.5%	0.82	Yes	0.96	7	2	0.85	0.231
50	Medical College of Georgia Hospital and Clinic, Augusta	27.0	0.0%	0.92	Yes	1.42	8	2	1.09	0.041

"Reputational score" is the percentage of board-certified AIDS specialists surveyed who named the hospital. "Hospitalwide mortality rate" is the ratio of actual to expected deaths overall (lower is better). "COTH member" indicates member of Council of Teaching Hospitals. "Interns and residents to beds" is the ratio of doctors in training to beds. "Technology score" is a specialty-specific index. "Discharge planning" indicates number of postdischarge services available. "R.N.'s to beds" is the ratio of full-time registered nurses to beds. "Board-certified internists to beds" is the ratio of these doctors to beds.

CANCER

Rank	Hospital	U.S. News index	Reputa-tional score	Cancer mortality rate	COTH member	Interns and residents to beds	Tech-nology score (of 12)	R.N.'s to beds	Board-certified oncologists to beds	Procedures to beds
1	Memorial Sloan-Kettering Cancer Center, New York	100.0	70.8%	0.97	Yes	0.38	9	1.37	0.083	7.93
2	University of Texas, M.D. Anderson Cancer Ctr., Houston	93.2	63.1%	0.27	Yes	0.70	11	1.88	0.010	7.18
3	Dana-Farber Cancer Institute, Boston	74.1	46.7%	0.01	No	0.49	4	1.58	0.964	12.91
4	Johns Hopkins Hospital, Baltimore	47.7	28.7%	0.53	Yes	0.73	11	1.43	0.011	1.57
5	Mayo Clinic, Rochester, Minn.	42.3	27.5%	0.57	Yes	0.24	8	0.77	0.026	3.03
6	Stanford University Hospital, Stanford, Calif.	30.9	15.3%	0.80	Yes	1.34	10	0.86	0.028	1.64
7	University of Washington Medical Center, Seattle	30.7	13.1%	0.58	Yes	1.05	9	2.06	0.039	2.11
8	Duke University Medical Center, Durham, N.C.	28.7	12.3%	0.71	Yes	0.91	12	1.61	0.028	2.76
9	University of Chicago Hospitals	25.1	8.1%	0.59	Yes	1.64	11	1.38	0.034	2.76
10	Roswell Park Cancer Institute, Buffalo	24.7	8.5%	0.52	No	0.68	9	2.58	0.000	14.09
11	University of California, San Francisco Medical Center	21.2	6.0%	0.59	Yes	1.03	11	1.82	0.021	0.92
12	Massachusetts General Hospital, Boston	21.1	7.3%	0.80	Yes	1.00	12	1.14	0.011	2.41
13	UCLA Medical Center, Los Angeles	19.4	4.4%	0.42	Yes	1.52	11	1.20	0.031	2.03
14	Hospital of the University of Pennsylvania, Philadelphia	19.2	4.0%	0.86	Yes	1.72	10	1.33	0.033	1.87
15	University of California, Davis Medical Center	19.2	0.8%	0.61	Yes	1.54	11	2.81	0.017	1.29
16	Indiana University Medical Center, Indianapolis	18.4	3.4%	0.57	Yes	1.10	11	1.86	0.022	1.31
17	UCSD Medical Center, San Diego	16.8	0.4%	0.54	Yes	1.65	8	2.17	0.058	1.66
18	University Hospital, Portland, Ore.	16.2	0.0%	0.40	Yes	1.54	9	2.31	0.017	1.45
19	Fox Chase Cancer Center, Philadelphia	16.1	3.7%	0.14	No	0.36	7	1.42	0.290	15.49
20	University Medical Center, Tucson, Ariz.	15.9	3.0%	0.71	Yes	0.74	9	1.73	0.053	1.51
21	University of Nebraska Medical Center, Omaha	15.9	2.8%	0.89	Yes	1.37	10	1.23	0.000	0.99
22	University of Wisconsin Hospital and Clinics, Madison	15.8	2.0%	0.62	Yes	1.30	11	1.24	0.039	2.14
23	Cleveland Clinic	15.8	1.9%	0.64	Yes	1.22	11	1.47	0.009	1.80
24	Vanderbilt University Hospital and Clinic, Nashville	15.6	1.9%	0.64	Yes	1.21	12	1.29	0.011	1.82
25	University Hospitals of Cleveland	15.5	0.0%	0.79	Yes	1.60	12	1.73	0.032	1.54
26	University of Pittsburgh-Presbyterian University Hospital	15.5	0.0%	0.58	Yes	1.48	8	2.10	0.062	1.71
27	University of Virginia Health Sciences Ctr., Charlottesville	15.3	0.0%	0.58	Yes	1.41	11	1.92	0.012	1.86
28	F.G. McGaw Hospital at Loyola University, Maywood, Ill.	15.1	0.4%	0.66	Yes	1.46	11	1.59	0.030	1.59
29	Mount Sinai Medical Center, New York	14.9	2.6%	1.05	Yes	0.99	9	1.50	0.010	2.45
30	University Hospitals, Oklahoma City	14.9	0.0%	0.65	Yes	1.60	11	1.56	0.029	0.86
31	University of North Carolina Hospitals, Chapel Hill	14.8	0.6%	0.90	Yes	1.41	10	1.71	0.013	1.28
32	Brigham and Women's Hospital, Boston	14.7	1.9%	0.69	Yes	1.49	10	0.79	0.066	1.45
33	St. Louis University Hospital	14.7	0.0%	0.82	Yes	1.89	10	1.33	0.016	1.61
34	University of Illinois Hospital and Clinics, Chicago	14.2	0.0%	0.65	Yes	1.29	9	1.95	0.015	0.65
35	Henry Ford Hospital, Detroit	14.1	0.5%	0.71	Yes	1.34	10	1.50	0.000	1.76
36	Yale-New Haven Hospital, New Haven, Conn.	14.1	1.3%	0.51	Yes	1.12	10	1.23	0.035	2.08
37	USC Kenneth Norris Cancer Hospital, Los Angeles	14.0	1.3%	0.88	No	0.40	8	1.37	0.400	17.13
38	Penn State's Milton S. Hershey Medical Ctr., Hershey	14.0	0.0%	0.81	Yes	1.55	9	1.57	0.007	2.15
39	Barnes Hospital, St. Louis	13.9	2.7%	0.65	Yes	0.89	11	0.82	0.000	1.66
40	University of Michigan Medical Center, Ann Arbor	13.9	1.6%	0.50	Yes	1.00	10	1.29	0.012	1.68
41	University Hospital of Arkansas, Little Rock	13.6	0.5%	0.65	Yes	1.11	5	2.01	0.000	2.41
42	University of Iowa Hospitals and Clinics, Iowa City	13.4	0.9%	0.66	Yes	0.96	11	1.34	0.037	1.42
43	University of Maryland Medical System, Baltimore	13.3	0.5%	0.84	Yes	0.96	11	1.67	0.029	0.95
44	North Carolina Baptist Hospital, Winston-Salem	13.3	0.6%	0.76	Yes	1.06	12	1.24	0.014	2.57
45	University of Utah Hospitals and Clinics, Salt Lake City	13.2	0.7%	0.68	Yes	0.88	9	1.73	0.028	0.95
46	Georgetown University Hospital, Washington, D.C.	13.2	0.6%	0.74	Yes	0.92	10	1.59	0.026	1.75
47	Medical College of Ohio Hospital, Toledo	13.1	0.5%	0.76	Yes	1.42	9	1.23	0.022	0.92
48	New England Medical Center, Boston	13.0	0.7%	0.76	Yes	1.07	7	1.66	0.012	1.40
49	George Washington University Hospital, Washington, D.C.	12.9	0.5%	0.97	Yes	1.40	9	1.16	0.049	1.51
50	University Hospital, Denver	12.9	2.2%	0.43	Yes	0.76	9	1.05	0.008	1.32

"Reputational score" is the percentage of board-certified cancer specialists surveyed who named the hospital. "Cancer mortality rate" is the ratio of actual to expected cancer deaths (lower is better). "COTH member" indicates member of Council of Teaching Hospitals. "Interns and residents to beds" is the ratio of doctors in training to beds. "Technology score" is a specialty-specific index. "R.N.'s to beds" is the ratio of full-time registered nurses to beds. "Board-certified oncologists to beds" is the ratio of these doctors to beds. "Procedures to beds" is the ratio of cancer-related procedures to beds.

NATIONAL RANKINGS

CARDIOLOGY

Rank	Hospital	U.S. News index	Reputa-tional score	Cardiology mortality rate	COTH member	Interns and residents to beds	Tech-nology score (of 10)	R.N.'s to beds	Board-certified cardiologists to beds	Procedures to beds
1	Cleveland Clinic	100.0	49.9%	0.90	Yes	1.22	10	1.47	0.035	9.03
2	Mayo Clinic, Rochester, Minn.	93.4	49.0%	0.82	Yes	0.24	8	0.77	0.053	6.57
3	Texas Heart Institute-St. Luke's Episcopal, Houston	81.4	24.6%	1.52	Yes	0.26	9	1.36	0.064	10.00
4	Massachusetts General Hospital, Boston	73.3	32.5%	0.71	Yes	1.00	10	1.14	0.034	7.24
5	Duke University Medical Center, Durham, N.C.	63.7	25.1%	0.85	Yes	0.91	10	1.61	0.054	6.30
6	Brigham and Women's Hospital, Boston	56.3	23.2%	1.03	Yes	1.49	9	0.79	0.071	5.70
7	Stanford University Hospital, Stanford, Calif.	54.1	20.3%	0.93	Yes	1.34	9	0.86	0.102	5.19
8	Emory University Hospital, Atlanta	48.3	17.6%	0.95	Yes	0.71	8	1.28	0.037	9.57
9	Johns Hopkins Hospital, Baltimore	40.5	15.6%	1.21	Yes	0.73	10	1.43	0.033	4.66
10	University of California, San Francisco Medical Center	37.0	8.4%	0.96	Yes	1.03	9	1.82	0.043	2.51
11	Columbia-Presbyterian Medical Center, New York	33.7	10.8%	1.16	Yes	0.85	10	1.05	0.044	3.76
12	UCLA Medical Center, Los Angeles	33.4	4.2%	0.68	Yes	1.52	10	1.20	0.034	3.68
13	University of Alabama Hospital at Birmingham	31.9	10.2%	1.17	Yes	0.82	9	0.92	0.040	6.48
14	Beth Israel Hospital, Boston	31.7	3.4%	0.87	Yes	0.57	9	1.93	0.087	10.50
15	UCSD Medical Center, San Diego	30.9	0.6%	0.80	Yes	1.65	7	2.17	0.100	3.04
16	University of Chicago Hospitals	29.7	1.0%	0.79	Yes	1.64	10	1.38	0.033	4.24
17	Methodist Hospital, Houston	29.6	8.6%	1.13	Yes	0.19	9	1.33	0.058	5.03
18	Cedars-Sinai Medical Center, Los Angeles	29.4	7.5%	1.06	Yes	0.51	9	0.83	0.113	6.95
19	Mount Sinai Medical Center, New York	29.1	2.0%	0.84	Yes	0.99	8	1.50	0.068	3.94
20	Barnes Hospital, St. Louis	28.8	6.9%	1.06	Yes	0.89	10	0.82	0.000	5.45
21	University Hospital, Portland, Ore.	28.6	0.0%	0.93	Yes	1.54	9	2.31	0.043	2.76
22	Hospital of the University of Pennsylvania, Philadelphia	28.4	0.8%	0.91	Yes	1.72	9	1.33	0.035	4.88
23	New York Hospital-Cornell Medical Center	28.3	4.7%	0.96	Yes	0.79	9	1.00	0.034	3.80
24	University of Washington Medical Center, Seattle	28.0	0.0%	0.75	Yes	1.05	8	2.06	0.132	4.35
25	University of California, Davis Medical Center	27.9	0.3%	1.02	Yes	1.54	9	2.81	0.017	3.22
26	Washington Hospital Center, Washington, D.C.	27.4	7.0%	1.13	Yes	0.49	9	0.90	0.106	8.91
27	New England Medical Center, Boston	27.1	0.6%	0.69	Yes	1.07	7	1.66	0.034	6.14
28	New York University Medical Center	26.7	3.7%	1.02	Yes	1.30	8	1.15	0.000	4.84
29	Georgetown University Hospital, Washington, D.C.	26.5	0.0%	0.87	Yes	0.92	9	1.59	0.114	4.45
30	University of Utah Hospitals and Clinics, Salt Lake City	26.1	0.0%	0.54	Yes	0.88	7	1.73	0.075	2.84
31	Henry Ford Hospital, Detroit	26.0	1.2%	0.96	Yes	1.34	9	1.50	0.000	7.47
32	University of Michigan Medical Center, Ann Arbor	25.9	3.9%	1.10	Yes	1.00	10	1.29	0.034	4.25
33	Thomas Jefferson University Hospital, Philadelphia	25.7	0.6%	0.91	Yes	0.96	9	1.44	0.047	5.18
34	Rush-Presbyterian-St. Luke's Medical Center, Chicago	25.6	0.8%	0.89	Yes	1.05	9	1.24	0.000	4.51
35	University Hospitals of Cleveland	25.0	0.0%	1.03	Yes	1.60	10	1.73	0.037	4.70
36	Cook County Hospital, Chicago	24.8	0.0%	0.62	Yes	1.00	7	1.43	0.021	2.27
37	Mount Sinai Medical Center, Cleveland	24.6	1.0%	0.81	Yes	0.76	8	0.86	0.024	8.29
38	Penn State's Milton S. Hershey Medical Ctr., Hershey	24.2	0.0%	1.02	Yes	1.55	8	1.57	0.034	6.51
39	Western Pennsylvania Hospital, Pittsburgh	24.2	0.0%	0.90	Yes	0.43	9	1.44	0.083	10.97
40	University of Pittsburgh-Presbyterian University Hospital	24.1	1.1%	1.19	Yes	1.48	8	2.10	0.056	6.32
41	North Carolina Baptist Hospital, Winston-Salem	23.8	1.1%	0.99	Yes	1.06	9	1.24	0.024	6.83
42	Fairfax Hospital, Falls Church, Va.	23.8	0.5%	0.88	Yes	0.15	9	1.34	0.099	8.00
43	Tulane University Hospital and Clinics, New Orleans	23.8	0.0%	0.83	Yes	0.76	9	0.88	0.059	3.40
44	F.G. McGaw Hospital at Loyola University, Maywood, Ill.	23.7	1.9%	1.23	Yes	1.46	9	1.59	0.128	8.23
45	St. Louis University Hospital	23.6	0.9%	1.22	Yes	1.89	10	1.33	0.092	10.57
46	Sinai Samaritan Medical Center, Milwaukee	23.6	0.0%	0.77	Yes	0.66	8	0.86	0.097	9.01
47	Temple University Hospital, Philadelphia	23.2	0.6%	1.03	Yes	1.25	9	1.15	0.092	5.62
48	William Beaumont Hospital, Royal Oak, Mich.	23.1	1.3%	1.04	Yes	0.63	10	1.46	0.046	10.28
49	Yale-New Haven Hospital, New Haven, Conn.	23.0	2.0%	1.14	Yes	1.12	9	1.23	0.081	7.27
50	Mary Imogene Bassett Hospital, Cooperstown, N.Y.	23.0	0.0%	0.84	Yes	0.22	6	1.69	0.026	8.04

"Reputational score" is the percentage of board-certified heart specialists surveyed who named the hospital. "Cardiology mortality rate" is the ratio of actual to expected cardiac deaths (lower is better). "COTH member" indicates member of Council of Teaching Hospitals. "Interns and residents to beds" is the ratio of doctors in training to beds. "Technology score" is a specialty-specific index. "R.N.'s to beds" is the ratio of full-time registered nurses to beds. "Board-certified cardiologists to beds" is the ratio of these doctors to beds. "Procedures to beds" is the ratio of cardiac-related procedures to beds.

ENDOCRINOLOGY

NATIONAL RANKINGS

Rank	Hospital	U.S. News index	Reputa-tional score	Endocrinology mortality rate	COTH member	Interns and residents to beds	Tech-nology score (of 11)	R.N.'s to beds	Board-certified internists to beds
1	Mayo Clinic, Rochester, Minn.	100.0	65.1%	0.48	Yes	0.24	8	0.77	0.060
2	Massachusetts General Hospital, Boston	92.0	58.2%	0.93	Yes	1.00	11	1.14	0.085
3	University of California, San Francisco Medical Center	52.2	24.0%	0.78	Yes	1.03	10	1.82	0.435
4	Johns Hopkins Hospital, Baltimore	41.8	18.4%	0.68	Yes	0.73	11	1.43	0.084
5	Barnes Hospital, St. Louis	39.1	17.8%	0.86	Yes	0.89	11	0.82	0.273
6	UCLA Medical Center, Los Angeles	37.9	14.1%	0.34	Yes	1.52	11	1.20	0.023
7	University of Chicago Hospitals	35.5	12.5%	0.78	Yes	1.64	11	1.38	0.074
8	University of Michigan Medical Center, Ann Arbor	34.9	12.8%	0.62	Yes	1.00	10	1.29	0.086
9	New England Deaconess Hospital, Boston	34.7	13.0%	0.72	Yes	1.08	10	1.33	0.089
10	University of Washington Medical Center, Seattle	34.2	11.3%	1.00	Yes	1.05	10	2.06	0.440
11	Brigham and Women's Hospital, Boston	33.5	13.1%	0.89	Yes	1.49	10	0.79	0.179
12	Parkland Memorial Hospital, Dallas	28.1	10.4%	1.00	Yes	1.35	10	0.93	0.039
13	Duke University Medical Center, Durham, N.C.	27.1	6.7%	0.69	Yes	0.91	11	1.61	0.081
14	Vanderbilt University Hospital and Clinic, Nashville	26.8	7.9%	0.93	Yes	1.21	11	1.29	0.171
15	University of Virginia Health Sciences Ctr., Charlottesville	26.3	6.0%	0.90	Yes	1.41	10	1.92	0.101
16	Beth Israel Hospital, Boston	25.9	5.0%	0.86	Yes	0.57	9	1.93	0.590
17	Stanford University Hospital, Stanford, Calif.	25.4	5.2%	0.38	Yes	1.34	11	0.86	0.147
18	University Hospital, Portland, Ore.	24.9	2.3%	0.73	Yes	1.54	9	2.31	0.164
19	University of Pittsburgh-Presbyterian University Hospital	24.3	3.1%	0.91	Yes	1.48	9	2.10	0.291
20	UCSD Medical Center, San Diego	22.9	0.8%	0.55	Yes	1.65	8	2.17	0.049
21	Columbia-Presbyterian Medical Center, New York	22.6	8.2%	1.35	Yes	0.85	10	1.05	0.111
22	Cleveland Clinic	22.5	5.5%	1.02	Yes	1.22	11	1.47	0.015
23	Hospital of the University of Pennsylvania, Philadelphia	22.5	2.4%	0.71	Yes	1.72	11	1.33	0.007
24	University of Texas, M.D. Anderson Cancer Ctr., Houston	21.7	2.2%	0.48	Yes	0.70	11	1.88	0.083
25	University of California, Davis Medical Center	20.7	0.0%	0.90	Yes	1.54	10	2.81	0.032
26	University of Illinois Hospital and Clinics, Chicago	20.5	0.4%	0.50	Yes	1.29	8	1.95	0.056
27	University of Minnesota Hospital and Clinic, Minneapolis	20.5	4.8%	0.78	Yes	0.59	10	0.86	0.133
28	University of Iowa Hospitals and Clinics, Iowa City	20.4	2.9%	0.76	Yes	0.96	11	1.34	0.053
29	University Hospitals, Oklahoma City	20.3	0.0%	0.64	Yes	1.60	10	1.56	0.040
30	Los Angeles County-USC Medical Center	20.3	1.7%	0.44	Yes	1.21	8	1.30	0.052
31	Boston City Hospital	20.0	0.0%	0.59	No	1.64	5	1.37	0.545
32	Ohio State University Medical Center, Columbus	19.9	3.2%	0.44	Yes	0.81	6	1.11	0.029
33	F.G. McGaw Hospital at Loyola University, Maywood, Ill.	19.9	0.0%	0.67	Yes	1.46	10	1.59	0.053
34	Medical College of Ohio Hospital, Toledo	19.3	0.0%	0.55	Yes	1.42	9	1.23	0.132
35	University of North Carolina Hospitals, Chapel Hill	19.1	1.2%	1.08	Yes	1.41	10	1.71	0.246
36	Loma Linda University Medical Center, Loma Linda, Calif.	18.9	0.0%	0.65	Yes	1.14	9	1.61	0.067
37	University of Massachusetts Medical Center, Worcester	18.9	1.0%	0.60	Yes	1.47	8	0.96	0.000
38	University Hospitals of Cleveland	18.7	0.0%	0.88	Yes	1.60	11	1.73	0.080
39	University of Wisconsin Hospital and Clinics, Madison	18.6	0.0%	0.61	Yes	1.30	11	1.24	0.037
40	Medical College of Georgia Hospital and Clinic, Augusta	18.4	0.0%	0.12	Yes	1.42	10	1.09	0.041
41	Rush-Presbyterian-St. Luke's Medical Center, Chicago	18.4	0.0%	0.70	Yes	1.05	10	1.24	0.224
42	New England Medical Center, Boston	18.2	0.9%	0.79	Yes	1.07	8	1.66	0.086
43	Boston University Medical Center-University Hospital	18.0	0.4%	0.65	Yes	0.96	9	0.85	0.231
44	University Hospital, Denver	17.9	2.2%	0.75	Yes	0.76	10	1.05	0.044
45	St. Louis University Hospital	17.9	0.0%	0.94	Yes	1.89	11	1.33	0.057
46	Emory University Hospital, Atlanta	17.8	1.2%	0.30	Yes	0.71	8	1.28	0.039
47	Baylor University Medical Center, Dallas	17.7	1.9%	0.67	Yes	0.29	8	1.38	0.093
48	Mount Sinai Medical Center, New York	17.7	2.7%	1.35	Yes	0.99	9	1.50	0.253
49	University Hospital, Albuquerque, N.M.	17.6	0.0%	1.01	Yes	1.20	6	1.82	0.373
50	Thomas Jefferson University Hospital, Philadelphia	17.5	0.5%	0.74	Yes	0.96	10	1.44	0.042

"Reputational score" is the percentage of board-certified endocrinology and diabetes specialists surveyed who named the hospital. "Endocrinology mortality rate" is the ratio of actual to expected deaths involving endocrine disorders (lower is better). "COTH member" indicates member of Council of Teaching Hospitals. "Interns and residents to beds" is the ratio of doctors in training to beds. "Technology score" is a specialty-specific index. "R.N.'s to beds" is the ratio of full-time registered nurses to beds. "Board-certified internists to beds" is the ratio of these doctors to beds.

GASTROENTEROLOGY

Rank	Hospital	U.S. News index	Reputational score	Gastro-enterology mortality rate	COTH member	Interns and residents to beds	Technology score (of 11)	R.N.'s to beds	Board-certified gastro-enterologists to beds	Procedures to beds
1	Mayo Clinic, Rochester, Minn.	100.0	59.8%	0.05	Yes	0.24	8	0.77	0.029	1.00
2	Johns Hopkins Hospital, Baltimore	64.8	33.4%	0.81	Yes	0.73	11	1.43	0.015	1.43
3	Massachusetts General Hospital, Boston	60.3	29.6%	0.71	Yes	1.00	11	1.14	0.014	2.89
4	Cleveland Clinic	53.0	24.1%	0.71	Yes	1.22	10	1.47	0.012	2.31
5	UCLA Medical Center, Los Angeles	51.9	23.1%	0.54	Yes	1.52	11	1.20	0.021	1.63
6	Duke University Medical Center, Durham, N.C.	51.5	24.2%	0.88	Yes	0.91	11	1.61	0.017	1.55
7	Mount Sinai Medical Center, New York	51.3	24.3%	0.91	Yes	0.99	9	1.50	0.037	2.23
8	University of California, San Francisco Medical Center	47.7	20.8%	0.71	Yes	1.03	10	1.82	0.048	1.11
9	University of Chicago Hospitals	40.6	15.1%	0.72	Yes	1.64	10	1.38	0.038	1.90
10	Brigham and Women's Hospital, Boston	33.4	12.2%	0.89	Yes	1.49	10	0.79	0.020	1.78
11	University of Pittsburgh-Presbyterian University Hospital	31.6	9.5%	0.97	Yes	1.48	8	2.10	0.056	2.18
12	Beth Israel Hospital, Boston	26.8	7.1%	0.79	Yes	0.57	9	1.93	0.041	3.48
13	Hospital of the University of Pennsylvania, Philadelphia	26.5	5.6%	0.84	Yes	1.72	11	1.33	0.017	1.82
14	University of Michigan Medical Center, Ann Arbor	25.3	6.9%	0.83	Yes	1.00	10	1.29	0.014	1.44
15	Baylor University Medical Center, Dallas	24.2	7.6%	0.80	Yes	0.29	8	1.38	0.008	2.44
16	Yale-New Haven Hospital, New Haven, Conn.	23.6	5.6%	0.85	Yes	1.12	9	1.23	0.050	1.92
17	Indiana University Medical Center, Indianapolis	21.8	5.6%	1.33	Yes	1.10	10	1.86	0.030	1.33
18	Barnes Hospital, St. Louis	21.4	6.1%	1.01	Yes	0.89	11	0.82	0.000	1.71
19	Georgetown University Hospital, Washington, D.C.	20.0	3.2%	0.86	Yes	0.92	10	1.59	0.040	1.56
20	Memorial Sloan-Kettering Cancer Center, New York	19.5	4.3%	0.83	Yes	0.38	8	1.37	0.011	2.58
21	Stanford University Hospital, Stanford, Calif.	19.3	2.1%	0.80	Yes	1.34	11	0.86	0.035	2.03
22	University of Virginia Health Sciences Ctr., Charlottesville	19.0	1.2%	0.95	Yes	1.41	10	1.92	0.009	1.95
23	Rush-Presbyterian-St. Luke's Medical Center, Chicago	18.4	2.0%	0.82	Yes	1.05	10	1.24	0.000	2.05
24	Cedars-Sinai Medical Center, Los Angeles	18.4	4.8%	1.02	Yes	0.51	9	0.83	0.037	3.02
25	University of Wisconsin Hospital and Clinics, Madison	18.3	2.0%	0.97	Yes	1.30	11	1.24	0.014	2.03
26	University Hospitals of Cleveland	17.7	0.0%	0.97	Yes	1.60	11	1.73	0.027	2.15
27	University of California, Davis Medical Center	17.6	0.0%	1.25	Yes	1.54	10	2.81	0.008	1.50
28	University of Miami, Jackson Memorial Hospital	17.4	3.5%	0.97	Yes	0.85	8	1.39	0.004	0.39
29	Shands Hospital at the University of Florida, Gainesville	17.0	3.2%	0.67	Yes	0.66	10	0.62	0.024	1.20
30	New York University Medical Center	16.8	1.6%	0.94	Yes	1.30	8	1.15	0.000	2.01
31	New England Deaconess Hospital, Boston	16.8	0.5%	0.68	Yes	1.08	9	1.33	0.020	2.68
32	Henry Ford Hospital, Detroit	16.7	0.0%	0.91	Yes	1.34	10	1.50	0.000	2.81
33	Vanderbilt University Hospital and Clinic, Nashville	16.7	0.5%	0.77	Yes	1.21	10	1.29	0.019	1.54
34	University of Texas, M.D. Anderson Cancer Ctr., Houston	16.5	0.6%	0.26	Yes	0.70	10	1.88	0.012	1.66
35	Thomas Jefferson University Hospital, Philadelphia	16.5	0.5%	0.65	Yes	0.96	10	1.44	0.024	2.09
36	William Beaumont Hospital, Royal Oak, Mich.	16.3	0.7%	0.82	Yes	0.63	10	1.46	0.019	3.26
37	New England Medical Center, Boston	16.2	1.3%	0.93	Yes	1.07	7	1.66	0.016	1.47
38	University of Maryland Medical System, Baltimore	16.1	0.4%	0.84	Yes	0.96	10	1.67	0.010	1.00
39	Penn State's Milton S. Hershey Medical Ctr., Hershey	16.0	0.0%	1.00	Yes	1.55	9	1.57	0.011	1.80
40	St. Louis University Hospital	15.9	0.0%	1.28	Yes	1.89	10	1.33	0.032	2.50
41	New York Hospital-Cornell Medical Center	15.9	2.3%	0.92	Yes	0.79	9	1.00	0.015	1.37
42	Roswell Park Cancer Institute, Buffalo	15.8	0.0%	0.21	No	0.68	9	2.58	0.000	4.46
43	Lahey Clinic Hospital, Burlington, Mass.	15.6	2.6%	0.89	No	0.51	10	1.22	0.029	4.77
44	University of Minnesota Hospital and Clinic, Minneapolis	15.6	2.0%	0.73	Yes	0.59	10	0.86	0.030	1.29
45	F.G. McGaw Hospital at Loyola University, Maywood, Ill.	15.6	0.0%	1.05	Yes	1.46	9	1.59	0.019	2.07
46	University of North Carolina Hospitals, Chapel Hill	15.6	0.8%	1.29	Yes	1.41	9	1.71	0.037	1.80
47	University of Iowa Hospitals and Clinics, Iowa City	15.6	1.1%	0.97	Yes	0.96	11	1.34	0.017	1.15
48	University of Massachusetts Medical Center, Worcester	15.3	0.0%	0.87	Yes	1.47	8	0.96	0.022	2.10
49	Medical University of South Carolina, Charleston	15.2	0.9%	1.15	Yes	1.42	9	1.39	0.011	1.14
50	Columbia-Presbyterian Medical Center, New York	15.1	2.4%	1.13	Yes	0.85	10	1.05	0.014	1.29

"Reputational score" is the percentage of board-certified gastroenterology specialists surveyed who named the hospital. "Gastroenterology mortality rate" is the ratio of actual to expected deaths involving digestive-tract disorders (lower is better). "COTH member" indicates member of Council of Teaching Hospitals. "Interns and residents to beds" is the ratio of doctors in training to beds. "Technology score" is a specialty-specific index. "R.N.'s to beds" is the ratio of full-time registered nurses to beds. "Board-certified gastroenterologists to beds" is the ratio of these doctors to beds. "Procedures to beds" is the ratio of gastroenterology-related procedures to beds.

The Top 50 Hospitals
GERIATRICS

Rank	Hospital	U.S. News index	Reputational score	Hospital-wide mortality rate	COTH member	Service mix (of 10)	Interns and residents to beds	Technology score (of 13)	R.N.'s to beds	Discharge planning (of 2)	Geriatric services (of 9)	Board-certified internists to beds
1	UCLA Medical Center, Los Angeles	100.0	27.9%	0.66	Yes	8	1.52	12	1.20	2	5	0.023
2	Massachusetts General Hospital, Boston	86.4	23.1%	0.88	Yes	8	1.00	13	1.14	2	4	0.085
3	Mount Sinai Medical Center, New York	85.9	24.3%	1.09	Yes	9	0.99	10	1.50	2	6	0.253
4	Duke University Medical Center, Durham, N.C.	77.0	19.5%	0.90	Yes	7	0.91	13	1.61	2	4	0.081
5	Beth Israel Hospital, Boston	69.9	15.7%	0.85	Yes	9	0.57	11	1.93	2	3	0.590
6	Johns Hopkins Hospital, Baltimore	66.5	16.9%	0.97	Yes	8	0.73	12	1.43	2	1	0.084
7	Mayo Clinic, Rochester, Minn.	57.7	14.0%	0.72	Yes	5	0.24	8	0.77	2	5	0.060
8	University of Michigan Medical Center, Ann Arbor	49.6	9.6%	0.98	Yes	9	1.00	12	1.29	2	8	0.086
9	University of Washington Medical Center, Seattle	47.3	7.2%	0.84	Yes	7	1.05	10	2.06	2	4	0.440
10	Brigham and Women's Hospital, Boston	45.9	7.8%	0.91	Yes	7	1.49	12	0.79	2	4	0.179
11	University of Chicago Hospitals	42.5	5.5%	0.80	Yes	8	1.64	12	1.38	2	7	0.074
12	Cleveland Clinic	42.0	5.8%	0.87	Yes	9	1.22	12	1.47	2	4	0.015
13	Stanford University Hospital, Stanford, Calif.	39.1	6.0%	0.90	Yes	4	1.34	12	0.86	2	1	0.147
14	University of California, San Francisco Medical Center	38.9	3.9%	0.89	Yes	7	1.03	12	1.82	2	6	0.435
15	New York University Medical Center	33.7	4.4%	0.98	Yes	4	1.30	10	1.15	2	1	0.360
16	Rush-Presbyterian-St. Luke's Medical Center, Chicago	32.8	2.2%	0.81	Yes	9	1.05	11	1.24	2	6	0.224
17	Barnes Hospital, St. Louis	32.5	3.4%	0.98	Yes	10	0.89	13	0.82	2	4	0.273
18	UCSD Medical Center, San Diego	32.1	1.8%	0.75	Yes	6	1.65	9	2.17	2	4	0.049
19	University of Wisconsin Hospital and Clinics, Madison	31.6	2.7%	0.95	Yes	9	1.30	11	1.24	2	5	0.037
20	Yale-New Haven Hospital, New Haven, Conn.	31.4	4.6%	1.06	Yes	5	1.12	11	1.23	2	3	0.094
21	University of Minnesota Hospital and Clinic, Minneapolis	31.2	2.9%	0.81	Yes	9	0.59	10	0.86	2	2	0.133
22	University Hospital, Portland, Ore.	31.2	1.1%	0.80	Yes	7	1.54	11	2.31	2	2	0.164
23	Hospital of the University of Pennsylvania, Philadelphia	30.3	2.1%	0.97	Yes	8	1.72	12	1.33	2	4	0.007
24	North Carolina Baptist Hospital, Winston-Salem	29.7	3.4%	1.07	Yes	8	1.06	13	1.24	2	5	0.042
25	New York Hospital-Cornell Medical Center	29.5	3.5%	1.07	Yes	9	0.79	11	1.00	2	6	0.113
26	Columbia-Presbyterian Medical Center, New York	29.1	5.3%	1.25	Yes	7	0.85	11	1.05	2	4	0.111
27	University Hospital, Denver	27.6	1.4%	0.89	Yes	6	0.76	10	1.05	2	7	0.044
28	Boston University Medical Center-University Hospital	26.9	1.3%	0.82	Yes	4	0.96	10	0.85	2	5	0.231
29	University of Illinois Hospital and Clinics, Chicago	26.9	0.0%	0.83	Yes	7	1.29	10	1.95	2	5	0.056
30	University Hospitals of Cleveland	26.9	1.4%	1.07	Yes	8	1.60	13	1.73	2	5	0.080
31	Montefiore Medical Center, Bronx, N.Y.	26.8	4.0%	1.19	Yes	7	0.53	11	1.28	2	5	0.095
32	University of Utah Hospitals and Clinics, Salt Lake City	26.7	0.7%	0.81	Yes	6	0.88	10	1.73	2	5	0.021
33	Northwestern Memorial Hospital, Chicago	26.6	1.6%	0.99	Yes	10	0.43	11	1.03	2	6	0.134
34	Thomas Jefferson University Hospital, Philadelphia	26.6	0.5%	0.85	Yes	8	0.96	11	1.44	2	3	0.042
35	St. Louis University Hospital	26.5	3.2%	1.24	Yes	6	1.89	12	1.33	2	5	0.057
36	Albert Einstein Medical Center, Philadelphia	26.2	2.3%	1.07	Yes	8	0.75	12	0.89	2	8	0.098
37	New England Medical Center, Boston	26.2	0.3%	0.86	Yes	8	1.07	10	1.66	2	1	0.086
38	Henry Ford Hospital, Detroit	26.0	0.0%	0.96	Yes	8	1.34	11	1.50	2	6	0.301
39	University of California, Davis Medical Center	26.0	0.0%	1.01	Yes	8	1.54	12	2.81	2	4	0.032
40	Jewish Hospital of St. Louis	26.0	1.0%	0.97	Yes	9	0.63	11	1.22	2	7	0.100
41	Mount Sinai Medical Center, Cleveland	25.7	0.4%	0.87	Yes	8	0.76	10	0.86	2	6	0.144
42	Baylor University Medical Center, Dallas	25.6	0.6%	0.89	Yes	8	0.29	11	1.38	2	4	0.093
43	University of Pittsburgh-Presbyterian University Hospital	25.0	1.5%	1.10	Yes	5	1.48	10	2.10	2	1	0.291
44	Georgetown University Hospital, Washington, D.C.	25.0	0.6%	0.97	Yes	8	0.92	11	1.59	2	3	0.140
45	California Pacific Medical Center, San Francisco	24.9	0.0%	0.87	Yes	8	0.33	13	1.19	2	5	0.197
46	Evanston Hospital, Evanston, Ill.	24.6	0.0%	0.79	Yes	8	0.26	11	1.18	2	7	0.160
47	Vanderbilt University Hospital and Clinic, Nashville	24.4	0.3%	1.01	Yes	8	1.21	12	1.29	2	7	0.171
48	University of Maryland Medical System, Baltimore	24.4	0.0%	0.98	Yes	8	0.96	12	1.67	2	3	0.281
49	Cook County Hospital, Chicago	24.3	0.0%	0.55	Yes	7	1.00	9	1.43	2	2	0.073
50	Hennepin County Medical Center, Minneapolis	24.2	0.0%	0.77	Yes	8	0.91	10	0.78	2	6	0.020

"Reputational score" is the percentage of board-certified geriatric specialists surveyed who named the hospital. "Hospitalwide mortality rate" is the ratio of actual to expected deaths overall (lower is better). "COTH member" indicates member of Council of Teaching Hospitals. "Service mix" indicates breadth of community services. "Interns and residents to beds" is the ratio of doctors in training to beds. "Technology score" is a specialty-specific index. "R.N.'s to beds" is the ratio of full-time registered nurses to beds. "Discharge planning" indicates number of postdischarge services available. "Geriatric services" is the number of geriatric services available. "Board-certified internists to beds" is the ratio of these doctors to beds.

The Top 50 Hospitals
GYNECOLOGY

Rank	Hospital	U.S. News index	Reputational score	Hospital-wide mortality rate	Interns and residents to beds	Technology score (of 10)	R.N.'s to beds	Board-certified OB-GYNs to beds	Procedures to beds
1	Johns Hopkins Hospital, Baltimore	100.0	29.5%	0.97	0.73	10	1.43	0.046	0.46
2	Mayo Clinic, Rochester, Minn.	95.4	30.0%	0.72	0.24	6	0.77	0.014	0.35
3	University of Texas, M.D. Anderson Cancer Ctr., Houston	85.9	22.5%	0.38	0.70	9	1.88	0.040	0.75
4	Brigham and Women's Hospital, Boston	80.9	20.9%	0.91	1.49	9	0.79	0.127	0.66
5	Massachusetts General Hospital, Boston	57.7	12.0%	0.88	1.00	10	1.14	0.046	0.53
6	Los Angeles County-USC Medical Center	55.9	11.7%	0.88	1.21	7	1.30	0.021	0.03
7	Duke University Medical Center, Durham, N.C.	53.9	10.2%	0.90	0.91	10	1.61	0.028	0.45
8	Cleveland Clinic	50.3	8.8%	0.87	1.22	9	1.47	0.009	0.48
9	University of Chicago Hospitals	49.2	7.2%	0.80	1.64	10	1.38	0.036	0.37
10	UCLA Medical Center, Los Angeles	49.1	7.8%	0.66	1.52	10	1.20	0.028	0.49
11	Memorial Sloan-Kettering Cancer Center, New York	45.6	9.4%	0.91	0.38	7	1.37	0.007	0.50
12	Parkland Memorial Hospital, Dallas	43.9	10.2%	1.22	1.35	9	0.93	0.024	0.11
13	Stanford University Hospital, Stanford, Calif.	43.0	6.1%	0.90	1.34	9	0.86	0.107	0.39
14	University of California, San Francisco Medical Center	42.6	5.3%	0.89	1.03	9	1.82	0.043	0.21
15	Hospital of the University of Pennsylvania, Philadelphia	39.7	4.5%	0.97	1.72	10	1.33	0.036	0.35
16	Yale-New Haven Hospital, New Haven, Conn.	38.4	5.9%	1.06	1.12	9	1.23	0.103	0.60
17	University of Washington Medical Center, Seattle	37.1	2.2%	0.84	1.05	9	2.06	0.093	0.59
18	Roswell Park Cancer Institute, Buffalo	36.1	2.5%	0.56	0.68	8	2.58	0.023	0.91
19	Beth Israel Hospital, Boston	35.3	3.0%	0.85	0.57	7	1.93	0.132	0.55
20	UCSD Medical Center, San Diego	35.0	0.8%	0.75	1.65	7	2.17	0.078	0.33
21	University of North Carolina Hospitals, Chapel Hill	33.8	4.5%	1.23	1.41	9	1.71	0.064	0.50
22	Thomas Jefferson University Hospital, Philadelphia	33.4	1.9%	0.85	0.96	9	1.44	0.102	0.41
23	University Hospital, Portland, Ore.	33.1	0.0%	0.80	1.54	8	2.31	0.055	0.38
24	University of California, Davis Medical Center	32.8	0.5%	1.01	1.54	9	2.81	0.025	0.36
25	Northwestern Memorial Hospital, Chicago	32.8	4.6%	0.99	0.43	9	1.03	0.088	0.44
26	Barnes Hospital, St. Louis	32.1	4.0%	0.98	0.89	9	0.82	0.071	0.56
27	Baylor University Medical Center, Dallas	32.0	4.0%	0.89	0.29	7	1.38	0.008	0.53
28	Rush-Presbyterian-St. Luke's Medical Center, Chicago	31.9	1.9%	0.81	1.05	9	1.24	0.060	0.33
29	New York Hospital-Cornell Medical Center	31.5	5.0%	1.07	0.79	8	1.00	0.055	0.23
30	University of Illinois Hospital and Clinics, Chicago	30.6	0.5%	0.83	1.29	7	1.95	0.039	0.28
31	New York University Medical Center	30.5	2.3%	0.98	1.30	8	1.15	0.074	0.36
32	Vanderbilt University Hospital and Clinic, Nashville	30.2	2.4%	1.01	1.21	10	1.29	0.024	0.39
33	Columbia-Presbyterian Medical Center, New York	29.9	5.2%	1.25	0.85	10	1.05	0.036	0.22
34	Georgetown University Hospital, Washington, D.C.	29.2	1.5%	0.97	0.92	9	1.59	0.056	0.40
35	University of Utah Hospitals and Clinics, Salt Lake City	28.4	0.4%	0.81	0.88	8	1.73	0.044	0.35
36	Mount Sinai Medical Center, New York	28.2	2.9%	1.09	0.99	7	1.50	0.061	0.28
37	University Hospitals, Oklahoma City	28.1	0.0%	0.98	1.60	8	1.56	0.095	0.19
38	University of Virginia Health Sciences Ctr., Charlottesville	28.1	2.2%	1.21	1.41	9	1.92	0.021	0.46
39	Cedars-Sinai Medical Center, Los Angeles	28.0	4.5%	1.13	0.51	8	0.83	0.094	0.48
40	University of Michigan Medical Center, Ann Arbor	27.8	1.6%	0.98	1.00	9	1.29	0.046	0.45
41	University of Wisconsin Hospital and Clinics, Madison	27.6	0.9%	0.95	1.30	9	1.24	0.027	0.31
42	University Hospitals of Cleveland	27.6	0.0%	1.07	1.60	10	1.73	0.083	0.42
43	Ohio State University Medical Center, Columbus	27.5	2.2%	0.94	0.81	7	1.11	0.041	0.12
44	Penn State's Milton S. Hershey Medical Ctr., Hershey	27.4	1.1%	1.03	1.55	8	1.57	0.021	0.61
45	University of Miami, Jackson Memorial Hospital	27.3	1.3%	1.12	0.85	7	1.39	0.018	0.18
46	Cook County Hospital, Chicago	27.1	0.6%	0.55	1.00	7	1.43	0.033	0.09
47	F.G. McGaw Hospital at Loyola University, Maywood, Ill.	26.9	1.3%	1.12	1.46	9	1.59	0.042	0.39
48	University Hospital, Denver	26.7	1.0%	0.89	0.76	9	1.05	0.028	0.46
49	Henry Ford Hospital, Detroit	26.6	0.0%	0.96	1.34	9	1.50	0.042	0.28
50	University Medical Center, Tucson, Ariz.	26.4	0.4%	0.97	0.74	8	1.73	0.103	0.60

"Reputational score" is the percentage of board-certified specialists in obstetrics and gynecology surveyed who named the hospital. "Hospitalwide mortality rate" is the ratio of actual to expected deaths overall (lower is better). "Interns and residents to beds" is the ratio of doctors in training to beds. "Technology score" is a specialty-specific index. "R.N.'s to beds" is the ratio of full-time registered nurses to beds. "Board-certified OB-GYNs to beds" is the ratio of these doctors to beds. "Procedures to beds" is the ratio of OB-GYN-related procedures to beds.

NEUROLOGY

Rank	Hospital	U.S. News index	Reputa-tional score	Neurology mortality rate	COTH member	Interns and residents to beds	Tech-nology score (of 9)	R.N.'s to beds	Board-certified neurologists to beds
1	Mayo Clinic, Rochester, Minn.	100.0	51.5%	0.72	Yes	0.24	6	0.77	0.035
2	Johns Hopkins Hospital, Baltimore	80.7	38.7%	0.84	Yes	0.73	9	1.43	0.014
3	University of California, San Francisco Medical Center	63.9	27.3%	0.91	Yes	1.03	8	1.82	0.029
4	Massachusetts General Hospital, Boston	61.8	28.6%	1.00	Yes	1.00	9	1.14	0.014
5	Columbia-Presbyterian Medical Center, New York	54.8	23.7%	1.02	Yes	0.85	9	1.05	0.040
6	UCLA Medical Center, Los Angeles	41.4	9.6%	0.69	Yes	1.52	9	1.20	0.056
7	Cleveland Clinic	40.6	10.6%	0.62	Yes	1.22	9	1.47	0.023
8	New York Hospital-Cornell Medical Center	40.2	12.8%	0.78	Yes	0.79	7	1.00	0.024
9	Barnes Hospital, St. Louis	39.6	12.5%	0.87	Yes	0.89	9	0.82	0.042
10	Hospital of the University of Pennsylvania, Philadelphia	36.1	9.2%	1.02	Yes	1.72	9	1.33	0.051
11	Duke University Medical Center, Durham, N.C.	33.2	8.6%	0.89	Yes	0.91	9	1.61	0.017
12	Brigham and Women's Hospital, Boston	31.1	5.3%	0.79	Yes	1.49	8	0.79	0.036
13	New York University Medical Center	28.6	3.7%	0.73	Yes	1.30	7	1.15	0.024
14	University of Illinois Hospital and Clinics, Chicago	27.7	2.4%	0.50	Yes	1.29	6	1.95	0.017
15	Stanford University Hospital, Stanford, Calif.	27.5	3.2%	0.79	Yes	1.34	9	0.86	0.031
16	University of Chicago Hospitals	27.3	1.5%	0.67	Yes	1.64	9	1.38	0.023
17	University of Washington Medical Center, Seattle	27.0	2.6%	0.89	Yes	1.05	8	2.06	0.047
18	Beth Israel Hospital, Boston	26.8	1.1%	0.82	Yes	0.57	7	1.93	0.087
19	Rush-Presbyterian-St. Luke's Medical Center, Chicago	26.7	2.4%	0.53	Yes	1.05	8	1.24	0.031
20	University of Pittsburgh-Presbyterian University Hospital	26.0	2.1%	1.05	Yes	1.48	7	2.10	0.066
21	University Hospital, Portland, Ore.	25.8	0.6%	0.95	Yes	1.54	7	2.31	0.063
22	Mount Sinai Medical Center, New York	25.4	1.9%	0.78	Yes	0.99	7	1.50	0.026
23	University of Iowa Hospitals and Clinics, Iowa City	24.9	4.6%	0.97	Yes	0.96	9	1.34	0.015
24	University of Michigan Medical Center, Ann Arbor	24.9	5.3%	1.02	Yes	1.00	8	1.29	0.014
25	Georgetown University Hospital, Washington, D.C.	24.7	1.1%	0.77	Yes	0.92	8	1.59	0.028
26	Thomas Jefferson University Hospital, Philadelphia	24.1	0.6%	0.59	Yes	0.96	8	1.44	0.031
27	University of Minnesota Hospital and Clinic, Minneapolis	23.8	1.6%	0.64	Yes	0.59	8	0.86	0.043
28	University Hospitals of Cleveland	23.7	0.0%	0.93	Yes	1.60	9	1.73	0.050
29	Medical College of Georgia Hospital and Clinic, Augusta	23.6	0.0%	0.70	Yes	1.42	8	1.09	0.030
30	University Hospitals, Oklahoma City	23.6	0.0%	0.80	Yes	1.60	8	1.56	0.017
31	Shands Hospital at the University of Florida, Gainesville	23.3	2.6%	0.57	Yes	0.66	8	0.62	0.019
32	Boston University Medical Center-University Hospital	23.2	0.0%	0.65	Yes	0.96	7	0.85	0.060
33	UCSD Medical Center, San Diego	23.1	0.4%	1.14	Yes	1.65	6	2.17	0.075
34	Temple University Hospital, Philadelphia	22.9	0.0%	0.75	Yes	1.25	8	1.15	0.025
35	Emory University Hospital, Atlanta	22.7	1.7%	0.81	Yes	0.71	6	1.28	0.030
36	Loma Linda University Medical Center, Loma Linda, Calif.	22.6	0.0%	0.78	Yes	1.14	7	1.61	0.018
37	George Washington University Hospital, Washington, D.C.	22.5	1.1%	1.06	Yes	1.40	8	1.16	0.076
38	University of California, Davis Medical Center	22.4	0.6%	1.07	Yes	1.54	8	2.81	0.017
39	New England Deaconess Hospital, Boston	22.3	0.0%	0.70	Yes	1.08	8	1.33	0.017
40	University of Maryland Medical System, Baltimore	22.2	1.9%	0.97	Yes	0.96	8	1.67	0.031
41	Northwestern Memorial Hospital, Chicago	21.8	2.0%	0.84	Yes	0.43	8	1.03	0.034
42	Harper Hospital, Detroit	21.5	1.0%	0.70	Yes	0.34	8	1.20	0.022
43	Strong Memorial Hospital-Rochester University, N.Y.	21.5	1.8%	1.09	Yes	1.00	8	1.45	0.057
44	University of Miami, Jackson Memorial Hospital	21.3	5.6%	1.28	Yes	0.85	6	1.39	0.016
45	Henry Ford Hospital, Detroit	20.9	0.2%	0.90	Yes	1.34	8	1.50	0.020
46	Western Pennsylvania Hospital, Pittsburgh	20.7	0.0%	0.65	Yes	0.43	7	1.44	0.024
47	University of Utah Hospitals and Clinics, Salt Lake City	20.7	0.6%	0.95	Yes	0.88	7	1.73	0.039
48	University Hospital, Denver	20.6	0.4%	0.75	Yes	0.76	8	1.05	0.008
49	University of Virginia Health Sciences Ctr., Charlottesville	20.4	1.2%	1.10	Yes	1.41	8	1.92	0.018
50	New England Medical Center, Boston	20.3	1.6%	0.98	Yes	1.07	6	1.66	0.014

"Reputational score" is the percentage of board-certified neurology specialists surveyed who named the hospital. "Neurology mortality rate" is the ratio of actual to expected neurology deaths (lower is better). "COTH member" indicates member of Council of Teaching Hospitals. "Interns and residents to beds" is the ratio of doctors in training to beds. "Technology score" is a specialty-specific index. "R.N.'s to beds" is the ratio of full-time registered nurses to beds. "Board-certified neurologists to beds" is the ratio of these doctors to beds.

ORTHOPEDICS

Rank	Hospital	U.S. News index	Reputa-tional score	Orthopedics mortality rate	COTH member	Interns and residents to beds	Tech-nology score (of 5)	R.N.'s to beds	Board-certified orthopedists to beds	Pro-cedures to beds
1	Mayo Clinic, Rochester, Minn.	100.0	41.7%	0.55	Yes	0.24	4	0.77	0.023	1.89
2	Hospital for Special Surgery, New York	95.9	36.6%	0.24	Yes	0.68	4	0.78	0.271	17.09
3	Massachusetts General Hospital, Boston	76.5	28.7%	0.72	Yes	1.00	5	1.14	0.026	2.29
4	Johns Hopkins Hospital, Baltimore	45.3	14.4%	0.80	Yes	0.73	5	1.43	0.026	1.11
5	Duke University Medical Center, Durham, N.C.	41.0	11.4%	0.75	Yes	0.91	5	1.61	0.016	1.54
6	UCLA Medical Center, Los Angeles	38.2	10.5%	0.93	Yes	1.52	5	1.20	0.015	1.72
7	Cleveland Clinic	37.7	8.8%	0.65	Yes	1.22	5	1.47	0.020	2.33
8	Hospital for Joint Diseases-Orthopedic Institute, New York	33.9	7.6%	0.11	Yes	0.27	4	1.26	0.277	9.68
9	University of Washington Medical Center, Seattle	31.3	5.9%	0.72	Yes	1.05	4	2.06	0.070	1.54
10	University of Iowa Hospitals and Clinics, Iowa City	31.2	7.9%	0.92	Yes	0.96	5	1.34	0.020	1.08
11	Hospital of the University of Pennsylvania, Philadelphia	28.7	3.9%	0.61	Yes	1.72	5	1.33	0.036	1.65
12	Stanford University Hospital, Stanford, Calif.	26.9	4.0%	0.63	Yes	1.34	5	0.86	0.068	2.34
13	University of Michigan Medical Center, Ann Arbor	25.0	5.7%	1.16	Yes	1.00	5	1.29	0.025	1.21
14	University of Texas, M.D. Anderson Cancer Ctr., Houston	24.4	2.9%	0.20	Yes	0.70	5	1.88	0.022	0.69
15	Brigham and Women's Hospital, Boston	23.7	3.6%	0.79	Yes	1.49	4	0.79	0.034	2.37
16	UCSD Medical Center, San Diego	23.1	1.0%	0.66	Yes	1.65	2	2.17	0.097	0.96
17	Thomas Jefferson University Hospital, Philadelphia	22.9	2.5%	0.61	Yes	0.96	4	1.44	0.034	1.73
18	Vanderbilt University Hospital and Clinic, Nashville	21.6	2.3%	0.80	Yes	1.21	5	1.29	0.018	1.62
19	University of Chicago Hospitals	21.4	0.5%	0.55	Yes	1.64	5	1.38	0.011	1.38
20	University of Wisconsin Hospital and Clinics, Madison	21.1	1.0%	0.57	Yes	1.30	5	1.24	0.014	1.66
21	Harborview Medical Center, Seattle	21.1	5.3%	1.24	Yes	0.37	2	1.73	0.049	1.21
22	University of California, Davis Medical Center	20.8	0.9%	1.10	Yes	1.54	4	2.81	0.021	1.42
23	University of North Carolina Hospitals, Chapel Hill	20.8	0.6%	0.68	Yes	1.41	4	1.71	0.018	1.21
24	Rush-Presbyterian-St. Luke's Medical Center, Chicago	20.4	2.0%	0.76	Yes	1.05	4	1.24	0.039	1.83
25	University Hospitals, Oklahoma City	20.1	0.0%	0.53	Yes	1.60	4	1.56	0.023	0.90
26	University of Pittsburgh-Presbyterian University Hospital	19.9	2.8%	1.79	Yes	1.48	3	2.10	0.103	1.80
27	New York University Medical Center	19.9	1.6%	0.78	Yes	1.30	4	1.15	0.032	1.28
28	Shands Hospital at the University of Florida, Gainesville	19.7	2.5%	0.29	Yes	0.66	4	0.62	0.017	1.48
29	Ohio State University Medical Center, Columbus	19.3	1.5%	0.62	Yes	0.81	4	1.11	0.018	0.90
30	Henry Ford Hospital, Detroit	19.2	1.0%	0.82	Yes	1.34	4	1.50	0.026	1.86
31	F.G. McGaw Hospital at Loyola University, Maywood, Ill.	19.2	0.0%	0.71	Yes	1.46	4	1.59	0.039	1.83
32	University of Minnesota Hospital and Clinic, Minneapolis	18.8	1.9%	0.35	Yes	0.59	4	0.86	0.016	1.55
33	University Hospitals and Clinics, Columbia, Mo.	18.8	0.8%	0.67	Yes	1.10	4	1.19	0.015	1.18
34	Medical College of Ohio Hospital, Toledo	18.8	0.0%	0.67	Yes	1.42	4	1.23	0.051	1.81
35	Beth Israel Hospital, Boston	18.7	0.3%	0.63	Yes	0.57	4	1.93	0.039	2.53
36	Bone and Joint Hospital, Oklahoma City	18.6	0.4%	0.49	No	0.04	0	0.63	0.157	43.45
37	Indiana University Medical Center, Indianapolis	18.1	0.3%	0.85	Yes	1.10	5	1.86	0.042	1.37
38	Medical College of Georgia Hospital and Clinic, Augusta	18.0	0.0%	0.50	Yes	1.42	4	1.09	0.014	0.59
39	Georgetown University Hospital, Washington, D.C.	18.0	1.4%	0.89	Yes	0.92	4	1.59	0.050	1.15
40	University Hosp.-SUNY Health Science Ctr., Syracuse, N.Y.	17.6	0.0%	0.78	Yes	1.30	3	1.61	0.086	2.50
41	Barnes Hospital, St. Louis	17.5	1.9%	0.90	Yes	0.89	5	0.82	0.017	1.34
42	University of Massachusetts Medical Center, Worcester	17.4	0.0%	0.68	Yes	1.47	3	0.96	0.059	1.62
43	Columbia-Presbyterian Medical Center, New York	17.3	3.5%	1.68	Yes	0.85	5	1.05	0.035	1.23
44	Emory University Hospital, Atlanta	17.3	2.3%	1.04	Yes	0.71	4	1.28	0.028	2.19
45	University Hospital, Portland, Ore.	17.2	0.0%	1.14	Yes	1.54	4	2.31	0.017	1.36
46	University Hospitals of Cleveland	17.2	0.0%	1.09	Yes	1.60	5	1.73	0.033	2.50
47	Allegheny General Hospital, Pittsburgh	16.7	1.4%	0.84	Yes	0.52	4	1.36	0.020	2.13
48	University of Virginia Health Sciences Ctr., Charlottesville	16.7	0.7%	1.24	Yes	1.41	4	1.92	0.007	1.75
49	Penn State's Milton S. Hershey Medical Ctr., Hershey	16.6	0.5%	1.10	Yes	1.55	4	1.57	0.016	1.71
50	University of Miami, Jackson Memorial Hospital	16.6	3.3%	1.40	Yes	0.85	2	1.39	0.024	0.28

"Reputational score" is the percentage of board-certified orthopedic specialists surveyed who named the hospital. "Orthopedics mortality rate" is the ratio of actual to expected orthopedic deaths (lower is better). "COTH member" indicates member of Council of Teaching Hospitals. "Interns and residents to beds" is the ratio of doctors in training to beds. "Technology score" is a specialty-specific index. "R.N.'s to beds" is the ratio of full-time registered nurses to beds. "Board-certified orthopedists to beds" is the ratio of these doctors to beds. "Procedures to beds" is the ratio of orthopedic-related procedures to beds.

The Top 50 Hospitals
OTOLARYNGOLOGY

Rank	Hospital	U.S. News index	Reputa-tional score	Hospital-wide mortality rate	COTH member	Interns and residents to beds	Tech-nology score (of 9)	R.N.'s to beds	Board-certified internists to beds	Procedures to beds
1	Johns Hopkins Hospital, Baltimore	100.0	27.0%	0.97	Yes	0.73	9	1.43	0.084	0.315
2	Massachusetts Eye and Ear Infirmary, Boston	91.3	18.4%	0.04	No	0.86	2	2.18	0.043	4.848
3	University of Iowa Hospitals and Clinics, Iowa City	89.8	23.7%	1.02	Yes	0.96	9	1.34	0.053	0.276
4	University of Michigan Medical Center, Ann Arbor	59.8	14.3%	0.98	Yes	1.00	8	1.29	0.086	0.274
5	UCLA Medical Center, Los Angeles	58.4	13.3%	0.66	Yes	1.52	9	1.20	0.023	0.316
6	Mayo Clinic, Rochester, Minn.	52.8	13.7%	0.72	Yes	0.24	6	0.77	0.089	0.222
7	Barnes Hospital, St. Louis	50.7	11.5%	0.98	Yes	0.89	9	0.82	0.273	0.261
8	University of Pittsburgh-Presbyterian University Hospital	47.0	8.5%	1.10	Yes	1.48	7	2.10	0.291	0.285
9	University of Texas, M.D. Anderson Cancer Ctr., Houston	42.7	8.6%	0.38	Yes	0.70	9	1.88	0.083	0.419
10	Cleveland Clinic	41.1	8.1%	0.87	Yes	1.22	9	1.47	0.015	0.231
11	Stanford University Hospital, Stanford, Calif.	39.5	7.7%	0.90	Yes	1.34	9	0.86	0.147	0.273
12	University of Virginia Health Sciences Ctr., Charlottesville	38.1	6.4%	1.21	Yes	1.41	8	1.92	0.101	0.357
13	Mount Sinai Medical Center, New York	37.5	6.8%	1.09	Yes	0.99	7	1.50	0.253	0.216
14	Vanderbilt University Hospital and Clinic, Nashville	36.7	6.5%	1.02	Yes	1.21	9	1.29	0.171	0.463
15	New York University Medical Center	33.2	5.1%	0.98	Yes	1.30	7	1.15	0.360	0.271
16	University of California, San Francisco Medical Center	32.9	4.4%	0.89	Yes	1.03	8	1.82	0.435	0.177
17	University of Washington Medical Center, Seattle	30.3	3.3%	0.84	Yes	1.05	8	2.06	0.440	0.225
18	Duke University Medical Center, Durham, N.C.	26.9	3.7%	0.90	Yes	0.91	9	1.61	0.081	0.126
19	University of Cincinnati Hospital	26.9	5.2%	1.11	Yes	0.78	0	1.10	0.074	0.246
20	Los Angeles County-USC Medical Center	26.7	3.9%	0.88	Yes	1.21	6	1.30	0.052	0.028
21	Manhattan Eye, Ear and Throat Hospital, New York	24.6	5.4%	0.01	No	0.86	1	0.53	0.181	1.833
22	University of North Carolina Hospitals, Chapel Hill	24.5	2.0%	1.23	Yes	1.41	8	1.71	0.246	0.235
23	University of Illinois Hospital and Clinics, Chicago	24.0	2.3%	0.83	Yes	1.29	6	1.95	0.056	0.228
24	University Hospital, Portland, Ore.	23.8	1.2%	0.80	Yes	1.54	7	2.31	0.164	0.374
25	Hospital of the University of Pennsylvania, Philadelphia	23.7	2.2%	0.97	Yes	1.72	9	1.33	0.007	0.315
26	University of Miami, Jackson Memorial Hospital	23.5	3.4%	1.11	Yes	0.85	6	1.39	0.046	0.078
27	Indiana University Medical Center, Indianapolis	22.3	1.9%	1.14	Yes	1.10	8	1.86	0.107	0.151
28	Northwestern Memorial Hospital, Chicago	22.1	3.4%	0.99	Yes	0.43	8	1.03	0.134	0.207
29	University Hospitals of Cleveland	21.9	1.2%	1.07	Yes	1.60	9	1.73	0.080	0.284
30	University of Minnesota Hospital and Clinic, Minneapolis	21.5	3.1%	0.81	Yes	0.59	8	0.86	0.133	0.267
31	University of Chicago Hospitals	21.3	1.3%	0.80	Yes	1.64	9	1.38	0.074	0.234
32	Parkland Memorial Hospital, Dallas	21.2	2.3%	1.22	Yes	1.35	8	0.93	0.039	0.050
33	F.G. McGaw Hospital at Loyola University, Maywood, Ill.	21.1	1.4%	1.12	Yes	1.46	8	1.59	0.053	0.314
34	Henry Ford Hospital, Detroit	20.8	0.9%	0.96	Yes	1.34	8	1.50	0.301	0.265
35	Beth Israel Hospital, Boston	20.7	0.7%	0.85	Yes	0.57	7	1.93	0.590	0.245
36	University of California, Davis Medical Center	20.5	0.0%	1.01	Yes	1.54	8	2.81	0.032	0.274
37	University of Maryland Medical System, Baltimore	19.9	1.0%	0.98	Yes	0.96	8	1.67	0.281	0.223
38	Columbia-Presbyterian Medical Center, New York	19.7	2.2%	1.25	Yes	0.85	8	1.05	0.111	0.130
39	University of Pittsburgh-Montefiore Hospital	19.6	2.4%	1.09	No	0.93	2	1.43	0.388	1.069
40	Yale-New Haven Hospital, New Haven, Conn.	19.5	1.6%	1.06	Yes	1.12	8	1.23	0.094	0.249
41	University Hosp.-SUNY Health Science Ctr., Syracuse, N.Y.	19.4	0.9%	1.28	Yes	1.30	7	1.61	0.160	0.550
42	University of Nebraska Medical Center, Omaha	19.3	0.9%	1.05	Yes	1.37	8	1.23	0.205	0.145
43	George Washington University Hospital, Washington, D.C.	19.3	0.9%	1.24	Yes	1.40	8	1.16	0.223	0.191
44	Medical Center of Louisiana at New Orleans	19.0	0.7%	1.15	Yes	1.39	5	0.91	0.457	0.094
45	UCSD Medical Center, San Diego	18.7	0.0%	0.75	Yes	1.65	6	2.17	0.049	0.163
46	New England Medical Center, Boston	18.5	1.1%	0.86	Yes	1.07	6	1.66	0.086	0.151
47	University of Texas Medical Branch Hospitals, Galveston	18.5	1.5%	1.16	Yes	1.09	8	1.19	0.068	0.072
48	Brigham and Women's Hospital, Boston	18.5	1.0%	0.91	Yes	1.49	8	0.79	0.179	0.153
49	North Carolina Baptist Hospital, Winston-Salem	18.4	1.4%	1.07	Yes	1.06	9	1.24	0.042	0.210
50	New York Eye and Ear Infirmary	18.1	3.3%	0.38	No	0.64	2	0.84	0.194	1.039

"Reputational score" is the percentage of board-certified otolaryngology specialists surveyed who named the hospital. "Hospitalwide mortality rate" is the ratio of actual to expected deaths overall (lower is better). "COTH member" indicates member of Council of Teaching Hospitals. "Interns and residents to beds" is the ratio of doctors in training to beds. "Technology score" is a specialty-specific index. "R.N.'s to beds" is the ratio of full-time registered nurses to beds. "Board-certified internists to beds" is the ratio of these doctors to beds. "Procedures to beds" is the ratio of otolaryngology-related procedures to beds.

RHEUMATOLOGY

Rank	Hospital	U.S. News index	Reputa-tional score	Hospital-wide mortality rate	COTH member	Interns and residents to beds	Tech-nology score (of 5)	R.N.'s to beds	Board-certified internists to beds
1	Mayo Clinic, Rochester, Minn.	100.0	38.7%	0.72	Yes	0.24	4	0.77	0.089
2	Johns Hopkins Hospital, Baltimore	75.3	26.6%	0.97	Yes	0.73	5	1.43	0.084
3	Brigham and Women's Hospital, Boston	73.3	25.0%	0.91	Yes	1.49	4	0.79	0.179
4	UCLA Medical Center, Los Angeles	60.4	18.6%	0.66	Yes	1.52	5	1.20	0.023
5	Hospital for Special Surgery, New York	53.3	17.4%	0.36	Yes	0.68	4	0.78	0.000
6	Duke University Medical Center, Durham, N.C.	48.0	13.5%	0.90	Yes	0.91	5	1.61	0.081
7	University of Alabama Hospital at Birmingham	46.7	15.3%	1.16	Yes	0.82	4	0.92	0.027
8	Cleveland Clinic	41.5	10.4%	0.87	Yes	1.22	5	1.47	0.015
9	New York University Medical Center	36.0	7.7%	0.98	Yes	1.30	4	1.15	0.360
10	University of Pittsburgh-Presbyterian University Hospital	35.8	7.2%	1.10	Yes	1.48	3	2.10	0.291
11	Stanford University Hospital, Stanford, Calif.	35.1	7.8%	0.90	Yes	1.34	5	0.86	0.147
12	Massachusetts General Hospital, Boston	33.7	7.4%	0.88	Yes	1.00	5	1.14	0.085
13	University of Michigan Medical Center, Ann Arbor	32.7	7.2%	0.98	Yes	1.00	5	1.29	0.086
14	University of Washington Medical Center, Seattle	31.5	4.1%	0.84	Yes	1.05	4	2.06	0.440
15	University of California, San Francisco Medical Center	30.4	4.2%	0.89	Yes	1.03	4	1.82	0.435
16	Beth Israel Hospital, Boston	27.1	2.5%	0.85	Yes	0.57	4	1.93	0.590
17	Yale-New Haven Hospital, New Haven, Conn.	26.9	5.1%	1.06	Yes	1.12	4	1.23	0.094
18	Barnes Hospital, St. Louis	26.0	4.4%	0.98	Yes	0.89	5	0.82	0.273
19	Hospital of the University of Pennsylvania, Philadelphia	25.6	3.2%	0.97	Yes	1.72	5	1.33	0.007
20	University of Chicago Hospitals	24.7	2.0%	0.80	Yes	1.64	5	1.38	0.074
21	Parkland Memorial Hospital, Dallas	24.7	4.8%	1.22	Yes	1.35	4	0.93	0.039
22	Hospital for Joint Diseases-Orthopedic Institute, New York	24.2	3.6%	0.10	Yes	0.27	4	1.26	0.227
23	UCSD Medical Center, San Diego	22.8	0.9%	0.75	Yes	1.65	2	2.17	0.049
24	University Hospital, Portland, Ore.	22.6	0.0%	0.80	Yes	1.54	4	2.31	0.164
25	Mount Sinai Medical Center, New York	22.3	2.6%	1.09	Yes	0.99	3	1.50	0.253
26	University Hospitals of Cleveland	22.0	1.5%	1.07	Yes	1.60	5	1.73	0.080
27	Henry Ford Hospital, Detroit	21.9	1.1%	0.96	Yes	1.34	4	1.50	0.301
28	University of Illinois Hospital and Clinics, Chicago	21.3	0.8%	0.83	Yes	1.29	3	1.95	0.056
29	University of California, Davis Medical Center	21.2	0.0%	1.01	Yes	1.54	4	2.81	0.032
30	University of Utah Hospitals and Clinics, Salt Lake City	21.1	1.6%	0.81	Yes	0.88	3	1.73	0.021
31	Medical University of South Carolina, Charleston	20.8	2.0%	1.07	Yes	1.42	4	1.39	0.022
32	Rush-Presbyterian-St. Luke's Medical Center, Chicago	20.7	0.9%	0.81	Yes	1.05	4	1.24	0.224
33	University of North Carolina Hospitals, Chapel Hill	20.7	1.3%	1.23	Yes	1.41	4	1.71	0.246
34	University of Texas, M.D. Anderson Cancer Ctr., Houston	20.3	0.7%	0.38	Yes	0.70	5	1.88	0.083
35	Thomas Jefferson University Hospital, Philadelphia	20.3	1.3%	0.85	Yes	0.96	4	1.44	0.042
36	George Washington University Hospital, Washington, D.C.	20.3	1.9%	1.24	Yes	1.40	4	1.16	0.223
37	Vanderbilt University Hospital and Clinic, Nashville	20.2	1.2%	1.02	Yes	1.21	5	1.29	0.171
38	University Medical Center, Tucson, Ariz.	20.0	1.6%	0.97	Yes	0.74	3	1.73	0.136
39	Green Hospital of Scripps Clinic, La Jolla, Calif.	19.9	3.1%	0.86	No	0.21	4	1.99	0.052
40	New England Medical Center, Boston	19.3	0.5%	0.86	Yes	1.07	3	1.66	0.086
41	University of Virginia Health Sciences Ctr., Charlottesville	19.1	0.7%	1.21	Yes	1.41	4	1.92	0.101
42	Indiana University Medical Center, Indianapolis	19.0	0.8%	1.14	Yes	1.10	5	1.86	0.107
43	University of Minnesota Hospital and Clinic, Minneapolis	18.7	1.4%	0.81	Yes	0.59	4	0.86	0.133
44	University of Iowa Hospitals and Clinics, Iowa City	18.6	1.2%	1.02	Yes	0.96	5	1.34	0.053
45	University of Maryland Medical System, Baltimore	18.4	0.0%	0.98	Yes	0.96	4	1.67	0.281
46	University Hospitals, Oklahoma City	18.4	0.0%	0.98	Yes	1.60	4	1.56	0.040
47	Georgetown University Hospital, Washington, D.C.	18.2	0.5%	0.97	Yes	0.92	4	1.59	0.140
48	University Hospital, Denver	17.9	1.1%	0.88	Yes	0.76	4	1.05	0.044
49	University Hospital of Arkansas, Little Rock	17.9	0.0%	1.11	Yes	1.11	4	2.01	0.175
50	University Hospital, Albuquerque, N.M.	17.8	0.0%	1.31	Yes	1.20	4	1.82	0.373

"Reputational score" is the percentage of board-certified rheumatology specialists surveyed who named the hospital. "Hospitalwide mortality rate" is the ratio of actual to expected deaths overall (lower is better). "COTH member" indicates member of Council of Teaching Hospitals. "Interns and residents to beds" is the ratio of doctors in training to beds. "Technology score" is a specialty-specific index. "R.N.'s to beds" is the ratio of full-time registered nurses to beds. "Board-certified internists to beds" is the ratio of these doctors to beds.

NATIONAL RANKINGS

UROLOGY

NATIONAL RANKINGS

Rank	Hospital	U.S. News index	Reputational score	Urology mortality rate	COTH member	Interns and residents to beds	Technology score (of 11)	R.N.'s to beds	Board-certified internists to beds	Procedures to beds
1	Johns Hopkins Hospital, Baltimore	100.0	63.5%	0.94	Yes	0.73	11	1.43	0.084	1.35
2	Mayo Clinic, Rochester, Minn.	89.7	56.6%	0.74	Yes	0.24	8	0.77	0.060	2.84
3	Cleveland Clinic	65.0	34.2%	0.62	Yes	1.22	10	1.47	0.015	1.59
4	UCLA Medical Center, Los Angeles	59.8	29.6%	0.46	Yes	1.52	11	1.20	0.023	2.36
5	Stanford University Hospital, Stanford, Calif.	46.6	22.5%	0.96	Yes	1.34	11	0.86	0.147	1.69
6	Duke University Medical Center, Durham, N.C.	44.1	19.8%	0.86	Yes	0.91	11	1.61	0.081	1.68
7	Massachusetts General Hospital, Boston	43.2	20.2%	0.92	Yes	1.00	11	1.14	0.085	2.02
8	Barnes Hospital, St. Louis	42.3	21.3%	1.08	Yes	0.89	11	0.82	0.273	1.52
9	University of Texas, M.D. Anderson Cancer Ctr., Houston	37.7	13.7%	0.51	Yes	0.70	10	1.88	0.083	1.76
10	Memorial Sloan-Kettering Cancer Center, New York	34.8	16.0%	0.98	Yes	0.38	8	1.37	0.074	2.26
11	Baylor University Medical Center, Dallas	28.8	9.4%	0.72	Yes	0.29	8	1.38	0.093	1.44
12	New York Hospital-Cornell Medical Center	28.6	10.3%	0.90	Yes	0.79	9	1.00	0.113	1.43
13	University of California, San Francisco Medical Center	28.1	8.2%	1.02	Yes	1.03	10	1.82	0.435	1.40
14	Indiana University Medical Center, Indianapolis	27.5	8.4%	1.13	Yes	1.10	10	1.86	0.107	1.40
15	University of Washington Medical Center, Seattle	26.9	4.9%	0.80	Yes	1.05	10	2.06	0.440	1.60
16	University of Pittsburgh-Presbyterian University Hospital	26.8	2.9%	0.73	Yes	1.48	8	2.10	0.291	2.86
17	Hospital of the University of Pennsylvania, Philadelphia	25.6	4.6%	0.87	Yes	1.72	11	1.33	0.007	2.56
18	University Hospital, Portland, Ore.	25.0	1.0%	0.53	Yes	1.54	9	2.31	0.164	2.08
19	University of California, Davis Medical Center	24.8	0.5%	0.47	Yes	1.54	10	2.81	0.032	1.24
20	Columbia-Presbyterian Medical Center, New York	23.9	7.4%	1.07	Yes	0.85	10	1.05	0.111	1.45
21	Emory University Hospital, Atlanta	23.8	4.8%	0.70	Yes	0.71	8	1.28	0.039	2.55
22	Brigham and Women's Hospital, Boston	23.4	6.3%	1.16	Yes	1.49	10	0.79	0.179	1.35
23	UCSD Medical Center, San Diego	23.0	0.5%	0.47	Yes	1.65	7	2.17	0.049	1.40
24	University of Michigan Medical Center, Ann Arbor	22.2	3.0%	0.77	Yes	1.00	10	1.29	0.086	1.30
25	University of Iowa Hospitals and Clinics, Iowa City	21.6	4.0%	0.92	Yes	0.96	11	1.34	0.053	1.30
26	Thomas Jefferson University Hospital, Philadelphia	21.3	1.8%	0.73	Yes	0.96	10	1.44	0.042	1.73
27	Lahey Clinic Hospital, Burlington, Mass.	21.1	7.1%	1.04	No	0.51	10	1.22	0.085	4.18
28	Parkland Memorial Hospital, Dallas	21.0	2.8%	0.81	Yes	1.35	9	0.93	0.039	0.71
29	Loma Linda University Medical Center, Loma Linda, Calif.	20.9	0.8%	0.67	Yes	1.14	9	1.61	0.067	1.52
30	University of Wisconsin Hospital and Clinics, Madison	20.8	0.5%	0.55	Yes	1.30	11	1.24	0.037	2.85
31	New England Deaconess Hospital, Boston	20.0	0.6%	0.69	Yes	1.08	9	1.33	0.089	1.87
32	University of Chicago Hospitals	19.8	1.1%	0.96	Yes	1.64	10	1.38	0.074	1.68
33	Penn State's Milton S. Hershey Medical Ctr., Hershey	19.8	0.6%	0.87	Yes	1.55	9	1.57	0.023	2.00
34	University of Virginia Health Sciences Ctr., Charlottesville	19.7	3.0%	1.51	Yes	1.41	10	1.92	0.101	1.80
35	Medical College of Georgia Hospital and Clinic, Augusta	19.5	0.0%	0.63	Yes	1.42	10	1.09	0.041	1.33
36	University of Massachusetts Medical Center, Worcester	19.3	0.6%	0.59	Yes	1.47	8	0.96	0.000	1.37
37	Roswell Park Cancer Institute, Buffalo	19.3	0.5%	0.26	No	0.68	9	2.58	0.109	2.05
38	University Hospital, Albuquerque, N.M.	19.2	0.0%	0.80	Yes	1.20	6	1.82	0.373	1.38
39	Beth Israel Hospital, Boston	19.1	0.0%	0.76	Yes	0.57	9	1.93	0.590	2.37
40	University of Minnesota Hospital and Clinic, Minneapolis	19.0	1.5%	0.73	Yes	0.59	10	0.86	0.133	2.14
41	Yale-New Haven Hospital, New Haven, Conn.	19.0	1.3%	0.85	Yes	1.12	9	1.23	0.094	1.49
42	New England Medical Center, Boston	18.7	0.0%	0.76	Yes	1.07	7	1.66	0.086	1.03
43	Rush-Presbyterian-St. Luke's Medical Center, Chicago	18.7	0.0%	0.79	Yes	1.05	10	1.24	0.224	1.92
44	Cook County Hospital, Chicago	18.7	0.6%	0.50	Yes	1.00	6	1.43	0.073	0.61
45	Henry Ford Hospital, Detroit	18.6	0.6%	1.02	Yes	1.34	10	1.50	0.301	2.29
46	Medical University of South Carolina, Charleston	18.6	0.7%	0.89	Yes	1.42	9	1.39	0.022	1.39
47	University of Utah Hospitals and Clinics, Salt Lake City	18.5	1.4%	0.89	Yes	0.88	9	1.73	0.021	1.20
48	Ochsner Foundation Hospital, New Orleans	18.5	2.0%	0.74	Yes	0.44	10	0.82	0.054	2.30
49	New York University Medical Center	18.4	2.5%	1.17	Yes	1.30	8	1.15	0.360	1.93
50	William Beaumont Hospital, Royal Oak, Mich.	18.2	1.4%	0.89	Yes	0.63	10	1.46	0.113	2.42

"Reputational score" is the percentage of board-certified urology specialists surveyed who named the hospital. "Urology mortality rate" is the ratio of actual to expected deaths involving urological disorders (lower is better). "COTH member" indicates member of Council of Teaching Hospitals. "Interns and residents to beds" is the ratio of doctors in training to beds. "Technology score" is a specialty-specific index. "R.N.'s to beds" is the ratio of full-time registered nurses to beds. "Board-certified internists to beds" is the ratio of these doctors to beds. "Procedures to beds" is the ratio of urology-related procedures to beds.

The Top 17 Hospitals
OPHTHALMOLOGY

Rank	Hospital	Reputa-tional score	Board-certified ophthalmologists to beds	Tech-nology score (of 26)	Procedures to beds	COTH member
1	Johns Hopkins Hospital (Wilmer Eye Institute), Baltimore	57.4%	0.027	25	15.5	Yes
2	University of Miami (Bascom Palmer Eye Institute)	53.7%	1.894	4	37.8	No
3	Wills Eye Hospital, Philadelphia	44.8%	1.100	3	44.5	No
4	Massachusetts Eye and Ear Infirmary, Boston	41.8%	0.024	4	78.4	No
5	UCLA Medical Ctr. (Jules Stein Eye Institute), Los Angeles	33.1%	0.048	25	14.6	Yes
6	University of Iowa Hospitals and Clinics, Iowa City	18.8%	0.023	24	25.5	Yes
7	Barnes Hospital, St. Louis	10.3%	0.057	23	11.1	Yes
8	University of California, San Francisco Medical Center	9.7%	0.090	25	18.3	Yes
9	Mayo Clinic, Rochester, Minn.	8.3%	0.015	18	21.5	Yes
10	Duke University Medical Center, Durham, N.C.	8.0%	0.018	25	15.3	Yes
11	Manhattan Eye, Ear and Throat Hospital, New York	6.8%	2.330	1	95.9	No
12	Doheny Eye Institute, Los Angeles	6.8%	0.762	0	31.3	No
13	New York Eye and Ear Infirmary	6.6%	2.631	3	52.2	No
14	University of Michigan Medical Center, Ann Arbor	5.4%	0.028	23	16.8	Yes
15	Baylor University Medical Center, Dallas	4.7%	0.019	20	19.3	Yes
16	Emory University Hospital, Atlanta	4.2%	0.030	16	17.2	Yes
17	University of Illinois Hospital and Clinics, Chicago	3.7%	0.022	19	13.7	Yes

The Top 23 Hospitals
PEDIATRICS

Rank	Hospital	Reputa-tional score	Board-certified pediatricians to beds	Tech-nology score (of 6)	R.N.'s to beds	COTH member
1	Children's Hospital, Boston	44.1%	0.307	5	1.60	Yes
2	Children's Hospital of Philadelphia	32.2%	0.133	4	1.89	Yes
3	Johns Hopkins Hospital, Baltimore	30.2%	0.069	6	1.43	Yes
4	Childrens Hospital Los Angeles	12.3%	0.051	0	1.45	No
5	Children's Hospital of Pittsburgh	9.1%	0.656	3	2.06	Yes
6	Children's National Medical Center, Washington, D.C.	8.6%	0.233	4	1.82	Yes
7	Univ. Hosps. of Cleveland (Rainbow Babies & Children's Hosp.)	8.0%	0.279	6	1.73	Yes
8	Children's Hospital, Denver	7.9%	0.468	5	1.74	No
9	Children's Hospital Medical Center, Cincinnati	7.7%	0.418	5	2.18	Yes
10	Children's Memorial Hospital, Chicago	6.3%	0.208	5	1.99	Yes
11	Children's Hospital and Medical Center, Seattle	6.2%	0.717	5	2.23	Yes
12	Mayo Clinic, Rochester, Minn.	6.1%	0.021	5	0.77	Yes
13	Columbia-Presbyterian Medical Center, New York	5.7%	0.179	6	1.05	Yes
14	Texas Children's Hospital, Houston	5.6%	0.411	4	1.97	Yes
15	UCLA Medical Center, Los Angeles	5.5%	0.128	5	1.20	Yes
16	University of California, San Francisco Medical Center	5.3%	0.233	5	1.82	Yes
17	Massachusetts General Hospital, Boston	5.2%	0.069	5	1.14	Yes
18	Stanford University Hospital, Stanford, Calif.	5.2%	0.145	3	0.86	Yes
19	Children's Medical Center of Dallas	4.7%	0.712	4	1.77	No
20	St. Jude Children's Research Hospital, Memphis	3.8%	0.687	2	3.62	No
21	St. Louis Children's Hospital	3.8%	0.783	5	1.70	Yes
22	University of Michigan Medical Center, Ann Arbor	3.3%	0.068	6	1.29	Yes
23	University of Washington Medical Center, Seattle	3.0%	0.231	5	2.06	Yes

"Reputational score" is the percentage of board-certified eye or pediatric specialists surveyed who named the hospital. "Board-certified ophthalmologists to beds" or "board-certified pediatricians to beds" is the ratio of these doctors to beds. "Technology score" is a specialty-specific index. "Procedures to beds" is the ratio of ophthalmology-related or pediatric-related procedures to beds. "COTH member" indicates member of Council of Teaching Hospitals. "R.N.'s to beds" is the ratio of full-time registered nurses to beds.

The Top 17 Hospitals
PSYCHIATRY

Rank	Hospital	Reputational score	Board-certified psychiatrists to beds	Discharge planning (of 2)	R.N.'s to beds	COTH member	Technology score (of 8)
1	C. F. Menninger Memorial Hospital, Topeka, Kan.	14.4%	0.172	2	0.48	No	6
2	Massachusetts General Hospital, Boston	14.1%	0.032	2	1.14	Yes	7
3	McLean Hospital, Belmont, Mass.	12.9%	0.370	2	0.66	No	8
4	Johns Hopkins Hospital, Baltimore	12.9%	0.032	2	1.43	Yes	8
5	New York Hospital-Cornell Medical Center	12.1%	0.227	2	1.00	Yes	8
6	Mayo Clinic, Rochester, Minn.	10.8%	0.024	2	0.77	Yes	8
7	Columbia-Presbyterian Medical Center, New York	9.2%	0.147	2	1.05	Yes	7
8	Sheppard and Enoch Pratt Hospital, Baltimore	8.6%	0.079	2	0.28	No	7
9	New York University Medical Center	7.9%	0.120	2	1.15	Yes	2
10	UCLA Neuropsychiatric Hospital, Los Angeles	6.7%	0.009	2	0.52	No	5
11	Duke University Medical Center, Durham, N.C.	6.4%	0.047	2	1.61	Yes	6
12	Yale-New Haven Hospital, New Haven, Conn.	5.8%	0.083	2	1.23	Yes	8
13	Institute of Living, Hartford, Conn.	5.0%	0.158	2	0.45	No	8
14	Hospital of the University of Pennsylvania, Philadelphia	5.0%	0.074	2	1.33	Yes	6
15	Mount Sinai Medical Center, New York	4.0%	0.136	2	1.50	Yes	7
16	Chestnut Lodge Hospital, Rockville, Md.	3.5%	0.040	0	0.34	No	4
17	Timberlawn Psychiatric Hospital, Dallas	3.2%	0.106	1	0.23	No	8

The Top 19 Hospitals
REHABILITATION

Rank	Hospital	Reputational score	Board-certified rehab. M.D.'s to beds	Discharge planning (of 2)	R.N.'s to beds	Geriatric services (of 9)	Technology score (of 10)
1	Rehabilitation Institute of Chicago	38.8%	0.094	1	0.52	1	7
2	University of Washington Medical Center, Seattle	30.5%	0.044	2	2.06	4	9
3	Mayo Clinic, Rochester, Minn.	27.0%	0.013	2	0.77	5	7
4	New York University Medical Center (Rusk Institute)	22.0%	0.023	2	1.15	1	8
5	Craig Hospital, Englewood, Colo.	17.8%	0.114	2	0.41	1	5
6	The Institute for Rehabilitation and Research, Houston	16.6%	0.011	1	0.35	0	6
7	L.A. County-Rancho Los Amigos Med. Ctr., Downey, Calif.	13.1%	0.004	2	1.01	6	9
8	Baylor University Medical Center, Dallas	12.7%	0.004	2	1.38	4	8
9	Ohio State University Medical Center, Columbus	11.2%	0.012	2	1.11	5	9
10	Thomas Jefferson University Hospital, Philadelphia	8.9%	0.033	2	1.44	3	9
11	University of Michigan Medical Center, Ann Arbor	8.6%	0.005	2	1.29	8	10
12	Kessler Institute for Rehabilitation, West Orange, N.J.	8.1%	0.102	2	0.50	1	6
13	Moss Rehabilitation Hospital, Philadelphia	6.8%	0.123	2	0.28	1	6
14	Spaulding Rehabilitation Institute, Boston	5.7%	0.004	2	1.14	4	9
15	Columbia-Presbyterian Medical Center, New York	5.0%	0.012	2	1.05	4	10
16	Northwestern Memorial Hospital, Chicago	4.8%	0.024	2	1.03	6	8
17	Johns Hopkins Hospital, Baltimore	4.4%	0.004	2	1.43	1	8
18	Mount Sinai Medical Center, New York	4.1%	0.009	2	1.50	6	9
19	National Rehabilitation Hospital, Washington, D.C.	3.0%	0.094	2	0.54	1	6

"Reputational score" is the percentage of board-certified psychiatrists or rehabilitation specialists surveyed who named the hospital. "Board-certified psychiatrists to beds" or "board-certified rehabilitation doctors to beds" is the ratio of these doctors to beds. "Discharge planning" indicates the number of postdischarge services available. "R.N.'s to beds" is the ratio of full-time registered nurses to beds. "COTH member" indicates member of Council of Teaching Hospitals. "Technology score" is a specialty-specific index. "Geriatric services" is the number of geriatric services.

AIDS

Natl. Rank	Hospital	U.S. News index	Reputa-tional score	Hospital-wide mortality rate	COTH member	Interns and residents to beds	Tech-nology score (of 11)	Discharge planning (of 2)	R.N.'s to beds	Board-certified internists to beds
	TIER TWO									
69	University of Alabama Hospital at Birmingham	26.0	3.0%	1.16	Yes	0.82	9	2	0.92	0.027
	TIER THREE									
	Carraway Methodist Medical Center, Birmingham	21.3	0.0%	1.10	Yes	0.38	6	2	1.08	0.054
	Mobile Infirmary Medical Center, Mobile	22.8	0.0%	0.86	No	0.00	8	2	0.84	0.039
	Montclair Baptist Medical Center, Birmingham	22.0	0.0%	0.99	Yes	0.06	7	2	0.73	0.044
	St. Vincent's Hospital, Birmingham	19.9	0.0%	1.01	No	0.00	6	2	0.89	0.058
	TIER FOUR									
	Baptist Medical Center, Montgomery	14.8	0.0%	1.41	No	0.02	5	2	0.76	0.040
	Baptist Memorial Hospital, Gadsden	17.1	0.0%	1.22	No	0.00	5	2	1.21	0.000
	Cooper Green Hospital, Birmingham	14.0	0.0%	1.41	No	0.22	5	1	0.61	0.000
	DCH Regional Medical Center, Tuscaloosa	18.9	0.0%	1.15	No	0.05	7	2	1.23	0.037
	Decatur General Hospital, Decatur	16.8	0.0%	1.29	No	0.00	6	2	1.15	0.051
	East Alabama Medical Center, Opelika	18.7	0.0%	1.12	No	0.00	7	2	0.90	0.043
	Huntsville Hospital, Huntsville	19.1	0.0%	1.11	No	0.12	7	2	0.92	0.055
	Lloyd Noland Hosp. and Ambulatory Center, Birmingham	13.8	0.0%	1.48	No	0.05	5	2	0.51	0.041
	Medical Center East, Birmingham	17.2	0.0%	1.19	No	0.10	4	2	0.97	0.069
	NE Alabama Regional Medical Center, Anniston	14.2	0.0%	1.53	No	0.00	6	2	0.80	0.018
	Princeton Baptist Medical Center, Birmingham	18.6	0.0%	1.25	Yes	0.09	6	2	0.85	0.076
	Providence Hospital, Mobile	19.6	0.0%	1.03	No	0.00	5	2	0.92	0.112
	Riverview Regional Medical Center, Gadsden	16.0	0.0%	1.22	No	0.00	6	2	0.26	0.018
	Southeast Alabama Medical Center, Dothan	16.4	0.0%	1.26	No	0.00	7	2	0.56	0.025
	University of South Alabama Medical Center, Mobile	18.6	0.0%	1.52	Yes	1.01	6	2	1.21	0.042

CANCER

Natl. Rank	Hospital	U.S. News index	Reputa-tional score	Cancer mortality rate	COTH member	Interns and residents to beds	Tech-nology score (of 12)	R.N.'s to beds	Board-certified oncologists to beds	Procedures to beds
	TIER THREE									
	Carraway Methodist Medical Center, Birmingham	8.1	0.0%	1.02	Yes	0.38	8	1.08	0.005	1.44
	DCH Regional Medical Center, Tuscaloosa	5.3	0.0%	0.89	No	0.05	9	1.23	0.004	1.36
	Montclair Baptist Medical Center, Birmingham	6.5	0.0%	0.76	Yes	0.06	9	0.73	0.003	0.89
	Princeton Baptist Medical Center, Birmingham	6.4	0.0%	1.10	Yes	0.09	7	0.85	0.006	2.86
81	University of Alabama Hospital at Birmingham	11.0	0.9%	0.71	Yes	0.82	9	0.92	0.029	1.09
	University of South Alabama Medical Center, Mobile	10.0	0.0%	1.11	Yes	1.01	7	1.21	0.012	0.61
	TIER FOUR									
	Baptist Medical Center, Montgomery	1.8	0.0%	1.32	No	0.02	3	0.76	0.011	0.89
	Baptist Memorial Hospital, Gadsden	3.7	0.0%	1.23	No	0.00	5	1.21	0.004	1.37
	Decatur General Hospital, Decatur	4.4	0.0%	0.81	No	0.00	7	1.15	0.010	0.98
	East Alabama Medical Center, Opelika	3.7	0.0%	0.94	No	0.00	7	0.90	0.010	1.38
	Huntsville Hospital, Huntsville	5.0	0.0%	0.90	No	0.12	10	0.92	0.012	1.37
	Lloyd Noland Hosp. and Ambulatory Center, Birmingham	1.5	0.0%	1.40	No	0.05	4	0.51	0.005	1.27
	Medical Center East, Birmingham	3.3	0.0%	1.23	No	0.10	5	0.97	0.010	1.28
	Mobile Infirmary Medical Center, Mobile	4.6	0.0%	0.75	No	0.00	10	0.84	0.000	1.71
	Montgomery Regional Medical Center, Montgomery	3.0	0.0%	1.09	No	0.05	4	1.00	0.006	1.13
	NE Alabama Regional Medical Center, Anniston	3.3	0.0%	0.96	No	0.00	7	0.80	0.011	1.24
	Providence Hospital, Mobile	4.0	0.0%	0.97	No	0.00	8	0.92	0.011	1.67
	Riverview Regional Medical Center, Gadsden	1.4	0.0%	0.94	No	0.00	6	0.26	0.004	0.70
	Southeast Alabama Medical Center, Dothan	3.2	0.0%	0.78	No	0.00	8	0.56	0.008	1.53
	St. Vincent's Hospital, Birmingham	3.6	0.0%	1.04	No	0.00	7	0.89	0.008	1.59

CARDIOLOGY

Natl. Rank	Hospital	U.S. News index	Reputa-tional score	Cardiology mortality rate	COTH member	Interns and residents to beds	Tech-nology score (of 10)	R.N.'s to beds	Board-certified cardiologists to beds	Procedures to beds
	TIER ONE									
13	University of Alabama Hospital at Birmingham	31.9	10.2%	1.17	Yes	0.82	9	0.92	0.040	6.48
	TIER THREE									
	Carraway Methodist Medical Center, Birmingham	16.8	0.0%	1.09	Yes	0.38	8	1.08	0.017	8.10
	Huntsville Hospital, Huntsville	14.2	0.0%	1.02	No	0.12	8	0.92	0.024	7.78
	Mobile Infirmary Medical Center, Mobile	17.1	0.0%	0.91	No	0.00	9	0.84	0.027	10.19
	Montclair Baptist Medical Center, Birmingham	15.0	0.0%	1.09	Yes	0.06	9	0.73	0.022	8.33
	Montgomery Regional Medical Center, Montgomery	14.8	0.0%	1.02	No	0.05	9	1.00	0.025	18.26
	Princeton Baptist Medical Center, Birmingham	15.4	0.0%	1.08	Yes	0.09	8	0.85	0.020	9.88
	Providence Hospital, Mobile	13.9	0.0%	1.04	No	0.00	7	0.92	0.049	10.79
	University of South Alabama Medical Center, Mobile	14.2	0.4%	1.50	Yes	1.01	9	1.21	0.033	2.55
	TIER FOUR									
	Baptist Medical Center, Montgomery	7.9	0.0%	1.28	No	0.02	6	0.76	0.021	5.41
	Baptist Memorial Hospital, Gadsden	9.8	0.0%	1.31	No	0.00	8	1.21	0.033	10.25
	DCH Regional Medical Center, Tuscaloosa	9.9	0.0%	1.26	No	0.05	7	1.23	0.013	7.05
	Decatur General Hospital, Decatur	6.2	0.0%	1.42	No	0.00	4	1.15	0.005	4.68
	East Alabama Medical Center, Opelika	12.4	0.0%	1.10	No	0.00	9	0.90	0.013	9.58
	Lloyd Noland Hosp. and Ambulatory Center, Birmingham	7.6	0.0%	1.24	No	0.05	5	0.51	0.009	9.26
	Medical Center East, Birmingham	8.8	0.0%	1.30	No	0.10	6	0.97	0.017	9.79
	NE Alabama Regional Medical Center, Anniston	7.5	0.0%	1.30	No	0.00	5	0.80	0.028	6.88
	Riverview Regional Medical Center, Gadsden	5.7	0.0%	1.41	No	0.00	9	0.26	0.021	7.01
	Selma Medical Center, Selma	9.5	0.0%	1.07	No	0.04	4	0.32	0.005	6.00
	Southeast Alabama Medical Center, Dothan	8.0	0.0%	1.33	No	0.00	9	0.56	0.028	10.99
	St. Vincent's Hospital, Birmingham	12.9	0.0%	1.06	No	0.00	9	0.89	0.014	6.22

ENDOCRINOLOGY

Natl. Rank	Hospital	U.S. News index	Reputa-tional score	Endocrinology mortality rate	COTH member	Interns and residents to beds	Tech-nology score (of 11)	R.N.'s to beds	Board-certified internists to beds
	TIER THREE								
	Carraway Methodist Medical Center, Birmingham	8.5	0.0%	1.62	Yes	0.38	8	1.08	0.054
	Mobile Infirmary Medical Center, Mobile	10.6	0.0%	0.62	No	0.00	10	0.84	0.039
	Montclair Baptist Medical Center, Birmingham	9.0	0.0%	1.05	Yes	0.06	9	0.73	0.044
	University of Alabama Hospital at Birmingham	11.9	1.3%	1.46	Yes	0.82	10	0.92	0.027
	University of South Alabama Medical Center, Mobile	11.0	0.0%	1.57	Yes	1.01	8	1.21	0.042
	TIER FOUR								
	Baptist Medical Center, Montgomery	3.2	0.0%	1.58	No	0.02	4	0.76	0.040
	Baptist Memorial Hospital, Gadsden	5.4	0.0%	1.31	No	0.00	6	1.21	0.000
	DCH Regional Medical Center, Tuscaloosa	5.3	0.0%	1.62	No	0.05	8	1.23	0.037
	Decatur General Hospital, Decatur	4.1	0.0%	2.03	No	0.00	8	1.15	0.051
	East Alabama Medical Center, Opelika	4.8	0.0%	1.44	No	0.00	8	0.90	0.043
	Huntsville Hospital, Huntsville	5.9	0.0%	1.32	No	0.12	9	0.92	0.055
	Lloyd Noland Hosp. and Ambulatory Center, Birmingham	3.7	0.0%	1.32	No	0.05	5	0.51	0.041
	Medical Center East, Birmingham	6.0	0.0%	1.15	No	0.10	5	0.97	0.069
	Montgomery Regional Medical Center, Montgomery	7.3	0.0%	0.96	No	0.05	6	1.00	0.063
	NE Alabama Regional Medical Center, Anniston	2.9	0.0%	2.03	No	0.00	8	0.80	0.018
	Princeton Baptist Medical Center, Birmingham	6.9	0.0%	1.72	Yes	0.09	8	0.85	0.076
	Providence Hospital, Mobile	5.3	0.0%	1.45	No	0.00	8	0.92	0.112
	Riverview Regional Medical Center, Gadsden	3.7	0.0%	1.18	No	0.00	7	0.26	0.018
	Selma Medical Center, Selma	2.8	0.0%	1.44	No	0.04	6	0.32	0.026
	Southeast Alabama Medical Center, Dothan	4.1	0.0%	1.37	No	0.00	9	0.56	0.025
	St. Vincent's Hospital, Birmingham	6.8	0.0%	0.99	No	0.00	7	0.89	0.058

GASTROENTEROLOGY

Natl. Rank	Hospital	U.S. News index	Reputational score	Gastroenterology mortality rate	COTH member	Interns and residents to beds	Technology score (of 11)	R.N.'s to beds	Board-certified gastroenterologists to beds	Procedures to beds
	TIER TWO									
52	University of Alabama Hospital at Birmingham	15.1	2.8%	1.12	Yes	0.82	9	0.92	0.014	1.34
	TIER THREE									
	Carraway Methodist Medical Center, Birmingham	11.0	0.0%	0.98	Yes	0.38	7	1.08	0.005	3.11
	Mobile Infirmary Medical Center, Mobile	8.7	0.0%	0.87	No	0.00	9	0.84	0.014	4.48
	Montclair Baptist Medical Center, Birmingham	8.3	0.0%	1.09	Yes	0.06	8	0.73	0.008	2.70
	Princeton Baptist Medical Center, Birmingham	8.6	0.0%	1.28	Yes	0.09	7	0.85	0.006	4.67
	Providence Hospital, Mobile	7.5	0.0%	0.99	No	0.00	7	0.92	0.023	4.70
	TIER FOUR									
	Baptist Medical Center, Montgomery	2.6	0.0%	1.62	No	0.02	5	0.76	0.011	2.78
	Baptist Memorial Hospital, Gadsden	6.1	0.0%	1.25	No	0.00	5	1.21	0.007	4.86
	DCH Regional Medical Center, Tuscaloosa	7.0	0.0%	1.20	No	0.05	8	1.23	0.007	4.01
	Decatur General Hospital, Decatur	5.2	0.0%	1.36	No	0.00	7	1.15	0.015	3.31
	East Alabama Medical Center, Opelika	6.0	0.0%	1.16	No	0.00	7	0.90	0.010	4.11
	Huntsville Hospital, Huntsville	5.4	0.0%	1.27	No	0.12	8	0.92	0.014	2.68
	Lloyd Noland Hosp. and Ambulatory Center, Birmingham	2.8	0.0%	1.80	No	0.05	5	0.51	0.005	4.69
	Medical Center East, Birmingham	4.9	0.0%	1.55	No	0.10	4	0.97	0.014	5.60
	Montgomery Regional Medical Center, Montgomery	5.8	0.0%	1.17	No	0.05	5	1.00	0.019	4.06
	NE Alabama Regional Medical Center, Anniston	3.1	0.0%	2.01	No	0.00	7	0.80	0.014	4.02
	Riverview Regional Medical Center, Gadsden	3.8	0.0%	1.10	No	0.00	6	0.26	0.007	2.87
	Selma Medical Center, Selma	3.5	0.0%	1.23	No	0.04	6	0.32	0.000	3.09
	Southeast Alabama Medical Center, Dothan	4.5	0.0%	1.49	No	0.00	9	0.56	0.010	4.23
	St. Vincent's Hospital, Birmingham	7.1	0.0%	0.89	No	0.00	6	0.89	0.017	3.26

GERIATRICS

Natl. Rank	Hospital	U.S. News index	Reputational score	Hospital-wide mortality rate	COTH member	Service mix	Interns and residents to beds	Technology score (of 13)	R.N.'s to beds	Discharge planning (of 2)	Geriatric services (of 9)	Board-certified internists to beds
	TIER TWO											
64	University of Alabama Hospital at Birmingham	23.0	1.6%	1.16	Yes	10	0.82	11	0.92	2	9	0.027
	TIER THREE											
	Carraway Methodist Medical Center, Birmingham	16.6	0.0%	1.10	Yes	6	0.38	11	1.08	2	4	0.054
	Mobile Infirmary Medical Center, Mobile	17.4	0.0%	0.86	No	4	0.00	11	0.84	2	1	0.039
	Montclair Baptist Medical Center, Birmingham	18.3	0.0%	0.99	Yes	6	0.06	12	0.73	2	5	0.044
	St. Vincent's Hospital, Birmingham	14.2	0.0%	1.01	No	4	0.00	10	0.89	2	3	0.058
	TIER FOUR											
	Baptist Medical Center, Montgomery	6.4	0.0%	1.41	No	7	0.02	6	0.76	2	3	0.040
	Baptist Memorial Hospital, Gadsden	8.4	0.0%	1.22	No	2	0.00	9	1.21	2	2	0.000
	DCH Regional Medical Center, Tuscaloosa	12.1	0.0%	1.15	No	5	0.05	11	1.23	2	3	0.037
	Decatur General Hospital, Decatur	8.4	0.0%	1.29	No	4	0.00	9	1.15	2	3	0.051
	East Alabama Medical Center, Opelika	11.2	0.0%	1.12	No	4	0.00	10	0.90	2	2	0.043
	Huntsville Hospital, Huntsville	12.1	0.0%	1.11	No	4	0.12	11	0.92	2	3	0.055
	Lloyd Noland Hosp. and Ambulatory Center, Birmingham	5.1	0.0%	1.48	No	5	0.05	7	0.51	2	6	0.041
	Medical Center East, Birmingham	9.5	0.0%	1.19	No	4	0.10	8	0.97	2	1	0.069
	Montgomery Regional Medical Center, Montgomery	10.7	0.0%	1.14	No	4	0.05	8	1.00	2	2	0.063
	NE Alabama Regional Medical Center, Anniston	4.5	0.0%	1.53	No	5	0.00	9	0.80	2	3	0.018
	Princeton Baptist Medical Center, Birmingham	11.4	0.0%	1.25	Yes	4	0.09	10	0.85	2	4	0.076
	Providence Hospital, Mobile	13.5	0.0%	1.03	No	3	0.00	10	0.92	2	2	0.112
	Riverview Regional Medical Center, Gadsden	7.7	0.0%	1.22	No	4	0.00	9	0.26	2	3	0.018
	Selma Medical Center, Selma	8.4	0.0%	1.16	No	4	0.04	6	0.32	2	2	0.026
	Southeast Alabama Medical Center, Dothan	9.0	0.0%	1.26	No	5	0.00	11	0.56	2	5	0.025

GYNECOLOGY

Natl. Rank	Hospital	U.S. News index	Reputational score	Hospital-wide mortality rate	Interns and residents to beds	Technology score (of 10)	R.N.'s to beds	Board-certified OB-GYNs to beds	Procedures to beds
	TIER THREE								
	Mobile Infirmary Medical Center, Mobile	19.3	0.0%	0.86	0.00	8	0.84	0.033	0.41
	Montclair Baptist Medical Center, Birmingham	14.6	0.0%	0.99	0.06	7	0.73	0.015	0.36
	Providence Hospital, Mobile	15.3	0.0%	1.03	0.00	6	0.92	0.092	0.34
	St. Vincent's Hospital, Birmingham	14.9	0.0%	1.01	0.00	7	0.89	0.033	0.84
	University of Alabama Hospital at Birmingham	20.9	1.7%	1.16	0.82	9	0.92	0.025	0.45
	TIER FOUR								
	Baptist Medical Center, Montgomery	5.3	0.0%	1.41	0.02	5	0.76	0.032	0.52
	Baptist Memorial Hospital, Gadsden	9.1	0.0%	1.22	0.00	4	1.21	0.015	0.40
	Carraway Methodist Medical Center, Birmingham	14.0	0.0%	1.10	0.38	6	1.08	0.007	0.25
	DCH Regional Medical Center, Tuscaloosa	12.9	0.0%	1.15	0.05	7	1.23	0.015	0.29
	East Alabama Medical Center, Opelika	12.2	0.0%	1.12	0.00	7	0.90	0.026	0.24
	Huntsville Hospital, Huntsville	13.9	0.0%	1.11	0.12	8	0.92	0.040	0.29
	Lloyd Noland Hosp. and Ambulatory Center, Birmingham	2.4	0.0%	1.48	0.05	4	0.51	0.023	0.54
	Medical Center East, Birmingham	8.4	0.0%	1.19	0.10	3	0.97	0.017	0.43
	NE Alabama Regional Medical Center, Anniston	4.4	0.0%	1.53	0.00	6	0.80	0.025	0.52
	Princeton Baptist Medical Center, Birmingham	9.2	0.0%	1.25	0.09	6	0.85	0.031	0.64
	Riverview Regional Medical Center, Gadsden	5.5	0.0%	1.22	0.00	5	0.26	0.011	0.30
	Selma Medical Center, Selma	7.1	0.0%	1.16	0.04	5	0.32	0.005	0.15
	Southeast Alabama Medical Center, Dothan	8.5	0.0%	1.26	0.00	8	0.56	0.022	0.35

NEUROLOGY

Natl. Rank	Hospital	U.S. News index	Reputational score	Neurology mortality rate	COTH member	Interns and residents to beds	Technology score (of 9)	R.N.'s to beds	Board-certified neurologists to beds
	TIER THREE								
	Carraway Methodist Medical Center, Birmingham	14.8	0.0%	0.89	Yes	0.38	6	1.08	0.002
	Mobile Infirmary Medical Center, Mobile	15.3	0.0%	0.76	No	0.00	8	0.84	0.017
	Montclair Baptist Medical Center, Birmingham	16.4	0.0%	0.77	Yes	0.06	7	0.73	0.007
	Providence Hospital, Mobile	12.5	0.0%	0.91	No	0.00	6	0.92	0.032
	University of Alabama Hospital at Birmingham	14.2	0.9%	1.18	Yes	0.82	8	0.92	0.015
	University of South Alabama Medical Center, Mobile	11.9	0.0%	1.38	Yes	1.01	6	1.21	0.018
	TIER FOUR								
	Baptist Medical Center, Montgomery	4.2	0.0%	1.34	No	0.02	4	0.76	0.005
	Baptist Memorial Hospital, Gadsden	8.5	0.0%	1.08	No	0.00	5	1.21	0.007
	DCH Regional Medical Center, Tuscaloosa	9.2	0.0%	1.06	No	0.05	6	1.23	0.006
	Huntsville Hospital, Huntsville	9.4	0.0%	1.08	No	0.12	7	0.92	0.016
	Lloyd Noland Hosp. and Ambulatory Center, Birmingham	3.3	0.0%	1.37	No	0.05	4	0.51	0.005
	Medical Center East, Birmingham	9.4	0.0%	1.00	No	0.10	3	0.97	0.014
	Montgomery Regional Medical Center, Montgomery	6.2	0.0%	1.28	No	0.05	5	1.00	0.013
	NE Alabama Regional Medical Center, Anniston	4.5	0.0%	1.37	No	0.00	6	0.80	0.004
	Princeton Baptist Medical Center, Birmingham	10.8	0.0%	1.04	Yes	0.09	6	0.85	0.003
	Riverview Regional Medical Center, Gadsden	6.7	0.0%	1.07	No	0.00	5	0.26	0.014
	Southeast Alabama Medical Center, Dothan	7.0	0.0%	1.13	No	0.00	7	0.56	0.010
	St. Vincent's Hospital, Birmingham	10.1	0.0%	0.94	No	0.00	6	0.89	0.006

ORTHOPEDICS

Natl. Rank Hospital	U.S. News index	Reputa-tional score	Orthopedics mortality rate	COTH member	Interns and residents to beds	Tech-nology score (of 5)	R.N.'s to beds	Board-certified orthopedists to beds	Pro-cedures to beds
TIER THREE									
Carraway Methodist Medical Center, Birmingham	11.0	0.0%	0.94	Yes	0.38	3	1.08	0.005	2.64
Decatur General Hospital, Decatur	9.5	0.0%	0.73	No	0.00	3	1.15	0.031	2.29
Medical Center East, Birmingham	8.6	0.0%	0.77	No	0.10	2	0.97	0.031	3.94
Montclair Baptist Medical Center, Birmingham	9.4	0.0%	0.96	Yes	0.06	4	0.73	0.013	2.21
University of Alabama Hospital at Birmingham	12.7	0.7%	1.08	Yes	0.82	4	0.92	0.008	1.25
TIER FOUR									
Baptist Medical Center, Montgomery	3.6	0.0%	1.47	No	0.02	3	0.76	0.021	3.07
Baptist Memorial Hospital, Gadsden	7.6	0.0%	0.93	No	0.00	3	1.21	0.015	3.11
DCH Regional Medical Center, Tuscaloosa	6.8	0.0%	1.03	No	0.05	3	1.23	0.015	2.03
East Alabama Medical Center, Opelika	7.8	0.0%	0.88	No	0.00	4	0.90	0.023	2.82
Huntsville Hospital, Huntsville	7.8	0.0%	0.85	No	0.12	3	0.92	0.024	2.27
Lloyd Noland Hosp. and Ambulatory Center, Birmingham	6.4	0.0%	0.84	No	0.05	3	0.51	0.018	1.90
NE Alabama Regional Medical Center, Anniston	3.5	0.0%	1.44	No	0.00	3	0.80	0.021	2.23
Princeton Baptist Medical Center, Birmingham	7.3	0.0%	1.27	Yes	0.09	3	0.85	0.014	2.33
Providence Hospital, Mobile	6.2	0.0%	1.00	No	0.00	2	0.92	0.080	3.86
Riverview Regional Medical Center, Gadsden	5.8	0.0%	0.88	No	0.00	4	0.26	0.007	1.85
Southeast Alabama Medical Center, Dothan	3.6	0.0%	1.44	No	0.00	4	0.56	0.025	2.48
St. Vincent's Hospital, Birmingham	5.8	0.0%	1.17	No	0.00	4	0.89	0.014	3.02

OTOLARYNGOLOGY

Natl. Rank Hospital	U.S. News index	Reputa-tional score	Hospital-wide mortality rate	COTH member	Interns and residents to beds	Tech-nology score (of 9)	R.N.'s to beds	Board-certified internists to beds	Procedures to beds
TIER THREE									
Carraway Methodist Medical Center, Birmingham	10.1	0.0%	1.10	Yes	0.38	6	1.08	0.054	0.219
Montclair Baptist Medical Center, Birmingham	8.0	0.0%	0.99	Yes	0.06	7	0.73	0.044	0.168
Princeton Baptist Medical Center, Birmingham	8.4	0.0%	1.25	Yes	0.09	6	0.85	0.076	0.222
University of Alabama Hospital at Birmingham	12.7	0.4%	1.16	Yes	0.82	8	0.92	0.027	0.271
University of South Alabama Medical Center, Mobile	12.6	0.0%	1.52	Yes	1.01	6	1.21	0.042	0.087
TIER FOUR									
Baptist Medical Center, Montgomery	3.1	0.0%	1.41	No	0.02	2	0.76	0.040	0.201
Baptist Memorial Hospital, Gadsden	4.8	0.0%	1.22	No	0.00	4	1.21	0.000	0.171
Cooper Green Hospital, Birmingham	3.1	0.0%	1.41	No	0.22	2	0.61	0.000	0.115
DCH Regional Medical Center, Tuscaloosa	6.0	0.0%	1.15	No	0.05	6	1.23	0.037	0.476
Decatur General Hospital, Decatur	5.5	0.0%	1.29	No	0.00	6	1.15	0.051	0.240
East Alabama Medical Center, Opelika	4.8	0.0%	1.12	No	0.00	6	0.90	0.043	0.302
Huntsville Hospital, Huntsville	5.7	0.0%	1.11	No	0.12	7	0.92	0.055	0.188
Lloyd Noland Hosp. and Ambulatory Center, Birmingham	2.8	0.0%	1.48	No	0.05	3	0.51	0.041	0.441
Medical Center East, Birmingham	4.7	0.0%	1.19	No	0.10	3	0.97	0.069	0.290
Mobile Infirmary Medical Center, Mobile	5.4	0.0%	0.86	No	0.00	8	0.84	0.039	0.298
Montgomery Regional Medical Center, Montgomery	4.9	0.0%	1.14	No	0.05	4	1.00	0.063	0.200
NE Alabama Regional Medical Center, Anniston	4.1	0.0%	1.53	No	0.00	6	0.80	0.018	0.339
Providence Hospital, Mobile	5.5	0.0%	1.03	No	0.00	6	0.92	0.112	0.278
Riverview Regional Medical Center, Gadsden	2.3	0.0%	1.22	No	0.00	5	0.26	0.018	0.125
Selma Medical Center, Selma	2.4	0.0%	1.16	No	0.04	4	0.32	0.026	0.313
Southeast Alabama Medical Center, Dothan	3.8	0.0%	1.26	No	0.00	7	0.56	0.025	0.378
St. Vincent's Hospital, Birmingham	4.7	0.0%	1.01	No	0.00	5	0.89	0.058	0.319
Vaughan Regional Medical Center, Selma	3.3	0.0%	1.30	No	0.00	1	0.88	0.049	0.262

RHEUMATOLOGY

Natl. Rank	Hospital	U.S. News index	Reputa-tional score	Hospital-wide mortality rate	COTH member	Interns and residents to beds	Tech-nology score (of 5)	R.N.'s to beds	Board-certified internists to beds
TIER ONE									
7	**University of Alabama Hospital at Birmingham**	**46.7**	15.3%	1.16	Yes	0.82	4	0.92	0.027
TIER THREE									
	Carraway Methodist Medical Center, Birmingham	12.9	0.5%	1.10	Yes	0.38	3	1.08	0.054
	East Alabama Medical Center, Opelika	9.7	0.8%	1.12	No	0.00	4	0.90	0.043
	Mobile Infirmary Medical Center, Mobile	10.2	0.0%	0.86	No	0.00	4	0.84	0.039
	Montclair Baptist Medical Center, Birmingham	11.2	0.0%	0.99	Yes	0.06	4	0.73	0.044
	St. Vincent's Hospital, Birmingham	9.7	0.4%	1.01	No	0.00	4	0.89	0.058
TIER FOUR									
	Baptist Medical Center, Montgomery	5.4	0.0%	1.41	No	0.02	3	0.76	0.040
	Baptist Memorial Hospital, Gadsden	7.3	0.0%	1.22	No	0.00	3	1.21	0.000
	DCH Regional Medical Center, Tuscaloosa	8.2	0.0%	1.15	No	0.05	3	1.23	0.037
	Decatur General Hospital, Decatur	7.1	0.0%	1.29	No	0.00	3	1.15	0.051
	Huntsville Hospital, Huntsville	8.0	0.0%	1.11	No	0.12	3	0.92	0.055
	Lloyd Noland Hosp. and Ambulatory Center, Birmingham	4.5	0.0%	1.48	No	0.05	3	0.51	0.041
	Medical Center East, Birmingham	7.2	0.0%	1.19	No	0.10	2	0.97	0.069
	Montgomery Regional Medical Center, Montgomery	8.3	0.0%	1.14	No	0.05	4	1.00	0.063
	NE Alabama Regional Medical Center, Anniston	4.8	0.0%	1.53	No	0.00	3	0.80	0.018
	Princeton Baptist Medical Center, Birmingham	9.5	0.0%	1.25	Yes	0.09	3	0.85	0.076
	Providence Hospital, Mobile	8.3	0.0%	1.03	No	0.00	2	0.92	0.112
	Riverview Regional Medical Center, Gadsden	5.3	0.0%	1.22	No	0.00	4	0.26	0.018
	Selma Medical Center, Selma	5.2	0.0%	1.16	No	0.04	2	0.32	0.026
	Southeast Alabama Medical Center, Dothan	6.0	0.0%	1.26	No	0.00	4	0.56	0.025

UROLOGY

Natl. Rank	Hospital	U.S. News index	Reputa-tional score	Urology mortality rate	COTH member	Interns and residents to beds	Tech-nology score (of 11)	R.N.'s to beds	Board-certified internists to beds	Procedures to beds
TIER THREE										
	Carraway Methodist Medical Center, Birmingham	11.2	0.0%	1.10	Yes	0.38	7	1.08	0.054	1.88
	Mobile Infirmary Medical Center, Mobile	8.7	0.0%	0.94	No	0.00	9	0.84	0.039	1.88
	Montclair Baptist Medical Center, Birmingham	10.0	0.0%	1.01	Yes	0.06	8	0.73	0.044	1.11
	Southeast Alabama Medical Center, Dothan	9.9	0.0%	0.80	No	0.00	9	0.56	0.025	3.02
	University of Alabama Hospital at Birmingham	13.4	0.0%	1.01	Yes	0.82	9	0.92	0.027	1.86
TIER FOUR										
	Baptist Medical Center, Montgomery	3.7	0.0%	1.51	No	0.02	5	0.76	0.040	1.41
	Baptist Memorial Hospital, Gadsden	4.5	0.0%	1.60	No	0.00	5	1.21	0.000	2.72
	DCH Regional Medical Center, Tuscaloosa	7.8	0.0%	1.15	No	0.05	8	1.23	0.037	1.98
	Decatur General Hospital, Decatur	6.5	0.0%	1.26	No	0.00	7	1.15	0.051	1.95
	East Alabama Medical Center, Opelika	4.1	0.0%	1.64	No	0.00	7	0.90	0.043	1.87
	Huntsville Hospital, Huntsville	8.0	0.0%	1.04	No	0.12	8	0.92	0.055	1.41
	Lloyd Noland Hosp. and Ambulatory Center, Birmingham	3.4	0.0%	1.53	No	0.05	5	0.51	0.041	2.42
	Medical Center East, Birmingham	4.2	0.0%	1.63	No	0.10	4	0.97	0.069	2.33
	Montgomery Regional Medical Center, Montgomery	7.6	0.0%	1.01	No	0.05	5	1.00	0.063	1.78
	NE Alabama Regional Medical Center, Anniston	3.3	0.0%	1.81	No	0.00	7	0.80	0.018	2.31
	Princeton Baptist Medical Center, Birmingham	6.4	0.0%	1.93	Yes	0.09	7	0.85	0.076	2.38
	Providence Hospital, Mobile	6.6	0.0%	1.23	No	0.00	7	0.92	0.112	2.10
	Riverview Regional Medical Center, Gadsden	3.4	0.0%	1.31	No	0.00	6	0.26	0.018	1.55
	Selma Medical Center, Selma	4.1	0.0%	1.29	No	0.04	6	0.32	0.026	2.19
	St. Vincent's Hospital, Birmingham	4.6	0.0%	1.46	No	0.00	6	0.89	0.058	1.65

AIDS

Natl. Rank	Hospital	U.S. News index	Reputa-tional score	Hospital-wide mortality rate	COTH member	Interns and residents to beds	Tech-nology score (of 11)	Discharge planning (of 2)	R.N.'s to beds	Board-certified internists to beds
	TIER FOUR									
	Providence Hospital, Anchorage	**19.3**	0.0%	1.09	No	0.00	7	1	1.23	0.126

CANCER

Natl. Rank	Hospital	U.S. News index	Reputa-tional score	Cancer mortality rate	COTH member	Interns and residents to beds	Tech-nology score (of 12)	R.N.'s to beds	Board-certified oncologists to beds	Procedures to beds
	TIER FOUR									
	Providence Hospital, Anchorage	**4.7**	0.0%	1.28	No	0.00	9	1.23	0.000	0.72

CARDIOLOGY

Natl. Rank	Hospital	U.S. News index	Reputa-tional score	Cardiology mortality rate	COTH member	Interns and residents to beds	Tech-nology score (of 10)	R.N.'s to beds	Board-certified cardiologists to beds	Procedures to beds
	TIER FOUR									
	Providence Hospital, Anchorage	**12.5**	0.0%	1.12	No	0.00	9	1.23	0.015	4.02

GASTROENTEROLOGY

Natl. Rank	Hospital	U.S. News index	Reputa-tional score	Gastro-enterology mortality rate	COTH member	Interns and residents to beds	Tech-nology score (of 11)	R.N.'s to beds	Board-certified gastro-enterologists to beds	Pro-cedures to beds
	TIER FOUR									
	Providence Hospital, Anchorage	**6.5**	0.0%	1.00	No	0.00	8	1.23	0.003	1.48

GERIATRICS

Natl. Rank	Hospital	U.S. News index	Reputa-tional score	Hospital-wide mortality rate	COTH member	Service mix	Interns and residents to beds	Tech-nology score (of 13)	R.N.'s to beds	Discharge planning (of 2)	Geriatric services (of 9)	Board-certified internists to beds
	TIER FOUR											
	Providence Hospital, Anchorage	**12.1**	0.0%	1.09	No	4	0.00	11	1.23	1	2	0.126

GYNECOLOGY

Natl. Rank	Hospital	U.S. News index	Reputa-tional score	Hospital-wide mortality rate	Interns and residents to beds	Tech-nology score (of 10)	R.N.'s to beds	Board-certified OB-GYNs to beds	Procedures to beds
	TIER THREE								
	Providence Hospital, Anchorage	**15.5**	0.0%	1.09	0.00	7	1.23	0.076	0.24

ORTHOPEDICS

Natl. Rank	Hospital	U.S. News index	Reputa-tional score	Orthopedics mortality rate	COTH member	Interns and residents to beds	Tech-nology score (of 5)	R.N.'s to beds	Board-certified orthopedists to beds	Pro-cedures to beds
	TIER THREE									
	Providence Hospital, Anchorage	**8.9**	0.0%	0.86	No	0.00	4	1.23	0.073	1.08

OTOLARYNGOLOGY

Natl. Rank	Hospital	U.S. News index	Reputa- tional score	Hospital- wide mortality rate	COTH member	Interns and residents to beds	Tech- nology score (of 9)	R.N.'s to beds	Board- certified internists to beds	Procedures to beds
TIER FOUR										
	Providence Hospital, Anchorage	6.5	0.0%	1.09	No	0.00	6	1.23	0.126	0.167

RHEUMATOLOGY

Natl. Rank	Hospital	U.S. News index	Reputa- tional score	Hospital- wide mortality rate	COTH member	Interns and residents to beds	Tech- nology score (of 5)	R.N.'s to beds	Board- certified internists to beds
TIER FOUR									
	Providence Hospital, Anchorage	8.6	0.0%	1.09	No	0.00	4	1.23	0.126

UROLOGY

Natl. Rank	Hospital	U.S. News index	Reputa- tional score	Urology mortality rate	COTH member	Interns and residents to beds	Tech- nology score (of 11)	R.N.'s to beds	Board- certified internists to beds	Procedures to beds
TIER THREE										
	Providence Hospital, Anchorage	8.9	0.0%	1.02	No	0.00	8	1.23	0.126	0.80

AIDS

Natl. Rank	Hospital	U.S. News index	Reputa-tional score	Hospital-wide mortality rate	COTH member	Interns and residents to beds	Technology score (of 11)	Discharge planning (of 2)	R.N.'s to beds	Board-certified internists to beds
	TIER TWO									
86	St. Joseph's Hospital and Medical Center, Phoenix	25.3	0.0%	1.02	Yes	0.60	8	2	1.61	0.228
66	University Medical Center, Tucson	26.2	0.0%	0.97	Yes	0.74	8	2	1.73	0.136
	TIER THREE									
	Flagstaff Medical Center, Flagstaff	22.4	0.0%	0.88	No	0.00	7	2	0.83	0.046
	Good Samaritan Regional Medical Center, Phoenix	23.1	0.0%	1.07	Yes	0.54	8	2	1.15	0.103
	John C. Lincoln Hospital and Health Center, Phoenix	20.4	0.0%	0.90	No	0.00	6	1	0.43	0.051
	Phoenix Baptist Hospital and Medical Center	20.2	0.0%	1.01	No	0.18	5	2	1.10	0.014
	Phoenix Memorial Hospital	22.3	0.0%	0.74	No	0.00	6	2	0.88	0.087
	Scottsdale Memorial Hospital-North, Scottsdale	20.8	0.0%	0.96	No	0.00	5	2	0.90	0.126
	TIER FOUR									
	Carondelet St. Mary's Hospital, Tucson	19.2	0.0%	1.09	No	0.00	6	2	0.91	0.155
	Maricopa Medical Center, Phoenix	19.6	0.0%	1.34	Yes	0.84	7	2	0.71	0.131
	Scottsdale Memorial Hospital, Scottsdale	18.5	0.0%	1.11	No	0.07	6	2	0.77	0.069
	Tucson Medical Center, Tucson	19.5	0.0%	1.17	Yes	0.08	7	2	0.61	0.095

CANCER

Natl. Rank	Hospital	U.S. News index	Reputa-tional score	Cancer mortality rate	COTH member	Interns and residents to beds	Technology score (of 12)	R.N.'s to beds	Board-certified oncologists to beds	Procedures to beds
	TIER TWO									
79	St. Joseph's Hospital and Medical Center, Phoenix	11.1	0.0%	1.08	Yes	0.60	11	1.61	0.005	1.73
20	University Medical Center, Tucson	15.9	3.0%	0.71	Yes	0.74	9	1.73	0.053	1.51
	TIER THREE									
	Good Samaritan Regional Medical Center, Phoenix	9.6	0.0%	0.77	Yes	0.54	10	1.15	0.007	1.14
	Tucson Medical Center, Tucson	6.0	0.0%	0.97	Yes	0.08	8	0.61	0.022	1.56
	TIER FOUR									
	Carondelet St. Mary's Hospital, Tucson	3.6	0.0%	0.75	No	0.00	5	0.91	0.028	1.82
	Flagstaff Medical Center, Flagstaff	4.7	0.0%	0.58	No	0.00	10	0.83	0.007	1.20
	John C. Lincoln Hospital and Health Center, Phoenix	1.9	0.0%	0.76	No	0.00	4	0.43	0.013	2.14
	Scottsdale Memorial Hospital, Scottsdale	2.8	0.0%	1.10	No	0.07	5	0.77	0.014	1.26
	Scottsdale Memorial Hospital-North, Scottsdale	4.0	0.0%	0.62	No	0.00	5	0.90	0.042	2.39

CARDIOLOGY

Natl. Rank	Hospital	U.S. News index	Reputa-tional score	Cardiology mortality rate	COTH member	Interns and residents to beds	Technology score (of 10)	R.N.'s to beds	Board-certified cardiologists to beds	Procedures to beds
	TIER TWO									
73	University Medical Center, Tucson	21.6	0.9%	1.10	Yes	0.74	8	1.73	0.043	7.12
	TIER THREE									
	Good Samaritan Regional Medical Center, Phoenix	18.2	0.0%	1.13	Yes	0.54	10	1.15	0.072	7.45
	John C. Lincoln Hospital and Health Center, Phoenix	14.6	0.0%	0.96	No	0.00	9	0.43	0.034	10.03
	St. Joseph's Hospital and Medical Center, Phoenix	18.4	1.2%	1.25	Yes	0.60	9	1.61	0.027	4.37
	TIER FOUR									
	Carondelet St. Mary's Hospital, Tucson	9.2	0.0%	1.35	No	0.00	9	0.91	0.057	12.24
	Phoenix Baptist Hospital and Medical Center	12.2	0.0%	1.20	No	0.18	8	1.10	0.063	6.53
	Scottsdale Memorial Hospital, Scottsdale	12.3	0.6%	1.15	No	0.07	9	0.77	0.030	8.01
	Scottsdale Memorial Hospital-North, Scottsdale	12.7	0.0%	1.10	No	0.00	7	0.90	0.142	8.90
	Tucson Medical Center, Tucson	13.0	0.0%	1.20	Yes	0.08	9	0.61	0.045	5.95

ENDOCRINOLOGY

Natl. Rank	Hospital	U.S. News index	Reputa-tional score	Endocrinology mortality rate	COTH member	Interns and residents to beds	Tech-nology score (of 11)	R.N.'s to beds	Board-certified internists to beds
TIER TWO										
64	Good Samaritan Regional Medical Center, Phoenix	16.2	0.0%	0.65	Yes	0.54	10	1.15	0.103
56	University Medical Center, Tucson	16.7	0.0%	0.80	Yes	0.74	9	1.73	0.136
TIER THREE										
	Carondelet St. Mary's Hospital, Tucson	10.4	0.0%	0.69	No	0.00	6	0.91	0.155
	John C. Lincoln Hospital and Health Center, Phoenix	8.6	0.0%	0.52	No	0.00	5	0.43	0.051
	Maricopa Medical Center, Phoenix	10.1	0.0%	1.28	Yes	0.84	5	0.71	0.131
	Scottsdale Memorial Hospital-North, Scottsdale	10.6	0.0%	0.61	No	0.00	6	0.90	0.126
86	St. Joseph's Hospital and Medical Center, Phoenix	14.2	0.0%	1.13	Yes	0.60	10	1.61	0.228
	Tucson Medical Center, Tucson	12.7	0.0%	0.65	Yes	0.08	8	0.61	0.095
TIER FOUR										
	Scottsdale Memorial Hospital, Scottsdale	6.2	0.0%	1.08	No	0.07	7	0.77	0.069

GASTROENTEROLOGY

Natl. Rank	Hospital	U.S. News index	Reputa-tional score	Gastro-enterology mortality rate	COTH member	Interns and residents to beds	Tech-nology score (of 11)	R.N.'s to beds	Board-certified gastro-enterologists to beds	Pro-cedures to beds
TIER TWO											
63	St. Joseph's Hospital and Medical Center, Phoenix	14.0	0.0%	0.95	Yes	0.60	10	1.61	0.029	2.76
TIER THREE											
	Carondelet St. Mary's Hospital, Tucson	7.9	0.0%	1.12	No	0.00	6	0.91	0.420	4.80
	Good Samaritan Regional Medical Center, Phoenix	10.8	0.0%	1.24	Yes	0.54	10	1.15	0.025	2.44
	Scottsdale Memorial Hospital-North, Scottsdale	8.2	0.0%	0.85	No	0.00	5	0.90	0.063	4.76
	Tucson Medical Center, Tucson	7.5	0.0%	1.28	Yes	0.08	8	0.61	0.022	3.27
80	University Medical Center, Tucson	12.9	0.0%	1.12	Yes	0.74	9	1.73	0.017	2.09
TIER FOUR											
	John C. Lincoln Hospital and Health Center, Phoenix	6.5	0.0%	0.98	No	0.00	6	0.43	0.008	5.33
	Phoenix Baptist Hospital and Medical Center	6.1	0.0%	1.09	No	0.18	4	1.10	0.018	3.26
	Scottsdale Memorial Hospital, Scottsdale	5.8	0.0%	1.09	No	0.07	6	0.77	0.017	3.64

GERIATRICS

Natl. Rank	Hospital	U.S. News index	Reputa-tional score	Hospital-wide mortality rate	COTH member	Service mix	Interns and residents to beds	Tech-nology score (of 13)	R.N.'s to beds	Discharge planning (of 2)	Geriatric services (of 9)	Board-certified internists to beds
TIER TWO													
87	St. Joseph's Hospital and Medical Center, Phoenix	21.8	0.3%	1.02	Yes	6	0.60	12	1.61	2	3	0.228
84	University Medical Center, Tucson	22.1	0.0%	0.97	Yes	7	0.74	10	1.73	2	1	0.136
TIER THREE													
	Good Samaritan Regional Medical Center, Phoenix	19.5	0.0%	1.07	Yes	7	0.54	13	1.15	2	6	0.103
	John C. Lincoln Hospital and Health Center, Phoenix	14.8	0.0%	0.90	No	4	0.00	7	0.43	1	2	0.051
	Phoenix Baptist Hospital and Medical Center	14.3	0.0%	1.01	No	5	0.18	7	1.10	2	1	0.014
	Scottsdale Memorial Hospital-North, Scottsdale	15.8	0.0%	0.96	No	5	0.00	7	0.90	2	2	0.126
TIER FOUR													
	Carondelet St. Mary's Hospital, Tucson	12.9	0.0%	1.09	No	6	0.00	8	0.91	2	2	0.155
	Maricopa Medical Center, Phoenix	10.9	0.0%	1.34	Yes	6	0.84	6	0.71	2	1	0.131
	Scottsdale Memorial Hospital, Scottsdale	11.9	0.0%	1.11	No	5	0.07	9	0.77	2	3	0.069
	Tucson Medical Center, Tucson	12.4	0.0%	1.17	Yes	5	0.08	10	0.61	2	2	0.095

GYNECOLOGY

Natl. Rank	Hospital	U.S. News index	Reputa- tional score	Hospital- wide mortality rate	Interns and residents to beds	Tech- nology score (of 10)	R.N.'s to beds	Board- certified OB-GYNs to beds	Procedures to beds
	TIER TWO								
70	St. Joseph's Hospital and Medical Center, Phoenix	23.6	0.0%	1.02	0.60	9	1.61	0.133	0.72
50	University Medical Center, Tucson	26.4	0.4%	0.97	0.74	8	1.73	0.103	0.60
	TIER THREE								
	Good Samaritan Regional Medical Center, Phoenix	19.7	0.4%	1.07	0.54	7	1.15	0.131	0.39
	John C. Lincoln Hospital and Health Center, Phoenix	15.2	0.0%	0.90	0.00	5	0.43	0.047	0.90
	Phoenix Baptist Hospital and Medical Center	14.7	0.0%	1.01	0.18	4	1.10	0.036	0.50
	Scottsdale Memorial Hospital-North, Scottsdale	16.0	0.0%	0.96	0.00	4	0.90	0.146	1.41
	TIER FOUR								
	Carondelet St. Mary's Hospital, Tucson	11.3	0.0%	1.09	0.00	5	0.91	0.019	0.22
	Maricopa Medical Center, Phoenix	10.6	0.0%	1.34	0.84	5	0.71	0.070	0.10
	Scottsdale Memorial Hospital, Scottsdale	10.4	0.0%	1.11	0.07	4	0.77	0.044	0.60
	Tucson Medical Center, Tucson	11.5	0.0%	1.17	0.08	7	0.61	0.087	0.76

NEUROLOGY

Natl. Rank	Hospital	U.S. News index	Reputa- tional score	Neurology mortality rate	COTH member	Interns and residents to beds	Tech- nology score (of 9)	R.N.'s to beds	Board- certified neurologists to beds
	TIER TWO								
82	Good Samaritan Regional Medical Center, Phoenix	17.9	0.0%	0.86	Yes	0.54	8	1.15	0.019
69	St. Joseph's Hospital and Medical Center, Phoenix	18.4	1.0%	1.08	Yes	0.60	8	1.61	0.039
51	University Medical Center, Tucson	19.8	0.0%	0.88	Yes	0.74	7	1.73	0.027
	TIER THREE								
	Carondelet St. Mary's Hospital, Tucson	11.4	0.0%	0.97	No	0.00	5	0.91	0.035
	Scottsdale Memorial Hospital-North, Scottsdale	11.3	0.0%	1.15	No	0.00	4	0.90	0.079
	TIER FOUR								
	John C. Lincoln Hospital and Health Center, Phoenix	9.5	0.0%	0.93	No	0.00	5	0.43	0.017
	Phoenix Baptist Hospital and Medical Center	9.0	0.0%	1.15	No	0.18	4	1.10	0.027
	Scottsdale Memorial Hospital, Scottsdale	8.5	0.0%	1.04	No	0.07	5	0.77	0.011
	Tucson Medical Center, Tucson	10.3	0.0%	1.13	Yes	0.08	6	0.61	0.024

ORTHOPEDICS

Natl. Rank	Hospital	U.S. News index	Reputa- tional score	Orthopedics mortality rate	COTH member	Interns and residents to beds	Tech- nology score (of 5)	R.N.'s to beds	Board- certified orthopedists to beds	Pro- cedures to beds
	TIER TWO									
72	St. Joseph's Hospital and Medical Center, Phoenix	14.9	0.0%	0.89	Yes	0.60	4	1.61	0.090	3.13
	TIER THREE									
	Good Samaritan Regional Medical Center, Phoenix	12.5	0.0%	1.08	Yes	0.54	5	1.15	0.100	2.37
	Maricopa Medical Center, Phoenix	9.9	0.0%	1.21	Yes	0.84	3	0.71	0.076	1.22
	Scottsdale Memorial Hospital-North, Scottsdale	11.0	0.0%	0.68	No	0.00	3	0.90	0.138	5.21
85	University Medical Center, Tucson	14.1	0.3%	1.04	Yes	0.74	3	1.73	0.040	2.57
	TIER FOUR									
	Carondelet St. Mary's Hospital, Tucson	7.0	0.0%	1.09	No	0.00	4	0.91	0.063	5.18
	Flagstaff Medical Center, Flagstaff	6.5	0.0%	1.04	No	0.00	4	0.83	0.040	3.15
	John C. Lincoln Hospital and Health Center, Phoenix	7.5	0.0%	0.84	No	0.00	4	0.43	0.047	4.10
	Phoenix Baptist Hospital and Medical Center	6.8	0.0%	1.11	No	0.18	3	1.10	0.059	2.82
	Scottsdale Memorial Hospital, Scottsdale	6.1	0.0%	1.13	No	0.07	4	0.77	0.033	3.24
	Tucson Medical Center, Tucson	7.6	0.0%	1.27	Yes	0.08	4	0.61	0.041	3.12

OTOLARYNGOLOGY

Natl. Rank	Hospital	U.S. News index	Reputational score	Hospital-wide mortality rate	COTH member	Interns and residents to beds	Technology score (of 9)	R.N.'s to beds	Board-certified internists to beds	Procedures to beds
TIER TWO										
	Good Samaritan Regional Medical Center, Phoenix	13.6	0.5%	1.07	Yes	0.54	8	1.15	0.103	0.172
77	St. Joseph's Hospital and Medical Center, Phoenix	14.7	0.0%	1.02	Yes	0.60	8	1.61	0.228	0.228
79	University Medical Center, Tucson	14.6	0.0%	0.97	Yes	0.74	7	1.73	0.136	0.209
TIER THREE										
	Maricopa Medical Center, Phoenix	10.4	0.0%	1.34	Yes	0.84	3	0.71	0.131	0.051
	Tucson Medical Center, Tucson	7.8	0.0%	1.17	Yes	0.08	6	0.61	0.095	0.172
TIER FOUR										
	Carondelet St. Mary's Hospital, Tucson	5.2	0.0%	1.09	No	0.00	4	0.91	0.155	0.325
	Flagstaff Medical Center, Flagstaff	5.4	0.0%	0.88	No	0.00	8	0.83	0.046	0.179
	John C. Lincoln Hospital and Health Center, Phoenix	2.8	0.0%	0.90	No	0.00	3	0.43	0.051	0.267
	Kino Community Hospital, Tucson	6.9	0.0%	1.41	No	1.05	0	0.67	0.104	0.130
	Phoenix Baptist Hospital and Medical Center	5.1	0.0%	1.01	No	0.18	3	1.10	0.014	0.108
	Phoenix Memorial Hospital	5.4	0.0%	0.74	No	0.00	6	0.88	0.087	0.064
	Scottsdale Memorial Hospital, Scottsdale	4.6	0.0%	1.11	No	0.07	5	0.77	0.069	0.262
	Scottsdale Memorial Hospital-North, Scottsdale	5.1	0.0%	0.96	No	0.00	4	0.90	0.126	0.377

RHEUMATOLOGY

Natl. Rank	Hospital	U.S. News index	Reputational score	Hospital-wide mortality rate	COTH member	Interns and residents to beds	Technology score (of 5)	R.N.'s to beds	Board-certified internists to beds
TIER TWO									
77	St. Joseph's Hospital and Medical Center, Phoenix	16.4	0.0%	1.02	Yes	0.60	4	1.61	0.228
38	University Medical Center, Tucson	20.0	1.6%	0.97	Yes	0.74	3	1.73	0.136
TIER THREE									
	Good Samaritan Regional Medical Center, Phoenix	14.1	0.0%	1.07	Yes	0.54	5	1.15	0.103
	Maricopa Medical Center, Phoenix	11.4	0.0%	1.34	Yes	0.84	3	0.71	0.131
	Tucson Medical Center, Tucson	9.9	0.0%	1.17	Yes	0.08	4	0.61	0.095
TIER FOUR									
	Carondelet St. Mary's Hospital, Tucson	9.0	0.0%	1.09	No	0.00	4	0.91	0.155
	John C. Lincoln Hospital and Health Center, Phoenix	7.7	0.0%	0.90	No	0.00	4	0.43	0.051
	Phoenix Baptist Hospital and Medical Center	9.3	0.0%	1.01	No	0.18	3	1.10	0.014
	Scottsdale Memorial Hospital, Scottsdale	8.0	0.0%	1.11	No	0.07	4	0.77	0.069
	Scottsdale Memorial Hospital-North, Scottsdale	9.5	0.0%	0.96	No	0.00	3	0.90	0.126

UROLOGY

Natl. Rank	Hospital	U.S. News index	Reputational score	Urology mortality rate	COTH member	Interns and residents to beds	Technology score (of 11)	R.N.'s to beds	Board-certified internists to beds	Procedures to beds
TIER TWO										
60	Good Samaritan Regional Medical Center, Phoenix	17.3	0.0%	0.69	Yes	0.54	10	1.15	0.103	1.82
71	University Medical Center, Tucson	16.4	0.6%	1.05	Yes	0.74	9	1.73	0.136	1.93
TIER THREE										
	Carondelet St. Mary's Hospital, Tucson	9.2	0.0%	0.93	No	0.00	6	0.91	0.155	2.63
	John C. Lincoln Hospital and Health Center, Phoenix	10.1	0.0%	0.51	No	0.00	6	0.43	0.051	3.23
	Maricopa Medical Center, Phoenix	11.7	0.0%	1.08	Yes	0.84	5	0.71	0.131	0.87
	Phoenix Baptist Hospital and Medical Center	10.4	0.0%	0.80	No	0.18	4	1.10	0.014	2.64
	Scottsdale Memorial Hospital-North, Scottsdale	12.1	0.0%	0.51	No	0.00	5	0.90	0.126	5.03
94	St. Joseph's Hospital and Medical Center, Phoenix	14.8	0.0%	1.09	Yes	0.60	10	1.61	0.228	1.71
	Tucson Medical Center, Tucson	13.9	0.0%	0.62	Yes	0.08	8	0.61	0.095	2.17
TIER FOUR										
	Scottsdale Memorial Hospital, Scottsdale	5.0	0.0%	1.37	No	0.07	6	0.77	0.069	1.57

AIDS

Natl. Rank	Hospital	U.S. News index	Reputational score	Hospital-wide mortality rate	COTH member	Interns and residents to beds	Technology score (of 11)	Discharge planning (of 2)	R.N.'s to beds	Board-certified internists to beds
	TIER THREE									
99	University Hospital of Arkansas, Little Rock	24.6	0.0%	1.11	Yes	1.11	6	2	2.01	0.175
	TIER FOUR									
	Baptist Medical Center, Little Rock	18.7	0.0%	1.04	No	0.01	4	2	0.81	0.049
	Baptist Memorial Medical Center, North Little Rock	15.1	0.0%	1.39	No	0.00	6	2	0.74	0.018
	HCA Doctor's Hospital, Little Rock	14.2	0.0%	1.35	No	0.00	5	1	0.59	0.023
	Jefferson Regional Medical Center, Pine Bluff	13.4	0.0%	1.56	No	0.04	6	2	0.42	0.008
	Medical Center of South Arkansas, El Dorado	12.3	0.0%	1.57	No	0.04	3	2	0.43	0.023
	Sparks Regional Medical Center, Fort Smith	13.8	0.0%	1.52	No	0.02	7	1	0.66	0.027
	Springdale Memorial Hospital, Springdale	13.0	0.0%	1.47	No	0.00	5	1	0.55	0.010
	St. Bernard's Regional Medical Center, Jonesboro	13.9	0.0%	1.60	No	0.04	7	2	0.62	0.031
	St. Edward Mercy Medical Center, Fort Smith	15.8	0.0%	1.23	No	0.00	6	1	0.57	0.052
	St. Michael Hospital, Texarkana	16.3	0.0%	1.19	No	0.00	6	1	0.63	0.049
	St. Vincent Infirmary Medical Center, Little Rock	17.3	0.0%	1.26	No	0.02	7	2	1.05	0.032

CANCER

Natl. Rank	Hospital	U.S. News index	Reputational score	Cancer mortality rate	COTH member	Interns and residents to beds	Technology score (of 12)	R.N.'s to beds	Board-certified oncologists to beds	Procedures to beds
	TIER TWO									
41	University Hospital of Arkansas, Little Rock	13.6	0.5%	0.65	Yes	1.11	5	2.01	0.000	2.41
	TIER FOUR									
	Baptist Medical Center, Little Rock	2.9	0.0%	1.02	No	0.01	4	0.81	0.010	3.20
	Baptist Memorial Medical Center, North Little Rock	3.2	0.0%	1.01	No	0.00	6	0.74	0.009	3.33
	HCA Doctor's Hospital, Little Rock	1.8	0.0%	1.15	No	0.00	4	0.59	0.020	1.17
	Jefferson Regional Medical Center, Pine Bluff	2.3	0.0%	1.21	No	0.04	8	0.42	0.002	0.87
	Medical Center of South Arkansas, El Dorado	0.7	0.0%	1.78	No	0.04	3	0.43	0.000	1.20
	Sparks Regional Medical Center, Fort Smith	3.1	0.0%	1.44	No	0.02	8	0.66	0.011	2.18
	Springdale Memorial Hospital, Springdale	1.9	0.0%	1.03	No	0.00	5	0.55	0.000	1.08
	St. Bernard's Regional Medical Center, Jonesboro	3.4	0.0%	1.21	No	0.04	9	0.62	0.009	1.76
	St. Edward Mercy Medical Center, Fort Smith	2.3	0.0%	1.36	No	0.00	6	0.57	0.020	1.86
	St. Joseph's Reg. Health Ctr., Hot Springs National Park	4.2	0.0%	1.19	No	0.00	8	0.87	0.007	4.42
	St. Michael Hospital, Texarkana	3.3	0.0%	1.02	No	0.00	8	0.63	0.008	2.28
	St. Vincent Infirmary Medical Center, Little Rock	3.9	0.0%	1.09	No	0.02	5	1.05	0.018	3.75
	Washington Regional Medical Center, Fayetteville	3.3	0.0%	0.96	No	0.05	3	1.08	0.014	2.07

CARDIOLOGY

Natl. Rank	Hospital	U.S. News index	Reputational score	Cardiology mortality rate	COTH member	Interns and residents to beds	Technology score (of 10)	R.N.'s to beds	Board-certified cardiologists to beds	Procedures to beds
	TIER THREE									
	St. Joseph's Reg. Health Ctr., Hot Springs National Park	17.7	0.0%	0.82	No	0.00	8	0.87	0.015	9.89
	TIER FOUR									
	Baptist Medical Center, Little Rock	13.3	0.4%	1.05	No	0.01	7	0.81	0.020	8.64
	Baptist Memorial Medical Center, North Little Rock	4.7	0.0%	1.50	No	0.00	5	0.74	0.014	6.39
	Jefferson Regional Medical Center, Pine Bluff	4.3	0.0%	1.51	No	0.04	8	0.42	0.000	4.09
	Medical Center of South Arkansas, El Dorado	1.5	0.0%	1.62	No	0.04	2	0.43	0.004	4.71
	Sparks Regional Medical Center, Fort Smith	4.6	0.0%	1.60	No	0.02	8	0.66	0.021	7.74
	Springdale Memorial Hospital, Springdale	4.2	0.0%	1.53	No	0.00	6	0.55	0.000	11.82
	St. Bernard's Regional Medical Center, Jonesboro	3.5	0.0%	1.79	No	0.04	9	0.62	0.022	11.95

Natl. Rank	Hospital	U.S. News index	Reputational score	Cardiology mortality rate	COTH member	Interns and residents to beds	Technology score (of 10)	R.N.'s to beds	Board-certified cardiologists to beds	Procedures to beds
	St. Edward Mercy Medical Center, Fort Smith	7.6	0.0%	1.32	No	0.00	8	0.57	0.023	9.60
	St. Michael Hospital, Texarkana	6.1	0.0%	1.43	No	0.00	8	0.63	0.012	8.72
	St. Vincent Infirmary Medical Center, Little Rock	10.1	0.0%	1.23	No	0.02	7	1.05	0.024	9.11
	Washington Regional Medical Center, Fayetteville	7.1	0.0%	1.38	No	0.05	5	1.08	0.005	7.03

ENDOCRINOLOGY

Natl. Rank	Hospital	U.S. News index	Reputational score	Endocrinology mortality rate	COTH member	Interns and residents to beds	Technology score (of 11)	R.N.'s to beds	Board-certified internists to beds
	TIER TWO								
59	University Hospital of Arkansas, Little Rock	16.4	0.0%	1.02	Yes	1.11	6	2.01	0.175
	TIER THREE								
	St. Joseph's Reg. Health Ctr., Hot Springs National Park	10.4	0.0%	0.56	No	0.00	9	0.87	0.033
	TIER FOUR								
	Baptist Medical Center, Little Rock	6.9	0.0%	0.87	No	0.01	4	0.81	0.049
	Baptist Memorial Medical Center, North Little Rock	5.4	0.0%	1.07	No	0.00	6	0.74	0.018
	Jefferson Regional Medical Center, Pine Bluff	3.2	0.0%	1.56	No	0.04	9	0.42	0.008
	Medical Center of South Arkansas, El Dorado	1.6	0.0%	1.87	No	0.04	4	0.43	0.023
	Sparks Regional Medical Center, Fort Smith	3.7	0.0%	1.57	No	0.02	8	0.66	0.027
	St. Bernard's Regional Medical Center, Jonesboro	3.0	0.0%	2.08	No	0.04	10	0.62	0.031
	St. Edward Mercy Medical Center, Fort Smith	4.8	0.0%	1.16	No	0.00	7	0.57	0.052
	St. Michael Hospital, Texarkana	4.1	0.0%	1.48	No	0.00	9	0.63	0.049
	St. Vincent Infirmary Medical Center, Little Rock	4.9	0.0%	1.35	No	0.02	5	1.05	0.032
	Washington Regional Medical Center, Fayetteville	8.1	0.0%	0.82	No	0.05	4	1.08	0.037

GASTROENTEROLOGY

Natl. Rank	Hospital	U.S. News index	Reputational score	Gastroenterology mortality rate	COTH member	Interns and residents to beds	Technology score (of 11)	R.N.'s to beds	Board-certified gastroenterologists to beds	Procedures to beds
	TIER FOUR									
	Baptist Medical Center, Little Rock	5.3	0.0%	1.07	No	0.01	5	0.81	0.017	3.27
	Baptist Memorial Medical Center, North Little Rock	4.8	0.0%	1.38	No	0.00	5	0.74	0.023	5.25
	HCA Doctor's Hospital, Little Rock	1.8	0.0%	1.56	No	0.00	5	0.59	0.036	1.72
	Jefferson Regional Medical Center, Pine Bluff	3.0	0.0%	1.52	No	0.04	8	0.42	0.004	2.75
	Medical Center of South Arkansas, El Dorado	0.5	0.0%	1.85	No	0.04	3	0.43	0.004	2.42
	Sparks Regional Medical Center, Fort Smith	3.4	0.0%	1.75	No	0.02	8	0.66	0.015	3.47
	Springdale Memorial Hospital, Springdale	3.0	0.0%	1.34	No	0.00	4	0.55	0.005	3.40
	St. Bernard's Regional Medical Center, Jonesboro	4.5	0.0%	1.61	No	0.04	9	0.62	0.006	4.43
	St. Edward Mercy Medical Center, Fort Smith	2.8	0.0%	1.72	No	0.00	6	0.57	0.020	3.89
	St. Joseph's Reg. Health Ctr., Hot Springs National Park	6.6	0.0%	1.12	No	0.00	8	0.87	0.007	4.31
	St. Michael Hospital, Texarkana	5.8	0.0%	1.16	No	0.00	8	0.63	0.008	4.25
	St. Vincent Infirmary Medical Center, Little Rock	5.2	0.0%	1.35	No	0.02	5	1.05	0.022	4.38
	Washington Regional Medical Center, Fayetteville	5.1	0.0%	1.41	No	0.05	4	1.08	0.014	5.01

GERIATRICS

Natl. Rank	Hospital	U.S. News index	Reputational score	Hospital-wide mortality rate	COTH member	Service mix	Interns and residents to beds	Technology score (of 13)	R.N.'s to beds	Discharge planning (of 2)	Geriatric services (of 9)	Board-certified internists to beds
	TIER THREE											
	St. Joseph's Reg. Health Ctr., Hot Springs National Park	17.6	0.0%	0.90	No	4	0.00	10	0.87	2	4	0.033
	University Hospital of Arkansas, Little Rock	19.7	0.0%	1.11	Yes	5	1.11	8	2.01	2	5	0.175

STATE RANKINGS ■ ARKANSAS

Natl. Rank	Hospital	U.S. News index	Reputa-tional score	Hospital-wide mortality rate	COTH member	Service mix	Interns and residents to beds	Tech-nology score (of 13)	R.N.'s to beds	Discharge planning (of 2)	Geriatric services (of 9)	Board-certified internists to beds
	TIER FOUR											
	Baptist Medical Center, Little Rock	**12.8**	0.0%	1.04	No	4	0.01	7	0.81	2	3	0.049
	Baptist Memorial Medical Center, North Little Rock	**5.3**	0.0%	1.39	No	4	0.00	8	0.74	2	2	0.018
	Jefferson Regional Medical Center, Pine Bluff	**4.2**	0.0%	1.56	No	7	0.04	10	0.42	2	2	0.008
	Medical Center of South Arkansas, El Dorado	**3.1**	0.0%	1.57	No	6	0.04	5	0.43	2	3	0.023
	Sparks Regional Medical Center, Fort Smith	**3.6**	0.0%	1.52	No	6	0.02	9	0.66	1	2	0.027
	Springdale Memorial Hospital, Springdale	**2.8**	0.0%	1.47	No	5	0.00	8	0.55	1	1	0.010
	St. Bernard's Regional Medical Center, Jonesboro	**3.7**	0.0%	1.60	No	5	0.04	11	0.62	2	2	0.031
	St. Edward Mercy Medical Center, Fort Smith	**7.4**	0.0%	1.23	No	6	0.00	8	0.57	1	1	0.052
	St. Michael Hospital, Texarkana	**8.6**	0.0%	1.19	No	4	0.00	10	0.63	1	4	0.049
	St. Vincent Infirmary Medical Center, Little Rock	**9.1**	0.0%	1.26	No	6	0.02	7	1.05	2	3	0.032
	Washington Regional Medical Center, Fayetteville	**7.8**	0.0%	1.28	No	5	0.05	5	1.08	2	2	0.037

GYNECOLOGY

Natl. Rank	Hospital	U.S. News index	Reputa-tional score	Hospital-wide mortality rate	Interns and residents to beds	Tech-nology score (of 10)	R.N.'s to beds	Board-certified OB-GYNs to beds	Procedures to beds
	TIER TWO								
84	**University Hospital of Arkansas, Little Rock**	**22.4**	0.4%	1.11	1.11	6	2.01	0.029	0.38
	TIER THREE								
	St. Joseph's Reg. Health Ctr., Hot Springs National Park	**17.5**	0.0%	0.90	0.00	7	0.87	0.007	0.42
	TIER FOUR								
	Baptist Medical Center, Little Rock	**11.5**	0.0%	1.04	0.01	4	0.81	0.019	0.42
	Baptist Memorial Medical Center, North Little Rock	**4.5**	0.0%	1.39	0.00	4	0.74	0.027	0.62
	Jefferson Regional Medical Center, Pine Bluff	**3.7**	0.0%	1.56	0.04	8	0.42	0.015	0.36
	Medical Center of South Arkansas, El Dorado	**0.0**	0.0%	1.57	0.04	3	0.43	0.011	0.36
	Sparks Regional Medical Center, Fort Smith	**4.8**	0.0%	1.52	0.02	7	0.66	0.027	0.47
	St. Bernard's Regional Medical Center, Jonesboro	**4.4**	0.0%	1.60	0.04	8	0.62	0.025	0.62
	St. Edward Mercy Medical Center, Fort Smith	**7.3**	0.0%	1.23	0.00	5	0.57	0.035	0.54
	St. Michael Hospital, Texarkana	**9.7**	0.0%	1.19	0.00	7	0.63	0.033	0.24
	St. Vincent Infirmary Medical Center, Little Rock	**8.5**	0.0%	1.26	0.02	4	1.05	0.044	0.66
	Washington Regional Medical Center, Fayetteville	**7.6**	0.0%	1.28	0.05	3	1.08	0.041	0.69

NEUROLOGY

Natl. Rank	Hospital	U.S. News index	Reputa-tional score	Neurology mortality rate	COTH member	Interns and residents to beds	Tech-nology score (of 9)	R.N.'s to beds	Board-certified neurologists to beds
	TIER THREE								
	St. Joseph's Reg. Health Ctr., Hot Springs National Park	**11.4**	0.0%	0.88	No	0.00	7	0.87	0.004
	TIER FOUR								
	Baptist Medical Center, Little Rock	**6.9**	0.0%	1.10	No	0.01	3	0.81	0.009
	Baptist Memorial Medical Center, North Little Rock	**4.2**	0.0%	1.42	No	0.00	4	0.74	0.018
	Jefferson Regional Medical Center, Pine Bluff	**1.4**	0.0%	1.73	No	0.04	7	0.42	0.002
	Medical Center of South Arkansas, El Dorado	**2.3**	0.0%	1.40	No	0.04	2	0.43	0.004
	Sparks Regional Medical Center, Fort Smith	**3.0**	0.0%	1.60	No	0.02	6	0.66	0.011
	St. Bernard's Regional Medical Center, Jonesboro	**6.8**	0.0%	1.17	No	0.04	8	0.62	0.006
	St. Edward Mercy Medical Center, Fort Smith	**9.2**	0.0%	0.96	No	0.00	5	0.57	0.015
	St. Michael Hospital, Texarkana	**5.9**	0.0%	1.25	No	0.00	7	0.63	0.012
	St. Vincent Infirmary Medical Center, Little Rock	**6.6**	0.0%	1.22	No	0.02	4	1.05	0.012
	Washington Regional Medical Center, Fayetteville	**5.8**	0.0%	1.33	No	0.05	4	1.08	0.014

ORTHOPEDICS

Natl. Rank	Hospital	U.S. News index	Reputa-tional score	Orthopedics mortality rate	COTH member	Interns and residents to beds	Tech-nology score (of 5)	R.N.'s to beds	Board-certified orthopedists to beds	Pro-cedures to beds
TIER TWO										
73	University Hospital of Arkansas, Little Rock	14.8	0.0%	1.19	Yes	1.11	4	2.01	0.025	1.78
TIER THREE										
	St. Joseph's Reg. Health Ctr., Hot Springs National Park	10.0	0.0%	0.47	No	0.00	3	0.87	0.015	3.44
TIER FOUR										
	Baptist Medical Center, Little Rock	7.7	0.0%	0.76	No	0.01	2	0.81	0.023	2.86
	Baptist Memorial Medical Center, North Little Rock	5.6	0.0%	1.04	No	0.00	3	0.74	0.023	3.37
	HCA Doctor's Hospital, Little Rock	2.8	0.0%	1.48	No	0.00	3	0.59	0.049	1.41
	Jefferson Regional Medical Center, Pine Bluff	5.4	0.0%	0.92	No	0.04	3	0.42	0.006	1.80
	Medical Center of South Arkansas, El Dorado	1.0	0.0%	1.51	No	0.04	1	0.43	0.011	1.89
	Sparks Regional Medical Center, Fort Smith	2.7	0.0%	1.93	No	0.02	4	0.66	0.015	2.89
	St. Bernard's Regional Medical Center, Jonesboro	4.3	0.0%	1.49	No	0.04	4	0.62	0.022	5.05
	St. Edward Mercy Medical Center, Fort Smith	4.4	0.0%	1.29	No	0.00	4	0.57	0.041	2.72
	St. Michael Hospital, Texarkana	6.3	0.0%	0.99	No	0.00	4	0.63	0.025	3.34
	St. Vincent Infirmary Medical Center, Little Rock	6.4	0.0%	1.08	No	0.02	3	1.05	0.040	3.67
	Washington Regional Medical Center, Fayetteville	7.7	0.0%	0.93	No	0.05	3	1.08	0.032	3.88

OTOLARYNGOLOGY

Natl. Rank	Hospital	U.S. News index	Reputa-tional score	Hospital-wide mortality rate	COTH member	Interns and residents to beds	Tech-nology score (of 9)	R.N.'s to beds	Board-certified internists to beds	Procedures to beds
TIER TWO										
52	University Hospital of Arkansas, Little Rock	17.6	0.4%	1.11	Yes	1.11	4	2.01	0.175	0.390
TIER FOUR										
	Baptist Medical Center, Little Rock	3.5	0.0%	1.03	No	0.01	2	0.81	0.049	0.176
	Baptist Memorial Medical Center, North Little Rock	3.4	0.0%	1.39	No	0.00	4	0.74	0.018	0.356
	HCA Doctor's Hospital, Little Rock	2.7	0.0%	1.35	No	0.00	3	0.59	0.023	0.109
	Jefferson Regional Medical Center, Pine Bluff	3.2	0.0%	1.56	No	0.04	7	0.42	0.008	0.160
	Medical Center of South Arkansas, El Dorado	2.0	0.0%	1.57	No	0.04	2	0.43	0.023	0.113
	Sparks Regional Medical Center, Fort Smith	3.8	0.0%	1.51	No	0.02	6	0.66	0.027	0.286
	Springdale Memorial Hospital, Springdale	2.4	0.0%	1.47	No	0.00	3	0.55	0.010	0.137
	St. Bernard's Regional Medical Center, Jonesboro	4.3	0.0%	1.60	No	0.04	8	0.62	0.031	0.585
	St. Edward Mercy Medical Center, Fort Smith	3.5	0.0%	1.23	No	0.00	5	0.57	0.052	0.187
	St. Joseph's Reg. Health Ctr., Hot Springs National Park	5.1	0.0%	0.90	No	0.00	7	0.87	0.033	0.153
	St. Michael Hospital, Texarkana	4.3	0.0%	1.19	No	0.00	7	0.63	0.049	0.305
	St. Vincent Infirmary Medical Center, Little Rock	4.3	0.0%	1.26	No	0.02	3	1.05	0.032	0.190
	Washington Regional Medical Center, Fayetteville	4.3	0.0%	1.28	No	0.05	2	1.08	0.037	0.333

RHEUMATOLOGY

Natl. Rank	Hospital	U.S. News index	Reputa-tional score	Hospital-wide mortality rate	COTH member	Interns and residents to beds	Tech-nology score (of 5)	R.N.'s to beds	Board-certified internists to beds
TIER TWO									
49	University Hospital of Arkansas, Little Rock	17.9	0.0%	1.11	Yes	1.11	4	2.01	0.175
TIER FOUR									
	Baptist Medical Center, Little Rock	7.5	0.0%	1.03	No	0.01	2	0.81	0.049
	Baptist Memorial Medical Center, North Little Rock	5.2	0.0%	1.39	No	0.00	3	0.74	0.018
	Jefferson Regional Medical Center, Pine Bluff	3.7	0.0%	1.56	No	0.04	3	0.42	0.008
	Medical Center of South Arkansas, El Dorado	2.9	0.0%	1.57	No	0.04	1	0.43	0.023
	Sparks Regional Medical Center, Fort Smith	4.1	0.0%	1.51	No	0.02	4	0.66	0.027
	Springdale Memorial Hospital, Springdale	2.8	0.0%	1.47	No	0.00	2	0.55	0.010
	St. Bernard's Regional Medical Center, Jonesboro	4.7	0.0%	1.60	No	0.04	4	0.62	0.031

Natl. Rank	Hospital	U.S. News index	Reputa-tional score	Hospital-wide mortality rate	COTH member	Interns and residents to beds	Tech-nology score (of 5)	R.N.'s to beds	Board-certified internists to beds
	St. Edward Mercy Medical Center, Fort Smith	5.4	0.0%	1.23	No	0.00	4	0.57	0.052
	St. Joseph's Reg. Health Ctr., Hot Springs National Park	9.3	0.0%	0.90	No	0.00	3	0.87	0.033
	St. Michael Hospital, Texarkana	5.7	0.0%	1.19	No	0.00	4	0.63	0.049
	St. Vincent Infirmary Medical Center, Little Rock	6.9	0.0%	1.26	No	0.02	3	1.05	0.032
	Washington Regional Medical Center, Fayetteville	7.0	0.0%	1.28	No	0.05	3	1.08	0.037

UROLOGY

Natl. Rank	Hospital	U.S. News index	Reputa-tional score	Urology mortality rate	COTH member	Interns and residents to beds	Tech-nology score (of 11)	R.N.'s to beds	Board-certified internists to beds	Procedures to beds
	TIER TWO									
82	University Hospital of Arkansas, Little Rock	15.8	0.0%	1.16	Yes	1.11	5	2.01	0.175	2.02
	TIER FOUR									
	Baptist Medical Center, Little Rock	6.2	0.0%	1.07	No	0.01	5	0.81	0.049	1.26
	Baptist Memorial Medical Center, North Little Rock	4.0	0.0%	1.45	No	0.00	5	0.74	0.018	2.51
	Jefferson Regional Medical Center, Pine Bluff	2.6	0.0%	1.84	No	0.04	8	0.42	0.008	2.22
	Medical Center of South Arkansas, El Dorado	1.9	0.0%	1.62	No	0.04	3	0.43	0.023	1.46
	Sparks Regional Medical Center, Fort Smith	3.6	0.0%	1.74	No	0.02	8	0.66	0.027	2.36
	Springdale Memorial Hospital, Springdale	2.8	0.0%	1.48	No	0.00	4	0.55	0.010	1.61
	St. Bernard's Regional Medical Center, Jonesboro	3.4	0.0%	1.98	No	0.04	9	0.62	0.031	3.04
	St. Edward Mercy Medical Center, Fort Smith	3.7	0.0%	1.52	No	0.00	6	0.57	0.052	2.28
	St. Joseph's Reg. Health Ctr., Hot Springs National Park	8.1	0.0%	1.00	No	0.00	8	0.87	0.033	2.77
	St. Michael Hospital, Texarkana	3.8	0.0%	1.68	No	0.00	8	0.63	0.049	2.30
	St. Vincent Infirmary Medical Center, Little Rock	4.1	0.0%	1.64	No	0.02	5	1.05	0.032	2.22
	Washington Regional Medical Center, Fayetteville	5.9	0.0%	1.23	No	0.05	4	1.08	0.037	2.36

AIDS

Natl. Rank	Hospital	U.S. News index	Reputational score	Hospital-wide mortality rate	COTH member	Interns and residents to beds	Technology score (of 11)	Discharge planning (of 2)	R.N.'s to beds	Board-certified internists to beds
TIER ONE										
1	San Francisco General Hospital Medical Center	100.0	59.1%	0.95	No	1.19	8	2	1.52	0.011
4	University of California, San Francisco Medical Center	55.0	19.4%	0.89	Yes	1.03	10	2	1.82	0.435
5	UCLA Medical Center, Los Angeles	54.2	19.7%	0.66	Yes	1.52	11	2	1.20	0.023
11	Stanford University Hospital, Stanford	35.4	6.1%	0.90	Yes	1.34	9	2	0.86	0.147
15	UCSD Medical Center, San Diego	33.6	2.8%	0.75	Yes	1.65	8	2	2.17	0.049
TIER TWO										
78	Cedars-Sinai Medical Center, Los Angeles	25.4	2.4%	1.13	Yes	0.51	10	2	0.83	0.086
74	Kaiser Foundation Hospital, Los Angeles	25.8	0.0%	0.86	No	0.63	9	2	1.42	0.134
36	Los Angeles County-Harbor-UCLA Medical Center	28.7	1.6%	0.91	No	1.53	8	2	1.33	0.148
28	Los Angeles County-USC Medical Center	29.8	1.9%	0.88	Yes	1.21	9	1	1.30	0.052
34	University of California, Davis Medical Center	28.8	0.0%	1.01	Yes	1.54	9	2	2.81	0.032
TIER THREE										
	Alta Bates Medical Center, Berkeley	20.1	0.0%	0.96	No	0.00	6	2	0.46	0.065
	Alvarado Hospital Medical Center, San Diego	21.4	0.0%	0.92	No	0.00	6	2	0.81	0.065
	Beverly Hospital, Montebello	21.6	0.0%	0.90	No	0.00	6	1	1.09	0.094
	Centinela Hospital Medical Center, Inglewood	20.9	0.0%	0.96	No	0.00	6	2	0.65	0.165
	Century City Hospital, Los Angeles	22.4	0.0%	0.82	No	0.00	6	2	0.76	0.144
	Davies Medical Center, San Francisco	22.7	0.7%	0.82	No	0.01	6	1	0.66	0.212
	Desert Hospital, Palm Springs	22.2	0.0%	0.85	No	0.07	5	2	1.00	0.069
	Downey Community Hospital, Downey	20.5	0.0%	0.92	No	0.00	6	1	0.65	0.076
	Eisenhower Memorial Hospital, Rancho Mirage	22.0	0.0%	0.86	No	0.00	7	2	0.95	0.054
	Encino-Tarzana Regional Medical Center, Tarzana	21.9	0.0%	0.78	No	0.00	6	2	0.66	0.065
	Fountain Valley Regional Hosp. Med. Ctr., Fountain Valley	20.5	0.0%	0.98	No	0.00	7	2	0.72	0.061
	Garfield Medical Center, Monterey Park	22.8	0.0%	0.90	No	0.00	6	2	1.16	0.161
	Glendale Adventist Medical Center, Glendale	20.4	0.0%	1.00	No	0.15	5	2	1.06	0.067
	Green Hospital of Scripps Clinic, La Jolla	24.0	0.0%	0.86	No	0.21	7	1	1.99	0.052
	Highland General Hospital, Oakland	22.7	0.0%	0.84	No	0.84	5	2	0.34	0.065
	Hoag Memorial Hospital Presbyterian, Newport Beach	22.2	0.0%	0.94	No	0.00	7	2	1.26	0.068
	Hospital of the Good Samaritan, Los Angeles	19.7	0.0%	1.19	Yes	0.04	7	2	0.98	0.067
	Huntington Memorial Hospital, Pasadena	20.6	0.2%	1.11	Yes	0.11	7	2	0.68	0.059
	Kaiser Foundation Hospital, Fontana	22.7	0.0%	0.88	No	0.08	6	2	1.05	0.078
	Kaiser Foundation Hospital, West Los Angeles	22.8	0.4%	0.89	No	0.06	5	2	0.86	0.156
	Kaiser Foundation Hospital, Oakland	19.9	0.0%	1.07	No	0.33	7	2	0.72	0.070
	Kaiser Foundation Hospital, Panorama City	22.2	0.0%	0.82	No	0.01	5	2	0.79	0.177
	Kaiser Foundation Hospital, Redwood City	22.4	0.0%	0.93	No	0.00	7	2	0.96	0.205
	Kaiser Foundation Hospital, San Diego	20.8	0.0%	0.92	No	0.09	6	1	0.70	0.099
	Kaiser Foundation Hospital, San Francisco	23.4	0.0%	0.82	No	0.31	8	2	0.74	0.067
	Kaiser Foundation Hospital, Santa Clara	23.8	0.0%	0.94	No	0.29	6	2	1.58	0.288
	Kaiser Foundation Hospital, Woodland Hills	23.8	0.0%	0.80	No	0.01	6	1	2.06	0.167
	L.A. County-Rancho Los Amigos Med. Ctr., Downey	22.5	0.0%	0.85	No	0.23	5	2	1.01	0.055
	Long Beach Community Hospital, Long Beach	21.1	0.0%	0.97	No	0.00	7	2	0.74	0.147
	Long Beach Memorial Medical Center, Long Beach	22.5	0.0%	1.00	Yes	0.18	8	2	0.80	0.037
	Los Angeles County-King-Drew Medical Center	23.0	0.3%	1.25	Yes	1.56	7	2	1.33	0.040
	Mercy General Hospital, Sacramento	22.2	0.0%	0.87	No	0.00	6	2	0.79	0.088
	Methodist Hospital of Southern California, Arcadia	21.8	0.0%	0.72	No	0.00	6	2	0.65	0.042
	Mills-Peninsula Hospitals, Burlingame	21.0	0.0%	0.92	No	0.00	6	2	0.49	0.086
	N.T. Enloe Memorial Hospital, Chico	20.2	0.0%	1.01	No	0.00	6	1	1.63	0.025
	Northridge Hospital Medical Center, Northridge	22.4	0.0%	0.95	No	0.09	7	2	0.87	0.290
	O'Connor Hospital, San Jose	19.8	0.0%	1.06	No	0.00	6	2	0.82	0.220
	Olive View Medical Center, Sylmar	22.7	0.0%	1.10	No	0.51	7	2	2.17	0.225
	Presbyterian Intercommunity Hospital, Whittier	20.2	0.2%	0.93	No	0.07	5	1	0.55	0.066

Natl. Rank	Hospital	U.S. News index	Reputa- tional score	Hospital- wide mortality rate	COTH member	Interns and residents to beds	Tech- nology score (of 11)	Discharge planning (of 2)	R.N.'s to beds	Board- certified internists to beds
	Queen of Angels-Hollywood Center, Hollywood	22.1	0.0%	0.85	No	0.00	6	2	0.72	0.098
	Queen of the Valley Hospital, Napa	22.2	0.0%	0.84	No	0.00	7	2	0.72	0.037
	Saddleback Memorial Medical Center, Laguna Hills	21.8	0.0%	0.83	No	0.01	4	2	1.05	0.073
	San Pedro Peninsula Hospital, San Pedro	20.8	0.0%	0.85	No	0.00	5	2	0.28	0.030
	Santa Clara Veterans Affairs Medical Center, San Jose	20.9	0.0%	1.29	No	0.67	10	2	1.83	0.095
	Santa Monica Hospital Medical Center, Santa Monica	23.8	0.0%	0.74	No	0.17	7	2	0.91	0.258
	Sequoia Hospital District, Redwood City	21.2	0.0%	0.86	No	0.00	6	1	0.60	0.106
	Seton Medical Center, Daly City	22.7	0.0%	0.52	No	0.00	5	2	1.14	0.158
	Sharp Memorial Hospital, San Diego	20.2	0.0%	1.02	No	0.00	5	2	1.40	0.052
	South Coast Medical Center, South Laguna	20.5	0.0%	0.93	No	0.00	7	1	0.52	0.063
	St. John's Hospital and Health Center, Santa Monica	22.0	0.2%	0.80	No	0.00	6	1	0.64	0.212
	St. Joseph Hospital, Orange	19.8	0.0%	1.09	No	0.01	7	2	0.92	0.206
	St. Joseph Medical Center, Burbank	22.0	0.0%	0.82	No	0.00	6	2	0.77	0.046
	St. Mary Medical Center, Long Beach	23.5	0.4%	0.86	No	0.15	8	2	0.73	0.042
	St. Mary's Hospital and Medical Center, San Francisco	22.3	0.0%	0.99	Yes	0.26	8	2	0.41	0.057
	St. Vincent Medical Center, Los Angeles	22.6	0.0%	0.85	No	0.01	7	2	0.84	0.076
	Torrance Memorial Medical Center, Torrance	22.8	0.0%	0.92	No	0.00	7	2	0.79	0.313
	Tri-City Medical Center, Oceanside	21.8	0.0%	0.82	No	0.01	6	2	0.63	0.058
	University of California, Irvine Medical Center, Orange	21.5	0.3%	1.19	Yes	0.54	7	2	1.29	0.038
	Washington Hospital, Fremont	22.3	0.0%	0.79	No	0.00	6	2	0.85	0.089
	White Memorial Medical Center, Los Angeles	22.6	0.0%	0.74	No	0.42	6	2	0.62	0.039
TIER FOUR										
	Antelope Valley Hospital Medical Center, Lancaster	16.2	0.0%	1.30	No	0.00	4	2	1.02	0.141
	Bakersfield Memorial Hospital, Bakersfield	17.3	0.0%	1.21	No	0.00	6	1	1.02	0.185
	Brookside Hospital, San Pablo	17.7	0.0%	1.06	No	0.00	5	2	0.20	0.057
	California Medical Center, Los Angeles	17.7	0.0%	1.16	No	0.13	5	1	1.18	0.107
	Community Hospital of Chula Vista, Chula Vista	17.5	0.0%	1.08	No	0.00	4	2	0.59	0.035
	Community Hospital, Santa Rosa	16.9	0.0%	1.27	No	0.53	6	2	0.50	0.014
	Community Memorial Hospital, Ventura	18.9	0.0%	1.02	No	0.00	6	1	0.85	0.038
	Dameron Hospital, Stockton	16.5	0.0%	1.27	No	0.00	5	2	0.76	0.175
	Fresno Community Hospital and Medical Center, Fresno	18.1	0.0%	1.17	No	0.00	7	2	0.88	0.069
	Glendale Memorial Hospital and Health Center, Glendale	18.6	0.0%	1.01	No	0.00	6	1	0.69	0.003
	Good Samaritan Hospital, San Jose	18.1	0.0%	1.20	No	0.00	7	2	0.52	0.288
	Grossmont Hospital, La Mesa	18.0	0.0%	1.12	No	0.00	6	2	0.73	0.023
	Hemet Valley Medical Center, Hemet	17.5	0.0%	1.07	No	0.00	5	1	0.64	0.024
	John Muir Medical Center, Walnut Creek	16.8	0.0%	1.15	No	0.01	4	1	0.88	0.095
	Kaiser Foundation Hospital, Walnut Creek	19.4	0.0%	0.96	No	0.02	4	2	0.42	0.055
	Kern Medical Center, Bakersfield	19.6	0.0%	1.33	Yes	0.93	4	1	1.40	0.222
	Loma Linda Community Hospital, Loma Linda	15.3	0.0%	1.21	No	0.06	4	1	0.52	0.050
	Marin General Hospital, Greenbrae	15.7	0.0%	1.18	No	0.00	4	1	0.37	0.139
	Martin Luther Hospital, Anaheim	19.3	0.0%	0.95	No	0.00	5	1	0.55	0.045
	Memorial Hospitals Association, Modesto	18.7	0.0%	1.12	No	0.00	6	2	1.10	0.043
	Merced Community Medical Center, Merced	17.2	0.0%	1.15	No	0.23	3	2	0.66	0.114
	Mercy Hospital and Medical Center, San Diego	18.6	0.0%	1.25	No	0.25	8	2	1.06	0.120
	Mercy Medical Center, Redding	15.2	0.0%	1.58	No	0.16	6	1	1.77	0.069
	Merrithew Memorial Hospital, Martinez	17.5	0.0%	1.17	No	0.21	4	2	1.11	0.015
	Natividad Medical Center, Salinas	16.7	0.0%	1.10	No	0.24	4	1	0.41	0.024
	Northbay Medical Center, Fairfield	15.0	0.0%	1.25	No	0.00	5	1	0.40	0.053
	Palomar Medical Center, Escondido	18.3	0.0%	1.09	No	0.00	6	2	0.73	0.012
	Riverside General Hospital-Medical Center, Riverside	14.0	0.0%	1.59	No	0.37	6	1	0.88	0.033
	Roseville Hospital, Roseville	17.3	0.0%	1.13	No	0.00	6	2	0.29	0.073
	Salinas Valley Memorial Hospital, Salinas	17.6	0.0%	1.11	No	0.00	6	2	0.28	0.094
	San Bernardino County Medical Center, San Bernardino	18.1	0.0%	1.51	No	0.66	7	2	2.02	0.051
	San Gabriel Valley Medical Center, San Gabriel	19.1	0.0%	1.09	No	0.00	7	2	0.56	0.180
	San Joaquin General Hospital, Stockton	13.5	0.0%	1.65	No	0.43	5	1	1.02	0.018
	San Jose Medical Center, San Jose	15.7	0.0%	1.31	No	0.12	7	1	0.61	0.066

STATE RANKINGS ■ CALIFORNIA

Natl. Rank	Hospital	U.S. News index	Reputa-tional score	Hospital-wide mortality rate	COTH member	Interns and residents to beds	Tech-nology score (of 11)	Discharge planning (of 2)	R.N.'s to beds	Board-certified internists to beds
	Santa Barbara Cottage Hospital, Santa Barbara	19.1	0.0%	1.07	No	0.25	4	1	0.94	0.253
	Santa Rosa Memorial Hospital, Santa Rosa	16.8	0.0%	1.17	No	0.00	5	2	0.26	0.160
	Scripps Memorial Hospital, La Jolla	19.2	0.0%	1.06	No	0.00	7	2	0.71	0.037
	St. Agnes Medical Center, Fresno	18.6	0.0%	1.17	No	0.00	7	2	0.92	0.164
	Stanislaus Medical Center, Modesto	19.3	0.0%	1.21	No	0.60	6	2	1.46	0.024
	St. Bernardine Medical Center, San Bernardino	17.0	0.0%	1.26	No	0.00	8	2	0.64	0.043
	St. Francis Medical Center, Lynwood	19.4	0.0%	1.02	No	0.00	6	2	0.70	0.038
	St. Francis Memorial Hospital, San Francisco	18.2	0.0%	1.03	No	0.06	6	1	0.41	0.063
	St. Joseph Hospital, Eureka	15.4	0.0%	1.37	No	0.00	7	2	0.48	0.059
	St. Joseph's Medical Center, Stockton	18.5	0.0%	1.09	No	0.00	6	2	0.71	0.063
	St. Jude Medical Center, Fullerton	19.2	0.0%	1.04	No	0.00	6	2	0.77	0.030
	Sutter General Hospital, Sacramento	19.3	0.0%	0.99	No	0.06	6	1	0.54	0.078
	USC Kenneth Norris Cancer Hospital, Los Angeles	16.6	0.0%	1.40	No	0.40	6	1	1.37	0.133
	Valley Medical Center of Fresno, Fresno	16.7	0.0%	1.57	Yes	0.80	7	1	0.71	0.034
	Western Medical Center, Santa Ana	19.5	0.0%	1.06	No	0.04	6	2	1.05	0.061

CANCER

Natl. Rank	Hospital	U.S. News index	Reputa-tional score	Cancer mortality rate	COTH member	Interns and residents to beds	Tech-nology score (of 12)	R.N.'s to beds	Board-certified oncologists to beds	Procedures to beds
	TIER ONE									
6	**Stanford University Hospital, Stanford**	30.9	15.3%	0.80	Yes	1.34	10	0.86	0.028	1.64
11	**University of California, San Francisco Medical Center**	21.2	6.0%	0.59	Yes	1.03	11	1.82	0.021	0.92
13	**UCLA Medical Center, Los Angeles**	19.4	4.4%	0.42	Yes	1.52	11	1.20	0.031	2.03
15	**University of California, Davis Medical Center**	19.2	0.8%	0.61	Yes	1.54	11	2.81	0.017	1.29
	TIER TWO									
54	**Loma Linda University Medical Center, Loma Linda**	12.8	0.0%	0.75	Yes	1.14	9	1.61	0.025	1.49
63	**Los Angeles County-USC Medical Center**	12.1	0.4%	0.73	Yes	1.21	8	1.30	0.006	0.13
17	**UCSD Medical Center, San Diego**	16.8	0.4%	0.54	Yes	1.65	8	2.17	0.058	1.66
37	**USC Kenneth Norris Cancer Hospital, Los Angeles**	14.0	1.3%	0.88	No	0.40	8	1.37	0.400	17.13
	TIER THREE									
	California Pacific Medical Center, San Francisco	9.9	0.0%	0.41	Yes	0.33	12	1.19	0.029	0.39
	Cedars-Sinai Medical Center, Los Angeles	8.3	0.5%	1.44	Yes	0.51	8	0.83	0.029	1.49
	City of Hope National Medical Center, Duarte	8.1	2.8%	0.99	No	0.15	7	0.70	0.052	5.19
	Green Hospital of Scripps Clinic, La Jolla	8.9	1.1%	0.86	No	0.21	6	1.99	0.006	3.19
	Hoag Memorial Hospital Presbyterian, Newport Beach	6.4	0.5%	0.75	No	0.00	9	1.26	0.029	2.41
	Hospital of the Good Samaritan, Los Angeles	6.8	0.0%	1.01	Yes	0.04	8	0.98	0.013	1.80
	Huntington Memorial Hospital, Pasadena	5.7	0.0%	1.48	Yes	0.11	8	0.68	0.006	0.94
	Kaiser Foundation Hospital, Los Angeles	8.4	0.0%	0.85	No	0.63	11	1.42	0.010	1.21
	Kaiser Foundation Hospital, Santa Clara	6.2	0.0%	0.88	No	0.29	5	1.58	0.011	2.30
	Kaiser Foundation Hospital, Woodland Hills	7.4	0.0%	0.56	No	0.01	6	2.06	0.032	2.06
	Kaweah Delta District Hospital, Visalia	6.4	0.0%	1.43	No	0.00	8	1.73	0.026	3.69
	Long Beach Memorial Medical Center, Long Beach	6.6	0.0%	0.98	Yes	0.18	8	0.80	0.007	1.16
	Mercy Medical Center, Redding	6.5	0.0%	1.56	No	0.16	7	1.77	0.010	2.88
	N.T. Enloe Memorial Hospital, Chico	6.5	0.0%	0.85	No	0.00	8	1.63	0.010	3.62
	Pomona Valley Hospital Medical Center, Pomona	5.3	0.0%	1.00	No	0.00	8	1.40	0.023	1.16
	Scripps Memorial Hospital, La Jolla	6.2	2.0%	0.93	No	0.00	9	0.71	0.012	1.16
	St. Mary's Hospital and Medical Center, San Francisco	5.7	0.0%	0.78	Yes	0.26	7	0.41	0.008	0.93
	University of California, Irvine Medical Center, Orange	10.2	0.6%	1.03	Yes	0.54	9	1.29	0.015	0.54
	TIER FOUR									
	Alta Bates Medical Center, Berkeley	2.5	0.0%	0.95	No	0.00	7	0.46	0.011	1.65
	Alvarado Hospital Medical Center, San Diego	3.4	0.0%	1.05	No	0.00	7	0.81	0.013	1.76
	Antelope Valley Hospital Medical Center, Lancaster	3.2	0.0%	1.06	No	0.00	5	1.02	0.011	0.69
	Bakersfield Memorial Hospital, Bakersfield	3.6	0.0%	0.98	No	0.00	6	1.02	0.013	1.13
	Beverly Hospital, Montebello	3.3	0.0%	1.23	No	0.00	5	1.09	0.005	1.13

Natl. Rank	Hospital	U.S. News index	Reputa-tional score	Cancer mortality rate	COTH member	Interns and residents to beds	Tech-nology score (of 12)	R.N.'s to beds	Board-certified oncologists to beds	Procedures to beds
	Brookside Hospital, San Pablo	1.4	0.0%	0.89	No	0.00	6	0.20	0.013	0.99
	California Medical Center, Los Angeles	4.7	0.0%	1.02	No	0.13	7	1.18	0.010	1.11
	Centinela Hospital Medical Center, Inglewood	2.8	0.0%	0.97	No	0.00	7	0.65	0.011	0.85
	Community Hospital of Chula Vista, Chula Vista	2.0	0.0%	1.33	No	0.00	5	0.59	0.010	1.62
	Community Memorial Hospital, Ventura	3.3	0.0%	0.80	No	0.00	5	0.85	0.019	1.96
	Dameron Hospital, Stockton	2.0	0.0%	1.35	No	0.00	4	0.76	0.000	1.35
	Daniel Freeman Memorial Hospital, Inglewood	1.3	0.0%	0.78	No	0.04	0	0.64	0.012	1.30
	Desert Hospital, Palm Springs	3.7	0.0%	0.83	No	0.07	5	1.00	0.014	1.19
	Downey Community Hospital, Downey	2.6	0.0%	0.87	No	0.00	4	0.65	0.043	2.39
	Eisenhower Memorial Hospital, Rancho Mirage	4.8	0.0%	0.78	No	0.00	8	0.95	0.029	3.03
	Encino-Tarzana Regional Medical Center, Tarzana	2.3	0.0%	1.00	No	0.00	5	0.66	0.015	1.10
	Fountain Valley Regional Hosp. Med. Ctr., Fountain Valley	2.5	0.0%	0.95	No	0.00	5	0.72	0.020	0.59
	Fresno Community Hospital and Medical Center, Fresno	4.3	0.0%	0.97	No	0.00	9	0.88	0.014	2.07
	Garfield Medical Center, Monterey Park	5.0	0.0%	0.75	No	0.00	7	1.16	0.058	1.66
	Glendale Adventist Medical Center, Glendale	4.5	0.0%	0.68	No	0.15	5	1.06	0.013	1.39
	Glendale Memorial Hospital and Health Center, Glendale	3.3	0.0%	0.75	No	0.00	7	0.69	0.009	1.10
	Good Samaritan Hospital, San Jose	3.2	0.0%	1.11	No	0.00	9	0.52	0.008	2.16
	Grossmont Hospital, La Mesa	2.9	0.0%	1.45	No	0.00	7	0.73	0.007	1.71
	Hemet Valley Medical Center, Hemet	2.8	0.0%	0.78	No	0.00	6	0.64	0.000	1.32
	Inter-Community Medical Center, Covina	2.3	0.0%	1.01	No	0.00	6	0.45	0.041	1.49
	John Muir Medical Center, Walnut Creek	2.6	0.0%	0.86	No	0.01	2	0.88	0.013	2.49
	Kaiser Foundation Hospital, Fontana	4.0	0.0%	0.77	No	0.08	5	1.05	0.011	1.24
	Kaiser Foundation Hospital, West Los Angeles	4.1	0.8%	0.82	No	0.06	4	0.86	0.014	1.42
	Kaiser Foundation Hospital, Oakland	3.6	0.0%	1.05	No	0.33	5	0.72	0.012	1.57
	Kaiser Foundation Hospital, Panorama City	2.2	0.0%	0.95	No	0.01	3	0.79	0.018	1.07
	Kaiser Foundation Hospital, Redwood City	3.6	0.0%	0.72	No	0.00	5	0.96	0.000	1.70
	Kaiser Foundation Hospital, Sacramento	2.0	0.0%	1.27	No	0.19	0	0.83	0.013	2.34
	Kaiser Foundation Hospital, San Diego	3.3	0.5%	0.93	No	0.09	4	0.70	0.015	1.74
	Kaiser Foundation Hospital, San Francisco	4.8	0.6%	0.96	No	0.31	6	0.74	0.012	1.69
	Kaiser Foundation Hospital, Walnut Creek	1.9	0.0%	0.76	No	0.02	4	0.42	0.006	2.30
	Little Company of Mary Hospital, Torrance	2.9	0.0%	0.95	No	0.00	7	0.64	0.017	1.17
	Long Beach Community Hospital, Long Beach	3.7	0.0%	0.72	No	0.00	8	0.74	0.006	1.14
	Marin General Hospital, Greenbrae	2.0	0.0%	0.93	No	0.00	6	0.37	0.021	1.48
	Memorial Hospitals Association, Modesto	4.3	0.0%	1.24	No	0.00	8	1.10	0.011	1.83
	Mercy General Hospital, Sacramento	2.4	0.0%	0.81	No	0.00	3	0.79	0.015	1.35
	Mercy Hospital and Medical Center, San Diego	4.9	0.0%	1.16	No	0.25	8	1.06	0.000	1.37
	Methodist Hospital of Southern California, Arcadia	3.0	0.0%	0.83	No	0.00	7	0.65	0.007	1.09
	Mills-Peninsula Hospitals, Burlingame	2.2	0.0%	0.86	No	0.00	6	0.49	0.012	0.52
	Mount Diablo Medical Center, Concord	2.0	0.0%	1.24	No	0.00	6	0.51	0.007	1.25
	Mount Zion Medical Center, San Francisco	2.1	0.0%	0.86	No	0.28	0	0.69	0.007	1.50
	Northridge Hospital Medical Center, Northridge	3.4	0.0%	1.43	No	0.09	7	0.87	0.012	0.98
	O'Connor Hospital, San Jose	3.8	0.0%	1.04	No	0.00	7	0.82	0.028	2.98
	Palomar Medical Center, Escondido	3.1	0.0%	0.96	No	0.00	7	0.73	0.012	0.94
	Presbyterian Intercommunity Hospital, Whittier	2.9	0.0%	0.73	No	0.07	6	0.55	0.013	1.06
	Queen of Angels-Hollywood Center, Hollywood	2.9	0.0%	0.99	No	0.00	7	0.72	0.005	0.61
	Queen of the Valley Hospital, Napa	4.2	0.0%	0.61	No	0.00	8	0.72	0.006	2.74
	Roseville Hospital, Roseville	2.1	0.0%	0.95	No	0.00	7	0.29	0.005	2.44
	Saddleback Memorial Medical Center, Laguna Hills	3.4	0.0%	0.92	No	0.01	4	1.05	0.027	1.34
	Salinas Valley Memorial Hospital, Salinas	2.1	0.0%	0.69	No	0.00	6	0.28	0.013	1.42
	San Antonio Community Hospital, Upland	4.1	0.0%	0.94	No	0.00	8	1.00	0.007	0.86
	San Gabriel Valley Medical Center, San Gabriel	2.8	0.0%	1.19	No	0.00	8	0.56	0.005	1.46
	San Jose Medical Center, San Jose	2.9	0.0%	1.27	No	0.12	7	0.61	0.013	0.73
	San Pedro Peninsula Hospital, San Pedro	1.6	0.0%	0.82	No	0.00	6	0.28	0.003	0.69
	Santa Barbara Cottage Hospital, Santa Barbara	3.5	0.0%	0.92	No	0.25	2	0.94	0.018	2.37
	Santa Monica Hospital Medical Center, Santa Monica	5.0	0.0%	0.43	No	0.17	8	0.91	0.000	1.84
	Santa Rosa Memorial Hospital, Santa Rosa	1.3	0.0%	1.23	No	0.00	5	0.26	0.013	2.64

Natl. Rank	Hospital	U.S. News index	Reputational score	Cancer mortality rate	COTH member	Interns and residents to beds	Technology score (of 12)	R.N.'s to beds	Board-certified oncologists to beds	Procedures to beds
	Sequoia Hospital District, Redwood City	3.3	0.0%	0.71	No	0.00	8	0.60	0.006	0.89
	Sharp Memorial Hospital, San Diego	4.8	0.0%	1.03	No	0.00	6	1.40	0.036	1.18
	St. Agnes Medical Center, Fresno	5.1	0.5%	1.00	No	0.00	8	0.92	0.022	3.59
	St. Bernardine Medical Center, San Bernardino	3.3	0.0%	1.03	No	0.00	9	0.64	0.006	0.81
	St. Francis Medical Center, Lynwood	3.9	0.0%	0.68	No	0.00	8	0.70	0.013	1.71
	St. Francis Memorial Hospital, San Francisco	2.3	0.0%	0.98	No	0.06	6	0.41	0.000	2.23
	St. John's Hospital and Health Center, Santa Monica	3.9	0.0%	0.77	No	0.00	8	0.64	0.037	2.68
	St. Joseph Hospital, Eureka	2.1	0.0%	1.36	No	0.00	6	0.48	0.012	2.48
	St. Joseph Hospital, Orange	3.7	0.0%	1.20	No	0.01	8	0.92	0.000	1.18
	St. Joseph Medical Center, Burbank	3.7	0.0%	0.62	No	0.00	7	0.77	0.008	1.28
	St. Joseph's Medical Center, Stockton	3.5	0.0%	1.08	No	0.00	8	0.71	0.006	2.42
	St. Jude Medical Center, Fullerton	4.1	0.0%	0.89	No	0.00	9	0.77	0.019	2.07
	St. Mary Medical Center, Long Beach	4.1	0.0%	0.75	No	0.15	8	0.73	0.008	0.68
	St. Vincent Medical Center, Los Angeles	4.3	0.0%	0.61	No	0.01	8	0.84	0.015	1.57
	Sutter General Hospital, Sacramento	2.1	0.0%	0.83	No	0.06	4	0.54	0.017	1.06
	Sutter Memorial Hospital, Sacramento	4.7	0.0%	1.09	No	0.03	7	1.18	0.017	2.88
	Torrance Memorial Medical Center, Torrance	3.8	0.0%	0.96	No	0.00	9	0.79	0.000	1.10
	Tri-City Medical Center, Oceanside	3.3	0.0%	0.62	No	0.01	6	0.63	0.008	2.23
	Washington Hospital, Fremont	3.4	0.0%	0.43	No	0.00	5	0.85	0.013	1.00
	Western Medical Center, Santa Ana	4.4	0.0%	0.81	No	0.04	7	1.05	0.027	0.80
	White Memorial Medical Center, Los Angeles	4.0	0.0%	0.58	No	0.42	5	0.62	0.000	0.96

CARDIOLOGY

Natl. Rank	Hospital	U.S. News index	Reputational score	Cardiology mortality rate	COTH member	Interns and residents to beds	Technology score (of 10)	R.N.'s to beds	Board-certified cardiologists to beds	Procedures to beds
	TIER ONE									
7	Stanford University Hospital, Stanford	54.1	20.3%	0.93	Yes	1.34	9	0.86	0.102	5.19
10	University of California, San Francisco Medical Center	37.0	8.4%	0.96	Yes	1.03	9	1.82	0.043	2.51
12	UCLA Medical Center, Los Angeles	33.4	4.2%	0.68	Yes	1.52	10	1.20	0.034	3.68
15	UCSD Medical Center, San Diego	30.9	0.6%	0.80	Yes	1.65	7	2.17	0.100	3.04
18	Cedars-Sinai Medical Center, Los Angeles	29.4	7.5%	1.06	Yes	0.51	9	0.83	0.113	6.95
	TIER TWO									
75	California Pacific Medical Center, San Francisco	21.5	0.4%	0.96	Yes	0.33	10	1.19	0.069	2.70
77	Kaiser Foundation Hospital, Los Angeles	21.4	0.0%	0.81	No	0.63	9	1.42	0.004	8.39
83	Loma Linda University Medical Center, Loma Linda	21.3	0.0%	1.12	Yes	1.14	9	1.61	0.072	4.43
25	University of California, Davis Medical Center	27.9	0.3%	1.02	Yes	1.54	9	2.81	0.017	3.22
	TIER THREE									
	Beverly Hospital, Montebello	14.1	0.0%	1.03	No	0.00	8	1.09	0.024	7.54
	Brookside Hospital, San Pablo	15.3	0.0%	0.85	No	0.00	7	0.20	0.017	7.47
	Community Memorial Hospital, Ventura	16.1	0.0%	0.95	No	0.00	9	0.85	0.038	8.22
	Desert Hospital, Palm Springs	18.1	0.0%	0.88	No	0.07	8	1.00	0.032	6.41
	Downey Community Hospital, Downey	18.3	0.0%	0.76	No	0.00	9	0.65	0.086	11.50
	Eisenhower Memorial Hospital, Rancho Mirage	18.8	0.0%	0.89	No	0.00	9	0.95	0.063	12.78
	Encino-Tarzana Regional Medical Center, Tarzana	16.6	0.0%	0.67	No	0.00	7	0.66	0.034	3.31
	Fresno Community Hospital and Medical Center, Fresno	13.9	0.0%	1.04	No	0.00	9	0.88	0.030	9.90
	Green Hospital of Scripps Clinic, La Jolla	19.3	0.6%	0.99	No	0.21	8	1.99	0.023	9.78
	Hemet Valley Medical Center, Hemet	14.0	0.0%	0.93	No	0.00	4	0.64	0.010	11.69
	Hospital of the Good Samaritan, Los Angeles	14.0	0.4%	1.23	Yes	0.04	9	0.98	0.032	8.97
	Huntington Memorial Hospital, Pasadena	14.9	0.0%	1.08	Yes	0.11	8	0.68	0.028	4.16
	Kaiser Foundation Hospital, Fontana	17.8	0.0%	0.78	No	0.08	6	1.05	0.013	10.16
	Kaiser Foundation Hospital, West Los Angeles	16.3	0.0%	0.85	No	0.06	3	0.86	0.014	10.08
	Kaiser Foundation Hospital, Panorama City	16.1	0.0%	0.70	No	0.01	4	0.79	0.014	8.84
	Kaiser Foundation Hospital, San Diego	16.1	0.0%	0.77	No	0.09	4	0.70	0.015	7.60
	Kaiser Foundation Hospital, San Francisco	19.1	0.0%	0.72	No	0.31	9	0.74	0.034	11.38

Natl. Rank	Hospital	U.S. News index	Reputational score	Cardiology mortality rate	COTH member	Interns and residents to beds	Technology score (of 10)	R.N.'s to beds	Board-certified cardiologists to beds	Procedures to beds
	Kaiser Foundation Hospital, Santa Clara	20.0	0.0%	0.77	No	0.29	6	1.58	0.019	7.71
	Kaiser Foundation Hospital, Walnut Creek	14.6	0.0%	0.78	No	0.02	2	0.42	0.018	8.60
	Kaiser Foundation Hospital, Woodland Hills	20.1	0.0%	0.87	No	0.01	4	2.06	0.026	9.79
	Little Company of Mary Hospital, Torrance	14.5	0.0%	0.99	No	0.00	8	0.64	0.087	7.01
	Long Beach Community Hospital, Long Beach	16.1	0.0%	0.93	No	0.00	9	0.74	0.029	6.41
	Long Beach Memorial Medical Center, Long Beach	18.3	0.0%	0.96	Yes	0.18	8	0.80	0.035	3.49
	Memorial Hospitals Association, Modesto	17.0	0.0%	0.92	No	0.00	8	1.10	0.032	6.20
	Mercy General Hospital, Sacramento	19.2	0.6%	0.88	No	0.00	8	0.79	0.121	12.28
	Mercy Hospital and Medical Center, San Diego	13.6	0.0%	1.11	No	0.25	8	1.06	0.043	6.17
	Methodist Hospital of Southern California, Arcadia	16.8	0.0%	0.65	No	0.00	7	0.65	0.039	5.34
	Mills-Peninsula Hospitals, Burlingame	14.6	0.0%	0.93	No	0.00	8	0.49	0.034	2.34
	Mount Diablo Medical Center, Concord	14.3	0.0%	0.99	No	0.00	8	0.51	0.078	11.36
	N.T. Enloe Memorial Hospital, Chico	17.1	0.0%	0.99	No	0.00	8	1.63	0.044	12.60
	Northridge Hospital Medical Center, Northridge	18.3	0.0%	0.78	No	0.09	8	0.87	0.056	4.52
	O'Connor Hospital, San Jose	17.5	0.6%	0.93	No	0.00	7	0.82	0.248	16.04
	Presbyterian Intercommunity Hospital, Whittier	15.9	0.0%	0.90	No	0.07	6	0.55	0.033	6.57
	Saddleback Memorial Medical Center, Laguna Hills	18.8	0.0%	0.82	No	0.01	7	1.05	0.059	11.44
	Santa Barbara Cottage Hospital, Santa Barbara	14.2	0.0%	1.05	No	0.25	7	0.94	0.048	6.19
	Santa Monica Hospital Medical Center, Santa Monica	18.4	0.0%	0.89	No	0.17	8	0.91	0.068	5.37
	Scripps Memorial Hospital, La Jolla	18.5	1.6%	0.92	No	0.00	8	0.71	0.042	4.92
	Sequoia Hospital District, Redwood City	16.9	0.0%	0.89	No	0.00	8	0.60	0.047	8.50
	Sharp Memorial Hospital, San Diego	20.0	0.6%	0.88	No	0.00	7	1.40	0.062	5.08
	St. Francis Memorial Hospital, San Francisco	15.1	0.0%	0.89	No	0.06	4	0.41	0.042	5.60
	St. John's Hospital and Health Center, Santa Monica	17.3	0.0%	0.89	No	0.00	8	0.64	0.074	6.41
	St. Joseph Medical Center, Burbank	16.9	0.0%	0.90	No	0.00	8	0.77	0.038	6.37
	St. Joseph's Medical Center, Stockton	14.7	0.0%	1.00	No	0.00	8	0.71	0.066	12.56
	St. Mary Medical Center, Long Beach	17.1	0.0%	0.86	No	0.15	7	0.73	0.024	3.01
	St. Mary's Hospital and Medical Center, San Francisco	17.1	0.0%	0.98	Yes	0.26	7	0.41	0.046	8.50
	St. Vincent Medical Center, Los Angeles	15.5	0.0%	0.97	No	0.01	8	0.84	0.073	5.41
	Sutter General Hospital, Sacramento	13.6	0.0%	0.96	No	0.06	3	0.54	0.100	4.78
	Sutter Memorial Hospital, Sacramento	20.4	0.6%	0.84	No	0.03	8	1.18	0.102	11.23
	Torrance Memorial Medical Center, Torrance	16.9	0.0%	0.86	No	0.00	7	0.79	0.019	5.42
	Tri-City Medical Center, Oceanside	16.7	0.0%	0.90	No	0.01	9	0.63	0.018	10.07
	Washington Hospital, Fremont	18.3	0.0%	0.85	No	0.00	7	0.85	0.067	12.56
	Western Medical Center, Santa Ana	15.7	0.0%	0.99	No	0.04	8	1.05	0.076	4.09
	White Memorial Medical Center, Los Angeles	17.8	0.0%	0.71	No	0.42	7	0.62	0.024	3.41
TIER FOUR										
	Alta Bates Medical Center, Berkeley	12.7	0.0%	0.99	No	0.00	7	0.46	0.018	5.55
	Alvarado Hospital Medical Center, San Diego	13.1	0.0%	1.04	No	0.00	7	0.81	0.035	9.25
	Antelope Valley Hospital Medical Center, Lancaster	8.8	0.0%	1.28	No	0.00	6	1.02	0.030	5.74
	Bakersfield Memorial Hospital, Bakersfield	11.1	0.0%	1.22	No	0.00	8	1.02	0.052	10.79
	California Medical Center, Los Angeles	12.5	0.0%	1.02	No	0.13	1	1.18	0.017	4.16
	Centinela Hospital Medical Center, Inglewood	12.6	0.0%	1.02	No	0.00	7	0.65	0.035	2.83
	Community Hospital of Chula Vista, Chula Vista	10.7	0.0%	1.08	No	0.00	5	0.59	0.035	4.58
	Dameron Hospital, Stockton	8.4	0.0%	1.31	No	0.00	8	0.76	0.033	8.19
	Daniel Freeman Memorial Hospital, Inglewood	12.4	0.0%	0.96	No	0.04	0	0.64	0.033	6.56
	Garfield Medical Center, Monterey Park	10.0	0.0%	1.28	No	0.00	8	1.16	0.049	4.15
	Glendale Adventist Medical Center, Glendale	12.4	0.0%	1.13	No	0.15	7	1.06	0.033	5.65
	Glendale Memorial Hospital and Health Center, Glendale	9.4	0.0%	1.19	No	0.00	8	0.69	0.006	6.28
	Good Samaritan Hospital, San Jose	9.4	0.6%	1.29	No	0.00	9	0.52	0.053	5.94
	Grossmont Hospital, La Mesa	11.3	0.0%	1.12	No	0.00	7	0.73	0.037	7.80
	Hoag Memorial Hospital Presbyterian, Newport Beach	13.2	0.0%	1.14	No	0.00	9	1.26	0.052	6.19
	Inter-Community Medical Center, Covina	13.2	0.0%	1.02	No	0.00	7	0.45	0.077	9.24
	John Muir Medical Center, Walnut Creek	10.5	0.0%	1.22	No	0.01	7	0.88	0.061	9.20
	Kaiser Foundation Hospital, Oakland	11.4	0.0%	1.09	No	0.33	3	0.72	0.027	6.42
	Kaiser Foundation Hospital, Sacramento	8.2	0.0%	1.23	No	0.19	0	0.83	0.033	9.47

Natl. Rank	Hospital	U.S. News index	Reputa-tional score	Cardiology mortality rate	COTH member	Interns and residents to beds	Tech-nology score (of 10)	R.N.'s to beds	Board-certified cardiologists to beds	Procedures to beds
	Kaweah Delta District Hospital, Visalia	10.2	0.0%	1.30	No	0.00	4	1.73	0.031	7.96
	Marin General Hospital, Greenbrae	10.0	0.0%	1.12	No	0.00	6	0.37	0.038	7.93
	Merced Community Medical Center, Merced	10.2	0.0%	1.12	No	0.23	3	0.66	0.019	7.28
	Mercy Medical Center, Redding	8.1	0.0%	1.62	No	0.16	8	1.77	0.025	6.43
	Mount Zion Medical Center, San Francisco	8.7	0.0%	1.15	No	0.28	0	0.69	0.017	4.21
	Palomar Medical Center, Escondido	11.3	0.0%	1.10	No	0.00	7	0.73	0.031	5.10
	Pomona Valley Hospital Medical Center, Pomona	11.8	0.0%	1.24	No	0.00	9	1.40	0.039	8.45
	Queen of Angels-Hollywood Center, Hollywood	13.0	0.0%	0.98	No	0.00	4	0.72	0.031	3.13
	Queen of the Valley Hospital, Napa	11.8	0.0%	1.11	No	0.00	8	0.72	0.031	11.48
	Roseville Hospital, Roseville	13.0	0.0%	0.99	No	0.00	8	0.29	0.028	9.30
	Salinas Valley Memorial Hospital, Salinas	9.3	0.0%	1.17	No	0.00	9	0.28	0.021	8.50
	San Antonio Community Hospital, Upland	12.4	0.0%	1.10	No	0.00	8	1.00	0.034	5.30
	San Gabriel Valley Medical Center, San Gabriel	10.2	0.0%	1.13	No	0.00	6	0.56	0.036	6.17
	San Jose Medical Center, San Jose	9.4	0.6%	1.27	No	0.12	7	0.61	0.033	5.72
	San Pedro Peninsula Hospital, San Pedro	8.4	0.0%	1.15	No	0.00	6	0.28	0.017	2.78
	Santa Rosa Memorial Hospital, Santa Rosa	8.5	0.0%	1.23	No	0.00	7	0.26	0.053	15.88
	St. Agnes Medical Center, Fresno	11.5	0.0%	1.22	No	0.00	10	0.92	0.059	14.79
	St. Bernardine Medical Center, San Bernardino	8.1	0.0%	1.34	No	0.00	10	0.64	0.036	4.96
	St. Francis Medical Center, Lynwood	12.8	0.0%	0.99	No	0.00	5	0.70	0.019	6.32
	St. Joseph Hospital, Eureka	5.4	0.0%	1.41	No	0.00	5	0.48	0.024	11.13
	St. Joseph Hospital, Orange	9.5	0.0%	1.23	No	0.01	9	0.92	0.000	4.09
	St. Jude Medical Center, Fullerton	11.3	0.0%	1.16	No	0.00	9	0.77	0.045	6.24

ENDOCRINOLOGY

Natl. Rank	Hospital	U.S. News index	Reputa-tional score	Endocrinology mortality rate	COTH member	Interns and residents to beds	Tech-nology score (of 11)	R.N.'s to beds	Board-certified internists to beds
TIER ONE									
3	University of California, San Francisco Medical Center	52.2	24.0%	0.78	Yes	1.03	10	1.82	0.435
6	UCLA Medical Center, Los Angeles	37.9	14.1%	0.34	Yes	1.52	11	1.20	0.023
17	Stanford University Hospital, Stanford	25.4	5.2%	0.38	Yes	1.34	11	0.86	0.147
20	UCSD Medical Center, San Diego	22.9	0.8%	0.55	Yes	1.65	8	2.17	0.049
25	University of California, Davis Medical Center	20.7	0.0%	0.90	Yes	1.54	10	2.81	0.032
TIER TWO									
58	California Pacific Medical Center, San Francisco	16.4	0.0%	0.26	Yes	0.33	11	1.19	0.197
81	Kaiser Foundation Hospital, Los Angeles	14.9	0.0%	0.31	No	0.63	10	1.42	0.134
36	Loma Linda University Medical Center, Loma Linda	18.9	0.0%	0.65	Yes	1.14	9	1.61	0.067
30	Los Angeles County-USC Medical Center	20.3	1.7%	0.44	Yes	1.21	8	1.30	0.052
TIER THREE									
	Alta Bates Medical Center, Berkeley	9.1	0.0%	0.48	No	0.00	7	0.46	0.065
	Alvarado Hospital Medical Center, San Diego	8.8	0.0%	0.77	No	0.00	8	0.81	0.065
	Beverly Hospital, Montebello	8.5	0.0%	0.88	No	0.00	7	1.09	0.094
	Cedars-Sinai Medical Center, Los Angeles	13.4	2.3%	1.19	Yes	0.51	9	0.83	0.086
	Community Memorial Hospital, Ventura	9.2	0.0%	0.69	No	0.00	6	0.85	0.038
	Desert Hospital, Palm Springs	9.5	0.0%	0.72	No	0.07	5	1.00	0.069
	Eisenhower Memorial Hospital, Rancho Mirage	8.4	0.0%	0.85	No	0.00	9	0.95	0.054
	Encino-Tarzana Regional Medical Center, Tarzana	9.5	0.0%	0.23	No	0.00	6	0.66	0.065
	Garfield Medical Center, Monterey Park	11.7	0.0%	0.61	No	0.00	7	1.16	0.161
	Glendale Memorial Hospital and Health Center, Glendale	8.6	0.0%	0.73	No	0.00	8	0.69	0.003
	Good Samaritan Hospital, San Jose	11.5	0.0%	0.61	No	0.00	10	0.52	0.288
	Hoag Memorial Hospital Presbyterian, Newport Beach	9.1	0.0%	0.88	No	0.00	9	1.26	0.068
	Inter-Community Medical Center, Covina	8.6	0.0%	0.91	No	0.00	6	0.45	0.418
	Kaiser Foundation Hospital, Fontana	10.9	0.0%	0.51	No	0.08	6	1.05	0.078
	Kaiser Foundation Hospital, West Los Angeles	9.1	0.0%	0.76	No	0.06	4	0.86	0.156
	Kaiser Foundation Hospital, Panorama City	10.1	0.0%	0.49	No	0.01	3	0.79	0.177

STATE RANKINGS ■ CALIFORNIA

Natl. Rank	Hospital	U.S. News index	Reputa-tional score	Endocrinology mortality rate	COTH member	Interns and residents to beds	Tech-nology score (of 11)	R.N.'s to beds	Board-certified internists to beds
	Kaiser Foundation Hospital, San Francisco	9.3	0.0%	0.76	No	0.31	6	0.74	0.067
85	Kaiser Foundation Hospital, Santa Clara	14.3	0.0%	0.41	No	0.29	5	1.58	0.288
	Little Company of Mary Hospital, Torrance	9.7	0.0%	0.58	No	0.00	8	0.64	0.049
	Long Beach Community Hospital, Long Beach	8.1	0.0%	0.89	No	0.00	9	0.74	0.147
	Long Beach Memorial Medical Center, Long Beach	13.1	0.0%	0.47	Yes	0.18	8	0.80	0.037
	Memorial Hospitals Association, Modesto	8.2	0.0%	0.89	No	0.00	8	1.10	0.043
	Mercy Medical Center, Redding	8.2	0.0%	1.35	No	0.16	8	1.77	0.069
	Mount Zion Medical Center, San Francisco	8.5	0.0%	0.70	No	0.28	0	0.69	0.041
	N.T. Enloe Memorial Hospital, Chico	12.2	0.0%	0.52	No	0.00	8	1.63	0.025
	Northridge Hospital Medical Center, Northridge	12.1	0.0%	0.47	No	0.09	7	0.87	0.290
	Pomona Valley Hospital Medical Center, Pomona	9.7	0.0%	0.85	No	0.00	9	1.40	0.057
	Queen of the Valley Hospital, Napa	10.0	0.0%	0.59	No	0.00	9	0.72	0.037
	Salinas Valley Memorial Hospital, Salinas	8.9	0.0%	0.52	No	0.00	7	0.28	0.094
	San Antonio Community Hospital, Upland	10.6	0.0%	0.68	No	0.00	9	1.00	0.068
	Santa Monica Hospital Medical Center, Santa Monica	12.0	0.0%	0.70	No	0.17	9	0.91	0.258
	Scripps Memorial Hospital, La Jolla	8.3	0.9%	0.95	No	0.00	10	0.71	0.037
	St. John's Hospital and Health Center, Santa Monica	11.1	0.0%	0.50	No	0.00	9	0.64	0.212
	St. Joseph Hospital, Orange	8.2	0.0%	1.01	No	0.01	9	0.92	0.206
	St. Jude Medical Center, Fullerton	10.3	0.0%	0.65	No	0.00	10	0.77	0.030
	St. Mary Medical Center, Long Beach	10.4	0.0%	0.51	No	0.15	8	0.73	0.042
	St. Mary's Hospital and Medical Center, San Francisco	11.4	0.0%	0.74	Yes	0.26	8	0.41	0.057
	St. Vincent Medical Center, Los Angeles	8.7	0.0%	0.81	No	0.01	9	0.84	0.076
	Sutter Memorial Hospital, Sacramento	11.1	0.0%	0.46	No	0.03	6	1.18	0.079
	Torrance Memorial Medical Center, Torrance	12.0	0.0%	0.67	No	0.00	9	0.79	0.313
	Valley Medical Center of Fresno, Fresno	8.8	0.0%	1.53	Yes	0.80	7	0.71	0.034
	Washington Hospital, Fremont	10.2	0.0%	0.26	No	0.00	6	0.85	0.089
	White Memorial Medical Center, Los Angeles	10.2	0.0%	0.62	No	0.42	4	0.62	0.039
TIER FOUR									
	Antelope Valley Hospital Medical Center, Lancaster	5.9	0.0%	1.26	No	0.00	5	1.02	0.141
	Bakersfield Memorial Hospital, Bakersfield	7.6	0.0%	1.06	No	0.00	7	1.02	0.185
	Brookside Hospital, San Pablo	4.8	0.0%	1.01	No	0.00	7	0.20	0.057
	California Medical Center, Los Angeles	5.9	0.0%	1.43	No	0.13	5	1.18	0.107
	Centinela Hospital Medical Center, Inglewood	5.9	0.0%	1.20	No	0.00	8	0.65	0.165
	Community Hospital of Chula Vista, Chula Vista	4.0	0.0%	1.29	No	0.00	6	0.59	0.035
	Dameron Hospital, Stockton	6.6	0.0%	1.03	No	0.00	5	0.76	0.175
	Daniel Freeman Memorial Hospital, Inglewood	4.5	0.0%	1.05	No	0.04	0	0.64	0.067
	Downey Community Hospital, Downey	5.1	0.0%	1.11	No	0.00	5	0.65	0.076
	Fresno Community Hospital and Medical Center, Fresno	7.5	0.0%	0.98	No	0.00	10	0.88	0.069
	Glendale Adventist Medical Center, Glendale	7.9	0.0%	0.98	No	0.15	7	1.06	0.067
	Grossmont Hospital, La Mesa	6.4	0.0%	0.95	No	0.00	7	0.73	0.023
	Hemet Valley Medical Center, Hemet	6.1	0.0%	0.95	No	0.00	7	0.64	0.024
	Hospital of the Good Samaritan, Los Angeles	8.1	0.0%	1.45	Yes	0.04	10	0.98	0.067
	Huntington Memorial Hospital, Pasadena	7.9	0.0%	1.23	Yes	0.11	8	0.68	0.059
	John Muir Medical Center, Walnut Creek	5.2	0.0%	1.17	No	0.01	3	0.88	0.095
	Kaiser Foundation Hospital, Oakland	7.8	0.0%	0.89	No	0.33	5	0.72	0.070
	Kaiser Foundation Hospital, Sacramento	2.8	0.0%	1.84	No	0.19	0	0.83	0.069
	Kaiser Foundation Hospital, San Diego	5.8	0.0%	1.10	No	0.09	5	0.70	0.099
	Kaiser Foundation Hospital, Walnut Creek	5.8	0.0%	0.86	No	0.02	3	0.42	0.055
	Kaweah Delta District Hospital, Visalia	6.7	0.0%	1.58	No	0.00	8	1.73	0.061
	Marin General Hospital, Greenbrae	3.3	0.0%	1.53	No	0.00	6	0.37	0.139
	Merced Community Medical Center, Merced	6.6	0.0%	0.96	No	0.23	2	0.66	0.114
	Mercy General Hospital, Sacramento	6.2	0.0%	0.99	No	0.00	4	0.79	0.088
	Mercy Hospital and Medical Center, San Diego	6.0	0.0%	1.56	No	0.25	7	1.06	0.120
	Methodist Hospital of Southern California, Arcadia	6.5	0.0%	0.95	No	0.00	8	0.65	0.042
	Mount Diablo Medical Center, Concord	4.6	0.0%	1.15	No	0.00	7	0.51	0.026
	O'Connor Hospital, San Jose	6.1	0.0%	1.35	No	0.00	8	0.82	0.220

STATE RANKINGS ■ CALIFORNIA

Natl. Rank	Hospital	U.S. News index	Reputa- tional score	Endocrinology mortality rate	COTH member	Interns and residents to beds	Tech- nology score (of 11)	R.N.'s to beds	Board- certified internists to beds
	Palomar Medical Center, Escondido	5.0	0.0%	1.20	No	0.00	8	0.73	0.012
	Presbyterian Intercommunity Hospital, Whittier	6.4	0.4%	1.05	No	0.07	8	0.55	0.066
	Queen of Angels-Hollywood Center, Hollywood	7.4	0.0%	0.91	No	0.00	8	0.72	0.098
	Roseville Hospital, Roseville	5.0	0.0%	1.06	No	0.00	8	0.29	0.073
	Saddleback Memorial Medical Center, Laguna Hills	6.5	0.0%	1.06	No	0.01	5	1.05	0.073
	San Gabriel Valley Medical Center, San Gabriel	7.3	0.0%	0.98	No	0.00	9	0.56	0.180
	San Jose Medical Center, San Jose	6.1	0.0%	1.08	No	0.12	8	0.61	0.066
	San Pedro Peninsula Hospital, San Pedro	4.2	0.0%	1.11	No	0.00	7	0.28	0.030
	Santa Barbara Cottage Hospital, Santa Barbara	8.1	0.0%	1.00	No	0.25	2	0.94	0.253
	Santa Rosa Memorial Hospital, Santa Rosa	7.5	0.0%	0.75	No	0.00	5	0.26	0.160
	Sequoia Hospital District, Redwood City	6.1	0.0%	1.07	No	0.00	8	0.60	0.106
	St. Agnes Medical Center, Fresno	7.4	0.0%	1.05	No	0.00	8	0.92	0.164
	St. Bernardine Medical Center, San Bernardino	4.4	0.0%	1.47	No	0.00	10	0.64	0.043
	St. Francis Medical Center, Lynwood	4.5	0.0%	1.36	No	0.00	8	0.70	0.038
	St. Francis Memorial Hospital, San Francisco	4.9	0.0%	1.13	No	0.06	7	0.41	0.063
	St. Joseph Hospital, Eureka	3.0	0.0%	1.69	No	0.00	8	0.48	0.059
	St. Joseph Medical Center, Burbank	6.5	0.0%	1.00	No	0.00	8	0.77	0.046
	St. Joseph's Medical Center, Stockton	8.0	0.0%	0.81	No	0.00	8	0.71	0.063
	Sutter General Hospital, Sacramento	6.1	0.0%	0.95	No	0.06	5	0.54	0.078
	Tri-City Medical Center, Oceanside	6.7	0.0%	0.92	No	0.01	7	0.63	0.058

GASTROENTEROLOGY

Natl. Rank	Hospital	U.S. News index	Reputa- tional score	Gastro- enterology mortality rate	COTH member	Interns and residents to beds	Tech- nology score (of 11)	R.N.'s to beds	Board- certified gastro- enterologists to beds	Pro- cedures to beds
TIER ONE										
5	UCLA Medical Center, Los Angeles	51.9	23.1%	0.54	Yes	1.52	11	1.20	0.021	1.63
8	University of California, San Francisco Medical Center	47.7	20.8%	0.71	Yes	1.03	10	1.82	0.048	1.11
TIER TWO										
24	Cedars-Sinai Medical Center, Los Angeles	18.4	4.8%	1.02	Yes	0.51	9	0.83	0.037	3.02
21	Stanford University Hospital, Stanford	19.3	2.1%	0.80	Yes	1.34	11	0.86	0.035	2.03
27	University of California, Davis Medical Center	17.6	0.0%	1.25	Yes	1.54	10	2.81	0.008	1.50
TIER THREE										
	Alvarado Hospital Medical Center, San Diego	8.5	0.0%	0.80	No	0.00	7	0.81	0.022	4.13
	California Pacific Medical Center, San Francisco	11.6	0.0%	0.92	Yes	0.33	11	1.19	0.042	0.94
	Eisenhower Memorial Hospital, Rancho Mirage	10.2	0.0%	0.81	No	0.00	8	0.95	0.025	6.01
	Glendale Adventist Medical Center, Glendale	8.3	0.0%	0.84	No	0.15	7	1.06	0.017	2.42
	Green Hospital of Scripps Clinic, La Jolla	11.6	0.0%	0.45	No	0.21	7	1.99	0.012	3.49
	Hoag Memorial Hospital Presbyterian, Newport Beach	9.6	0.0%	0.74	No	0.00	9	1.26	0.031	3.03
	Hospital of the Good Samaritan, Los Angeles	7.7	0.0%	1.40	Yes	0.04	9	0.98	0.016	2.68
	Kaiser Foundation Hospital, Fontana	8.2	0.0%	0.86	No	0.08	6	1.05	0.022	3.52
	Kaiser Foundation Hospital, Los Angeles	11.6	0.0%	0.82	No	0.63	9	1.42	0.002	2.20
	Kaiser Foundation Hospital, San Francisco	8.5	0.0%	0.66	No	0.31	6	0.74	0.018	3.09
	Kaiser Foundation Hospital, Santa Clara	10.0	0.0%	0.73	No	0.29	4	1.58	0.007	3.55
96	Kaiser Foundation Hospital, Woodland Hills	11.9	0.0%	0.60	No	0.01	8	2.06	0.038	4.35
	Kaweah Delta District Hospital, Visalia	7.7	0.0%	1.46	No	0.00	8	1.73	0.015	5.44
77	Loma Linda University Medical Center, Loma Linda	13.1	0.0%	1.32	Yes	1.14	9	1.61	0.018	2.06
	Long Beach Memorial Medical Center, Long Beach	9.8	0.0%	0.88	Yes	0.18	8	0.80	0.014	1.57
	Mercy Medical Center, Redding	7.8	0.0%	1.37	No	0.16	7	1.77	0.020	4.21
	Methodist Hospital of Southern California, Arcadia	7.4	0.0%	0.72	No	0.00	7	0.65	0.013	2.87
	N.T. Enloe Memorial Hospital, Chico	9.2	0.0%	1.07	No	0.00	7	1.63	0.020	5.81
	O'Connor Hospital, San Jose	8.8	0.0%	0.97	No	0.00	7	0.82	0.035	7.02
	Presbyterian Intercommunity Hospital, Whittier	7.6	0.0%	0.74	No	0.07	7	0.55	0.017	3.16
	Queen of the Valley Hospital, Napa	9.5	0.0%	0.77	No	0.00	9	0.72	0.013	5.14

Natl. Rank Hospital	U.S. News index	Reputa-tional score	Gastro-enterology mortality rate	COTH member	Interns and residents to beds	Tech-nology score (of 11)	R.N.'s to beds	Board-certified gastro-enterologists to beds	Pro-cedures to beds
Saddleback Memorial Medical Center, Laguna Hills	7.8	0.0%	0.86	No	0.01	4	1.05	0.041	4.16
Santa Monica Hospital Medical Center, Santa Monica	8.9	0.0%	0.61	No	0.17	8	0.91	0.027	2.78
Scripps Memorial Hospital, La Jolla	7.7	0.0%	0.78	No	0.00	9	0.71	0.014	2.17
St. Agnes Medical Center, Fresno	8.4	0.0%	1.07	No	0.00	7	0.92	0.043	6.97
St. Francis Medical Center, Lynwood	7.4	0.0%	0.80	No	0.00	7	0.70	0.016	2.70
St. John's Hospital and Health Center, Santa Monica	8.1	0.0%	0.60	No	0.00	8	0.64	0.034	3.56
St. Joseph Medical Center, Burbank	8.0	0.0%	0.75	No	0.00	8	0.77	0.015	2.86
St. Jude Medical Center, Fullerton	8.0	0.0%	0.89	No	0.00	10	0.77	0.026	3.21
St. Mary's Hospital and Medical Center, San Francisco	8.4	0.0%	0.97	Yes	0.26	7	0.41	0.016	2.00
Sutter General Hospital, Sacramento	7.4	0.0%	0.71	No	0.06	6	0.54	0.025	3.39
Tri-City Medical Center, Oceanside	8.2	0.0%	0.78	No	0.01	6	0.63	0.013	4.92
Washington Hospital, Fremont	8.2	0.0%	0.64	No	0.00	6	0.85	0.022	3.96
TIER FOUR									
Alta Bates Medical Center, Berkeley	4.7	0.0%	1.06	No	0.00	7	0.46	0.016	2.60
Antelope Valley Hospital Medical Center, Lancaster	2.2	0.0%	1.76	No	0.00	4	1.02	0.011	2.26
Bakersfield Memorial Hospital, Bakersfield	6.4	0.0%	1.03	No	0.00	6	1.02	0.022	3.36
Beverly Hospital, Montebello	6.3	0.0%	1.09	No	0.00	6	1.09	0.005	3.72
Brookside Hospital, San Pablo	3.0	0.0%	1.24	No	0.00	6	0.20	0.017	2.96
California Medical Center, Los Angeles	4.0	0.0%	1.35	No	0.13	4	1.18	0.000	1.83
Centinela Hospital Medical Center, Inglewood	6.3	0.0%	0.86	No	0.00	7	0.65	0.032	1.64
Community Hospital of Chula Vista, Chula Vista	3.0	0.0%	1.22	No	0.00	5	0.59	0.021	1.72
Community Memorial Hospital, Ventura	5.7	0.0%	1.10	No	0.00	5	0.85	0.024	4.16
Dameron Hospital, Stockton	4.2	0.0%	1.19	No	0.00	4	0.76	0.014	3.36
Daniel Freeman Memorial Hospital, Inglewood	5.3	0.0%	0.70	No	0.04	0	0.64	0.018	2.74
Desert Hospital, Palm Springs	7.1	0.0%	0.88	No	0.07	5	1.00	0.017	2.79
Downey Community Hospital, Downey	6.0	0.0%	1.05	No	0.00	5	0.65	0.043	4.75
Encino-Tarzana Regional Medical Center, Tarzana	6.4	0.0%	0.76	No	0.00	6	0.66	0.022	1.66
Fresno Community Hospital and Medical Center, Fresno	4.7	0.0%	1.67	No	0.00	9	0.88	0.017	4.18
Glendale Memorial Hospital and Health Center, Glendale	6.3	0.0%	0.93	No	0.00	7	0.69	0.009	2.77
Good Samaritan Hospital, San Jose	4.4	0.0%	1.30	No	0.00	9	0.52	0.018	2.87
Grossmont Hospital, La Mesa	5.7	0.0%	1.10	No	0.00	6	0.73	0.018	4.07
Hemet Valley Medical Center, Hemet	5.4	0.0%	1.12	No	0.00	6	0.64	0.010	4.12
Huntington Memorial Hospital, Pasadena	7.1	0.0%	1.24	Yes	0.11	8	0.68	0.014	1.73
Inter-Community Medical Center, Covina	3.0	0.0%	1.45	No	0.00	5	0.45	0.026	3.86
John Muir Medical Center, Walnut Creek	5.5	0.0%	1.29	No	0.01	4	0.88	0.035	5.60
Kaiser Foundation Hospital, West Los Angeles	6.7	0.0%	0.91	No	0.06	3	0.86	0.014	4.20
Kaiser Foundation Hospital, Oakland	7.3	0.0%	1.00	No	0.33	5	0.72	0.019	4.25
Kaiser Foundation Hospital, Panorama City	6.6	0.0%	0.67	No	0.01	3	0.79	0.018	3.00
Kaiser Foundation Hospital, Sacramento	4.0	0.0%	1.44	No	0.19	0	0.83	0.016	5.44
Kaiser Foundation Hospital, San Diego	6.7	0.0%	1.04	No	0.09	6	0.70	0.012	4.83
Kaiser Foundation Hospital, Walnut Creek	6.5	0.0%	0.77	No	0.02	2	0.42	0.012	4.73
Little Company of Mary Hospital, Torrance	5.5	0.0%	1.02	No	0.00	7	0.64	0.032	2.60
Long Beach Community Hospital, Long Beach	5.5	0.0%	1.11	No	0.00	8	0.74	0.010	2.89
Marin General Hospital, Greenbrae	5.2	0.0%	0.98	No	0.00	5	0.37	0.025	3.81
Memorial Hospitals Association, Modesto	5.3	0.0%	1.23	No	0.00	7	1.10	0.016	2.57
Mercy General Hospital, Sacramento	7.1	0.0%	0.78	No	0.00	5	0.79	0.028	2.67
Mercy Hospital and Medical Center, San Diego	5.0	0.0%	1.48	No	0.25	6	1.06	0.022	2.93
Mills-Peninsula Hospitals, Burlingame	4.6	0.0%	1.06	No	0.00	8	0.49	0.016	1.72
Mount Diablo Medical Center, Concord	4.7	0.0%	1.13	No	0.00	7	0.51	0.019	3.20
Mount Zion Medical Center, San Francisco	6.0	0.0%	0.81	No	0.28	0	0.69	0.007	2.22
Northridge Hospital Medical Center, Northridge	6.6	0.0%	0.89	No	0.09	6	0.87	0.039	1.74
Palomar Medical Center, Escondido	4.9	0.0%	1.11	No	0.00	7	0.73	0.014	2.36
Pomona Valley Hospital Medical Center, Pomona	6.6	0.0%	1.34	No	0.00	9	1.40	0.013	3.44
Queen of Angels-Hollywood Center, Hollywood	5.2	0.0%	1.00	No	0.00	7	0.72	0.018	1.75
Roseville Hospital, Roseville	6.5	0.0%	0.96	No	0.00	8	0.29	0.009	4.64

Natl. Rank	Hospital	U.S. News index	Reputational score	Gastro-enterology mortality rate	COTH member	Interns and residents to beds	Technology score (of 11)	R.N.'s to beds	Board-certified gastro-enterologists to beds	Pro-cedures to beds
	Salinas Valley Memorial Hospital, Salinas	4.2	0.0%	1.33	No	0.00	7	0.28	0.004	4.97
	San Antonio Community Hospital, Upland	6.9	0.0%	0.95	No	0.00	8	1.00	0.010	2.34
	San Gabriel Valley Medical Center, San Gabriel	6.0	0.0%	1.02	No	0.00	9	0.56	0.014	2.83
	San Jose Medical Center, San Jose	4.6	0.0%	1.20	No	0.12	7	0.61	0.017	2.35
	Santa Barbara Cottage Hospital, Santa Barbara	6.5	0.0%	0.96	No	0.25	2	0.94	0.015	3.56
	Santa Rosa Memorial Hospital, Santa Rosa	5.8	0.0%	0.97	No	0.00	5	0.26	0.018	5.24
	Sequoia Hospital District, Redwood City	6.1	0.0%	0.89	No	0.00	7	0.60	0.018	2.22
	Sharp Memorial Hospital, San Diego	5.8	0.0%	1.16	No	0.00	6	1.40	0.026	2.15
	St. Bernardine Medical Center, San Bernardino	4.2	0.0%	1.25	No	0.00	9	0.64	0.009	1.81
	St. Francis Memorial Hospital, San Francisco	4.1	0.0%	1.15	No	0.06	6	0.41	0.016	2.71
	St. Joseph Hospital, Eureka	5.8	0.0%	1.36	No	0.00	7	0.48	0.012	6.98
	St. Joseph Hospital, Orange	7.2	0.0%	0.94	No	0.01	9	0.92	0.000	2.53
	St. Joseph's Medical Center, Stockton	7.1	0.0%	1.00	No	0.00	7	0.71	0.016	5.12
	St. Mary Medical Center, Long Beach	3.5	0.0%	1.49	No	0.15	8	0.73	0.014	1.39
	St. Vincent Medical Center, Los Angeles	7.1	0.0%	0.93	No	0.01	8	0.84	0.024	3.02
	Sutter Memorial Hospital, Sacramento	7.2	0.0%	0.83	No	0.03	5	1.18	0.025	1.63
	Torrance Memorial Medical Center, Torrance	5.4	0.0%	1.15	No	0.00	9	0.79	0.009	2.29

GERIATRICS

Natl. Rank	Hospital	U.S. News index	Reputational score	Hospital-wide mortality rate	COTH member	Service mix	Interns and residents to beds	Technology score (of 13)	R.N.'s to beds	Discharge planning (of 2)	Geriatric services (of 9)	Board-certified internists to beds
TIER ONE												
1	UCLA Medical Center, Los Angeles	100.0	27.9%	0.66	Yes	8	1.52	12	1.20	2	5	0.023
13	Stanford University Hospital, Stanford	39.1	6.0%	0.90	Yes	4	1.34	12	0.86	2	1	0.147
14	University of California, San Francisco Medical Center	38.9	3.9%	0.89	Yes	7	1.03	12	1.82	2	6	0.435
18	UCSD Medical Center, San Diego	32.1	1.8%	0.75	Yes	6	1.65	9	2.17	2	4	0.049
TIER TWO												
45	California Pacific Medical Center, San Francisco	24.9	0.0%	0.87	Yes	8	0.33	13	1.19	2	5	0.197
68	Kaiser Foundation Hospital, Los Angeles	22.7	0.0%	0.86	No	8	0.63	12	1.42	2	2	0.134
39	University of California, Davis Medical Center	26.0	0.0%	1.01	Yes	8	1.54	12	2.81	2	4	0.032
TIER THREE												
	Alta Bates Medical Center, Berkeley	16.4	0.0%	0.96	No	8	0.00	9	0.46	2	3	0.065
	Alvarado Hospital Medical Center, San Diego	16.2	0.0%	0.92	No	3	0.00	9	0.81	2	3	0.065
	Beverly Hospital, Montebello	15.5	0.0%	0.90	No	2	0.00	9	1.09	1	1	0.094
	Cedars-Sinai Medical Center, Los Angeles	19.9	1.0%	1.13	Yes	9	0.51	11	0.83	2	4	0.086
	Centinela Hospital Medical Center, Inglewood	15.6	0.0%	0.96	No	5	0.00	9	0.65	2	1	0.165
	Desert Hospital, Palm Springs	19.2	0.0%	0.85	No	7	0.07	8	1.00	2	3	0.069
	Downey Community Hospital, Downey	14.9	0.0%	0.92	No	4	0.00	7	0.65	1	3	0.076
	Eisenhower Memorial Hospital, Rancho Mirage	17.1	0.0%	0.86	No	4	0.00	11	0.95	1	3	0.054
	Encino-Tarzana Regional Medical Center, Tarzana	18.0	0.0%	0.78	No	6	0.00	8	0.66	2	3	0.065
	Garfield Medical Center, Monterey Park	18.4	0.0%	0.90	No	4	0.00	8	1.16	2	3	0.161
	Glendale Adventist Medical Center, Glendale	15.5	0.0%	1.00	No	6	0.15	9	1.06	2	1	0.067
	Hoag Memorial Hospital Presbyterian, Newport Beach	18.1	0.0%	0.94	No	5	0.00	12	1.26	2	3	0.068
	Huntington Memorial Hospital, Pasadena	15.0	0.0%	1.11	Yes	6	0.11	10	0.68	2	5	0.059
	Kaiser Foundation Hospital, Fontana	18.3	0.0%	0.88	No	6	0.08	7	1.05	2	1	0.078
	Kaiser Foundation Hospital, West Los Angeles	17.9	0.0%	0.89	No	6	0.06	4	0.86	2	2	0.156
	Kaiser Foundation Hospital, Oakland	14.8	0.0%	1.07	No	10	0.33	5	0.72	2	3	0.070
	Kaiser Foundation Hospital, Panorama City	17.9	0.0%	0.82	No	7	0.01	4	0.79	2	1	0.177
	Kaiser Foundation Hospital, Redwood City	17.4	0.0%	0.93	No	5	0.00	7	0.96	2	3	0.205
	Kaiser Foundation Hospital, San Diego	16.1	0.0%	0.92	No	7	0.09	5	0.70	1	3	0.099
	Kaiser Foundation Hospital, San Francisco	19.0	0.0%	0.82	No	7	0.31	8	0.74	2	2	0.067
	Kaiser Foundation Hospital, Santa Clara	19.5	0.0%	0.94	No	5	0.29	6	1.58	2	4	0.288
	Little Company of Mary Hospital, Torrance	14.9	0.0%	0.89	No	2	0.00	10	0.64	1	1	0.049

Natl. Rank	Hospital	U.S. News index	Reputational score	Hospital-wide mortality rate	COTH member	Service mix	Interns and residents to beds	Technology score (of 13)	R.N.'s to beds	Discharge planning (of 2)	Geriatric services (of 9)	Board-certified internists to beds
96	Loma Linda University Medical Center, Loma Linda	20.6	0.4%	1.07	Yes	6	1.14	12	1.61	2	1	0.067
	Long Beach Community Hospital, Long Beach	16.5	0.0%	0.97	No	4	0.00	11	0.74	2	6	0.147
	Long Beach Memorial Medical Center, Long Beach	19.4	0.0%	1.00	Yes	8	0.18	10	0.80	2	7	0.037
	Mercy General Hospital, Sacramento	17.3	0.0%	0.87	No	4	0.00	6	0.79	2	4	0.088
	Methodist Hospital of Southern California, Arcadia	18.1	0.0%	0.72	No	5	0.00	9	0.65	2	5	0.042
	Mills-Peninsula Hospitals, Burlingame	18.1	0.0%	0.92	No	6	0.00	10	0.49	2	6	0.086
	Northridge Hospital Medical Center, Northridge	19.1	0.0%	0.95	No	7	0.09	8	0.87	2	6	0.290
	O'Connor Hospital, San Jose	14.9	0.0%	1.06	No	6	0.00	9	0.82	2	5	0.220
	Presbyterian Intercommunity Hospital, Whittier	14.2	0.0%	0.93	No	4	0.07	8	0.55	1	1	0.066
	Queen of Angels-Hollywood Center, Hollywood	17.1	0.0%	0.85	No	4	0.00	9	0.72	2	1	0.098
	Queen of the Valley Hospital, Napa	17.5	0.0%	0.84	No	4	0.00	10	0.72	2	3	0.037
	Saddleback Memorial Medical Center, Laguna Hills	18.3	0.0%	0.83	No	6	0.01	7	1.05	2	2	0.073
	San Antonio Community Hospital, Upland	15.8	0.0%	0.96	No	5	0.00	10	1.00	2	1	0.068
	San Pedro Peninsula Hospital, San Pedro	18.2	0.0%	0.85	No	7	0.00	9	0.28	2	5	0.030
	Santa Monica Hospital Medical Center, Santa Monica	18.7	0.0%	0.74	No	3	0.17	10	0.91	2	2	0.258
	Sequoia Hospital District, Redwood City	16.9	0.0%	0.86	No	5	0.00	11	0.60	1	2	0.106
	Sharp Memorial Hospital, San Diego	14.6	0.0%	1.02	No	6	0.00	7	1.40	2	1	0.052
	St. Joseph Hospital, Orange	14.4	0.0%	1.09	No	6	0.01	11	0.92	2	4	0.206
	St. Joseph Medical Center, Burbank	18.7	0.0%	0.82	No	6	0.00	10	0.77	2	4	0.046
	St. Jude Medical Center, Fullerton	15.0	0.0%	1.04	No	6	0.00	11	0.77	2	6	0.030
	St. Mary Medical Center, Long Beach	19.6	0.0%	0.86	No	6	0.15	9	0.73	2	7	0.042
	St. Mary's Hospital and Medical Center, San Francisco	18.4	0.0%	0.99	Yes	7	0.26	9	0.41	2	6	0.057
	St. Vincent Medical Center, Los Angeles	17.9	0.0%	0.85	No	5	0.01	9	0.84	2	2	0.076
	Sutter Memorial Hospital, Sacramento	17.0	0.0%	0.91	No	6	0.03	9	1.18	1	1	0.079
	Torrance Memorial Medical Center, Torrance	17.5	0.0%	0.92	No	4	0.00	9	0.79	2	1	0.313
	Tri-City Medical Center, Oceanside	18.3	0.0%	0.82	No	6	0.01	9	0.63	2	4	0.058
	Washington Hospital, Fremont	16.5	0.0%	0.79	No	3	0.00	7	0.85	2	1	0.089
	White Memorial Medical Center, Los Angeles	17.9	0.0%	0.74	No	5	0.42	6	0.62	2	3	0.039
	TIER FOUR											
	Antelope Valley Hospital Medical Center, Lancaster	9.1	0.0%	1.30	No	7	0.00	7	1.02	2	2	0.141
	Brookside Hospital, San Pablo	11.2	0.0%	1.06	No	4	0.00	9	0.20	2	2	0.057
	California Medical Center, Los Angeles	9.5	0.0%	1.16	No	5	0.13	5	1.18	1	1	0.107
	Community Hospital of Chula Vista, Chula Vista	10.1	0.0%	1.08	No	3	0.00	7	0.59	2	1	0.035
	Community Memorial Hospital, Ventura	11.5	0.0%	1.02	No	3	0.00	8	0.85	1	2	0.038
	Dameron Hospital, Stockton	7.8	0.0%	1.27	No	3	0.00	7	0.76	2	3	0.175
	Fresno Community Hospital and Medical Center, Fresno	11.7	0.0%	1.17	No	6	0.00	11	0.88	2	4	0.069
	Glendale Memorial Hospital and Health Center, Glendale	12.7	0.0%	1.01	No	6	0.00	10	0.69	1	1	0.003
	Good Samaritan Hospital, San Jose	12.2	0.0%	1.20	No	8	0.00	11	0.52	2	3	0.288
	Grossmont Hospital, La Mesa	11.5	0.0%	1.12	No	6	0.00	9	0.73	2	2	0.023
	Hemet Valley Medical Center, Hemet	9.9	0.0%	1.07	No	3	0.00	9	0.64	1	1	0.024
	Hospital of the Good Samaritan, Los Angeles	12.7	0.0%	1.19	Yes	5	0.04	11	0.98	2	2	0.067
	John Muir Medical Center, Walnut Creek	8.5	0.0%	1.15	No	4	0.01	5	0.88	1	1	0.095
	Kaiser Foundation Hospital, Walnut Creek	12.6	0.0%	0.96	No	3	0.02	3	0.42	2	1	0.055
	Kaweah Delta District Hospital, Visalia	8.0	0.0%	1.33	No	5	0.00	10	1.73	1	1	0.061
	Marin General Hospital, Greenbrae	9.3	0.0%	1.18	No	6	0.00	9	0.37	1	3	0.139
	Memorial Hospitals Association, Modesto	12.7	0.0%	1.12	No	6	0.00	11	1.10	2	2	0.043
	Mercy Hospital and Medical Center, San Diego	10.8	0.0%	1.25	No	5	0.25	9	1.06	2	5	0.120
	Mercy Medical Center, Redding	5.1	0.0%	1.58	No	4	0.16	11	1.77	1	2	0.069
	Mount Diablo Medical Center, Concord	12.6	0.0%	1.05	No	5	0.00	9	0.51	2	3	0.026
	Palomar Medical Center, Escondido	12.4	0.0%	1.09	No	6	0.00	9	0.73	2	4	0.012
	Pomona Valley Hospital Medical Center, Pomona	11.7	0.0%	1.12	No	3	0.00	11	1.40	2	1	0.057
	Roseville Hospital, Roseville	10.9	0.0%	1.13	No	6	0.00	10	0.29	2	3	0.073
	Salinas Valley Memorial Hospital, Salinas	10.2	0.0%	1.11	No	4	0.00	9	0.28	2	2	0.094
	San Gabriel Valley Medical Center, San Gabriel	11.9	0.0%	1.09	No	4	0.00	10	0.56	2	2	0.180
	San Jose Medical Center, San Jose	7.6	0.0%	1.31	No	6	0.12	9	0.61	1	5	0.066
	Santa Rosa Memorial Hospital, Santa Rosa	8.2	0.0%	1.17	No	3	0.00	6	0.26	2	2	0.160

STATE RANKINGS ■ CALIFORNIA

Natl. Rank	Hospital	U.S. News index	Reputa-tional score	Hospital-wide mortality rate	COTH member	Service mix	Interns and residents to beds	Tech-nology score (of 13)	R.N.'s to beds	Discharge planning (of 2)	Geriatric services (of 9)	Board-certified internists to beds
	Scripps Memorial Hospital, La Jolla	13.1	0.0%	1.06	No	6	0.00	10	0.71	2	2	0.037
	St. Agnes Medical Center, Fresno	12.2	0.0%	1.17	No	5	0.00	11	0.92	2	5	0.164
	St. Bernardine Medical Center, San Bernardino	9.9	0.0%	1.26	No	8	0.00	12	0.64	2	2	0.043
	St. Francis Medical Center, Lynwood	12.4	0.0%	1.02	No	3	0.00	8	0.70	2	2	0.038
	St. Francis Memorial Hospital, San Francisco	11.4	0.0%	1.03	No	5	0.06	9	0.41	1	1	0.063
	St. Joseph's Medical Center, Stockton	12.1	0.0%	1.09	No	4	0.00	11	0.71	2	3	0.063
	Sutter General Hospital, Sacramento	11.2	0.0%	0.99	No	2	0.06	5	0.54	1	2	0.078

GYNECOLOGY

Natl. Rank	Hospital	U.S. News index	Reputa-tional score	Hospital-wide mortality rate	Interns and residents to beds	Tech-nology score (of 10)	R.N.'s to beds	Board-certified OB-GYNs to beds	Procedures to beds
	TIER ONE								
6	Los Angeles County-USC Medical Center	55.9	11.7%	0.88	1.21	7	1.30	0.021	0.03
10	UCLA Medical Center, Los Angeles	49.1	7.8%	0.66	1.52	10	1.20	0.028	0.49
13	Stanford University Hospital, Stanford	43.0	6.1%	0.90	1.34	9	0.86	0.107	0.39
14	University of California, San Francisco Medical Center	42.6	5.3%	0.89	1.03	9	1.82	0.043	0.21
20	UCSD Medical Center, San Diego	35.0	0.8%	0.75	1.65	7	2.17	0.078	0.33
24	University of California, Davis Medical Center	32.8	0.5%	1.01	1.54	9	2.81	0.025	0.36
	TIER TWO								
56	California Pacific Medical Center, San Francisco	25.3	0.0%	0.87	0.33	10	1.19	0.133	0.12
39	Cedars-Sinai Medical Center, Los Angeles	28.0	4.5%	1.13	0.51	8	0.83	0.094	0.48
59	Green Hospital of Scripps Clinic, La Jolla	25.0	0.4%	0.86	0.21	6	1.99	0.035	1.06
54	Kaiser Foundation Hospital, Los Angeles	26.0	0.0%	0.86	0.63	9	1.42	0.060	0.35
79	Kaiser Foundation Hospital, Woodland Hills	22.6	0.0%	0.80	0.01	6	2.06	0.006	0.54
77	Santa Monica Hospital Medical Center, Santa Monica	23.0	0.4%	0.74	0.17	8	0.91	0.139	0.50
	TIER THREE								
	Alta Bates Medical Center, Berkeley	15.0	0.0%	0.96	0.00	7	0.46	0.054	0.40
	Alvarado Hospital Medical Center, San Diego	17.3	0.0%	0.92	0.00	7	0.81	0.035	0.47
	Beverly Hospital, Montebello	17.5	0.0%	0.90	0.00	5	1.09	0.024	0.48
	Centinela Hospital Medical Center, Inglewood	16.3	0.0%	0.96	0.00	7	0.65	0.069	0.20
	Desert Hospital, Palm Springs	17.7	0.0%	0.85	0.07	4	1.00	0.046	0.31
	Downey Community Hospital, Downey	15.9	0.0%	0.92	0.00	6	0.65	0.032	0.88
	Eisenhower Memorial Hospital, Rancho Mirage	19.0	0.0%	0.86	0.00	7	0.95	0.029	0.90
95	Hoag Memorial Hospital Presbyterian, Newport Beach	21.4	0.4%	0.94	0.00	7	1.26	0.104	0.66
	Kaiser Foundation Hospital, Fontana	19.8	0.0%	0.88	0.08	6	1.05	0.062	0.36
	Kaiser Foundation Hospital, West Los Angeles	17.6	0.0%	0.89	0.06	4	0.86	0.066	0.29
	Kaiser Foundation Hospital, Panorama City	17.4	0.0%	0.82	0.01	5	0.79	0.050	0.33
	Kaiser Foundation Hospital, San Diego	17.6	0.0%	0.92	0.09	6	0.70	0.087	0.60
	Kaiser Foundation Hospital, San Francisco	19.0	0.0%	0.82	0.31	6	0.74	0.043	0.38
	Kaiser Foundation Hospital, Santa Clara	21.0	0.0%	0.94	0.29	5	1.58	0.082	0.61
	Long Beach Community Hospital, Long Beach	16.2	0.0%	0.97	0.00	8	0.74	0.038	0.36
	Long Beach Memorial Medical Center, Long Beach	17.3	0.5%	1.00	0.18	7	0.80	0.055	0.41
	Mercy General Hospital, Sacramento	16.7	0.0%	0.87	0.00	4	0.79	0.053	0.39
	Methodist Hospital of Southern California, Arcadia	17.7	0.0%	0.72	0.00	7	0.65	0.029	0.48
	N.T. Enloe Memorial Hospital, Chico	18.4	0.0%	1.01	0.00	7	1.63	0.044	0.70
	Northridge Hospital Medical Center, Northridge	17.9	0.0%	0.95	0.09	6	0.87	0.130	0.23
	O'Connor Hospital, San Jose	15.0	0.0%	1.06	0.00	7	0.82	0.177	1.18
	Pomona Valley Hospital Medical Center, Pomona	15.9	0.0%	1.12	0.00	8	1.40	0.062	0.61
	Presbyterian Intercommunity Hospital, Whittier	16.5	0.0%	0.93	0.07	7	0.55	0.046	0.50
	Queen of Angels-Hollywood Center, Hollywood	18.6	0.0%	0.85	0.00	7	0.72	0.054	0.18
	Queen of the Valley Hospital, Napa	18.6	0.0%	0.84	0.00	8	0.72	0.025	0.54
	Saddleback Memorial Medical Center, Laguna Hills	18.3	0.0%	0.83	0.01	3	1.05	0.109	0.45
	San Antonio Community Hospital, Upland	18.4	0.0%	0.96	0.00	7	1.00	0.108	0.40
	Scripps Memorial Hospital, La Jolla	14.4	0.0%	1.06	0.00	8	0.71	0.065	0.34

Natl. Rank	Hospital	U.S. News index	Reputa-tional score	Hospital-wide mortality rate	Interns and residents to beds	Technology score (of 10)	R.N.'s to beds	Board-certified OB-GYNs to beds	Procedures to beds
	Sequoia Hospital District, Redwood City	17.4	0.0%	0.86	0.00	6	0.60	0.059	0.36
	Sharp Memorial Hospital, San Diego	17.7	0.0%	1.02	0.00	6	1.40	0.143	0.50
	St. Francis Medical Center, Lynwood	14.5	0.0%	1.02	0.00	8	0.70	0.029	0.21
	St. John's Hospital and Health Center, Santa Monica	20.0	0.0%	0.80	0.00	8	0.64	0.146	0.44
	St. Joseph Hospital, Orange	14.3	0.0%	1.09	0.01	7	0.92	0.081	0.55
	St. Joseph Medical Center, Burbank	19.2	0.3%	0.82	0.00	7	0.77	0.038	0.32
	St. Jude Medical Center, Fullerton	16.0	0.0%	1.04	0.00	9	0.77	0.071	0.57
	St. Mary Medical Center, Long Beach	19.0	0.4%	0.86	0.15	6	0.73	0.026	0.18
	St. Vincent Medical Center, Los Angeles	18.1	0.0%	0.85	0.01	7	0.84	0.012	0.26
	Sutter Memorial Hospital, Sacramento	19.4	0.0%	0.91	0.03	5	1.18	0.113	0.99
	Torrance Memorial Medical Center, Torrance	19.6	0.0%	0.92	0.00	8	0.79	0.153	0.32
	Tri-City Medical Center, Oceanside	17.2	0.0%	0.82	0.01	6	0.63	0.042	0.74
	Washington Hospital, Fremont	19.0	0.0%	0.79	0.00	6	0.85	0.080	0.39
	White Memorial Medical Center, Los Angeles	17.8	0.0%	0.74	0.42	5	0.62	0.021	0.17
TIER FOUR									
	Antelope Valley Hospital Medical Center, Lancaster	7.4	0.0%	1.30	0.00	4	1.02	0.033	0.37
	Bakersfield Memorial Hospital, Bakersfield	11.2	0.0%	1.21	0.00	6	1.02	0.069	0.71
	Brookside Hospital, San Pablo	8.9	0.0%	1.06	0.00	5	0.20	0.017	0.17
	California Medical Center, Los Angeles	12.3	0.0%	1.16	0.13	5	1.18	0.054	0.40
	Community Hospital of Chula Vista, Chula Vista	10.0	0.0%	1.08	0.00	5	0.59	0.017	0.15
	Community Memorial Hospital, Ventura	13.8	0.0%	1.02	0.00	5	0.85	0.067	0.85
	Dameron Hospital, Stockton	8.3	0.0%	1.27	0.00	5	0.76	0.076	0.81
	Fresno Community Hospital and Medical Center, Fresno	12.9	0.0%	1.17	0.00	9	0.88	0.044	0.45
	Glendale Memorial Hospital and Health Center, Glendale	13.0	0.0%	1.01	0.00	6	0.69	0.022	0.26
	Good Samaritan Hospital, San Jose	11.8	0.0%	1.20	0.00	9	0.52	0.095	0.56
	Grossmont Hospital, La Mesa	11.3	0.0%	1.12	0.00	6	0.73	0.046	0.62
	Hemet Valley Medical Center, Hemet	10.5	0.0%	1.07	0.00	5	0.64	0.010	0.41
	Huntington Memorial Hospital, Pasadena	12.5	0.0%	1.11	0.11	7	0.68	0.048	0.41
	Inter-Community Medical Center, Covina	11.5	0.0%	1.11	0.00	6	0.45	0.134	0.50
	John Muir Medical Center, Walnut Creek	11.2	0.0%	1.15	0.01	4	0.88	0.160	0.57
	Kaiser Foundation Hospital, Oakland	12.9	0.0%	1.07	0.33	5	0.72	0.039	0.68
	Kaiser Foundation Hospital, Walnut Creek	11.7	0.0%	0.96	0.02	3	0.42	0.031	0.57
	Kaweah Delta District Hospital, Visalia	12.5	0.0%	1.33	0.00	7	1.73	0.051	0.69
	Marin General Hospital, Greenbrae	8.3	0.0%	1.18	0.00	5	0.37	0.072	0.43
	Memorial Hospitals Association, Modesto	12.7	0.0%	1.12	0.00	6	1.10	0.038	0.43
	Mercy Hospital and Medical Center, San Diego	12.6	0.0%	1.25	0.25	7	1.06	0.082	0.39
	Mercy Medical Center, Redding	9.7	0.0%	1.58	0.16	6	1.77	0.064	1.12
	Mount Diablo Medical Center, Concord	12.1	0.0%	1.05	0.00	6	0.51	0.052	0.24
	Palomar Medical Center, Escondido	12.2	0.0%	1.09	0.00	7	0.73	0.033	0.35
	Roseville Hospital, Roseville	8.8	0.0%	1.13	0.00	6	0.29	0.041	0.41
	Salinas Valley Memorial Hospital, Salinas	7.8	0.0%	1.11	0.00	4	0.28	0.038	0.64
	San Gabriel Valley Medical Center, San Gabriel	11.1	0.0%	1.09	0.00	7	0.56	0.014	0.35
	San Jose Medical Center, San Jose	7.6	0.0%	1.31	0.12	6	0.61	0.046	0.24
	Santa Barbara Cottage Hospital, Santa Barbara	13.3	0.0%	1.07	0.25	4	0.94	0.057	0.78
	Santa Rosa Memorial Hospital, Santa Rosa	8.4	0.0%	1.17	0.00	6	0.26	0.062	0.60
	St. Agnes Medical Center, Fresno	12.3	0.0%	1.17	0.00	6	0.92	0.121	1.12
	St. Bernardine Medical Center, San Bernardino	9.5	0.0%	1.26	0.00	9	0.64	0.019	0.21
	St. Francis Memorial Hospital, San Francisco	11.3	0.0%	1.03	0.06	5	0.41	0.042	0.17
	St. Joseph's Medical Center, Stockton	11.9	0.0%	1.09	0.00	6	0.71	0.047	0.75
	St. Mary's Hospital and Medical Center, San Francisco	13.8	0.0%	0.99	0.26	6	0.41	0.030	0.13

NEUROLOGY

Natl. Rank	Hospital	U.S. News index	Reputa-tional score	Neurology mortality rate	COTH member	Interns and residents to beds	Tech-nology score (of 9)	R.N.'s to beds	Board-certified neurologists to beds
	TIER ONE								
3	University of California, San Francisco Medical Center	63.9	27.3%	0.91	Yes	1.03	8	1.82	0.029
6	UCLA Medical Center, Los Angeles	41.4	9.6%	0.69	Yes	1.52	9	1.20	0.056
15	Stanford University Hospital, Stanford	27.5	3.2%	0.79	Yes	1.34	9	0.86	0.031
	TIER TWO								
54	California Pacific Medical Center, San Francisco	19.7	0.0%	0.73	Yes	0.33	9	1.19	0.015
85	Green Hospital of Scripps Clinic, La Jolla	17.9	0.0%	0.77	No	0.21	6	1.99	0.012
70	Kaiser Foundation Hospital, Los Angeles	18.4	0.0%	0.59	No	0.63	8	1.42	0.010
36	Loma Linda University Medical Center, Loma Linda	22.6	0.0%	0.78	Yes	1.14	7	1.61	0.018
33	UCSD Medical Center, San Diego	23.1	0.4%	1.14	Yes	1.65	6	2.17	0.075
38	University of California, Davis Medical Center	22.4	0.6%	1.07	Yes	1.54	8	2.81	0.017
	TIER THREE								
	Alvarado Hospital Medical Center, San Diego	11.0	0.0%	0.91	No	0.00	6	0.81	0.013
	Cedars-Sinai Medical Center, Los Angeles	11.9	0.0%	1.14	Yes	0.51	7	0.83	0.016
	Centinela Hospital Medical Center, Inglewood	13.9	0.0%	0.64	No	0.00	6	0.65	0.011
	Desert Hospital, Palm Springs	14.4	0.0%	0.73	No	0.07	4	1.00	0.011
	Eisenhower Memorial Hospital, Rancho Mirage	15.8	0.0%	0.69	No	0.00	7	0.95	0.025
	Glendale Adventist Medical Center, Glendale	15.2	0.0%	0.56	No	0.15	5	1.06	0.013
	Glendale Memorial Hospital and Health Center, Glendale	13.8	0.0%	0.71	No	0.00	6	0.69	0.009
	Good Samaritan Hospital, San Jose	14.7	0.0%	0.73	No	0.00	8	0.52	0.020
	Hemet Valley Medical Center, Hemet	11.0	0.0%	0.85	No	0.00	5	0.64	0.007
	Hoag Memorial Hospital Presbyterian, Newport Beach	13.9	0.0%	0.89	No	0.00	7	1.26	0.029
	Hospital of the Good Samaritan, Los Angeles	14.1	0.0%	0.93	Yes	0.04	8	0.98	0.013
	Huntington Memorial Hospital, Pasadena	12.2	0.0%	0.94	Yes	0.11	6	0.68	0.005
	Kaiser Foundation Hospital, Fontana	14.8	0.0%	0.75	No	0.08	5	1.05	0.011
	Kaiser Foundation Hospital, West Los Angeles	13.9	0.0%	0.60	No	0.06	3	0.86	0.014
	Kaiser Foundation Hospital, Oakland	12.9	0.0%	0.84	No	0.33	4	0.72	0.016
	Kaiser Foundation Hospital, Redwood City	14.8	0.0%	0.55	No	0.00	6	0.96	0.013
	Kaiser Foundation Hospital, San Diego	14.6	0.0%	0.63	No	0.09	5	0.70	0.020
	Kaiser Foundation Hospital, San Francisco	13.8	0.0%	0.80	No	0.31	5	0.74	0.012
	Kaiser Foundation Hospital, Woodland Hills	16.7	0.0%	0.81	No	0.01	6	2.06	0.019
	Kaweah Delta District Hospital, Visalia	12.5	0.0%	0.98	No	0.00	6	1.73	0.020
	Little Company of Mary Hospital, Torrance	14.6	0.0%	0.70	No	0.00	6	0.64	0.023
	Long Beach Community Hospital, Long Beach	12.7	0.0%	0.83	No	0.00	7	0.74	0.010
	Long Beach Memorial Medical Center, Long Beach	11.1	0.0%	1.05	Yes	0.18	6	0.80	0.008
	Mercy General Hospital, Sacramento	14.4	0.0%	0.50	No	0.00	4	0.79	0.023
	Methodist Hospital of Southern California, Arcadia	14.2	0.0%	0.53	No	0.00	6	0.65	0.016
	N.T. Enloe Memorial Hospital, Chico	14.2	0.0%	0.86	No	0.00	6	1.63	0.015
	Northridge Hospital Medical Center, Northridge	12.1	0.0%	0.99	No	0.09	5	0.87	0.048
	Pomona Valley Hospital Medical Center, Pomona	12.4	0.0%	0.94	No	0.00	7	1.40	0.015
	Queen of Angels-Hollywood Center, Hollywood	14.2	0.0%	0.70	No	0.00	6	0.72	0.013
	Queen of the Valley Hospital, Napa	14.0	0.0%	0.74	No	0.00	7	0.72	0.006
	Saddleback Memorial Medical Center, Laguna Hills	13.3	0.0%	0.81	No	0.01	3	1.05	0.018
	San Antonio Community Hospital, Upland	12.0	0.0%	0.91	No	0.00	7	1.00	0.017
93	San Francisco General Hospital Medical Center	17.5	1.5%	0.96	No	1.19	4	1.52	0.014
	Santa Monica Hospital Medical Center, Santa Monica	16.2	0.0%	0.58	No	0.17	7	0.91	0.024
	Sequoia Hospital District, Redwood City	12.6	0.0%	0.80	No	0.00	6	0.60	0.009
	St. Francis Medical Center, Lynwood	12.0	0.0%	0.83	No	0.00	6	0.70	0.006
	St. John's Hospital and Health Center, Santa Monica	13.9	0.0%	0.77	No	0.00	7	0.64	0.013
	St. Joseph Hospital, Orange	12.7	0.0%	0.86	No	0.01	7	0.92	0.013
	St. Joseph Medical Center, Burbank	13.7	0.0%	0.63	No	0.00	6	0.77	0.004
	St. Jude Medical Center, Fullerton	11.7	0.0%	0.92	No	0.00	8	0.77	0.019
	St. Mary Medical Center, Long Beach	14.1	0.0%	0.77	No	0.15	6	0.73	0.008
	St. Mary's Hospital and Medical Center, San Francisco	12.6	0.0%	0.93	Yes	0.26	6	0.41	0.011

Natl. Rank	Hospital	U.S. News index	Reputa-tional score	Neurology mortality rate	COTH member	Interns and residents to beds	Tech-nology score (of 9)	R.N.'s to beds	Board-certified neurologists to beds
	St. Vincent Medical Center, Los Angeles	14.5	0.0%	0.51	No	0.01	7	0.84	0.009
	Torrance Memorial Medical Center, Torrance	14.6	0.0%	0.73	No	0.00	7	0.79	0.013
	Tri-City Medical Center, Oceanside	13.5	0.0%	0.77	No	0.01	5	0.63	0.013
	Washington Hospital, Fremont	12.8	0.0%	0.82	No	0.00	6	0.85	0.009
TIER FOUR									
	Alta Bates Medical Center, Berkeley	8.2	0.0%	0.99	No	0.00	6	0.46	0.007
	Antelope Valley Hospital Medical Center, Lancaster	6.5	0.0%	1.18	No	0.00	3	1.02	0.011
	Bakersfield Memorial Hospital, Bakersfield	6.7	0.0%	1.23	No	0.00	5	1.02	0.013
	Beverly Hospital, Montebello	10.8	0.0%	0.93	No	0.00	5	1.09	0.009
	Brookside Hospital, San Pablo	6.7	0.0%	1.06	No	0.00	5	0.20	0.013
	California Medical Center, Los Angeles	8.8	0.0%	1.05	No	0.13	3	1.18	0.007
	Community Memorial Hospital, Ventura	8.5	0.0%	1.03	No	0.00	5	0.85	0.010
	Dameron Hospital, Stockton	6.3	0.0%	1.21	No	0.00	4	0.76	0.019
	Daniel Freeman Memorial Hospital, Inglewood	9.9	0.0%	0.86	No	0.04	0	0.64	0.012
	Downey Community Hospital, Downey	10.8	0.0%	0.89	No	0.00	5	0.65	0.016
	Fresno Community Hospital and Medical Center, Fresno	9.0	0.0%	1.07	No	0.00	8	0.88	0.011
	Grossmont Hospital, La Mesa	7.7	0.0%	1.07	No	0.00	5	0.73	0.011
	Inter-Community Medical Center, Covina	8.3	0.0%	1.05	No	0.00	4	0.45	0.031
	John Muir Medical Center, Walnut Creek	6.9	0.0%	1.18	No	0.01	3	0.88	0.022
	Kaiser Foundation Hospital, Panorama City	10.5	0.0%	0.88	No	0.01	3	0.79	0.011
	Kaiser Foundation Hospital, Sacramento	5.9	0.0%	1.18	No	0.19	0	0.83	0.013
	Kaiser Foundation Hospital, Santa Clara	9.1	0.0%	1.21	No	0.29	4	1.58	0.015
	Marin General Hospital, Greenbrae	4.2	0.0%	1.25	No	0.00	4	0.37	0.008
	Mercy Hospital and Medical Center, San Diego	9.8	0.0%	1.08	No	0.25	6	1.06	0.014
	Mercy Medical Center, Redding	6.1	0.0%	1.68	No	0.16	6	1.77	0.015
	Mills-Peninsula Hospitals, Burlingame	9.2	0.0%	0.96	No	0.00	6	0.49	0.014
	Mount Diablo Medical Center, Concord	9.9	0.0%	0.92	No	0.00	6	0.51	0.011
	Mount Zion Medical Center, San Francisco	9.5	0.0%	0.90	No	0.28	0	0.69	0.007
	O'Connor Hospital, San Jose	9.5	0.0%	1.00	No	0.00	6	0.82	0.014
	Palomar Medical Center, Escondido	8.1	0.0%	1.05	No	0.00	6	0.73	0.007
	Presbyterian Intercommunity Hospital, Whittier	8.4	0.0%	1.04	No	0.07	6	0.55	0.013
	Roseville Hospital, Roseville	3.5	0.0%	1.37	No	0.00	6	0.29	0.009
	Salinas Valley Memorial Hospital, Salinas	6.7	0.0%	1.07	No	0.00	5	0.28	0.013
	San Gabriel Valley Medical Center, San Gabriel	10.2	0.0%	0.95	No	0.00	7	0.56	0.018
	San Jose Medical Center, San Jose	7.4	0.0%	1.13	No	0.12	6	0.61	0.013
	Santa Barbara Cottage Hospital, Santa Barbara	9.0	0.0%	1.05	No	0.25	2	0.94	0.018
	Santa Rosa Memorial Hospital, Santa Rosa	2.5	0.0%	1.37	No	0.00	4	0.26	0.004
	Scripps Memorial Hospital, La Jolla	7.2	0.0%	1.19	No	0.00	8	0.71	0.014
	Sharp Memorial Hospital, San Diego	10.5	0.0%	1.09	No	0.00	5	1.40	0.031
	St. Agnes Medical Center, Fresno	7.1	0.0%	1.38	No	0.00	6	0.92	0.040
	St. Bernardine Medical Center, San Bernardino	8.8	0.0%	1.00	No	0.00	8	0.64	0.002
	St. Francis Memorial Hospital, San Francisco	5.4	0.0%	1.20	No	0.06	5	0.41	0.011
	St. Joseph's Medical Center, Stockton	7.3	0.0%	1.13	No	0.00	6	0.71	0.013
	Sutter General Hospital, Sacramento	8.7	0.0%	1.03	No	0.06	4	0.54	0.025

ORTHOPEDICS

Natl. Rank	Hospital	U.S. News index	Reputa-tional score	Orthopedics mortality rate	COTH member	Interns and residents to beds	Tech-nology score (of 5)	R.N.'s to beds	Board-certified orthopedists to beds	Pro-cedures to beds
TIER ONE										
6	UCLA Medical Center, Los Angeles	38.2	10.5%	0.93	Yes	1.52	5	1.20	0.015	1.72
12	Stanford University Hospital, Stanford	26.9	4.0%	0.63	Yes	1.34	5	0.86	0.068	2.34
16	UCSD Medical Center, San Diego	23.1	1.0%	0.66	Yes	1.65	2	2.17	0.097	0.96
22	University of California, Davis Medical Center	20.8	0.9%	1.10	Yes	1.54	4	2.81	0.021	1.42

Natl. Rank	Hospital	U.S. News index	Reputational score	Orthopedics mortality rate	COTH member	Interns and residents to beds	Technology score (of 5)	R.N.'s to beds	Board-certified orthopedists to beds	Procedures to beds
	TIER TWO									
70	Green Hospital of Scripps Clinic, La Jolla	15.1	0.0%	0.55	No	0.21	4	1.99	0.029	6.24
57	Loma Linda University Medical Center, Loma Linda	16.0	0.0%	0.89	Yes	1.14	4	1.61	0.035	1.58
55	University of California, San Francisco Medical Center	16.2	1.0%	1.17	Yes	1.03	4	1.82	0.031	1.23
	TIER THREE									
	Alta Bates Medical Center, Berkeley	9.5	0.7%	0.65	No	0.00	2	0.46	0.025	2.00
	Alvarado Hospital Medical Center, San Diego	8.3	0.0%	0.78	No	0.00	3	0.81	0.026	3.91
	California Pacific Medical Center, San Francisco	12.4	0.0%	0.94	Yes	0.33	5	1.19	0.060	1.08
97	Cedars-Sinai Medical Center, Los Angeles	13.2	1.5%	1.17	Yes	0.51	4	0.83	0.062	2.08
	Century City Hospital, Los Angeles	10.3	0.0%	0.56	No	0.00	2	0.76	0.235	3.05
	Community Memorial Hospital, Ventura	11.2	0.0%	0.26	No	0.00	4	0.85	0.043	5.24
	Desert Hospital, Palm Springs	9.2	0.0%	0.74	No	0.07	3	1.00	0.032	2.58
	Downey Community Hospital, Downey	10.4	0.0%	0.64	No	0.00	4	0.65	0.059	3.87
	Eisenhower Memorial Hospital, Rancho Mirage	12.6	0.3%	0.55	No	0.00	4	0.95	0.042	7.18
	Encino-Tarzana Regional Medical Center, Tarzana	8.6	0.0%	0.68	No	0.00	3	0.66	0.028	1.26
	Hoag Memorial Hospital Presbyterian, Newport Beach	9.4	0.0%	0.86	No	0.00	4	1.26	0.086	3.04
	Hospital of the Good Samaritan, Los Angeles	8.9	0.0%	1.13	Yes	0.04	4	0.98	0.029	2.08
	Kaiser Foundation Hospital, Fontana	11.2	0.0%	0.46	No	0.08	4	1.05	0.027	2.38
100	Kaiser Foundation Hospital, Los Angeles	13.1	0.0%	0.71	No	0.63	4	1.42	0.018	1.59
	Kaiser Foundation Hospital, West Los Angeles	9.2	0.0%	0.58	No	0.06	2	0.86	0.033	1.74
	Kaiser Foundation Hospital, Oakland	8.6	0.7%	0.98	No	0.33	3	0.72	0.035	2.97
	Kaiser Foundation Hospital, San Diego	9.0	0.0%	0.79	No	0.09	4	0.70	0.047	4.16
	Kaiser Foundation Hospital, Santa Clara	12.6	0.0%	0.62	No	0.29	3	1.58	0.022	2.14
	Kaiser Foundation Hospital, Woodland Hills	12.7	0.0%	0.75	No	0.01	4	2.06	0.032	3.57
	Kaweah Delta District Hospital, Visalia	8.2	0.0%	1.12	No	0.00	3	1.73	0.036	4.67
	Long Beach Community Hospital, Long Beach	10.1	0.0%	0.45	No	0.00	4	0.74	0.022	2.59
	Long Beach Memorial Medical Center, Long Beach	10.6	0.0%	0.82	Yes	0.18	3	0.80	0.033	1.66
	Mercy General Hospital, Sacramento	8.4	0.0%	0.77	No	0.00	3	0.79	0.053	2.90
	Mercy Hospital and Medical Center, San Diego	8.8	0.0%	0.96	No	0.25	4	1.06	0.070	3.35
	Methodist Hospital of Southern California, Arcadia	9.3	0.0%	0.62	No	0.00	3	0.65	0.029	2.76
	Mills-Peninsula Hospitals, Burlingame	8.6	0.0%	0.60	No	0.00	3	0.49	0.024	1.51
	Mount Diablo Medical Center, Concord	8.8	0.0%	0.63	No	0.00	3	0.51	0.044	1.95
	N.T. Enloe Memorial Hospital, Chico	12.7	0.0%	0.50	No	0.00	3	1.63	0.069	4.98
	Pomona Valley Hospital Medical Center, Pomona	9.5	0.0%	0.85	No	0.00	4	1.40	0.036	2.32
	San Antonio Community Hospital, Upland	9.4	0.0%	0.75	No	0.00	4	1.00	0.044	1.70
	Santa Barbara Cottage Hospital, Santa Barbara	8.7	0.0%	0.82	No	0.25	2	0.94	0.054	4.42
	Santa Monica Hospital Medical Center, Santa Monica	11.3	0.0%	0.56	No	0.17	4	0.91	0.071	2.19
	Sharp Memorial Hospital, San Diego	10.5	0.0%	0.73	No	0.00	3	1.40	0.078	2.37
	St. John's Hospital and Health Center, Santa Monica	10.1	0.0%	0.50	No	0.00	3	0.64	0.106	4.43
	St. Joseph Medical Center, Burbank	9.4	0.0%	0.48	No	0.00	3	0.77	0.023	1.98
	St. Jude Medical Center, Fullerton	8.9	0.3%	0.83	No	0.00	4	0.77	0.052	2.61
	St. Mary Medical Center, Long Beach	9.6	0.0%	0.48	No	0.15	3	0.73	0.022	0.99
	St. Mary's Hospital and Medical Center, San Francisco	9.2	0.0%	0.91	Yes	0.26	3	0.41	0.033	2.45
	Sutter General Hospital, Sacramento	8.7	0.0%	0.79	No	0.06	3	0.54	0.097	6.25
	Tri-City Medical Center, Oceanside	10.2	0.0%	0.63	No	0.01	4	0.63	0.016	4.02
	TIER FOUR									
	Antelope Valley Hospital Medical Center, Lancaster	7.7	0.0%	0.78	No	0.00	2	1.02	0.030	1.69
	Bakersfield Memorial Hospital, Bakersfield	4.3	0.0%	1.72	No	0.00	4	1.02	0.052	2.97
	Beverly Hospital, Montebello	6.1	0.0%	1.05	No	0.00	3	1.09	0.024	1.81
	Brookside Hospital, San Pablo	2.5	0.0%	1.14	No	0.00	2	0.20	0.017	1.68
	Centinela Hospital Medical Center, Inglewood	6.6	0.5%	1.07	No	0.00	3	0.65	0.096	3.30
	Community Hospital of Chula Vista, Chula Vista	3.7	0.0%	1.00	No	0.00	1	0.59	0.014	1.37
	Dameron Hospital, Stockton	6.7	0.0%	0.89	No	0.00	3	0.76	0.057	1.86
	Fountain Valley Regional Hosp. Med. Ctr., Fountain Valley	5.2	0.0%	1.13	No	0.00	4	0.72	0.034	1.16
	Fresno Community Hospital and Medical Center, Fresno	4.8	0.0%	1.32	No	0.00	4	0.88	0.030	2.04
	Glendale Adventist Medical Center, Glendale	6.2	0.0%	1.04	No	0.15	2	1.06	0.030	2.39

Natl. Rank	Hospital	U.S. News index	Reputational score	Orthopedics mortality rate	COTH member	Interns and residents to beds	Technology score (of 5)	R.N.'s to beds	Board-certified orthopedists to beds	Procedures to beds
	Glendale Memorial Hospital and Health Center, Glendale	7.2	0.0%	0.80	No	0.00	3	0.69	0.019	1.59
	Good Samaritan Hospital, San Jose	4.9	0.5%	1.41	No	0.00	4	0.52	0.083	2.14
	Grossmont Hospital, La Mesa	7.0	0.0%	0.87	No	0.00	3	0.73	0.034	3.18
	Hemet Valley Medical Center, Hemet	3.3	0.0%	1.29	No	0.00	2	0.64	0.010	3.51
	Huntington Memorial Hospital, Pasadena	7.9	0.0%	1.08	Yes	0.11	3	0.68	0.013	2.12
	Inter-Community Medical Center, Covina	2.4	0.0%	1.47	No	0.00	2	0.45	0.088	2.98
	John Muir Medical Center, Walnut Creek	3.6	0.0%	1.65	No	0.01	2	0.88	0.087	5.26
	Kaiser Foundation Hospital, Panorama City	5.5	0.0%	1.04	No	0.01	3	0.79	0.021	2.16
	Kaiser Foundation Hospital, Redwood City	7.2	0.0%	1.16	No	0.00	5	0.96	0.033	4.82
	Kaiser Foundation Hospital, San Francisco	6.7	0.0%	1.08	No	0.31	4	0.74	0.034	1.85
	Kaiser Foundation Hospital, Walnut Creek	7.0	0.0%	0.76	No	0.02	2	0.42	0.031	3.72
	Little Company of Mary Hospital, Torrance	8.1	0.0%	0.75	No	0.00	3	0.64	0.101	1.58
	Marin General Hospital, Greenbrae	1.3	0.0%	1.47	No	0.00	1	0.37	0.051	2.92
	Memorial Hospitals Association, Modesto	3.5	0.0%	1.73	No	0.00	3	1.10	0.029	2.37
	Mercy Medical Center, Redding	5.7	0.0%	2.00	No	0.16	3	1.77	0.049	3.82
	Northridge Hospital Medical Center, Northridge	5.4	0.0%	1.31	No	0.09	4	0.87	0.094	1.42
	O'Connor Hospital, San Jose	8.0	0.0%	0.90	No	0.00	3	0.82	0.142	5.06
	Orthopaedic Hospital, Los Angeles	6.9	0.7%	1.02	No	0.13	3	0.55	0.033	2.45
	Palomar Medical Center, Escondido	5.9	0.0%	0.97	No	0.00	3	0.73	0.026	2.32
	Presbyterian Intercommunity Hospital, Whittier	7.8	0.0%	0.72	No	0.07	2	0.55	0.033	2.58
	Queen of Angels-Hollywood Center, Hollywood	6.8	0.0%	0.84	No	0.00	3	0.72	0.021	1.20
	Queen of the Valley Hospital, Napa	7.1	0.0%	0.95	No	0.00	4	0.72	0.037	4.31
	Roseville Hospital, Roseville	4.8	0.0%	0.98	No	0.00	3	0.29	0.032	3.15
	Saddleback Memorial Medical Center, Laguna Hills	6.3	0.0%	1.04	No	0.01	2	1.05	0.073	4.34
	Salinas Valley Memorial Hospital, Salinas	3.0	0.0%	1.42	No	0.00	4	0.28	0.026	2.64
	San Gabriel Valley Medical Center, San Gabriel	5.4	0.0%	1.08	No	0.00	4	0.56	0.027	2.93
	San Jose Medical Center, San Jose	7.8	0.0%	0.76	No	0.12	3	0.61	0.033	1.11
	San Pedro Peninsula Hospital, San Pedro	7.3	0.0%	0.44	No	0.00	2	0.28	0.023	1.19
	Santa Rosa Memorial Hospital, Santa Rosa	4.3	0.3%	1.27	No	0.00	3	0.26	0.049	5.67
	Scripps Memorial Hospital, La Jolla	6.9	0.3%	1.01	No	0.00	4	0.71	0.042	2.19
	Sequoia Hospital District, Redwood City	7.5	0.0%	0.78	No	0.00	3	0.60	0.059	1.97
	St. Agnes Medical Center, Fresno	7.1	0.0%	1.20	No	0.00	5	0.92	0.071	5.06
	St. Bernardine Medical Center, San Bernardino	5.0	0.0%	1.24	No	0.00	5	0.64	0.009	1.86
	St. Francis Medical Center, Lynwood	8.0	0.0%	0.73	No	0.00	3	0.70	0.013	1.38
	St. Francis Memorial Hospital, San Francisco	2.9	0.0%	1.32	No	0.06	2	0.41	0.068	2.94
	St. Joseph Hospital, Eureka	3.1	0.0%	1.52	No	0.00	3	0.48	0.059	4.44
	St. Joseph Hospital, Orange	7.3	0.0%	1.00	No	0.01	4	0.92	0.089	2.85
	St. Joseph's Medical Center, Stockton	7.0	0.0%	0.89	No	0.00	3	0.71	0.050	3.66
	St. Vincent Medical Center, Los Angeles	7.5	0.0%	0.88	No	0.01	4	0.84	0.027	1.73
	Torrance Memorial Medical Center, Torrance	4.7	0.0%	1.24	No	0.00	3	0.79	0.100	1.63
	Washington Hospital, Fremont	5.3	0.0%	1.09	No	0.00	3	0.85	0.031	2.13

OTOLARYNGOLOGY

Natl. Rank	Hospital	U.S. News index	Reputational score	Hospital-wide mortality rate	COTH member	Interns and residents to beds	Technology score (of 9)	R.N.'s to beds	Board-certified internists to beds	Procedures to beds
	TIER ONE									
5	UCLA Medical Center, Los Angeles	58.4	13.3%	0.66	Yes	1.52	9	1.20	0.023	0.316
11	Stanford University Hospital, Stanford	39.5	7.7%	0.90	Yes	1.34	9	0.86	0.147	0.273
16	University of California, San Francisco Medical Center	32.9	4.4%	0.89	Yes	1.03	8	1.82	0.435	0.177
20	Los Angeles County-USC Medical Center	26.7	3.9%	0.88	Yes	1.21	6	1.30	0.052	0.028
36	University of California, Davis Medical Center	20.5	0.0%	1.01	Yes	1.54	8	2.81	0.032	0.274
	TIER TWO									
	Kern Medical Center, Bakersfield	13.7	0.0%	1.33	Yes	0.93	3	1.40	0.222	0.067
58	Loma Linda University Medical Center, Loma Linda	16.8	0.5%	1.07	Yes	1.14	7	1.61	0.067	0.183

Natl. Rank	Hospital	U.S. News index	Reputational score	Hospital-wide mortality rate	COTH member	Interns and residents to beds	Technology score (of 9)	R.N.'s to beds	Board-certified internists to beds	Procedures to beds
76	Los Angeles County-King-Drew Medical Center	14.7	0.0%	1.25	Yes	1.56	4	1.33	0.040	0.028
45	UCSD Medical Center, San Diego	18.7	0.0%	0.75	Yes	1.65	6	2.17	0.049	0.163
TIER THREE										
	California Pacific Medical Center, San Francisco	12.5	0.0%	0.87	Yes	0.33	9	1.19	0.197	0.069
	Cedars-Sinai Medical Center, Los Angeles	12.9	0.8%	1.13	Yes	0.51	7	0.83	0.086	0.225
	Good Samaritan Hospital, San Jose	7.8	0.5%	1.20	No	0.00	8	0.52	0.288	0.153
	Green Hospital of Scripps Clinic, La Jolla	9.0	0.0%	0.86	No	0.21	5	1.99	0.052	0.277
	Hospital of the Good Samaritan, Los Angeles	10.4	0.4%	1.19	Yes	0.04	8	0.98	0.067	0.152
	Huntington Memorial Hospital, Pasadena	7.9	0.0%	1.11	Yes	0.11	6	0.68	0.059	0.113
	Kaiser Foundation Hospital, Los Angeles	10.4	0.0%	0.86	No	0.63	8	1.42	0.134	0.172
	Kaiser Foundation Hospital, Santa Clara	9.4	0.0%	0.94	No	0.29	3	1.58	0.288	0.221
	Kaiser Foundation Hospital, Woodland Hills	9.5	0.0%	0.80	No	0.01	5	2.06	0.167	0.256
	Kaweah Delta District Hospital, Visalia	7.4	0.0%	1.33	No	0.00	6	1.73	0.061	0.153
	Long Beach Memorial Medical Center, Long Beach	8.4	0.0%	1.00	Yes	0.18	6	0.80	0.037	0.096
	Los Angeles County-Harbor-UCLA Medical Center	13.2	0.0%	0.91	No	1.53	6	1.33	0.148	0.067
	Mercy Hospital and Medical Center, San Diego	7.8	0.4%	1.25	No	0.25	5	1.06	0.120	0.197
	Mercy Medical Center, Redding	8.1	0.0%	1.58	No	0.16	6	1.77	0.069	0.281
	N.T. Enloe Memorial Hospital, Chico	7.0	0.0%	1.01	No	0.00	6	1.63	0.025	0.335
	Northridge Hospital Medical Center, Northridge	7.0	0.0%	0.95	No	0.09	5	0.87	0.290	0.111
	Olive View Medical Center, Sylmar	11.7	0.0%	1.09	No	0.51	4	2.17	0.225	0.021
	San Bernardino County Medical Center, San Bernardino	10.1	0.0%	1.50	No	0.66	4	2.02	0.051	0.021
	San Francisco General Hospital Medical Center	11.5	0.4%	0.95	No	1.19	3	1.52	0.011	0.131
	Santa Clara Veterans Affairs Medical Center, San Jose	11.2	0.0%	1.29	No	0.67	8	1.83	0.095	0.070
	Santa Monica Hospital Medical Center, Santa Monica	7.9	0.0%	0.74	No	0.17	7	0.91	0.258	0.132
	Scripps Memorial Hospital, La Jolla	7.0	0.7%	1.06	No	0.00	8	0.71	0.037	0.141
	Sharp Memorial Hospital, San Diego	7.4	0.4%	1.02	No	0.00	5	1.40	0.052	0.073
	Stanislaus Medical Center, Modesto	8.1	0.0%	1.21	No	0.60	4	1.46	0.024	0.119
	St. Mary's Hospital and Medical Center, San Francisco	7.6	0.0%	0.99	Yes	0.26	6	0.41	0.057	0.076
	St. Vincent Medical Center, Los Angeles	8.4	0.9%	0.85	No	0.01	7	0.84	0.076	0.313
	Torrance Memorial Medical Center, Torrance	7.2	0.0%	0.92	No	0.00	7	0.79	0.313	0.234
	USC Kenneth Norris Cancer Hospital, Los Angeles	10.0	0.5%	1.40	No	0.40	6	1.37	0.133	0.083
	University of California, Irvine Medical Center, Orange	11.2	0.0%	1.19	Yes	0.54	6	1.29	0.038	0.098
	Valley Medical Center of Fresno, Fresno	9.9	0.0%	1.57	Yes	0.80	5	0.71	0.034	0.081
TIER FOUR										
	Alta Bates Medical Center, Berkeley	3.5	0.0%	0.96	No	0.00	5	0.46	0.065	0.138
	Alvarado Hospital Medical Center, San Diego	4.9	0.0%	0.92	No	0.00	6	0.81	0.065	0.212
	Antelope Valley Hospital Medical Center, Lancaster	5.0	0.0%	1.30	No	0.00	3	1.02	0.141	0.167
	Bakersfield Memorial Hospital, Bakersfield	6.0	0.0%	1.21	No	0.00	5	1.02	0.185	0.134
	Beverly Hospital, Montebello	5.7	0.0%	0.90	No	0.00	5	1.09	0.094	0.170
	Brookside Hospital, San Pablo	2.5	0.0%	1.06	No	0.00	5	0.20	0.057	0.170
	California Medical Center, Los Angeles	6.4	0.0%	1.16	No	0.13	5	1.18	0.107	0.124
	Centinela Hospital Medical Center, Inglewood	5.2	0.0%	0.96	No	0.00	6	0.65	0.165	0.117
	Century City Hospital, Los Angeles	5.2	0.0%	0.82	No	0.00	5	0.76	0.144	0.170
	City of Hope National Medical Center, Duarte	6.2	0.0%	0.91	No	0.15	6	0.70	0.190	0.118
	Community Hospital of Chula Vista, Chula Vista	3.2	0.0%	1.08	No	0.00	4	0.59	0.035	0.101
	Community Hospital, Santa Rosa	5.0	0.0%	1.26	No	0.53	5	0.50	0.014	0.103
	Community Memorial Hospital, Ventura	4.1	0.0%	1.02	No	0.00	4	0.85	0.038	0.205
	Dameron Hospital, Stockton	4.5	0.0%	1.27	No	0.00	3	0.76	0.175	0.123
	Daniel Freeman Memorial Hospital, Inglewood	2.8	0.0%	0.91	No	0.04	0	0.64	0.067	0.130
	Davies Medical Center, San Francisco	5.2	0.0%	0.82	No	0.01	4	0.66	0.212	0.101
	Desert Hospital, Palm Springs	5.0	0.0%	0.85	No	0.07	3	1.00	0.069	0.181
	Downey Community Hospital, Downey	3.6	0.0%	0.92	No	0.00	3	0.65	0.076	0.292
	Eisenhower Memorial Hospital, Rancho Mirage	5.6	0.0%	0.86	No	0.00	7	0.95	0.054	0.339
	Encino-Tarzana Regional Medical Center, Tarzana	4.0	0.0%	0.78	No	0.00	4	0.66	0.065	0.062
	Fountain Valley Regional Hosp. Med. Ctr., Fountain Valley	3.6	0.0%	0.98	No	0.00	3	0.72	0.061	0.044
	Fresno Community Hospital and Medical Center, Fresno	5.5	0.0%	1.17	No	0.00	8	0.88	0.069	0.140

Natl. Rank	Hospital	U.S. News index	Reputational score	Hospital-wide mortality rate	COTH member	Interns and residents to beds	Technology score (of 9)	R.N.'s to beds	Board-certified internists to beds	Procedures to beds
	Garfield Medical Center, Monterey Park	6.8	0.0%	0.90	No	0.00	6	1.16	0.161	0.049
	Glendale Adventist Medical Center, Glendale	5.9	0.0%	1.00	No	0.15	5	1.06	0.067	0.170
	Glendale Memorial Hospital and Health Center, Glendale	3.9	0.0%	1.02	No	0.00	6	0.69	0.003	0.139
	Grossmont Hospital, La Mesa	3.8	0.0%	1.11	No	0.00	5	0.73	0.023	0.189
	Hemet Valley Medical Center, Hemet	3.6	0.0%	1.07	No	0.00	5	0.64	0.024	0.210
	Highland General Hospital, Oakland	5.7	0.0%	0.84	No	0.84	2	0.34	0.065	0.104
	Hoag Memorial Hospital Presbyterian, Newport Beach	6.5	0.0%	0.94	No	0.00	7	1.26	0.068	0.206
	Inter-Community Medical Center, Covina	6.3	0.0%	1.11	No	0.00	5	0.45	0.418	0.201
	John C. Fremont Hospital, Mariposa	1.2	0.0%	0.70	No	0.00	0	0.29	0.000	0.118
	John Muir Medical Center, Walnut Creek	3.8	0.0%	1.15	No	0.01	1	0.88	0.095	0.398
	Kaiser Foundation Hospital, Fontana	5.5	0.0%	0.88	No	0.08	4	1.05	0.078	0.240
	Kaiser Foundation Hospital, West Los Angeles	5.0	0.0%	0.88	No	0.06	2	0.86	0.156	0.431
	Kaiser Foundation Hospital, Oakland	6.2	0.4%	1.07	No	0.33	3	0.72	0.070	0.393
	Kaiser Foundation Hospital, Panorama City	4.8	0.0%	0.82	No	0.01	2	0.79	0.177	0.206
	Kaiser Foundation Hospital, Redwood City	6.0	0.0%	0.93	No	0.00	4	0.96	0.205	0.291
	Kaiser Foundation Hospital, Sacramento	3.8	0.0%	1.33	No	0.19	0	0.83	0.069	0.339
	Kaiser Foundation Hospital, San Diego	4.3	0.0%	0.92	No	0.09	3	0.70	0.099	0.248
	Kaiser Foundation Hospital, San Francisco	5.4	0.0%	0.82	No	0.31	4	0.74	0.067	0.171
	Kaiser Foundation Hospital, Walnut Creek	2.8	0.0%	0.96	No	0.02	3	0.42	0.055	0.227
	L.A. County-Rancho Los Amigos Med. Ctr., Downey	5.3	0.0%	0.83	No	0.23	2	1.01	0.055	0.005
	Little Company of Mary Hospital, Torrance	4.2	0.0%	0.89	No	0.00	6	0.64	0.049	0.165
	Loma Linda Community Hospital, Loma Linda	2.4	0.0%	1.21	No	0.06	1	0.52	0.050	0.075
	Long Beach Community Hospital, Long Beach	5.6	0.0%	0.97	No	0.00	7	0.74	0.147	0.163
	Marin General Hospital, Greenbrae	3.4	0.0%	1.18	No	0.00	4	0.37	0.139	0.160
	Martin Luther Hospital, Anaheim	3.6	0.0%	0.95	No	0.00	5	0.55	0.045	0.020
	Memorial Hospitals Association, Modesto	5.4	0.0%	1.11	No	0.00	6	1.10	0.043	0.129
	Merced Community Medical Center, Merced	3.9	0.0%	1.15	No	0.23	0	0.66	0.114	0.190
	Mercy General Hospital, Sacramento	3.9	0.0%	0.87	No	0.00	2	0.79	0.088	0.232
	Merrithew Memorial Hospital, Martinez	4.6	0.0%	1.18	No	0.21	1	1.11	0.015	0.160
	Methodist Hospital of Southern California, Arcadia	4.3	0.0%	0.71	No	0.00	6	0.65	0.042	0.169
	Mills-Peninsula Hospitals, Burlingame	4.0	0.0%	0.92	No	0.00	6	0.49	0.086	0.048
	Mount Diablo Medical Center, Concord	3.2	0.0%	1.05	No	0.00	5	0.51	0.026	0.163
	Mount Zion Medical Center, San Francisco	3.6	0.0%	1.07	No	0.28	0	0.69	0.041	0.241
	Natividad Medical Center, Salinas	2.6	0.0%	1.11	No	0.24	1	0.41	0.024	0.024
	Northbay Medical Center, Fairfield	3.0	0.0%	1.25	No	0.00	5	0.40	0.053	0.035
	O'Connor Hospital, San Jose	6.1	0.0%	1.06	No	0.00	6	0.82	0.220	0.248
	Palomar Medical Center, Escondido	4.0	0.0%	1.09	No	0.00	6	0.73	0.012	0.109
	Pomona Valley Hospital Medical Center, Pomona	6.7	0.0%	1.12	No	0.00	7	1.40	0.057	0.216
	Presbyterian Intercommunity Hospital, Whittier	4.4	0.0%	0.93	No	0.07	6	0.55	0.066	0.228
	Queen of Angels-Hollywood Center, Hollywood	4.9	0.0%	0.85	No	0.00	6	0.72	0.098	0.122
	Queen of the Valley Hospital, Napa	4.7	0.0%	0.84	No	0.00	7	0.72	0.037	0.244
	Riverside General Hospital-Medical Center, Riverside	4.5	0.0%	1.59	No	0.37	1	0.88	0.033	0.025
	Roseville Hospital, Roseville	3.2	0.0%	1.13	No	0.00	6	0.29	0.073	0.294
	Saddleback Memorial Medical Center, Laguna Hills	5.0	0.0%	0.83	No	0.01	3	1.05	0.073	0.209
	Salinas Valley Memorial Hospital, Salinas	3.1	0.0%	1.11	No	0.00	5	0.28	0.094	0.349
	San Antonio Community Hospital, Upland	5.7	0.0%	0.96	No	0.00	7	1.00	0.068	0.054
	San Gabriel Valley Medical Center, San Gabriel	5.2	0.0%	1.09	No	0.00	7	0.56	0.180	0.329
	San Joaquin General Hospital, Stockton	5.0	0.0%	1.64	No	0.43	1	1.02	0.018	0.090
	San Jose Medical Center, San Jose	4.4	0.0%	1.31	No	0.12	6	0.61	0.066	0.106
	San Pedro Peninsula Hospital, San Pedro	2.7	0.0%	0.85	No	0.00	5	0.28	0.030	0.057
	Santa Barbara Cottage Hospital, Santa Barbara	6.3	0.0%	1.07	No	0.25	1	0.94	0.253	0.190
	Santa Rosa Memorial Hospital, Santa Rosa	3.2	0.0%	1.17	No	0.00	4	0.26	0.160	0.280
	Selma District Hospital, Selma	1.2	0.0%	1.14	No	0.00	1	0.32	0.000	0.092
	Sequoia Hospital District, Redwood City	4.6	0.0%	0.86	No	0.00	6	0.60	0.106	0.153
	Seton Medical Center, Daly City	6.5	0.0%	0.50	No	0.00	5	1.14	0.158	0.007
	South Coast Medical Center, South Laguna	4.2	0.0%	0.93	No	0.00	7	0.52	0.063	0.063

Natl. Rank	Hospital	U.S. News index	Reputational score	Hospital-wide mortality rate	COTH member	Interns and residents to beds	Technology score (of 9)	R.N.'s to beds	Board-certified internists to beds	Procedures to beds
	St. Agnes Medical Center, Fresno	5.9	0.0%	1.17	No	0.00	6	0.92	0.164	0.260
	St. Bernardine Medical Center, San Bernardino	4.5	0.0%	1.26	No	0.00	8	0.64	0.043	0.122
	St. Francis Medical Center, Lynwood	4.5	0.0%	1.02	No	0.00	7	0.70	0.038	0.130
	St. Francis Memorial Hospital, San Francisco	3.5	0.0%	1.03	No	0.06	5	0.41	0.063	0.216
	St. John's Hospital and Health Center, Santa Monica	6.0	0.0%	0.80	No	0.00	7	0.64	0.212	0.254
	St. Joseph Hospital, Eureka	3.5	0.0%	1.37	No	0.00	6	0.48	0.059	0.341
	St. Joseph Hospital, Orange	6.6	0.0%	1.09	No	0.01	7	0.92	0.206	0.102
	St. Joseph Medical Center, Burbank	4.7	0.0%	0.82	No	0.00	6	0.77	0.046	0.249
	St. Joseph's Medical Center, Stockton	4.4	0.0%	1.09	No	0.00	6	0.71	0.063	0.235
	St. Jude Medical Center, Fullerton	6.2	0.4%	1.04	No	0.00	8	0.77	0.030	0.116
	St. Mary Medical Center, Long Beach	5.0	0.0%	0.86	No	0.15	6	0.73	0.042	0.113
	Sutter General Hospital, Sacramento	3.5	0.0%	0.99	No	0.06	3	0.54	0.078	0.169
	Sutter Memorial Hospital, Sacramento	5.7	0.0%	0.91	No	0.03	4	1.18	0.079	0.139
	Tri-City Medical Center, Oceanside	4.1	0.0%	0.82	No	0.01	5	0.63	0.058	0.275
	Washington Hospital, Fremont	4.8	0.0%	0.79	No	0.00	4	0.85	0.089	0.133
	Western Medical Center, Santa Ana	5.3	0.0%	1.06	No	0.04	5	1.05	0.061	0.167
	White Memorial Medical Center, Los Angeles	5.0	0.0%	0.74	No	0.42	3	0.62	0.039	0.068

RHEUMATOLOGY

Natl. Rank	Hospital	U.S. News index	Reputational score	Hospital-wide mortality rate	COTH member	Interns and residents to beds	Technology score (of 5)	R.N.'s to beds	Board-certified internists to beds
	TIER ONE								
4	UCLA Medical Center, Los Angeles	60.4	18.6%	0.66	Yes	1.52	5	1.20	0.023
11	Stanford University Hospital, Stanford	35.1	7.8%	0.90	Yes	1.34	5	0.86	0.147
15	University of California, San Francisco Medical Center	30.4	4.2%	0.89	Yes	1.03	4	1.82	0.435
23	UCSD Medical Center, San Diego	22.8	0.9%	0.75	Yes	1.65	2	2.17	0.049
	TIER TWO								
81	California Pacific Medical Center, San Francisco	16.1	0.0%	0.87	Yes	0.33	5	1.19	0.197
39	Green Hospital of Scripps Clinic, La Jolla	19.9	3.1%	0.86	No	0.21	4	1.99	0.052
74	Loma Linda University Medical Center, Loma Linda	16.5	0.0%	1.07	Yes	1.14	4	1.61	0.067
29	University of California, Davis Medical Center	21.2	0.0%	1.01	Yes	1.54	4	2.81	0.032
	TIER THREE								
	Cedars-Sinai Medical Center, Los Angeles	14.5	1.1%	1.13	Yes	0.51	4	0.83	0.086
	Desert Hospital, Palm Springs	10.8	0.0%	0.85	No	0.07	3	1.00	0.069
	Encino-Tarzana Regional Medical Center, Tarzana	9.7	0.0%	0.78	No	0.00	3	0.66	0.065
	Garfield Medical Center, Monterey Park	11.0	0.0%	0.90	No	0.00	3	1.16	0.161
	Hoag Memorial Hospital Presbyterian, Newport Beach	10.7	0.0%	0.94	No	0.00	4	1.26	0.068
	Hospital of the Good Samaritan, Los Angeles	10.4	0.0%	1.19	Yes	0.04	4	0.98	0.067
	Huntington Memorial Hospital, Pasadena	9.9	0.0%	1.11	Yes	0.11	3	0.68	0.059
	Kaiser Foundation Hospital, Fontana	11.0	0.0%	0.88	No	0.08	4	1.05	0.078
	Kaiser Foundation Hospital, Los Angeles	10.1	0.0%	0.88	No	0.06	2	0.86	0.156
	Kaiser Foundation Hospital, West Los Angeles	14.4	0.0%	0.86	No	0.63	4	1.42	0.134
	Kaiser Foundation Hospital, Panorama City	10.9	0.0%	0.82	No	0.01	3	0.79	0.177
	Kaiser Foundation Hospital, Redwood City	11.4	0.0%	0.93	No	0.00	5	0.96	0.205
	Kaiser Foundation Hospital, San Francisco	11.4	0.0%	0.82	No	0.31	4	0.74	0.067
	Kaiser Foundation Hospital, Santa Clara	13.5	0.0%	0.94	No	0.29	3	1.58	0.288
	Kaiser Foundation Hospital, Woodland Hills	13.6	0.0%	0.80	No	0.01	4	2.06	0.167
	Long Beach Memorial Medical Center, Long Beach	11.2	0.0%	1.00	Yes	0.18	3	0.80	0.037
	Mercy General Hospital, Sacramento	9.9	0.0%	0.87	No	0.00	3	0.79	0.088
	Northridge Hospital Medical Center, Northridge	11.4	0.0%	0.95	No	0.09	4	0.87	0.290
	Queen of Angels-Hollywood Center, Hollywood	10.0	0.0%	0.85	No	0.00	3	0.72	0.098
	Queen of the Valley Hospital, Napa	10.1	0.0%	0.84	No	0.00	4	0.72	0.037
	Saddleback Memorial Medical Center, Laguna Hills	10.4	0.0%	0.83	No	0.01	2	1.05	0.073
	San Antonio Community Hospital, Upland	9.7	0.0%	0.96	No	0.00	4	1.00	0.068

Natl. Rank	Hospital	U.S. News index	Reputa-tional score	Hospital-wide mortality rate	COTH member	Interns and residents to beds	Tech-nology score (of 5)	R.N.'s to beds	Board-certified internists to beds
	Santa Monica Hospital Medical Center, Santa Monica	12.8	0.0%	0.74	No	0.17	4	0.91	0.258
	Scripps Memorial Hospital, La Jolla	10.9	1.4%	1.06	No	0.00	4	0.71	0.037
	Sharp Memorial Hospital, San Diego	10.5	0.4%	1.02	No	0.00	3	1.40	0.052
	St. John's Hospital and Health Center, Santa Monica	9.7	0.0%	0.80	No	0.00	3	0.64	0.212
	St. Joseph Medical Center, Burbank	9.9	0.0%	0.82	No	0.00	3	0.77	0.046
	St. Mary Medical Center, Long Beach	9.9	0.0%	0.86	No	0.15	3	0.73	0.042
	St. Mary's Hospital and Medical Center, San Francisco	10.6	0.0%	0.99	Yes	0.26	3	0.41	0.057
	St. Vincent Medical Center, Los Angeles	10.6	0.0%	0.85	No	0.01	4	0.84	0.076
	Torrance Memorial Medical Center, Torrance	11.0	0.0%	0.92	No	0.00	3	0.79	0.313
	Tri-City Medical Center, Oceanside	10.1	0.0%	0.82	No	0.01	4	0.63	0.058
	Washington Hospital, Fremont	10.4	0.0%	0.79	No	0.00	3	0.85	0.089
	White Memorial Medical Center, Los Angeles	10.7	0.0%	0.74	No	0.42	3	0.62	0.039
TIER FOUR									
	Alta Bates Medical Center, Berkeley	7.3	0.0%	0.96	No	0.00	2	0.46	0.065
	Alvarado Hospital Medical Center, San Diego	9.1	0.0%	0.92	No	0.00	3	0.81	0.065
	Antelope Valley Hospital Medical Center, Lancaster	6.9	0.0%	1.30	No	0.00	2	1.02	0.141
	Bakersfield Memorial Hospital, Bakersfield	7.6	0.0%	1.21	No	0.00	4	1.02	0.185
	Beverly Hospital, Montebello	9.3	0.0%	0.90	No	0.00	3	1.09	0.094
	Brookside Hospital, San Pablo	5.7	0.0%	1.06	No	0.00	2	0.20	0.057
	California Medical Center, Los Angeles	6.9	0.0%	1.16	No	0.13	1	1.18	0.107
	Centinela Hospital Medical Center, Inglewood	9.1	0.0%	0.96	No	0.00	3	0.65	0.165
	Community Hospital of Chula Vista, Chula Vista	5.9	0.0%	1.08	No	0.00	1	0.59	0.035
	Community Memorial Hospital, Ventura	7.5	0.0%	1.02	No	0.00	4	0.85	0.038
	Dameron Hospital, Stockton	7.1	0.0%	1.27	No	0.00	3	0.76	0.175
	Daniel Freeman Memorial Hospital, Inglewood	5.6	0.0%	0.91	No	0.04	0	0.64	0.067
	Downey Community Hospital, Downey	8.2	0.0%	0.92	No	0.00	4	0.65	0.076
	Eisenhower Memorial Hospital, Rancho Mirage	9.5	0.0%	0.86	No	0.00	4	0.95	0.054
	Fresno Community Hospital and Medical Center, Fresno	7.7	0.0%	1.17	No	0.00	4	0.88	0.069
	Glendale Adventist Medical Center, Glendale	9.1	0.0%	1.00	No	0.15	2	1.06	0.067
	Glendale Memorial Hospital and Health Center, Glendale	6.4	0.0%	1.02	No	0.00	3	0.69	0.003
	Good Samaritan Hospital, San Jose	8.1	0.0%	1.20	No	0.00	4	0.52	0.288
	Grossmont Hospital, La Mesa	6.9	0.0%	1.11	No	0.00	3	0.73	0.023
	Hemet Valley Medical Center, Hemet	5.6	0.0%	1.07	No	0.00	2	0.64	0.024
	Inter-Community Medical Center, Covina	7.6	0.0%	1.11	No	0.00	2	0.45	0.418
	John Muir Medical Center, Walnut Creek	6.2	0.0%	1.15	No	0.01	2	0.88	0.095
	Kaiser Foundation Hospital, Oakland	8.6	0.0%	1.07	No	0.33	3	0.72	0.070
	Kaiser Foundation Hospital, Sacramento	3.4	0.0%	1.33	No	0.19	0	0.83	0.069
	Kaiser Foundation Hospital, San Diego	8.8	0.0%	0.92	No	0.09	4	0.70	0.099
	Kaiser Foundation Hospital, Walnut Creek	7.3	0.0%	0.96	No	0.02	2	0.42	0.055
	Kaweah Delta District Hospital, Visalia	7.5	0.0%	1.33	No	0.00	3	1.73	0.061
	Little Company of Mary Hospital, Torrance	7.9	0.0%	0.89	No	0.00	3	0.64	0.049
	Long Beach Community Hospital, Long Beach	9.5	0.0%	0.97	No	0.00	4	0.74	0.147
	Marin General Hospital, Greenbrae	4.4	0.0%	1.18	No	0.00	1	0.37	0.139
	Memorial Hospitals Association, Modesto	8.0	0.0%	1.11	No	0.00	3	1.10	0.043
	Mercy Hospital and Medical Center, San Diego	8.8	0.0%	1.25	No	0.25	4	1.06	0.120
	Mercy Medical Center, Redding	7.0	0.0%	1.58	No	0.16	3	1.77	0.069
	Methodist Hospital of Southern California, Arcadia	9.5	0.0%	0.71	No	0.00	3	0.65	0.042
	Mills-Peninsula Hospitals, Burlingame	8.5	0.0%	0.92	No	0.00	3	0.49	0.086
	Mount Diablo Medical Center, Concord	6.9	0.0%	1.05	No	0.00	3	0.51	0.026
	Mount Zion Medical Center, San Francisco	4.7	0.0%	1.07	No	0.28	0	0.69	0.041
	N.T. Enloe Memorial Hospital, Chico	9.1	0.0%	1.01	No	0.00	3	1.63	0.025
	O'Connor Hospital, San Jose	9.0	0.0%	1.06	No	0.00	3	0.82	0.220
	Palomar Medical Center, Escondido	7.0	0.0%	1.09	No	0.00	3	0.73	0.012
	Pomona Valley Hospital Medical Center, Pomona	9.3	0.0%	1.12	No	0.00	4	1.40	0.057
	Presbyterian Intercommunity Hospital, Whittier	7.2	0.0%	0.93	No	0.07	2	0.55	0.066
	Roseville Hospital, Roseville	6.0	0.0%	1.13	No	0.00	3	0.29	0.073

Natl. Rank	Hospital	U.S. News index	Reputational score	Hospital-wide mortality rate	COTH member	Interns and residents to beds	Technology score (of 5)	R.N.'s to beds	Board-certified internists to beds
	Salinas Valley Memorial Hospital, Salinas	6.7	0.0%	1.11	No	0.00	4	0.28	0.094
	San Gabriel Valley Medical Center, San Gabriel	8.2	0.0%	1.09	No	0.00	4	0.56	0.180
	San Jose Medical Center, San Jose	5.0	0.0%	1.31	No	0.12	3	0.61	0.066
	San Pedro Peninsula Hospital, San Pedro	7.9	0.0%	0.85	No	0.00	2	0.28	0.030
	Santa Barbara Cottage Hospital, Santa Barbara	8.9	0.0%	1.07	No	0.25	2	0.94	0.253
	Santa Rosa Memorial Hospital, Santa Rosa	6.3	0.0%	1.17	No	0.00	3	0.26	0.160
	Sequoia Hospital District, Redwood City	8.6	0.0%	0.86	No	0.00	3	0.60	0.106
	St. Agnes Medical Center, Fresno	9.0	0.0%	1.17	No	0.00	5	0.92	0.164
	St. Bernardine Medical Center, San Bernardino	6.7	0.0%	1.26	No	0.00	5	0.64	0.043
	St. Francis Medical Center, Lynwood	7.7	0.0%	1.02	No	0.00	3	0.70	0.038
	St. Francis Memorial Hospital, San Francisco	5.7	0.0%	1.03	No	0.06	2	0.41	0.063
	St. Joseph Hospital, Orange	9.4	0.0%	1.09	No	0.01	4	0.92	0.206
	St. Joseph's Medical Center, Stockton	7.3	0.0%	1.09	No	0.00	3	0.71	0.063
	St. Jude Medical Center, Fullerton	8.1	0.0%	1.04	No	0.00	4	0.77	0.030
	Sutter General Hospital, Sacramento	7.0	0.0%	0.99	No	0.06	3	0.54	0.078
	Sutter Memorial Hospital, Sacramento	9.4	0.0%	0.91	No	0.03	3	1.18	0.079

UROLOGY

Natl. Rank	Hospital	U.S. News index	Reputational score	Urology mortality rate	COTH member	Interns and residents to beds	Technology score (of 11)	R.N.'s to beds	Board-certified internists to beds	Procedures to beds
	TIER ONE									
4	UCLA Medical Center, Los Angeles	59.8	29.6%	0.46	Yes	1.52	11	1.20	0.023	2.36
5	Stanford University Hospital, Stanford	46.6	22.5%	0.96	Yes	1.34	11	0.86	0.147	1.69
13	University of California, San Francisco Medical Center	28.1	8.2%	1.02	Yes	1.03	10	1.82	0.435	1.40
19	University of California, Davis Medical Center	24.8	0.5%	0.47	Yes	1.54	10	2.81	0.032	1.24
23	UCSD Medical Center, San Diego	23.0	0.5%	0.47	Yes	1.65	7	2.17	0.049	1.40
	TIER TWO									
63	California Pacific Medical Center, San Francisco	16.9	0.0%	0.74	Yes	0.33	11	1.19	0.197	1.13
29	Loma Linda University Medical Center, Loma Linda	20.9	0.8%	0.67	Yes	1.14	9	1.61	0.067	1.52
66	USC Kenneth Norris Cancer Hospital, Los Angeles	16.6	1.1%	0.80	No	0.40	7	1.37	0.133	8.72
	TIER THREE									
	Alta Bates Medical Center, Berkeley	8.6	0.0%	0.84	No	0.00	7	0.46	0.065	2.27
	Alvarado Hospital Medical Center, San Diego	11.2	0.0%	0.70	No	0.00	7	0.81	0.065	2.51
	Cedars-Sinai Medical Center, Los Angeles	10.1	0.0%	1.42	Yes	0.51	9	0.83	0.086	2.23
	Daniel Freeman Memorial Hospital, Inglewood	8.9	0.0%	0.71	No	0.04	0	0.64	0.067	1.82
	Desert Hospital, Palm Springs	11.1	0.0%	0.57	No	0.07	5	1.00	0.069	1.63
	Downey Community Hospital, Downey	10.8	0.0%	0.64	No	0.00	5	0.65	0.076	3.90
	Eisenhower Memorial Hospital, Rancho Mirage	12.3	0.0%	0.70	No	0.00	8	0.95	0.054	4.13
	Encino-Tarzana Regional Medical Center, Tarzana	10.2	0.0%	0.39	No	0.00	6	0.66	0.065	1.20
	Garfield Medical Center, Monterey Park	11.0	0.0%	0.79	No	0.00	6	1.16	0.161	1.20
	Glendale Adventist Medical Center, Glendale	10.9	0.0%	0.81	No	0.15	7	1.06	0.067	1.46
	Glendale Memorial Hospital and Health Center, Glendale	10.3	0.0%	0.68	No	0.00	7	0.69	0.003	1.92
93	Green Hospital of Scripps Clinic, La Jolla	14.8	0.0%	0.71	No	0.21	7	1.99	0.052	2.62
	Hoag Memorial Hospital Presbyterian, Newport Beach	10.0	0.0%	0.92	No	0.00	9	1.26	0.068	1.59
	Kaiser Foundation Hospital, Fontana	9.2	0.0%	0.92	No	0.08	6	1.05	0.078	2.09
	Kaiser Foundation Hospital, Los Angeles	11.0	0.0%	0.60	No	0.06	3	0.86	0.156	2.15
	Kaiser Foundation Hospital, West Los Angeles	14.0	0.0%	0.84	No	0.63	9	1.42	0.134	1.68
	Kaiser Foundation Hospital, San Francisco	8.6	0.0%	0.95	No	0.31	6	0.74	0.067	1.52
	Kaiser Foundation Hospital, Santa Clara	13.7	0.0%	0.70	No	0.29	4	1.58	0.288	1.89
	Kaiser Foundation Hospital, Woodland Hills	12.9	0.0%	0.93	No	0.01	8	2.06	0.167	3.49
	Kaweah Delta District Hospital, Visalia	9.2	0.0%	1.20	No	0.00	8	1.73	0.061	3.46
	Little Company of Mary Hospital, Torrance	9.3	0.0%	0.80	No	0.00	7	0.64	0.049	1.67
	Long Beach Community Hospital, Long Beach	10.8	0.0%	0.78	No	0.00	8	0.74	0.147	1.53
	Long Beach Memorial Medical Center, Long Beach	13.7	0.0%	0.75	Yes	0.18	8	0.80	0.037	1.09

Natl. Rank	Hospital	U.S. News index	Reputational score	Urology mortality rate	COTH member	Interns and residents to beds	Technology score (of 11)	R.N.'s to beds	Board-certified internists to beds	Procedures to beds
	Merced Community Medical Center, Merced	10.5	0.0%	0.45	No	0.23	2	0.66	0.114	2.00
	Methodist Hospital of Southern California, Arcadia	10.3	0.0%	0.52	No	0.00	7	0.65	0.042	1.23
	N.T. Enloe Memorial Hospital, Chico	9.4	0.0%	1.02	No	0.00	7	1.63	0.025	2.47
	Pomona Valley Hospital Medical Center, Pomona	8.6	0.0%	1.14	No	0.00	9	1.40	0.057	2.12
	Presbyterian Intercommunity Hospital, Whittier	10.6	0.0%	0.49	No	0.07	7	0.55	0.066	1.76
	Queen of Angels-Hollywood Center, Hollywood	10.1	0.0%	0.78	No	0.00	7	0.72	0.098	1.57
	Queen of the Valley Hospital, Napa	11.3	0.0%	0.38	No	0.00	9	0.72	0.037	2.42
	Saddleback Memorial Medical Center, Laguna Hills	10.1	0.0%	0.77	No	0.01	4	1.05	0.073	1.52
	San Antonio Community Hospital, Upland	9.1	0.0%	0.91	No	0.00	8	1.00	0.068	1.14
	Santa Barbara Cottage Hospital, Santa Barbara	11.5	0.0%	0.53	No	0.25	2	0.94	0.253	2.14
	Santa Clara Veterans Affairs Medical Center, San Jose	9.7	0.0%	1.51	No	0.67	9	1.83	0.095	0.68
	Santa Monica Hospital Medical Center, Santa Monica	12.8	0.0%	0.68	No	0.17	8	0.91	0.258	2.08
	Sequoia Hospital District, Redwood City	8.6	0.0%	0.86	No	0.00	7	0.60	0.106	1.02
	St. Francis Memorial Hospital, San Francisco	8.7	0.0%	0.80	No	0.06	6	0.41	0.063	1.33
	St. John's Hospital and Health Center, Santa Monica	11.1	0.0%	0.75	No	0.00	8	0.64	0.212	1.93
	St. Joseph Hospital, Orange	9.7	0.5%	0.99	No	0.01	9	0.92	0.206	1.66
	St. Mary Medical Center, Long Beach	9.4	0.0%	0.85	No	0.15	8	0.73	0.042	0.97
	St. Mary's Hospital and Medical Center, San Francisco	11.6	0.0%	0.83	Yes	0.26	7	0.41	0.057	1.07
	Tri-City Medical Center, Oceanside	10.5	0.0%	0.71	No	0.01	6	0.63	0.058	2.62
	Washington Hospital, Fremont	11.0	0.0%	0.69	No	0.00	6	0.85	0.089	1.72
	White Memorial Medical Center, Los Angeles	10.5	0.0%	0.62	No	0.42	3	0.62	0.039	1.28
TIER FOUR										
	Antelope Valley Hospital Medical Center, Lancaster	4.2	0.0%	1.65	No	0.00	4	1.02	0.141	1.70
	Bakersfield Memorial Hospital, Bakersfield	6.7	0.0%	1.24	No	0.00	6	1.02	0.185	1.71
	Beverly Hospital, Montebello	7.7	0.0%	1.08	No	0.00	6	1.09	0.094	2.18
	Brookside Hospital, San Pablo	6.2	0.0%	0.96	No	0.00	6	0.20	0.057	1.83
	California Medical Center, Los Angeles	7.5	0.0%	1.10	No	0.13	4	1.18	0.107	1.34
	Centinela Hospital Medical Center, Inglewood	6.7	0.0%	1.11	No	0.00	7	0.65	0.165	1.01
	Community Hospital of Chula Vista, Chula Vista	6.8	0.0%	0.93	No	0.00	5	0.59	0.035	1.14
	Community Memorial Hospital, Ventura	5.5	0.0%	1.23	No	0.00	5	0.85	0.038	2.57
	Dameron Hospital, Stockton	7.7	0.0%	0.98	No	0.00	4	0.76	0.175	2.47
	Fresno Community Hospital and Medical Center, Fresno	4.5	0.0%	1.80	No	0.00	9	0.88	0.069	2.64
	Good Samaritan Hospital, San Jose	7.7	0.0%	1.02	No	0.00	9	0.52	0.288	1.43
	Grossmont Hospital, La Mesa	8.1	0.0%	0.88	No	0.00	6	0.73	0.023	1.98
	Hemet Valley Medical Center, Hemet	5.4	0.0%	1.18	No	0.00	6	0.64	0.024	2.25
	Hospital of the Good Samaritan, Los Angeles	7.8	0.0%	1.55	Yes	0.04	9	0.98	0.067	1.11
	Huntington Memorial Hospital, Pasadena	7.8	0.0%	1.36	Yes	0.11	8	0.68	0.059	0.98
	Inter-Community Medical Center, Covina	6.3	0.0%	1.05	No	0.00	5	0.45	0.418	1.63
	John Muir Medical Center, Walnut Creek	7.6	0.0%	1.00	No	0.01	4	0.88	0.095	2.91
	Kaiser Foundation Hospital, Oakland	7.7	0.0%	1.04	No	0.33	5	0.72	0.070	2.11
	Kaiser Foundation Hospital, Panorama City	7.5	0.0%	0.96	No	0.01	3	0.79	0.177	2.04
	Kaiser Foundation Hospital, Redwood City	7.9	0.0%	1.06	No	0.00	6	0.96	0.205	2.05
	Kaiser Foundation Hospital, Sacramento	4.6	0.0%	1.37	No	0.19	0	0.83	0.069	3.66
	Kaiser Foundation Hospital, San Diego	7.8	0.0%	1.01	No	0.09	6	0.70	0.099	2.78
	Kaiser Foundation Hospital, Walnut Creek	8.2	0.0%	0.77	No	0.02	2	0.42	0.055	2.41
	Marin General Hospital, Greenbrae	6.5	0.0%	0.99	No	0.00	5	0.37	0.139	1.73
	Memorial Hospitals Association, Modesto	8.0	0.0%	1.02	No	0.00	7	1.10	0.043	1.68
	Mercy General Hospital, Sacramento	8.5	0.0%	0.87	No	0.00	5	0.79	0.088	1.67
	Mercy Hospital and Medical Center, San Diego	6.2	0.0%	1.48	No	0.25	6	1.06	0.120	1.80
	Mercy Medical Center, Redding	7.0	0.0%	1.75	No	0.16	7	1.77	0.069	2.76
	Mills-Peninsula Hospitals, Burlingame	7.3	0.0%	0.96	No	0.00	8	0.49	0.086	0.78
	Mount Diablo Medical Center, Concord	6.3	0.0%	1.02	No	0.00	7	0.51	0.026	1.43
	Mount Zion Medical Center, San Francisco	5.9	0.0%	1.01	No	0.28	0	0.69	0.041	1.27
	Northridge Hospital Medical Center, Northridge	7.3	0.0%	1.11	No	0.09	6	0.87	0.290	1.16
	O'Connor Hospital, San Jose	5.9	0.0%	1.44	No	0.00	7	0.82	0.220	3.44
	Palomar Medical Center, Escondido	4.3	0.0%	1.44	No	0.00	7	0.73	0.012	1.96

Natl. Rank	Hospital	U.S. News index	Reputa-tional score	Urology mortality rate	COTH member	Interns and residents to beds	Tech-nology score (of 11)	R.N.'s to beds	Board-certified internists to beds	Procedures to beds
	Roseville Hospital, Roseville	7.6	0.0%	0.92	No	0.00	8	0.29	0.073	2.36
	Salinas Valley Memorial Hospital, Salinas	8.5	0.0%	0.84	No	0.00	7	0.28	0.094	2.52
	San Gabriel Valley Medical Center, San Gabriel	5.6	0.0%	1.38	No	0.00	9	0.56	0.180	1.94
	San Jose Medical Center, San Jose	5.9	0.0%	1.20	No	0.12	7	0.61	0.066	1.52
	San Pedro Peninsula Hospital, San Pedro	7.5	0.0%	0.83	No	0.00	6	0.28	0.030	1.24
	Santa Rosa Memorial Hospital, Santa Rosa	4.3	0.0%	1.35	No	0.00	5	0.26	0.160	3.02
	Scripps Memorial Hospital, La Jolla	5.9	0.5%	1.34	No	0.00	9	0.71	0.037	1.19
	Sharp Memorial Hospital, San Diego	4.6	0.0%	1.80	No	0.00	6	1.40	0.052	1.63
	St. Agnes Medical Center, Fresno	7.4	0.0%	1.25	No	0.00	7	0.92	0.164	4.03
	St. Bernardine Medical Center, San Bernardino	3.5	0.0%	1.73	No	0.00	9	0.64	0.043	1.23
	St. Francis Medical Center, Lynwood	5.2	0.0%	1.26	No	0.00	7	0.70	0.038	1.69
	St. Joseph Hospital, Eureka	3.2	0.0%	1.76	No	0.00	7	0.48	0.059	3.12
	St. Joseph Medical Center, Burbank	7.8	0.0%	0.98	No	0.00	8	0.77	0.046	1.45
	St. Joseph's Medical Center, Stockton	6.1	0.0%	1.20	No	0.00	7	0.71	0.063	2.51
	St. Jude Medical Center, Fullerton	7.8	0.0%	1.04	No	0.00	10	0.77	0.030	2.06
	St. Vincent Medical Center, Los Angeles	7.4	0.0%	1.14	No	0.01	8	0.84	0.076	3.53
	Sutter General Hospital, Sacramento	5.7	0.0%	1.18	No	0.06	6	0.54	0.078	2.24
	Sutter Memorial Hospital, Sacramento	7.0	0.0%	1.11	No	0.03	5	1.18	0.079	0.79
	Torrance Memorial Medical Center, Torrance	7.7	0.0%	1.11	No	0.00	9	0.79	0.313	1.58
	Western Medical Center, Santa Ana	7.8	0.5%	1.09	No	0.04	6	1.05	0.061	1.36

AIDS

Natl. Rank	Hospital	U.S. News index	Reputa- tional score	Hospital- wide mortality rate	COTH member	Interns and residents to beds	Tech- nology score (of 11)	Discharge planning (of 2)	R.N.'s to beds	Board- certified internists to beds
	TIER TWO									
42	University Hospital, Denver	28.1	1.1%	0.89	Yes	0.76	9	2	1.05	0.044
	TIER THREE									
	Boulder Community Hospital, Boulder	20.9	0.0%	0.94	No	0.00	5	2	0.77	0.144
	Denver Health and Hospitals	21.9	0.3%	1.08	No	0.58	7	2	1.39	0.106
	Lutheran Medical Center, Wheat Ridge	22.7	0.0%	0.80	No	0.00	6	2	1.13	0.080
	Memorial Hospital, Colorado Springs	20.0	0.0%	1.12	No	0.00	8	2	1.51	0.027
	National Jewish Center, Denver	23.9	1.0%	0.74	No	0.00	3	2	0.62	0.533
	Porter Memorial Hospital, Denver	21.7	0.0%	0.98	No	0.02	8	2	0.80	0.207
	Poudre Valley Hospital, Fort Collins	19.8	0.0%	0.95	No	0.10	6	2	0.13	0.029
	Presbyterian-St. Luke's Medical Center, Denver	19.7	0.0%	1.17	Yes	0.07	7	2	0.75	0.071
	Rose Medical Center, Denver	20.4	0.4%	1.04	No	0.15	5	2	1.00	0.100
	St. Anthony Hospital Central, Denver	19.7	0.0%	1.02	No	0.03	5	2	0.74	0.176
	St. Joseph Hospital, Denver	24.2	0.0%	0.43	No	0.40	7	2	1.11	0.165
	St. Mary's Hospital and Medical Center, Grand Junction	21.6	0.0%	0.96	No	0.16	7	2	1.06	0.033
	Swedish Medical Center, Englewood	23.3	0.0%	0.99	No	0.02	7	2	1.01	0.642
	TIER FOUR									
	Mercy Medical Center, Denver	17.4	0.0%	1.16	No	0.31	4	2	0.70	0.053
	North Colorado Medical Center, Greeley	18.2	0.0%	1.13	No	0.16	6	2	0.78	0.022
	Penrose-St. Francis Health System, Colorado Springs	17.7	0.0%	1.11	No	0.01	6	2	0.41	0.047
	St. Mary-Corwin Regional Medical Center, Pueblo	16.2	0.0%	1.27	No	0.12	5	2	0.73	0.055

CANCER

Natl. Rank	Hospital	U.S. News index	Reputa- tional score	Cancer mortality rate	COTH member	Interns and residents to beds	Tech- nology score (of 12)	R.N.'s to beds	Board- certified oncologists to beds	Procedures to beds
	TIER TWO									
50	University Hospital, Denver	12.9	2.2%	0.43	Yes	0.76	9	1.05	0.008	1.32
	TIER THREE									
	Memorial Hospital, Colorado Springs	6.3	0.0%	0.81	No	0.00	10	1.51	0.016	0.87
	Presbyterian-St. Luke's Medical Center, Denver	6.4	0.0%	0.94	Yes	0.07	9	0.75	0.007	0.67
	St. Joseph Hospital, Denver	6.7	0.0%	0.26	No	0.40	9	1.11	0.022	1.18
	St. Mary's Hospital and Medical Center, Grand Junction	5.3	0.0%	0.96	No	0.16	9	1.06	0.014	1.74
	TIER FOUR									
	Boulder Community Hospital, Boulder	3.1	0.0%	0.70	No	0.00	5	0.77	0.014	1.06
	Lutheran Medical Center, Wheat Ridge	4.1	0.0%	0.52	No	0.00	4	1.13	0.013	2.13
	Mercy Medical Center, Denver	2.5	0.0%	1.19	No	0.31	2	0.70	0.022	0.93
	North Colorado Medical Center, Greeley	3.8	0.0%	1.04	No	0.16	7	0.78	0.011	1.49
	Penrose-St. Francis Health System, Colorado Springs	2.1	0.0%	1.11	No	0.01	7	0.41	0.008	1.19
	Porter Memorial Hospital, Denver	4.2	0.0%	0.78	No	0.02	9	0.80	0.014	1.28
	Poudre Valley Hospital, Fort Collins	1.9	0.0%	0.70	No	0.10	6	0.13	0.013	1.38
	Rose Medical Center, Denver	4.1	0.0%	0.66	No	0.15	4	1.00	0.016	1.29
	St. Anthony Hospital Central, Denver	3.6	0.0%	0.79	No	0.03	7	0.74	0.019	1.43
	St. Mary-Corwin Regional Medical Center, Pueblo	3.7	0.0%	0.92	No	0.12	7	0.73	0.016	1.86
	Swedish Medical Center, Englewood	5.2	0.0%	0.33	No	0.02	8	1.01	0.084	1.03

CARDIOLOGY

Natl. Rank	Hospital	U.S. News index	Reputa-tional score	Cardiology mortality rate	COTH member	Interns and residents to beds	Tech-nology score (of 10)	R.N.'s to beds	Board-certified cardiologists to beds	Procedures to beds
	TIER TWO									
69	University Hospital, Denver	21.9	0.4%	0.94	Yes	0.76	8	1.05	0.016	5.17
	TIER THREE									
	Boulder Community Hospital, Boulder	16.9	0.0%	0.88	No	0.00	7	0.77	0.029	4.43
	Lutheran Medical Center, Wheat Ridge	14.3	0.0%	1.05	No	0.00	8	1.13	0.048	7.16
	Memorial Hospital, Colorado Springs	15.4	0.0%	1.04	No	0.00	9	1.51	0.038	5.59
	St. Anthony Hospital Central, Denver	13.8	0.0%	1.01	No	0.03	7	0.74	0.044	6.73
	St. Joseph Hospital, Denver	20.2	0.0%	0.37	No	0.40	9	1.11	0.034	7.26
	St. Mary's Hospital and Medical Center, Grand Junction	16.8	0.0%	0.95	No	0.16	9	1.06	0.019	7.95
	Swedish Medical Center, Englewood	14.0	0.0%	1.03	No	0.02	6	1.01	0.123	4.65
	TIER FOUR									
	Mercy Medical Center, Denver	7.7	0.0%	1.38	No	0.31	6	0.70	0.035	4.76
	North Colorado Medical Center, Greeley	12.0	0.0%	1.10	No	0.16	7	0.78	0.022	7.85
	Penrose-St. Francis Health System, Colorado Springs	9.8	0.0%	1.14	No	0.01	8	0.41	0.027	4.53
	Porter Memorial Hospital, Denver	12.1	0.0%	1.10	No	0.02	8	0.80	0.038	7.24
	Poudre Valley Hospital, Fort Collins	13.2	0.0%	0.97	No	0.10	8	0.13	0.021	6.93
	Presbyterian-St. Luke's Medical Center, Denver	13.2	0.0%	1.16	Yes	0.07	8	0.75	0.023	4.70
	Rose Medical Center, Denver	9.8	0.0%	1.28	No	0.15	7	1.00	0.044	5.92
	St. Mary-Corwin Regional Medical Center, Pueblo	5.1	0.0%	1.53	No	0.12	6	0.73	0.023	4.91

ENDOCRINOLOGY

Natl. Rank	Hospital	U.S. News index	Reputa-tional score	Endocrinology mortality rate	COTH member	Interns and residents to beds	Tech-nology score (of 11)	R.N.'s to beds	Board-certified internists to beds
	TIER TWO								
44	University Hospital, Denver	17.9	2.2%	0.75	Yes	0.76	10	1.05	0.044
	TIER THREE								
	Lutheran Medical Center, Wheat Ridge	9.3	0.0%	0.76	No	0.00	5	1.13	0.080
	Penrose-St. Francis Health System, Colorado Springs	9.1	0.0%	0.58	No	0.01	8	0.41	0.047
	Presbyterian-St. Luke's Medical Center, Denver	9.1	0.0%	1.08	Yes	0.07	9	0.75	0.071
	Rose Medical Center, Denver	10.8	0.4%	0.70	No	0.15	5	1.00	0.100
	St. Joseph Hospital, Denver	13.5	0.0%	0.44	No	0.40	10	1.11	0.165
	St. Mary's Hospital and Medical Center, Grand Junction	11.1	0.0%	0.69	No	0.16	10	1.06	0.033
	Swedish Medical Center, Englewood	10.9	0.0%	1.12	No	0.02	9	1.01	0.642
	TIER FOUR								
	Memorial Hospital, Colorado Springs	7.0	0.0%	1.37	No	0.00	10	1.51	0.027
	Mercy Medical Center, Denver	7.0	0.0%	0.91	No	0.31	3	0.70	0.053
	North Colorado Medical Center, Greeley	6.2	0.0%	1.11	No	0.16	8	0.78	0.022
	Porter Memorial Hospital, Denver	7.1	0.0%	1.12	No	0.02	8	0.80	0.207
	Poudre Valley Hospital, Fort Collins	3.0	0.0%	1.31	No	0.10	6	0.13	0.029
	St. Anthony Hospital Central, Denver	7.2	0.0%	1.00	No	0.03	7	0.74	0.176
	St. Mary-Corwin Regional Medical Center, Pueblo	5.7	0.0%	1.21	No	0.12	8	0.73	0.055

GASTROENTEROLOGY

Natl. Rank	Hospital	U.S. News index	Reputa-tional score	Gastro-enterology mortality rate	COTH member	Interns and residents to beds	Tech-nology score (of 11)	R.N.'s to beds	Board-certified gastro-enterologists to beds	Pro-cedures to beds
	TIER THREE									
	Lutheran Medical Center, Wheat Ridge	9.3	0.0%	0.75	No	0.00	6	1.13	0.019	4.71
	Presbyterian-St. Luke's Medical Center, Denver	7.8	0.0%	1.11	Yes	0.07	8	0.75	0.011	1.77
	St. Joseph Hospital, Denver	11.1	0.0%	0.50	No	0.40	10	1.11	0.030	3.28
	St. Mary's Hospital and Medical Center, Grand Junction	9.2	0.0%	0.93	No	0.16	9	1.06	0.014	4.29

Natl. Rank	Hospital	U.S. News index	Reputational score	Gastro-enterology mortality rate	COTH member	Interns and residents to beds	Technology score (of 11)	R.N.'s to beds	Board-certified gastro-enterologists to beds	Procedures to beds
	TIER FOUR									
	Boulder Community Hospital, Boulder	6.1	0.0%	0.90	No	0.00	5	0.77	0.019	2.60
	Memorial Hospital, Colorado Springs	6.1	0.0%	1.37	No	0.00	9	1.51	0.011	2.32
	Mercy Medical Center, Denver	3.3	0.0%	1.64	No	0.31	3	0.70	0.022	3.43
	North Colorado Medical Center, Greeley	6.5	0.0%	1.13	No	0.16	7	0.78	0.011	4.27
	Penrose-St. Francis Health System, Colorado Springs	3.2	0.0%	1.35	No	0.01	7	0.41	0.006	2.76
	Porter Memorial Hospital, Denver	4.9	0.0%	1.23	No	0.02	7	0.80	0.000	3.15
	Poudre Valley Hospital, Fort Collins	6.0	0.4%	0.93	No	0.10	6	0.13	0.013	3.44
	Rose Medical Center, Denver	6.3	0.0%	1.06	No	0.15	5	1.00	0.036	3.22
	St. Anthony Hospital Central, Denver	5.0	0.0%	1.20	No	0.03	6	0.74	0.011	3.81
	St. Mary-Corwin Regional Medical Center, Pueblo	4.6	0.0%	1.56	No	0.12	8	0.73	0.007	3.91
	Swedish Medical Center, Englewood	6.9	0.0%	1.08	No	0.02	9	1.01	0.045	3.00

GERIATRICS

Natl. Rank	Hospital	U.S. News index	Reputational score	Hospital-wide mortality rate	COTH member	Service mix	Interns and residents to beds	Technology score (of 13)	R.N.'s to beds	Discharge planning (of 2)	Geriatric services (of 9)	Board-certified internists to beds
	TIER TWO											
89	St. Joseph Hospital, Denver	21.7	0.0%	0.43	No	6	0.40	11	1.11	2	6	0.165
27	University Hospital, Denver	27.6	1.4%	0.89	Yes	6	0.76	10	1.05	2	7	0.044
	TIER THREE											
	Boulder Community Hospital, Boulder	16.4	0.0%	0.94	No	6	0.00	6	0.77	2	2	0.144
	Lutheran Medical Center, Wheat Ridge	18.8	0.0%	0.80	No	6	0.00	7	1.13	2	3	0.080
	Porter Memorial Hospital, Denver	17.0	0.0%	0.98	No	8	0.02	9	0.80	2	2	0.207
	Poudre Valley Hospital, Fort Collins	14.9	0.0%	0.95	No	5	0.10	8	0.13	2	4	0.029
	Presbyterian-St. Luke's Medical Center, Denver	14.9	0.0%	1.17	Yes	7	0.07	11	0.75	2	7	0.071
	Rose Medical Center, Denver	14.1	0.0%	1.04	No	6	0.15	6	1.00	2	2	0.100
	St. Anthony Hospital Central, Denver	13.9	0.0%	1.02	No	4	0.03	9	0.74	2	2	0.176
	St. Mary's Hospital and Medical Center, Grand Junction	18.0	0.0%	0.96	No	7	0.16	11	1.06	2	4	0.033
	Swedish Medical Center, Englewood	20.1	0.0%	0.99	No	6	0.02	10	1.01	2	7	0.642
	TIER FOUR											
	Memorial Hospital, Colorado Springs	13.7	0.0%	1.12	No	5	0.00	11	1.51	2	5	0.027
	Mercy Medical Center, Denver	10.2	0.0%	1.16	No	4	0.31	4	0.70	2	5	0.053
	North Colorado Medical Center, Greeley	11.5	0.0%	1.13	No	6	0.16	9	0.78	2	2	0.022
	Penrose-St. Francis Health System, Colorado Springs	12.8	0.0%	1.11	No	7	0.01	10	0.41	2	6	0.047
	St. Mary-Corwin Regional Medical Center, Pueblo	9.8	0.0%	1.27	No	7	0.12	8	0.73	2	5	0.055

GYNECOLOGY

Natl. Rank	Hospital	U.S. News index	Reputational score	Hospital-wide mortality rate	Interns and residents to beds	Technology score (of 10)	R.N.'s to beds	Board-certified OB-GYNs to beds	Procedures to beds
	TIER TWO								
64	St. Joseph Hospital, Denver	24.4	0.0%	0.43	0.40	9	1.11	0.092	0.60
48	University Hospital, Denver	26.7	1.0%	0.89	0.76	9	1.05	0.028	0.46
	TIER THREE								
	Boulder Community Hospital, Boulder	16.5	0.0%	0.94	0.00	5	0.77	0.096	0.38
	Lutheran Medical Center, Wheat Ridge	19.5	0.0%	0.80	0.00	5	1.13	0.080	0.62
	Memorial Hospital, Colorado Springs	17.0	0.0%	1.12	0.00	9	1.51	0.057	0.29
	Porter Memorial Hospital, Denver	16.9	0.0%	0.98	0.02	7	0.80	0.095	0.29
	Rose Medical Center, Denver	15.6	0.0%	1.04	0.15	5	1.00	0.196	0.58
	St. Mary's Hospital and Medical Center, Grand Junction	18.9	0.0%	0.96	0.16	9	1.06	0.019	0.50
	Swedish Medical Center, Englewood	18.4	0.0%	0.99	0.02	8	1.01	0.271	0.62

Natl. Rank Hospital	U.S. News index	Reputational score	Hospital-wide mortality rate	Interns and residents to beds	Technology score (of 10)	R.N.'s to beds	Board-certified OB-GYNs to beds	Procedures to beds
TIER FOUR								
Mercy Medical Center, Denver	9.6	0.0%	1.16	0.31	3	0.70	0.058	0.27
North Colorado Medical Center, Greeley	11.4	0.0%	1.13	0.16	6	0.78	0.030	0.41
Penrose-St. Francis Health System, Colorado Springs	9.8	0.0%	1.11	0.01	6	0.41	0.036	0.36
Poudre Valley Hospital, Fort Collins	13.0	0.0%	0.95	0.10	5	0.13	0.059	0.54
Presbyterian-St. Luke's Medical Center, Denver	12.8	0.0%	1.17	0.07	8	0.75	0.080	0.41
St. Anthony Hospital Central, Denver	12.7	0.0%	1.02	0.03	5	0.74	0.030	0.26
St. Mary-Corwin Regional Medical Center, Pueblo	8.4	0.0%	1.27	0.12	6	0.73	0.029	0.30

NEUROLOGY

Natl. Rank Hospital	U.S. News index	Reputational score	Neurology mortality rate	COTH member	Interns and residents to beds	Technology score (of 9)	R.N.'s to beds	Board-certified neurologists to beds
TIER TWO								
48 University Hospital, Denver	20.6	0.4%	0.75	Yes	0.76	8	1.05	0.008
TIER THREE								
Lutheran Medical Center, Wheat Ridge	15.8	0.0%	0.56	No	0.00	5	1.13	0.026
Memorial Hospital, Colorado Springs	14.2	0.0%	0.90	No	0.00	8	1.51	0.022
Porter Memorial Hospital, Denver	14.5	0.0%	0.81	No	0.02	6	0.80	0.033
Presbyterian-St. Luke's Medical Center, Denver	15.9	0.0%	0.79	Yes	0.07	7	0.75	0.007
Rose Medical Center, Denver	15.8	0.0%	0.67	No	0.15	4	1.00	0.028
100 St. Joseph Hospital, Denver	17.0	0.0%	0.41	No	0.40	8	1.11	0.012
Swedish Medical Center, Englewood	13.2	0.0%	1.14	No	0.02	7	1.01	0.087
TIER FOUR								
North Colorado Medical Center, Greeley	6.2	0.0%	1.25	No	0.16	6	0.78	0.007
Penrose-St. Francis Health System, Colorado Springs	6.9	0.0%	1.09	No	0.01	6	0.41	0.009
Poudre Valley Hospital, Fort Collins	6.1	0.0%	1.08	No	0.10	5	0.13	0.008
St. Anthony Hospital Central, Denver	8.4	0.0%	1.07	No	0.03	5	0.74	0.019
St. Mary's Hospital and Medical Center, Grand Junction	9.8	0.0%	1.10	No	0.16	8	1.06	0.014
St. Mary-Corwin Regional Medical Center, Pueblo	8.3	0.0%	1.10	No	0.12	6	0.73	0.016

ORTHOPEDICS

Natl. Rank Hospital	U.S. News index	Reputational score	Orthopedics mortality rate	COTH member	Interns and residents to beds	Technology score (of 5)	R.N.'s to beds	Board-certified orthopedists to beds	Procedures to beds
TIER TWO									
63 University Hospital, Denver	15.6	0.0%	0.69	Yes	0.76	4	1.05	0.020	1.89
TIER THREE									
Boulder Community Hospital, Boulder	9.7	0.0%	0.56	No	0.00	3	0.77	0.043	2.58
Lutheran Medical Center, Wheat Ridge	12.6	0.5%	0.57	No	0.00	3	1.13	0.093	4.87
Mercy Medical Center, Denver	10.0	0.0%	0.62	No	0.31	2	0.70	0.049	2.62
Porter Memorial Hospital, Denver	8.3	0.0%	0.84	No	0.02	4	0.80	0.079	2.52
Poudre Valley Hospital, Fort Collins	8.7	0.0%	0.73	No	0.10	4	0.13	0.038	5.79
Presbyterian-St. Luke's Medical Center, Denver	8.2	0.0%	1.19	Yes	0.07	4	0.75	0.034	2.37
St. Anthony Hospital Central, Denver	9.0	0.0%	0.68	No	0.03	2	0.74	0.047	3.06
86 St. Joseph Hospital, Denver	13.8	0.5%	0.59	No	0.40	4	1.11	0.054	2.94
St. Mary's Hospital and Medical Center, Grand Junction	8.2	0.0%	1.07	No	0.16	4	1.06	0.047	5.86
Swedish Medical Center, Englewood	10.3	0.0%	0.78	No	0.02	4	1.01	0.187	3.28
TIER FOUR									
Memorial Hospital, Colorado Springs	6.3	0.0%	1.45	No	0.00	4	1.51	0.076	2.07
North Colorado Medical Center, Greeley	7.9	0.0%	0.89	No	0.16	3	0.78	0.049	4.60
Penrose-St. Francis Health System, Colorado Springs	3.8	0.0%	1.22	No	0.01	3	0.41	0.052	2.98
Rose Medical Center, Denver	7.1	0.0%	1.00	No	0.15	3	1.00	0.052	2.77
St. Mary-Corwin Regional Medical Center, Pueblo	4.1	0.0%	1.28	No	0.12	2	0.73	0.033	3.67

OTOLARYNGOLOGY

Natl. Rank	Hospital	U.S. News index	Reputa-tional score	Hospital-wide mortality rate	COTH member	Interns and residents to beds	Tech-nology score (of 9)	R.N.'s to beds	Board-certified internists to beds	Procedures to beds
TIER TWO										
99	University Hospital, Denver	13.8	0.5%	0.88	Yes	0.76	8	1.05	0.044	0.348
TIER THREE										
	Denver Health and Hospitals	8.0	0.0%	1.08	No	0.58	2	1.39	0.106	0.115
	Memorial Hospital, Colorado Springs	7.1	0.0%	1.12	No	0.00	8	1.51	0.027	0.095
	National Jewish Center, Denver	10.4	0.8%	0.74	No	0.00	2	0.62	0.533	5.086
	Presbyterian-St. Luke's Medical Center, Denver	8.3	0.0%	1.17	Yes	0.07	7	0.75	0.071	0.123
	St. Joseph Hospital, Denver	9.0	0.0%	0.43	No	0.40	8	1.11	0.165	0.253
	Swedish Medical Center, Englewood	10.7	0.0%	0.99	No	0.02	7	1.01	0.642	0.371
TIER FOUR										
	Boulder Community Hospital, Boulder	4.8	0.0%	0.94	No	0.00	4	0.77	0.144	0.215
	Lutheran Medical Center, Wheat Ridge	5.3	0.0%	0.80	No	0.00	3	1.13	0.080	0.304
	Mercy Medical Center, Denver	4.1	0.0%	1.17	No	0.31	1	0.70	0.053	0.168
	North Colorado Medical Center, Greeley	4.9	0.0%	1.14	No	0.16	6	0.78	0.022	0.423
	Penrose-St. Francis Health System, Colorado Springs	3.4	0.0%	1.11	No	0.01	6	0.41	0.047	0.193
	Porter Memorial Hospital, Denver	6.4	0.0%	0.98	No	0.02	7	0.80	0.207	0.337
	Poudre Valley Hospital, Fort Collins	2.3	0.0%	0.95	No	0.10	4	0.13	0.029	0.286
	Rose Medical Center, Denver	5.4	0.0%	1.03	No	0.15	3	1.00	0.100	0.208
	St. Anthony Hospital Central, Denver	5.6	0.0%	1.02	No	0.03	6	0.74	0.176	0.214
	St. Mary's Hospital and Medical Center, Grand Junction	6.5	0.0%	0.96	No	0.16	8	1.06	0.033	0.519
	St. Mary-Corwin Regional Medical Center, Pueblo	4.8	0.0%	1.27	No	0.12	6	0.73	0.055	0.358

RHEUMATOLOGY

Natl. Rank	Hospital	U.S. News index	Reputa-tional score	Hospital-wide mortality rate	COTH member	Interns and residents to beds	Tech-nology score (of 5)	R.N.'s to beds	Board-certified internists to beds
TIER TWO									
48	University Hospital, Denver	17.9	1.1%	0.88	Yes	0.76	4	1.05	0.044
TIER THREE									
	Lutheran Medical Center, Wheat Ridge	11.1	0.0%	0.80	No	0.00	3	1.13	0.080
	Porter Memorial Hospital, Denver	10.1	0.0%	0.98	No	0.02	4	0.80	0.207
	Presbyterian-St. Luke's Medical Center, Denver	10.1	0.0%	1.17	Yes	0.07	4	0.75	0.071
	Rose Medical Center, Denver	10.1	0.4%	1.03	No	0.15	3	1.00	0.100
	St. Joseph Hospital, Denver	13.4	0.0%	0.43	No	0.40	4	1.11	0.165
	St. Mary's Hospital and Medical Center, Grand Junction	10.1	0.0%	0.96	No	0.16	4	1.06	0.033
	Swedish Medical Center, Englewood	13.7	0.0%	0.99	No	0.02	4	1.01	0.642
TIER FOUR									
	Boulder Community Hospital, Boulder	9.4	0.0%	0.94	No	0.00	3	0.77	0.144
	Memorial Hospital, Colorado Springs	9.4	0.0%	1.12	No	0.00	4	1.51	0.027
	Mercy Medical Center, Denver	7.2	0.0%	1.17	No	0.31	2	0.70	0.053
	North Colorado Medical Center, Greeley	7.4	0.0%	1.14	No	0.16	3	0.78	0.022
	Penrose-St. Francis Health System, Colorado Springs	6.3	0.0%	1.11	No	0.01	3	0.41	0.047
	Poudre Valley Hospital, Fort Collins	7.5	0.0%	0.95	No	0.10	4	0.13	0.029
	St. Anthony Hospital Central, Denver	8.4	0.0%	1.02	No	0.03	2	0.74	0.176
	St. Mary-Corwin Regional Medical Center, Pueblo	6.0	0.0%	1.27	No	0.12	2	0.73	0.055

UROLOGY

Natl. Rank	Hospital	U.S. News index	Reputa-tional score	Urology mortality rate	COTH member	Interns and residents to beds	Tech-nology score (of 11)	R.N.'s to beds	Board-certified internists to beds	Procedures to beds
TIER TWO										
84	University Hospital, Denver	15.3	2.5%	1.24	Yes	0.76	9	1.05	0.044	1.80
TIER THREE										
	Boulder Community Hospital, Boulder	10.9	0.0%	0.57	No	0.00	5	0.77	0.144	1.70
	Lutheran Medical Center, Wheat Ridge	11.9	0.0%	0.63	No	0.00	6	1.13	0.080	2.51
	Memorial Hospital, Colorado Springs	9.6	0.0%	0.98	No	0.00	9	1.51	0.027	0.98
	North Colorado Medical Center, Greeley	9.8	0.0%	0.82	No	0.16	7	0.78	0.022	1.94
	Porter Memorial Hospital, Denver	11.6	0.0%	0.65	No	0.02	7	0.80	0.207	1.68
	Rose Medical Center, Denver	11.7	0.0%	0.64	No	0.15	5	1.00	0.100	1.81
99	St. Joseph Hospital, Denver	14.4	0.0%	0.36	No	0.40	10	1.11	0.165	1.44
	St. Mary's Hospital and Medical Center, Grand Junction	11.4	0.0%	0.81	No	0.16	9	1.06	0.033	2.19
	Swedish Medical Center, Englewood	12.6	0.0%	0.63	No	0.02	9	1.01	0.642	1.50
TIER FOUR										
	Mercy Medical Center, Denver	7.8	0.0%	0.93	No	0.31	3	0.70	0.053	1.34
	Penrose-St. Francis Health System, Colorado Springs	3.8	0.0%	1.39	No	0.01	7	0.41	0.047	1.20
	Poudre Valley Hospital, Fort Collins	8.3	0.0%	0.79	No	0.10	6	0.13	0.029	2.12
	Presbyterian-St. Luke's Medical Center, Denver	8.1	0.0%	1.34	Yes	0.07	8	0.75	0.071	1.24
	St. Anthony Hospital Central, Denver	8.0	0.0%	0.98	No	0.03	6	0.74	0.176	1.63
	St. Mary-Corwin Regional Medical Center, Pueblo	4.2	0.0%	1.70	No	0.12	8	0.73	0.055	1.73

AIDS

Natl. Rank	Hospital	U.S. News index	Reputa-tional score	Hospital-wide mortality rate	COTH member	Interns and residents to beds	Tech-nology score (of 11)	Discharge planning (of 2)	R.N.'s to beds	Board-certified internists to beds
	TIER TWO									
38	Yale-New Haven Hospital, New Haven	28.6	2.6%	1.06	Yes	1.12	10	2	1.23	0.094
	TIER THREE									
	Danbury Hospital, Danbury	22.2	0.0%	0.99	Yes	0.11	7	2	0.50	0.138
	Greenwich Hospital, Greenwich	20.7	0.0%	1.04	No	0.23	5	2	1.40	0.108
	Hartford Hospital, Hartford	21.0	0.0%	1.11	Yes	0.36	8	1	0.87	0.086
	Hospital of St. Raphael, New Haven	24.3	0.0%	0.97	Yes	0.44	7	2	1.36	0.082
	New Britain General Hospital, New Britain	20.7	0.0%	1.08	Yes	0.17	7	2	0.53	0.083
	St. Francis Hospital and Medical Center, Hartford	21.6	0.0%	1.11	Yes	0.45	8	2	0.65	0.103
	St. Mary's Hospital, Waterbury	20.8	0.0%	1.10	Yes	0.36	6	2	0.74	0.070
	Stamford Hospital, Stamford	20.8	0.0%	1.15	Yes	0.29	7	2	0.99	0.087
	University of Connecticut Health Center, Farmington	22.8	0.4%	1.10	Yes	0.56	7	2	0.65	0.293
	TIER FOUR									
	Bridgeport Hospital, Bridgeport	18.8	0.0%	1.40	Yes	0.35	8	2	1.06	0.059
	Griffin Hospital, Derby	17.7	0.0%	1.15	No	0.24	5	2	0.69	0.036
	Middlesex Hospital, Middletown	16.8	0.0%	1.18	No	0.16	6	1	0.69	0.031
	Mount Sinai Hospital, Hartford	19.2	0.0%	1.11	No	0.21	6	2	0.98	0.097
	Norwalk Hospital, Norwalk	18.1	0.0%	1.25	No	0.31	6	2	0.98	0.175
	Waterbury Hospital, Waterbury	17.1	0.0%	1.25	No	0.35	6	2	0.64	0.058

CANCER

Natl. Rank	Hospital	U.S. News index	Reputa-tional score	Cancer mortality rate	COTH member	Interns and residents to beds	Tech-nology score (of 12)	R.N.'s to beds	Board-certified oncologists to beds	Procedures to beds
	TIER TWO									
36	Yale-New Haven Hospital, New Haven	14.1	1.3%	0.51	Yes	1.12	10	1.23	0.035	2.08
	TIER THREE									
	Bridgeport Hospital, Bridgeport	7.8	0.0%	1.28	Yes	0.35	8	1.06	0.007	1.56
	Danbury Hospital, Danbury	5.6	0.0%	0.85	Yes	0.11	8	0.50	0.013	0.41
	Greenwich Hospital, Greenwich	5.3	0.0%	1.46	No	0.23	6	1.40	0.017	1.88
	Hartford Hospital, Hartford	8.1	0.5%	1.15	Yes	0.36	9	0.87	0.006	1.18
	Hospital of St. Raphael, New Haven	9.7	0.0%	0.67	Yes	0.44	8	1.36	0.020	1.54
	New Britain General Hospital, New Britain	6.0	0.0%	1.01	Yes	0.17	8	0.53	0.012	1.76
	St. Francis Hospital and Medical Center, Hartford	7.6	0.0%	0.86	Yes	0.45	9	0.65	0.011	1.35
	St. Mary's Hospital, Waterbury	6.8	0.0%	1.26	Yes	0.36	7	0.74	0.020	2.18
	Stamford Hospital, Stamford	7.8	0.0%	1.21	Yes	0.29	9	0.99	0.025	1.47
	TIER FOUR									
	Griffin Hospital, Derby	2.2	0.0%	1.09	No	0.24	2	0.69	0.006	1.24
	Middlesex Hospital, Middletown	3.3	0.0%	1.84	No	0.16	7	0.69	0.013	2.13
	Mount Sinai Hospital, Hartford	4.0	0.0%	0.66	No	0.21	4	0.98	0.004	0.74
	Norwalk Hospital, Norwalk	4.7	0.0%	1.34	No	0.31	7	0.98	0.013	1.72
	St. Vincent's Medical Center, Bridgeport	3.9	0.0%	1.31	Yes	0.17	0	0.70	0.013	1.54
	Waterbury Hospital, Waterbury	3.8	0.0%	1.45	No	0.35	7	0.64	0.015	1.49

CARDIOLOGY

Natl. Rank	Hospital	U.S. News index	Reputa-tional score	Cardiology mortality rate	COTH member	Interns and residents to beds	Tech-nology score (of 10)	R.N.'s to beds	Board-certified cardiologists to beds	Procedures to beds
	TIER TWO									
49	Yale-New Haven Hospital, New Haven	23.0	2.0%	1.14	Yes	1.12	9	1.23	0.081	7.27
	TIER THREE									
	Danbury Hospital, Danbury	16.3	0.0%	0.96	Yes	0.11	5	0.50	0.039	2.86
	Greenwich Hospital, Greenwich	16.4	0.0%	0.98	No	0.23	5	1.40	0.040	6.89
	Griffin Hospital, Derby	13.6	0.0%	1.00	No	0.24	4	0.69	0.036	9.12
	Hartford Hospital, Hartford	16.3	0.0%	1.09	Yes	0.36	8	0.87	0.032	6.36
	Hospital of St. Raphael, New Haven	20.1	0.0%	1.03	Yes	0.44	8	1.36	0.082	12.65
	Middlesex Hospital, Middletown	15.6	0.0%	0.93	No	0.16	5	0.69	0.031	10.03
	Mount Sinai Hospital, Hartford	17.8	0.0%	0.85	No	0.21	5	0.98	0.036	4.78
	New Britain General Hospital, New Britain	14.7	0.0%	1.08	Yes	0.17	7	0.53	0.039	7.86
	St. Francis Hospital and Medical Center, Hartford	20.7	0.3%	0.95	Yes	0.45	9	0.65	0.054	10.05
	St. Mary's Hospital, Waterbury	14.2	0.0%	1.14	Yes	0.36	5	0.74	0.027	10.43
	Stamford Hospital, Stamford	14.0	0.0%	1.20	Yes	0.29	6	0.99	0.047	5.89
	TIER FOUR									
	Bridgeport Hospital, Bridgeport	12.5	0.0%	1.36	Yes	0.35	8	1.06	0.028	8.89
	Norwalk Hospital, Norwalk	12.2	0.0%	1.12	No	0.31	5	0.98	0.026	7.55
	St. Vincent's Medical Center, Bridgeport	12.0	0.0%	1.14	Yes	0.17	0	0.70	0.031	11.99
	Waterbury Hospital, Waterbury	11.3	0.0%	1.13	No	0.35	5	0.64	0.027	8.27

ENDOCRINOLOGY

Natl. Rank	Hospital	U.S. News index	Reputa-tional score	Endocrinology mortality rate	COTH member	Interns and residents to beds	Tech-nology score (of 11)	R.N.'s to beds	Board-certified internists to beds
	TIER TWO								
54	Yale-New Haven Hospital, New Haven	17.2	3.3%	1.36	Yes	1.12	10	1.23	0.094
	TIER THREE								
	Hartford Hospital, Hartford	8.7	0.4%	1.58	Yes	0.36	8	0.87	0.086
	Hospital of St. Raphael, New Haven	10.7	0.0%	1.32	Yes	0.44	8	1.36	0.082
	St. Francis Hospital and Medical Center, Hartford	9.2	0.0%	1.31	Yes	0.45	9	0.65	0.103
	St. Mary's Hospital, Waterbury	10.5	0.0%	0.98	Yes	0.36	8	0.74	0.070
	Stamford Hospital, Stamford	8.5	0.0%	1.67	Yes	0.29	10	0.99	0.087
	Waterbury Hospital, Waterbury	9.4	0.0%	0.77	No	0.35	8	0.64	0.058
	TIER FOUR								
	Bridgeport Hospital, Bridgeport	7.8	0.0%	1.89	Yes	0.35	8	1.06	0.059
	Greenwich Hospital, Greenwich	7.7	0.0%	1.25	No	0.23	6	1.40	0.108
	Griffin Hospital, Derby	4.3	0.0%	1.39	No	0.24	4	0.69	0.036
	Middlesex Hospital, Middletown	4.1	0.0%	1.64	No	0.16	8	0.69	0.031
	Mount Sinai Hospital, Hartford	4.5	0.0%	1.73	No	0.21	4	0.98	0.097
	New Britain General Hospital, New Britain	7.0	0.0%	1.52	Yes	0.17	9	0.53	0.083
	Norwalk Hospital, Norwalk	6.5	0.0%	1.61	No	0.31	8	0.98	0.175
	St. Vincent's Medical Center, Bridgeport	5.9	0.0%	1.44	Yes	0.17	0	0.70	0.066

GASTROENTEROLOGY

Natl. Rank	Hospital	U.S. News index	Reputa-tional score	Gastro-enterology mortality rate	COTH member	Interns and residents to beds	Tech-nology score (of 11)	R.N.'s to beds	Board-certified gastro-enterologists to beds	Pro-cedures to beds
	TIER ONE									
16	Yale-New Haven Hospital, New Haven	23.6	5.6%	0.85	Yes	1.12	9	1.23	0.050	1.92
	TIER TWO									
60	Hospital of St. Raphael, New Haven	14.2	0.0%	0.80	Yes	0.44	7	1.36	0.033	4.41

Natl. Rank	Hospital	U.S. News index	Reputational score	Gastro-enterology mortality rate	COTH member	Interns and residents to beds	Technology score (of 11)	R.N.'s to beds	Board-certified gastro-enterologists to beds	Pro-cedures to beds
	T I E R T H R E E									
	Bridgeport Hospital, Bridgeport	9.4	0.0%	1.23	Yes	0.35	7	1.06	0.009	3.23
	Greenwich Hospital, Greenwich	7.5	0.0%	1.12	No	0.23	5	1.40	0.028	3.70
	Hartford Hospital, Hartford	10.2	0.0%	0.98	Yes	0.36	7	0.87	0.016	2.66
	New Britain General Hospital, New Britain	10.1	0.0%	0.91	Yes	0.17	8	0.53	0.012	3.61
	Norwalk Hospital, Norwalk	8.3	0.0%	1.01	No	0.31	7	0.98	0.040	4.08
	St. Francis Hospital and Medical Center, Hartford	9.4	0.0%	1.17	Yes	0.45	8	0.65	0.018	3.09
	St. Mary's Hospital, Waterbury	11.2	0.0%	1.00	Yes	0.36	7	0.74	0.030	5.05
	Stamford Hospital, Stamford	10.9	0.0%	1.00	Yes	0.29	9	0.99	0.032	2.90
	T I E R F O U R									
	Danbury Hospital, Danbury	5.4	0.0%	1.48	Yes	0.11	8	0.50	0.033	1.12
	Griffin Hospital, Derby	6.0	0.0%	1.10	No	0.24	4	0.69	0.018	4.33
	Middlesex Hospital, Middletown	7.2	0.0%	1.13	No	0.16	7	0.69	0.018	5.71
	Mount Sinai Hospital, Hartford	4.2	0.0%	1.34	No	0.21	4	0.98	0.024	2.21
	St. Vincent's Medical Center, Bridgeport	6.4	0.0%	1.21	Yes	0.17	0	0.70	0.018	3.93
	Waterbury Hospital, Waterbury	5.6	0.0%	1.38	No	0.35	7	0.64	0.027	3.84

GERIATRICS

Natl. Rank	Hospital	U.S. News index	Reputational score	Hospital-wide mortality rate	COTH member	Service mix	Interns and residents to beds	Technology score (of 13)	R.N.'s to beds	Discharge planning (of 2)	Geriatric services (of 9)	Board-certified internists to beds
	T I E R O N E											
20	Yale-New Haven Hospital, New Haven	31.4	4.6%	1.06	Yes	5	1.12	11	1.23	2	3	0.094
	T I E R T W O											
88	Hospital of St. Raphael, New Haven	21.7	0.0%	0.97	Yes	7	0.44	11	1.36	2	6	0.082
	T I E R T H R E E											
	Greenwich Hospital, Greenwich	16.5	0.0%	1.04	No	8	0.23	7	1.40	2	3	0.108
	Hartford Hospital, Hartford	16.1	0.0%	1.11	Yes	8	0.36	11	0.87	1	5	0.086
	New Britain General Hospital, New Britain	16.3	0.0%	1.08	Yes	7	0.17	11	0.53	2	5	0.083
	St. Francis Hospital and Medical Center, Hartford	17.8	0.0%	1.11	Yes	9	0.45	12	0.65	2	5	0.103
	St. Mary's Hospital, Waterbury	14.8	0.0%	1.10	Yes	5	0.36	10	0.74	2	2	0.070
	Stamford Hospital, Stamford	15.5	0.0%	1.15	Yes	7	0.29	10	0.99	2	4	0.087
	T I E R F O U R											
	Bridgeport Hospital, Bridgeport	11.0	0.0%	1.40	Yes	7	0.35	10	1.06	2	3	0.059
	Griffin Hospital, Derby	9.9	0.0%	1.15	No	5	0.24	4	0.69	2	2	0.036
	Middlesex Hospital, Middletown	9.1	0.0%	1.18	No	6	0.16	9	0.69	1	1	0.031
	Mount Sinai Hospital, Hartford	13.6	0.0%	1.11	No	7	0.21	6	0.98	2	5	0.097
	Norwalk Hospital, Norwalk	11.9	0.0%	1.25	No	7	0.31	9	0.98	2	5	0.175
	Waterbury Hospital, Waterbury	9.1	0.0%	1.25	No	5	0.35	9	0.64	2	2	0.058

GYNECOLOGY

Natl. Rank	Hospital	U.S. News index	Reputational score	Hospital-wide mortality rate	Interns and residents to beds	Technology score (of 10)	R.N.'s to beds	Board-certified OB-GYNs to beds	Procedures to beds
	T I E R O N E								
16	Yale-New Haven Hospital, New Haven	38.4	5.9%	1.06	1.12	9	1.23	0.103	0.60
	T I E R T H R E E								
	Greenwich Hospital, Greenwich	16.4	0.0%	1.04	0.23	5	1.40	0.045	0.46
	Hartford Hospital, Hartford	14.5	0.0%	1.11	0.36	7	0.87	0.053	0.41
	Hospital of St. Raphael, New Haven	19.2	0.0%	0.97	0.44	6	1.36	0.029	0.28
	St. Francis Hospital and Medical Center, Hartford	15.1	0.0%	1.11	0.45	8	0.65	0.067	0.48
	Stamford Hospital, Stamford	15.7	0.0%	1.15	0.29	9	0.99	0.072	0.33

Natl. Rank	Hospital	U.S. News index	Reputational score	Hospital-wide mortality rate	Interns and residents to beds	Technology score (of 10)	R.N.'s to beds	Board-certified OB-GYNs to beds	Procedures to beds
	TIER FOUR								
	Bridgeport Hospital, Bridgeport	9.6	0.0%	1.40	0.35	7	1.06	0.028	0.37
	Griffin Hospital, Derby	9.5	0.0%	1.15	0.24	4	0.69	0.024	0.50
	Middlesex Hospital, Middletown	10.2	0.0%	1.18	0.16	6	0.69	0.036	0.62
	Mount Sinai Hospital, Hartford	13.6	0.0%	1.11	0.21	5	0.98	0.085	0.25
	New Britain General Hospital, New Britain	13.9	0.0%	1.08	0.17	8	0.53	0.068	0.69
	Norwalk Hospital, Norwalk	11.9	0.0%	1.25	0.31	7	0.98	0.053	0.29
	St. Mary's Hospital, Waterbury	12.7	0.0%	1.10	0.36	6	0.74	0.020	0.37
	Waterbury Hospital, Waterbury	9.4	0.0%	1.25	0.35	6	0.64	0.033	0.35

NEUROLOGY

Natl. Rank	Hospital	U.S. News index	Reputational score	Neurology mortality rate	COTH member	Interns and residents to beds	Technology score (of 9)	R.N.'s to beds	Board-certified neurologists to beds
	TIER TWO								
62	Yale-New Haven Hospital, New Haven	18.9	1.2%	1.13	Yes	1.12	8	1.23	0.042
	TIER THREE								
	Greenwich Hospital, Greenwich	11.1	0.0%	1.02	No	0.23	4	1.40	0.017
	Hartford Hospital, Hartford	11.3	0.0%	1.09	Yes	0.36	6	0.87	0.008
	Hospital of St. Raphael, New Haven	13.8	0.0%	1.05	Yes	0.44	6	1.36	0.014
	St. Francis Hospital and Medical Center, Hartford	14.6	0.0%	0.89	Yes	0.45	7	0.65	0.007
	St. Mary's Hospital, Waterbury	12.6	0.0%	0.98	Yes	0.36	6	0.74	0.007
	TIER FOUR								
	Bridgeport Hospital, Bridgeport	7.3	0.0%	1.59	Yes	0.35	6	1.06	0.009
	Middlesex Hospital, Middletown	5.6	0.0%	1.31	No	0.16	6	0.69	0.009
	New Britain General Hospital, New Britain	7.7	0.0%	1.32	Yes	0.17	7	0.53	0.009
	Norwalk Hospital, Norwalk	8.8	0.0%	1.15	No	0.31	6	0.98	0.013
	St. Vincent's Medical Center, Bridgeport	6.9	0.0%	1.25	Yes	0.17	0	0.70	0.013
	Stamford Hospital, Stamford	10.9	0.0%	1.21	Yes	0.29	8	0.99	0.014
	Waterbury Hospital, Waterbury	7.6	0.0%	1.14	No	0.35	6	0.64	0.006

ORTHOPEDICS

Natl. Rank	Hospital	U.S. News index	Reputational score	Orthopedics mortality rate	COTH member	Interns and residents to beds	Technology score (of 5)	R.N.'s to beds	Board-certified orthopedists to beds	Procedures to beds
	TIER TWO									
60	Yale-New Haven Hospital, New Haven	15.7	1.2%	1.11	Yes	1.12	4	1.23	0.040	1.27
	TIER THREE									
	Danbury Hospital, Danbury	8.8	0.0%	0.88	Yes	0.11	3	0.50	0.039	0.71
	Greenwich Hospital, Greenwich	8.3	0.0%	0.98	No	0.23	2	1.40	0.040	4.26
	Hartford Hospital, Hartford	8.9	0.0%	1.16	Yes	0.36	3	0.87	0.016	2.40
	Hospital of St. Raphael, New Haven	11.3	0.0%	1.06	Yes	0.44	3	1.36	0.041	2.86
	New Britain General Hospital, New Britain	8.7	0.0%	1.06	Yes	0.17	4	0.53	0.036	2.58
	St. Francis Hospital and Medical Center, Hartford	8.8	0.0%	1.25	Yes	0.45	4	0.65	0.027	2.11
	University of Connecticut Health Center, Farmington	11.1	0.0%	0.85	Yes	0.56	3	0.65	0.026	1.64
	TIER FOUR									
	Bridgeport Hospital, Bridgeport	7.3	0.0%	1.74	Yes	0.35	3	1.06	0.024	2.32
	Griffin Hospital, Derby	2.1	0.0%	2.28	No	0.24	3	0.69	0.018	2.16
	Middlesex Hospital, Middletown	4.4	0.0%	1.41	No	0.16	3	0.69	0.027	4.13
	Mount Sinai Hospital, Hartford	6.4	0.0%	1.06	No	0.21	3	0.98	0.032	1.27
	Norwalk Hospital, Norwalk	5.9	0.0%	1.27	No	0.31	3	0.98	0.030	2.79
	St. Mary's Hospital, Waterbury	7.9	0.0%	1.37	Yes	0.36	3	0.74	0.030	3.24
	Stamford Hospital, Stamford	7.4	0.0%	1.75	Yes	0.29	4	0.99	0.040	1.51
	Waterbury Hospital, Waterbury	4.3	0.0%	1.53	No	0.35	3	0.64	0.027	3.62

OTOLARYNGOLOGY

Natl. Rank	Hospital	U.S. News index	Reputa-tional score	Hospital-wide mortality rate	COTH member	Interns and residents to beds	Tech-nology score (of 9)	R.N.'s to beds	Board-certified internists to beds	Procedures to beds
TIER TWO										
40	Yale-New Haven Hospital, New Haven	19.5	1.6%	1.06	Yes	1.12	8	1.23	0.094	0.249
TIER THREE										
	Bridgeport Hospital, Bridgeport	9.8	0.0%	1.40	Yes	0.35	6	1.06	0.059	0.247
	Danbury Hospital, Danbury	8.3	0.0%	0.99	Yes	0.11	7	0.50	0.138	0.109
	Greenwich Hospital, Greenwich	7.6	0.0%	1.04	No	0.23	5	1.40	0.108	0.307
	Hartford Hospital, Hartford	9.6	0.0%	1.11	Yes	0.36	6	0.87	0.086	0.213
	Hospital of St. Raphael, New Haven	11.6	0.0%	0.97	Yes	0.44	6	1.36	0.082	0.388
	New Britain General Hospital, New Britain	8.1	0.0%	1.08	Yes	0.17	7	0.53	0.083	0.214
	Norwalk Hospital, Norwalk	7.3	0.0%	1.25	No	0.31	6	0.98	0.175	0.304
	St. Francis Hospital and Medical Center, Hartford	9.8	0.0%	1.11	Yes	0.45	7	0.65	0.103	0.233
	St. Mary's Hospital, Waterbury	9.1	0.0%	1.10	Yes	0.36	6	0.74	0.070	0.282
	Stamford Hospital, Stamford	10.3	0.0%	1.15	Yes	0.29	8	0.99	0.087	0.238
	University of Connecticut Health Center, Farmington	11.5	0.0%	1.10	Yes	0.56	6	0.65	0.293	0.237
TIER FOUR										
	Griffin Hospital, Derby	3.9	0.0%	1.15	No	0.24	2	0.69	0.036	0.436
	Middlesex Hospital, Middletown	4.6	0.0%	1.18	No	0.16	6	0.69	0.031	0.228
	Mount Sinai Hospital, Hartford	6.4	0.4%	1.11	No	0.21	2	0.98	0.097	0.113
	St. Vincent's Medical Center, Bridgeport	6.5	0.0%	1.20	Yes	0.17	0	0.70	0.066	0.263
	Waterbury Hospital, Waterbury	5.4	0.0%	1.25	No	0.35	6	0.64	0.058	0.288

RHEUMATOLOGY

Natl. Rank	Hospital	U.S. News index	Reputa-tional score	Hospital-wide mortality rate	COTH member	Interns and residents to beds	Tech-nology score (of 5)	R.N.'s to beds	Board-certified internists to beds
TIER ONE									
17	Yale-New Haven Hospital, New Haven	26.9	5.1%	1.06	Yes	1.12	4	1.23	0.094
TIER THREE									
	Bridgeport Hospital, Bridgeport	10.0	0.0%	1.40	Yes	0.35	3	1.06	0.059
	Danbury Hospital, Danbury	11.0	0.0%	0.99	Yes	0.11	3	0.50	0.138
	Greenwich Hospital, Greenwich	10.2	0.0%	1.04	No	0.23	2	1.40	0.108
	Hartford Hospital, Hartford	10.4	0.0%	1.11	Yes	0.36	3	0.87	0.086
	Hospital of St. Raphael, New Haven	14.1	0.0%	0.97	Yes	0.44	3	1.36	0.082
	New Britain General Hospital, New Britain	10.5	0.0%	1.08	Yes	0.17	4	0.53	0.083
	St. Francis Hospital and Medical Center, Hartford	11.7	0.0%	1.11	Yes	0.45	4	0.65	0.103
	St. Mary's Hospital, Waterbury	11.0	0.0%	1.10	Yes	0.36	3	0.74	0.070
	Stamford Hospital, Stamford	11.6	0.0%	1.15	Yes	0.29	4	0.99	0.087
TIER FOUR									
	Griffin Hospital, Derby	7.4	0.0%	1.15	No	0.24	3	0.69	0.036
	Middlesex Hospital, Middletown	5.9	0.0%	1.18	No	0.16	3	0.69	0.031
	Mount Sinai Hospital, Hartford	8.8	0.0%	1.11	No	0.21	3	0.98	0.097
	Norwalk Hospital, Norwalk	8.8	0.0%	1.25	No	0.31	3	0.98	0.175
	St. Vincent's Medical Center, Bridgeport	6.2	0.0%	1.20	Yes	0.17	0	0.70	0.066
	Waterbury Hospital, Waterbury	7.1	0.0%	1.25	No	0.35	3	0.64	0.058

UROLOGY

Natl. Rank	Hospital	U.S. News index	Reputa-tional score	Urology mortality rate	COTH member	Interns and residents to beds	Tech-nology score (of 11)	R.N.'s to beds	Board-certified internists to beds	Procedures to beds
TIER TWO										
89	Stamford Hospital, Stamford	15.1	0.0%	0.76	Yes	0.29	9	0.99	0.087	1.58
41	Yale-New Haven Hospital, New Haven	19.0	1.3%	0.85	Yes	1.12	9	1.23	0.094	1.49
TIER THREE										
	Bridgeport Hospital, Bridgeport	9.4	0.0%	1.39	Yes	0.35	7	1.06	0.059	1.79
	Greenwich Hospital, Greenwich	11.6	0.0%	0.82	No	0.23	5	1.40	0.108	1.82
	Hartford Hospital, Hartford	10.1	0.0%	1.19	Yes	0.36	7	0.87	0.086	1.50
	Hospital of St. Raphael, New Haven	13.1	0.0%	1.03	Yes	0.44	7	1.36	0.082	2.41
	St. Francis Hospital and Medical Center, Hartford	9.6	0.0%	1.29	Yes	0.45	8	0.65	0.103	1.42
	St. Mary's Hospital, Waterbury	10.9	0.0%	1.08	Yes	0.36	7	0.74	0.070	2.65
TIER FOUR										
	Griffin Hospital, Derby	3.6	0.0%	1.63	No	0.24	4	0.69	0.036	1.92
	Middlesex Hospital, Middletown	4.8	0.0%	1.51	No	0.16	7	0.69	0.031	2.60
	Mount Sinai Hospital, Hartford	7.7	0.0%	1.04	No	0.21	4	0.98	0.097	1.31
	New Britain General Hospital, New Britain	7.7	0.0%	1.45	Yes	0.17	8	0.53	0.083	2.26
	Norwalk Hospital, Norwalk	7.7	0.0%	1.28	No	0.31	7	0.98	0.175	1.88
	St. Vincent's Medical Center, Bridgeport	7.0	0.0%	1.21	Yes	0.17	0	0.70	0.066	1.61
	Waterbury Hospital, Waterbury	8.5	0.0%	0.99	No	0.35	7	0.64	0.058	2.15

AIDS

Natl. Rank	Hospital	U.S. News index	Reputa- tional score	Hospital- wide mortality rate	COTH member	Interns and residents to beds	Tech- nology score (of 11)	Discharge planning (of 2)	R.N.'s to beds	Board- certified internists to beds
	TIER THREE									
	Medical Center of Delaware, Wilmington	22.4	0.3%	1.09	Yes	0.44	7	2	1.21	0.060
	TIER FOUR									
	St. Francis Hospital, Wilmington	16.0	0.0%	1.25	No	0.08	5	1	0.76	0.117

CANCER

Natl. Rank	Hospital	U.S. News index	Reputa- tional score	Cancer mortality rate	COTH member	Interns and residents to beds	Tech- nology score (of 12)	R.N.'s to beds	Board- certified oncologists to beds	Procedures to beds
	TIER THREE									
	Medical Center of Delaware, Wilmington	8.6	0.0%	1.05	Yes	0.44	8	1.21	0.001	1.79
	TIER FOUR									
	St. Francis Hospital, Wilmington	2.5	0.0%	0.87	No	0.08	3	0.76	0.027	1.11

CARDIOLOGY

Natl. Rank	Hospital	U.S. News index	Reputa- tional score	Cardiology mortality rate	COTH member	Interns and residents to beds	Tech- nology score (of 10)	R.N.'s to beds	Board- certified cardiologists to beds	Procedures to beds
	TIER THREE									
	Medical Center of Delaware, Wilmington	18.2	0.0%	1.04	Yes	0.44	7	1.21	0.025	7.90
	TIER FOUR									
	St. Francis Hospital, Wilmington	11.9	0.0%	1.10	No	0.08	5	0.76	0.084	8.22

ENDOCRINOLOGY

Natl. Rank	Hospital	U.S. News index	Reputa- tional score	Endocrinology mortality rate	COTH member	Interns and residents to beds	Tech- nology score (of 11)	R.N.'s to beds	Board- certified internists to beds
	TIER THREE								
	Medical Center of Delaware, Wilmington	10.1	0.0%	1.32	Yes	0.44	8	1.21	0.060
	TIER FOUR								
	St. Francis Hospital, Wilmington	4.4	0.0%	1.44	No	0.08	4	0.76	0.117

GASTROENTEROLOGY

Natl. Rank	Hospital	U.S. News index	Reputa- tional score	Gastro- enterology mortality rate	COTH member	Interns and residents to beds	Tech- nology score (of 11)	R.N.'s to beds	Board- certified gastro- enterologists to beds	Pro- cedures to beds
	TIER THREE									
	Medical Center of Delaware, Wilmington	10.8	0.0%	1.06	Yes	0.44	7	1.21	0.010	2.82
	TIER FOUR									
	St. Francis Hospital, Wilmington	5.5	0.0%	1.07	No	0.08	4	0.76	0.036	3.70

GERIATRICS

Natl. Rank	Hospital	U.S. News index	Reputational score	Hospital-wide mortality rate	COTH member	Service mix	Interns and residents to beds	Technology score (of 13)	R.N.'s to beds	Discharge planning (of 2)	Geriatric services (of 9)	Board-certified internists to beds
TIER THREE												
	Medical Center of Delaware, Wilmington	16.3	0.0%	1.09	Yes	6	0.44	9	1.21	2	2	0.060
TIER FOUR												
	St. Francis Hospital, Wilmington	6.8	0.0%	1.25	No	4	0.08	5	0.76	1	2	0.117

GYNECOLOGY

Natl. Rank	Hospital	U.S. News index	Reputational score	Hospital-wide mortality rate	Interns and residents to beds	Technology score (of 10)	R.N.'s to beds	Board-certified OB-GYNs to beds	Procedures to beds
TIER THREE									
	Medical Center of Delaware, Wilmington	16.7	0.0%	1.09	0.44	7	1.21	0.051	0.49
TIER FOUR									
	St. Francis Hospital, Wilmington	7.9	0.0%	1.25	0.08	4	0.76	0.054	0.29

NEUROLOGY

Natl. Rank	Hospital	U.S. News index	Reputational score	Neurology mortality rate	COTH member	Interns and residents to beds	Technology score (of 9)	R.N.'s to beds	Board-certified neurologists to beds
TIER THREE									
	Medical Center of Delaware, Wilmington	11.6	0.0%	1.16	Yes	0.44	6	1.21	0.007
TIER FOUR									
	St. Francis Hospital, Wilmington	8.1	0.0%	1.16	No	0.08	4	0.76	0.033

ORTHOPEDICS

Natl. Rank	Hospital	U.S. News index	Reputational score	Orthopedics mortality rate	COTH member	Interns and residents to beds	Technology score (of 5)	R.N.'s to beds	Board-certified orthopedists to beds	Procedures to beds
TIER THREE										
	Medical Center of Delaware, Wilmington	12.3	0.0%	0.79	Yes	0.44	2	1.21	0.025	1.85
TIER FOUR										
	St. Francis Hospital, Wilmington	3.3	0.0%	1.74	No	0.08	3	0.76	0.069	3.14

OTOLARYNGOLOGY

Natl. Rank	Hospital	U.S. News index	Reputational score	Hospital-wide mortality rate	COTH member	Interns and residents to beds	Technology score (of 9)	R.N.'s to beds	Board-certified internists to beds	Procedures to beds
TIER THREE										
	Medical Center of Delaware, Wilmington	10.8	0.0%	1.09	Yes	0.44	6	1.21	0.060	0.216
TIER FOUR										
	St. Francis Hospital, Wilmington	4.1	0.0%	1.25	No	0.08	2	0.76	0.117	0.315

RHEUMATOLOGY

Natl. Rank	Hospital	U.S. News index	Reputational score	Hospital-wide mortality rate	COTH member	Interns and residents to beds	Technology score (of 5)	R.N.'s to beds	Board-certified internists to beds
TIER THREE									
	Medical Center of Delaware, Wilmington	12.0	0.0%	1.09	Yes	0.44	2	1.21	0.060
TIER FOUR									
	St. Francis Hospital, Wilmington	6.0	0.0%	1.25	No	0.08	3	0.76	0.117

UROLOGY

Natl. Rank	Hospital	U.S. News index	Reputa- tional score	Urology mortality rate	COTH member	Interns and residents to beds	Tech- nology score (of 11)	R.N.'s to beds	Board- certified internists to beds	Procedures to beds
	TIER THREE									
	Medical Center of Delaware, Wilmington	**9.8**	0.0%	1.41	Yes	0.44	7	1.21	0.060	1.42
	TIER FOUR									
	St. Francis Hospital, Wilmington	**3.2**	0.0%	1.89	No	0.08	4	0.76	0.117	2.46

AIDS

Natl. Rank	Hospital	U.S. News index	Reputa-tional score	Hospital-wide mortality rate	COTH member	Interns and residents to beds	Tech-nology score (of 11)	Discharge planning (of 2)	R.N.'s to beds	Board-certified internists to beds
TIER TWO										
35	Georgetown University Hospital	28.8	1.6%	0.97	Yes	0.92	9	2	1.59	0.140
TIER THREE										
	George Washington University Hospital	23.3	0.3%	1.24	Yes	1.40	7	2	1.16	0.223
	Howard University Hospital	22.4	0.0%	1.19	Yes	1.14	8	2	1.13	0.033
TIER FOUR										
	District of Columbia General Hospital	16.3	0.0%	1.52	No	0.67	6	2	1.10	0.092
	Greater Southeast Community Hospital	16.8	0.0%	1.23	No	0.11	5	2	0.77	0.071
	Providence Hospital	14.9	0.0%	1.44	No	0.33	6	1	0.89	0.020
	Sibley Memorial Hospital	18.4	0.0%	1.04	No	0.02	5	2	0.52	0.036
	Washington Hospital Center	18.8	0.0%	1.36	Yes	0.49	7	2	0.90	0.054

CANCER

Natl. Rank	Hospital	U.S. News index	Reputa-tional score	Cancer mortality rate	COTH member	Interns and residents to beds	Tech-nology score (of 12)	R.N.'s to beds	Board-certified oncologists to beds	Procedures to beds
TIER TWO										
49	George Washington University Hospital	12.9	0.5%	0.97	Yes	1.40	9	1.16	0.049	1.51
46	Georgetown University Hospital	13.2	0.6%	0.74	Yes	0.92	10	1.59	0.026	1.75
77	Howard University Hospital	11.3	0.0%	1.17	Yes	1.14	11	1.13	0.005	0.67
TIER THREE										
	Washington Hospital Center	7.8	0.0%	1.21	Yes	0.49	8	0.90	0.014	1.09
TIER FOUR										
	Greater Southeast Community Hospital	2.4	0.0%	1.24	No	0.11	4	0.77	0.012	0.58
	Providence Hospital	3.2	0.0%	1.42	No	0.33	3	0.89	0.018	0.99
	Sibley Memorial Hospital	2.1	0.0%	1.09	No	0.02	5	0.52	0.011	2.11

CARDIOLOGY

Natl. Rank	Hospital	U.S. News index	Reputa-tional score	Cardiology mortality rate	COTH member	Interns and residents to beds	Tech-nology score (of 10)	R.N.'s to beds	Board-certified cardiologists to beds	Procedures to beds
TIER TWO										
29	Georgetown University Hospital	26.5	0.0%	0.87	Yes	0.92	9	1.59	0.114	4.45
87	Howard University Hospital	21.3	0.6%	1.07	Yes	1.14	10	1.13	0.021	3.46
26	Washington Hospital Center	27.4	7.0%	1.13	Yes	0.49	9	0.90	0.106	8.91
TIER THREE										
	George Washington University Hospital	20.3	0.5%	1.20	Yes	1.40	9	1.16	0.096	4.33
TIER FOUR										
	Greater Southeast Community Hospital	10.8	0.0%	1.10	No	0.11	4	0.77	0.032	3.51
	Providence Hospital	6.4	0.0%	1.49	No	0.33	4	0.89	0.032	6.42
	Sibley Memorial Hospital	10.8	0.0%	1.05	No	0.02	3	0.52	0.047	4.83

ENDOCRINOLOGY

Natl. Rank	Hospital	U.S. News index	Reputa- tional score	Endocrinology mortality rate	COTH member	Interns and residents to beds	Tech- nology score (of 11)	R.N.'s to beds	Board- certified internists to beds
	TIER TWO								
67	George Washington University Hospital	16.0	0.9%	1.31	Yes	1.40	10	1.16	0.223
69	Georgetown University Hospital	15.8	0.7%	1.07	Yes	0.92	10	1.59	0.140
	TIER THREE								
98	Howard University Hospital	13.6	0.0%	1.11	Yes	1.14	11	1.13	0.033
	TIER FOUR								
	District of Columbia General Hospital	7.0	0.0%	1.66	No	0.67	7	1.10	0.092
	Greater Southeast Community Hospital	5.1	0.0%	1.29	No	0.11	6	0.77	0.071
	Providence Hospital	4.6	0.0%	1.53	No	0.33	4	0.89	0.020
	Sibley Memorial Hospital	5.4	0.0%	1.00	No	0.02	6	0.52	0.036
	Washington Hospital Center	8.1	0.0%	1.87	Yes	0.49	9	0.90	0.054

GASTROENTEROLOGY

Natl. Rank	Hospital	U.S. News index	Reputa- tional score	Gastro- enterology mortality rate	COTH member	Interns and residents to beds	Tech- nology score (of 11)	R.N.'s to beds	Board- certified gastro- enterologists to beds	Pro- cedures to beds
	TIER ONE									
19	Georgetown University Hospital	20.0	3.2%	0.86	Yes	0.92	10	1.59	0.040	1.56
	TIER THREE									
75	George Washington University Hospital	13.2	0.0%	1.33	Yes	1.40	9	1.16	0.064	2.23
	TIER FOUR									
	Greater Southeast Community Hospital	2.6	0.0%	1.58	No	0.11	6	0.77	0.016	1.48
	Providence Hospital	3.1	0.0%	1.94	No	0.33	4	0.89	0.018	3.01
	Sibley Memorial Hospital	5.8	0.0%	0.99	No	0.02	6	0.52	0.028	3.74
	Washington Hospital Center	7.0	0.0%	1.87	Yes	0.49	8	0.90	0.029	1.66

GERIATRICS

Natl. Rank	Hospital	U.S. News index	Reputa- tional score	Hospital- wide mortality rate	COTH member	Service mix	Interns and residents to beds	Tech- nology score (of 13)	R.N.'s to beds	Discharge planning (of 2)	Geriatric services (of 9)	Board- certified internists to beds
	TIER TWO											
44	Georgetown University Hospital	25.0	0.6%	0.97	Yes	8	0.92	11	1.59	2	3	0.140
	TIER THREE											
	George Washington University Hospital	19.7	1.8%	1.24	Yes	3	1.40	11	1.16	2	1	0.223
	Howard University Hospital	15.6	0.0%	1.19	Yes	5	1.14	13	1.13	2	1	0.033
	TIER FOUR											
	Greater Southeast Community Hospital	9.6	0.0%	1.23	No	6	0.11	7	0.77	2	3	0.071
	Providence Hospital	5.2	0.0%	1.44	No	6	0.33	4	0.89	1	4	0.020
	Sibley Memorial Hospital	12.0	0.0%	1.04	No	4	0.02	7	0.52	2	3	0.036
	Washington Hospital Center	12.0	0.0%	1.36	Yes	7	0.49	11	0.90	2	4	0.054

GYNECOLOGY

Natl. Rank	Hospital	U.S. News index	Reputa- tional score	Hospital- wide mortality rate	Interns and residents to beds	Tech- nology score (of 10)	R.N.'s to beds	Board- certified OB-GYNs to beds	Procedures to beds
	TIER TWO								
34	Georgetown University Hospital	29.2	1.5%	0.97	0.92	9	1.59	0.056	0.40
	TIER THREE								
92	George Washington University Hospital	21.9	0.9%	1.24	1.40	8	1.16	0.167	0.27
	Howard University Hospital	19.1	0.0%	1.19	1.14	10	1.13	0.035	0.16

Natl. Rank	Hospital	U.S. News index	Reputational score	Hospital-wide mortality rate	Interns and residents to beds	Technology score (of 10)	R.N.'s to beds	Board-certified OB-GYNs to beds	Procedures to beds
	TIER FOUR								
	Greater Southeast Community Hospital	8.9	0.0%	1.23	0.11	5	0.77	0.045	0.11
	Providence Hospital	7.4	0.0%	1.44	0.33	5	0.89	0.058	0.23
	Sibley Memorial Hospital	12.1	0.0%	1.04	0.02	5	0.52	0.075	0.41
	Washington Hospital Center	11.6	0.0%	1.36	0.49	8	0.90	0.062	0.21

NEUROLOGY

Natl. Rank	Hospital	U.S. News index	Reputational score	Neurology mortality rate	COTH member	Interns and residents to beds	Technology score (of 9)	R.N.'s to beds	Board-certified neurologists to beds
	TIER ONE								
25	Georgetown University Hospital	24.7	1.1%	0.77	Yes	0.92	8	1.59	0.028
	TIER TWO								
37	George Washington University Hospital	22.5	1.1%	1.06	Yes	1.40	8	1.16	0.076
	TIER THREE								
	Howard University Hospital	13.2	0.3%	1.34	Yes	1.14	9	1.13	0.009
	TIER FOUR								
	Greater Southeast Community Hospital	7.6	0.0%	1.13	No	0.11	5	0.77	0.014
	Providence Hospital	9.2	0.0%	1.08	No	0.33	4	0.89	0.018
	Sibley Memorial Hospital	9.1	0.0%	0.95	No	0.02	5	0.52	0.011
	Washington Hospital Center	10.0	0.5%	1.40	Yes	0.49	7	0.90	0.013

ORTHOPEDICS

Natl. Rank	Hospital	U.S. News index	Reputational score	Orthopedics mortality rate	COTH member	Interns and residents to beds	Technology score (of 5)	R.N.'s to beds	Board-certified orthopedists to beds	Procedures to beds
	TIER TWO									
39	Georgetown University Hospital	18.0	1.4%	0.89	Yes	0.92	4	1.59	0.050	1.15
	TIER THREE									
	George Washington University Hospital	12.5	0.0%	1.45	Yes	1.40	4	1.16	0.042	1.53
	TIER FOUR									
	Greater Southeast Community Hospital	3.3	0.0%	1.51	No	0.11	3	0.77	0.028	0.71
	Providence Hospital	4.8	0.0%	1.58	No	0.33	4	0.89	0.009	1.29
	Sibley Memorial Hospital	5.7	0.0%	0.92	No	0.02	2	0.52	0.072	3.54
	Washington Hospital Center	7.9	0.0%	1.62	Yes	0.49	4	0.90	0.017	0.89

OTOLARYNGOLOGY

Natl. Rank	Hospital	U.S. News index	Reputational score	Hospital-wide mortality rate	COTH member	Interns and residents to beds	Technology score (of 9)	R.N.'s to beds	Board-certified internists to beds	Procedures to beds
	TIER TWO									
43	George Washington University Hospital	19.3	0.9%	1.24	Yes	1.40	8	1.16	0.223	0.191
73	Georgetown University Hospital	15.2	0.0%	0.97	Yes	0.92	8	1.59	0.140	0.212
96	Howard University Hospital	13.8	0.0%	1.19	Yes	1.14	9	1.13	0.033	0.121
	TIER THREE									
	District of Columbia General Hospital	7.9	0.0%	1.52	No	0.67	5	1.10	0.092	0.053
	Washington Hospital Center	10.1	0.0%	1.36	Yes	0.49	7	0.90	0.054	0.248
	TIER FOUR									
	Greater Southeast Community Hospital	4.4	0.0%	1.23	No	0.11	4	0.77	0.071	0.101
	Providence Hospital	4.8	0.0%	1.44	No	0.33	3	0.89	0.020	0.211
	Sibley Memorial Hospital	3.1	0.0%	1.04	No	0.02	4	0.52	0.036	0.384

RHEUMATOLOGY

Natl. Rank	Hospital	U.S. News index	Reputational score	Hospital-wide mortality rate	COTH member	Interns and residents to beds	Technology score (of 5)	R.N.'s to beds	Board-certified internists to beds
	TIER TWO								
36	George Washington University Hospital	20.3	1.9%	1.24	Yes	1.40	4	1.16	0.223
47	Georgetown University Hospital	18.2	0.5%	0.97	Yes	0.92	4	1.59	0.140
	TIER THREE								
	Howard University Hospital	14.5	0.0%	1.19	Yes	1.14	5	1.13	0.033
	Washington Hospital Center	10.6	0.0%	1.36	Yes	0.49	4	0.90	0.054
	TIER FOUR								
	Greater Southeast Community Hospital	6.9	0.0%	1.23	No	0.11	3	0.77	0.071
	Providence Hospital	5.9	0.0%	1.44	No	0.33	4	0.89	0.020
	Sibley Memorial Hospital	6.6	0.0%	1.04	No	0.02	2	0.52	0.036

UROLOGY

Natl. Rank	Hospital	U.S. News index	Reputational score	Urology mortality rate	COTH member	Interns and residents to beds	Technology score (of 11)	R.N.'s to beds	Board-certified internists to beds	Procedures to beds
	TIER TWO									
75	Howard University Hospital	16.2	0.0%	0.90	Yes	1.14	10	1.13	0.033	1.04
	TIER THREE									
95	George Washington University Hospital	14.8	0.7%	1.49	Yes	1.40	9	1.16	0.223	1.75
	Georgetown University Hospital	14.3	0.8%	1.55	Yes	0.92	10	1.59	0.140	1.68
	Washington Hospital Center	11.5	1.4%	1.39	Yes	0.49	8	0.90	0.054	1.70
	TIER FOUR									
	Greater Southeast Community Hospital	5.6	0.0%	1.25	No	0.11	6	0.77	0.071	1.07
	Providence Hospital	3.6	0.0%	1.97	No	0.33	4	0.89	0.020	2.77
	Sibley Memorial Hospital	5.6	0.0%	1.10	No	0.02	6	0.52	0.036	1.85

STATE RANKINGS ■ DISTRICT OF COLUMBIA

AIDS

Natl. Rank	Hospital	U.S. News index	Reputa-tional score	Hospital-wide mortality rate	COTH member	Interns and residents to beds	Tech-nology score (of 11)	Discharge planning (of 2)	R.N.'s to beds	Board-certified internists to beds
	TIER ONE									
6	**University of Miami, Jackson Memorial Hospital**	**42.8**	15.4%	1.12	Yes	0.85	8	2	1.39	0.046
	TIER TWO									
76	**Shands Hospital at the University of Florida, Gainesville**	**25.7**	0.5%	0.90	Yes	0.66	8	2	0.62	0.007
71	**Tampa General Hospital, Tampa**	**25.9**	0.5%	0.88	Yes	0.00	9	2	1.09	0.081
	TIER THREE									
	Alachua General Hospital, Gainesville	**19.9**	0.0%	0.95	No	0.04	5	2	0.56	0.017
	Baptist Hospital of Miami	**23.5**	0.0%	0.90	No	0.00	8	2	1.45	0.029
	Baptist Medical Center, Jacksonville	**21.0**	0.0%	0.95	No	0.01	6	2	0.99	0.040
	Bayfront Medical Center, St. Petersburg	**19.8**	0.0%	1.10	No	0.17	7	2	1.01	0.110
	Boca Raton Community Hospital, Boca Raton	**22.5**	0.0%	0.65	No	0.00	7	2	0.85	0.059
	Bon Secours-St. Joseph Hospital, Port Charlotte	**21.8**	0.0%	0.89	No	0.00	7	2	0.36	0.113
	Broward General Medical Center, Fort Lauderdale	**20.3**	0.0%	1.03	No	0.00	8	2	0.80	0.073
	Cedars Medical Center, Miami	**21.1**	0.0%	0.94	No	0.05	6	2	0.86	0.047
	Florida Hospital Medical Center, Orlando	**23.0**	0.0%	0.92	No	0.09	8	2	1.30	0.036
	Florida Medical Center Hospital, Fort Lauderdale	**21.2**	0.0%	0.83	No	0.00	5	2	0.52	0.039
	H. Lee Moffitt Cancer Center, Tampa	**23.6**	0.0%	0.68	No	0.35	5	2	1.49	0.070
	HCA Medical Center Hospital-Largo, Largo	**22.2**	0.0%	0.86	No	0.00	6	2	0.86	0.059
	Halifax Medical Center, Daytona Beach	**21.2**	0.0%	0.96	No	0.07	7	2	0.89	0.043
	Holy Cross Hospital, Fort Lauderdale	**21.0**	0.0%	0.97	No	0.00	6	2	0.89	0.162
	JFK Medical Center, Atlantis	**20.0**	0.0%	1.01	No	0.00	6	2	0.83	0.089
	Jupiter Medical Center, Jupiter	**21.5**	0.0%	0.80	No	0.00	6	1	0.71	0.135
	Lee Memorial Hospital, Fort Myers	**22.1**	0.0%	0.90	No	0.00	7	2	0.87	0.036
	Martin Memorial Medical Center, Stuart	**22.2**	0.0%	0.92	No	0.00	6	2	1.33	0.049
	Mease Hospital Dunedin, Dunedin	**22.2**	0.0%	0.89	No	0.00	6	2	0.87	0.079
	Memorial Hospital, Hollywood	**20.5**	0.0%	1.03	No	0.00	8	2	0.94	0.072
	Mercy Hospital, Miami	**23.6**	0.0%	0.86	No	0.00	9	2	1.16	0.027
	Mount Sinai Medical Center, Miami Beach	**23.0**	0.0%	1.05	Yes	0.43	9	2	0.94	0.047
	Naples Community Hospital, Naples	**22.6**	0.0%	0.88	No	0.00	7	2	0.95	0.040
	North Broward Medical Center, Pompano Beach	**21.0**	0.0%	0.98	No	0.00	6	2	0.88	0.212
	Orlando Regional Medical Center, Orlando	**21.5**	0.0%	1.10	Yes	0.27	6	2	1.25	0.087
	Parkway Regional Medical Center, North Miami Beach	**21.3**	0.0%	0.81	No	0.03	6	1	0.83	0.022
	Sarasota Memorial Hospital, Sarasota	**21.0**	0.3%	0.95	No	0.00	6	2	0.76	0.045
	South Miami Hospital	**22.7**	0.0%	0.85	No	0.00	8	2	0.78	0.027
	St. Anthony's Hospital, St. Petersburg	**20.1**	0.0%	0.95	No	0.00	6	2	0.40	0.053
	St. Joseph's Hospital, Tampa	**20.0**	0.0%	1.08	No	0.00	9	2	0.85	0.060
	St. Luke's Hospital, Jacksonville	**21.0**	0.0%	0.91	No	0.00	6	1	0.78	0.110
	St. Mary's Hospital, West Palm Beach	**21.0**	0.0%	0.99	No	0.00	8	1	1.30	0.058
	St. Vincent's Medical Center, Jacksonville	**22.4**	0.0%	0.85	No	0.07	7	2	0.67	0.053
	Tallahassee Memorial Regional Medical Ctr., Tallahassee	**20.7**	0.0%	0.98	No	0.09	8	2	0.50	0.036
	Wuesthoff Hospital, Rockledge	**21.8**	0.0%	0.83	No	0.00	6	2	0.76	0.018
	TIER FOUR									
	Baptist Hospital, Pensacola	**18.4**	0.0%	1.10	No	0.00	7	2	0.66	0.015
	Bay Medical Center, Panama City	**18.3**	0.0%	1.08	No	0.00	7	1	0.77	0.026
	Bethesda Memorial Hospital, Boynton Beach	**18.3**	0.0%	1.02	No	0.00	5	1	0.68	0.025
	HCA L.W. Blake Hospital, Bradenton	**17.5**	0.0%	1.06	No	0.00	5	1	0.58	0.044
	HCA West Florida Regional Medical Center, Pensacola	**18.8**	0.0%	1.04	No	0.00	7	1	0.73	0.024
	Holmes Regional Medical Center, Melbourne	**17.9**	0.0%	1.18	No	0.00	7	2	0.96	0.023
	Lakeland Regional Medical Center, Lakeland	**15.5**	0.0%	1.26	No	0.00	6	1	0.57	0.044
	Manatee Memorial Hospital, Bradenton	**17.2**	0.0%	1.11	No	0.00	6	1	0.61	0.029
	Memorial Hospital-Ormond Beach, Ormond Beach	**14.7**	0.0%	1.47	No	0.00	6	2	0.88	0.020
	Memorial Medical Center of Jacksonville, Jacksonville	**18.9**	0.0%	1.15	No	0.00	8	2	0.99	0.068

Natl. Rank	Hospital	U.S. News index	Reputa- tional score	Hospital- wide mortality rate	COTH member	Interns and residents to beds	Tech- nology score (of 11)	Discharge planning (of 2)	R.N.'s to beds	Board- certified internists to beds
	Morton Plant Hospital, Clearwater	17.9	0.0%	1.07	No	0.00	6	1	0.61	0.051
	Palms of Pasadena Hospital, St. Petersburg	19.1	0.0%	1.00	No	0.00	6	2	0.41	0.016
	Sacred Heart Hospital of Pensacola, Pensacola	18.8	0.0%	1.10	No	0.08	7	2	0.75	0.023
	University Community Hospital, Tampa	17.3	0.0%	1.25	No	0.00	7	2	0.88	0.076
	University Medical Center, Jacksonville	19.1	0.0%	1.41	Yes	0.47	8	2	1.24	0.016
	Winter Haven Hospital, Winter Haven	19.6	0.0%	1.00	No	0.00	6	2	0.58	0.036
	Winter Park Memorial Hospital, Winter Park	19.4	0.0%	0.99	No	0.00	6	2	0.36	0.073

CANCER

Natl. Rank	Hospital	U.S. News index	Reputa- tional score	Cancer mortality rate	COTH member	Interns and residents to beds	Tech- nology score (of 12)	R.N.'s to beds	Board- certified oncologists to beds	Procedures to beds
	TIER TWO									
74	H. Lee Moffitt Cancer Center, Tampa	11.3	1.5%	0.71	No	0.35	7	1.49	0.158	9.54
	TIER THREE									
	Baptist Hospital of Miami	6.8	0.5%	0.83	No	0.00	10	1.45	0.024	1.33
	Florida Hospital Medical Center, Orlando	6.1	0.0%	0.79	No	0.09	10	1.30	0.009	1.18
	Martin Memorial Medical Center, Stuart	5.7	0.0%	0.66	No	0.00	7	1.33	0.019	3.16
	Mount Sinai Medical Center, Miami Beach	8.5	0.0%	0.82	Yes	0.43	9	0.94	0.016	1.51
	Orlando Regional Medical Center, Orlando	8.4	0.0%	1.02	Yes	0.27	9	1.25	0.006	1.23
	Shands Hospital at the University of Florida, Gainesville	9.9	0.5%	0.54	Yes	0.66	11	0.62	0.030	1.16
	St. Mary's Hospital, West Palm Beach	5.5	0.0%	0.81	No	0.00	9	1.30	0.021	0.99
	Tampa General Hospital, Tampa	8.3	0.0%	0.63	Yes	0.00	11	1.09	0.009	1.43
	University Medical Center, Jacksonville	8.6	0.0%	1.04	Yes	0.47	8	1.24	0.004	0.64
87	University of Miami, Jackson Memorial Hospital	10.7	0.0%	0.95	Yes	0.85	9	1.39	0.015	0.60
	TIER FOUR									
	Alachua General Hospital, Gainesville	2.7	0.0%	0.39	No	0.04	5	0.56	0.005	1.01
	Baptist Hospital, Pensacola	3.5	0.0%	0.75	No	0.00	8	0.66	0.011	1.10
	Baptist Medical Center, Jacksonville	3.9	0.0%	0.70	No	0.01	6	0.99	0.012	0.75
	Bay Medical Center, Panama City	3.3	0.0%	1.10	No	0.00	8	0.77	0.007	1.00
	Bayfront Medical Center, St. Petersburg	5.0	0.0%	0.91	No	0.17	9	1.01	0.008	1.00
	Bethesda Memorial Hospital, Boynton Beach	3.1	0.0%	0.72	No	0.00	6	0.68	0.006	1.54
	Boca Raton Community Hospital, Boca Raton	4.8	0.0%	0.57	No	0.00	8	0.85	0.021	3.61
	Bon Secours-St. Joseph Hospital, Port Charlotte	2.2	0.0%	0.56	No	0.00	5	0.36	0.005	1.98
	Broward General Medical Center, Fort Lauderdale	4.3	0.0%	0.81	No	0.00	10	0.80	0.009	0.64
	Florida Medical Center Hospital, Fort Lauderdale	3.4	0.0%	0.65	No	0.00	8	0.52	0.035	0.75
	HCA L.W. Blake Hospital, Bradenton	2.5	0.0%	0.97	No	0.00	6	0.58	0.008	1.69
	HCA Medical Center Hospital-Largo, Largo	4.0	0.0%	0.63	No	0.00	6	0.86	0.031	1.98
	HCA West Florida Regional Medical Center, Pensacola	3.8	0.0%	0.79	No	0.00	9	0.73	0.007	0.94
	Halifax Medical Center, Daytona Beach	4.0	0.0%	0.80	No	0.07	7	0.89	0.006	1.35
	Holmes Regional Medical Center, Melbourne	4.4	0.0%	1.09	No	0.00	9	0.96	0.010	2.33
	Holy Cross Hospital, Fort Lauderdale	3.9	0.0%	0.85	No	0.00	7	0.89	0.020	1.69
	JFK Medical Center, Atlantis	3.5	0.0%	1.00	No	0.00	7	0.83	0.024	1.64
	Jupiter Medical Center, Jupiter	4.0	0.0%	0.66	No	0.00	8	0.71	0.000	2.42
	Lakeland Regional Medical Center, Lakeland	3.3	0.0%	0.99	No	0.00	8	0.57	0.008	3.09
	Lee Memorial Hospital, Fort Myers	3.3	0.0%	0.75	No	0.00	5	0.87	0.014	1.42
	Manatee Memorial Hospital, Bradenton	2.8	0.0%	0.91	No	0.00	7	0.61	0.008	1.01
	Mease Hospital Dunedin, Dunedin	3.1	0.0%	0.83	No	0.00	5	0.87	0.018	1.09
	Memorial Hospital, Hollywood	4.8	0.0%	0.77	No	0.00	10	0.94	0.010	1.16
	Memorial Hospital-Ormond Beach, Ormond Beach	2.5	0.0%	0.91	No	0.00	3	0.88	0.015	1.13
	Memorial Medical Center of Jacksonville, Jacksonville	3.6	0.0%	0.75	No	0.00	5	0.99	0.014	1.30
	Mercy Hospital, Miami	5.2	0.0%	0.83	No	0.00	9	1.16	0.011	1.87
	Morton Plant Hospital, Clearwater	3.9	0.5%	0.85	No	0.00	8	0.61	0.005	1.63
	Naples Community Hospital, Naples	4.8	0.0%	0.63	No	0.00	8	0.95	0.014	2.36
	North Broward Medical Center, Pompano Beach	4.2	0.0%	0.73	No	0.00	8	0.88	0.010	1.22

Natl. Rank Hospital	U.S. News index	Reputational score	Cancer mortality rate	COTH member	Interns and residents to beds	Technology score (of 12)	R.N.'s to beds	Board-certified oncologists to beds	Procedures to beds
Palms of Pasadena Hospital, St. Petersburg	3.0	0.0%	0.86	No	0.00	9	0.41	0.006	1.78
Parkway Regional Medical Center, North Miami Beach	3.4	0.0%	0.41	No	0.03	5	0.83	0.009	1.36
Sacred Heart Hospital of Pensacola, Pensacola	3.8	0.0%	0.97	No	0.08	8	0.75	0.013	1.53
Sarasota Memorial Hospital, Sarasota	3.2	0.0%	0.74	No	0.00	5	0.76	0.009	2.60
South Miami Hospital	4.1	0.0%	0.69	No	0.00	8	0.78	0.032	1.19
St. Anthony's Hospital, St. Petersburg	2.5	0.0%	0.92	No	0.00	8	0.40	0.002	1.26
St. Joseph's Hospital, Tampa	4.4	0.0%	1.09	No	0.00	10	0.85	0.012	1.98
St. Luke's Hospital, Jacksonville	3.3	0.0%	0.47	No	0.00	5	0.78	0.000	2.11
St. Vincent's Medical Center, Jacksonville	4.3	0.0%	0.59	No	0.07	9	0.67	0.004	1.29
Tallahassee Memorial Regional Medical Ctr., Tallahassee	3.8	0.0%	0.83	No	0.09	10	0.50	0.007	1.14
University Community Hospital, Tampa	3.5	0.0%	1.24	No	0.00	8	0.88	0.013	0.88
Winter Haven Hospital, Winter Haven	3.4	0.0%	0.73	No	0.00	8	0.58	0.002	1.71
Winter Park Memorial Hospital, Winter Park	3.0	0.0%	0.64	No	0.00	8	0.36	0.010	1.72
Wuesthoff Hospital, Rockledge	3.0	0.0%	0.78	No	0.00	5	0.76	0.022	1.13

CARDIOLOGY

Natl. Rank Hospital	U.S. News index	Reputational score	Cardiology mortality rate	COTH member	Interns and residents to beds	Technology score (of 10)	R.N.'s to beds	Board-certified cardiologists to beds	Procedures to beds
TIER TWO									
84 Shands Hospital at the University of Florida, Gainesville	21.3	0.9%	0.95	Yes	0.66	9	0.62	0.028	2.50
66 Tampa General Hospital, Tampa	21.9	0.0%	0.86	Yes	0.00	9	1.09	0.064	6.06
81 University of Miami, Jackson Memorial Hospital	21.4	0.0%	0.96	Yes	0.85	7	1.39	0.008	0.93
TIER THREE									
Baptist Hospital of Miami	18.1	0.0%	0.94	No	0.00	8	1.45	0.077	5.91
Baptist Medical Center, Jacksonville	17.6	0.0%	0.86	No	0.01	7	0.99	0.032	4.15
Boca Raton Community Hospital, Boca Raton	17.9	0.0%	0.63	No	0.00	7	0.85	0.046	13.70
Bon Secours-St. Joseph Hospital, Port Charlotte	15.7	0.0%	0.88	No	0.00	5	0.36	0.047	9.23
Broward General Medical Center, Fort Lauderdale	14.6	0.0%	0.98	No	0.00	9	0.80	0.021	3.87
Cedars Medical Center, Miami	17.1	0.0%	0.92	No	0.05	8	0.86	0.086	6.01
Florida Hospital Medical Center, Orlando	19.2	0.0%	0.89	No	0.09	9	1.30	0.032	10.14
Florida Medical Center Hospital, Fort Lauderdale	14.5	0.0%	0.98	No	0.00	7	0.52	0.129	11.03
HCA Medical Center Hospital-Largo, Largo	16.2	0.0%	0.96	No	0.00	8	0.86	0.113	15.19
Halifax Medical Center, Daytona Beach	14.1	0.0%	0.99	No	0.07	7	0.89	0.016	3.27
Holy Cross Hospital, Fort Lauderdale	15.5	0.0%	0.98	No	0.00	8	0.89	0.053	8.58
JFK Medical Center, Atlantis	14.9	0.0%	1.00	No	0.00	8	0.83	0.051	11.77
Jupiter Medical Center, Jupiter	16.8	0.0%	0.84	No	0.00	4	0.71	0.090	8.99
Lee Memorial Hospital, Fort Myers	18.2	0.0%	0.86	No	0.00	9	0.87	0.034	8.27
Martin Memorial Medical Center, Stuart	18.6	0.0%	0.82	No	0.00	6	1.33	0.026	12.92
Mease Hospital Dunedin, Dunedin	17.3	0.0%	0.78	No	0.00	6	0.87	0.040	7.26
Memorial Hospital, Hollywood	14.9	0.0%	0.99	No	0.00	9	0.94	0.029	6.18
Mercy Hospital, Miami	18.4	0.0%	0.92	No	0.00	9	1.16	0.073	9.04
Mount Sinai Medical Center, Miami Beach	18.0	0.0%	1.08	Yes	0.43	9	0.94	0.060	9.14
Naples Community Hospital, Naples	17.5	0.0%	0.86	No	0.00	7	0.95	0.012	10.03
North Broward Medical Center, Pompano Beach	15.5	0.0%	0.93	No	0.00	5	0.88	0.031	8.40
Orlando Regional Medical Center, Orlando	16.4	0.0%	1.08	Yes	0.27	6	1.25	0.023	5.80
Parkway Regional Medical Center, North Miami Beach	18.2	0.0%	0.80	No	0.03	7	0.83	0.074	8.80
Sarasota Memorial Hospital, Sarasota	17.2	0.0%	0.91	No	0.00	9	0.76	0.039	12.14
South Miami Hospital	15.8	0.0%	0.96	No	0.00	9	0.78	0.118	5.27
St. Luke's Hospital, Jacksonville	15.6	0.0%	0.99	No	0.00	9	0.78	0.138	10.81
St. Mary's Hospital, West Palm Beach	18.2	0.0%	0.90	No	0.00	7	1.30	0.049	4.31
St. Vincent's Medical Center, Jacksonville	18.0	0.0%	0.84	No	0.07	9	0.67	0.040	8.84
University Medical Center, Jacksonville	13.6	0.0%	1.32	Yes	0.47	8	1.24	0.024	3.36
Winter Haven Hospital, Winter Haven	14.2	0.0%	0.94	No	0.00	6	0.58	0.014	9.69
Wuesthoff Hospital, Rockledge	18.1	0.0%	0.79	No	0.00	9	0.76	0.043	8.65

Natl. Rank	Hospital	U.S. News index	Reputational score	Cardiology mortality rate	COTH member	Interns and residents to beds	Technology score (of 10)	R.N.'s to beds	Board-certified cardiologists to beds	Procedures to beds
	TIER FOUR									
	Alachua General Hospital, Gainesville	11.7	0.0%	1.05	No	0.04	7	0.56	0.015	5.73
	Baptist Hospital, Pensacola	12.6	0.0%	1.03	No	0.00	8	0.66	0.021	3.91
	Bay Medical Center, Panama City	10.7	0.0%	1.14	No	0.00	7	0.77	0.017	9.21
	Bayfront Medical Center, St. Petersburg	13.5	0.0%	1.07	No	0.17	7	1.01	0.040	5.25
	Bethesda Memorial Hospital, Boynton Beach	12.7	0.0%	0.99	No	0.00	4	0.68	0.025	6.33
	HCA L.W. Blake Hospital, Bradenton	12.6	0.0%	1.02	No	0.00	7	0.58	0.018	9.11
	HCA West Florida Regional Medical Center, Pensacola	10.2	0.0%	1.17	No	0.00	9	0.73	0.011	5.39
	Holmes Regional Medical Center, Melbourne	11.5	0.0%	1.18	No	0.00	9	0.96	0.033	15.38
	Lakeland Regional Medical Center, Lakeland	5.4	0.0%	1.51	No	0.00	8	0.57	0.018	11.54
	Manatee Memorial Hospital, Bradenton	12.8	0.0%	1.02	No	0.00	8	0.61	0.016	6.45
	Memorial Hospital-Ormond Beach, Ormond Beach	3.8	0.0%	1.96	No	0.00	9	0.88	0.068	12.65
	Memorial Medical Center of Jacksonville, Jacksonville	9.5	0.0%	1.31	No	0.00	9	0.99	0.031	9.59
	Morton Plant Hospital, Clearwater	11.1	0.0%	1.12	No	0.00	8	0.61	0.029	8.26
	Palms of Pasadena Hospital, St. Petersburg	11.0	0.0%	1.05	No	0.00	6	0.41	0.016	8.49
	Sacred Heart Hospital of Pensacola, Pensacola	10.3	0.0%	1.21	No	0.08	9	0.75	0.018	7.79
	St. Anthony's Hospital, St. Petersburg	9.7	0.0%	1.09	No	0.00	5	0.40	0.018	5.98
	St. Joseph's Hospital, Tampa	12.8	0.0%	1.07	No	0.00	9	0.85	0.023	7.31
	Tallahassee Memorial Regional Medical Ctr., Tallahassee	9.4	0.0%	1.20	No	0.09	8	0.50	0.026	5.89
	University Community Hospital, Tampa	8.0	0.0%	1.40	No	0.00	9	0.88	0.045	6.37
	Winter Park Memorial Hospital, Winter Park	12.4	0.0%	1.01	No	0.00	7	0.36	0.043	4.52

ENDOCRINOLOGY

Natl. Rank	Hospital	U.S. News index	Reputational score	Endocrinology mortality rate	COTH member	Interns and residents to beds	Technology score (of 11)	R.N.'s to beds	Board-certified internists to beds
	TIER TWO								
62	University of Miami, Jackson Memorial Hospital	16.2	1.0%	0.83	Yes	0.85	8	1.39	0.046
	TIER THREE								
	Baptist Hospital, Pensacola	8.8	0.0%	0.72	No	0.00	9	0.66	0.015
	Boca Raton Community Hospital, Boca Raton	9.2	0.0%	0.76	No	0.00	9	0.85	0.059
	Florida Hospital Medical Center, Orlando	8.4	0.0%	0.99	No	0.09	9	1.30	0.036
	HCA Medical Center Hospital-Largo, Largo	10.0	0.0%	0.55	No	0.00	6	0.86	0.059
	Jupiter Medical Center, Jupiter	10.7	0.0%	0.61	No	0.00	9	0.71	0.135
	Mercy Hospital, Miami	8.5	0.0%	0.91	No	0.00	10	1.16	0.027
	Mount Sinai Medical Center, Miami Beach	10.3	0.0%	1.18	Yes	0.43	10	0.94	0.047
	Naples Community Hospital, Naples	10.7	0.0%	0.57	No	0.00	9	0.95	0.040
	North Broward Medical Center, Pompano Beach	8.6	0.0%	0.95	No	0.00	9	0.88	0.212
	Orlando Regional Medical Center, Orlando	10.5	0.0%	1.16	Yes	0.27	8	1.25	0.087
	Shands Hospital at the University of Florida, Gainesville	12.8	1.4%	0.99	Yes	0.66	10	0.62	0.007
	South Miami Hospital	10.1	0.0%	0.23	No	0.00	9	0.78	0.027
	St. Joseph's Hospital, Tampa	8.9	0.0%	0.80	No	0.00	10	0.85	0.060
	St. Mary's Hospital, West Palm Beach	9.0	0.0%	0.90	No	0.00	9	1.30	0.058
	St. Vincent's Medical Center, Jacksonville	10.3	0.0%	0.60	No	0.07	9	0.67	0.053
	Tallahassee Memorial Regional Medical Ctr., Tallahassee	8.2	0.0%	0.77	No	0.09	9	0.50	0.036
89	Tampa General Hospital, Tampa	14.1	0.0%	0.57	Yes	0.00	10	1.09	0.081
	University Medical Center, Jacksonville	8.6	0.0%	1.82	Yes	0.47	8	1.24	0.016
	TIER FOUR								
	Alachua General Hospital, Gainesville	3.8	0.0%	1.32	No	0.04	6	0.56	0.017
	Baptist Hospital of Miami	7.2	0.0%	1.26	No	0.00	10	1.45	0.029
	Baptist Medical Center, Jacksonville	5.4	0.0%	1.23	No	0.01	6	0.99	0.040
	Bay Medical Center, Panama City	6.5	0.0%	1.02	No	0.00	9	0.77	0.026
	Bayfront Medical Center, St. Petersburg	7.2	0.0%	1.20	No	0.17	9	1.01	0.110
	Bethesda Memorial Hospital, Boynton Beach	3.2	0.0%	1.68	No	0.00	7	0.68	0.025
	Bon Secours-St. Joseph Hospital, Port Charlotte	6.8	0.0%	0.83	No	0.00	6	0.36	0.113

Natl. Rank	Hospital	U.S. News index	Reputa-tional score	Endocrinology mortality rate	COTH member	Interns and residents to beds	Tech-nology score (of 11)	R.N.'s to beds	Board-certified internists to beds
	Broward General Medical Center, Fort Lauderdale	5.3	0.0%	1.39	No	0.00	10	0.80	0.073
	Cedars Medical Center, Miami	6.0	0.0%	1.16	No	0.05	8	0.86	0.047
	Florida Medical Center Hospital, Fort Lauderdale	5.4	0.0%	1.02	No	0.00	7	0.52	0.039
	HCA L.W. Blake Hospital, Bradenton	3.7	0.0%	1.43	No	0.00	7	0.58	0.044
	HCA West Florida Regional Medical Center, Pensacola	7.2	0.0%	0.90	No	0.00	9	0.73	0.024
	Halifax Medical Center, Daytona Beach	7.3	0.0%	0.96	No	0.07	8	0.89	0.043
	Holmes Regional Medical Center, Melbourne	5.6	0.0%	1.32	No	0.00	10	0.96	0.023
	Holy Cross Hospital, Fort Lauderdale	7.4	0.0%	1.05	No	0.00	8	0.89	0.162
	JFK Medical Center, Atlantis	6.5	0.0%	1.08	No	0.00	8	0.83	0.089
	Lakeland Regional Medical Center, Lakeland	4.7	0.0%	1.23	No	0.00	8	0.57	0.044
	Lee Memorial Hospital, Fort Myers	6.0	0.0%	1.05	No	0.00	6	0.87	0.036
	Manatee Memorial Hospital, Bradenton	7.0	0.0%	0.86	No	0.00	8	0.61	0.029
	Martin Memorial Medical Center, Stuart	7.2	0.0%	1.14	No	0.00	8	1.33	0.049
	Mease Hospital Dunedin, Dunedin	6.6	0.0%	1.03	No	0.00	7	0.87	0.079
	Memorial Hospital, Hollywood	6.1	0.0%	1.26	No	0.00	10	0.94	0.072
	Memorial Medical Center of Jacksonville, Jacksonville	5.3	0.0%	1.35	No	0.00	7	0.99	0.068
	Morton Plant Hospital, Clearwater	6.8	0.0%	0.93	No	0.00	9	0.61	0.051
	Palms of Pasadena Hospital, St. Petersburg	7.2	0.0%	0.80	No	0.00	9	0.41	0.016
	Parkway Regional Medical Center, North Miami Beach	7.6	0.0%	0.83	No	0.03	6	0.83	0.022
	Sacred Heart Hospital of Pensacola, Pensacola	6.1	0.0%	1.08	No	0.08	8	0.75	0.023
	Sarasota Memorial Hospital, Sarasota	5.7	0.0%	1.06	No	0.00	6	0.76	0.045
	St. Anthony's Hospital, St. Petersburg	5.2	0.0%	1.10	No	0.00	9	0.40	0.053
	St. Luke's Hospital, Jacksonville	6.5	0.0%	1.02	No	0.00	6	0.78	0.110
	University Community Hospital, Tampa	5.3	0.0%	1.41	No	0.00	9	0.88	0.076
	Winter Haven Hospital, Winter Haven	5.7	0.0%	1.04	No	0.00	8	0.58	0.036
	Winter Park Memorial Hospital, Winter Park	4.5	0.0%	1.20	No	0.00	8	0.36	0.073
	Wuesthoff Hospital, Rockledge	7.9	0.0%	0.77	No	0.00	6	0.76	0.018

GASTROENTEROLOGY

Natl. Rank	Hospital	U.S. News index	Reputa-tional score	Gastro-enterology mortality rate	COTH member	Interns and residents to beds	Tech-nology score (of 11)	R.N.'s to beds	Board-certified gastro-enterologists to beds	Pro-cedures to beds
	TIER TWO									
29	Shands Hospital at the University of Florida, Gainesville	17.0	3.2%	0.67	Yes	0.66	10	0.62	0.024	1.20
28	University of Miami, Jackson Memorial Hospital	17.4	3.5%	0.97	Yes	0.85	8	1.39	0.004	0.39
	TIER THREE									
	Baptist Hospital of Miami	8.6	0.0%	0.91	No	0.00	9	1.45	0.044	2.11
	Bay Medical Center, Panama City	7.5	0.0%	0.88	No	0.00	8	0.77	0.013	3.33
	Boca Raton Community Hospital, Boca Raton	9.7	0.0%	0.67	No	0.00	8	0.85	0.026	5.38
	Florida Hospital Medical Center, Orlando	9.3	0.0%	0.83	No	0.09	9	1.30	0.015	2.34
	HCA Medical Center Hospital-Largo, Largo	9.7	0.0%	0.77	No	0.00	5	0.86	0.066	6.66
	Holmes Regional Medical Center, Melbourne	8.0	0.0%	1.04	No	0.00	9	0.96	0.016	5.04
	Jupiter Medical Center, Jupiter	9.0	0.0%	0.71	No	0.00	8	0.71	0.051	4.65
	Lee Memorial Hospital, Fort Myers	8.1	0.0%	0.79	No	0.00	6	0.87	0.022	3.72
	Martin Memorial Medical Center, Stuart	9.4	0.0%	1.01	No	0.00	7	1.33	0.030	6.50
	Mease Hospital Dunedin, Dunedin	8.0	0.0%	0.81	No	0.00	6	0.87	0.032	3.38
	Mercy Hospital, Miami	7.7	0.0%	1.02	No	0.00	9	1.16	0.030	3.27
	Mount Sinai Medical Center, Miami Beach	11.1	0.0%	0.96	Yes	0.43	9	0.94	0.025	2.15
	Naples Community Hospital, Naples	8.8	0.0%	0.95	No	0.00	8	0.95	0.019	5.73
	Orlando Regional Medical Center, Orlando	9.7	0.0%	1.15	Yes	0.27	8	1.25	0.007	2.29
	Parkway Regional Medical Center, North Miami Beach	7.7	0.0%	0.72	No	0.03	6	0.83	0.028	2.88
	St. Anthony's Hospital, St. Petersburg	7.7	0.0%	0.81	No	0.00	8	0.40	0.018	3.83
	St. Luke's Hospital, Jacksonville	8.5	0.0%	0.83	No	0.00	7	0.78	0.060	4.24
	St. Vincent's Medical Center, Jacksonville	8.3	0.0%	0.77	No	0.07	9	0.67	0.013	2.91

Natl. Rank	Hospital	U.S. News index	Reputational score	Gastroenterology mortality rate	COTH member	Interns and residents to beds	Technology score (of 11)	R.N.'s to beds	Board-certified gastroenterologists to beds	Procedures to beds
	Tampa General Hospital, Tampa	10.8	0.0%	0.95	Yes	0.00	9	1.09	0.020	3.46
	TIER FOUR									
	Alachua General Hospital, Gainesville	4.8	0.0%	1.01	No	0.04	5	0.56	0.012	2.61
	Baptist Hospital, Pensacola	4.2	0.0%	1.26	No	0.00	9	0.66	0.008	1.86
	Baptist Medical Center, Jacksonville	5.4	0.0%	0.98	No	0.01	5	0.99	0.018	1.62
	Bayfront Medical Center, St. Petersburg	7.0	0.0%	1.03	No	0.17	8	1.01	0.011	2.43
	Bethesda Memorial Hospital, Boynton Beach	6.0	0.0%	0.94	No	0.00	6	0.68	0.011	3.12
	Bon Secours-St. Joseph Hospital, Port Charlotte	3.9	0.0%	1.22	No	0.00	5	0.36	0.009	4.26
	Broward General Medical Center, Fort Lauderdale	4.2	0.0%	1.29	No	0.00	10	0.80	0.010	0.93
	Cedars Medical Center, Miami	5.7	0.0%	1.04	No	0.05	7	0.86	0.044	1.93
	Florida Medical Center Hospital, Fort Lauderdale	5.6	0.0%	0.94	No	0.00	6	0.52	0.068	2.63
	HCA L.W. Blake Hospital, Bradenton	6.1	0.0%	1.03	No	0.00	6	0.58	0.005	4.76
	HCA West Florida Regional Medical Center, Pensacola	3.9	0.0%	1.30	No	0.00	8	0.73	0.007	1.84
	Halifax Medical Center, Daytona Beach	5.8	0.0%	1.07	No	0.07	8	0.89	0.016	1.93
	Holy Cross Hospital, Fort Lauderdale	6.9	0.0%	1.03	No	0.00	8	0.89	0.045	3.50
	JFK Medical Center, Atlantis	5.5	0.0%	1.15	No	0.00	7	0.83	0.030	3.33
	Lakeland Regional Medical Center, Lakeland	7.2	0.0%	0.90	No	0.00	7	0.57	0.014	4.38
	Manatee Memorial Hospital, Bradenton	4.9	0.0%	1.11	No	0.00	7	0.61	0.000	2.96
	Memorial Hospital, Hollywood	6.1	0.0%	1.04	No	0.00	9	0.94	0.015	1.78
	Memorial Hospital-Ormond Beach, Ormond Beach	3.5	0.0%	1.56	No	0.00	5	0.88	0.049	3.35
	Memorial Medical Center of Jacksonville, Jacksonville	5.3	0.0%	1.23	No	0.00	6	0.99	0.017	3.63
	Morton Plant Hospital, Clearwater	6.0	0.0%	1.01	No	0.00	8	0.61	0.015	3.17
	North Broward Medical Center, Pompano Beach	5.1	0.0%	1.29	No	0.00	8	0.88	0.042	2.92
	Palms of Pasadena Hospital, St. Petersburg	6.9	0.0%	0.94	No	0.00	8	0.41	0.016	4.61
	Sacred Heart Hospital of Pensacola, Pensacola	6.0	0.0%	1.08	No	0.08	7	0.75	0.010	3.31
	Sarasota Memorial Hospital, Sarasota	6.3	0.0%	0.99	No	0.00	6	0.76	0.017	3.78
	South Miami Hospital	6.5	0.0%	0.92	No	0.00	8	0.78	0.043	1.85
	St. Joseph's Hospital, Tampa	7.1	0.4%	1.05	No	0.00	9	0.85	0.020	2.82
	St. Mary's Hospital, West Palm Beach	6.4	0.0%	1.14	No	0.00	9	1.30	0.037	1.77
	Tallahassee Memorial Regional Medical Ctr., Tallahassee	5.4	0.0%	1.04	No	0.09	8	0.50	0.010	2.45
	University Community Hospital, Tampa	4.9	0.0%	1.22	No	0.00	8	0.88	0.018	2.15
	Winter Haven Hospital, Winter Haven	5.4	0.0%	1.16	No	0.00	7	0.58	0.007	4.40
	Winter Park Memorial Hospital, Winter Park	5.5	0.0%	0.96	No	0.00	7	0.36	0.030	3.08
	Wuesthoff Hospital, Rockledge	6.6	0.0%	0.93	No	0.00	6	0.76	0.014	3.59

GERIATRICS

Natl. Rank	Hospital	U.S. News index	Reputational score	Hospital-wide mortality rate	COTH member	Service mix	Interns and residents to beds	Technology score (of 13)	R.N.'s to beds	Discharge planning (of 2)	Geriatric services (of 9)	Board-certified internists to beds
	TIER TWO											
86	Mercy Hospital, Miami	21.9	0.5%	0.86	No	8	0.00	11	1.16	2	4	0.027
57	Shands Hospital at the University of Florida, Gainesville	23.4	0.9%	0.90	Yes	5	0.66	12	0.62	2	1	0.007
76	University of Miami, Jackson Memorial Hospital	22.4	1.3%	1.12	Yes	8	0.85	10	1.39	2	6	0.046
	TIER THREE											
	Alachua General Hospital, Gainesville	15.1	0.0%	0.95	No	4	0.04	7	0.56	2	5	0.017
	Baptist Hospital of Miami	20.0	0.4%	0.90	No	5	0.00	10	1.45	2	2	0.029
	Baptist Medical Center, Jacksonville	17.0	0.0%	0.95	No	8	0.01	7	0.99	2	2	0.040
	Boca Raton Community Hospital, Boca Raton	17.5	0.0%	0.65	No	4	0.00	11	0.85	2	1	0.059
	Bon Secours-St. Joseph Hospital, Port Charlotte	16.3	0.0%	0.89	No	4	0.00	7	0.36	2	2	0.113
	Cedars Medical Center, Miami	19.3	0.5%	0.94	No	6	0.05	11	0.86	2	5	0.047
	Florida Hospital Medical Center, Orlando	19.2	0.0%	0.92	No	5	0.09	12	1.30	2	5	0.036
	Florida Medical Center Hospital, Fort Lauderdale	16.6	0.0%	0.83	No	4	0.00	9	0.52	2	2	0.039
	HCA Medical Center Hospital-Largo, Largo	16.7	0.0%	0.86	No	3	0.00	9	0.86	2	1	0.059
	Halifax Medical Center, Daytona Beach	16.7	0.0%	0.96	No	7	0.07	10	0.89	2	2	0.043

Natl. Rank	Hospital	U.S. News index	Reputa-tional score	Hospital-wide mortality rate	COTH member	Service mix	Interns and residents to beds	Tech-nology score (of 13)	R.N.'s to beds	Discharge planning (of 2)	Geriatric services (of 9)	Board-certified internists to beds
	Holy Cross Hospital, Fort Lauderdale	16.0	0.0%	0.97	No	4	0.00	10	0.89	2	3	0.162
	JFK Medical Center, Atlantis	14.3	0.0%	1.01	No	5	0.00	10	0.83	2	1	0.089
	Lee Memorial Hospital, Fort Myers	18.2	0.0%	0.90	No	5	0.00	8	0.87	2	6	0.036
	Martin Memorial Medical Center, Stuart	18.0	0.0%	0.92	No	5	0.00	10	1.33	2	2	0.049
	Mease Hospital Dunedin, Dunedin	17.5	0.0%	0.89	No	4	0.00	9	0.87	2	2	0.079
	Memorial Hospital, Hollywood	14.7	0.0%	1.03	No	6	0.00	11	0.94	2	2	0.072
	Mount Sinai Medical Center, Miami Beach	20.0	0.0%	1.05	Yes	9	0.43	11	0.94	2	8	0.047
	Naples Community Hospital, Naples	18.3	0.0%	0.88	No	5	0.00	11	0.95	2	2	0.040
	North Broward Medical Center, Pompano Beach	16.4	0.0%	0.98	No	5	0.00	9	0.88	2	4	0.212
	Orlando Regional Medical Center, Orlando	16.1	0.0%	1.10	Yes	6	0.27	10	1.25	2	2	0.087
	Sarasota Memorial Hospital, Sarasota	16.7	0.0%	0.95	No	6	0.00	8	0.76	2	5	0.045
	South Miami Hospital	17.9	0.0%	0.85	No	5	0.00	11	0.78	2	2	0.027
	St. Anthony's Hospital, St. Petersburg	15.5	0.0%	0.95	No	5	0.00	9	0.40	2	4	0.053
	St. Vincent's Medical Center, Jacksonville	18.2	0.0%	0.85	No	5	0.07	12	0.67	2	2	0.053
	Tallahassee Memorial Regional Medical Ctr., Tallahassee	16.9	0.0%	0.98	No	7	0.09	11	0.50	2	6	0.036
95	Tampa General Hospital, Tampa	20.8	0.0%	0.88	Yes	5	0.00	12	1.09	2	1	0.081
	Winter Haven Hospital, Winter Haven	14.7	0.0%	1.00	No	6	0.00	11	0.58	2	2	0.036
	Winter Park Memorial Hospital, Winter Park	14.9	0.0%	0.99	No	5	0.00	11	0.36	2	5	0.073
	Wuesthoff Hospital, Rockledge	18.6	0.0%	0.83	No	7	0.00	8	0.76	2	4	0.018
TIER FOUR												
	Baptist Hospital, Pensacola	13.0	0.0%	1.10	No	6	0.00	11	0.66	2	6	0.015
	Bay Medical Center, Panama City	11.0	0.0%	1.08	No	5	0.00	10	0.77	1	1	0.026
	Bayfront Medical Center, St. Petersburg	13.1	0.0%	1.10	No	4	0.17	12	1.01	2	2	0.110
	Bethesda Memorial Hospital, Boynton Beach	13.2	0.0%	1.02	No	7	0.00	9	0.68	1	2	0.025
	Broward General Medical Center, Fort Lauderdale	13.5	0.0%	1.03	No	4	0.00	12	0.80	2	1	0.073
	HCA West Florida Regional Medical Center, Pensacola	13.0	0.0%	1.04	No	5	0.00	12	0.73	1	4	0.024
	Holmes Regional Medical Center, Melbourne	10.1	0.0%	1.18	No	4	0.00	11	0.96	2	2	0.023
	Manatee Memorial Hospital, Bradenton	10.2	0.0%	1.11	No	4	0.00	10	0.61	1	4	0.029
	Memorial Hospital-Ormond Beach, Ormond Beach	4.0	0.0%	1.47	No	4	0.00	7	0.88	2	1	0.020
	Memorial Medical Center of Jacksonville, Jacksonville	10.5	0.0%	1.15	No	5	0.00	8	0.99	2	1	0.068
	Morton Plant Hospital, Clearwater	11.7	0.0%	1.07	No	5	0.00	10	0.61	1	4	0.051
	Palms of Pasadena Hospital, St. Petersburg	13.0	0.0%	1.00	No	4	0.00	11	0.41	2	1	0.016
	Sacred Heart Hospital of Pensacola, Pensacola	11.0	0.0%	1.10	No	3	0.08	10	0.75	2	2	0.023
	St. Joseph's Hospital, Tampa	13.5	0.0%	1.08	No	6	0.00	11	0.85	2	3	0.060
	University Community Hospital, Tampa	9.1	0.0%	1.25	No	4	0.00	11	0.88	2	3	0.076
	University Medical Center, Jacksonville	10.7	0.0%	1.41	Yes	7	0.47	10	1.24	2	1	0.016

GYNECOLOGY

Natl. Rank	Hospital	U.S. News index	Reputa-tional score	Hospital-wide mortality rate	Interns and residents to beds	Tech-nology score (of 10)	R.N.'s to beds	Board-certified OB-GYNs to beds	Procedures to beds
TIER TWO									
72	Baptist Hospital of Miami	23.5	0.0%	0.90	0.00	9	1.45	0.086	0.28
68	Shands Hospital at the University of Florida, Gainesville	23.7	0.8%	0.90	0.66	9	0.62	0.032	0.53
85	Tampa General Hospital, Tampa	22.3	0.4%	0.88	0.00	9	1.09	0.040	0.50
45	University of Miami, Jackson Memorial Hospital	27.3	1.3%	1.12	0.85	7	1.39	0.018	0.18
TIER THREE									
	Baptist Medical Center, Jacksonville	17.6	0.0%	0.95	0.01	7	0.99	0.052	0.35
	Bayfront Medical Center, St. Petersburg	17.0	0.4%	1.10	0.17	8	1.01	0.083	0.67
	Boca Raton Community Hospital, Boca Raton	19.0	0.0%	0.65	0.00	7	0.85	0.051	0.72
	Bon Secours-St. Joseph Hospital, Port Charlotte	14.1	0.0%	0.89	0.00	4	0.36	0.028	1.01
	Broward General Medical Center, Fort Lauderdale	15.6	0.0%	1.03	0.00	9	0.80	0.035	0.15
	Cedars Medical Center, Miami	16.1	0.0%	0.94	0.05	6	0.86	0.022	0.33
	Florida Hospital Medical Center, Orlando	20.6	0.0%	0.92	0.09	8	1.30	0.036	0.34
	Florida Medical Center Hospital, Fort Lauderdale	16.5	0.0%	0.83	0.00	6	0.52	0.033	0.16

Natl. Rank Hospital	U.S. News index	Reputa-tional score	Hospital-wide mortality rate	Interns and residents to beds	Tech-nology score (of 10)	R.N.'s to beds	Board-certified OB-GYNs to beds	Procedures to beds
HCA Medical Center Hospital-Largo, Largo	17.0	0.0%	0.86	0.00	5	0.86	0.023	0.67
Halifax Medical Center, Daytona Beach	15.0	0.0%	0.96	0.07	5	0.89	0.023	0.39
Holy Cross Hospital, Fort Lauderdale	16.2	0.0%	0.97	0.00	7	0.89	0.038	0.50
JFK Medical Center, Atlantis	14.1	0.0%	1.01	0.00	6	0.83	0.030	0.30
Jupiter Medical Center, Jupiter	18.4	0.0%	0.80	0.00	7	0.71	0.051	0.87
Martin Memorial Medical Center, Stuart	19.5	0.0%	0.92	0.00	6	1.33	0.060	0.95
Mease Hospital Dunedin, Dunedin	18.2	0.0%	0.89	0.00	6	0.87	0.047	0.41
Memorial Hospital, Hollywood	16.5	0.0%	1.03	0.00	9	0.94	0.047	0.25
Mercy Hospital, Miami	21.0	0.0%	0.86	0.00	8	1.16	0.048	0.63
Mount Sinai Medical Center, Miami Beach	17.4	0.0%	1.05	0.43	9	0.94	0.028	0.27
Naples Community Hospital, Naples	19.0	0.0%	0.88	0.00	7	0.95	0.028	0.82
North Broward Medical Center, Pompano Beach	15.0	0.0%	0.98	0.00	7	0.88	0.003	0.17
Orlando Regional Medical Center, Orlando	15.9	0.0%	1.10	0.27	7	1.25	0.050	0.32
Parkway Regional Medical Center, North Miami Beach	18.2	0.0%	0.81	0.03	6	0.83	0.046	0.23
Sarasota Memorial Hospital, Sarasota	15.4	0.0%	0.95	0.00	6	0.76	0.032	0.70
South Miami Hospital	20.4	0.3%	0.85	0.00	8	0.78	0.056	0.22
St. Anthony's Hospital, St. Petersburg	14.4	0.0%	0.95	0.00	7	0.40	0.030	0.41
St. Joseph's Hospital, Tampa	14.1	0.0%	1.08	0.00	8	0.85	0.046	0.31
St. Luke's Hospital, Jacksonville	16.7	0.0%	0.91	0.00	6	0.78	0.032	0.92
St. Mary's Hospital, West Palm Beach	18.9	0.0%	0.99	0.00	8	1.30	0.070	0.22
St. Vincent's Medical Center, Jacksonville	18.0	0.0%	0.85	0.07	7	0.67	0.027	0.36
Tallahassee Memorial Regional Medical Ctr., Tallahassee	15.3	0.0%	0.98	0.09	8	0.50	0.031	0.36
Wuesthoff Hospital, Rockledge	16.6	0.0%	0.83	0.00	5	0.76	0.022	0.36
TIER FOUR								
Alachua General Hospital, Gainesville	14.0	0.0%	0.95	0.04	5	0.56	0.037	0.20
Baptist Hospital, Pensacola	11.3	0.0%	1.10	0.00	7	0.66	0.017	0.23
Bay Medical Center, Panama City	12.3	0.0%	1.08	0.00	7	0.77	0.010	0.22
Bethesda Memorial Hospital, Boynton Beach	13.3	0.0%	1.02	0.00	5	0.68	0.069	0.44
HCA L.W. Blake Hospital, Bradenton	10.5	0.0%	1.06	0.00	5	0.58	0.018	0.62
HCA West Florida Regional Medical Center, Pensacola	13.1	0.0%	1.04	0.00	7	0.73	0.011	0.26
Holmes Regional Medical Center, Melbourne	12.6	0.0%	1.18	0.00	9	0.96	0.025	0.42
Lakeland Regional Medical Center, Lakeland	8.4	0.4%	1.26	0.00	6	0.57	0.030	1.13
Manatee Memorial Hospital, Bradenton	11.2	0.0%	1.11	0.00	7	0.61	0.029	0.33
Memorial Hospital-Ormond Beach, Ormond Beach	4.4	0.0%	1.47	0.00	5	0.88	0.015	0.42
Memorial Medical Center of Jacksonville, Jacksonville	11.6	0.0%	1.15	0.00	6	0.99	0.045	0.40
Morton Plant Hospital, Clearwater	12.6	0.0%	1.07	0.00	8	0.61	0.016	0.40
Palms of Pasadena Hospital, St. Petersburg	13.7	0.4%	1.00	0.00	7	0.41	0.013	0.39
Sacred Heart Hospital of Pensacola, Pensacola	12.3	0.0%	1.10	0.08	7	0.75	0.026	0.40
University Community Hospital, Tampa	10.4	0.0%	1.25	0.00	7	0.88	0.065	0.23
University Medical Center, Jacksonville	10.7	0.0%	1.41	0.47	7	1.24	0.028	0.37
Winter Haven Hospital, Winter Haven	13.8	0.0%	1.00	0.00	7	0.58	0.024	0.60
Winter Park Memorial Hospital, Winter Park	14.0	0.0%	0.99	0.00	7	0.36	0.070	0.38

NEUROLOGY

Natl. Rank Hospital	U.S. News index	Reputa-tional score	Neurology mortality rate	COTH member	Interns and residents to beds	Tech-nology score (of 9)	R.N.'s to beds	Board-certified neurologists to beds
TIER TWO								
81 Baptist Hospital of Miami	18.0	0.0%	0.59	No	0.00	8	1.45	0.033
83 Mount Sinai Medical Center, Miami Beach	17.9	0.3%	0.83	Yes	0.43	8	0.94	0.014
31 Shands Hospital at the University of Florida, Gainesville	23.3	2.6%	0.57	Yes	0.66	8	0.62	0.019
44 University of Miami, Jackson Memorial Hospital	21.3	5.6%	1.28	Yes	0.85	6	1.39	0.016
TIER THREE								
Alachua General Hospital, Gainesville	11.8	0.0%	0.86	No	0.04	5	0.56	0.022
Baptist Hospital, Pensacola	12.5	0.0%	0.82	No	0.00	7	0.66	0.006

Natl. Rank	Hospital	U.S. News index	Reputa-tional score	Neurology mortality rate	COTH member	Interns and residents to beds	Tech-nology score (of 9)	R.N.'s to beds	Board-certified neurologists to beds
	Baptist Medical Center, Jacksonville	12.1	0.0%	0.84	No	0.01	5	0.99	0.006
	Boca Raton Community Hospital, Boca Raton	15.1	0.0%	0.60	No	0.00	7	0.85	0.018
	Cedars Medical Center, Miami	15.2	0.0%	0.73	No	0.05	6	0.86	0.020
	Florida Medical Center Hospital, Fort Lauderdale	13.5	0.0%	0.66	No	0.00	5	0.52	0.015
	HCA Medical Center Hospital-Largo, Largo	14.2	0.0%	0.68	No	0.00	5	0.86	0.012
	HCA West Florida Regional Medical Center, Pensacola	13.8	0.0%	0.78	No	0.00	7	0.73	0.011
	Holy Cross Hospital, Fort Lauderdale	13.4	0.0%	0.89	No	0.00	6	0.89	0.040
	JFK Medical Center, Atlantis	13.0	0.0%	0.80	No	0.00	6	0.83	0.008
	Jupiter Medical Center, Jupiter	15.7	0.0%	0.62	No	0.00	7	0.71	0.032
	Lee Memorial Hospital, Fort Myers	12.0	0.0%	0.84	No	0.00	5	0.87	0.008
	Martin Memorial Medical Center, Stuart	11.2	0.0%	0.95	No	0.00	6	1.33	0.007
	Mease Hospital Dunedin, Dunedin	12.0	0.0%	0.85	No	0.00	5	0.87	0.011
	Memorial Hospital, Hollywood	14.2	0.0%	0.81	No	0.00	8	0.94	0.015
	Memorial Medical Center of Jacksonville, Jacksonville	11.9	0.0%	0.88	No	0.00	6	0.99	0.011
	Mercy Hospital, Miami	15.9	0.0%	0.69	No	0.00	8	1.16	0.013
	Naples Community Hospital, Naples	11.4	0.0%	0.95	No	0.00	7	0.95	0.021
	North Broward Medical Center, Pompano Beach	13.3	0.0%	0.81	No	0.00	7	0.88	0.010
	Orlando Regional Medical Center, Orlando	12.0	0.0%	1.09	Yes	0.27	6	1.25	0.007
	Parkway Regional Medical Center, North Miami Beach	15.0	0.0%	0.65	No	0.03	5	0.83	0.025
	Sacred Heart Hospital of Pensacola, Pensacola	12.6	0.0%	0.81	No	0.08	6	0.75	0.005
	South Miami Hospital	16.3	0.0%	0.68	No	0.00	7	0.78	0.038
	St. Mary's Hospital, West Palm Beach	14.1	0.0%	0.87	No	0.00	7	1.30	0.026
	St. Vincent's Medical Center, Jacksonville	14.3	0.0%	0.76	No	0.07	7	0.67	0.009
	Tallahassee Memorial Regional Medical Ctr., Tallahassee	12.8	0.0%	0.80	No	0.09	7	0.50	0.008
	Tampa General Hospital, Tampa	14.2	0.0%	0.95	Yes	0.00	8	1.09	0.018
	Wuesthoff Hospital, Rockledge	13.8	0.0%	0.75	No	0.00	5	0.76	0.011
TIER FOUR									
	Bay Medical Center, Panama City	9.5	0.0%	1.03	No	0.00	7	0.77	0.020
	Bayfront Medical Center, St. Petersburg	10.4	0.0%	0.99	No	0.17	7	1.01	0.005
	Bethesda Memorial Hospital, Boynton Beach	10.8	0.0%	0.87	No	0.00	5	0.68	0.008
	Broward General Medical Center, Fort Lauderdale	10.5	0.0%	0.97	No	0.00	8	0.80	0.014
	Florida Hospital Medical Center, Orlando	10.6	0.0%	1.00	No	0.09	7	1.30	0.004
	HCA L.W. Blake Hospital, Bradenton	7.8	0.0%	1.00	No	0.00	5	0.58	0.003
	Halifax Medical Center, Daytona Beach	10.1	0.0%	0.97	No	0.07	6	0.89	0.010
	Holmes Regional Medical Center, Melbourne	9.1	0.0%	1.11	No	0.00	8	0.96	0.018
	Lakeland Regional Medical Center, Lakeland	5.8	0.0%	1.19	No	0.00	6	0.57	0.006
	Manatee Memorial Hospital, Bradenton	10.0	0.0%	0.92	No	0.00	6	0.61	0.008
	Memorial Hospital-Ormond Beach, Ormond Beach	6.4	0.0%	1.20	No	0.00	5	0.88	0.010
	Morton Plant Hospital, Clearwater	8.2	0.0%	1.03	No	0.00	7	0.61	0.004
	Palms of Pasadena Hospital, St. Petersburg	10.8	0.0%	0.86	No	0.00	7	0.41	0.006
	Sarasota Memorial Hospital, Sarasota	7.5	0.0%	1.07	No	0.00	5	0.76	0.007
	St. Anthony's Hospital, St. Petersburg	9.6	0.0%	0.94	No	0.00	7	0.40	0.012
	St. Joseph's Hospital, Tampa	10.2	0.0%	1.03	No	0.00	8	0.85	0.020
	St. Luke's Hospital, Jacksonville	9.4	0.0%	1.10	No	0.00	6	0.78	0.037
	University Community Hospital, Tampa	9.8	0.0%	1.02	No	0.00	7	0.88	0.016
	University Medical Center, Jacksonville	10.7	0.0%	1.23	Yes	0.47	6	1.24	0.004
	Winter Haven Hospital, Winter Haven	8.8	0.0%	0.99	No	0.00	6	0.58	0.012
	Winter Park Memorial Hospital, Winter Park	6.5	0.0%	1.10	No	0.00	6	0.36	0.010

ORTHOPEDICS

Natl. Rank	Hospital	U.S. News index	Reputa- tional score	Orthopedics mortality rate	COTH member	Interns and residents to beds	Tech- nology score (of 5)	R.N.'s to beds	Board- certified orthopedists to beds	Pro- cedures to beds
	TIER TWO									
28	Shands Hospital at the University of Florida, Gainesville	19.7	2.5%	0.29	Yes	0.66	4	0.62	0.017	1.48
50	University of Miami, Jackson Memorial Hospital	16.6	3.3%	1.40	Yes	0.85	2	1.39	0.024	0.28
	TIER THREE									
	Baptist Hospital of Miami	9.6	0.0%	0.84	No	0.00	4	1.45	0.040	1.85
	Bayfront Medical Center, St. Petersburg	8.9	0.0%	0.85	No	0.17	4	1.01	0.035	1.83
	Boca Raton Community Hospital, Boca Raton	11.0	0.0%	0.59	No	0.00	4	0.85	0.046	4.66
	HCA L.W. Blake Hospital, Bradenton	8.3	0.0%	0.70	No	0.00	2	0.58	0.026	4.41
	HCA Medical Center Hospital-Largo, Largo	10.3	0.0%	0.60	No	0.00	3	0.86	0.051	4.19
	Holy Cross Hospital, Fort Lauderdale	8.5	0.0%	0.81	No	0.00	3	0.89	0.043	4.81
	Lee Memorial Hospital, Fort Myers	8.5	0.0%	0.83	No	0.00	4	0.87	0.017	3.98
	Martin Memorial Medical Center, Stuart	11.0	0.0%	0.70	No	0.00	3	1.33	0.030	4.52
	Mease Hospital Dunedin, Dunedin	10.6	0.0%	0.59	No	0.00	4	0.87	0.018	3.06
	Memorial Hospital, Hollywood	9.1	0.0%	0.75	No	0.00	4	0.94	0.026	1.29
	Memorial Medical Center of Jacksonville, Jacksonville	8.4	0.0%	0.90	No	0.00	5	0.99	0.031	2.08
	Mercy Hospital, Miami	8.4	0.0%	0.89	No	0.00	4	1.16	0.032	2.16
	Mount Sinai Medical Center, Miami Beach	10.9	0.0%	1.03	Yes	0.43	4	0.94	0.030	2.48
96	Orlando Regional Medical Center, Orlando	13.2	0.0%	0.69	Yes	0.27	2	1.25	0.037	1.71
	Parkway Regional Medical Center, North Miami Beach	10.3	0.0%	0.67	No	0.03	4	0.83	0.037	2.18
	Sarasota Memorial Hospital, Sarasota	8.2	0.0%	0.85	No	0.00	4	0.76	0.029	4.30
	St. Luke's Hospital, Jacksonville	9.4	0.0%	0.80	No	0.00	4	0.78	0.064	5.77
	St. Mary's Hospital, West Palm Beach	9.1	0.0%	0.85	No	0.00	4	1.30	0.040	2.07
	Tallahassee Memorial Regional Medical Ctr., Tallahassee	8.9	0.0%	0.52	No	0.09	3	0.50	0.016	1.76
	Tampa General Hospital, Tampa	11.7	0.4%	0.92	Yes	0.00	4	1.09	0.031	3.08
	Winter Park Memorial Hospital, Winter Park	9.0	0.0%	0.69	No	0.00	4	0.36	0.083	2.61
	TIER FOUR									
	Alachua General Hospital, Gainesville	6.0	0.0%	0.89	No	0.04	3	0.56	0.015	1.79
	Baptist Hospital, Pensacola	5.5	0.0%	1.04	No	0.00	4	0.66	0.011	1.29
	Baptist Medical Center, Jacksonville	8.1	0.0%	0.80	No	0.01	3	0.99	0.042	1.11
	Bay Medical Center, Panama City	4.8	0.0%	1.21	No	0.00	4	0.77	0.013	1.38
	Bethesda Memorial Hospital, Boynton Beach	6.2	0.0%	0.85	No	0.00	2	0.68	0.022	2.77
	Bon Secours-St. Joseph Hospital, Port Charlotte	6.0	0.0%	0.86	No	0.00	3	0.36	0.014	3.16
	Broward General Medical Center, Fort Lauderdale	5.3	0.0%	1.11	No	0.00	4	0.80	0.019	0.74
	Cedars Medical Center, Miami	6.5	0.0%	0.97	No	0.05	3	0.86	0.059	1.82
	Florida Hospital Medical Center, Orlando	7.7	0.0%	1.07	No	0.09	4	1.30	0.032	2.36
	Florida Medical Center Hospital, Fort Lauderdale	5.1	0.0%	0.89	No	0.00	2	0.52	0.020	1.54
	HCA West Florida Regional Medical Center, Pensacola	7.1	0.0%	0.89	No	0.00	4	0.73	0.011	2.34
	Halifax Medical Center, Daytona Beach	5.2	0.0%	1.19	No	0.07	3	0.89	0.029	2.43
	Holmes Regional Medical Center, Melbourne	6.7	0.0%	1.08	No	0.00	4	0.96	0.029	3.74
	JFK Medical Center, Atlantis	7.4	0.0%	0.86	No	0.00	3	0.83	0.038	3.21
	Jupiter Medical Center, Jupiter	8.0	0.0%	0.82	No	0.00	3	0.71	0.090	3.78
	Lakeland Regional Medical Center, Lakeland	5.7	0.0%	0.98	No	0.00	3	0.57	0.022	3.79
	Manatee Memorial Hospital, Bradenton	7.5	0.0%	0.77	No	0.00	3	0.61	0.020	2.29
	Memorial Hospital-Ormond Beach, Ormond Beach	7.3	0.0%	0.95	No	0.00	4	0.88	0.059	2.35
	Morton Plant Hospital, Clearwater	7.6	0.0%	0.77	No	0.00	3	0.61	0.015	3.11
	Naples Community Hospital, Naples	8.1	0.0%	0.92	No	0.00	4	0.95	0.019	5.10
	North Broward Medical Center, Pompano Beach	6.4	0.0%	0.97	No	0.00	3	0.88	0.021	2.89
	Palms of Pasadena Hospital, St. Petersburg	6.2	0.0%	0.90	No	0.00	3	0.41	0.016	4.97
	Sacred Heart Hospital of Pensacola, Pensacola	6.5	0.0%	1.00	No	0.08	4	0.75	0.015	1.87
	South Miami Hospital	5.2	0.0%	1.18	No	0.00	4	0.78	0.040	1.55
	St. Anthony's Hospital, St. Petersburg	5.3	0.0%	0.95	No	0.00	3	0.40	0.041	2.66
	St. Joseph's Hospital, Tampa	6.8	0.0%	0.97	No	0.00	4	0.85	0.022	2.20
	St. Vincent's Medical Center, Jacksonville	6.0	0.0%	1.03	No	0.07	4	0.67	0.017	2.00

Natl. Rank	Hospital	U.S. News index	Reputational score	Orthopedics mortality rate	COTH member	Interns and residents to beds	Technology score (of 5)	R.N.'s to beds	Board-certified orthopedists to beds	Procedures to beds
	University Community Hospital, Tampa	5.2	0.0%	1.24	No	0.00	4	0.88	0.022	2.13
	Winter Haven Hospital, Winter Haven	6.9	0.0%	0.86	No	0.00	3	0.58	0.017	4.55
	Wuesthoff Hospital, Rockledge	6.0	0.0%	1.05	No	0.00	4	0.76	0.018	2.43

OTOLARYNGOLOGY

Natl. Rank	Hospital	U.S. News index	Reputational score	Hospital-wide mortality rate	COTH member	Interns and residents to beds	Technology score (of 9)	R.N.'s to beds	Board-certified internists to beds	Procedures to beds
TIER ONE										
26	University of Miami, Jackson Memorial Hospital	23.5	3.4%	1.11	Yes	0.85	6	1.39	0.046	0.078
TIER TWO										
82	Shands Hospital at the University of Florida, Gainesville	14.5	1.4%	0.90	Yes	0.66	8	0.62	0.007	0.228
TIER THREE										
	Baptist Hospital of Miami	7.1	0.0%	0.90	No	0.00	8	1.45	0.029	0.084
	H. Lee Moffitt Cancer Center, Tampa	8.3	0.0%	0.68	No	0.35	5	1.49	0.070	0.658
	Mount Sinai Medical Center, Miami Beach	10.4	0.0%	1.05	Yes	0.43	8	0.94	0.047	0.160
	Orlando Regional Medical Center, Orlando	10.5	0.0%	1.10	Yes	0.27	6	1.25	0.087	0.148
	Tampa General Hospital, Tampa	9.6	0.0%	0.88	Yes	0.00	8	1.09	0.081	0.162
	University Medical Center, Jacksonville	10.4	0.0%	1.41	Yes	0.47	6	1.24	0.016	0.150
TIER FOUR										
	Alachua General Hospital, Gainesville	3.2	0.0%	0.95	No	0.04	4	0.56	0.017	0.159
	Baptist Hospital, Pensacola	4.1	0.0%	1.10	No	0.00	7	0.66	0.015	0.090
	Baptist Medical Center, Jacksonville	6.0	0.3%	0.95	No	0.01	5	0.99	0.040	0.088
	Bay Medical Center, Panama City	4.6	0.0%	1.07	No	0.00	7	0.77	0.026	0.159
	Bayfront Medical Center, St. Petersburg	6.6	0.0%	1.10	No	0.17	7	1.01	0.110	0.104
	Bethesda Memorial Hospital, Boynton Beach	3.7	0.0%	1.02	No	0.00	5	0.68	0.025	0.152
	Boca Raton Community Hospital, Boca Raton	5.4	0.0%	0.65	No	0.00	7	0.85	0.059	0.241
	Bon Secours-St. Joseph Hospital, Port Charlotte	3.3	0.0%	0.89	No	0.00	4	0.36	0.113	0.142
	Broward General Medical Center, Fort Lauderdale	5.3	0.0%	1.03	No	0.00	8	0.80	0.073	0.059
	Cedars Medical Center, Miami	5.0	0.0%	0.94	No	0.05	6	0.86	0.047	0.118
	Florida Hospital Medical Center, Orlando	6.7	0.0%	0.92	No	0.09	7	1.30	0.036	0.102
	Florida Medical Center Hospital, Fort Lauderdale	3.8	0.0%	0.83	No	0.00	6	0.52	0.039	0.107
	HCA L.W. Blake Hospital, Bradenton	3.6	0.0%	1.06	No	0.00	5	0.58	0.044	0.178
	HCA Medical Center Hospital-Largo, Largo	4.5	0.0%	0.85	No	0.00	4	0.86	0.059	0.371
	HCA West Florida Regional Medical Center, Pensacola	4.4	0.0%	1.04	No	0.00	7	0.73	0.024	0.117
	Halifax Medical Center, Daytona Beach	5.1	0.0%	0.96	No	0.07	6	0.89	0.043	0.097
	Holmes Regional Medical Center, Melbourne	5.3	0.0%	1.18	No	0.00	8	0.96	0.023	0.328
	Holy Cross Hospital, Fort Lauderdale	5.9	0.0%	0.97	No	0.00	6	0.89	0.162	0.121
	JFK Medical Center, Atlantis	5.0	0.0%	1.01	No	0.00	6	0.83	0.089	0.136
	Jupiter Medical Center, Jupiter	5.6	0.0%	0.80	No	0.00	7	0.71	0.135	0.237
	Lakeland Regional Medical Center, Lakeland	3.7	0.0%	1.26	No	0.00	6	0.57	0.044	0.244
	Lee Memorial Hospital, Fort Myers	4.3	0.0%	0.90	No	0.00	4	0.87	0.036	0.244
	Manatee Memorial Hospital, Bradenton	3.8	0.0%	1.11	No	0.00	6	0.61	0.029	0.131
	Martin Memorial Medical Center, Stuart	6.3	0.0%	0.92	No	0.00	6	1.33	0.049	0.363
	Mease Hospital Dunedin, Dunedin	4.9	0.0%	0.89	No	0.00	5	0.87	0.079	0.165
	Memorial Hospital, Hollywood	5.8	0.0%	1.03	No	0.00	8	0.94	0.072	0.076
	Memorial Hospital-Ormond Beach, Ormond Beach	3.5	0.0%	1.47	No	0.00	3	0.88	0.020	0.122
	Memorial Medical Center of Jacksonville, Jacksonville	5.0	0.0%	1.15	No	0.00	5	0.99	0.068	0.156
	Mercy Hospital, Miami	6.2	0.0%	0.86	No	0.00	8	1.16	0.027	0.113
	Morton Plant Hospital, Clearwater	4.3	0.0%	1.07	No	0.00	7	0.61	0.051	0.138
	Naples Community Hospital, Naples	5.4	0.0%	0.88	No	0.00	7	0.95	0.040	0.268
	North Broward Medical Center, Pompano Beach	6.5	0.0%	0.98	No	0.00	7	0.88	0.212	0.149
	Palms of Pasadena Hospital, St. Petersburg	3.4	0.0%	1.00	No	0.00	7	0.41	0.016	0.165
	Parkway Regional Medical Center, North Miami Beach	4.2	0.0%	0.81	No	0.03	4	0.83	0.022	0.080
	Sacred Heart Hospital of Pensacola, Pensacola	4.5	0.0%	1.10	No	0.08	6	0.75	0.023	0.237

Natl. Rank	Hospital	U.S. News index	Reputa-tional score	Hospital-wide mortality rate	COTH member	Interns and residents to beds	Tech-nology score (of 9)	R.N.'s to beds	Board-certified internists to beds	Procedures to beds
	Sarasota Memorial Hospital, Sarasota	4.0	0.0%	0.95	No	0.00	4	0.76	0.045	0.236
	South Miami Hospital	4.8	0.0%	0.85	No	0.00	7	0.78	0.027	0.075
	St. Anthony's Hospital, St. Petersburg	3.7	0.0%	0.95	No	0.00	7	0.40	0.053	0.141
	St. Joseph's Hospital, Tampa	5.4	0.0%	1.08	No	0.00	8	0.85	0.060	0.119
	St. Luke's Hospital, Jacksonville	4.6	0.0%	0.91	No	0.00	4	0.78	0.110	0.454
	St. Mary's Hospital, West Palm Beach	6.5	0.0%	0.99	No	0.00	7	1.30	0.058	0.100
	St. Vincent's Medical Center, Jacksonville	5.0	0.0%	0.84	No	0.07	7	0.67	0.053	0.170
	Tallahassee Memorial Regional Medical Ctr., Tallahassee	4.2	0.0%	0.97	No	0.09	7	0.50	0.036	0.148
	University Community Hospital, Tampa	5.2	0.0%	1.25	No	0.00	7	0.88	0.076	0.177
	Winter Haven Hospital, Winter Haven	3.9	0.0%	1.00	No	0.00	6	0.58	0.036	0.329
	Winter Park Memorial Hospital, Winter Park	3.5	0.0%	0.99	No	0.00	6	0.36	0.073	0.153
	Wuesthoff Hospital, Rockledge	3.8	0.0%	0.83	No	0.00	4	0.76	0.018	0.155

RHEUMATOLOGY

Natl. Rank	Hospital	U.S. News index	Reputa-tional score	Hospital-wide mortality rate	COTH member	Interns and residents to beds	Tech-nology score (of 5)	R.N.'s to beds	Board-certified internists to beds
	TIER THREE								
	Baptist Hospital of Miami	11.3	0.0%	0.90	No	0.00	4	1.45	0.029
	Boca Raton Community Hospital, Boca Raton	10.6	0.0%	0.65	No	0.00	4	0.85	0.059
	Florida Hospital Medical Center, Orlando	13.0	0.9%	0.92	No	0.09	4	1.30	0.036
	HCA Medical Center Hospital-Largo, Largo	10.0	0.0%	0.85	No	0.00	3	0.86	0.059
	Holy Cross Hospital, Fort Lauderdale	9.6	0.0%	0.97	No	0.00	3	0.89	0.162
	Lee Memorial Hospital, Fort Myers	9.7	0.0%	0.90	No	0.00	4	0.87	0.036
	Martin Memorial Medical Center, Stuart	10.4	0.0%	0.92	No	0.00	3	1.33	0.049
	Mease Hospital Dunedin, Dunedin	10.2	0.0%	0.89	No	0.00	4	0.87	0.079
	Mercy Hospital, Miami	11.0	0.0%	0.86	No	0.00	4	1.16	0.027
	Mount Sinai Medical Center, Miami Beach	12.5	0.0%	1.05	Yes	0.43	4	0.94	0.047
	Naples Community Hospital, Naples	10.3	0.0%	0.88	No	0.00	4	0.95	0.040
	North Broward Medical Center, Pompano Beach	10.9	0.5%	0.98	No	0.00	3	0.88	0.212
	Orlando Regional Medical Center, Orlando	11.7	0.0%	1.10	Yes	0.27	2	1.25	0.087
98	Shands Hospital at the University of Florida, Gainesville	15.0	0.7%	0.90	Yes	0.66	4	0.62	0.007
	South Miami Hospital	10.1	0.0%	0.85	No	0.00	4	0.78	0.027
	St. Vincent's Medical Center, Jacksonville	10.3	0.0%	0.84	No	0.07	4	0.67	0.053
	Tampa General Hospital, Tampa	13.4	0.0%	0.88	Yes	0.00	4	1.09	0.081
	University Medical Center, Jacksonville	10.4	0.0%	1.41	Yes	0.47	3	1.24	0.016
88	University of Miami, Jackson Memorial Hospital	15.6	0.9%	1.11	Yes	0.85	2	1.39	0.046
	Wuesthoff Hospital, Rockledge	10.1	0.0%	0.83	No	0.00	4	0.76	0.018
	TIER FOUR								
	Alachua General Hospital, Gainesville	7.9	0.0%	0.95	No	0.04	3	0.56	0.017
	Baptist Hospital, Pensacola	7.2	0.0%	1.10	No	0.00	4	0.66	0.015
	Baptist Medical Center, Jacksonville	9.1	0.0%	0.95	No	0.01	3	0.99	0.040
	Bay Medical Center, Panama City	6.8	0.0%	1.07	No	0.00	4	0.77	0.026
	Bayfront Medical Center, St. Petersburg	9.4	0.0%	1.10	No	0.17	4	1.01	0.110
	Bethesda Memorial Hospital, Boynton Beach	6.1	0.0%	1.02	No	0.00	2	0.68	0.025
	Bon Secours-St. Joseph Hospital, Port Charlotte	8.6	0.0%	0.89	No	0.00	3	0.36	0.113
	Broward General Medical Center, Fort Lauderdale	8.6	0.0%	1.03	No	0.00	4	0.80	0.073
	Cedars Medical Center, Miami	9.1	0.0%	0.94	No	0.05	3	0.86	0.047
	Florida Medical Center Hospital, Fort Lauderdale	8.7	0.0%	0.83	No	0.00	2	0.52	0.039
	HCA L.W. Blake Hospital, Bradenton	5.6	0.0%	1.06	No	0.00	2	0.58	0.044
	HCA West Florida Regional Medical Center, Pensacola	7.0	0.0%	1.04	No	0.00	4	0.73	0.024
	Halifax Medical Center, Daytona Beach	9.0	0.0%	0.96	No	0.07	3	0.89	0.043
	Holmes Regional Medical Center, Melbourne	7.5	0.0%	1.18	No	0.00	4	0.96	0.023
	JFK Medical Center, Atlantis	8.5	0.0%	1.01	No	0.00	3	0.83	0.089
	Jupiter Medical Center, Jupiter	9.3	0.0%	0.80	No	0.00	3	0.71	0.135

Natl. Rank	Hospital	U.S. News index	Reputa-tional score	Hospital-wide mortality rate	COTH member	Interns and residents to beds	Tech-nology score (of 5)	R.N.'s to beds	Board-certified internists to beds
	Lakeland Regional Medical Center, Lakeland	5.7	0.5%	1.26	No	0.00	3	0.57	0.044
	Manatee Memorial Hospital, Bradenton	5.7	0.0%	1.11	No	0.00	3	0.61	0.029
	Memorial Hospital, Hollywood	9.0	0.0%	1.03	No	0.00	4	0.94	0.072
	Memorial Hospital-Ormond Beach, Ormond Beach	5.7	0.0%	1.47	No	0.00	4	0.88	0.020
	Memorial Medical Center of Jacksonville, Jacksonville	8.5	0.0%	1.15	No	0.00	5	0.99	0.068
	Morton Plant Hospital, Clearwater	6.1	0.0%	1.07	No	0.00	3	0.61	0.051
	Palms of Pasadena Hospital, St. Petersburg	6.9	0.0%	1.00	No	0.00	3	0.41	0.016
	Parkway Regional Medical Center, North Miami Beach	9.4	0.0%	0.81	No	0.03	4	0.83	0.022
	Sacred Heart Hospital of Pensacola, Pensacola	7.8	0.0%	1.10	No	0.08	4	0.75	0.023
	Sarasota Memorial Hospital, Sarasota	9.0	0.0%	0.95	No	0.00	4	0.76	0.045
	St. Anthony's Hospital, St. Petersburg	7.6	0.0%	0.95	No	0.00	3	0.40	0.053
	St. Joseph's Hospital, Tampa	8.2	0.0%	1.08	No	0.00	4	0.85	0.060
	St. Luke's Hospital, Jacksonville	8.9	0.0%	0.91	No	0.00	4	0.78	0.110
	St. Mary's Hospital, West Palm Beach	9.1	0.0%	0.99	No	0.00	4	1.30	0.058
	Tallahassee Memorial Regional Medical Ctr., Tallahassee	7.9	0.0%	0.97	No	0.09	3	0.50	0.036
	University Community Hospital, Tampa	7.2	0.0%	1.25	No	0.00	4	0.88	0.076
	Winter Haven Hospital, Winter Haven	8.6	0.5%	1.00	No	0.00	3	0.58	0.036
	Winter Park Memorial Hospital, Winter Park	7.8	0.0%	0.99	No	0.00	4	0.36	0.073

UROLOGY

Natl. Rank	Hospital	U.S. News index	Reputa-tional score	Urology mortality rate	COTH member	Interns and residents to beds	Tech-nology score (of 11)	R.N.'s to beds	Board-certified internists to beds	Procedures to beds
	TIER TWO									
77	Shands Hospital at the University of Florida, Gainesville	16.1	1.8%	0.86	Yes	0.66	10	0.62	0.007	1.46
76	University of Miami, Jackson Memorial Hospital	16.2	2.1%	1.10	Yes	0.85	8	1.39	0.046	0.46
	TIER THREE									
	Baptist Hospital of Miami	10.3	0.0%	0.90	No	0.00	9	1.45	0.029	1.12
	Baptist Medical Center, Jacksonville	10.5	0.0%	0.71	No	0.01	5	0.99	0.040	0.89
	Boca Raton Community Hospital, Boca Raton	11.7	0.0%	0.64	No	0.00	8	0.85	0.059	3.08
	Bon Secours-St. Joseph Hospital, Port Charlotte	8.8	0.0%	0.79	No	0.00	5	0.36	0.113	2.26
	Broward General Medical Center, Fort Lauderdale	11.5	0.0%	0.72	No	0.00	10	0.80	0.073	0.82
	Cedars Medical Center, Miami	9.3	0.0%	0.87	No	0.05	7	0.86	0.047	2.09
	Florida Hospital Medical Center, Orlando	10.0	0.0%	0.94	No	0.09	9	1.30	0.036	1.46
	H. Lee Moffitt Cancer Center, Tampa	13.8	0.0%	0.38	No	0.35	6	1.49	0.070	2.33
	HCA Medical Center Hospital-Largo, Largo	10.4	0.0%	0.75	No	0.00	5	0.86	0.059	2.54
	Holy Cross Hospital, Fort Lauderdale	8.7	0.0%	0.99	No	0.00	8	0.89	0.162	1.68
	Jupiter Medical Center, Jupiter	9.3	0.0%	0.92	No	0.00	8	0.71	0.135	3.18
	Lee Memorial Hospital, Fort Myers	10.3	0.0%	0.76	No	0.00	6	0.87	0.036	1.91
	Martin Memorial Medical Center, Stuart	11.4	0.0%	0.82	No	0.00	7	1.33	0.049	3.70
	Mease Hospital Dunedin, Dunedin	8.9	0.0%	0.87	No	0.00	6	0.87	0.079	1.50
	Memorial Medical Center of Jacksonville, Jacksonville	10.7	0.0%	0.76	No	0.00	6	0.99	0.068	1.82
	Morton Plant Hospital, Clearwater	8.7	0.0%	0.87	No	0.00	8	0.61	0.051	1.99
96	Mount Sinai Medical Center, Miami Beach	14.6	0.0%	0.79	Yes	0.43	9	0.94	0.047	1.18
	Orlando Regional Medical Center, Orlando	12.2	0.0%	1.03	Yes	0.27	8	1.25	0.087	1.37
	Parkway Regional Medical Center, North Miami Beach	9.5	0.0%	0.80	No	0.03	6	0.83	0.022	1.61
	Sarasota Memorial Hospital, Sarasota	10.8	0.0%	0.71	No	0.00	6	0.76	0.045	2.86
	South Miami Hospital	10.7	0.0%	0.64	No	0.00	8	0.78	0.027	1.02
	St. Mary's Hospital, West Palm Beach	10.5	0.0%	0.87	No	0.00	9	1.30	0.058	1.12
	St. Vincent's Medical Center, Jacksonville	11.3	0.0%	0.72	No	0.07	9	0.67	0.053	1.70
	Tampa General Hospital, Tampa	9.7	0.0%	1.25	Yes	0.00	9	1.09	0.081	1.77
	Winter Haven Hospital, Winter Haven	10.5	0.0%	0.74	No	0.00	7	0.58	0.036	2.91
	Wuesthoff Hospital, Rockledge	9.2	0.0%	0.81	No	0.00	6	0.76	0.018	2.10
	TIER FOUR									
	Alachua General Hospital, Gainesville	3.2	0.0%	1.48	No	0.04	5	0.56	0.017	1.38

Natl. Rank	Hospital	U.S. News index	Reputa-tional score	Urology mortality rate	COTH member	Interns and residents to beds	Tech-nology score (of 11)	R.N.'s to beds	Board-certified internists to beds	Procedures to beds
	Baptist Hospital, Pensacola	4.2	0.0%	1.50	No	0.00	9	0.66	0.015	1.15
	Bay Medical Center, Panama City	4.8	0.0%	1.43	No	0.00	8	0.77	0.026	2.09
	Bayfront Medical Center, St. Petersburg	7.2	0.0%	1.25	No	0.17	8	1.01	0.110	1.16
	Bethesda Memorial Hospital, Boynton Beach	4.7	0.0%	1.29	No	0.00	6	0.68	0.025	1.81
	Florida Medical Center Hospital, Fort Lauderdale	7.1	0.0%	0.91	No	0.00	6	0.52	0.039	1.18
	HCA L.W. Blake Hospital, Bradenton	7.6	0.0%	0.90	No	0.00	6	0.58	0.044	1.81
	HCA West Florida Regional Medical Center, Pensacola	5.2	0.0%	1.28	No	0.00	8	0.73	0.024	0.96
	Halifax Medical Center, Daytona Beach	6.8	0.0%	1.15	No	0.07	8	0.89	0.043	1.10
	Holmes Regional Medical Center, Melbourne	6.7	0.0%	1.28	No	0.00	9	0.96	0.023	3.14
	JFK Medical Center, Atlantis	7.9	0.0%	1.01	No	0.00	7	0.83	0.089	2.15
	Lakeland Regional Medical Center, Lakeland	5.2	0.0%	1.28	No	0.00	7	0.57	0.044	2.92
	Manatee Memorial Hospital, Bradenton	3.8	0.0%	1.46	No	0.00	7	0.61	0.029	1.35
	Memorial Hospital, Hollywood	7.7	0.0%	1.06	No	0.00	9	0.94	0.072	0.77
	Memorial Hospital-Ormond Beach, Ormond Beach	3.7	0.0%	1.68	No	0.00	5	0.88	0.020	3.22
	Mercy Hospital, Miami	8.3	0.0%	1.06	No	0.00	9	1.16	0.027	1.79
	Naples Community Hospital, Naples	6.6	0.0%	1.25	No	0.00	8	0.95	0.040	2.92
	North Broward Medical Center, Pompano Beach	5.5	0.0%	1.52	No	0.00	8	0.88	0.212	1.83
	Palms of Pasadena Hospital, St. Petersburg	6.6	0.0%	0.99	No	0.00	8	0.41	0.016	1.88
	Sacred Heart Hospital of Pensacola, Pensacola	4.6	0.0%	1.44	No	0.08	7	0.75	0.023	1.60
	St. Anthony's Hospital, St. Petersburg	5.9	0.0%	1.10	No	0.00	8	0.40	0.053	1.55
	St. Joseph's Hospital, Tampa	5.2	0.0%	1.50	No	0.00	9	0.85	0.060	1.79
	St. Luke's Hospital, Jacksonville	6.4	0.0%	1.25	No	0.00	7	0.78	0.110	2.96
	Tallahassee Memorial Regional Medical Ctr., Tallahassee	8.0	0.0%	0.92	No	0.09	8	0.50	0.036	1.80
	University Community Hospital, Tampa	6.3	0.0%	1.20	No	0.00	8	0.88	0.076	0.95
	University Medical Center, Jacksonville	8.1	0.0%	1.82	Yes	0.47	7	1.24	0.016	0.88
	Winter Park Memorial Hospital, Winter Park	6.5	0.0%	1.00	No	0.00	7	0.36	0.073	1.63

AIDS

Natl. Rank	Hospital	U.S. News index	Reputa-tional score	Hospital-wide mortality rate	COTH member	Interns and residents to beds	Tech-nology score (of 11)	Discharge planning (of 2)	R.N.'s to beds	Board-certified internists to beds
TIER TWO										
72	Emory University Hospital, Atlanta	25.9	0.3%	0.92	Yes	0.71	7	2	1.28	0.039
50	Medical College of Georgia Hospital and Clinic, Augusta	27.0	0.0%	0.92	Yes	1.42	8	2	1.09	0.041
TIER THREE										
	Crawford Long Hospital at Emory University, Atlanta	22.1	0.0%	0.99	Yes	0.00	6	1	1.09	0.208
	Grady Memorial Hospital, Atlanta	21.2	1.2%	1.32	Yes	0.60	9	2	0.45	0.142
	Memorial Medical Center, Savannah	19.7	0.0%	1.19	Yes	0.25	7	2	0.79	0.048
	Northside Hospital, Atlanta	20.8	0.0%	1.06	No	0.00	6	2	1.35	0.263
	South Fulton Medical Center, Eastpoint	20.2	0.0%	1.00	No	0.00	7	2	0.80	0.023
	West Paces Medical Center, Atlanta	21.2	0.0%	0.90	No	0.00	5	2	0.64	0.065
TIER FOUR										
	Athens Regional Medical Center, Athens	18.1	0.0%	1.11	No	0.00	6	2	0.72	0.020
	De Kalb Medical Center, Decatur	18.4	0.0%	1.15	No	0.00	7	2	0.90	0.082
	Floyd Medical Center, Rome	16.1	0.0%	1.33	No	0.15	5	2	1.05	0.033
	Georgia Baptist Medical Center, Atlanta	19.1	0.0%	1.33	Yes	0.25	6	2	0.58	0.408
	Gwinnett Hospital System, Lawrenceville	18.1	0.0%	1.15	No	0.00	6	2	1.05	0.033
	Hamilton Medical Center, Dalton	16.1	0.0%	1.26	No	0.00	6	2	0.53	0.030
	John D. Archbold Memorial Hospital, Thomasville	19.5	0.0%	1.05	No	0.00	8	2	0.60	0.031
	Kennestone Hospital, Marietta	19.4	0.0%	1.13	No	0.00	8	2	1.22	0.032
	Medical Center of Central Georgia, Macon	18.5	0.6%	1.30	Yes	0.23	5	2	0.75	0.032
	Northeast Georgia Medical Center, Gainesville	15.5	0.0%	1.30	No	0.00	5	2	0.67	0.021
	Phoebe Putney Memorial Hospital, Albany	16.3	0.0%	1.31	No	0.00	6	2	0.92	0.041
	Piedmont Hospital, Atlanta	16.8	0.0%	1.21	No	0.01	6	1	1.02	0.073
	St. Francis Hospital, Columbus	13.9	0.0%	1.43	No	0.00	5	1	0.69	0.098
	St. Joseph's Hospital of Atlanta	19.1	0.0%	1.14	No	0.00	6	1	1.98	0.066
	The Medical Center, Columbus	13.9	0.0%	1.44	No	0.11	7	1	0.34	0.015
	University Hospital, Augusta	15.2	0.0%	1.50	No	0.07	7	2	1.00	0.034
	West Georgia Medical Center, La Grange	16.1	0.0%	1.22	No	0.00	7	1	0.47	0.034

CANCER

Natl. Rank	Hospital	U.S. News index	Reputa-tional score	Cancer mortality rate	COTH member	Interns and residents to beds	Tech-nology score (of 12)	R.N.'s to beds	Board-certified oncologists to beds	Procedures to beds
TIER TWO										
70	Emory University Hospital, Atlanta	11.5	1.2%	0.76	Yes	0.71	7	1.28	0.026	2.42
51	Medical College of Georgia Hospital and Clinic, Augusta	12.9	0.0%	0.56	Yes	1.42	11	1.09	0.008	1.14
TIER THREE										
	Crawford Long Hospital at Emory University, Atlanta	6.6	0.6%	0.93	Yes	0.00	4	1.09	0.000	1.57
	Grady Memorial Hospital, Atlanta	7.6	0.0%	1.03	Yes	0.60	11	0.45	0.000	0.36
	Kennestone Hospital, Marietta	5.4	0.0%	0.88	No	0.00	10	1.22	0.010	1.21
	Medical Center of Central Georgia, Macon	5.4	0.0%	0.83	Yes	0.23	3	0.75	0.006	1.25
	Memorial Medical Center, Savannah	7.3	0.0%	1.02	Yes	0.25	10	0.79	0.007	0.98
	Northside Hospital, Atlanta	5.4	0.0%	0.88	No	0.00	8	1.35	0.026	1.35
	St. Joseph's Hospital of Atlanta	7.0	0.0%	1.08	No	0.00	7	1.98	0.064	2.22
TIER FOUR										
	Athens Regional Medical Center, Athens	3.4	0.0%	1.04	No	0.00	8	0.72	0.007	1.66
	De Kalb Medical Center, Decatur	4.1	0.0%	0.85	No	0.00	8	0.90	0.015	1.55
	Floyd Medical Center, Rome	3.5	0.0%	1.41	No	0.15	5	1.05	0.010	0.82
	Gwinnett Hospital System, Lawrenceville	3.7	0.0%	1.22	No	0.00	7	1.05	0.015	0.76
	Hamilton Medical Center, Dalton	2.3	0.0%	1.29	No	0.00	7	0.53	0.007	1.47
	John D. Archbold Memorial Hospital, Thomasville	3.5	0.0%	1.07	No	0.00	10	0.60	0.008	1.46

Natl. Rank	Hospital	U.S. News index	Reputa-tional score	Cancer mortality rate	COTH member	Interns and residents to beds	Tech-nology score (of 12)	R.N.'s to beds	Board-certified oncologists to beds	Procedures to beds
	Northeast Georgia Medical Center, Gainesville	2.5	0.0%	1.13	No	0.00	6	0.67	0.003	1.10
	Phoebe Putney Memorial Hospital, Albany	3.5	0.0%	1.25	No	0.00	7	0.92	0.010	1.70
	Piedmont Hospital, Atlanta	4.5	0.0%	0.89	No	0.01	8	1.02	0.013	1.94
	South Fulton Medical Center, Eastpoint	3.7	0.0%	0.87	No	0.00	8	0.80	0.011	1.20
	South Georgia Medical Center, Valdosta	3.2	0.0%	1.15	No	0.00	8	0.73	0.003	1.08
	St. Francis Hospital, Columbus	2.1	0.0%	1.03	No	0.00	4	0.69	0.008	1.15
	The Medical Center, Columbus	2.4	0.0%	1.76	No	0.11	9	0.34	0.010	0.57
	University Hospital, Augusta	3.6	0.0%	1.18	No	0.07	6	1.00	0.007	1.16
	West Georgia Medical Center, La Grange	2.4	0.0%	1.13	No	0.00	8	0.47	0.005	0.91
	West Paces Medical Center, Atlanta	2.2	0.0%	0.61	No	0.00	3	0.64	0.014	0.80

CARDIOLOGY

Natl. Rank	Hospital	U.S. News index	Reputa-tional score	Cardiology mortality rate	COTH member	Interns and residents to beds	Tech-nology score (of 10)	R.N.'s to beds	Board-certified cardiologists to beds	Procedures to beds
TIER ONE										
8	Emory University Hospital, Atlanta	48.3	17.6%	0.95	Yes	0.71	8	1.28	0.037	9.57
TIER TWO										
74	Crawford Long Hospital at Emory University, Atlanta	21.5	2.6%	0.98	Yes	0.00	8	1.09	0.000	8.77
TIER THREE										
	Grady Memorial Hospital, Atlanta	17.6	0.0%	0.99	Yes	0.60	9	0.45	0.000	2.02
	John D. Archbold Memorial Hospital, Thomasville	16.4	0.0%	0.83	No	0.00	8	0.60	0.004	6.03
	Medical College of Georgia Hospital and Clinic, Augusta	17.4	0.0%	1.25	Yes	1.42	8	1.09	0.020	2.30
	Memorial Medical Center, Savannah	14.9	0.0%	1.12	Yes	0.25	8	0.79	0.028	5.46
	Northside Hospital, Atlanta	14.3	0.0%	1.02	No	0.00	6	1.35	0.033	2.89
	South Fulton Medical Center, Eastpoint	13.9	0.0%	0.98	No	0.00	6	0.80	0.037	5.98
	St. Joseph's Hospital of Atlanta	18.1	2.1%	1.17	No	0.00	8	1.98	0.168	21.89
TIER FOUR										
	Athens Regional Medical Center, Athens	12.9	0.0%	1.04	No	0.00	8	0.72	0.013	9.44
	De Kalb Medical Center, Decatur	13.3	0.0%	1.05	No	0.00	7	0.90	0.050	6.20
	Floyd Medical Center, Rome	7.4	0.0%	1.36	No	0.15	3	1.05	0.030	5.33
	Georgia Baptist Medical Center, Atlanta	9.7	0.0%	1.34	Yes	0.25	6	0.58	0.000	5.22
	Gwinnett Hospital System, Lawrenceville	12.8	0.0%	1.07	No	0.00	6	1.05	0.036	7.48
	Hamilton Medical Center, Dalton	8.1	0.0%	1.21	No	0.00	6	0.53	0.011	6.77
	Kennestone Hospital, Marietta	12.0	0.0%	1.15	No	0.00	8	1.22	0.026	5.81
	Medical Center of Central Georgia, Macon	9.8	0.0%	1.45	Yes	0.23	7	0.75	0.023	9.89
	Northeast Georgia Medical Center, Gainesville	7.5	0.0%	1.25	No	0.00	5	0.67	0.006	5.57
	Phoebe Putney Memorial Hospital, Albany	6.4	0.0%	1.47	No	0.00	8	0.92	0.012	5.82
	Piedmont Hospital, Atlanta	10.4	0.0%	1.24	No	0.01	9	1.02	0.032	5.99
	South Georgia Medical Center, Valdosta	4.1	0.0%	1.55	No	0.00	6	0.73	0.000	5.65
	St. Francis Hospital, Columbus	6.7	0.0%	1.45	No	0.00	8	0.69	0.038	10.06
	St. Joseph's Hospital, Savannah	7.2	0.0%	1.31	No	0.00	8	0.56	0.000	7.90
	The Medical Center, Columbus	5.8	0.0%	1.33	No	0.11	5	0.34	0.017	2.49
	University Hospital, Augusta	5.4	0.0%	1.65	No	0.07	8	1.00	0.024	7.58
	West Georgia Medical Center, La Grange	7.9	0.0%	1.19	No	0.00	5	0.47	0.005	5.46

ENDOCRINOLOGY

Natl. Rank	Hospital	U.S. News index	Reputational score	Endocrinology mortality rate	COTH member	Interns and residents to beds	Technology score (of 11)	R.N.'s to beds	Board-certified internists to beds
	TIER TWO								
46	Emory University Hospital, Atlanta	17.8	1.2%	0.30	Yes	0.71	8	1.28	0.039
40	Medical College of Georgia Hospital and Clinic, Augusta	18.4	0.0%	0.12	Yes	1.42	10	1.09	0.041
	TIER THREE								
	Crawford Long Hospital at Emory University, Atlanta	8.9	0.0%	1.29	Yes	0.00	5	1.09	0.208
	Georgia Baptist Medical Center, Atlanta	9.0	0.0%	1.58	Yes	0.25	6	0.58	0.408
	Grady Memorial Hospital, Atlanta	10.0	0.0%	1.21	Yes	0.60	10	0.45	0.142
	John D. Archbold Memorial Hospital, Thomasville	8.5	0.0%	0.77	No	0.00	11	0.60	0.031
	Medical Center of Central Georgia, Macon	8.2	0.0%	1.06	Yes	0.23	3	0.75	0.032
	St. Joseph's Hospital of Atlanta	9.2	0.0%	1.12	No	0.00	8	1.98	0.066
	St. Joseph's Hospital, Savannah	9.0	0.0%	0.49	No	0.00	6	0.56	0.032
	TIER FOUR								
	Athens Regional Medical Center, Athens	5.2	0.0%	1.21	No	0.00	9	0.72	0.020
	De Kalb Medical Center, Decatur	5.2	0.0%	1.45	No	0.00	9	0.90	0.082
	Floyd Medical Center, Rome	5.7	0.0%	1.30	No	0.15	6	1.05	0.033
	Gwinnett Hospital System, Lawrenceville	4.4	0.0%	1.71	No	0.00	8	1.05	0.033
	Hamilton Medical Center, Dalton	2.9	0.0%	1.71	No	0.00	8	0.53	0.030
	Kennestone Hospital, Marietta	6.3	0.0%	1.40	No	0.00	11	1.22	0.032
	Memorial Medical Center, Savannah	7.3	0.0%	1.69	Yes	0.25	9	0.79	0.048
	Northeast Georgia Medical Center, Gainesville	5.0	0.0%	1.15	No	0.00	7	0.67	0.021
	Northside Hospital, Atlanta	6.4	0.0%	1.91	No	0.00	8	1.35	0.263
	Phoebe Putney Memorial Hospital, Albany	4.8	0.0%	1.43	No	0.00	8	0.92	0.041
	Piedmont Hospital, Atlanta	7.3	0.0%	1.06	No	0.01	9	1.02	0.073
	South Fulton Medical Center, Eastpoint	6.0	0.0%	1.11	No	0.00	9	0.80	0.023
	South Georgia Medical Center, Valdosta	4.4	0.0%	1.43	No	0.00	9	0.73	0.024
	St. Francis Hospital, Columbus	2.4	0.0%	2.14	No	0.00	5	0.69	0.098
	The Medical Center, Columbus	3.6	0.0%	1.39	No	0.11	8	0.34	0.015
	University Hospital, Augusta	3.9	0.0%	1.78	No	0.07	6	1.00	0.034
	West Georgia Medical Center, La Grange	5.0	0.0%	1.10	No	0.00	8	0.47	0.034
	West Paces Medical Center, Atlanta	6.8	0.0%	0.86	No	0.00	5	0.64	0.065

GASTROENTEROLOGY

Natl. Rank	Hospital	U.S. News index	Reputational score	Gastroenterology mortality rate	COTH member	Interns and residents to beds	Technology score (of 11)	R.N.'s to beds	Board-certified gastroenterologists to beds	Procedures to beds
	TIER TWO									
55	Emory University Hospital, Atlanta	14.6	1.1%	0.90	Yes	0.71	8	1.28	0.013	1.90
65	Medical College of Georgia Hospital and Clinic, Augusta	13.9	0.4%	1.18	Yes	1.42	10	1.09	0.014	1.01
	TIER THREE									
	Crawford Long Hospital at Emory University, Atlanta	11.0	0.0%	0.76	Yes	0.00	6	1.09	0.000	3.41
	Grady Memorial Hospital, Atlanta	8.1	0.0%	1.19	Yes	0.60	9	0.45	0.000	0.64
	John D. Archbold Memorial Hospital, Thomasville	8.7	0.0%	0.85	No	0.00	11	0.60	0.004	3.90
	Memorial Medical Center, Savannah	8.3	0.0%	1.23	Yes	0.25	9	0.79	0.009	1.94
	St. Joseph's Hospital of Atlanta	10.3	0.0%	0.90	No	0.00	7	1.98	0.052	3.88
	TIER FOUR									
	Athens Regional Medical Center, Athens	6.3	0.0%	1.10	No	0.00	9	0.72	0.013	3.63
	De Kalb Medical Center, Decatur	6.1	0.0%	1.16	No	0.00	8	0.90	0.017	3.60
	Floyd Medical Center, Rome	4.2	0.0%	1.44	No	0.15	5	1.05	0.010	2.51
	Georgia Baptist Medical Center, Atlanta	6.6	0.0%	1.29	Yes	0.25	6	0.58	0.000	2.04
	Gwinnett Hospital System, Lawrenceville	4.6	0.0%	1.41	No	0.00	7	1.05	0.012	2.95
	Hamilton Medical Center, Dalton	4.9	0.0%	1.21	No	0.00	7	0.53	0.007	4.09
	Kennestone Hospital, Marietta	6.7	0.0%	1.33	No	0.00	11	1.22	0.014	3.32
	Medical Center of Central Georgia, Macon	5.4	0.0%	1.50	Yes	0.23	3	0.75	0.009	2.18

Natl. Rank	Hospital	U.S. News index	Reputational score	Gastroenterology mortality rate	COTH member	Interns and residents to beds	Technology score (of 11)	R.N.'s to beds	Board-certified gastroenterologists to beds	Procedures to beds
	Northeast Georgia Medical Center, Gainesville	2.6	0.0%	1.71	No	0.00	6	0.67	0.009	3.05
	Northside Hospital, Atlanta	6.6	0.0%	1.05	No	0.00	7	1.35	0.037	1.95
	Phoebe Putney Memorial Hospital, Albany	4.1	0.0%	1.44	No	0.00	7	0.92	0.007	2.84
	Piedmont Hospital, Atlanta	6.3	0.0%	1.15	No	0.01	8	1.02	0.017	3.31
	South Fulton Medical Center, Eastpoint	6.6	0.0%	0.97	No	0.00	8	0.80	0.017	2.78
	South Georgia Medical Center, Valdosta	2.9	0.0%	2.17	No	0.00	8	0.73	0.007	3.93
	St. Francis Hospital, Columbus	3.1	0.0%	1.57	No	0.00	5	0.69	0.030	3.56
	St. Joseph's Hospital, Savannah	3.8	0.0%	1.25	No	0.00	6	0.56	0.000	2.95
	The Medical Center, Columbus	1.5	0.0%	1.64	No	0.11	7	0.34	0.008	1.12
	University Hospital, Augusta	3.5	0.0%	1.58	No	0.07	5	1.00	0.006	2.87
	West Georgia Medical Center, La Grange	4.5	0.0%	1.17	No	0.00	8	0.47	0.005	2.82

GERIATRICS

Natl. Rank	Hospital	U.S. News index	Reputational score	Hospital-wide mortality rate	COTH member	Service mix	Interns and residents to beds	Technology score (of 13)	R.N.'s to beds	Discharge planning (of 2)	Geriatric services (of 9)	Board-certified internists to beds
	**TIER TWO**											
74	Emory University Hospital, Atlanta	22.4	0.6%	0.92	Yes	4	0.71	10	1.28	2	1	0.039
54	Medical College of Georgia Hospital and Clinic, Augusta	24.0	0.0%	0.92	Yes	6	1.42	12	1.09	2	3	0.041
	**TIER THREE**											
	John D. Archbold Memorial Hospital, Thomasville	15.2	0.0%	1.05	No	9	0.00	12	0.60	2	4	0.031
	Northside Hospital, Atlanta	17.0	0.0%	1.06	No	9	0.00	11	1.35	2	2	0.263
	West Paces Medical Center, Atlanta	16.9	0.0%	0.90	No	6	0.00	6	0.64	2	1	0.065
	**TIER FOUR**											
	Athens Regional Medical Center, Athens	10.8	0.0%	1.11	No	4	0.00	10	0.72	2	1	0.020
	De Kalb Medical Center, Decatur	11.3	0.0%	1.15	No	5	0.00	11	0.90	2	2	0.082
	Floyd Medical Center, Rome	8.2	0.0%	1.33	No	6	0.15	7	1.05	2	3	0.033
	Georgia Baptist Medical Center, Atlanta	10.0	0.0%	1.33	Yes	3	0.25	8	0.58	2	1	0.408
	Grady Memorial Hospital, Atlanta	12.3	0.0%	1.32	Yes	8	0.60	12	0.45	2	1	0.142
	Gwinnett Hospital System, Lawrenceville	10.5	0.0%	1.15	No	4	0.00	9	1.05	2	2	0.033
	Hamilton Medical Center, Dalton	9.1	0.0%	1.26	No	7	0.00	10	0.53	2	3	0.030
	Kennestone Hospital, Marietta	11.9	0.0%	1.13	No	4	0.00	12	1.22	2	2	0.032
	Medical Center of Central Georgia, Macon	10.9	0.0%	1.30	Yes	8	0.23	5	0.75	2	3	0.032
	Memorial Medical Center, Savannah	13.7	0.0%	1.19	Yes	8	0.25	11	0.79	2	1	0.048
	Northeast Georgia Medical Center, Gainesville	8.4	0.0%	1.30	No	7	0.00	9	0.67	2	3	0.021
	Phoebe Putney Memorial Hospital, Albany	9.4	0.0%	1.31	No	7	0.00	10	0.92	2	4	0.041
	Piedmont Hospital, Atlanta	7.8	0.0%	1.21	No	3	0.01	10	1.02	1	1	0.073
	South Fulton Medical Center, Eastpoint	13.7	0.0%	1.00	No	4	0.00	10	0.80	2	1	0.023
	South Georgia Medical Center, Valdosta	4.9	0.0%	1.51	No	4	0.00	10	0.73	2	5	0.024
	St. Francis Hospital, Columbus	4.0	0.0%	1.43	No	4	0.00	7	0.69	1	3	0.098
	St. Joseph's Hospital of Atlanta	11.1	0.0%	1.14	No	3	0.00	10	1.98	1	1	0.066
	St. Joseph's Hospital, Savannah	9.9	0.0%	1.14	No	4	0.00	8	0.56	2	3	0.032
	The Medical Center, Columbus	4.2	0.0%	1.44	No	6	0.11	10	0.34	1	2	0.015
	University Hospital, Augusta	5.0	0.0%	1.50	No	6	0.07	7	1.00	2	1	0.034
	West Georgia Medical Center, La Grange	7.8	0.0%	1.22	No	6	0.00	9	0.47	1	2	0.034

GYNECOLOGY

Natl. Rank	Hospital	U.S. News index	Reputa- tional score	Hospital- wide mortality rate	Interns and residents to beds	Tech- nology score (of 10)	R.N.'s to beds	Board- certified OB-GYNs to beds	Procedures to beds
TIER TWO									
52	Medical College of Georgia Hospital and Clinic, Augusta	26.1	0.0%	0.92	1.42	9	1.09	0.026	0.40
TIER THREE									
	Crawford Long Hospital at Emory University, Atlanta	16.2	0.0%	0.99	0.00	6	1.09	0.046	30.33
	Kennestone Hospital, Marietta	16.0	0.0%	1.13	0.00	10	1.22	0.048	0.40
	Northside Hospital, Atlanta	18.3	0.4%	1.06	0.00	7	1.35	0.174	0.67
	South Fulton Medical Center, Eastpoint	15.0	0.0%	1.00	0.00	7	0.80	0.037	0.30
	St. Joseph's Hospital of Atlanta	15.7	0.0%	1.14	0.00	6	1.98	0.029	0.55
TIER FOUR									
	Athens Regional Medical Center, Athens	13.2	0.0%	1.11	0.00	8	0.72	0.062	0.41
	De Kalb Medical Center, Decatur	13.3	0.0%	1.15	0.00	8	0.90	0.075	0.49
	Floyd Medical Center, Rome	7.9	0.0%	1.33	0.15	4	1.05	0.046	0.44
	Georgia Baptist Medical Center, Atlanta	8.3	0.0%	1.33	0.25	5	0.58	0.101	0.34
	Grady Memorial Hospital, Atlanta	10.4	0.0%	1.32	0.60	9	0.45	0.025	0.12
	Gwinnett Hospital System, Lawrenceville	12.6	0.0%	1.15	0.00	7	1.05	0.045	0.21
	Hamilton Medical Center, Dalton	7.5	0.0%	1.26	0.00	6	0.53	0.041	0.44
	John D. Archbold Memorial Hospital, Thomasville	13.8	0.0%	1.05	0.00	9	0.60	0.023	0.64
	Medical Center of Central Georgia, Macon	7.4	0.0%	1.30	0.23	4	0.75	0.043	0.25
	Memorial Medical Center, Savannah	12.1	0.0%	1.19	0.25	8	0.79	0.030	0.38
	Northeast Georgia Medical Center, Gainesville	6.8	0.0%	1.30	0.00	5	0.67	0.047	0.52
	Phoebe Putney Memorial Hospital, Albany	8.9	0.0%	1.31	0.00	7	0.92	0.034	0.47
	Piedmont Hospital, Atlanta	12.0	0.0%	1.21	0.01	8	1.02	0.045	0.57
	South Georgia Medical Center, Valdosta	5.6	0.0%	1.51	0.00	8	0.73	0.021	0.48
	St. Francis Hospital, Columbus	3.9	0.0%	1.43	0.00	4	0.69	0.034	0.29
	St. Joseph's Hospital, Savannah	9.2	0.0%	1.14	0.00	5	0.56	0.039	0.22
	The Medical Center, Columbus	4.7	0.0%	1.44	0.11	7	0.34	0.028	0.16
	University Hospital, Augusta	6.0	0.0%	1.50	0.07	6	1.00	0.030	0.33
	West Georgia Medical Center, La Grange	7.5	0.0%	1.22	0.00	6	0.47	0.021	0.29

NEUROLOGY

Natl. Rank	Hospital	U.S. News index	Reputa- tional score	Neurology mortality rate	COTH member	Interns and residents to beds	Tech- nology score (of 9)	R.N.'s to beds	Board- certified neurologists to beds
TIER TWO									
35	Emory University Hospital, Atlanta	22.7	1.7%	0.81	Yes	0.71	6	1.28	0.030
29	Medical College of Georgia Hospital and Clinic, Augusta	23.6	0.0%	0.70	Yes	1.42	8	1.09	0.030
TIER THREE									
	Crawford Long Hospital at Emory University, Atlanta	14.2	0.0%	0.89	Yes	0.00	5	1.09	0.013
	Memorial Medical Center, Savannah	11.4	0.0%	1.10	Yes	0.25	7	0.79	0.015
	Northside Hospital, Atlanta	12.2	0.0%	0.94	No	0.00	6	1.35	0.020
	St. Joseph's Hospital of Atlanta	11.4	0.7%	1.19	No	0.00	6	1.98	0.020
TIER FOUR									
	Athens Regional Medical Center, Athens	7.7	0.0%	1.11	No	0.00	7	0.72	0.010
	De Kalb Medical Center, Decatur	8.1	0.0%	1.13	No	0.00	7	0.90	0.013
	Floyd Medical Center, Rome	6.3	0.0%	1.26	No	0.15	4	1.05	0.007
	Grady Memorial Hospital, Atlanta	9.2	0.0%	1.36	Yes	0.60	8	0.45	0.016
	Gwinnett Hospital System, Lawrenceville	5.9	0.0%	1.32	No	0.00	6	1.05	0.009
	Hamilton Medical Center, Dalton	5.2	0.0%	1.22	No	0.00	6	0.53	0.004
	Kennestone Hospital, Marietta	8.7	0.0%	1.22	No	0.00	9	1.22	0.016
	Medical Center of Central Georgia, Macon	8.2	0.6%	1.33	Yes	0.23	3	0.75	0.011
	Northeast Georgia Medical Center, Gainesville	5.3	0.0%	1.21	No	0.00	5	0.67	0.003
	Phoebe Putney Memorial Hospital, Albany	8.6	0.0%	1.03	No	0.00	6	0.92	0.005
	Piedmont Hospital, Atlanta	8.0	0.0%	1.17	No	0.01	7	1.02	0.013

Natl. Rank	Hospital	U.S. News index	Reputational score	Neurology mortality rate	COTH member	Interns and residents to beds	Technology score (of 9)	R.N.'s to beds	Board-certified neurologists to beds
	South Fulton Medical Center, Eastpoint	10.5	0.0%	0.93	No	0.00	7	0.80	0.006
	St. Francis Hospital, Columbus	4.3	0.0%	1.32	No	0.00	4	0.69	0.008
	The Medical Center, Columbus	5.1	0.0%	1.22	No	0.11	6	0.34	0.005
	University Hospital, Augusta	5.8	0.0%	1.28	No	0.07	5	1.00	0.006
	West Georgia Medical Center, La Grange	4.7	0.0%	1.24	No	0.00	6	0.47	0.003

ORTHOPEDICS

Natl. Rank	Hospital	U.S. News index	Reputational score	Orthopedics mortality rate	COTH member	Interns and residents to beds	Technology score (of 5)	R.N.'s to beds	Board-certified orthopedists to beds	Procedures to beds
	TIER TWO									
44	Emory University Hospital, Atlanta	17.3	2.3%	1.04	Yes	0.71	4	1.28	0.028	2.19
38	Medical College of Georgia Hospital and Clinic, Augusta	18.0	0.0%	0.50	Yes	1.42	4	1.09	0.014	0.59
	TIER THREE									
	Crawford Long Hospital at Emory University, Atlanta	9.1	0.0%	1.11	Yes	0.00	4	1.09	0.027	1.69
	Grady Memorial Hospital, Atlanta	9.8	1.0%	1.39	Yes	0.60	4	0.45	0.021	0.34
88	Hughston Sports Medicine Hospital, Columbus	13.8	1.1%	0.17	No	0.00	2	0.52	0.150	13.12
	Kennestone Hospital, Marietta	8.9	0.0%	0.91	No	0.00	5	1.22	0.026	2.01
	Memorial Medical Center, Savannah	8.6	0.0%	1.09	Yes	0.25	3	0.79	0.017	1.92
	Northside Hospital, Atlanta	11.0	0.0%	0.47	No	0.00	3	1.35	0.048	1.42
	St. Joseph's Hospital of Atlanta	9.2	0.4%	1.16	No	0.00	3	1.98	0.069	2.55
	TIER FOUR									
	Athens Regional Medical Center, Athens	7.2	0.0%	0.84	No	0.00	3	0.72	0.033	3.17
	De Kalb Medical Center, Decatur	5.9	0.0%	1.13	No	0.00	4	0.90	0.022	2.42
	Floyd Medical Center, Rome	3.8	0.0%	1.48	No	0.15	2	1.05	0.016	1.85
	Gwinnett Hospital System, Lawrenceville	6.5	0.0%	0.99	No	0.00	3	1.05	0.039	1.70
	Hamilton Medical Center, Dalton	5.6	0.0%	0.91	No	0.00	3	0.53	0.015	1.47
	John D. Archbold Memorial Hospital, Thomasville	3.7	0.0%	1.66	No	0.00	5	0.60	0.008	3.29
	Medical Center of Central Georgia, Macon	7.2	0.0%	1.23	Yes	0.23	2	0.75	0.028	2.51
	Northeast Georgia Medical Center, Gainesville	5.4	0.0%	0.92	No	0.00	2	0.67	0.018	1.83
	Phoebe Putney Memorial Hospital, Albany	7.5	0.0%	0.83	No	0.00	3	0.92	0.022	1.54
	Piedmont Hospital, Atlanta	6.5	0.0%	1.16	No	0.01	4	1.02	0.028	3.88
	South Fulton Medical Center, Eastpoint	6.5	0.0%	0.97	No	0.00	4	0.80	0.017	1.85
	South Georgia Medical Center, Valdosta	4.5	0.0%	1.27	No	0.00	4	0.73	0.007	2.09
	St. Francis Hospital, Columbus	4.3	0.0%	1.21	No	0.00	3	0.69	0.056	1.87
	St. Joseph's Hospital, Savannah	6.5	0.0%	0.90	No	0.00	3	0.56	0.046	3.77
	The Medical Center, Columbus	2.5	0.3%	1.60	No	0.11	3	0.34	0.031	0.61
	University Hospital, Augusta	5.3	0.0%	1.14	No	0.07	3	1.00	0.007	1.07
	West Georgia Medical Center, La Grange	3.3	0.0%	1.22	No	0.00	3	0.47	0.008	1.34
	West Paces Medical Center, Atlanta	3.2	0.0%	1.38	No	0.00	3	0.64	0.024	1.45

OTOLARYNGOLOGY

Natl. Rank	Hospital	U.S. News index	Reputational score	Hospital-wide mortality rate	COTH member	Interns and residents to beds	Technology score (of 9)	R.N.'s to beds	Board-certified internists to beds	Procedures to beds
	TIER TWO									
75	Medical College of Georgia Hospital and Clinic, Augusta	14.8	0.0%	0.92	Yes	1.42	8	1.09	0.041	0.343
	TIER THREE									
	Crawford Long Hospital at Emory University, Atlanta	12.4	0.0%	0.99	Yes	0.00	3	1.09	0.208	0.330
	Emory University Hospital, Atlanta	12.0	0.0%	0.92	Yes	0.71	6	1.28	0.039	0.344
	Georgia Baptist Medical Center, Atlanta	10.3	0.0%	1.33	Yes	0.25	4	0.58	0.408	0.094
	Grady Memorial Hospital, Atlanta	10.2	0.0%	1.32	Yes	0.60	8	0.45	0.142	0.059
	Memorial Medical Center, Savannah	8.9	0.0%	1.19	Yes	0.25	7	0.79	0.048	0.212
	Northside Hospital, Atlanta	8.1	0.0%	1.06	No	0.00	6	1.35	0.263	0.128

Natl. Rank	Hospital	U.S. News index	Reputa- tional score	Hospital- wide mortality rate	COTH member	Interns and residents to beds	Tech- nology score (of 9)	R.N.'s to beds	Board- certified internists to beds	Procedures to beds
	St. Joseph's Hospital of Atlanta	8.3	0.0%	1.14	No	0.00	6	1.98	0.066	0.214
	University Hospital, Augusta	7.1	0.8%	1.50	No	0.07	4	1.00	0.034	0.131
TIER FOUR										
	Athens Regional Medical Center, Athens	5.5	0.4%	1.11	No	0.00	7	0.72	0.020	0.226
	De Kalb Medical Center, Decatur	5.4	0.0%	1.15	No	0.00	7	0.90	0.082	0.190
	Floyd Medical Center, Rome	5.1	0.0%	1.33	No	0.15	4	1.05	0.033	0.171
	Gwinnett Hospital System, Lawrenceville	5.1	0.0%	1.15	No	0.00	6	1.05	0.033	0.167
	Hamilton Medical Center, Dalton	3.5	0.0%	1.26	No	0.00	6	0.53	0.030	0.276
	Hughston Sports Medicine Hospital, Columbus	2.4	0.0%	0.20	No	0.00	2	0.52	0.000	0.010
	John D. Archbold Memorial Hospital, Thomasville	4.7	0.0%	1.05	No	0.00	9	0.60	0.031	0.251
	Kennestone Hospital, Marietta	6.5	0.0%	1.13	No	0.00	9	1.22	0.032	0.253
	Medical Center of Central Georgia, Macon	6.8	0.0%	1.30	Yes	0.23	1	0.75	0.032	0.200
	Northeast Georgia Medical Center, Gainesville	3.5	0.0%	1.30	No	0.00	5	0.67	0.021	0.154
	Phoebe Putney Memorial Hospital, Albany	4.7	0.0%	1.31	No	0.00	6	0.92	0.041	0.111
	Piedmont Hospital, Atlanta	5.7	0.0%	1.21	No	0.01	7	1.02	0.073	0.143
	South Fulton Medical Center, Eastpoint	4.7	0.0%	1.00	No	0.00	7	0.80	0.023	0.140
	South Georgia Medical Center, Valdosta	4.2	0.0%	1.51	No	0.00	7	0.73	0.024	0.274
	Southwest Hospital and Medical Center, Atlanta	2.8	0.0%	1.10	No	0.13	0	0.61	0.052	0.052
	St. Francis Hospital, Columbus	3.6	0.0%	1.43	No	0.00	3	0.69	0.098	0.267
	St. Joseph's Hospital, Savannah	3.1	0.0%	1.14	No	0.00	4	0.56	0.032	0.291
	The Medical Center, Columbus	3.1	0.0%	1.44	No	0.11	6	0.34	0.015	0.089
	West Georgia Medical Center, La Grange	3.3	0.0%	1.22	No	0.00	6	0.47	0.034	0.149
	West Paces Medical Center, Atlanta	3.5	0.0%	0.90	No	0.00	3	0.64	0.065	0.276

RHEUMATOLOGY

Natl. Rank	Hospital	U.S. News index	Reputa- tional score	Hospital- wide mortality rate	COTH member	Interns and residents to beds	Tech- nology score (of 5)	R.N.'s to beds	Board- certified internists to beds
TIER TWO									
54	Emory University Hospital, Atlanta	17.6	1.0%	0.92	Yes	0.71	4	1.28	0.039
62	Medical College of Georgia Hospital and Clinic, Augusta	17.1	0.0%	0.92	Yes	1.42	4	1.09	0.041
TIER THREE									
	Crawford Long Hospital at Emory University, Atlanta	12.2	0.0%	0.99	Yes	0.00	4	1.09	0.208
	Georgia Baptist Medical Center, Atlanta	11.2	0.0%	1.33	Yes	0.25	3	0.58	0.408
	Grady Memorial Hospital, Atlanta	10.6	0.0%	1.32	Yes	0.60	4	0.45	0.142
	Memorial Medical Center, Savannah	10.0	0.0%	1.19	Yes	0.25	3	0.79	0.048
	Northside Hospital, Atlanta	10.7	0.0%	1.06	No	0.00	3	1.35	0.263
TIER FOUR									
	Athens Regional Medical Center, Athens	6.9	0.0%	1.11	No	0.00	3	0.72	0.020
	De Kalb Medical Center, Decatur	8.0	0.0%	1.15	No	0.00	4	0.90	0.082
	Floyd Medical Center, Rome	6.5	0.0%	1.33	No	0.15	2	1.05	0.033
	Gwinnett Hospital System, Lawrenceville	7.5	0.0%	1.15	No	0.00	3	1.05	0.033
	Hamilton Medical Center, Dalton	5.5	0.0%	1.26	No	0.00	3	0.53	0.030
	John D. Archbold Memorial Hospital, Thomasville	8.0	0.0%	1.05	No	0.00	5	0.60	0.031
	Kennestone Hospital, Marietta	9.1	0.0%	1.13	No	0.00	5	1.22	0.032
	Medical Center of Central Georgia, Macon	8.6	0.0%	1.30	Yes	0.23	2	0.75	0.032
	Northeast Georgia Medical Center, Gainesville	5.1	0.0%	1.30	No	0.00	2	0.67	0.021
	Phoebe Putney Memorial Hospital, Albany	6.3	0.0%	1.31	No	0.00	3	0.92	0.041
	Piedmont Hospital, Atlanta	6.8	0.0%	1.21	No	0.01	4	1.02	0.073
	South Fulton Medical Center, Eastpoint	8.5	0.0%	1.00	No	0.00	4	0.80	0.023
	South Georgia Medical Center, Valdosta	5.2	0.0%	1.51	No	0.00	4	0.73	0.024
	St. Francis Hospital, Columbus	4.5	0.0%	1.43	No	0.00	3	0.69	0.098
	St. Joseph's Hospital of Atlanta	9.3	0.0%	1.14	No	0.00	3	1.98	0.066
	St. Joseph's Hospital, Savannah	6.4	0.0%	1.14	No	0.00	3	0.56	0.032
	The Medical Center, Columbus	3.3	0.0%	1.44	No	0.11	3	0.34	0.015

Natl. Rank	Hospital	U.S. News index	Reputational score	Hospital-wide mortality rate	COTH member	Interns and residents to beds	Technology score (of 5)	R.N.'s to beds	Board-certified internists to beds
	University Hospital, Augusta	5.8	0.0%	1.50	No	0.07	3	1.00	0.034
	West Georgia Medical Center, La Grange	4.6	0.0%	1.22	No	0.00	3	0.47	0.034
	West Paces Medical Center, Atlanta	9.0	0.0%	0.90	No	0.00	3	0.64	0.065

UROLOGY

Natl. Rank	Hospital	U.S. News index	Reputational score	Urology mortality rate	COTH member	Interns and residents to beds	Technology score (of 11)	R.N.'s to beds	Board-certified internists to beds	Procedures to beds
	TIER ONE									
21	Emory University Hospital, Atlanta	23.8	4.8%	0.70	Yes	0.71	8	1.28	0.039	2.55
	TIER TWO									
35	Medical College of Georgia Hospital and Clinic, Augusta	19.5	0.0%	0.63	Yes	1.42	10	1.09	0.041	1.33
	TIER THREE									
	Crawford Long Hospital at Emory University, Atlanta	12.1	1.3%	1.13	Yes	0.00	6	1.09	0.208	2.28
	Grady Memorial Hospital, Atlanta	10.8	0.5%	1.25	Yes	0.60	9	0.45	0.142	0.92
	Medical Center of Central Georgia, Macon	9.3	0.0%	1.02	Yes	0.23	3	0.75	0.032	1.55
	Memorial Medical Center, Savannah	9.5	0.0%	1.22	Yes	0.25	9	0.79	0.048	1.23
	St. Joseph's Hospital of Atlanta	10.5	0.7%	1.13	No	0.00	7	1.98	0.066	1.97
	St. Joseph's Hospital, Savannah	9.2	0.0%	0.76	No	0.00	6	0.56	0.032	1.24
	West Paces Medical Center, Atlanta	9.9	0.0%	0.35	No	0.00	5	0.64	0.065	1.43
	TIER FOUR									
	Athens Regional Medical Center, Athens	4.1	0.0%	1.71	No	0.00	9	0.72	0.020	2.85
	De Kalb Medical Center, Decatur	7.8	0.0%	1.06	No	0.00	8	0.90	0.082	1.97
	Floyd Medical Center, Rome	3.4	0.0%	1.99	No	0.15	5	1.05	0.033	1.67
	Georgia Baptist Medical Center, Atlanta	7.7	0.0%	1.46	Yes	0.25	6	0.58	0.408	1.27
	Gwinnett Hospital System, Lawrenceville	5.8	0.0%	1.33	No	0.00	7	1.05	0.033	1.90
	Hamilton Medical Center, Dalton	5.9	0.0%	1.09	No	0.00	7	0.53	0.030	1.87
	John D. Archbold Memorial Hospital, Thomasville	6.5	0.0%	1.22	No	0.00	11	0.60	0.031	2.69
	Kennestone Hospital, Marietta	5.8	0.0%	1.68	No	0.00	11	1.22	0.032	1.72
	Northeast Georgia Medical Center, Gainesville	1.8	0.0%	2.11	No	0.00	6	0.67	0.021	1.52
	Northside Hospital, Atlanta	8.2	0.0%	1.17	No	0.00	7	1.35	0.263	1.46
	Phoebe Putney Memorial Hospital, Albany	3.5	0.0%	1.83	No	0.00	7	0.92	0.041	1.53
	Piedmont Hospital, Atlanta	5.5	0.0%	1.52	No	0.01	8	1.02	0.073	2.17
	South Fulton Medical Center, Eastpoint	5.1	0.0%	1.36	No	0.00	8	0.80	0.023	1.87
	South Georgia Medical Center, Valdosta	3.8	0.0%	1.68	No	0.00	8	0.73	0.024	2.11
	St. Francis Hospital, Columbus	6.8	0.0%	1.05	No	0.00	5	0.69	0.098	2.51
	The Medical Center, Columbus	3.1	0.0%	1.49	No	0.11	7	0.34	0.015	0.66
	University Hospital, Augusta	3.9	0.0%	1.62	No	0.07	5	1.00	0.034	1.27
	West Georgia Medical Center, La Grange	2.5	0.0%	1.83	No	0.00	8	0.47	0.034	1.35

AIDS

Natl. Rank	Hospital	U.S. News index	Reputa-tional score	Hospital-wide mortality rate	COTH member	Interns and residents to beds	Tech-nology score (of 11)	Discharge planning (of 2)	R.N.'s to beds	Board-certified internists to beds
	TIER THREE									
	Kapiolani Medical Center at Pali Momi, Aiea, Hawaii	21.5	0.0%	1.07	No	0.00	5	2	1.99	0.293
	St. Raub Clinic and Hospital, Honolulu	20.4	0.0%	0.92	No	0.03	5	2	0.32	0.091
	TIER FOUR									
	Kaiser Foundation Hospital, Honolulu	17.2	0.0%	1.40	No	0.28	7	2	1.12	0.171
	Kuakini Medical Center, Honolulu	18.1	0.0%	1.29	No	0.13	7	2	1.33	0.117
	Queen's Medical Center, Honolulu	19.1	0.0%	1.40	Yes	0.13	9	2	1.02	0.177
	St. Francis Medical Center, Honolulu	18.8	0.0%	1.37	No	0.11	6	2	1.12	0.659

CANCER

Natl. Rank	Hospital	U.S. News index	Reputa-tional score	Cancer mortality rate	COTH member	Interns and residents to beds	Tech-nology score (of 12)	R.N.'s to beds	Board-certified oncologists to beds	Procedures to beds
	TIER THREE									
	Kuakini Medical Center, Honolulu	5.3	0.0%	1.51	No	0.13	8	1.33	0.015	2.19
	Queen's Medical Center, Honolulu	7.5	0.0%	1.10	Yes	0.13	9	1.02	0.019	2.20
	TIER FOUR									
	Kaiser Foundation Hospital, Honolulu	4.9	0.0%	1.10	No	0.28	5	1.12	0.007	3.97
	St. Francis Medical Center, Honolulu	4.5	0.0%	1.22	No	0.11	7	1.12	0.022	1.42
	St. Raub Clinic and Hospital, Honolulu	2.0	0.0%	0.83	No	0.03	4	0.32	0.014	3.87

CARDIOLOGY

Natl. Rank	Hospital	U.S. News index	Reputa-tional score	Cardiology mortality rate	COTH member	Interns and residents to beds	Tech-nology score (of 10)	R.N.'s to beds	Board-certified cardiologists to beds	Procedures to beds
	TIER FOUR									
	Kaiser Foundation Hospital, Honolulu	9.8	0.0%	1.30	No	0.28	6	1.12	0.015	11.06
	Kuakini Medical Center, Honolulu	12.3	0.0%	1.23	No	0.13	9	1.33	0.046	8.33
	Queen's Medical Center, Honolulu	12.9	0.0%	1.30	Yes	0.13	9	1.02	0.045	6.12
	St. Francis Medical Center, Honolulu	7.7	0.0%	1.53	No	0.11	8	1.12	0.102	6.63
	St. Raub Clinic and Hospital, Honolulu	12.2	0.0%	1.02	No	0.03	7	0.32	0.028	8.73

ENDOCRINOLOGY

Natl. Rank	Hospital	U.S. News index	Reputa-tional score	Endocrinology mortality rate	COTH member	Interns and residents to beds	Tech-nology score (of 11)	R.N.'s to beds	Board-certified internists to beds
	TIER THREE								
	Queen's Medical Center, Honolulu	9.4	0.0%	1.37	Yes	0.13	9	1.02	0.177
	St. Francis Medical Center, Honolulu	8.9	0.0%	1.93	No	0.11	8	1.12	0.659
	St. Raub Clinic and Hospital, Honolulu	8.6	0.0%	0.49	No	0.03	5	0.32	0.091
	TIER FOUR								
	Kaiser Foundation Hospital, Honolulu	7.0	0.0%	1.37	No	0.28	6	1.12	0.171
	Kuakini Medical Center, Honolulu	6.7	0.0%	1.57	No	0.13	9	1.33	0.117

GASTROENTEROLOGY

Natl. Rank	Hospital	U.S. News index	Reputational score	Gastroenterology mortality rate	COTH member	Interns and residents to beds	Technology score (of 11)	R.N.'s to beds	Board-certified gastroenterologists to beds	Procedures to beds
	TIER THREE									
	Kuakini Medical Center, Honolulu	**9.2**	0.0%	1.03	No	0.13	8	1.33	0.036	5.11
	Queen's Medical Center, Honolulu	**8.4**	0.0%	1.24	Yes	0.13	8	1.02	0.027	2.38
	TIER FOUR									
	Kaiser Foundation Hospital, Honolulu	**6.9**	0.0%	1.24	No	0.28	6	1.12	0.011	4.30
	St. Francis Medical Center, Honolulu	**5.3**	0.0%	1.44	No	0.11	7	1.12	0.031	3.24
	St. Raub Clinic and Hospital, Honolulu	**6.7**	0.0%	0.83	No	0.03	4	0.32	0.021	4.71

GERIATRICS

Natl. Rank	Hospital	U.S. News index	Reputational score	Hospital-wide mortality rate	COTH member	Service mix	Interns and residents to beds	Technology score (of 13)	R.N.'s to beds	Discharge planning (of 2)	Geriatric services (of 9)	Board-certified internists to beds
	TIER THREE											
	St. Raub Clinic and Hospital, Honolulu	**16.1**	0.0%	0.92	No	5	0.03	7	0.32	2	4	0.091
	TIER FOUR											
	Kaiser Foundation Hospital, Honolulu	**9.7**	0.0%	1.40	No	8	0.28	7	1.12	2	5	0.171
	Kuakini Medical Center, Honolulu	**11.1**	0.8%	1.29	No	3	0.13	11	1.33	2	1	0.117
	Queen's Medical Center, Honolulu	**10.7**	0.0%	1.40	Yes	5	0.13	12	1.02	2	4	0.177
	St. Francis Medical Center, Honolulu	**11.4**	0.0%	1.37	No	6	0.11	9	1.12	2	3	0.659

GYNECOLOGY

Natl. Rank	Hospital	U.S. News index	Reputational score	Hospital-wide mortality rate	Interns and residents to beds	Technology score (of 10)	R.N.'s to beds	Board-certified OB-GYNs to beds	Procedures to beds
	TIER FOUR								
	Kaiser Foundation Hospital, Honolulu	**9.4**	0.0%	1.40	0.28	6	1.12	0.056	0.79
	Kuakini Medical Center, Honolulu	**11.5**	0.0%	1.29	0.13	7	1.33	0.031	0.10
	Queen's Medical Center, Honolulu	**9.4**	0.0%	1.40	0.13	7	1.02	0.072	0.44
	St. Francis Medical Center, Honolulu	**8.7**	0.0%	1.37	0.11	6	1.12	0.040	0.07
	St. Raub Clinic and Hospital, Honolulu	**12.3**	0.0%	0.92	0.03	3	0.32	0.035	0.46

NEUROLOGY

Natl. Rank	Hospital	U.S. News index	Reputational score	Neurology mortality rate	COTH member	Interns and residents to beds	Technology score (of 9)	R.N.'s to beds	Board-certified neurologists to beds
	TIER THREE								
	St. Raub Clinic and Hospital, Honolulu	**12.5**	0.0%	0.79	No	0.03	3	0.32	0.028
	TIER FOUR								
	Kaiser Foundation Hospital, Honolulu	**5.3**	0.0%	1.47	No	0.28	5	1.12	0.007
	Kuakini Medical Center, Honolulu	**7.8**	0.0%	1.28	No	0.13	7	1.33	0.010
	Queen's Medical Center, Honolulu	**7.5**	0.0%	1.47	Yes	0.13	7	1.02	0.008
	St. Francis Medical Center, Honolulu	**10.8**	0.0%	1.08	No	0.11	6	1.12	0.035

STATE RANKINGS ■ HAWAII

ORTHOPEDICS

Natl. Rank	Hospital	U.S. News index	Reputa-tional score	Orthopedics mortality rate	COTH member	Interns and residents to beds	Tech-nology score (of 5)	R.N.'s to beds	Board-certified orthopedists to beds	Pro-cedures to beds
	TIER FOUR									
	Kaiser Foundation Hospital, Honolulu	5.7	0.0%	1.64	No	0.28	4	1.12	0.026	3.87
	Kuakini Medical Center, Honolulu	6.1	0.0%	1.52	No	0.13	4	1.33	0.051	3.06
	Queen's Medical Center, Honolulu	7.4	0.0%	1.64	Yes	0.13	4	1.02	0.051	2.14
	St. Raub Clinic and Hospital, Honolulu	3.9	0.0%	1.04	No	0.03	2	0.32	0.028	2.97

OTOLARYNGOLOGY

Natl. Rank	Hospital	U.S. News index	Reputa-tional score	Hospital-wide mortality rate	COTH member	Interns and residents to beds	Tech-nology score (of 9)	R.N.'s to beds	Board-certified internists to beds	Procedures to beds
	TIER THREE									
	Kapiolani Medical Center at Pali Momi, Aiea, Hawaii	9.5	0.0%	1.07	No	0.00	3	1.99	0.293	0.480
	Kuakini Medical Center, Honolulu	7.4	0.0%	1.28	No	0.13	7	1.33	0.117	0.357
	Queen's Medical Center, Honolulu	10.1	0.0%	1.40	Yes	0.13	7	1.02	0.177	0.218
	St. Francis Medical Center, Honolulu	11.0	0.0%	1.37	No	0.11	6	1.12	0.659	0.186
	TIER FOUR									
	Kaiser Foundation Hospital, Honolulu	6.9	0.0%	1.40	No	0.28	4	1.12	0.171	0.394
	St. Raub Clinic and Hospital, Honolulu	2.9	0.0%	0.92	No	0.03	3	0.32	0.091	0.357

RHEUMATOLOGY

Natl. Rank	Hospital	U.S. News index	Reputa-tional score	Hospital-wide mortality rate	COTH member	Interns and residents to beds	Tech-nology score (of 5)	R.N.'s to beds	Board-certified internists to beds
	TIER THREE								
	Queen's Medical Center, Honolulu	10.5	0.0%	1.40	Yes	0.13	4	1.02	0.177
	St. Francis Medical Center, Honolulu	11.9	0.0%	1.37	No	0.11	4	1.12	0.659
	TIER FOUR								
	Kaiser Foundation Hospital, Honolulu	8.7	0.0%	1.40	No	0.28	4	1.12	0.171
	Kuakini Medical Center, Honolulu	8.9	0.0%	1.28	No	0.13	4	1.33	0.117
	St. Raub Clinic and Hospital, Honolulu	7.7	0.0%	0.92	No	0.03	2	0.32	0.091

UROLOGY

Natl. Rank	Hospital	U.S. News index	Reputa-tional score	Urology mortality rate	COTH member	Interns and residents to beds	Tech-nology score (of 11)	R.N.'s to beds	Board-certified internists to beds	Procedures to beds
	TIER THREE									
	Kaiser Foundation Hospital, Honolulu	9.0	0.0%	1.11	No	0.28	6	1.12	0.171	2.70
	Kuakini Medical Center, Honolulu	10.3	0.0%	0.96	No	0.13	8	1.33	0.117	1.62
	Queen's Medical Center, Honolulu	11.0	0.0%	1.11	Yes	0.13	8	1.02	0.177	1.50
	TIER FOUR									
	St. Francis Medical Center, Honolulu	7.7	0.0%	1.26	No	0.11	7	1.12	0.659	2.50
	St. Raub Clinic and Hospital, Honolulu	3.8	0.0%	1.35	No	0.03	4	0.32	0.091	3.04

AIDS

Natl. Rank	Hospital	U.S. News index	Reputational score	Hospital-wide mortality rate	COTH member	Interns and residents to beds	Technology score (of 11)	Discharge planning (of 2)	R.N.'s to beds	Board-certified internists to beds
	TIER THREE									
	St. Luke's Regional Medical Center, Boise	20.0	0.0%	1.17	No	0.02	8	2	1.87	0.034
	TIER FOUR									
	Bannock Regional Medical Center, Pocatello	17.0	0.0%	1.17	No	0.00	7	2	0.25	0.029
	Kootenai Medical Center, Coeur d'Alene	18.6	0.0%	1.06	No	0.00	5	2	0.82	0.037
	Magic Valley Regional Medical Center, Twin Falls	16.6	0.0%	1.29	No	0.00	7	2	0.80	0.044
	St. Alphonsus Regional Medical Center, Boise	16.9	0.0%	1.26	No	0.04	6	2	1.03	0.027
	St. Joseph Regional Medical Center, Lewiston	16.2	0.0%	1.34	No	0.00	7	2	0.80	0.056

CANCER

Natl. Rank	Hospital	U.S. News index	Reputational score	Cancer mortality rate	COTH member	Interns and residents to beds	Technology score (of 12)	R.N.'s to beds	Board-certified oncologists to beds	Procedures to beds
	TIER THREE									
	St. Luke's Regional Medical Center, Boise	7.4	0.0%	1.30	No	0.02	10	1.87	0.026	3.10
	TIER FOUR									
	Eastern Idaho Regional Medical Center Falls	4.2	0.0%	0.63	No	0.00	5	1.15	0.004	1.04
	Kootenai Medical Center, Coeur d'Alene	3.4	0.0%	1.13	No	0.00	6	0.82	0.011	3.62
	St. Alphonsus Regional Medical Center, Boise	3.9	0.0%	0.56	No	0.04	5	1.03	0.004	0.91
	St. Joseph Regional Medical Center, Lewiston	3.8	0.0%	1.30	No	0.00	8	0.80	0.024	3.22

CARDIOLOGY

Natl. Rank	Hospital	U.S. News index	Reputational score	Cardiology mortality rate	COTH member	Interns and residents to beds	Technology score (of 10)	R.N.'s to beds	Board-certified cardiologists to beds	Procedures to beds
	TIER THREE									
	Eastern Idaho Regional Medical Center Falls	13.8	0.0%	1.03	No	0.00	8	1.15	0.011	4.30
	St. Luke's Regional Medical Center, Boise	14.7	0.0%	1.16	No	0.02	9	1.87	0.045	11.42
	TIER FOUR									
	Kootenai Medical Center, Coeur d'Alene	8.7	0.0%	1.24	No	0.00	6	0.82	0.016	7.14
	Magic Valley Regional Medical Center, Twin Falls	9.9	0.0%	1.12	No	0.00	4	0.80	0.007	6.09
	St. Alphonsus Regional Medical Center, Boise	9.7	0.0%	1.26	No	0.04	7	1.03	0.046	4.69
	St. Joseph Regional Medical Center, Lewiston	8.8	0.0%	1.20	No	0.00	5	0.80	0.008	7.02

ENDOCRINOLOGY

Natl. Rank	Hospital	U.S. News index	Reputational score	Endocrinology mortality rate	COTH member	Interns and residents to beds	Technology score (of 11)	R.N.'s to beds	Board-certified internists to beds
	TIER THREE								
	Kootenai Medical Center, Coeur d'Alene	9.9	0.0%	0.31	No	0.00	7	0.82	0.037
	St. Alphonsus Regional Medical Center, Boise	10.3	0.0%	0.48	No	0.04	6	1.03	0.027
	St. Luke's Regional Medical Center, Boise	9.6	0.0%	1.04	No	0.02	10	1.87	0.034

GASTROENTEROLOGY

Natl. Rank	Hospital	U.S. News index	Reputational score	Gastroenterology mortality rate	COTH member	Interns and residents to beds	Technology score (of 11)	R.N.'s to beds	Board-certified gastroenterologists to beds	Procedures to beds
	TIER THREE									
	St. Luke's Regional Medical Center, Boise	**8.1**	0.0%	1.33	No	0.02	10	1.87	0.022	3.37
	TIER FOUR									
	Eastern Idaho Regional Medical Center Falls	**6.3**	0.0%	1.04	No	0.00	6	1.15	0.004	2.88
	Kootenai Medical Center, Coeur d'Alene	**7.1**	0.0%	0.99	No	0.00	6	0.82	0.011	5.01
	Magic Valley Regional Medical Center, Twin Falls	**4.6**	0.0%	1.34	No	0.00	7	0.80	0.000	3.64
	St. Alphonsus Regional Medical Center, Boise	**5.5**	0.0%	1.18	No	0.04	6	1.03	0.015	3.18
	St. Joseph Regional Medical Center, Lewiston	**5.7**	0.0%	1.51	No	0.00	8	0.80	0.024	5.90

GERIATRICS

Natl. Rank	Hospital	U.S. News index	Reputational score	Hospital-wide mortality rate	COTH member	Service mix	Interns and residents to beds	Technology score (of 13)	R.N.'s to beds	Discharge planning (of 2)	Geriatric services (of 9)	Board-certified internists to beds
	TIER FOUR											
	Kootenai Medical Center, Coeur d'Alene	**12.2**	0.0%	1.06	No	4	0.00	9	0.82	2	2	0.037
	St. Alphonsus Regional Medical Center, Boise	**9.6**	0.0%	1.26	No	6	0.04	7	1.03	2	5	0.027
	St. Joseph Regional Medical Center, Lewiston	**7.5**	0.0%	1.34	No	6	0.00	9	0.80	2	2	0.056
	St. Luke's Regional Medical Center, Boise	**13.4**	0.0%	1.17	No	5	0.02	11	1.87	2	5	0.034

GYNECOLOGY

Natl. Rank	Hospital	U.S. News index	Reputational score	Hospital-wide mortality rate	Interns and residents to beds	Technology score (of 10)	R.N.'s to beds	Board-certified OB-GYNs to beds	Procedures to beds
	TIER THREE								
	Eastern Idaho Regional Medical Center Falls	**14.7**	0.0%	1.06	0.00	7	1.15	0.026	0.37
	St. Luke's Regional Medical Center, Boise	**18.1**	0.0%	1.17	0.02	9	1.87	0.079	0.96
	TIER FOUR								
	Kootenai Medical Center, Coeur d'Alene	**11.8**	0.0%	1.06	0.00	5	0.82	0.027	0.74
	St. Alphonsus Regional Medical Center, Boise	**8.6**	0.0%	1.26	0.04	5	1.03	0.019	0.33
	St. Joseph Regional Medical Center, Lewiston	**7.8**	0.0%	1.34	0.00	7	0.80	0.032	0.64

NEUROLOGY

Natl. Rank	Hospital	U.S. News index	Reputational score	Neurology mortality rate	COTH member	Interns and residents to beds	Technology score (of 9)	R.N.'s to beds	Board-certified neurologists to beds
	TIER THREE								
	Eastern Idaho Regional Medical Center Falls	**11.3**	0.0%	0.91	No	0.00	6	1.15	0.004
	St. Luke's Regional Medical Center, Boise	**13.2**	0.0%	1.00	No	0.02	8	1.87	0.019
	TIER FOUR								
	Kootenai Medical Center, Coeur d'Alene	**10.7**	0.0%	0.90	No	0.00	5	0.82	0.011
	St. Alphonsus Regional Medical Center, Boise	**9.3**	0.0%	1.15	No	0.04	5	1.03	0.038
	St. Joseph Regional Medical Center, Lewiston	**7.2**	0.0%	1.25	No	0.00	7	0.80	0.024

ORTHOPEDICS

Natl. Rank	Hospital	U.S. News index	Reputa-tional score	Orthopedics mortality rate	COTH member	Interns and residents to beds	Tech-nology score (of 5)	R.N.'s to beds	Board-certified orthopedists to beds	Pro-cedures to beds
TIER THREE										
	Eastern Idaho Regional Medical Center Falls	8.8	0.0%	0.84	No	0.00	4	1.15	0.022	2.46
	St. Alphonsus Regional Medical Center, Boise	8.8	0.0%	0.94	No	0.04	4	1.03	0.073	6.17
	St. Luke's Regional Medical Center, Boise	8.3	0.0%	1.26	No	0.02	4	1.87	0.045	3.70
TIER FOUR										
	Kootenai Medical Center, Coeur d'Alene	7.1	0.0%	0.90	No	0.00	3	0.82	0.021	4.16
	Magic Valley Regional Medical Center, Twin Falls	3.2	0.0%	1.73	No	0.00	3	0.80	0.015	4.79
	St. Joseph Regional Medical Center, Lewiston	6.8	0.0%	1.03	No	0.00	4	0.80	0.048	4.28

OTOLARYNGOLOGY

Natl. Rank	Hospital	U.S. News index	Reputa-tional score	Hospital-wide mortality rate	COTH member	Interns and residents to beds	Tech-nology score (of 9)	R.N.'s to beds	Board-certified internists to beds	Procedures to beds
TIER THREE										
	St. Luke's Regional Medical Center, Boise	8.3	0.0%	1.17	No	0.02	8	1.87	0.034	0.191
TIER FOUR										
	Bannock Regional Medical Center, Pocatello	2.6	0.0%	1.17	No	0.00	6	0.25	0.029	0.058
	Eastern Idaho Regional Medical Center Falls	4.8	0.0%	1.06	No	0.00	4	1.15	0.011	0.160
	Kootenai Medical Center, Coeur d'Alene	4.3	0.0%	1.06	No	0.00	5	0.82	0.037	0.321
	Magic Valley Regional Medical Center, Twin Falls	5.7	0.4%	1.29	No	0.00	6	0.80	0.044	0.368
	St. Alphonsus Regional Medical Center, Boise	4.6	0.0%	1.26	No	0.04	4	1.03	0.027	0.207
	St. Joseph Regional Medical Center, Lewiston	4.8	0.0%	1.34	No	0.00	7	0.80	0.056	0.468

RHEUMATOLOGY

Natl. Rank	Hospital	U.S. News index	Reputa-tional score	Hospital-wide mortality rate	COTH member	Interns and residents to beds	Tech-nology score (of 5)	R.N.'s to beds	Board-certified internists to beds
TIER THREE									
	St. Luke's Regional Medical Center, Boise	10.1	0.0%	1.17	No	0.02	4	1.87	0.034
TIER FOUR									
	Eastern Idaho Regional Medical Center Falls	7.8	0.0%	1.06	No	0.00	4	1.15	0.011
	Kootenai Medical Center, Coeur d'Alene	7.7	0.0%	1.06	No	0.00	3	0.82	0.037
	St. Alphonsus Regional Medical Center, Boise	7.3	0.0%	1.26	No	0.04	4	1.03	0.027
	St. Joseph Regional Medical Center, Lewiston	6.4	0.0%	1.34	No	0.00	4	0.80	0.056

UROLOGY

Natl. Rank	Hospital	U.S. News index	Reputa-tional score	Urology mortality rate	COTH member	Interns and residents to beds	Tech-nology score (of 11)	R.N.'s to beds	Board-certified internists to beds	Procedures to beds
TIER THREE										
	St. Alphonsus Regional Medical Center, Boise	11.3	0.0%	0.71	No	0.04	6	1.03	0.027	2.14
TIER FOUR										
	Eastern Idaho Regional Medical Center Falls	4.9	0.0%	1.50	No	0.00	6	1.15	0.011	2.13
	Kootenai Medical Center, Coeur d'Alene	5.5	0.0%	1.27	No	0.00	6	0.82	0.037	2.54
	St. Joseph Regional Medical Center, Lewiston	2.2	0.0%	2.69	No	0.00	8	0.80	0.056	2.42
	St. Luke's Regional Medical Center, Boise	8.1	0.0%	1.44	No	0.02	10	1.87	0.034	1.59

AIDS

Natl. Rank	Hospital	U.S. News index	Reputational score	Hospital-wide mortality rate	COTH member	Interns and residents to beds	Technology score (of 11)	Discharge planning (of 2)	R.N.'s to beds	Board-certified internists to beds
	TIER ONE									
17	Northwestern Memorial Hospital, Chicago	32.7	6.4%	0.99	Yes	0.43	9	2	1.03	0.134
18	Rush-Presbyterian-St. Luke's Medical Center, Chicago	32.3	2.9%	0.81	Yes	1.05	10	2	1.24	0.224
	TIER TWO									
29	Cook County Hospital, Chicago	29.5	1.3%	0.55	Yes	1.00	9	2	1.43	0.073
77	Evanston Hospital, Evanston	25.6	0.0%	0.79	Yes	0.26	7	2	1.18	0.160
87	F.G. McGaw Hospital at Loyola University, Maywood	25.1	0.0%	1.12	Yes	1.46	9	2	1.59	0.053
81	St. John's Hospital, Springfield	25.4	0.4%	0.90	Yes	0.22	8	2	0.76	0.123
30	University of Chicago Hospitals	29.5	0.2%	0.80	Yes	1.64	9	2	1.38	0.074
32	University of Illinois Hospital and Clinics, Chicago	29.3	0.0%	0.83	Yes	1.29	9	2	1.95	0.056
	TIER THREE									
	Alexian Brothers Medical Center, Elk Grove Village	23.0	0.0%	0.82	No	0.00	7	2	0.96	0.118
	Columbus Hospital, Chicago	22.1	0.0%	0.97	No	0.40	7	2	0.82	0.144
	Edgewater Medical Center, Chicago	20.6	0.0%	0.81	No	0.26	4	1	0.42	0.064
	Elmhurst Memorial Hospital, Elmhurst	20.9	0.0%	1.00	No	0.00	7	2	1.01	0.111
	Good Samaritan Hospital, Downers Grove	21.3	0.0%	0.88	No	0.00	6	1	0.66	0.089
	Gottlieb Memorial Hospital, Melrose Park	21.0	0.0%	0.94	No	0.01	6	2	0.64	0.099
	Grant Hospital of Chicago	21.3	0.0%	0.71	No	0.24	5	1	0.63	0.090
	Hinsdale Hospital, Hinsdale	21.8	0.0%	0.92	No	0.12	7	2	0.69	0.062
	Holy Family Hospital, Des Plaines	21.8	0.0%	0.91	No	0.01	5	2	1.14	0.055
	Illinois Masonic Medical Center, Chicago	22.7	0.0%	1.00	Yes	0.43	9	1	0.73	0.068
	Ingalls Memorial Hospital, Harvey	20.6	0.0%	0.93	No	0.00	6	2	0.42	0.066
	La Grange Memorial Health System, La Grange	20.3	0.0%	0.96	No	0.12	5	2	0.60	0.065
	Louis A. Weiss Memorial Hospital, Chicago	23.6	0.0%	0.87	No	0.37	7	2	0.63	0.227
	Lutheran General Healthsystem, Park Ridge	23.0	0.0%	0.99	Yes	0.42	7	2	0.82	0.076
	MacNeal Hospital, Berwyn	21.8	0.0%	0.95	Yes	0.28	4	1	1.05	0.052
	Memorial Medical Center, Springfield	22.2	0.4%	1.05	Yes	0.28	6	2	0.89	0.115
	Mercy Hospital and Medical Center, Chicago	22.3	0.0%	1.03	Yes	0.38	7	2	0.90	0.035
	Michael Reese Hospital and Medical Center, Chicago	23.1	0.0%	0.90	Yes	0.36	3	1	1.28	0.064
	Northwest Community Hospital, Arlington Heights	21.5	0.0%	0.94	No	0.00	7	2	0.72	0.113
	Oak Park Hospital, Oak Park	20.7	0.0%	0.89	No	0.00	6	1	0.44	0.067
	Rush North Shore Medical Center, Skokie	20.8	0.0%	1.01	No	0.22	4	2	0.93	0.296
	St. Anthony Medical Center, Rockford	20.7	0.0%	1.02	No	0.04	6	2	1.48	0.038
	St. Anthony's Health Center, Alton	21.7	0.0%	0.90	No	0.00	7	1	0.85	0.092
	St. Elizabeth Medical Center, Granite City	19.7	0.0%	0.98	No	0.00	6	2	0.52	0.012
	St. Elizabeth's Hospital, Belleville	20.9	0.0%	0.82	No	0.04	6	1	0.53	0.023
	St. Francis Hospital, Evanston	20.1	0.0%	0.99	No	0.36	7	1	0.57	0.071
	St. Francis Medical Center, Peoria	20.5	0.0%	1.05	No	0.29	8	2	0.90	0.036
	St. James Hospital and Health Center, Chicago Heights	20.8	0.0%	0.83	No	0.00	5	1	0.45	0.136
	St. Joseph Hospital and Health Care Center, Chicago	20.6	0.0%	1.04	No	0.32	8	2	0.66	0.071
	Swedish American Hospital, Rockford	20.7	0.0%	0.98	No	0.03	7	2	0.65	0.090
	Swedish Covenant Hospital, Chicago	20.1	0.0%	1.01	No	0.14	6	2	0.72	0.070
	West Suburban Hospital Medical Center, Oak Park	20.8	0.0%	0.98	No	0.28	6	2	0.82	0.051
	TIER FOUR									
	Blessing Hospital, Quincy	17.5	0.0%	1.16	No	0.04	5	2	0.84	0.043
	Carle Foundation Hospital, Urbana	17.2	0.0%	1.11	No	0.05	4	2	0.53	0.043
	Central Du Page Hospital, Winfield	18.6	0.0%	1.07	No	0.00	5	2	0.81	0.077
	Christ Hospital and Medical Center, Oak Lawn	17.5	0.0%	1.22	No	0.33	7	2	0.52	0.040
	Copley Memorial Hospital, Aurora	16.9	0.0%	1.23	No	0.00	6	2	0.68	0.104
	Covenant Medical Center, Urbana	18.1	0.0%	1.17	No	0.04	7	2	0.79	0.054
	Decatur Memorial Hospital, Decatur	19.3	0.0%	1.04	No	0.03	7	2	0.48	0.077
	Little Company of Mary Hospital, Evergreen Park	19.3	0.0%	1.09	No	0.03	7	2	1.01	0.029

Natl. Rank	Hospital	U.S. News index	Reputa- tional score	Hospital- wide mortality rate	COTH member	Interns and residents to beds	Tech- nology score (of 11)	Discharge planning (of 2)	R.N.'s to beds	Board- certified internists to beds
	Memorial Hospital of Carbondale, Carbondale	17.8	0.0%	1.15	No	0.16	6	1	1.07	0.040
	Mercy Center for Health Care Services, Aurora	17.2	0.0%	1.14	No	0.00	4	2	0.56	0.149
	Methodist Medical Center of Illinois, Peoria	16.6	0.0%	1.48	No	0.06	8	2	1.36	0.102
	Mount Sinai Hospital Medical Center, Chicago	18.5	0.0%	1.26	Yes	0.54	5	2	0.72	0.000
	Oak Forest Hospital of Cook County, Oak Forest	8.9	0.0%	2.35	No	0.00	4	2	0.25	0.036
	Ravenswood Hospital Medical Center, Chicago	19.5	0.0%	1.07	No	0.30	5	2	0.98	0.063
	Resurrection Medical Center, Chicago	17.9	0.0%	1.07	No	0.08	5	2	0.38	0.029
	Riverside Medical Center, Kankakee	14.0	0.0%	1.52	No	0.00	6	2	0.62	0.024
	Rockford Memorial Hospital, Rockford	18.0	0.0%	1.22	No	0.01	9	2	0.80	0.025
	Sherman Hospital, Elgin	19.5	0.0%	1.02	No	0.00	6	1	0.95	0.123
	St. Joseph Medical Center, Bloomington	18.0	0.0%	1.04	No	0.00	5	1	0.73	0.032
	St. Joseph Medical Center, Joliet	17.5	0.0%	1.23	No	0.00	7	2	1.06	0.028
	St. Mary Hospital, Quincy	18.2	0.0%	1.08	No	0.09	5	1	0.93	0.104
	St. Mary of Nazareth Hospital Center, Chicago	17.4	0.0%	1.24	No	0.17	6	2	1.08	0.007
	St. Mary's Hospital of Kankakee, Kankakee	16.6	0.0%	1.26	No	0.00	7	2	0.60	0.052
	St. Mary's Hospital, Decatur	17.2	0.0%	1.10	No	0.01	6	1	0.52	0.030
	Trinity Medical Center, Moline	16.0	0.0%	1.35	No	0.00	7	2	0.80	0.032

CANCER

Natl. Rank	Hospital	U.S. News index	Reputa- tional score	Cancer mortality rate	COTH member	Interns and residents to beds	Tech- nology score (of 12)	R.N.'s to beds	Board- certified oncologists to beds	Procedures to beds
TIER ONE										
9	University of Chicago Hospitals	25.1	8.1%	0.59	Yes	1.64	11	1.38	0.034	2.76
TIER TWO										
71	Cook County Hospital, Chicago	11.5	0.0%	0.30	Yes	1.00	8	1.43	0.009	0.47
28	F.G. McGaw Hospital at Loyola University, Maywood	15.1	0.4%	0.66	Yes	1.46	11	1.59	0.030	1.59
58	Rush-Presbyterian-St. Luke's Medical Center, Chicago	12.4	0.4%	0.64	Yes	1.05	10	1.24	0.000	1.64
34	University of Illinois Hospital and Clinics, Chicago	14.2	0.0%	0.65	Yes	1.29	9	1.95	0.015	0.65
TIER THREE										
	Columbus Hospital, Chicago	5.8	0.0%	0.63	No	0.40	9	0.82	0.000	1.58
	Evanston Hospital, Evanston	8.8	0.0%	0.79	Yes	0.26	9	1.18	0.018	2.11
	Illinois Masonic Medical Center, Chicago	7.5	0.0%	0.73	Yes	0.43	8	0.73	0.016	0.49
	Lutheran General Healthsystem, Park Ridge	8.1	0.0%	1.05	Yes	0.42	10	0.82	0.013	1.46
	MacNeal Hospital, Berwyn	6.3	0.0%	0.89	Yes	0.28	3	1.05	0.009	1.08
	Memorial Medical Center, Springfield	6.9	0.0%	1.20	Yes	0.28	7	0.89	0.010	1.96
	Mercy Hospital and Medical Center, Chicago	7.8	0.0%	0.91	Yes	0.38	8	0.90	0.006	1.81
	Methodist Medical Center of Illinois, Peoria	5.6	0.0%	1.34	No	0.06	9	1.36	0.019	2.07
	Michael Reese Hospital and Medical Center, Chicago	7.0	0.0%	0.83	Yes	0.36	2	1.28	0.014	0.84
	Mount Sinai Hospital Medical Center, Chicago	7.1	0.0%	0.97	Yes	0.54	7	0.72	0.000	0.47
	Northwestern Memorial Hospital, Chicago	9.7	1.0%	1.06	Yes	0.43	9	1.03	0.017	1.59
	St. Anthony Medical Center, Rockford	5.8	0.0%	0.67	No	0.04	7	1.48	0.005	1.50
	St. John's Hospital, Springfield	6.9	0.0%	0.82	Yes	0.22	8	0.76	0.010	1.36
TIER FOUR										
	Alexian Brothers Medical Center, Elk Grove Village	4.2	0.0%	0.67	No	0.00	7	0.96	0.013	0.82
	Blessing Hospital, Quincy	3.3	0.0%	1.14	No	0.04	6	0.84	0.005	2.28
	Carle Foundation Hospital, Urbana	1.2	0.0%	1.05	No	0.05	2	0.53	0.007	1.21
	Central Du Page Hospital, Winfield	2.5	0.0%	0.90	No	0.00	4	0.81	0.009	0.99
	Christ Hospital and Medical Center, Oak Lawn	4.1	0.0%	1.04	No	0.33	9	0.52	0.004	1.42
	Copley Memorial Hospital, Aurora	3.1	0.0%	1.19	No	0.00	7	0.68	0.022	2.48
	Covenant Medical Center, Urbana	3.8	0.0%	1.28	No	0.04	9	0.79	0.004	1.85
	Decatur Memorial Hospital, Decatur	3.3	0.4%	0.99	No	0.03	8	0.48	0.009	1.60
	Edgewater Medical Center, Chicago	2.8	0.0%	0.78	No	0.26	5	0.42	0.000	1.32
	Elmhurst Memorial Hospital, Elmhurst	4.3	0.0%	0.93	No	0.00	8	1.01	0.000	1.80
	Good Samaritan Hospital, Downers Grove	2.8	0.0%	0.65	No	0.00	5	0.66	0.006	1.06

STATE RANKINGS ■ ILLINOIS

Natl. Rank	Hospital	U.S. News index	Reputational score	Cancer mortality rate	COTH member	Interns and residents to beds	Technology score (of 12)	R.N.'s to beds	Board-certified oncologists to beds	Procedures to beds
	Gottlieb Memorial Hospital, Melrose Park	2.8	0.0%	0.65	No	0.01	5	0.64	0.012	1.10
	Grant Hospital of Chicago	3.1	0.0%	0.70	No	0.24	4	0.63	0.006	0.74
	Hinsdale Hospital, Hinsdale	3.7	0.0%	1.04	No	0.12	8	0.69	0.021	1.21
	Holy Family Hospital, Des Plaines	4.2	0.0%	0.75	No	0.01	5	1.14	0.033	1.16
	Ingalls Memorial Hospital, Harvey	2.8	0.0%	0.80	No	0.00	8	0.42	0.011	1.53
	La Grange Memorial Health System, La Grange	2.8	0.0%	0.85	No	0.12	5	0.60	0.004	1.94
	Little Company of Mary Hospital, Evergreen Park	4.4	0.0%	0.97	No	0.03	8	1.01	0.012	1.65
	Louis A. Weiss Memorial Hospital, Chicago	4.6	0.0%	0.47	No	0.37	6	0.63	0.034	1.93
	Memorial Hospital, Belleville	2.2	0.0%	0.89	No	0.02	5	0.58	0.002	1.08
	Mercy Center for Health Care Services, Aurora	1.3	0.0%	0.87	No	0.00	2	0.56	0.019	0.82
	Northwest Community Hospital, Arlington Heights	3.6	0.0%	0.93	No	0.00	8	0.72	0.015	1.90
	Oak Park Hospital, Oak Park	2.9	0.0%	0.63	No	0.00	7	0.44	0.010	1.51
	Ravenswood Hospital Medical Center, Chicago	4.4	0.0%	0.97	No	0.30	6	0.98	0.006	0.86
	Resurrection Medical Center, Chicago	2.2	0.0%	0.93	No	0.08	6	0.38	0.009	1.57
	Riverside Medical Center, Kankakee	2.3	0.0%	1.66	No	0.00	7	0.62	0.006	0.95
	Rockford Memorial Hospital, Rockford	3.7	0.0%	1.16	No	0.01	9	0.80	0.009	1.05
	Rush North Shore Medical Center, Skokie	4.4	0.0%	0.72	No	0.22	4	0.93	0.046	2.48
	Sherman Hospital, Elgin	3.2	0.0%	1.07	No	0.00	6	0.95	0.000	0.89
	St. Anthony's Health Center, Alton	3.1	0.0%	1.19	No	0.00	6	0.85	0.005	2.25
	St. Elizabeth Medical Center, Granite City	1.2	0.0%	1.03	No	0.00	3	0.52	0.009	0.76
	St. Elizabeth's Hospital, Belleville	2.6	0.0%	0.63	No	0.04	5	0.53	0.013	1.09
	St. Francis Hospital, Evanston	4.6	0.0%	0.70	No	0.36	8	0.57	0.007	1.61
	St. Francis Medical Center, Peoria	5.2	0.0%	1.16	No	0.29	10	0.90	0.011	1.11
	St. James Hospital and Health Center, Chicago Heights	2.3	0.0%	0.80	No	0.00	6	0.45	0.018	1.04
	St. Joseph Hospital and Health Care Center, Chicago	4.4	0.0%	0.68	No	0.32	7	0.66	0.012	0.95
	St. Joseph Medical Center, Bloomington	3.3	0.0%	0.95	No	0.00	7	0.73	0.013	1.88
	St. Joseph Medical Center, Joliet	4.5	0.0%	1.12	No	0.00	9	1.06	0.013	1.28
	St. Mary Hospital, Quincy	3.2	0.0%	0.98	No	0.09	4	0.93	0.009	1.77
	St. Mary of Nazareth Hospital Center, Chicago	4.6	0.0%	0.92	No	0.17	7	1.08	0.011	0.83
	St. Mary's Hospital of Kankakee, Kankakee	2.8	0.0%	1.24	No	0.00	8	0.60	0.009	1.08
	St. Mary's Hospital, Decatur	2.0	0.0%	1.22	No	0.01	6	0.52	0.008	0.76
	Swedish American Hospital, Rockford	3.5	0.0%	0.88	No	0.03	8	0.65	0.010	1.99
	Swedish Covenant Hospital, Chicago	4.4	0.4%	0.98	No	0.14	7	0.72	0.004	3.02
	Trinity Medical Center, Moline	3.5	0.0%	1.64	No	0.00	9	0.80	0.011	1.25
	West Suburban Hospital Medical Center, Oak Park	4.7	0.0%	0.62	No	0.28	7	0.82	0.005	0.89

CARDIOLOGY

Natl. Rank	Hospital	U.S. News index	Reputational score	Cardiology mortality rate	COTH member	Interns and residents to beds	Technology score (of 10)	R.N.'s to beds	Board-certified cardiologists to beds	Procedures to beds
TIER ONE										
16	University of Chicago Hospitals	29.7	1.0%	0.79	Yes	1.64	10	1.38	0.033	4.24
TIER TWO										
36	Cook County Hospital, Chicago	24.8	0.0%	0.62	Yes	1.00	7	1.43	0.021	2.27
53	Evanston Hospital, Evanston	22.9	0.0%	0.64	Yes	0.26	9	1.18	0.045	7.06
44	F.G. McGaw Hospital at Loyola University, Maywood	23.7	1.9%	1.23	Yes	1.46	9	1.59	0.128	8.23
71	Michael Reese Hospital and Medical Center, Chicago	21.8	0.0%	0.82	Yes	0.36	5	1.28	0.036	2.56
65	Northwestern Memorial Hospital, Chicago	21.9	0.4%	0.94	Yes	0.43	9	1.03	0.061	4.52
34	Rush-Presbyterian-St. Luke's Medical Center, Chicago	25.6	0.8%	0.89	Yes	1.05	9	1.24	0.000	4.51
89	St. John's Hospital, Springfield	21.2	0.0%	0.82	Yes	0.22	8	0.76	0.032	10.21
67	University of Illinois Hospital and Clinics, Chicago	21.9	0.0%	1.09	Yes	1.29	7	1.95	0.022	2.85
TIER THREE										
	Alexian Brothers Medical Center, Elk Grove Village	17.9	0.0%	0.84	No	0.00	8	0.96	0.034	4.84
	Columbus Hospital, Chicago	15.6	0.0%	0.99	No	0.40	6	0.82	0.064	4.53
	Edgewater Medical Center, Chicago	17.0	0.0%	0.83	No	0.26	6	0.42	0.035	9.24

Natl. Rank	Hospital	U.S. News index	Reputa-tional score	Cardiology mortality rate	COTH member	Interns and residents to beds	Tech-nology score (of 10)	R.N.'s to beds	Board-certified cardiologists to beds	Procedures to beds
	Elmhurst Memorial Hospital, Elmhurst	14.5	0.0%	1.00	No	0.00	9	1.01	0.000	8.80
	Good Samaritan Hospital, Downers Grove	16.5	0.0%	0.92	No	0.00	8	0.66	0.101	8.47
	Gottlieb Memorial Hospital, Melrose Park	14.1	0.0%	0.99	No	0.01	8	0.64	0.032	7.62
	Grant Hospital of Chicago	17.5	0.0%	0.78	No	0.24	7	0.63	0.032	5.04
	Hinsdale Hospital, Hinsdale	15.6	0.0%	0.96	No	0.12	9	0.69	0.050	4.25
	Holy Family Hospital, Des Plaines	17.7	0.0%	0.90	No	0.01	6	1.14	0.096	5.68
	Illinois Masonic Medical Center, Chicago	19.1	0.0%	0.98	Yes	0.43	8	0.73	0.068	3.36
	La Grange Memorial Health System, La Grange	16.6	0.0%	0.91	No	0.12	8	0.60	0.040	8.98
	Louis A. Weiss Memorial Hospital, Chicago	17.8	0.0%	0.85	No	0.37	6	0.63	0.034	6.27
	Lutheran General Healthsystem, Park Ridge	15.2	0.0%	1.16	Yes	0.42	8	0.82	0.039	6.14
98	MacNeal Hospital, Berwyn	20.8	0.0%	0.80	Yes	0.28	5	1.05	0.016	7.55
	Memorial Hospital, Belleville	16.8	0.0%	0.59	No	0.02	8	0.58	0.026	6.23
	Memorial Medical Center, Springfield	17.0	0.0%	1.05	Yes	0.28	8	0.89	0.033	7.89
	Mercy Hospital and Medical Center, Chicago	16.7	0.0%	1.07	Yes	0.38	8	0.90	0.021	5.38
	Northwest Community Hospital, Arlington Heights	16.0	0.0%	0.91	No	0.00	8	0.72	0.015	9.20
	Rush North Shore Medical Center, Skokie	16.2	0.0%	0.94	No	0.22	4	0.93	0.071	7.97
	St. Anthony's Health Center, Alton	16.8	0.0%	0.80	No	0.00	6	0.85	0.022	5.90
	St. Elizabeth's Hospital, Belleville	17.0	0.0%	0.73	No	0.04	8	0.53	0.036	7.09
	St. Francis Hospital, Evanston	16.4	0.0%	0.97	No	0.36	9	0.57	0.055	8.25
	St. Francis Medical Center, Peoria	16.2	0.0%	0.97	No	0.29	9	0.90	0.021	6.63
	St. James Hospital and Health Center, Chicago Heights	15.4	0.0%	0.87	No	0.00	5	0.45	0.021	6.82
	St. Joseph Medical Center, Bloomington	13.7	0.0%	1.00	No	0.00	7	0.73	0.032	7.84
	Swedish Covenant Hospital, Chicago	15.9	0.0%	0.90	No	0.14	5	0.72	0.021	6.22
	West Suburban Hospital Medical Center, Oak Park	15.3	0.0%	0.96	No	0.28	7	0.82	0.008	4.33
	TIER FOUR									
	Blessing Hospital, Quincy	7.2	0.0%	1.31	No	0.04	4	0.84	0.010	7.34
	Carle Foundation Hospital, Urbana	9.1	0.0%	1.15	No	0.05	6	0.53	0.007	3.62
	Central Du Page Hospital, Winfield	12.7	0.0%	1.04	No	0.00	8	0.81	0.015	5.15
	Christ Hospital and Medical Center, Oak Lawn	8.6	0.0%	1.30	No	0.33	8	0.52	0.015	7.16
	Copley Memorial Hospital, Aurora	9.1	0.0%	1.24	No	0.00	7	0.68	0.049	5.70
	Covenant Medical Center, Urbana	8.5	0.0%	1.29	No	0.04	8	0.79	0.008	8.54
	Decatur Memorial Hospital, Decatur	7.3	0.0%	1.22	No	0.03	4	0.48	0.014	4.95
	Ingalls Memorial Hospital, Harvey	11.2	0.0%	1.07	No	0.00	8	0.42	0.021	6.57
	Little Company of Mary Hospital, Evergreen Park	12.0	0.0%	1.08	No	0.03	5	1.01	0.027	7.12
	Mercy Center for Health Care Services, Aurora	6.3	0.0%	1.36	No	0.00	6	0.56	0.034	4.13
	Methodist Medical Center of Illinois, Peoria	11.3	0.0%	1.30	No	0.06	9	1.36	0.059	7.41
	Oak Park Hospital, Oak Park	12.5	0.0%	1.00	No	0.00	4	0.44	0.159	6.40
	Ravenswood Hospital Medical Center, Chicago	12.2	0.0%	1.13	No	0.30	7	0.98	0.018	4.21
	Resurrection Medical Center, Chicago	10.3	0.0%	1.04	No	0.08	3	0.38	0.016	5.47
	Riverside Medical Center, Kankakee	10.0	0.0%	1.12	No	0.00	6	0.62	0.015	4.90
	Rockford Memorial Hospital, Rockford	11.8	0.0%	1.10	No	0.01	9	0.80	0.014	5.18
	Sherman Hospital, Elgin	11.6	0.0%	1.14	No	0.00	9	0.95	0.018	6.70
	St. Anthony Medical Center, Rockford	12.1	0.0%	1.23	No	0.04	9	1.48	0.019	12.34
	St. Elizabeth Medical Center, Granite City	7.2	0.0%	1.26	No	0.00	6	0.52	0.009	4.40
	St. Joseph Hospital and Health Care Center, Chicago	11.8	0.0%	1.12	No	0.32	7	0.66	0.032	4.13
	St. Joseph Medical Center, Joliet	13.1	0.0%	1.09	No	0.00	9	1.06	0.026	6.81
	St. Mary of Nazareth Hospital Center, Chicago	12.5	0.0%	1.15	No	0.17	8	1.08	0.039	5.24
	St. Mary's Hospital of Kankakee, Kankakee	8.9	0.0%	1.19	No	0.00	6	0.60	0.022	6.57
	St. Mary's Hospital, Decatur	6.6	0.0%	1.26	No	0.01	4	0.52	0.011	4.24
	Swedish American Hospital, Rockford	10.5	0.0%	1.15	No	0.03	8	0.65	0.021	8.10
	Trinity Medical Center, Moline	10.7	0.0%	1.12	No	0.00	7	0.80	0.011	4.50

ENDOCRINOLOGY

Natl. Rank	Hospital	U.S. News index	Reputa- tional score	Endocrinology mortality rate	COTH member	Interns and residents to beds	Tech- nology score (of 11)	R.N.'s to beds	Board- certified internists to beds
	TIER ONE								
7	University of Chicago Hospitals	35.5	12.5%	0.78	Yes	1.64	11	1.38	0.074
26	University of Illinois Hospital and Clinics, Chicago	20.5	0.4%	0.50	Yes	1.29	8	1.95	0.056
	TIER TWO								
55	Cook County Hospital, Chicago	16.7	0.4%	0.77	Yes	1.00	7	1.43	0.073
76	Evanston Hospital, Evanston	15.1	0.0%	0.70	Yes	0.26	10	1.18	0.160
33	F.G. McGaw Hospital at Loyola University, Maywood	19.9	0.0%	0.67	Yes	1.46	10	1.59	0.053
65	Northwestern Memorial Hospital, Chicago	16.0	0.8%	0.71	Yes	0.43	10	1.03	0.134
41	Rush-Presbyterian-St. Luke's Medical Center, Chicago	18.4	0.0%	0.70	Yes	1.05	10	1.24	0.224
	TIER THREE								
	Alexian Brothers Medical Center, Elk Grove Village	11.1	0.0%	0.48	No	0.00	8	0.96	0.118
	Central Du Page Hospital, Winfield	8.2	0.0%	0.78	No	0.00	5	0.81	0.077
	Columbus Hospital, Chicago	8.2	0.0%	1.11	No	0.40	9	0.82	0.144
	Covenant Medical Center, Urbana	8.3	0.0%	0.85	No	0.04	10	0.79	0.054
	Edgewater Medical Center, Chicago	8.5	0.0%	0.74	No	0.26	6	0.42	0.064
	Good Samaritan Hospital, Downers Grove	8.9	0.0%	0.71	No	0.00	6	0.66	0.089
	Grant Hospital of Chicago	10.4	0.0%	0.41	No	0.24	6	0.63	0.090
	Illinois Masonic Medical Center, Chicago	11.1	0.0%	0.91	Yes	0.43	8	0.73	0.068
	Louis A. Weiss Memorial Hospital, Chicago	11.8	0.0%	0.65	No	0.37	6	0.63	0.227
	Lutheran General Healthsystem, Park Ridge	11.8	0.0%	0.89	Yes	0.42	9	0.82	0.076
	MacNeal Hospital, Berwyn	9.5	0.0%	1.06	Yes	0.28	4	1.05	0.052
	Memorial Hospital, Belleville	9.0	0.0%	0.36	No	0.02	6	0.58	0.022
87	Memorial Medical Center, Springfield	14.2	0.0%	0.66	Yes	0.28	8	0.89	0.115
	Mercy Hospital and Medical Center, Chicago	11.1	0.0%	0.93	Yes	0.38	8	0.90	0.035
91	Michael Reese Hospital and Medical Center, Chicago	14.1	0.0%	0.67	Yes	0.36	3	1.28	0.064
	Rush North Shore Medical Center, Skokie	9.8	0.0%	0.85	No	0.22	4	0.93	0.296
	St. Anthony Medical Center, Rockford	9.2	0.0%	0.88	No	0.04	7	1.48	0.038
	St. Anthony's Health Center, Alton	10.4	0.0%	0.11	No	0.00	7	0.85	0.092
	St. Elizabeth's Hospital, Belleville	9.0	0.0%	0.38	No	0.04	6	0.53	0.023
	St. Francis Hospital, Evanston	10.0	0.0%	0.73	No	0.36	9	0.57	0.071
	St. James Hospital and Health Center, Chicago Heights	9.6	0.0%	0.46	No	0.00	7	0.45	0.136
	St. John's Hospital, Springfield	12.5	0.0%	0.77	Yes	0.22	9	0.76	0.123
	St. Joseph Hospital and Health Care Center, Chicago	11.0	0.0%	0.53	No	0.32	8	0.66	0.071
	TIER FOUR								
	Blessing Hospital, Quincy	5.3	0.0%	1.23	No	0.04	7	0.84	0.043
	Carle Foundation Hospital, Urbana	4.8	0.0%	1.00	No	0.05	2	0.53	0.043
	Christ Hospital and Medical Center, Oak Lawn	5.0	0.0%	1.37	No	0.33	8	0.52	0.040
	Decatur Memorial Hospital, Decatur	5.6	0.0%	1.07	No	0.03	8	0.48	0.077
	Elmhurst Memorial Hospital, Elmhurst	6.6	0.0%	1.22	No	0.00	9	1.01	0.111
	Gottlieb Memorial Hospital, Melrose Park	5.9	0.0%	1.04	No	0.01	6	0.64	0.099
	Hinsdale Hospital, Hinsdale	6.3	0.0%	1.11	No	0.12	9	0.69	0.062
	Holy Family Hospital, Des Plaines	6.0	0.0%	1.22	No	0.01	6	1.14	0.055
	Ingalls Memorial Hospital, Harvey	6.6	0.0%	0.91	No	0.00	9	0.42	0.066
	La Grange Memorial Health System, La Grange	6.0	0.0%	1.03	No	0.12	6	0.60	0.065
	Little Company of Mary Hospital, Evergreen Park	6.4	0.0%	1.12	No	0.03	8	1.01	0.029
	Memorial Hospital of Carbondale, Carbondale	6.7	0.0%	1.20	No	0.16	8	1.07	0.040
	Mercy Center for Health Care Services, Aurora	3.4	0.0%	1.45	No	0.00	2	0.56	0.149
	Methodist Medical Center of Illinois, Peoria	7.1	0.0%	1.40	No	0.06	10	1.36	0.102
	Mount Sinai Hospital Medical Center, Chicago	7.9	0.0%	1.56	Yes	0.54	8	0.72	0.000
	Northwest Community Hospital, Arlington Heights	6.2	0.0%	1.15	No	0.00	9	0.72	0.113
	Oak Park Hospital, Oak Park	4.0	0.0%	1.35	No	0.00	8	0.44	0.067
	Ravenswood Hospital Medical Center, Chicago	7.2	0.0%	1.13	No	0.30	7	0.98	0.063
	Resurrection Medical Center, Chicago	6.6	0.0%	0.85	No	0.08	7	0.38	0.029
	Riverside Medical Center, Kankakee	3.2	0.0%	1.70	No	0.00	8	0.62	0.024

Natl. Rank Hospital	U.S. News index	Reputa- tional score	Endocrinology mortality rate	COTH member	Interns and residents to beds	Tech- nology score (of 11)	R.N.'s to beds	Board- certified internists to beds
Rockford Memorial Hospital, Rockford	6.5	0.0%	1.02	No	0.01	9	0.80	0.025
Sherman Hospital, Elgin	6.5	0.0%	1.11	No	0.00	6	0.95	0.123
St. Elizabeth Medical Center, Granite City	8.1	0.0%	0.41	No	0.00	3	0.52	0.012
St. Francis Medical Center, Peoria	8.0	0.0%	1.03	No	0.29	10	0.90	0.036
St. Joseph Medical Center, Joliet	5.6	0.0%	1.42	No	0.00	10	1.06	0.028
St. Mary of Nazareth Hospital Center, Chicago	3.4	0.0%	2.63	No	0.17	8	1.08	0.007
St. Mary's Hospital of Kankakee, Kankakee	3.5	0.0%	1.69	No	0.00	9	0.60	0.052
St. Mary's Hospital, Decatur	6.6	0.0%	0.84	No	0.01	6	0.52	0.030
Swedish American Hospital, Rockford	6.2	0.0%	1.06	No	0.03	8	0.65	0.090
Swedish Covenant Hospital, Chicago	7.1	0.0%	0.98	No	0.14	8	0.72	0.070
Trinity Medical Center, Moline	5.1	0.0%	1.36	No	0.00	10	0.80	0.032
West Suburban Hospital Medical Center, Oak Park	7.2	0.0%	1.07	No	0.28	8	0.82	0.051

GASTROENTEROLOGY

Natl. Rank Hospital	U.S. News index	Reputa- tional score	Gastro- enterology mortality rate	COTH member	Interns and residents to beds	Tech- nology score (of 11)	R.N.'s to beds	Board- certified gastro- enterologists to beds	Pro- cedures to beds
TIER ONE									
9 University of Chicago Hospitals	40.6	15.1%	0.72	Yes	1.64	10	1.38	0.038	1.90
TIER TWO									
66 Cook County Hospital, Chicago	13.8	0.0%	0.39	Yes	1.00	6	1.43	0.010	0.54
45 F.G. McGaw Hospital at Loyola University, Maywood	15.6	0.0%	1.05	Yes	1.46	9	1.59	0.019	2.07
57 Northwestern Memorial Hospital, Chicago	14.3	1.0%	0.73	Yes	0.43	10	1.03	0.028	1.94
23 Rush-Presbyterian-St. Luke's Medical Center, Chicago	18.4	2.0%	0.82	Yes	1.05	10	1.24	0.000	2.05
TIER THREE									
Columbus Hospital, Chicago	7.9	0.0%	0.96	No	0.40	8	0.82	0.047	2.14
Edgewater Medical Center, Chicago	7.7	0.0%	0.84	No	0.26	5	0.42	0.017	4.31
Elmhurst Memorial Hospital, Elmhurst	7.7	0.0%	0.96	No	0.00	8	1.01	0.000	3.74
78 Evanston Hospital, Evanston	13.0	0.0%	0.85	Yes	0.26	9	1.18	0.013	3.96
Hinsdale Hospital, Hinsdale	7.8	0.0%	0.75	No	0.12	8	0.69	0.025	2.06
Holy Family Hospital, Des Plaines	7.4	0.0%	0.89	No	0.01	5	1.14	0.030	3.19
Illinois Masonic Medical Center, Chicago	9.5	0.0%	0.94	Yes	0.43	7	0.73	0.016	1.02
Louis A. Weiss Memorial Hospital, Chicago	8.1	0.0%	0.68	No	0.37	5	0.63	0.021	2.96
83 Lutheran General Healthsystem, Park Ridge	12.8	0.4%	0.74	Yes	0.42	8	0.82	0.020	2.80
MacNeal Hospital, Berwyn	9.8	0.0%	0.97	Yes	0.28	4	1.05	0.009	3.22
Memorial Medical Center, Springfield	8.8	0.0%	1.23	Yes	0.28	8	0.89	0.012	2.80
Mercy Hospital and Medical Center, Chicago	11.0	0.0%	0.87	Yes	0.38	7	0.90	0.008	2.26
Michael Reese Hospital and Medical Center, Chicago	10.5	0.6%	0.90	Yes	0.36	3	1.28	0.020	1.13
St. Anthony Medical Center, Rockford	7.7	0.0%	1.09	No	0.04	7	1.48	0.019	3.60
St. Francis Hospital, Evanston	8.3	0.0%	0.73	No	0.36	8	0.57	0.009	2.09
St. John's Hospital, Springfield	10.0	0.0%	0.94	Yes	0.22	8	0.76	0.012	2.66
West Suburban Hospital Medical Center, Oak Park	7.5	0.0%	0.90	No	0.28	7	0.82	0.008	2.14
TIER FOUR									
Alexian Brothers Medical Center, Elk Grove Village	6.4	0.0%	0.95	No	0.00	7	0.96	0.029	2.05
Blessing Hospital, Quincy	6.6	0.0%	1.14	No	0.04	7	0.84	0.010	4.89
Carle Foundation Hospital, Urbana	2.4	0.0%	1.16	No	0.05	2	0.53	0.009	1.65
Central Du Page Hospital, Winfield	3.4	0.0%	1.33	No	0.00	4	0.81	0.021	2.82
Christ Hospital and Medical Center, Oak Lawn	5.2	0.0%	1.22	No	0.33	7	0.52	0.008	2.70
Copley Memorial Hospital, Aurora	4.7	0.0%	1.22	No	0.00	7	0.68	0.033	3.13
Covenant Medical Center, Urbana	6.6	0.0%	1.15	No	0.04	9	0.79	0.000	4.26
Decatur Memorial Hospital, Decatur	7.1	0.0%	0.79	No	0.03	7	0.48	0.009	3.00
Good Samaritan Hospital, Downers Grove	6.8	0.0%	0.85	No	0.00	5	0.66	0.076	3.01
Gottlieb Memorial Hospital, Melrose Park	4.1	0.0%	1.21	No	0.01	6	0.64	0.024	2.64
Grant Hospital of Chicago	7.2	0.0%	0.69	No	0.24	5	0.63	0.015	2.18

Natl. Rank	Hospital	U.S. News index	Reputa- tional score	Gastro- enterology mortality rate	COTH member	Interns and residents to beds	Tech- nology score (of 11)	R.N.'s to beds	Board- certified gastro- enterologists to beds	Pro- cedures to beds
	Ingalls Memorial Hospital, Harvey	5.1	0.0%	1.03	No	0.00	8	0.42	0.009	2.63
	La Grange Memorial Health System, La Grange	6.8	0.0%	0.93	No	0.12	5	0.60	0.049	4.12
	Little Company of Mary Hospital, Evergreen Park	6.4	0.0%	1.13	No	0.03	7	1.01	0.029	3.75
	Memorial Hospital of Carbondale, Carbondale	6.9	0.0%	1.12	No	0.16	7	1.07	0.000	3.59
	Memorial Hospital, Belleville	5.8	0.0%	0.90	No	0.02	5	0.58	0.004	2.92
	Mercy Center for Health Care Services, Aurora	5.0	0.0%	0.85	No	0.00	2	0.56	0.019	2.34
	Methodist Medical Center of Illinois, Peoria	5.2	0.0%	1.66	No	0.06	9	1.36	0.017	2.69
	Northwest Community Hospital, Arlington Heights	7.3	0.0%	0.97	No	0.00	8	0.72	0.007	4.40
	Oak Park Hospital, Oak Park	7.2	0.0%	0.81	No	0.00	7	0.44	0.041	3.30
	Ravenswood Hospital Medical Center, Chicago	6.1	0.0%	1.12	No	0.30	6	0.98	0.012	2.16
	Resurrection Medical Center, Chicago	4.1	0.0%	1.18	No	0.08	6	0.38	0.013	3.07
	Riverside Medical Center, Kankakee	1.1	0.0%	2.29	No	0.00	7	0.62	0.003	2.10
	Rockford Memorial Hospital, Rockford	3.8	0.0%	1.45	No	0.01	8	0.80	0.009	2.31
	Rush North Shore Medical Center, Skokie	6.7	0.0%	1.05	No	0.22	4	0.93	0.067	3.86
	Sherman Hospital, Elgin	5.4	0.0%	1.05	No	0.00	5	0.95	0.009	2.78
	St. Anthony's Health Center, Alton	6.9	0.0%	0.98	No	0.00	8	0.85	0.011	3.34
	St. Elizabeth Medical Center, Granite City	2.8	0.0%	1.15	No	0.00	3	0.52	0.009	2.01
	St. Elizabeth's Hospital, Belleville	5.1	0.0%	1.01	No	0.04	5	0.53	0.008	3.26
	St. Francis Medical Center, Peoria	6.7	0.0%	1.15	No	0.29	9	0.90	0.007	2.25
	St. James Hospital and Health Center, Chicago Heights	4.9	0.0%	1.01	No	0.00	6	0.45	0.006	2.87
	St. Joseph Hospital and Health Care Center, Chicago	6.1	0.0%	1.03	No	0.32	7	0.66	0.016	1.90
	St. Joseph Medical Center, Bloomington	4.8	0.0%	1.24	No	0.00	7	0.73	0.025	3.27
	St. Joseph Medical Center, Joliet	5.9	0.0%	1.30	No	0.00	9	1.06	0.006	3.40
	St. Mary of Nazareth Hospital Center, Chicago	6.4	0.0%	1.07	No	0.17	7	1.08	0.018	1.96
	St. Mary's Hospital of Kankakee, Kankakee	4.6	0.0%	1.29	No	0.00	9	0.60	0.004	2.93
	St. Mary's Hospital, Decatur	3.1	0.0%	1.28	No	0.01	5	0.52	0.005	2.63
	Swedish American Hospital, Rockford	7.3	0.0%	0.89	No	0.03	7	0.65	0.024	3.81
	Swedish Covenant Hospital, Chicago	5.6	0.0%	1.14	No	0.14	7	0.72	0.007	3.11
	Trinity Medical Center, Moline	3.3	0.0%	1.79	No	0.00	9	0.80	0.011	2.53

GERIATRICS

Natl. Rank	Hospital	U.S. News index	Reputa- tional score	Hospital- wide mortality rate	COTH member	Service mix	Interns and residents to beds	Tech- nology score (of 13)	R.N.'s to beds	Discharge planning (of 2)	Geriatric services (of 9)	Board- certified internists to beds
TIER ONE												
11	University of Chicago Hospitals	42.5	5.5%	0.80	Yes	8	1.64	12	1.38	2	7	0.074
16	Rush-Presbyterian-St. Luke's Medical Center, Chicago	32.8	2.2%	0.81	Yes	9	1.05	11	1.24	2	6	0.224
TIER TWO												
49	Cook County Hospital, Chicago	24.3	0.0%	0.55	Yes	7	1.00	9	1.43	2	2	0.073
46	Evanston Hospital, Evanston	24.6	0.0%	0.79	Yes	8	0.26	11	1.18	2	7	0.160
55	F.G. McGaw Hospital at Loyola University, Maywood	23.9	1.0%	1.12	Yes	9	1.46	12	1.59	2	5	0.053
80	Lutheran General Healthsystem, Park Ridge	22.2	0.6%	0.99	Yes	7	0.42	11	0.82	2	8	0.076
90	Michael Reese Hospital and Medical Center, Chicago	21.7	0.5%	0.90	Yes	7	0.36	5	1.28	1	2	0.064
33	Northwestern Memorial Hospital, Chicago	26.6	1.6%	0.99	Yes	10	0.43	11	1.03	2	6	0.134
60	St. John's Hospital, Springfield	23.2	0.0%	0.90	Yes	8	0.22	10	0.76	2	7	0.123
29	University of Illinois Hospital and Clinics, Chicago	26.9	0.0%	0.83	Yes	7	1.29	10	1.95	2	5	0.056
TIER THREE												
	Alexian Brothers Medical Center, Elk Grove Village	18.9	0.0%	0.82	No	5	0.00	9	0.96	2	4	0.118
	Columbus Hospital, Chicago	17.4	0.0%	0.97	No	6	0.40	9	0.82	2	3	0.144
	Edgewater Medical Center, Chicago	15.0	0.0%	0.81	No	3	0.26	7	0.42	1	1	0.064
	Elmhurst Memorial Hospital, Elmhurst	16.7	0.0%	1.00	No	6	0.00	11	1.01	2	5	0.111
	Good Samaritan Hospital, Downers Grove	16.6	0.0%	0.88	No	5	0.00	7	0.66	1	4	0.089
	Gottlieb Memorial Hospital, Melrose Park	17.9	0.0%	0.94	No	7	0.01	7	0.64	2	7	0.099
	Grant Hospital of Chicago	17.3	0.0%	0.71	No	6	0.24	8	0.63	1	2	0.090

Natl. Rank	Hospital	U.S. News index	Reputa- tional score	Hospital- wide mortality rate	COTH member	Service mix	Interns and residents to beds	Tech- nology score (of 13)	R.N.'s to beds	Discharge planning (of 2)	Geriatric services (of 9)	Board- certified internists to beds
	Hinsdale Hospital, Hinsdale	17.5	0.0%	0.92	No	5	0.12	11	0.69	2	3	0.062
	Holy Family Hospital, Des Plaines	17.8	0.0%	0.91	No	6	0.01	8	1.14	2	1	0.055
	Illinois Masonic Medical Center, Chicago	18.5	0.0%	1.00	Yes	10	0.43	10	0.73	1	2	0.068
	Ingalls Memorial Hospital, Harvey	17.5	0.0%	0.93	No	8	0.00	10	0.42	2	3	0.066
	La Grange Memorial Health System, La Grange	14.1	0.0%	0.96	No	2	0.12	8	0.60	2	2	0.065
	Little Company of Mary Hospital, Evergreen Park	14.4	0.0%	1.09	No	7	0.03	10	1.01	2	6	0.029
	Louis A. Weiss Memorial Hospital, Chicago	18.6	0.0%	0.87	No	4	0.37	7	0.63	2	3	0.227
	MacNeal Hospital, Berwyn	17.8	0.0%	0.95	Yes	7	0.28	6	1.05	1	1	0.052
	Memorial Medical Center, Springfield	17.8	0.0%	1.05	Yes	8	0.28	10	0.89	2	3	0.115
	Mercy Hospital and Medical Center, Chicago	18.6	0.0%	1.03	Yes	7	0.38	10	0.90	2	6	0.035
	Northwest Community Hospital, Arlington Heights	17.4	0.0%	0.94	No	6	0.00	11	0.72	2	3	0.113
	Ravenswood Hospital Medical Center, Chicago	14.7	0.0%	1.07	No	8	0.30	8	0.98	2	2	0.063
	Rush North Shore Medical Center, Skokie	15.9	0.0%	1.01	No	5	0.22	6	0.93	2	3	0.296
	St. Anthony Medical Center, Rockford	14.6	0.0%	1.02	No	4	0.04	9	1.48	2	2	0.038
	St. Anthony's Health Center, Alton	18.4	0.0%	0.90	No	7	0.00	8	0.85	1	6	0.092
	St. Elizabeth Medical Center, Granite City	14.5	0.0%	0.98	No	7	0.00	4	0.52	2	4	0.012
	St. Elizabeth's Hospital, Belleville	16.0	0.0%	0.82	No	6	0.04	7	0.53	1	2	0.023
	St. Francis Hospital, Evanston	15.4	0.0%	0.99	No	7	0.36	11	0.57	1	3	0.071
	St. Francis Medical Center, Peoria	15.7	0.0%	1.05	No	7	0.29	11	0.90	2	5	0.036
	St. James Hospital and Health Center, Chicago Heights	15.7	0.0%	0.83	No	4	0.00	9	0.45	1	1	0.136
	St. Joseph Hospital and Health Care Center, Chicago	15.3	0.0%	1.04	No	6	0.32	9	0.66	2	6	0.071
	Swedish American Hospital, Rockford	16.4	0.0%	0.98	No	6	0.03	10	0.65	2	5	0.090
	Swedish Covenant Hospital, Chicago	15.7	0.0%	1.01	No	7	0.14	9	0.72	2	4	0.070
	West Suburban Hospital Medical Center, Oak Park	17.4	0.0%	0.98	No	7	0.28	9	0.82	2	6	0.051
	**TIER FOUR**											
	Blessing Hospital, Quincy	11.4	0.0%	1.16	No	5	0.04	9	0.84	2	5	0.043
	Carle Foundation Hospital, Urbana	10.0	0.0%	1.11	No	6	0.05	3	0.53	2	1	0.043
	Central Du Page Hospital, Winfield	12.2	0.0%	1.07	No	4	0.00	7	0.81	2	4	0.077
	Christ Hospital and Medical Center, Oak Lawn	10.8	0.0%	1.22	No	7	0.33	11	0.52	2	3	0.040
	Copley Memorial Hospital, Aurora	7.9	0.0%	1.23	No	3	0.00	9	0.68	2	1	0.104
	Covenant Medical Center, Urbana	11.2	0.0%	1.17	No	6	0.04	10	0.79	2	3	0.054
	Decatur Memorial Hospital, Decatur	13.2	0.0%	1.04	No	6	0.03	9	0.48	2	2	0.077
	Mercy Center for Health Care Services, Aurora	10.2	0.0%	1.14	No	5	0.00	3	0.56	2	4	0.149
	Methodist Medical Center of Illinois, Peoria	8.8	0.0%	1.48	No	7	0.06	12	1.36	2	5	0.102
	Resurrection Medical Center, Chicago	12.2	0.0%	1.07	No	6	0.08	8	0.38	2	3	0.029
	Riverside Medical Center, Kankakee	6.2	0.0%	1.52	No	7	0.00	10	0.62	2	6	0.024
	Rockford Memorial Hospital, Rockford	10.7	0.0%	1.22	No	8	0.01	11	0.80	2	2	0.025
	Sherman Hospital, Elgin	13.3	0.0%	1.02	No	5	0.00	9	0.95	1	2	0.123
	St. Joseph Medical Center, Joliet	10.8	0.0%	1.23	No	7	0.00	11	1.06	2	3	0.028
	St. Mary of Nazareth Hospital Center, Chicago	10.0	0.0%	1.24	No	5	0.17	10	1.08	2	3	0.007
	St. Mary's Hospital of Kankakee, Kankakee	8.4	0.0%	1.26	No	5	0.00	10	0.60	2	3	0.052
	St. Mary's Hospital, Decatur	9.6	0.0%	1.10	No	5	0.01	6	0.52	1	3	0.030
	Trinity Medical Center, Moline	8.7	0.0%	1.35	No	7	0.00	10	0.80	2	5	0.032

GYNECOLOGY

Natl. Rank	Hospital	U.S. News index	Reputa- tional score	Hospital- wide mortality rate	Interns and residents to beds	Tech- nology score (of 10)	R.N.'s to beds	Board- certified OB-GYNs to beds	Procedures to beds
	**TIER ONE**								
9	University of Chicago Hospitals	49.2	7.2%	0.80	1.64	10	1.38	0.036	0.37
25	Northwestern Memorial Hospital, Chicago	32.8	4.6%	0.99	0.43	9	1.03	0.088	0.44
28	Rush-Presbyterian-St. Luke's Medical Center, Chicago	31.9	1.9%	0.81	1.05	9	1.24	0.060	0.33
30	University of Illinois Hospital and Clinics, Chicago	30.6	0.5%	0.83	1.29	7	1.95	0.039	0.28

Natl. Rank	Hospital	U.S. News index	Reputational score	Hospital-wide mortality rate	Interns and residents to beds	Technology score (of 10)	R.N.'s to beds	Board-certified OB-GYNs to beds	Procedures to beds
	TIER TWO								
46	**Cook County Hospital, Chicago**	**27.1**	0.6%	0.55	1.00	7	1.43	0.033	0.09
67	**Evanston Hospital, Evanston**	**23.9**	0.0%	0.79	0.26	9	1.18	0.086	0.34
47	**F.G. McGaw Hospital at Loyola University, Maywood**	**26.9**	1.3%	1.12	1.46	9	1.59	0.042	0.39
	TIER THREE								
	Alexian Brothers Medical Center, Elk Grove Village	18.7	0.0%	0.82	0.00	6	0.96	0.047	0.22
	Columbus Hospital, Chicago	19.1	0.0%	0.97	0.40	8	0.82	0.067	0.29
	Edgewater Medical Center, Chicago	15.7	0.0%	0.81	0.26	4	0.42	0.029	0.20
	Elmhurst Memorial Hospital, Elmhurst	15.8	0.0%	1.00	0.00	7	1.01	0.031	0.28
	Good Samaritan Hospital, Downers Grove	17.3	0.0%	0.88	0.00	5	0.66	0.073	0.31
	Gottlieb Memorial Hospital, Melrose Park	15.3	0.0%	0.94	0.01	5	0.64	0.060	0.21
	Grant Hospital of Chicago	17.8	0.0%	0.71	0.24	4	0.63	0.084	0.15
	Hinsdale Hospital, Hinsdale	18.4	0.0%	0.92	0.12	8	0.69	0.050	0.38
	Holy Family Hospital, Des Plaines	17.2	0.0%	0.91	0.01	4	1.14	0.041	0.30
	Illinois Masonic Medical Center, Chicago	17.0	0.0%	1.00	0.43	7	0.73	0.060	0.08
	Ingalls Memorial Hospital, Harvey	15.5	0.0%	0.93	0.00	7	0.42	0.043	0.27
	Louis A. Weiss Memorial Hospital, Chicago	17.7	0.0%	0.87	0.37	5	0.63	0.026	0.30
	Lutheran General Healthsystem, Park Ridge	19.9	0.4%	0.99	0.42	8	0.82	0.080	0.31
	MacNeal Hospital, Berwyn	17.0	0.6%	0.95	0.28	3	1.05	0.028	0.30
	Memorial Hospital, Belleville	15.8	0.0%	0.75	0.02	5	0.58	0.020	0.33
	Memorial Medical Center, Springfield	14.7	0.0%	1.05	0.28	6	0.89	0.046	0.63
	Mercy Hospital and Medical Center, Chicago	15.5	0.0%	1.03	0.38	6	0.90	0.033	0.13
93	Michael Reese Hospital and Medical Center, Chicago	21.8	0.8%	0.90	0.36	4	1.28	0.039	0.10
	Northwest Community Hospital, Arlington Heights	17.1	0.0%	0.94	0.00	7	0.72	0.064	0.52
	Oak Park Hospital, Oak Park	15.6	0.0%	0.89	0.00	6	0.44	0.015	0.18
	Rush North Shore Medical Center, Skokie	15.0	0.0%	1.01	0.22	3	0.93	0.117	0.30
	Sherman Hospital, Elgin	14.3	0.0%	1.02	0.00	6	0.95	0.035	0.33
	St. Anthony Medical Center, Rockford	16.5	0.0%	1.02	0.04	6	1.48	0.024	0.39
	St. Anthony's Health Center, Alton	18.2	0.0%	0.90	0.00	7	0.85	0.033	0.39
	St. Elizabeth's Hospital, Belleville	15.6	0.0%	0.82	0.04	5	0.53	0.015	0.24
	St. Francis Hospital, Evanston	15.1	0.0%	0.99	0.36	7	0.57	0.011	0.17
	St. Francis Medical Center, Peoria	16.2	0.0%	1.05	0.29	9	0.90	0.016	0.32
	St. James Hospital and Health Center, Chicago Heights	15.4	0.0%	0.83	0.00	5	0.45	0.030	0.30
	St. John's Hospital, Springfield	19.8	0.0%	0.90	0.22	8	0.76	0.042	0.28
	St. Joseph Hospital and Health Care Center, Chicago	14.2	0.0%	1.04	0.32	6	0.66	0.045	0.19
	Swedish American Hospital, Rockford	14.2	0.0%	0.98	0.03	6	0.65	0.028	0.60
	West Suburban Hospital Medical Center, Oak Park	15.7	0.0%	0.98	0.28	6	0.82	0.024	0.25
	TIER FOUR								
	Blessing Hospital, Quincy	9.7	0.0%	1.16	0.04	5	0.84	0.019	0.59
	Carle Foundation Hospital, Urbana	7.9	0.0%	1.11	0.05	3	0.53	0.013	0.26
	Central Du Page Hospital, Winfield	12.4	0.0%	1.07	0.00	5	0.81	0.068	0.34
	Christ Hospital and Medical Center, Oak Lawn	10.1	0.0%	1.22	0.33	7	0.52	0.035	0.23
	Copley Memorial Hospital, Aurora	8.4	0.0%	1.23	0.00	5	0.68	0.060	0.24
	Covenant Medical Center, Urbana	11.3	0.0%	1.17	0.04	8	0.79	0.015	0.55
	Decatur Memorial Hospital, Decatur	11.4	0.0%	1.04	0.03	6	0.48	0.017	0.36
	La Grange Memorial Health System, La Grange	13.9	0.0%	0.96	0.12	4	0.60	0.045	0.39
	Little Company of Mary Hospital, Evergreen Park	13.6	0.0%	1.09	0.03	7	1.01	0.034	0.37
	Mercy Center for Health Care Services, Aurora	8.0	0.0%	1.14	0.00	3	0.56	0.053	0.15
	Methodist Medical Center of Illinois, Peoria	9.8	0.0%	1.48	0.06	8	1.36	0.055	0.56
	Ravenswood Hospital Medical Center, Chicago	13.7	0.0%	1.07	0.30	5	0.98	0.030	0.19
	Resurrection Medical Center, Chicago	10.0	0.0%	1.07	0.08	5	0.38	0.026	0.26
	Riverside Medical Center, Kankakee	3.7	0.0%	1.52	0.00	6	0.62	0.024	0.31
	Rockford Memorial Hospital, Rockford	10.4	0.0%	1.22	0.01	8	0.80	0.025	0.37
	St. Elizabeth Medical Center, Granite City	11.4	0.0%	0.98	0.00	4	0.52	0.003	0.20
	St. Joseph Medical Center, Joliet	11.7	0.0%	1.23	0.00	8	1.06	0.043	0.25
	St. Mary of Nazareth Hospital Center, Chicago	10.6	0.0%	1.24	0.17	6	1.08	0.025	0.13

Natl. Rank	Hospital	U.S. News index	Reputational score	Hospital-wide mortality rate	Interns and residents to beds	Technology score (of 10)	R.N.'s to beds	Board-certified OB-GYNs to beds	Procedures to beds
	St. Mary's Hospital of Kankakee, Kankakee	8.3	0.0%	1.26	0.00	7	0.60	0.035	0.30
	St. Mary's Hospital, Decatur	9.3	0.0%	1.10	0.01	5	0.52	0.016	0.29
	Swedish Covenant Hospital, Chicago	13.9	0.0%	1.01	0.14	6	0.72	0.021	0.26
	Trinity Medical Center, Moline	8.7	0.0%	1.35	0.00	8	0.80	0.043	0.43

NEUROLOGY

Natl. Rank	Hospital	U.S. News index	Reputational score	Neurology mortality rate	COTH member	Interns and residents to beds	Technology score (of 9)	R.N.'s to beds	Board-certified neurologists to beds
	TIER ONE								
14	University of Illinois Hospital and Clinics, Chicago	27.7	2.4%	0.50	Yes	1.29	6	1.95	0.017
16	University of Chicago Hospitals	27.3	1.5%	0.67	Yes	1.64	9	1.38	0.023
19	Rush-Presbyterian-St. Luke's Medical Center, Chicago	26.7	2.4%	0.53	Yes	1.05	8	1.24	0.031
	TIER TWO								
68	Evanston Hospital, Evanston	18.4	0.0%	0.80	Yes	0.26	8	1.18	0.020
72	Lutheran General Healthsystem, Park Ridge	18.3	0.0%	0.70	Yes	0.42	7	0.82	0.013
41	Northwestern Memorial Hospital, Chicago	21.8	2.0%	0.84	Yes	0.43	8	1.03	0.034
	TIER THREE								
	Alexian Brothers Medical Center, Elk Grove Village	15.3	0.0%	0.70	No	0.00	6	0.96	0.021
	Columbus Hospital, Chicago	16.6	0.0%	0.60	No	0.40	7	0.82	0.023
	Edgewater Medical Center, Chicago	12.9	0.0%	0.79	No	0.26	4	0.42	0.012
90	F.G. McGaw Hospital at Loyola University, Maywood	17.6	0.0%	1.14	Yes	1.46	8	1.59	0.023
	Good Samaritan Hospital, Downers Grove	13.9	0.0%	0.59	No	0.00	5	0.66	0.016
	Gottlieb Memorial Hospital, Melrose Park	13.4	0.0%	0.66	No	0.01	5	0.64	0.008
	Grant Hospital of Chicago	13.4	0.0%	0.59	No	0.24	4	0.63	0.003
	Hinsdale Hospital, Hinsdale	14.5	0.0%	0.74	No	0.12	7	0.69	0.009
	Holy Family Hospital, Des Plaines	14.6	0.0%	0.71	No	0.01	4	1.14	0.011
	Illinois Masonic Medical Center, Chicago	14.5	0.0%	0.90	Yes	0.43	6	0.73	0.013
	Ingalls Memorial Hospital, Harvey	13.6	0.0%	0.69	No	0.00	7	0.42	0.011
	La Grange Memorial Health System, La Grange	11.3	0.0%	0.84	No	0.12	4	0.60	0.008
	Little Company of Mary Hospital, Evergreen Park	13.9	0.0%	0.80	No	0.03	6	1.01	0.010
	Louis A. Weiss Memorial Hospital, Chicago	13.9	0.0%	0.80	No	0.37	4	0.63	0.021
	MacNeal Hospital, Berwyn	15.4	0.0%	0.81	Yes	0.28	3	1.05	0.005
	Memorial Hospital, Belleville	13.2	0.0%	0.58	No	0.02	5	0.58	0.007
	Memorial Medical Center, Springfield	13.9	0.2%	0.97	Yes	0.28	6	0.89	0.017
89	Mercy Hospital and Medical Center, Chicago	17.7	0.0%	0.76	Yes	0.38	6	0.90	0.008
98	Michael Reese Hospital and Medical Center, Chicago	17.0	0.0%	0.81	Yes	0.36	3	1.28	0.013
	Mount Sinai Hospital Medical Center, Chicago	13.1	0.0%	0.97	Yes	0.54	6	0.72	0.006
	Oak Park Hospital, Oak Park	13.6	0.0%	0.76	No	0.00	6	0.44	0.015
	Rush North Shore Medical Center, Skokie	15.1	0.0%	0.80	No	0.22	3	0.93	0.037
	St. Anthony Medical Center, Rockford	14.4	0.0%	0.84	No	0.04	6	1.48	0.014
	St. Anthony's Health Center, Alton	13.8	0.0%	0.78	No	0.00	7	0.85	0.005
	St. Elizabeth's Hospital, Belleville	13.0	0.0%	0.67	No	0.04	5	0.53	0.005
	St. James Hospital and Health Center, Chicago Heights	12.5	0.0%	0.70	No	0.00	5	0.45	0.003
	St. John's Hospital, Springfield	16.8	0.0%	0.81	Yes	0.22	7	0.76	0.019
	St. Joseph Hospital and Health Care Center, Chicago	14.3	0.0%	0.79	No	0.32	6	0.66	0.014
	St. Mary of Nazareth Hospital Center, Chicago	12.1	0.0%	0.95	No	0.17	6	1.08	0.021
	TIER FOUR								
	Blessing Hospital, Quincy	6.9	0.0%	1.13	No	0.04	5	0.84	0.005
	Carle Foundation Hospital, Urbana	6.4	0.0%	1.06	No	0.05	2	0.53	0.006
	Central Du Page Hospital, Winfield	9.0	0.0%	0.98	No	0.00	4	0.81	0.009
	Christ Hospital and Medical Center, Oak Lawn	8.6	0.0%	1.03	No	0.33	6	0.52	0.004
	Covenant Medical Center, Urbana	8.4	0.0%	1.07	No	0.04	8	0.79	0.004
	Decatur Memorial Hospital, Decatur	8.8	0.0%	0.98	No	0.03	6	0.48	0.011
	Elmhurst Memorial Hospital, Elmhurst	9.7	0.0%	1.00	No	0.00	7	1.01	0.005

STATE RANKINGS ■ ILLINOIS

Natl. Rank	Hospital	U.S. News index	Reputa-tional score	Neurology mortality rate	COTH member	Interns and residents to beds	Technology score (of 9)	R.N.'s to beds	Board-certified neurologists to beds
	Methodist Medical Center of Illinois, Peoria	8.0	0.0%	1.32	No	0.06	8	1.36	0.017
	Northwest Community Hospital, Arlington Heights	10.7	0.0%	0.94	No	0.00	7	0.72	0.017
	Ravenswood Hospital Medical Center, Chicago	9.7	0.0%	1.04	No	0.30	5	0.98	0.009
	Resurrection Medical Center, Chicago	9.5	0.0%	0.91	No	0.08	5	0.38	0.007
	Riverside Medical Center, Kankakee	3.3	0.0%	1.48	No	0.00	6	0.62	0.006
	Rockford Memorial Hospital, Rockford	6.0	0.0%	1.25	No	0.01	7	0.80	0.005
	Sherman Hospital, Elgin	9.0	0.0%	1.01	No	0.00	5	0.95	0.009
	St. Elizabeth Medical Center, Granite City	10.6	0.0%	0.83	No	0.00	3	0.52	0.006
	St. Francis Hospital, Evanston	9.4	0.0%	1.01	No	0.36	7	0.57	0.002
	St. Francis Medical Center, Peoria	9.0	0.0%	1.15	No	0.29	8	0.90	0.012
	St. Joseph Medical Center, Bloomington	5.4	0.0%	1.27	No	0.00	6	0.73	0.006
	St. Joseph Medical Center, Joliet	5.6	0.0%	1.42	No	0.00	8	1.06	0.009
	St. Mary's Hospital of Kankakee, Kankakee	9.5	0.0%	0.96	No	0.00	7	0.60	0.009
	St. Mary's Hospital, Decatur	10.0	0.0%	0.88	No	0.01	4	0.52	0.008
	Swedish American Hospital, Rockford	10.9	0.0%	0.89	No	0.03	6	0.65	0.010
	Swedish Covenant Hospital, Chicago	9.4	0.0%	1.04	No	0.14	6	0.72	0.018
	Trinity Medical Center, Moline	8.0	0.0%	1.11	No	0.00	8	0.80	0.007
	West Suburban Hospital Medical Center, Oak Park	10.1	0.0%	0.98	No	0.28	6	0.82	0.005

ORTHOPEDICS

Natl. Rank	Hospital	U.S. News index	Reputa-tional score	Orthopedics mortality rate	COTH member	Interns and residents to beds	Technology score (of 5)	R.N.'s to beds	Board-certified orthopedists to beds	Pro-cedures to beds
TIER ONE										
19	University of Chicago Hospitals	21.4	0.5%	0.55	Yes	1.64	5	1.38	0.011	1.38
TIER TWO										
31	F.G. McGaw Hospital at Loyola University, Maywood	19.2	0.0%	0.71	Yes	1.46	4	1.59	0.039	1.83
24	Rush-Presbyterian-St. Luke's Medical Center, Chicago	20.4	2.0%	0.76	Yes	1.05	4	1.24	0.039	1.83
TIER THREE										
	Alexian Brothers Medical Center, Elk Grove Village	9.1	0.0%	0.76	No	0.00	4	0.96	0.037	1.31
	Evanston Hospital, Evanston	13.0	0.0%	0.81	Yes	0.26	4	1.18	0.034	2.91
	Good Samaritan Hospital, Downers Grove	10.2	0.0%	0.57	No	0.00	4	0.66	0.079	2.18
	Grant Hospital of Chicago	9.5	0.0%	0.20	No	0.24	3	0.63	0.012	0.84
	Holy Family Hospital, Des Plaines	10.5	0.0%	0.64	No	0.01	3	1.14	0.033	1.89
	Illinois Masonic Medical Center, Chicago	10.9	0.0%	0.82	Yes	0.43	3	0.73	0.017	0.49
	Louis A. Weiss Memorial Hospital, Chicago	9.7	0.0%	0.47	No	0.37	2	0.63	0.047	1.76
	Lutheran General Healthsystem, Park Ridge	10.3	0.0%	0.95	Yes	0.42	3	0.82	0.023	2.24
	MacNeal Hospital, Berwyn	8.8	0.0%	1.09	Yes	0.28	2	1.05	0.016	2.12
	Memorial Hospital, Belleville	9.2	0.0%	0.70	No	0.02	4	0.58	0.013	2.56
	Memorial Medical Center, Springfield	9.9	0.0%	1.00	Yes	0.28	3	0.89	0.025	2.96
	Mercy Hospital and Medical Center, Chicago	8.4	0.0%	1.22	Yes	0.38	3	0.90	0.014	1.09
	Michael Reese Hospital and Medical Center, Chicago	10.6	0.0%	0.86	Yes	0.36	1	1.28	0.028	0.65
	Northwest Community Hospital, Arlington Heights	9.7	0.0%	0.71	No	0.00	4	0.72	0.056	3.33
	Northwestern Memorial Hospital, Chicago	12.4	0.4%	0.96	Yes	0.43	4	1.03	0.027	2.12
	Rush North Shore Medical Center, Skokie	8.9	0.0%	0.77	No	0.22	2	0.93	0.071	2.94
	St. Anthony Medical Center, Rockford	10.7	0.0%	0.77	No	0.04	4	1.48	0.029	2.38
	St. Elizabeth Medical Center, Granite City	8.4	0.0%	0.54	No	0.00	3	0.52	0.003	0.97
	St. Elizabeth's Hospital, Belleville	9.4	0.0%	0.67	No	0.04	4	0.53	0.015	2.24
	St. Francis Medical Center, Peoria	8.3	0.0%	0.91	No	0.29	4	0.90	0.012	2.00
	St. John's Hospital, Springfield	10.7	0.0%	0.89	Yes	0.22	4	0.76	0.022	2.40
	St. Joseph Hospital and Health Care Center, Chicago	8.3	0.0%	0.79	No	0.32	3	0.66	0.028	1.35
TIER FOUR										
	Blessing Hospital, Quincy	6.0	0.0%	0.96	No	0.04	2	0.84	0.019	3.24
	Carle Foundation Hospital, Urbana	6.0	0.0%	0.82	No	0.05	2	0.53	0.011	1.84
	Central Du Page Hospital, Winfield	4.5	0.0%	1.29	No	0.00	3	0.81	0.047	3.31

Natl. Rank	Hospital	U.S. News index	Reputa-tional score	Orthopedics mortality rate	COTH member	Interns and residents to beds	Tech-nology score (of 5)	R.N.'s to beds	Board-certified orthopedists to beds	Pro-cedures to beds
	Christ Hospital and Medical Center, Oak Lawn	5.1	0.0%	1.14	No	0.33	3	0.52	0.013	1.85
	Columbus Hospital, Chicago	6.7	0.0%	1.05	No	0.40	3	0.82	0.043	1.25
	Copley Memorial Hospital, Aurora	7.4	0.0%	0.81	No	0.00	3	0.68	0.049	2.23
	Covenant Medical Center, Urbana	7.3	0.0%	0.92	No	0.04	4	0.79	0.008	3.26
	Decatur Memorial Hospital, Decatur	2.5	0.0%	1.51	No	0.03	3	0.48	0.014	2.38
	Elmhurst Memorial Hospital, Elmhurst	7.8	0.0%	0.91	No	0.00	4	1.01	0.018	2.79
	Gottlieb Memorial Hospital, Melrose Park	5.6	0.0%	1.04	No	0.01	4	0.64	0.028	1.59
	Hinsdale Hospital, Hinsdale	7.0	0.0%	0.95	No	0.12	4	0.69	0.025	2.33
	Ingalls Memorial Hospital, Harvey	7.3	0.0%	0.74	No	0.00	3	0.42	0.026	1.72
	La Grange Memorial Health System, La Grange	5.8	0.0%	1.00	No	0.12	3	0.60	0.020	2.82
	Little Company of Mary Hospital, Evergreen Park	7.4	0.0%	0.89	No	0.03	3	1.01	0.017	2.46
	Memorial Hospital of Carbondale, Carbondale	5.7	0.0%	1.22	No	0.16	3	1.07	0.013	2.27
	Mercy Center for Health Care Services, Aurora	4.2	0.0%	1.06	No	0.00	2	0.56	0.034	2.20
	Methodist Medical Center of Illinois, Peoria	7.1	0.0%	1.35	No	0.06	5	1.36	0.045	2.83
	Oak Park Hospital, Oak Park	8.1	0.0%	0.72	No	0.00	3	0.44	0.087	2.17
	Resurrection Medical Center, Chicago	5.1	0.0%	0.88	No	0.08	2	0.38	0.012	1.67
	Riverside Medical Center, Kankakee	5.0	0.0%	1.02	No	0.00	3	0.62	0.012	1.81
	Rockford Memorial Hospital, Rockford	5.2	0.0%	1.22	No	0.01	4	0.80	0.014	2.48
	Sherman Hospital, Elgin	6.5	0.0%	1.03	No	0.00	4	0.95	0.018	1.83
	St. Anthony's Health Center, Alton	5.9	0.0%	1.12	No	0.00	4	0.85	0.027	2.42
	St. Francis Hospital, Evanston	7.3	0.0%	0.93	No	0.36	4	0.57	0.011	1.45
	St. James Hospital and Health Center, Chicago Heights	3.8	0.0%	1.02	No	0.00	2	0.45	0.012	1.70
	St. Joseph Medical Center, Bloomington	6.2	0.0%	0.94	No	0.00	3	0.73	0.025	2.51
	St. Joseph Medical Center, Joliet	4.5	0.0%	1.49	No	0.00	4	1.06	0.017	1.48
	St. Mary's Hospital of Kankakee, Kankakee	5.6	0.0%	1.02	No	0.00	4	0.60	0.017	1.87
	St. Mary's Hospital, Decatur	6.3	0.0%	0.85	No	0.01	3	0.52	0.014	2.08
	Swedish American Hospital, Rockford	6.2	0.0%	0.93	No	0.03	3	0.65	0.028	2.61
	Swedish Covenant Hospital, Chicago	5.5	0.0%	1.07	No	0.14	3	0.72	0.025	2.16
	Trinity Medical Center, Moline	8.1	0.0%	0.81	No	0.00	4	0.80	0.029	1.72
	West Suburban Hospital Medical Center, Oak Park	6.9	0.0%	0.97	No	0.28	3	0.82	0.019	1.70

OTOLARYNGOLOGY

Natl. Rank	Hospital	U.S. News index	Reputa-tional score	Hospital-wide mortality rate	COTH member	Interns and residents to beds	Tech-nology score (of 9)	R.N.'s to beds	Board-certified internists to beds	Procedures to beds
TIER ONE										
23	University of Illinois Hospital and Clinics, Chicago	24.0	2.3%	0.83	Yes	1.29	6	1.95	0.056	0.228
28	Northwestern Memorial Hospital, Chicago	22.1	3.4%	0.99	Yes	0.43	8	1.03	0.134	0.207
31	University of Chicago Hospitals	21.3	1.3%	0.80	Yes	1.64	9	1.38	0.074	0.234
33	F.G. McGaw Hospital at Loyola University, Maywood	21.1	1.4%	1.12	Yes	1.46	8	1.59	0.053	0.314
TIER TWO										
71	Cook County Hospital, Chicago	15.2	0.4%	0.55	Yes	1.00	6	1.43	0.073	0.082
67	Rush-Presbyterian-St. Luke's Medical Center, Chicago	15.5	0.0%	0.81	Yes	1.05	8	1.24	0.224	0.185
TIER THREE										
	Columbus Hospital, Chicago	7.4	0.0%	0.97	No	0.40	7	0.82	0.144	0.127
	Evanston Hospital, Evanston	11.7	0.0%	0.79	Yes	0.26	8	1.18	0.160	0.373
	Illinois Masonic Medical Center, Chicago	9.4	0.0%	1.00	Yes	0.43	6	0.73	0.068	0.129
	Lutheran General Healthsystem, Park Ridge	10.0	0.0%	0.99	Yes	0.42	7	0.82	0.076	0.167
	MacNeal Hospital, Berwyn	8.6	0.0%	0.95	Yes	0.28	2	1.05	0.052	0.194
	Memorial Medical Center, Springfield	9.7	0.0%	1.05	Yes	0.28	6	0.89	0.115	0.232
	Mercy Hospital and Medical Center, Chicago	9.4	0.0%	1.03	Yes	0.38	6	0.90	0.035	0.131
	Methodist Medical Center of Illinois, Peoria	7.3	0.0%	1.48	No	0.06	8	1.36	0.102	0.137
	Michael Reese Hospital and Medical Center, Chicago	9.5	0.0%	0.90	Yes	0.36	1	1.28	0.064	0.075
	Mount Sinai Hospital Medical Center, Chicago	9.1	0.0%	1.26	Yes	0.54	6	0.72	0.000	0.087
	St. John's Hospital, Springfield	9.5	0.0%	0.90	Yes	0.22	7	0.76	0.123	0.242

Natl. Rank	Hospital	U.S. News index	Reputa-tional score	Hospital-wide mortality rate	COTH member	Interns and residents to beds	Tech-nology score (of 9)	R.N.'s to beds	Board-certified internists to beds	Procedures to beds
	TIER FOUR									
	Alexian Brothers Medical Center, Elk Grove Village	**5.9**	0.0%	0.82	No	0.00	6	0.96	0.118	0.176
	Blessing Hospital, Quincy	**4.5**	0.0%	1.15	No	0.04	5	0.84	0.043	0.507
	Carle Foundation Hospital, Urbana	**2.4**	0.0%	1.11	No	0.05	1	0.53	0.043	0.115
	Central Du Page Hospital, Winfield	**4.0**	0.0%	1.07	No	0.00	3	0.81	0.077	0.195
	Christ Hospital and Medical Center, Oak Lawn	**4.8**	0.0%	1.22	No	0.33	6	0.52	0.040	0.184
	Copley Memorial Hospital, Aurora	**4.6**	0.0%	1.23	No	0.00	6	0.68	0.104	0.137
	Covenant Medical Center, Urbana	**5.3**	0.0%	1.17	No	0.04	8	0.79	0.054	0.479
	Decatur Memorial Hospital, Decatur	**4.0**	0.0%	1.04	No	0.03	6	0.48	0.077	0.350
	Edgewater Medical Center, Chicago	**4.3**	0.0%	0.81	No	0.26	4	0.42	0.064	0.387
	Elmhurst Memorial Hospital, Elmhurst	**6.1**	0.0%	1.00	No	0.00	7	1.01	0.111	0.325
	Good Samaritan Hospital, Downers Grove	**4.1**	0.0%	0.88	No	0.00	4	0.66	0.089	0.168
	Gottlieb Memorial Hospital, Melrose Park	**4.1**	0.0%	0.94	No	0.01	4	0.64	0.099	0.147
	Grant Hospital of Chicago	**5.1**	0.0%	0.71	No	0.24	4	0.63	0.090	0.110
	Hinsdale Hospital, Hinsdale	**5.2**	0.0%	0.92	No	0.12	7	0.69	0.062	0.310
	Holy Family Hospital, Des Plaines	**5.3**	0.0%	0.91	No	0.01	4	1.14	0.055	0.232
	Ingalls Memorial Hospital, Harvey	**3.9**	0.0%	0.93	No	0.00	7	0.42	0.066	0.215
	La Grange Memorial Health System, La Grange	**4.1**	0.0%	0.96	No	0.12	4	0.60	0.065	0.267
	Little Company of Mary Hospital, Evergreen Park	**5.2**	0.0%	1.09	No	0.03	6	1.01	0.029	0.328
	Louis A. Weiss Memorial Hospital, Chicago	**6.9**	0.0%	0.87	No	0.37	5	0.63	0.227	0.227
	Memorial Hospital of Carbondale, Carbondale	**5.9**	0.0%	1.15	No	0.16	6	1.07	0.040	0.280
	Memorial Hospital, Belleville	**3.5**	0.0%	0.76	No	0.02	4	0.58	0.022	0.256
	Mercy Center for Health Care Services, Aurora	**3.2**	0.0%	1.14	No	0.00	1	0.56	0.149	0.088
	Northwest Community Hospital, Arlington Heights	**5.3**	0.0%	0.94	No	0.00	7	0.72	0.113	0.365
	Oak Forest Hospital of Cook County, Oak Forest	**0.9**	0.0%	2.35	No	0.00	1	0.25	0.036	0.003
	Oak Park Hospital, Oak Park	**3.8**	0.0%	0.89	No	0.00	6	0.44	0.067	0.138
	Ravenswood Hospital Medical Center, Chicago	**6.1**	0.0%	1.07	No	0.30	5	0.98	0.063	0.147
	Resurrection Medical Center, Chicago	**3.1**	0.0%	1.07	No	0.08	5	0.38	0.029	0.203
	Riverside Medical Center, Kankakee	**3.6**	0.0%	1.52	No	0.00	6	0.62	0.024	0.207
	Rockford Memorial Hospital, Rockford	**4.6**	0.0%	1.22	No	0.01	7	0.80	0.025	0.134
	Rush North Shore Medical Center, Skokie	**6.9**	0.0%	1.00	No	0.22	2	0.93	0.296	0.242
	Sherman Hospital, Elgin	**6.7**	0.5%	1.02	No	0.00	4	0.95	0.123	0.223
	St. Anthony Medical Center, Rockford	**6.5**	0.0%	1.02	No	0.04	5	1.48	0.038	0.319
	St. Anthony's Health Center, Alton	**5.0**	0.0%	0.90	No	0.00	5	0.85	0.092	0.293
	St. Elizabeth Medical Center, Granite City	**2.3**	0.0%	0.98	No	0.00	2	0.52	0.012	0.227
	St. Elizabeth's Hospital, Belleville	**3.4**	0.0%	0.82	No	0.04	4	0.53	0.023	0.246
	St. Francis Hospital, Evanston	**5.8**	0.0%	0.99	No	0.36	7	0.57	0.071	0.155
	St. Francis Medical Center, Peoria	**6.5**	0.0%	1.05	No	0.29	8	0.90	0.036	0.174
	St. James Hospital and Health Center, Chicago Heights	**4.2**	0.0%	0.83	No	0.00	5	0.45	0.136	0.214
	St. Joseph Hospital and Health Care Center, Chicago	**5.6**	0.0%	1.04	No	0.32	6	0.66	0.071	0.219
	St. Joseph Medical Center, Bloomington	**4.2**	0.0%	1.04	No	0.00	6	0.73	0.032	0.146
	St. Joseph Medical Center, Joliet	**5.7**	0.0%	1.23	No	0.00	8	1.06	0.028	0.300
	St. Mary Hospital, Quincy	**4.9**	0.0%	1.09	No	0.09	3	0.93	0.104	0.358
	St. Mary of Nazareth Hospital Center, Chicago	**5.6**	0.0%	1.24	No	0.17	6	1.08	0.007	0.109
	St. Mary's Hospital of Kankakee, Kankakee	**4.1**	0.0%	1.26	No	0.00	7	0.60	0.052	0.235
	St. Mary's Hospital, Decatur	**3.0**	0.0%	1.10	No	0.01	4	0.52	0.030	0.232
	Swedish American Hospital, Rockford	**4.6**	0.0%	0.98	No	0.03	6	0.65	0.090	0.259
	Swedish Covenant Hospital, Chicago	**5.1**	0.0%	1.01	No	0.14	6	0.72	0.070	0.179
	Trinity Medical Center, Moline	**4.8**	0.0%	1.34	No	0.00	8	0.80	0.032	0.137
	West Suburban Hospital Medical Center, Oak Park	**5.8**	0.0%	0.98	No	0.28	6	0.82	0.051	0.097

RHEUMATOLOGY

Natl. Rank	Hospital	U.S. News index	Reputa- tional score	Hospital- wide mortality rate	COTH member	Interns and residents to beds	Tech- nology score (of 5)	R.N.'s to beds	Board- certified internists to beds
	TIER ONE								
20	**University of Chicago Hospitals**	24.7	2.0%	0.80	Yes	1.64	5	1.38	0.074
	TIER TWO								
56	**Cook County Hospital, Chicago**	17.5	0.0%	0.55	Yes	1.00	3	1.43	0.073
64	**F.G. McGaw Hospital at Loyola University, Maywood**	16.9	0.0%	1.12	Yes	1.46	4	1.59	0.053
82	**Northwestern Memorial Hospital, Chicago**	16.1	1.0%	0.99	Yes	0.43	4	1.03	0.134
32	**Rush-Presbyterian-St. Luke's Medical Center, Chicago**	20.7	0.9%	0.81	Yes	1.05	4	1.24	0.224
28	**University of Illinois Hospital and Clinics, Chicago**	21.3	0.8%	0.83	Yes	1.29	3	1.95	0.056
	TIER THREE								
	Alexian Brothers Medical Center, Elk Grove Village	11.4	0.0%	0.82	No	0.00	4	0.96	0.118
	Columbus Hospital, Chicago	10.5	0.0%	0.97	No	0.40	3	0.82	0.144
	Elmhurst Memorial Hospital, Elmhurst	9.7	0.0%	1.00	No	0.00	4	1.01	0.111
89	**Evanston Hospital, Evanston**	15.6	0.0%	0.79	Yes	0.26	4	1.18	0.160
	Grant Hospital of Chicago	9.6	0.0%	0.71	No	0.24	3	0.63	0.090
	Hinsdale Hospital, Hinsdale	9.6	0.0%	0.92	No	0.12	4	0.69	0.062
	Holy Family Hospital, Des Plaines	10.1	0.0%	0.91	No	0.01	3	1.14	0.055
	Illinois Masonic Medical Center, Chicago	11.0	0.0%	1.00	Yes	0.43	3	0.73	0.068
	Louis A. Weiss Memorial Hospital, Chicago	11.2	0.0%	0.87	No	0.37	2	0.63	0.227
85	**Lutheran General Healthsystem, Park Ridge**	15.7	1.5%	0.99	Yes	0.42	3	0.82	0.076
	MacNeal Hospital, Berwyn	11.2	0.0%	0.95	Yes	0.28	2	1.05	0.052
	Memorial Medical Center, Springfield	11.8	0.0%	1.05	Yes	0.28	3	0.89	0.115
	Mercy Hospital and Medical Center, Chicago	11.8	0.0%	1.03	Yes	0.38	3	0.90	0.035
	Michael Reese Hospital and Medical Center, Chicago	12.3	0.0%	0.90	Yes	0.36	1	1.28	0.064
	Rush North Shore Medical Center, Skokie	10.6	0.0%	1.00	No	0.22	2	0.93	0.296
	St. Anthony Medical Center, Rockford	10.3	0.0%	1.02	No	0.04	4	1.48	0.038
	St. John's Hospital, Springfield	13.3	0.0%	0.90	Yes	0.22	4	0.76	0.123
	TIER FOUR								
	Blessing Hospital, Quincy	6.7	0.0%	1.15	No	0.04	2	0.84	0.043
	Carle Foundation Hospital, Urbana	6.3	0.0%	1.11	No	0.05	2	0.53	0.043
	Central Du Page Hospital, Winfield	7.8	0.0%	1.07	No	0.00	3	0.81	0.077
	Christ Hospital and Medical Center, Oak Lawn	6.8	0.0%	1.22	No	0.33	3	0.52	0.040
	Copley Memorial Hospital, Aurora	6.6	0.0%	1.23	No	0.00	3	0.68	0.104
	Covenant Medical Center, Urbana	7.5	0.0%	1.17	No	0.04	4	0.79	0.054
	Decatur Memorial Hospital, Decatur	7.3	0.0%	1.04	No	0.03	3	0.48	0.077
	Edgewater Medical Center, Chicago	8.4	0.0%	0.81	No	0.26	2	0.42	0.064
	Good Samaritan Hospital, Downers Grove	8.9	0.0%	0.88	No	0.00	4	0.66	0.089
	Gottlieb Memorial Hospital, Melrose Park	9.3	0.0%	0.94	No	0.01	4	0.64	0.099
	Ingalls Memorial Hospital, Harvey	8.0	0.0%	0.93	No	0.00	3	0.42	0.066
	La Grange Memorial Health System, La Grange	8.6	0.0%	0.96	No	0.12	3	0.60	0.065
	Little Company of Mary Hospital, Evergreen Park	8.0	0.0%	1.09	No	0.03	3	1.01	0.029
	Memorial Hospital, Belleville	8.7	0.0%	0.76	No	0.02	4	0.58	0.022
	Mercy Center for Health Care Services, Aurora	6.7	0.0%	1.14	No	0.00	2	0.56	0.149
	Methodist Medical Center of Illinois, Peoria	8.2	0.0%	1.48	No	0.06	5	1.36	0.102
	Northwest Community Hospital, Arlington Heights	9.5	0.0%	0.94	No	0.00	4	0.72	0.113
	Oak Park Hospital, Oak Park	7.5	0.0%	0.89	No	0.00	3	0.44	0.067
	Ravenswood Hospital Medical Center, Chicago	9.1	0.0%	1.07	No	0.30	3	0.98	0.063
	Resurrection Medical Center, Chicago	6.2	0.0%	1.07	No	0.08	2	0.38	0.029
	Riverside Medical Center, Kankakee	4.4	0.0%	1.52	No	0.00	3	0.62	0.024
	Rockford Memorial Hospital, Rockford	7.7	0.4%	1.22	No	0.01	4	0.80	0.025
	Sherman Hospital, Elgin	8.4	0.0%	1.02	No	0.00	4	0.95	0.123
	St. Anthony's Health Center, Alton	9.1	0.0%	0.90	No	0.00	4	0.85	0.092
	St. Elizabeth Medical Center, Granite City	7.4	0.0%	0.98	No	0.00	3	0.52	0.012
	St. Elizabeth's Hospital, Belleville	8.6	0.0%	0.82	No	0.04	4	0.53	0.023
	St. Francis Hospital, Evanston	8.4	0.0%	0.99	No	0.36	4	0.57	0.071

Natl. Rank	Hospital	U.S. News index	Reputa-tional score	Hospital-wide mortality rate	COTH member	Interns and residents to beds	Tech-nology score (of 5)	R.N.'s to beds	Board-certified internists to beds
	St. Francis Medical Center, Peoria	9.3	0.0%	1.05	No	0.29	4	0.90	0.036
	St. James Hospital and Health Center, Chicago Heights	8.2	0.0%	0.83	No	0.00	2	0.45	0.136
	St. Joseph Hospital and Health Care Center, Chicago	8.7	0.0%	1.04	No	0.32	3	0.66	0.071
	St. Joseph Medical Center, Joliet	7.5	0.0%	1.23	No	0.00	4	1.06	0.028
	St. Mary of Nazareth Hospital Center, Chicago	7.4	0.0%	1.24	No	0.17	3	1.08	0.007
	St. Mary's Hospital of Kankakee, Kankakee	6.3	0.0%	1.26	No	0.00	4	0.60	0.052
	St. Mary's Hospital, Decatur	5.5	0.0%	1.10	No	0.01	3	0.52	0.030
	Swedish American Hospital, Rockford	8.4	0.0%	0.98	No	0.03	3	0.65	0.090
	Swedish Covenant Hospital, Chicago	8.5	0.0%	1.01	No	0.14	3	0.72	0.070
	Trinity Medical Center, Moline	6.2	0.0%	1.34	No	0.00	4	0.80	0.032
	West Suburban Hospital Medical Center, Oak Park	9.3	0.0%	0.98	No	0.28	3	0.82	0.051

UROLOGY

Natl. Rank	Hospital	U.S. News index	Reputa-tional score	Urology mortality rate	COTH member	Interns and residents to beds	Tech-nology score (of 11)	R.N.'s to beds	Board-certified internists to beds	Procedures to beds
	TIER TWO									
44	Cook County Hospital, Chicago	18.7	0.6%	0.50	Yes	1.00	6	1.43	0.073	0.61
65	F.G. McGaw Hospital at Loyola University, Maywood	16.8	0.5%	1.17	Yes	1.46	9	1.59	0.053	1.90
52	Northwestern Memorial Hospital, Chicago	17.7	4.5%	1.20	Yes	0.43	10	1.03	0.134	1.52
43	Rush-Presbyterian-St. Luke's Medical Center, Chicago	18.7	0.0%	0.79	Yes	1.05	10	1.24	0.224	1.92
32	University of Chicago Hospitals	19.8	1.1%	0.96	Yes	1.64	10	1.38	0.074	1.68
62	University of Illinois Hospital and Clinics, Chicago	17.2	0.0%	0.99	Yes	1.29	7	1.95	0.056	1.11
	TIER THREE									
	Columbus Hospital, Chicago	9.6	0.0%	1.04	No	0.40	8	0.82	0.144	2.28
	Edgewater Medical Center, Chicago	10.5	0.0%	0.60	No	0.26	5	0.42	0.064	2.30
	Elmhurst Memorial Hospital, Elmhurst	9.2	0.0%	0.95	No	0.00	8	1.01	0.111	1.83
	Evanston Hospital, Evanston	12.6	0.0%	1.05	Yes	0.26	9	1.18	0.160	1.78
	Grant Hospital of Chicago	11.1	0.0%	0.46	No	0.24	5	0.63	0.090	2.25
	Holy Family Hospital, Des Plaines	8.6	0.0%	0.93	No	0.01	5	1.14	0.055	1.75
	Illinois Masonic Medical Center, Chicago	9.3	0.0%	1.25	Yes	0.43	7	0.73	0.068	0.69
	Little Company of Mary Hospital, Evergreen Park	11.0	0.0%	0.76	No	0.03	7	1.01	0.029	2.38
	Louis A. Weiss Memorial Hospital, Chicago	11.7	0.0%	0.66	No	0.37	5	0.63	0.227	1.46
	Lutheran General Healthsystem, Park Ridge	11.2	0.0%	1.07	Yes	0.42	8	0.82	0.076	1.47
	Memorial Hospital, Belleville	9.6	0.0%	0.59	No	0.02	5	0.58	0.022	1.42
	Memorial Medical Center, Springfield	10.9	0.0%	1.14	Yes	0.28	8	0.89	0.115	2.10
	Mercy Hospital and Medical Center, Chicago	12.2	0.0%	0.91	Yes	0.38	7	0.90	0.035	1.36
97	Michael Reese Hospital and Medical Center, Chicago	14.6	0.0%	0.67	Yes	0.36	3	1.28	0.064	0.78
	Mount Sinai Hospital Medical Center, Chicago	8.9	0.0%	1.31	Yes	0.54	7	0.72	0.000	0.83
	Rush North Shore Medical Center, Skokie	10.8	0.0%	0.80	No	0.22	4	0.93	0.296	2.09
	Sherman Hospital, Elgin	11.1	0.0%	0.56	No	0.00	5	0.95	0.123	1.39
	St. Elizabeth Medical Center, Granite City	8.7	0.0%	0.56	No	0.00	3	0.52	0.012	1.30
	St. Elizabeth's Hospital, Belleville	9.5	0.0%	0.73	No	0.04	5	0.53	0.023	1.53
	St. Francis Medical Center, Peoria	9.2	0.0%	0.98	No	0.29	9	0.90	0.036	1.37
	St. James Hospital and Health Center, Chicago Heights	10.2	0.0%	0.60	No	0.00	6	0.45	0.136	1.55
	St. John's Hospital, Springfield	12.2	0.0%	0.91	Yes	0.22	8	0.76	0.123	1.33
	Swedish American Hospital, Rockford	11.0	0.0%	0.73	No	0.03	7	0.65	0.090	2.14
	TIER FOUR									
	Alexian Brothers Medical Center, Elk Grove Village	6.0	0.0%	1.32	No	0.00	7	0.96	0.118	1.40
	Blessing Hospital, Quincy	7.7	0.0%	1.06	No	0.04	7	0.84	0.043	3.28
	Carle Foundation Hospital, Urbana	2.7	0.0%	1.40	No	0.05	2	0.53	0.043	0.97
	Central Du Page Hospital, Winfield	5.8	0.0%	1.10	No	0.00	4	0.81	0.077	1.12
	Christ Hospital and Medical Center, Oak Lawn	4.5	0.0%	1.52	No	0.33	7	0.52	0.040	1.36
	Copley Memorial Hospital, Aurora	3.9	0.0%	1.65	No	0.00	7	0.68	0.104	1.53
	Covenant Medical Center, Urbana	5.8	0.0%	1.33	No	0.04	9	0.79	0.054	1.66

Natl. Rank	Hospital	U.S. News index	Reputa-tional score	Urology mortality rate	COTH member	Interns and residents to beds	Tech-nology score (of 11)	R.N.'s to beds	Board-certified internists to beds	Procedures to beds
	Decatur Memorial Hospital, Decatur	4.7	0.0%	1.31	No	0.03	7	0.48	0.077	1.62
	Good Samaritan Hospital, Downers Grove	7.4	0.0%	0.95	No	0.00	5	0.66	0.089	1.81
	Gottlieb Memorial Hospital, Melrose Park	6.0	0.0%	1.13	No	0.01	6	0.64	0.099	1.38
	Hinsdale Hospital, Hinsdale	4.1	0.0%	1.68	No	0.12	8	0.69	0.062	1.20
	Ingalls Memorial Hospital, Harvey	5.8	0.0%	1.11	No	0.00	8	0.42	0.066	1.33
	La Grange Memorial Health System, La Grange	7.5	0.0%	0.95	No	0.12	5	0.60	0.065	2.22
	MacNeal Hospital, Berwyn	8.4	0.0%	1.38	Yes	0.28	4	1.05	0.052	2.09
	Memorial Hospital of Carbondale, Carbondale	3.8	0.0%	2.18	No	0.16	7	1.07	0.040	2.23
	Methodist Medical Center of Illinois, Peoria	5.1	0.0%	2.15	No	0.06	9	1.36	0.102	1.82
	Northwest Community Hospital, Arlington Heights	5.5	0.0%	1.38	No	0.00	8	0.72	0.113	2.04
	Oak Park Hospital, Oak Park	8.1	0.0%	0.88	No	0.00	7	0.44	0.067	2.06
	Ravenswood Hospital Medical Center, Chicago	5.2	0.0%	1.58	No	0.30	6	0.98	0.063	1.02
	Resurrection Medical Center, Chicago	3.0	0.0%	1.54	No	0.08	6	0.38	0.029	1.70
	Riverside Medical Center, Kankakee	3.8	0.0%	1.46	No	0.00	7	0.62	0.024	1.39
	Rockford Memorial Hospital, Rockford	4.2	0.0%	1.53	No	0.01	8	0.80	0.025	1.04
	St. Anthony Medical Center, Rockford	7.9	0.0%	1.18	No	0.04	7	1.48	0.038	1.81
	St. Anthony's Health Center, Alton	6.3	0.0%	1.27	No	0.00	8	0.85	0.092	2.19
	St. Francis Hospital, Evanston	6.1	0.0%	1.31	No	0.36	8	0.57	0.071	1.24
	St. Joseph Hospital and Health Care Center, Chicago	7.1	0.0%	1.13	No	0.32	7	0.66	0.071	1.07
	St. Joseph Medical Center, Joliet	5.4	0.0%	1.50	No	0.00	9	1.06	0.028	1.62
	St. Mary of Nazareth Hospital Center, Chicago	3.9	0.0%	1.93	No	0.17	7	1.08	0.007	1.15
	St. Mary's Hospital of Kankakee, Kankakee	4.2	0.0%	1.58	No	0.00	9	0.60	0.052	1.84
	St. Mary's Hospital, Decatur	3.0	0.0%	1.50	No	0.01	5	0.52	0.030	1.35
	Swedish Covenant Hospital, Chicago	5.4	0.0%	1.38	No	0.14	7	0.72	0.070	2.13
	Trinity Medical Center, Moline	3.3	0.0%	1.95	No	0.00	9	0.80	0.032	1.47
	West Suburban Hospital Medical Center, Oak Park	8.5	0.0%	0.99	No	0.28	7	0.82	0.051	1.69

AIDS

Natl. Rank	Hospital	U.S. News index	Reputational score	Hospital-wide mortality rate	COTH member	Interns and residents to beds	Technology score (of 11)	Discharge planning (of 2)	R.N.'s to beds	Board-certified internists to beds
	TIER TWO									
70	Indiana University Medical Center, Indianapolis	26.0	0.3%	1.14	Yes	1.10	11	2	1.86	0.107
89	William N. Wishard Memorial Hospital, Indianapolis	25.1	0.0%	0.90	Yes	0.38	6	2	1.20	0.123
	TIER THREE									
	Caylor-Nickel Medical Center, Bluffton	21.1	0.0%	0.79	No	0.00	6	2	0.26	0.025
	Columbus Regional Hospital, Columbus	21.9	0.0%	0.86	No	0.00	5	2	1.00	0.035
	TIER FOUR									
	Ball Memorial Hospital, Muncie	16.7	0.0%	1.23	No	0.24	7	2	0.23	0.014
	Bloomington Hospital, Bloomington	18.4	0.0%	1.03	No	0.00	6	1	0.61	0.033
	Deaconess Hospital, Evansville	17.7	0.0%	1.23	No	0.05	7	2	1.04	0.043
	Floyd Memorial Hospital, New Albany	18.6	0.0%	1.05	No	0.00	6	2	0.56	0.011
	Good Samaritan Hospital, Vincennes	17.2	0.0%	1.14	No	0.00	6	1	0.86	0.021
	Lafayette Home Hospital, Lafayette	15.9	0.0%	1.34	No	0.00	6	2	0.80	0.084
	Lakeshore Health System, East Chicago	15.9	0.0%	1.28	No	0.00	6	2	0.60	0.007
	Lutheran Hospital of Indiana, Fort Wayne	17.7	0.0%	1.20	No	0.05	6	2	1.06	0.021
	Memorial Hospital of South Bend, South Bend	17.5	0.0%	1.30	No	0.09	7	2	1.30	0.042
	Methodist Hospitals, Gary	17.8	0.0%	1.06	No	0.03	6	1	0.58	0.011
	Parkview Memorial Hospital, Fort Wayne	18.5	0.0%	1.07	No	0.01	6	2	0.72	0.012
	Porter Memorial Hospital, Valparaiso	17.4	0.0%	1.13	No	0.00	6	1	0.89	0.024
	Reid Hospital and Health Care Services, Richmond	19.0	0.0%	1.07	No	0.00	7	2	0.69	0.043
	St. Anthony Medical Center, Crown Point	14.7	0.0%	1.37	No	0.00	7	1	0.58	0.027
	St. Elizabeth Hospital Medical Center, Lafayette	18.4	0.0%	1.09	No	0.00	7	1	0.90	0.052
	St. Francis Hospital and Health Centers, Beech Grove	18.6	0.0%	1.17	No	0.09	7	2	1.20	0.014
	St. Joseph Medical Center, Fort Wayne	16.4	0.0%	1.18	No	0.02	4	2	0.63	0.030
	St. Joseph's Medical Center, South Bend	18.2	0.0%	1.24	No	0.12	7	2	1.26	0.068
	St. Margaret Mercy Health Centers, Hammond	16.4	0.0%	1.25	No	0.00	6	2	0.54	0.089
	St. Mary's Medical Center, Evansville	18.9	0.0%	0.97	No	0.06	6	1	0.32	0.026
	St. Vincent Hospital and Health Center, Indianapolis	17.4	0.0%	1.32	No	0.22	7	2	1.13	0.086
	Union Hospital, Terre Haute	18.7	0.0%	1.17	No	0.08	6	2	1.53	0.017
	Welborn Memorial Baptist Hospital, Evansville	15.2	0.0%	1.49	No	0.01	8	2	0.74	0.046

CANCER

Natl. Rank	Hospital	U.S. News index	Reputational score	Cancer mortality rate	COTH member	Interns and residents to beds	Technology score (of 12)	R.N.'s to beds	Board-certified oncologists to beds	Procedures to beds
	TIER ONE									
16	Indiana University Medical Center, Indianapolis	18.4	3.4%	0.57	Yes	1.10	11	1.86	0.022	1.31
	TIER THREE									
	Methodist Hospital of Indiana, Indianapolis	10.2	0.0%	1.06	Yes	0.36	10	1.68	0.009	1.47
	St. Joseph's Medical Center, South Bend	5.4	0.0%	1.40	No	0.12	9	1.26	0.012	1.86
	St. Vincent Hospital and Health Center, Indianapolis	5.4	0.0%	1.15	No	0.22	9	1.13	0.009	1.42
	Union Hospital, Terre Haute	5.8	0.0%	0.91	No	0.08	7	1.53	0.003	2.30
	William N. Wishard Memorial Hospital, Indianapolis	7.1	0.0%	0.85	Yes	0.38	3	1.20	0.027	0.64
	TIER FOUR									
	Ball Memorial Hospital, Muncie	3.9	0.5%	0.85	No	0.24	9	0.23	0.004	1.49
	Bloomington Hospital, Bloomington	3.1	0.0%	1.08	No	0.00	8	0.61	0.004	1.88
	Columbus Regional Hospital, Columbus	3.9	0.0%	0.85	No	0.00	7	1.00	0.005	0.98
	Community Hospitals, Indianapolis	2.4	0.0%	1.11	No	0.21	0	0.99	0.011	1.13
	Deaconess Hospital, Evansville	4.7	0.0%	0.78	No	0.05	8	1.04	0.002	1.56
	Floyd Memorial Hospital, New Albany	2.9	0.0%	0.80	No	0.00	7	0.56	0.004	1.45
	Good Samaritan Hospital, Vincennes	4.1	0.0%	0.73	No	0.00	7	0.86	0.000	3.04

Natl. Rank	Hospital	U.S. News index	Reputational score	Cancer mortality rate	COTH member	Interns and residents to beds	Technology score (of 12)	R.N.'s to beds	Board-certified oncologists to beds	Procedures to beds
	Lafayette Home Hospital, Lafayette	2.5	0.0%	1.13	No	0.00	5	0.80	0.000	0.84
	Lakeshore Health System, East Chicago	2.8	0.0%	1.11	No	0.00	8	0.60	0.005	0.64
	Lutheran Hospital of Indiana, Fort Wayne	4.3	0.0%	0.86	No	0.05	7	1.06	0.013	1.04
	Memorial Hospital of South Bend, South Bend	5.1	0.0%	1.31	No	0.09	8	1.30	0.016	1.41
	Methodist Hospitals, Gary	2.7	0.0%	0.88	No	0.03	7	0.58	0.013	0.29
	Parkview Memorial Hospital, Fort Wayne	3.9	0.0%	0.64	No	0.01	8	0.72	0.007	1.26
	Porter Memorial Hospital, Valparaiso	3.4	0.0%	0.82	No	0.00	6	0.89	0.003	0.92
	Reid Hospital and Health Care Services, Richmond	3.1	0.0%	1.26	No	0.00	8	0.69	0.006	1.73
	St. Anthony Medical Center, Crown Point	2.8	0.0%	1.16	No	0.00	8	0.58	0.018	0.71
	St. Elizabeth Hospital Medical Center, Lafayette	3.9	0.0%	1.10	No	0.00	8	0.90	0.008	1.81
	St. Francis Hospital and Health Centers, Beech Grove	4.6	0.0%	1.55	No	0.09	8	1.20	0.009	1.44
	St. Joseph Medical Center, Fort Wayne	1.9	0.0%	0.49	No	0.02	2	0.63	0.004	0.98
	St. Margaret Mercy Health Centers, Hammond	2.5	0.0%	1.08	No	0.00	7	0.54	0.016	0.80
	St. Mary's Medical Center, Evansville	2.6	0.0%	0.84	No	0.06	8	0.32	0.002	1.29
	Terre Haute Regional Hospital, Terre Haute	2.3	0.0%	0.96	No	0.00	6	0.58	0.004	0.88
	Welborn Memorial Baptist Hospital, Evansville	3.8	0.0%	1.15	No	0.01	10	0.74	0.003	1.14

CARDIOLOGY

Natl. Rank	Hospital	U.S. News index	Reputational score	Cardiology mortality rate	COTH member	Interns and residents to beds	Technology score (of 10)	R.N.'s to beds	Board-certified cardiologists to beds	Procedures to beds
TIER TWO										
54	Indiana University Medical Center, Indianapolis	22.8	3.3%	1.36	Yes	1.10	10	1.86	0.047	2.54
62	William N. Wishard Memorial Hospital, Indianapolis	22.1	0.0%	0.69	Yes	0.38	5	1.20	0.059	3.00
TIER THREE										
	Columbus Regional Hospital, Columbus	14.8	0.0%	0.94	No	0.00	4	1.00	0.015	7.98
	Methodist Hospital of Indiana, Indianapolis	15.9	0.0%	1.23	Yes	0.36	8	1.68	0.027	6.55
	Methodist Hospitals, Gary	16.3	0.0%	0.79	No	0.03	7	0.58	0.029	1.96
	St. Francis Hospital and Health Centers, Beech Grove	14.6	0.0%	1.06	No	0.09	9	1.20	0.033	8.83
TIER FOUR										
	Ball Memorial Hospital, Muncie	6.2	0.0%	1.38	No	0.24	8	0.23	0.008	6.69
	Bloomington Hospital, Bloomington	13.2	0.0%	0.99	No	0.00	7	0.61	0.015	6.80
	Community Hospitals, Indianapolis	9.8	0.0%	1.15	No	0.21	0	0.99	0.034	4.96
	Deaconess Hospital, Evansville	10.6	0.0%	1.25	No	0.05	9	1.04	0.025	10.68
	Floyd Memorial Hospital, New Albany	8.6	0.0%	1.18	No	0.00	5	0.56	0.011	7.84
	Good Samaritan Hospital, Vincennes	4.5	0.0%	1.58	No	0.00	6	0.86	0.010	7.14
	Lafayette Home Hospital, Lafayette	6.9	0.0%	1.34	No	0.00	6	0.80	0.018	4.32
	Lakeshore Health System, East Chicago	7.8	0.0%	1.27	No	0.00	7	0.60	0.021	4.81
	Lutheran Hospital of Indiana, Fort Wayne	8.3	0.0%	1.42	No	0.05	7	1.06	0.059	8.74
	Memorial Hospital of South Bend, South Bend	11.9	0.0%	1.21	No	0.09	8	1.30	0.047	6.29
	Parkview Memorial Hospital, Fort Wayne	9.0	0.0%	1.22	No	0.01	6	0.72	0.033	6.92
	Porter Memorial Hospital, Valparaiso	7.3	0.0%	1.38	No	0.00	8	0.89	0.011	5.88
	Reid Hospital and Health Care Services, Richmond	12.6	0.0%	1.02	No	0.00	7	0.69	0.006	7.88
	St. Anthony Medical Center, Crown Point	7.6	0.0%	1.37	No	0.00	9	0.58	0.052	5.26
	St. Elizabeth Hospital Medical Center, Lafayette	10.8	0.0%	1.18	No	0.00	9	0.90	0.016	8.33
	St. Joseph Medical Center, Fort Wayne	8.4	0.0%	1.28	No	0.02	7	0.63	0.034	8.78
	St. Joseph's Medical Center, South Bend	10.6	0.0%	1.29	No	0.12	8	1.26	0.035	8.50
	St. Margaret Mercy Health Centers, Hammond	9.2	0.0%	1.22	No	0.00	9	0.54	0.035	4.90
	St. Mary's Medical Center, Evansville	9.7	0.0%	1.13	No	0.06	8	0.32	0.013	5.13
	St. Vincent Hospital and Health Center, Indianapolis	12.5	2.3%	1.49	No	0.22	9	1.13	0.059	10.44
	Terre Haute Regional Hospital, Terre Haute	9.4	0.0%	1.16	No	0.00	7	0.58	0.018	4.37
	Union Hospital, Terre Haute	12.1	0.0%	1.20	No	0.08	7	1.53	0.010	10.48
	Welborn Memorial Baptist Hospital, Evansville	6.5	0.0%	1.44	No	0.01	9	0.74	0.014	4.73

STATE RANKINGS ■ INDIANA

ENDOCRINOLOGY

Natl. Rank Hospital	U.S. News index	Reputa-tional score	Endocrinology mortality rate	COTH member	Interns and residents to beds	Tech-nology score (of 11)	R.N.'s to beds	Board-certified internists to beds
TIER TWO								
60 Indiana University Medical Center, Indianapolis	16.3	0.5%	1.14	Yes	1.10	10	1.86	0.107
TIER THREE								
Howard Community Hospital, Kokomo	10.0	0.0%	0.56	No	0.00	7	0.83	0.039
Methodist Hospital of Indiana, Indianapolis	12.4	0.5%	1.20	Yes	0.36	9	1.68	0.044
St. Elizabeth Hospital Medical Center, Lafayette	10.6	0.0%	0.57	No	0.00	9	0.90	0.052
St. Joseph's Medical Center, South Bend	8.2	0.0%	1.04	No	0.12	8	1.26	0.068
St. Mary's Medical Center, Evansville	9.1	0.0%	0.43	No	0.06	9	0.32	0.026
Terre Haute Regional Hospital, Terre Haute	8.2	0.0%	0.73	No	0.00	7	0.58	0.022
William N. Wishard Memorial Hospital, Indianapolis	10.4	0.0%	1.12	Yes	0.38	4	1.20	0.123
TIER FOUR								
Ball Memorial Hospital, Muncie	3.5	0.0%	1.52	No	0.24	9	0.23	0.014
Bloomington Hospital, Bloomington	6.7	0.0%	0.90	No	0.00	8	0.61	0.033
Columbus Regional Hospital, Columbus	8.1	0.0%	0.87	No	0.00	8	1.00	0.035
Community Hospitals, Indianapolis	7.1	0.0%	0.92	No	0.21	0	0.99	0.085
Deaconess Hospital, Evansville	6.7	0.0%	1.14	No	0.05	9	1.04	0.043
Floyd Memorial Hospital, New Albany	3.7	0.0%	1.40	No	0.00	8	0.56	0.011
Good Samaritan Hospital, Vincennes	6.7	0.0%	0.98	No	0.00	8	0.86	0.021
Lafayette Home Hospital, Lafayette	5.0	0.0%	1.27	No	0.00	6	0.80	0.084
Lakeshore Health System, East Chicago	4.2	0.0%	1.35	No	0.00	9	0.60	0.007
Lutheran Hospital of Indiana, Fort Wayne	6.8	0.0%	1.01	No	0.05	6	1.06	0.021
Memorial Hospital of South Bend, South Bend	4.9	0.0%	1.97	No	0.09	8	1.30	0.042
Methodist Hospitals, Gary	4.6	0.0%	1.22	No	0.03	8	0.58	0.011
Parkview Memorial Hospital, Fort Wayne	4.8	0.0%	1.25	No	0.01	8	0.72	0.012
Porter Memorial Hospital, Valparaiso	5.9	0.0%	1.09	No	0.00	7	0.89	0.024
Reid Hospital and Health Care Services, Richmond	7.9	0.0%	0.82	No	0.00	9	0.69	0.043
St. Anthony Medical Center, Crown Point	4.2	0.0%	1.38	No	0.00	9	0.58	0.027
St. Francis Hospital and Health Centers, Beech Grove	7.6	0.0%	1.04	No	0.09	9	1.20	0.014
St. Joseph Medical Center, Fort Wayne	3.5	0.0%	1.30	No	0.02	3	0.63	0.030
St. Margaret Mercy Health Centers, Hammond	3.9	0.0%	1.51	No	0.00	8	0.54	0.089
St. Vincent Hospital and Health Center, Indianapolis	7.6	0.0%	1.23	No	0.22	10	1.13	0.086
Union Hospital, Terre Haute	6.8	0.0%	1.32	No	0.08	7	1.53	0.017
Welborn Memorial Baptist Hospital, Evansville	4.8	0.0%	1.43	No	0.01	10	0.74	0.046

GASTROENTEROLOGY

Natl. Rank Hospital	U.S. News index	Reputa-tional score	Gastro-enterology mortality rate	COTH member	Interns and residents to beds	Tech-nology score (of 11)	R.N.'s to beds	Board-certified gastro-enterologists to beds	Pro-cedures to beds
TIER ONE									
17 Indiana University Medical Center, Indianapolis	21.8	5.6%	1.33	Yes	1.10	10	1.86	0.030	1.33
TIER THREE									
Columbus Regional Hospital, Columbus	8.7	0.0%	0.82	No	0.00	7	1.00	0.010	3.79
Methodist Hospital of Indiana, Indianapolis	11.5	0.0%	1.15	Yes	0.36	9	1.68	0.009	2.56
St. Francis Hospital and Health Centers, Beech Grove	7.6	0.0%	1.08	No	0.09	8	1.20	0.014	3.78
Union Hospital, Terre Haute	7.4	0.0%	1.22	No	0.08	6	1.53	0.007	4.48
TIER FOUR									
Ball Memorial Hospital, Muncie	4.4	0.0%	1.28	No	0.24	8	0.23	0.006	3.16
Bloomington Hospital, Bloomington	7.3	0.0%	0.90	No	0.00	7	0.61	0.015	4.41
Community Hospitals, Indianapolis	4.4	0.0%	1.06	No	0.21	0	0.99	0.015	2.25
Deaconess Hospital, Evansville	5.6	0.0%	1.39	No	0.05	8	1.04	0.013	3.79
Floyd Memorial Hospital, New Albany	4.8	0.0%	1.22	No	0.00	7	0.56	0.004	3.92
Good Samaritan Hospital, Vincennes	6.6	0.0%	1.08	No	0.00	8	0.86	0.003	3.91
Lafayette Home Hospital, Lafayette	2.0	0.0%	1.93	No	0.00	6	0.80	0.011	2.43

Natl. Rank	Hospital	U.S. News index	Reputa- tional score	Gastro- enterology mortality rate	COTH member	Interns and residents to beds	Tech- nology score (of 11)	R.N.'s to beds	Board- certified gastro- enterologists to beds	Pro- cedures to beds
	Lakeshore Health System, East Chicago	3.7	0.0%	1.26	No	0.00	8	0.60	0.007	1.69
	Lutheran Hospital of Indiana, Fort Wayne	5.9	0.0%	1.14	No	0.05	7	1.06	0.008	2.75
	Memorial Hospital of South Bend, South Bend	4.6	0.0%	1.60	No	0.09	7	1.30	0.010	2.55
	Parkview Memorial Hospital, Fort Wayne	4.6	0.0%	1.18	No	0.01	7	0.72	0.010	2.51
	Porter Memorial Hospital, Valparaiso	6.3	0.0%	0.94	No	0.00	6	0.89	0.005	2.78
	Reid Hospital and Health Care Services, Richmond	3.8	0.0%	1.63	No	0.00	8	0.69	0.006	3.77
	St. Anthony Medical Center, Crown Point	3.7	0.0%	1.28	No	0.00	8	0.58	0.009	1.93
	St. Elizabeth Hospital Medical Center, Lafayette	6.1	0.0%	1.07	No	0.00	8	0.90	0.012	2.90
	St. Joseph Medical Center, Fort Wayne	1.4	0.0%	1.75	No	0.02	3	0.63	0.011	2.76
	St. Joseph's Medical Center, South Bend	6.3	0.0%	1.46	No	0.12	8	1.26	0.009	4.01
	St. Margaret Mercy Health Centers, Hammond	3.4	0.0%	1.35	No	0.00	8	0.54	0.012	1.96
	St. Mary's Medical Center, Evansville	3.6	0.0%	1.21	No	0.06	8	0.32	0.011	1.87
	St. Vincent Hospital and Health Center, Indianapolis	5.7	0.0%	1.40	No	0.22	9	1.13	0.013	2.13
	Welborn Memorial Baptist Hospital, Evansville	3.5	0.0%	1.64	No	0.01	9	0.74	0.006	2.51

GERIATRICS

Natl. Rank	Hospital	U.S. News index	Reputa- tional score	Hospital- wide mortality rate	COTH member	Service mix	Interns and residents to beds	Tech- nology score (of 13)	R.N.'s to beds	Discharge planning (of 2)	Geriatric services (of 9)	Board- certified internists to beds
TIER TWO												
69	William N. Wishard Memorial Hospital, Indianapolis	22.7	0.0%	0.90	Yes	7	0.38	5	1.20	2	6	0.123
TIER THREE												
	Columbus Regional Hospital, Columbus	18.7	0.0%	0.86	No	6	0.00	8	1.00	2	4	0.035
	Indiana University Medical Center, Indianapolis	20.0	0.0%	1.14	Yes	8	1.10	13	1.86	2	2	0.107
	Methodist Hospital of Indiana, Indianapolis	19.4	0.6%	1.16	Yes	8	0.36	11	1.68	2	6	0.044
	St. Mary's Medical Center, Evansville	14.4	0.0%	0.97	No	7	0.06	10	0.32	1	3	0.026
TIER FOUR												
	Ball Memorial Hospital, Muncie	9.0	0.0%	1.23	No	6	0.24	11	0.23	2	2	0.014
	Bloomington Hospital, Bloomington	13.3	0.0%	1.03	No	6	0.00	10	0.61	1	5	0.033
	Deaconess Hospital, Evansville	11.7	0.0%	1.23	No	8	0.05	11	1.04	2	4	0.043
	Floyd Memorial Hospital, New Albany	12.1	0.0%	1.05	No	4	0.00	9	0.56	2	3	0.011
	Good Samaritan Hospital, Vincennes	9.2	0.0%	1.14	No	5	0.00	8	0.86	1	1	0.021
	Lafayette Home Hospital, Lafayette	6.9	0.0%	1.34	No	4	0.00	7	0.80	2	4	0.084
	Lakeshore Health System, East Chicago	7.6	0.0%	1.28	No	6	0.00	9	0.60	2	1	0.007
	Lutheran Hospital of Indiana, Fort Wayne	10.6	0.0%	1.20	No	6	0.05	8	1.06	2	3	0.021
	Memorial Hospital of South Bend, South Bend	11.1	0.0%	1.30	No	8	0.09	10	1.30	2	5	0.042
	Methodist Hospitals, Gary	11.3	0.0%	1.06	No	6	0.03	9	0.58	1	2	0.011
	Parkview Memorial Hospital, Fort Wayne	12.6	0.0%	1.07	No	7	0.01	8	0.72	2	2	0.012
	Reid Hospital and Health Care Services, Richmond	13.3	0.0%	1.07	No	6	0.00	11	0.69	2	3	0.043
	St. Elizabeth Hospital Medical Center, Lafayette	11.4	0.0%	1.09	No	5	0.00	11	0.90	1	2	0.052
	St. Francis Hospital and Health Centers, Beech Grove	13.5	0.0%	1.17	No	7	0.09	11	1.20	2	7	0.014
	St. Joseph Medical Center, Fort Wayne	8.0	0.0%	1.18	No	3	0.02	5	0.63	2	2	0.030
	St. Joseph's Medical Center, South Bend	10.6	0.0%	1.24	No	3	0.12	11	1.26	2	6	0.068
	St. Margaret Mercy Health Centers, Hammond	9.1	0.0%	1.25	No	6	0.00	10	0.54	2	3	0.089
	St. Vincent Hospital and Health Center, Indianapolis	10.5	0.0%	1.32	No	7	0.22	11	1.13	2	4	0.086
	Terre Haute Regional Hospital, Terre Haute	9.4	0.0%	1.15	No	4	0.00	9	0.58	2	1	0.022
	Union Hospital, Terre Haute	11.5	0.0%	1.17	No	5	0.08	9	1.53	2	2	0.017
	Welborn Memorial Baptist Hospital, Evansville	5.5	0.0%	1.49	No	5	0.01	11	0.74	2	3	0.046

GYNECOLOGY

Natl. Rank	Hospital	U.S. News index	Reputational score	Hospital-wide mortality rate	Interns and residents to beds	Technology score (of 10)	R.N.'s to beds	Board-certified OB-GYNs to beds	Procedures to beds
	TIER TWO								
53	Indiana University Medical Center, Indianapolis	26.0	1.3%	1.14	1.10	9	1.86	0.043	0.49
	TIER THREE								
	Columbus Regional Hospital, Columbus	18.5	0.0%	0.86	0.00	6	1.00	0.030	0.61
	Methodist Hospital of Indiana, Indianapolis	18.2	0.5%	1.16	0.36	8	1.68	0.018	0.32
	St. Mary's Medical Center, Evansville	14.2	0.0%	0.97	0.06	8	0.32	0.021	0.33
	William N. Wishard Memorial Hospital, Indianapolis	20.2	0.0%	0.90	0.38	5	1.20	0.045	0.24
	TIER FOUR								
	Ball Memorial Hospital, Muncie	8.5	0.0%	1.23	0.24	8	0.23	0.012	0.46
	Bloomington Hospital, Bloomington	12.6	0.0%	1.03	0.00	6	0.61	0.037	0.68
	Deaconess Hospital, Evansville	10.8	0.0%	1.23	0.05	7	1.04	0.027	0.33
	Floyd Memorial Hospital, New Albany	11.2	0.0%	1.05	0.00	6	0.56	0.008	0.40
	Good Samaritan Hospital, Vincennes	11.0	0.0%	1.14	0.00	7	0.86	0.003	0.39
	Lafayette Home Hospital, Lafayette	7.3	0.0%	1.34	0.00	6	0.80	0.042	0.44
	Lakeshore Health System, East Chicago	7.4	0.0%	1.28	0.00	7	0.60	0.007	0.12
	Lutheran Hospital of Indiana, Fort Wayne	11.3	0.0%	1.20	0.05	7	1.06	0.016	0.56
	Memorial Hospital of South Bend, South Bend	11.3	0.0%	1.30	0.09	7	1.30	0.042	0.49
	Methodist Hospitals, Gary	12.2	0.0%	1.06	0.03	7	0.58	0.027	0.10
	Parkview Memorial Hospital, Fort Wayne	12.4	0.0%	1.07	0.01	7	0.72	0.021	0.35
	Porter Memorial Hospital, Valparaiso	11.0	0.0%	1.13	0.00	6	0.89	0.016	0.34
	Reid Hospital and Health Care Services, Richmond	12.0	0.0%	1.07	0.00	7	0.69	0.009	0.26
	St. Anthony Medical Center, Crown Point	6.3	0.0%	1.37	0.00	7	0.58	0.030	0.14
	St. Elizabeth Hospital Medical Center, Lafayette	13.3	0.0%	1.09	0.00	7	0.90	0.048	0.32
	St. Francis Hospital and Health Centers, Beech Grove	13.6	0.0%	1.17	0.09	8	1.20	0.030	0.46
	St. Joseph Medical Center, Fort Wayne	6.6	0.0%	1.18	0.02	3	0.63	0.007	0.22
	St. Joseph's Medical Center, South Bend	12.2	0.0%	1.24	0.12	7	1.26	0.041	0.46
	St. Margaret Mercy Health Centers, Hammond	8.2	0.0%	1.25	0.00	7	0.54	0.037	0.20
	St. Vincent Hospital and Health Center, Indianapolis	13.5	0.5%	1.32	0.22	9	1.13	0.046	0.44
	Terre Haute Regional Hospital, Terre Haute	8.6	0.0%	1.15	0.00	5	0.58	0.018	0.35
	Union Hospital, Terre Haute	13.2	0.0%	1.17	0.08	6	1.53	0.017	0.57
	Welborn Memorial Baptist Hospital, Evansville	6.7	0.0%	1.49	0.01	9	0.74	0.020	0.57

NEUROLOGY

Natl. Rank	Hospital	U.S. News index	Reputational score	Neurology mortality rate	COTH member	Interns and residents to beds	Technology score (of 9)	R.N.'s to beds	Board-certified neurologists to beds
	TIER TWO								
76	Indiana University Medical Center, Indianapolis	18.1	0.9%	1.16	Yes	1.10	8	1.86	0.018
	TIER THREE								
	Columbus Regional Hospital, Columbus	15.7	0.0%	0.53	No	0.00	6	1.00	0.025
	Community Hospitals, Indianapolis	13.8	0.0%	0.70	No	0.21	0	0.99	0.013
	Floyd Memorial Hospital, New Albany	13.6	0.0%	0.70	No	0.00	6	0.56	0.011
	Methodist Hospital of Indiana, Indianapolis	14.5	0.0%	1.05	Yes	0.36	7	1.68	0.010
	Methodist Hospitals, Gary	12.1	0.0%	0.83	No	0.03	6	0.58	0.011
	Parkview Memorial Hospital, Fort Wayne	11.1	0.0%	0.89	No	0.01	6	0.72	0.013
	William N. Wishard Memorial Hospital, Indianapolis	14.6	0.0%	1.02	Yes	0.38	4	1.20	0.037
	TIER FOUR								
	Ball Memorial Hospital, Muncie	4.5	0.0%	1.31	No	0.24	7	0.23	0.002
	Bloomington Hospital, Bloomington	7.7	0.0%	1.05	No	0.00	6	0.61	0.007
	Deaconess Hospital, Evansville	8.0	0.0%	1.16	No	0.05	7	1.04	0.009
	Good Samaritan Hospital, Vincennes	8.6	0.0%	1.04	No	0.00	7	0.86	0.003
	Lakeshore Health System, East Chicago	5.6	0.0%	1.22	No	0.00	7	0.60	0.003
	Lutheran Hospital of Indiana, Fort Wayne	10.1	0.0%	0.99	No	0.05	6	1.06	0.008

Natl. Rank	Hospital	U.S. News index	Reputational score	Neurology mortality rate	COTH member	Interns and residents to beds	Technology score (of 9)	R.N.'s to beds	Board-certified neurologists to beds
	Memorial Hospital of South Bend, South Bend	6.3	0.0%	1.35	No	0.09	6	1.30	0.005
	Reid Hospital and Health Care Services, Richmond	9.0	0.0%	0.98	No	0.00	7	0.69	0.003
	St. Anthony Medical Center, Crown Point	5.6	0.0%	1.25	No	0.00	7	0.58	0.009
	St. Elizabeth Hospital Medical Center, Lafayette	10.7	0.0%	0.95	No	0.00	7	0.90	0.012
	St. Francis Hospital and Health Centers, Beech Grove	9.6	0.0%	1.04	No	0.09	7	1.20	0.002
	St. Joseph Medical Center, Fort Wayne	9.9	0.0%	0.88	No	0.02	3	0.63	0.007
	St. Joseph's Medical Center, South Bend	7.6	0.0%	1.23	No	0.12	6	1.26	0.006
	St. Margaret Mercy Health Centers, Hammond	4.3	0.0%	1.33	No	0.00	6	0.54	0.006
	St. Mary's Medical Center, Evansville	10.7	0.0%	0.87	No	0.06	7	0.32	0.008
	St. Vincent Hospital and Health Center, Indianapolis	10.2	0.0%	1.09	No	0.22	8	1.13	0.013
	Welborn Memorial Baptist Hospital, Evansville	6.1	0.0%	1.28	No	0.01	8	0.74	0.009

ORTHOPEDICS

Natl. Rank	Hospital	U.S. News index	Reputational score	Orthopedics mortality rate	COTH member	Interns and residents to beds	Technology score (of 5)	R.N.'s to beds	Board-certified orthopedists to beds	Procedures to beds
	TIER TWO									
37	Indiana University Medical Center, Indianapolis	18.1	0.3%	0.85	Yes	1.10	5	1.86	0.042	1.37
79	William N. Wishard Memorial Hospital, Indianapolis	14.5	0.0%	0.31	Yes	0.38	3	1.20	0.056	0.77
	TIER THREE									
	Lakeshore Health System, East Chicago	8.4	0.0%	0.67	No	0.00	3	0.60	0.007	0.93
	Methodist Hospital of Indiana, Indianapolis	12.0	0.6%	1.20	Yes	0.36	3	1.68	0.019	2.31
	St. Elizabeth Hospital Medical Center, Lafayette	10.6	0.0%	0.50	No	0.00	4	0.90	0.028	2.57
	St. Mary's Medical Center, Evansville	8.4	0.0%	0.57	No	0.06	3	0.32	0.017	1.99
	St. Vincent Hospital and Health Center, Indianapolis	8.3	1.1%	1.40	No	0.22	4	1.13	0.032	2.73
	Union Hospital, Terre Haute	9.8	0.0%	0.75	No	0.08	2	1.53	0.017	2.46
	TIER FOUR									
	Ball Memorial Hospital, Muncie	4.3	0.0%	1.24	No	0.24	4	0.23	0.008	2.88
	Bloomington Hospital, Bloomington	5.2	0.0%	1.12	No	0.00	4	0.61	0.026	2.45
	Columbus Regional Hospital, Columbus	6.8	0.0%	0.90	No	0.00	2	1.00	0.030	3.49
	Deaconess Hospital, Evansville	6.9	0.0%	1.09	No	0.05	4	1.04	0.031	3.24
	Floyd Memorial Hospital, New Albany	5.1	0.0%	0.99	No	0.00	3	0.56	0.011	1.94
	Good Samaritan Hospital, Vincennes	7.3	0.0%	0.92	No	0.00	4	0.86	0.014	3.01
	Lafayette Home Hospital, Lafayette	6.9	0.0%	0.96	No	0.00	4	0.80	0.028	2.46
	Lutheran Hospital of Indiana, Fort Wayne	5.0	0.0%	1.21	No	0.05	2	1.06	0.029	3.43
	Memorial Hospital of South Bend, South Bend	6.5	0.0%	1.18	No	0.09	3	1.30	0.044	2.76
	Parkview Memorial Hospital, Fort Wayne	6.1	0.6%	1.05	No	0.01	2	0.72	0.021	3.51
	Porter Memorial Hospital, Valparaiso	7.1	0.0%	0.94	No	0.00	4	0.89	0.014	2.10
	Reid Hospital and Health Care Services, Richmond	3.7	0.0%	1.47	No	0.00	4	0.69	0.009	2.14
	St. Anthony Medical Center, Crown Point	6.1	0.0%	0.95	No	0.00	4	0.58	0.018	1.93
	St. Francis Hospital and Health Centers, Beech Grove	4.9	0.0%	1.67	No	0.09	4	1.20	0.023	2.65
	St. Joseph Medical Center, Fort Wayne	4.5	0.0%	1.03	No	0.02	2	0.63	0.019	2.32
	St. Joseph's Medical Center, South Bend	6.5	0.0%	1.27	No	0.12	3	1.26	0.038	4.51
	St. Margaret Mercy Health Centers, Hammond	4.5	0.0%	1.16	No	0.00	4	0.54	0.025	1.17
	Terre Haute Regional Hospital, Terre Haute	2.6	0.0%	1.28	No	0.00	2	0.58	0.007	1.22
	Welborn Memorial Baptist Hospital, Evansville	2.5	0.0%	1.96	No	0.01	4	0.74	0.011	1.79

OTOLARYNGOLOGY

Natl. Rank	Hospital	U.S. News index	Reputa-tional score	Hospital-wide mortality rate	COTH member	Interns and residents to beds	Tech-nology score (of 9)	R.N.'s to beds	Board-certified internists to beds	Procedures to beds
	TIER ONE									
27	**Indiana University Medical Center, Indianapolis**	**22.3**	1.9%	1.14	Yes	1.10	8	1.86	0.107	0.151
	TIER TWO									
81	**Methodist Hospital of Indiana, Indianapolis**	**14.6**	0.8%	1.16	Yes	0.36	7	1.68	0.044	0.277
	TIER THREE									
	St. Vincent Hospital and Health Center, Indianapolis	7.2	0.0%	1.32	No	0.22	8	1.13	0.086	0.126
	William N. Wishard Memorial Hospital, Indianapolis	10.1	0.0%	0.90	Yes	0.38	2	1.20	0.123	0.126
	TIER FOUR									
	Ball Memorial Hospital, Muncie	3.6	0.0%	1.23	No	0.24	7	0.23	0.014	0.239
	Bloomington Hospital, Bloomington	3.9	0.0%	1.03	No	0.00	6	0.61	0.033	0.278
	Caylor-Nickel Medical Center, Bluffton	3.0	0.0%	0.79	No	0.00	6	0.26	0.025	0.145
	Columbus Regional Hospital, Columbus	5.3	0.0%	0.86	No	0.00	6	1.00	0.035	0.485
	Community Hospitals, Indianapolis	4.6	0.0%	1.02	No	0.21	0	0.99	0.085	0.191
	Deaconess Hospital, Evansville	5.6	0.0%	1.23	No	0.05	7	1.04	0.043	0.416
	Floyd Memorial Hospital, New Albany	3.5	0.0%	1.05	No	0.00	6	0.56	0.011	0.444
	Good Samaritan Hospital, Vincennes	4.5	0.0%	1.14	No	0.00	6	0.86	0.021	0.388
	Howard Community Hospital, Kokomo	4.3	0.0%	1.00	No	0.00	5	0.83	0.039	0.157
	Lafayette Home Hospital, Lafayette	4.1	0.0%	1.34	No	0.00	4	0.80	0.084	0.235
	Lakeshore Health System, East Chicago	3.7	0.0%	1.28	No	0.00	7	0.60	0.007	0.135
	Lutheran Hospital of Indiana, Fort Wayne	4.7	0.0%	1.20	No	0.05	4	1.06	0.021	0.237
	Memorial Hospital of South Bend, South Bend	6.3	0.0%	1.30	No	0.09	6	1.30	0.042	0.229
	Methodist Hospitals, Gary	3.7	0.0%	1.06	No	0.03	6	0.58	0.011	0.069
	Parkview Memorial Hospital, Fort Wayne	4.1	0.0%	1.08	No	0.01	6	0.72	0.012	0.183
	Porter Memorial Hospital, Valparaiso	4.3	0.0%	1.13	No	0.00	5	0.89	0.024	0.236
	Reid Hospital and Health Care Services, Richmond	4.5	0.0%	1.07	No	0.00	7	0.69	0.043	0.368
	St. Anthony Medical Center, Crown Point	3.8	0.0%	1.38	No	0.00	7	0.58	0.027	0.158
	St. Elizabeth Hospital Medical Center, Lafayette	5.2	0.0%	1.09	No	0.00	7	0.90	0.052	0.187
	St. Francis Hospital and Health Centers, Beech Grove	6.1	0.0%	1.17	No	0.09	7	1.20	0.014	0.231
	St. Joseph Medical Center, Fort Wayne	2.5	0.0%	1.18	No	0.02	1	0.63	0.030	0.187
	St. Joseph's Medical Center, South Bend	6.5	0.0%	1.24	No	0.12	6	1.26	0.068	0.242
	St. Margaret Mercy Health Centers, Hammond	4.0	0.0%	1.26	No	0.00	6	0.54	0.089	0.133
	St. Mary's Medical Center, Evansville	3.5	0.0%	0.97	No	0.06	7	0.32	0.026	0.108
	Terre Haute Regional Hospital, Terre Haute	3.3	0.0%	1.15	No	0.00	5	0.58	0.022	0.083
	Union Hospital, Terre Haute	6.5	0.0%	1.17	No	0.08	5	1.53	0.017	0.265
	Welborn Memorial Baptist Hospital, Evansville	4.7	0.0%	1.49	No	0.01	8	0.74	0.046	0.169

RHEUMATOLOGY

Natl. Rank	Hospital	U.S. News index	Reputa-tional score	Hospital-wide mortality rate	COTH member	Interns and residents to beds	Tech-nology score (of 5)	R.N.'s to beds	Board-certified internists to beds
	TIER TWO								
42	**Indiana University Medical Center, Indianapolis**	**19.0**	0.8%	1.14	Yes	1.10	5	1.86	0.107
	TIER THREE								
	Columbus Regional Hospital, Columbus	9.7	0.0%	0.86	No	0.00	2	1.00	0.035
	Methodist Hospital of Indiana, Indianapolis	12.9	0.0%	1.16	Yes	0.36	3	1.68	0.044
	William N. Wishard Memorial Hospital, Indianapolis	14.5	0.0%	0.90	Yes	0.38	3	1.20	0.123
	TIER FOUR								
	Ball Memorial Hospital, Muncie	5.9	0.0%	1.23	No	0.24	4	0.23	0.014
	Bloomington Hospital, Bloomington	6.8	0.0%	1.03	No	0.00	4	0.61	0.033
	Community Hospitals, Indianapolis	6.1	0.0%	1.02	No	0.21	0	0.99	0.085
	Deaconess Hospital, Evansville	7.7	0.0%	1.23	No	0.05	4	1.04	0.043
	Floyd Memorial Hospital, New Albany	6.9	0.0%	1.05	No	0.00	3	0.56	0.011
	Good Samaritan Hospital, Vincennes	6.5	0.0%	1.14	No	0.00	4	0.86	0.021

Natl. Rank	Hospital	U.S. News index	Reputa-tional score	Hospital-wide mortality rate	COTH member	Interns and residents to beds	Tech-nology score (of 5)	R.N.'s to beds	Board-certified internists to beds
	Lafayette Home Hospital, Lafayette	6.6	0.0%	1.34	No	0.00	4	0.80	0.084
	Lakeshore Health System, East Chicago	5.4	0.0%	1.28	No	0.00	3	0.60	0.007
	Lutheran Hospital of Indiana, Fort Wayne	6.9	0.0%	1.20	No	0.05	2	1.06	0.021
	Memorial Hospital of South Bend, South Bend	7.6	0.0%	1.30	No	0.09	3	1.30	0.042
	Methodist Hospitals, Gary	5.9	0.0%	1.06	No	0.03	3	0.58	0.011
	Parkview Memorial Hospital, Fort Wayne	6.7	0.0%	1.08	No	0.01	2	0.72	0.012
	Porter Memorial Hospital, Valparaiso	6.7	0.0%	1.13	No	0.00	4	0.89	0.024
	Reid Hospital and Health Care Services, Richmond	7.7	0.0%	1.07	No	0.00	4	0.69	0.043
	St. Anthony Medical Center, Crown Point	4.4	0.0%	1.38	No	0.00	4	0.58	0.027
	St. Elizabeth Hospital Medical Center, Lafayette	7.2	0.0%	1.09	No	0.00	4	0.90	0.052
	St. Francis Hospital and Health Centers, Beech Grove	8.4	0.0%	1.17	No	0.09	4	1.20	0.014
	St. Joseph Medical Center, Fort Wayne	5.8	0.0%	1.18	No	0.02	2	0.63	0.030
	St. Joseph's Medical Center, South Bend	8.2	0.0%	1.24	No	0.12	3	1.26	0.068
	St. Margaret Mercy Health Centers, Hammond	6.4	0.0%	1.26	No	0.00	4	0.54	0.089
	St. Mary's Medical Center, Evansville	6.2	0.0%	0.97	No	0.06	3	0.32	0.026
	St. Vincent Hospital and Health Center, Indianapolis	8.3	0.0%	1.32	No	0.22	4	1.13	0.086
	Terre Haute Regional Hospital, Terre Haute	5.8	0.0%	1.15	No	0.00	2	0.58	0.022
	Union Hospital, Terre Haute	8.3	0.0%	1.17	No	0.08	2	1.53	0.017
	Welborn Memorial Baptist Hospital, Evansville	5.5	0.0%	1.49	No	0.01	4	0.74	0.046

UROLOGY

Natl. Rank	Hospital	U.S. News index	Reputa-tional score	Urology mortality rate	COTH member	Interns and residents to beds	Tech-nology score (of 11)	R.N.'s to beds	Board-certified internists to beds	Procedures to beds
TIER ONE										
14	Indiana University Medical Center, Indianapolis	27.5	8.4%	1.13	Yes	1.10	10	1.86	0.107	1.40
TIER THREE										
	Bloomington Hospital, Bloomington	10.4	0.0%	0.47	No	0.00	7	0.61	0.033	2.24
	Columbus Regional Hospital, Columbus	10.6	0.0%	0.79	No	0.00	7	1.00	0.035	2.65
	Lutheran Hospital of Indiana, Fort Wayne	9.7	0.0%	0.85	No	0.05	7	1.06	0.021	1.74
	Methodist Hospital of Indiana, Indianapolis	12.9	1.1%	1.37	Yes	0.36	9	1.68	0.044	1.47
	Parkview Memorial Hospital, Fort Wayne	8.8	0.0%	0.82	No	0.01	7	0.72	0.012	1.09
	Union Hospital, Terre Haute	8.6	0.0%	1.08	No	0.08	6	1.53	0.017	2.24
	William N. Wishard Memorial Hospital, Indianapolis	12.5	0.0%	0.93	Yes	0.38	4	1.20	0.123	0.92
TIER FOUR										
	Ball Memorial Hospital, Muncie	4.2	0.0%	1.44	No	0.24	8	0.23	0.014	2.14
	Community Hospitals, Indianapolis	6.6	0.0%	1.03	No	0.21	0	0.99	0.085	1.23
	Deaconess Hospital, Evansville	5.6	0.0%	1.47	No	0.05	8	1.04	0.043	1.90
	Floyd Memorial Hospital, New Albany	2.8	0.0%	1.71	No	0.00	7	0.56	0.011	1.77
	Good Samaritan Hospital, Vincennes	7.1	0.0%	1.07	No	0.00	8	0.86	0.021	1.90
	Howard Community Hospital, Kokomo	5.0	0.0%	1.43	No	0.00	8	0.83	0.039	1.89
	Lafayette Home Hospital, Lafayette	4.4	0.0%	1.46	No	0.00	6	0.80	0.084	1.39
	Lakeshore Health System, East Chicago	2.9	0.0%	1.70	No	0.00	8	0.60	0.007	0.96
	Memorial Hospital of South Bend, South Bend	5.0	0.0%	1.69	No	0.09	7	1.30	0.042	1.06
	Methodist Hospitals, Gary	8.0	0.0%	0.87	No	0.03	8	0.58	0.011	0.53
	Porter Memorial Hospital, Valparaiso	6.8	0.0%	1.06	No	0.00	6	0.89	0.024	1.94
	Reid Hospital and Health Care Services, Richmond	5.2	0.0%	1.33	No	0.00	8	0.69	0.043	1.89
	St. Anthony Medical Center, Crown Point	2.2	0.0%	2.03	No	0.00	8	0.58	0.027	1.23
	St. Elizabeth Hospital Medical Center, Lafayette	6.7	0.0%	1.16	No	0.00	8	0.90	0.052	1.55
	St. Francis Hospital and Health Centers, Beech Grove	7.8	0.0%	1.13	No	0.09	8	1.20	0.014	1.98
	St. Joseph Medical Center, Fort Wayne	6.9	0.0%	0.90	No	0.02	3	0.63	0.030	1.56
	St. Joseph's Medical Center, South Bend	7.7	0.0%	1.25	No	0.12	8	1.26	0.068	2.03
	St. Margaret Mercy Health Centers, Hammond	4.2	0.0%	1.49	No	0.00	8	0.54	0.089	1.27

Natl. Rank	Hospital	U.S. News index	Reputa- tional score	Urology mortality rate	COTH member	Interns and residents to beds	Tech- nology score (of 11)	R.N.'s to beds	Board- certified internists to beds	Procedures to beds
	St. Mary's Medical Center, Evansville	5.6	0.0%	1.10	No	0.06	8	0.32	0.026	1.10
	St. Vincent Hospital and Health Center, Indianapolis	7.3	0.0%	1.35	No	0.22	9	1.13	0.086	1.17
	Welborn Memorial Baptist Hospital, Evansville	4.3	0.0%	1.60	No	0.01	9	0.74	0.046	1.36

AIDS

Natl. Rank	Hospital	U.S. News index	Reputa-tional score	Hospital-wide mortality rate	COTH member	Interns and residents to beds	Tech-nology score (of 11)	Discharge planning (of 2)	R.N.'s to beds	Board-certified internists to beds
			TIER TWO							
51	University of Iowa Hospitals and Clinics City	27.0	1.2%	1.02	Yes	0.96	10	2	1.34	0.053
			TIER THREE							
	Iowa Lutheran Hospital, Des Moines	19.7	0.0%	1.02	No	0.08	6	2	0.71	0.069
	Mary Greeley Medical Center, Ames	20.1	0.0%	0.98	No	0.00	7	1	0.85	0.069
			TIER FOUR							
	Allen Memorial Hospital, Waterloo	17.7	0.0%	1.17	No	0.02	6	2	0.84	0.047
	Broadlawns Medical Center, Des Moines	16.5	0.0%	1.10	No	0.22	3	1	0.51	0.015
	Burlington Medical Center, Burlington	18.2	0.0%	1.06	No	0.00	7	2	0.14	0.010
	Covenant Medical Center, Waterloo	17.2	0.0%	1.13	No	0.02	6	2	0.28	0.016
	Iowa Methodist Medical Center, Des Moines	17.5	0.0%	1.25	No	0.11	7	2	0.85	0.092
	Jennie Edmundson Memorial Hospital, Council Bluffs	15.3	0.0%	1.36	No	0.00	7	2	0.42	0.035
	Marian Health Center, Sioux City	19.6	0.0%	1.00	No	0.01	6	2	0.67	0.015
	Mercy Health Center, Dubuque	17.3	0.0%	1.10	No	0.00	6	1	0.55	0.042
	Mercy Hospital Medical Center, Des Moines	18.2	0.0%	1.06	No	0.00	6	1	0.79	0.037
	Mercy Hospital, Davenport	17.2	0.0%	1.19	No	0.02	5	2	1.00	0.019
	Mercy Hospital City	15.6	0.0%	1.20	No	0.02	5	0	0.84	0.050
	Mercy Medical Center, Cedar Rapids	17.0	0.0%	1.25	No	0.04	8	2	0.62	0.020
	St. Joseph Mercy Hospital, Mason City	16.8	0.0%	1.19	No	0.12	6	1	0.83	0.038
	St. Luke's Hospital, Davenport	17.3	0.0%	1.21	No	0.04	6	2	0.82	0.066
	St. Luke's Regional Medical Center, Sioux City	18.0	0.0%	1.13	No	0.02	7	2	0.60	0.024

CANCER

Natl. Rank	Hospital	U.S. News index	Reputa-tional score	Cancer mortality rate	COTH member	Interns and residents to beds	Tech-nology score (of 12)	R.N.'s to beds	Board-certified oncologists to beds	Procedures to beds
			TIER TWO							
42	University of Iowa Hospitals and Clinics City	13.4	0.9%	0.66	Yes	0.96	11	1.34	0.037	1.42
			TIER FOUR							
	Allen Memorial Hospital, Waterloo	3.0	0.0%	0.88	No	0.02	5	0.84	0.009	1.32
	Burlington Medical Center, Burlington	1.9	0.0%	1.04	No	0.00	9	0.14	0.005	0.82
	Covenant Medical Center, Waterloo	1.5	0.0%	1.39	No	0.02	7	0.28	0.003	0.94
	Iowa Lutheran Hospital, Des Moines	3.0	0.0%	0.80	No	0.08	5	0.71	0.009	1.43
	Iowa Methodist Medical Center, Des Moines	4.3	0.0%	0.98	No	0.11	8	0.85	0.011	2.16
	Jennie Edmundson Memorial Hospital, Council Bluffs	2.7	0.0%	0.87	No	0.00	8	0.42	0.008	1.51
	Marian Health Center, Sioux City	3.3	0.0%	0.93	No	0.01	8	0.67	0.004	1.47
	Mary Greeley Medical Center, Ames	3.5	0.0%	1.14	No	0.00	7	0.85	0.014	2.12
	Mercy Health Center, Dubuque	1.9	0.0%	0.96	No	0.00	5	0.55	0.005	0.70
	Mercy Hospital Medical Center, Des Moines	3.0	0.0%	1.16	No	0.00	6	0.79	0.007	2.22
	Mercy Hospital, Davenport	2.7	0.0%	1.34	No	0.02	4	1.00	0.011	0.87
	Mercy Hospital City	2.8	0.0%	1.16	No	0.02	5	0.84	0.004	1.52
	Mercy Medical Center, Cedar Rapids	3.0	0.0%	1.21	No	0.04	8	0.62	0.011	0.92
	St. Joseph Mercy Hospital, Mason City	4.0	0.0%	0.87	No	0.12	7	0.83	0.008	1.66
	St. Luke's Hospital, Davenport	3.5	0.0%	1.32	No	0.04	7	0.82	0.013	2.38
	St. Luke's Methodist Hospital, Cedar Rapids	3.4	0.0%	1.06	No	0.04	5	1.04	0.011	0.73
	St. Luke's Regional Medical Center, Sioux City	3.0	0.0%	0.91	No	0.02	7	0.60	0.005	1.82

CARDIOLOGY

Natl. Rank	Hospital	U.S. News index	Reputa-tional score	Cardiology mortality rate	COTH member	Interns and residents to beds	Tech-nology score (of 10)	R.N.'s to beds	Board-certified cardiologists to beds	Procedures to beds
	TIER THREE									
	Mercy Hospital Medical Center, Des Moines	13.6	0.0%	1.04	No	0.00	8	0.79	0.035	12.81
	University of Iowa Hospitals and Clinics City	18.2	0.0%	1.20	Yes	0.96	10	1.34	0.038	3.23
	TIER FOUR									
	Allen Memorial Hospital, Waterloo	8.8	0.0%	1.30	No	0.02	8	0.84	0.019	11.23
	Burlington Medical Center, Burlington	10.4	0.0%	1.03	No	0.00	7	0.14	0.005	3.16
	Covenant Medical Center, Waterloo	9.7	0.0%	1.04	No	0.02	4	0.28	0.000	3.98
	Iowa Lutheran Hospital, Des Moines	10.4	0.0%	1.21	No	0.08	8	0.71	0.057	5.44
	Iowa Methodist Medical Center, Des Moines	10.3	0.4%	1.27	No	0.11	7	0.85	0.061	5.71
	Jennie Edmundson Memorial Hospital, Council Bluffs	3.7	0.0%	1.57	No	0.00	7	0.42	0.024	4.35
	Marian Health Center, Sioux City	10.1	0.0%	1.16	No	0.01	8	0.67	0.015	5.86
	Mary Greeley Medical Center, Ames	12.0	0.0%	1.06	No	0.00	7	0.85	0.005	5.09
	Mercy Health Center, Dubuque	8.1	0.0%	1.25	No	0.00	8	0.55	0.008	5.96
	Mercy Hospital, Davenport	10.1	0.0%	1.19	No	0.02	6	1.00	0.030	3.80
	Mercy Hospital City	7.6	0.0%	1.34	No	0.02	7	0.84	0.013	7.98
	Mercy Medical Center, Cedar Rapids	7.1	0.0%	1.31	No	0.04	7	0.62	0.014	3.66
	St. Joseph Mercy Hospital, Mason City	11.2	0.0%	1.15	No	0.12	8	0.83	0.008	9.20
	St. Luke's Hospital, Davenport	9.4	0.0%	1.27	No	0.04	7	0.82	0.040	11.83
	St. Luke's Methodist Hospital, Cedar Rapids	13.4	0.0%	1.04	No	0.04	7	1.04	0.017	5.52
	St. Luke's Regional Medical Center, Sioux City	8.1	0.0%	1.24	No	0.02	7	0.60	0.019	3.62

ENDOCRINOLOGY

Natl. Rank	Hospital	U.S. News index	Reputa-tional score	Endocrinology mortality rate	COTH member	Interns and residents to beds	Tech-nology score (of 11)	R.N.'s to beds	Board-certified internists to beds
	TIER TWO								
28	University of Iowa Hospitals and Clinics City	20.4	2.9%	0.76	Yes	0.96	11	1.34	0.053
	TIER THREE								
	Iowa Lutheran Hospital, Des Moines	9.9	0.0%	0.61	No	0.08	6	0.71	0.069
	Marian Health Center, Sioux City	9.6	0.0%	0.55	No	0.01	8	0.67	0.015
	Mary Greeley Medical Center, Ames	10.4	0.0%	0.64	No	0.00	8	0.85	0.069
	TIER FOUR								
	Allen Memorial Hospital, Waterloo	4.2	0.0%	1.48	No	0.02	6	0.84	0.047
	Covenant Medical Center, Waterloo	2.0	0.0%	1.72	No	0.02	7	0.28	0.016
	Iowa Methodist Medical Center, Des Moines	4.5	0.0%	1.74	No	0.11	8	0.85	0.092
	Mercy Health Center, Dubuque	4.1	0.0%	1.26	No	0.00	6	0.55	0.042
	Mercy Hospital Medical Center, Des Moines	6.0	0.0%	1.02	No	0.00	6	0.79	0.037
	Mercy Hospital, Davenport	5.7	0.0%	1.04	No	0.02	3	1.00	0.019
	Mercy Medical Center, Cedar Rapids	3.7	0.0%	1.51	No	0.04	8	0.62	0.020
	St. Joseph Mercy Hospital, Mason City	3.8	0.0%	1.91	No	0.12	8	0.83	0.038
	St. Luke's Methodist Hospital, Cedar Rapids	5.6	0.0%	1.16	No	0.04	5	1.04	0.019
	St. Luke's Regional Medical Center, Sioux City	2.9	0.0%	1.73	No	0.02	7	0.60	0.024

GASTROENTEROLOGY

Natl. Rank	Hospital	U.S. News index	Reputa-tional score	Gastro-enterology mortality rate	COTH member	Interns and residents to beds	Tech-nology score (of 11)	R.N.'s to beds	Board-certified gastro-enterologists to beds	Pro-cedures to beds
	TIER TWO									
47	University of Iowa Hospitals and Clinics City	15.6	1.1%	0.97	Yes	0.96	11	1.34	0.017	1.15
	TIER THREE									
	Allen Memorial Hospital, Waterloo	7.5	0.0%	0.99	No	0.02	7	0.84	0.005	4.99
	Mary Greeley Medical Center, Ames	8.4	0.0%	0.84	No	0.00	7	0.85	0.009	4.24

Natl. Rank	Hospital	U.S. News index	Reputa-tional score	Gastro-enterology mortality rate	COTH member	Interns and residents to beds	Tech-nology score (of 11)	R.N.'s to beds	Board-certified gastro-enterologists to beds	Pro-cedures to beds
	TIER FOUR									
	Burlington Medical Center, Burlington	6.1	0.0%	0.81	No	0.00	9	0.14	0.000	1.78
	Covenant Medical Center, Waterloo	2.4	0.0%	1.38	No	0.02	6	0.28	0.005	2.60
	Iowa Lutheran Hospital, Des Moines	6.6	0.0%	0.86	No	0.08	6	0.71	0.006	2.33
	Iowa Methodist Medical Center, Des Moines	4.5	0.0%	1.35	No	0.11	7	0.85	0.009	2.42
	Jennie Edmundson Memorial Hospital, Council Bluffs	2.5	0.0%	1.66	No	0.00	9	0.42	0.008	2.14
	Marian Health Center, Sioux City	3.8	0.0%	1.37	No	0.01	8	0.67	0.009	2.22
	Mercy Health Center, Dubuque	6.7	0.0%	0.81	No	0.00	6	0.55	0.003	2.66
	Mercy Hospital Medical Center, Des Moines	5.1	0.0%	1.27	No	0.00	6	0.79	0.009	4.40
	Mercy Hospital, Davenport	3.7	0.0%	1.30	No	0.02	3	1.00	0.015	2.70
	Mercy Hospital City	6.4	0.0%	0.99	No	0.02	5	0.84	0.008	4.13
	Mercy Medical Center, Cedar Rapids	3.5	0.0%	1.41	No	0.04	7	0.62	0.011	2.56
	St. Joseph Mercy Hospital, Mason City	6.4	0.0%	1.14	No	0.12	7	0.83	0.004	4.23
	St. Luke's Hospital, Davenport	5.3	0.0%	1.17	No	0.04	7	0.82	0.018	3.10
	St. Luke's Methodist Hospital, Cedar Rapids	6.9	0.0%	0.89	No	0.04	5	1.04	0.009	2.65
	St. Luke's Regional Medical Center, Sioux City	5.6	0.0%	1.02	No	0.02	7	0.60	0.011	3.01

GERIATRICS

Natl. Rank	Hospital	U.S. News index	Reputa-tional score	Hospital-wide mortality rate	COTH member	Service mix	Interns and residents to beds	Tech-nology score (of 13)	R.N.'s to beds	Discharge planning (of 2)	Geriatric services (of 9)	Board-certified internists to beds
	TIER TWO											
67	**University of Iowa Hospitals and Clinics City**	22.8	0.5%	1.02	Yes	8	0.96	12	1.34	2	4	0.053
	TIER THREE											
	Marian Health Center, Sioux City	14.8	0.0%	1.00	No	5	0.01	11	0.67	2	4	0.015
	Mary Greeley Medical Center, Ames	14.5	0.0%	0.98	No	7	0.00	9	0.85	1	1	0.069
	St. Luke's Methodist Hospital, Cedar Rapids	18.5	0.0%	0.94	No	9	0.04	7	1.04	2	5	0.019
	TIER FOUR											
	Allen Memorial Hospital, Waterloo	11.3	0.0%	1.17	No	7	0.02	7	0.84	2	4	0.047
	Burlington Medical Center, Burlington	11.9	0.0%	1.06	No	6	0.00	10	0.14	2	2	0.010
	Covenant Medical Center, Waterloo	10.9	0.0%	1.13	No	7	0.02	7	0.28	2	4	0.016
	Iowa Lutheran Hospital, Des Moines	13.4	0.0%	1.02	No	5	0.08	7	0.71	2	2	0.069
	Iowa Methodist Medical Center, Des Moines	11.2	0.0%	1.25	No	7	0.11	9	0.85	2	7	0.092
	Jennie Edmundson Memorial Hospital, Council Bluffs	7.0	0.0%	1.36	No	6	0.00	11	0.42	2	3	0.035
	Mercy Health Center, Dubuque	10.5	0.0%	1.10	No	5	0.00	7	0.55	1	5	0.042
	Mercy Hospital Medical Center, Des Moines	12.5	0.0%	1.06	No	6	0.00	7	0.79	1	6	0.037
	Mercy Hospital, Davenport	9.5	0.0%	1.19	No	5	0.02	5	1.00	2	3	0.019
	Mercy Hospital City	7.1	0.0%	1.20	No	5	0.02	7	0.84	0	2	0.050
	Mercy Medical Center, Cedar Rapids	10.4	0.0%	1.25	No	8	0.04	9	0.62	2	6	0.020
	St. Joseph Mercy Hospital, Mason City	10.1	0.0%	1.19	No	5	0.12	10	0.83	1	6	0.038
	St. Luke's Hospital, Davenport	8.9	0.0%	1.21	No	4	0.04	9	0.82	2	1	0.066
	St. Luke's Regional Medical Center, Sioux City	11.1	0.0%	1.13	No	5	0.02	9	0.60	2	4	0.024

GYNECOLOGY

Natl. Rank	Hospital	U.S. News index	Reputa-tional score	Hospital-wide mortality rate	Interns and residents to beds	Tech-nology score (of 10)	R.N.'s to beds	Board-certified OB-GYNs to beds	Procedures to beds
	TIER TWO								
60	**University of Iowa Hospitals and Clinics City**	24.8	0.8%	1.02	0.96	10	1.34	0.021	0.26
	TIER THREE								
	Mary Greeley Medical Center, Ames	16.2	0.0%	0.98	0.00	8	0.85	0.028	0.61
	St. Luke's Methodist Hospital, Cedar Rapids	15.5	0.0%	0.94	0.04	4	1.04	0.028	0.40

Natl. Rank	Hospital	U.S. News index	Reputational score	Hospital-wide mortality rate	Interns and residents to beds	Technology score (of 10)	R.N.'s to beds	Board-certified OB-GYNs to beds	Procedures to beds
	TIER FOUR								
	Allen Memorial Hospital, Waterloo	9.3	0.0%	1.17	0.02	5	0.84	0.014	0.51
	Burlington Medical Center, Burlington	10.7	0.0%	1.06	0.00	8	0.14	0.013	0.16
	Covenant Medical Center, Waterloo	8.4	0.0%	1.13	0.02	6	0.28	0.016	0.32
	Iowa Lutheran Hospital, Des Moines	12.6	0.0%	1.02	0.08	5	0.71	0.024	0.33
	Iowa Methodist Medical Center, Des Moines	9.9	0.0%	1.25	0.11	7	0.85	0.030	0.33
	Jennie Edmundson Memorial Hospital, Council Bluffs	5.4	0.0%	1.36	0.00	7	0.42	0.016	0.28
	Marian Health Center, Sioux City	13.3	0.0%	1.00	0.01	6	0.67	0.015	0.19
	Mercy Health Center, Dubuque	10.3	0.0%	1.10	0.00	6	0.55	0.021	0.26
	Mercy Hospital Medical Center, Des Moines	12.0	0.0%	1.06	0.00	6	0.79	0.012	0.42
	Mercy Hospital, Davenport	9.4	0.0%	1.19	0.02	3	1.00	0.068	0.16
	Mercy Hospital City	9.1	0.0%	1.20	0.02	5	0.84	0.029	0.39
	Mercy Medical Center, Cedar Rapids	8.6	0.0%	1.25	0.04	7	0.62	0.032	0.22
	St. Joseph Mercy Hospital, Mason City	10.8	0.0%	1.19	0.12	7	0.83	0.023	0.46
	St. Luke's Hospital, Davenport	10.8	0.0%	1.21	0.04	7	0.82	0.053	0.77
	St. Luke's Regional Medical Center, Sioux City	9.9	0.0%	1.13	0.02	6	0.60	0.019	0.48

NEUROLOGY

Natl. Rank	Hospital	U.S. News index	Reputational score	Neurology mortality rate	COTH member	Interns and residents to beds	Technology score (of 9)	R.N.'s to beds	Board-certified neurologists to beds
	TIER ONE								
23	University of Iowa Hospitals and Clinics City	24.9	4.6%	0.97	Yes	0.96	9	1.34	0.015
	TIER THREE								
	Allen Memorial Hospital, Waterloo	11.2	0.0%	0.89	No	0.02	5	0.84	0.014
	Burlington Medical Center, Burlington	12.6	0.0%	0.64	No	0.00	8	0.14	0.003
	Iowa Lutheran Hospital, Des Moines	13.5	0.0%	0.78	No	0.08	5	0.71	0.009
	Mary Greeley Medical Center, Ames	14.1	0.0%	0.79	No	0.00	7	0.85	0.014
	Mercy Hospital City	11.4	0.0%	0.87	No	0.02	4	0.84	0.013
	St. Luke's Hospital, Davenport	12.8	0.0%	0.83	No	0.04	6	0.82	0.013
	St. Luke's Methodist Hospital, Cedar Rapids	14.1	0.0%	0.65	No	0.04	3	1.04	0.011
	TIER FOUR								
	Iowa Methodist Medical Center, Des Moines	9.6	0.0%	1.00	No	0.11	6	0.85	0.009
	Jennie Edmundson Memorial Hospital, Council Bluffs	6.6	0.0%	1.11	No	0.00	7	0.42	0.004
	Marian Health Center, Sioux City	8.8	0.0%	1.00	No	0.01	6	0.67	0.009
	Mercy Health Center, Dubuque	6.2	0.0%	1.11	No	0.00	5	0.55	0.003
	Mercy Hospital Medical Center, Des Moines	10.0	0.0%	0.92	No	0.00	5	0.79	0.007
	Mercy Hospital, Davenport	10.0	0.0%	0.94	No	0.02	3	1.00	0.011
	Mercy Medical Center, Cedar Rapids	9.1	0.0%	1.02	No	0.04	7	0.62	0.014
	St. Joseph Mercy Hospital, Mason City	7.0	0.0%	1.19	No	0.12	6	0.83	0.008
	St. Luke's Regional Medical Center, Sioux City	9.0	0.0%	0.96	No	0.02	5	0.60	0.008

ORTHOPEDICS

Natl. Rank	Hospital	U.S. News index	Reputational score	Orthopedics mortality rate	COTH member	Interns and residents to beds	Technology score (of 5)	R.N.'s to beds	Board-certified orthopedists to beds	Procedures to beds
	TIER ONE									
10	University of Iowa Hospitals and Clinics City	31.2	7.9%	0.92	Yes	0.96	5	1.34	0.020	1.08
	TIER THREE									
	Iowa Lutheran Hospital, Des Moines	10.3	0.0%	0.56	No	0.08	4	0.71	0.042	2.22
	Marian Health Center, Sioux City	9.2	0.0%	0.63	No	0.01	3	0.67	0.015	2.23
	Mercy Health Center, Dubuque	9.5	0.0%	0.50	No	0.00	4	0.55	0.023	2.24
	St. Joseph Mercy Hospital, Mason City	10.7	0.0%	0.57	No	0.12	3	0.83	0.030	4.87
	St. Luke's Methodist Hospital, Cedar Rapids	8.8	0.0%	0.73	No	0.04	2	1.04	0.034	2.60

Natl. Rank	Hospital	U.S. News index	Reputational score	Orthopedics mortality rate	COTH member	Interns and residents to beds	Technology score (of 5)	R.N.'s to beds	Board-certified orthopedists to beds	Procedures to beds
	TIER FOUR									
	Allen Memorial Hospital, Waterloo	7.7	0.0%	0.93	No	0.02	4	0.84	0.019	4.55
	Burlington Medical Center, Burlington	2.1	0.0%	1.47	No	0.00	4	0.14	0.008	1.70
	Covenant Medical Center, Waterloo	5.3	0.0%	0.82	No	0.02	2	0.28	0.016	1.80
	Iowa Methodist Medical Center, Des Moines	5.1	0.0%	1.25	No	0.11	3	0.85	0.023	3.37
	Jennie Edmundson Memorial Hospital, Council Bluffs	6.3	0.0%	0.93	No	0.00	4	0.42	0.012	3.91
	Mary Greeley Medical Center, Ames	6.1	0.0%	1.14	No	0.00	4	0.85	0.019	4.32
	Mercy Hospital Medical Center, Des Moines	6.0	0.0%	1.00	No	0.00	3	0.79	0.021	3.29
	Mercy Hospital, Davenport	6.7	0.0%	1.02	No	0.02	3	1.00	0.030	3.83
	Mercy Hospital City	4.8	0.0%	1.28	No	0.02	3	0.84	0.029	4.25
	Mercy Medical Center, Cedar Rapids	5.9	0.0%	1.04	No	0.04	4	0.62	0.034	2.46
	St. Luke's Hospital, Davenport	6.3	0.0%	0.99	No	0.04	3	0.82	0.044	2.80
	St. Luke's Regional Medical Center, Sioux City	7.0	0.0%	0.92	No	0.02	4	0.60	0.024	4.02

OTOLARYNGOLOGY

Natl. Rank	Hospital	U.S. News index	Reputational score	Hospital-wide mortality rate	COTH member	Interns and residents to beds	Technology score (of 9)	R.N.'s to beds	Board-certified internists to beds	Procedures to beds
	TIER ONE									
3	University of Iowa Hospitals and Clinics City	89.8	23.7%	1.02	Yes	0.96	9	1.34	0.053	0.276
	TIER FOUR									
	Allen Memorial Hospital, Waterloo	4.1	0.0%	1.16	No	0.02	4	0.84	0.047	0.272
	Broadlawns Medical Center, Des Moines	2.5	0.0%	1.09	No	0.22	0	0.51	0.015	0.055
	Burlington Medical Center, Burlington	2.8	0.0%	1.06	No	0.00	8	0.14	0.010	0.095
	Covenant Medical Center, Waterloo	2.4	0.0%	1.13	No	0.02	5	0.28	0.016	0.153
	Iowa Lutheran Hospital, Des Moines	4.2	0.0%	1.02	No	0.08	4	0.71	0.069	0.137
	Iowa Methodist Medical Center, Des Moines	5.4	0.0%	1.25	No	0.11	6	0.85	0.092	0.195
	Jennie Edmundson Memorial Hospital, Council Bluffs	3.4	0.0%	1.36	No	0.00	7	0.42	0.035	0.173
	Marian Health Center, Sioux City	4.0	0.0%	1.00	No	0.01	6	0.67	0.015	0.111
	Mary Greeley Medical Center, Ames	5.0	0.0%	0.98	No	0.00	6	0.85	0.069	0.495
	Mercy Health Center, Dubuque	3.2	0.0%	1.10	No	0.00	4	0.55	0.042	0.201
	Mercy Hospital Medical Center, Des Moines	3.9	0.0%	1.06	No	0.00	4	0.79	0.037	0.571
	Mercy Hospital, Davenport	3.8	0.0%	1.19	No	0.02	2	1.00	0.019	0.121
	Mercy Hospital City	4.2	0.0%	1.20	No	0.02	4	0.84	0.050	0.404
	Mercy Medical Center, Cedar Rapids	3.8	0.0%	1.25	No	0.04	6	0.62	0.020	0.216
	St. Joseph Mercy Hospital, Mason City	5.0	0.0%	1.19	No	0.12	6	0.83	0.038	0.308
	St. Luke's Hospital, Davenport	4.8	0.0%	1.20	No	0.04	6	0.82	0.066	0.173
	St. Luke's Methodist Hospital, Cedar Rapids	4.5	0.0%	0.94	No	0.04	3	1.04	0.019	0.183
	St. Luke's Regional Medical Center, Sioux City	3.5	0.0%	1.13	No	0.02	5	0.60	0.024	0.140

RHEUMATOLOGY

Natl. Rank	Hospital	U.S. News index	Reputational score	Hospital-wide mortality rate	COTH member	Interns and residents to beds	Technology score (of 5)	R.N.'s to beds	Board-certified internists to beds
	TIER TWO								
44	University of Iowa Hospitals and Clinics City	18.6	1.2%	1.02	Yes	0.96	5	1.34	0.053
	TIER FOUR								
	Allen Memorial Hospital, Waterloo	7.5	0.0%	1.16	No	0.02	4	0.84	0.047
	Burlington Medical Center, Burlington	6.1	0.0%	1.06	No	0.00	4	0.14	0.010
	Covenant Medical Center, Waterloo	5.2	0.0%	1.13	No	0.02	2	0.28	0.016
	Iowa Lutheran Hospital, Des Moines	8.6	0.0%	1.02	No	0.08	4	0.71	0.069
	Iowa Methodist Medical Center, Des Moines	7.2	0.0%	1.25	No	0.11	3	0.85	0.092
	Jennie Edmundson Memorial Hospital, Council Bluffs	5.1	0.0%	1.36	No	0.00	4	0.42	0.035
	Marian Health Center, Sioux City	7.7	0.0%	1.00	No	0.01	3	0.67	0.015

Natl. Rank	Hospital	U.S. News index	Reputational score	Hospital-wide mortality rate	COTH member	Interns and residents to beds	Technology score (of 5)	R.N.'s to beds	Board-certified internists to beds
	Mary Greeley Medical Center, Ames	8.1	0.0%	0.98	No	0.00	4	0.85	0.069
	Mercy Health Center, Dubuque	6.1	0.0%	1.10	No	0.00	4	0.55	0.042
	Mercy Hospital Medical Center, Des Moines	6.6	0.0%	1.06	No	0.00	3	0.79	0.037
	Mercy Hospital, Davenport	7.1	0.0%	1.19	No	0.02	3	1.00	0.019
	Mercy Hospital City	4.9	0.0%	1.20	No	0.02	3	0.84	0.050
	Mercy Medical Center, Cedar Rapids	6.3	0.0%	1.25	No	0.04	4	0.62	0.020
	St. Joseph Mercy Hospital, Mason City	6.1	0.0%	1.19	No	0.12	3	0.83	0.038
	St. Luke's Hospital, Davenport	6.9	0.0%	1.20	No	0.04	3	0.82	0.066
	St. Luke's Methodist Hospital, Cedar Rapids	8.9	0.0%	0.94	No	0.04	2	1.04	0.019
	St. Luke's Regional Medical Center, Sioux City	7.0	0.0%	1.13	No	0.02	4	0.60	0.024

UROLOGY

Natl. Rank	Hospital	U.S. News index	Reputational score	Urology mortality rate	COTH member	Interns and residents to beds	Technology score (of 11)	R.N.'s to beds	Board-certified internists to beds	Procedures to beds
	TIER ONE									
25	University of Iowa Hospitals and Clinics City	21.6	4.0%	0.92	Yes	0.96	11	1.34	0.053	1.30
	TIER THREE									
	Marian Health Center, Sioux City	10.5	0.0%	0.56	No	0.01	8	0.67	0.015	1.56
	TIER FOUR									
	Allen Memorial Hospital, Waterloo	6.2	0.0%	1.23	No	0.02	7	0.84	0.047	2.60
	Burlington Medical Center, Burlington	7.2	0.0%	0.86	No	0.00	9	0.14	0.010	0.86
	Covenant Medical Center, Waterloo	5.3	0.0%	1.04	No	0.02	6	0.28	0.016	1.43
	Iowa Lutheran Hospital, Des Moines	6.4	0.0%	1.10	No	0.08	6	0.71	0.069	1.27
	Iowa Methodist Medical Center, Des Moines	6.6	0.0%	1.21	No	0.11	7	0.85	0.092	1.51
	Jennie Edmundson Memorial Hospital, Council Bluffs	2.1	0.0%	2.04	No	0.00	9	0.42	0.035	1.09
	Mary Greeley Medical Center, Ames	5.4	0.0%	1.43	No	0.00	7	0.85	0.069	3.19
	Mercy Health Center, Dubuque	4.1	0.0%	1.33	No	0.00	6	0.55	0.042	1.19
	Mercy Hospital Medical Center, Des Moines	4.2	0.0%	1.49	No	0.00	6	0.79	0.037	2.15
	Mercy Hospital City	3.9	0.0%	1.53	No	0.02	5	0.84	0.050	1.74
	Mercy Medical Center, Cedar Rapids	4.3	0.0%	1.37	No	0.04	7	0.62	0.020	1.29
	St. Joseph Mercy Hospital, Mason City	4.6	0.0%	1.57	No	0.12	7	0.83	0.038	1.99
	St. Luke's Hospital, Davenport	3.6	0.0%	1.82	No	0.04	7	0.82	0.066	1.58
	St. Luke's Methodist Hospital, Cedar Rapids	5.5	0.0%	1.27	No	0.04	5	1.04	0.019	1.51
	St. Luke's Regional Medical Center, Sioux City	4.0	0.0%	1.46	No	0.02	7	0.60	0.024	1.84

AIDS

Natl. Rank / Hospital	U.S. News index	Reputa-tional score	Hospital-wide mortality rate	COTH member	Interns and residents to beds	Tech-nology score (of 11)	Discharge planning (of 2)	R.N.'s to beds	Board-certified internists to beds
TIER THREE									
Overland Park Regional Medical Center, Overland Park	20.7	0.0%	0.83	No	0.00	4	2	0.41	0.063
St. John's Regional Health Center, Salina	20.3	0.0%	0.99	No	0.01	7	2	0.71	0.044
University of Kansas Hospital, Kansas City	22.5	0.0%	1.19	Yes	1.21	9	2	0.81	0.043
TIER FOUR									
Asbury-Salina Regional Medical Center, Salina	15.0	0.0%	1.36	No	0.04	5	2	0.62	0.039
Mount Carmel Medical Center, Pittsburg	17.3	0.0%	1.15	No	0.00	7	2	0.28	0.025
Providence Medical Center, Kansas City	18.0	0.0%	1.13	No	0.00	5	2	1.02	0.052
St. Francis Hospital and Medical Center, Topeka	19.1	0.0%	1.13	No	0.01	6	2	1.37	0.057
St. Francis Regional Medical Center, Wichita	16.1	0.0%	1.44	No	0.20	9	2	0.65	0.025
St. Joseph Medical Center, Wichita	15.2	0.0%	1.43	No	0.08	8	1	0.91	0.024
St. Ormont-Vail Regional Medical Center, Topeka	18.5	0.0%	1.07	No	0.01	5	2	0.80	0.057

CANCER

Natl. Rank / Hospital	U.S. News index	Reputa-tional score	Cancer mortality rate	COTH member	Interns and residents to beds	Tech-nology score (of 12)	R.N.'s to beds	Board-certified oncologists to beds	Procedures to beds
TIER THREE									
St. Francis Hospital and Medical Center, Topeka	5.4	0.0%	0.87	No	0.01	8	1.37	0.013	1.64
University of Kansas Hospital, Kansas City	10.2	0.0%	0.95	Yes	1.21	8	0.81	0.011	1.57
TIER FOUR									
Asbury-Salina Regional Medical Center, Salina	2.6	0.0%	1.01	No	0.04	6	0.62	0.006	1.19
Bethany Medical Center, Kansas City	2.9	0.0%	0.74	No	0.05	6	0.58	0.003	1.31
HCA Wesley Medical Center, Wichita	5.2	0.0%	1.00	No	0.15	9	1.10	0.000	1.79
Mount Carmel Medical Center, Pittsburg	1.7	0.0%	1.11	No	0.00	7	0.28	0.000	1.21
Overland Park Regional Medical Center, Overland Park	1.1	0.0%	0.91	No	0.00	3	0.41	0.015	0.57
Providence Medical Center, Kansas City	4.1	0.0%	0.69	No	0.00	6	1.02	0.014	1.46
St. Francis Regional Medical Center, Wichita	3.8	0.0%	1.52	No	0.20	9	0.65	0.014	1.13
St. John's Regional Health Center, Salina	3.2	0.0%	0.91	No	0.01	7	0.71	0.006	1.26
St. Joseph Medical Center, Wichita	4.2	0.0%	1.28	No	0.08	9	0.91	0.016	0.88
St. Ormont-Vail Regional Medical Center, Topeka	2.5	0.0%	0.90	No	0.01	4	0.80	0.014	0.76

CARDIOLOGY

Natl. Rank / Hospital	U.S. News index	Reputa-tional score	Cardiology mortality rate	COTH member	Interns and residents to beds	Tech-nology score (of 10)	R.N.'s to beds	Board-certified cardiologists to beds	Procedures to beds
TIER THREE									
Bethany Medical Center, Kansas City	15.8	0.0%	0.87	No	0.05	6	0.58	0.003	4.86
Overland Park Regional Medical Center, Overland Park	15.0	0.0%	0.89	No	0.00	6	0.41	0.037	2.97
University of Kansas Hospital, Kansas City	14.5	0.5%	1.43	Yes	1.21	9	0.81	0.019	2.86
TIER FOUR									
Asbury-Salina Regional Medical Center, Salina	5.8	0.0%	1.35	No	0.04	5	0.62	0.000	4.69
HCA Wesley Medical Center, Wichita	8.7	0.0%	1.38	No	0.15	9	1.10	0.002	7.85
Mount Carmel Medical Center, Pittsburg	3.1	0.0%	1.46	No	0.00	4	0.28	0.000	5.15
Providence Medical Center, Kansas City	10.8	0.0%	1.16	No	0.00	6	1.02	0.028	7.04
St. Francis Hospital and Medical Center, Topeka	11.9	0.0%	1.19	No	0.01	8	1.37	0.029	7.42
St. Francis Regional Medical Center, Wichita	9.9	0.0%	1.27	No	0.20	9	0.65	0.031	10.14
St. Joseph Medical Center, Wichita	5.4	0.0%	1.69	No	0.08	9	0.91	0.049	5.55
St. Ormont-Vail Regional Medical Center, Topeka	11.2	0.0%	1.12	No	0.01	7	0.80	0.029	5.42

ENDOCRINOLOGY

Natl. Rank	Hospital	U.S. News index	Reputa-tional score	Endocrinology mortality rate	COTH member	Interns and residents to beds	Tech-nology score (of 11)	R.N.'s to beds	Board-certified internists to beds
	TIER TWO								
71	University of Kansas Hospital, Kansas City	15.7	0.3%	0.77	Yes	1.21	9	0.81	0.043
	TIER THREE								
	HCA Wesley Medical Center, Wichita	10.1	0.0%	0.91	No	0.15	9	1.10	0.232
	TIER FOUR								
	Bethany Medical Center, Kansas City	7.6	0.0%	0.80	No	0.05	7	0.58	0.032
	Providence Medical Center, Kansas City	5.9	0.0%	1.21	No	0.00	7	1.02	0.052
	St. Francis Hospital and Medical Center, Topeka	6.5	0.0%	1.40	No	0.01	9	1.37	0.057
	St. Francis Regional Medical Center, Wichita	3.9	0.0%	1.77	No	0.20	9	0.65	0.025
	St. Joseph Medical Center, Wichita	4.7	0.0%	1.57	No	0.08	9	0.91	0.024
	St. Ormont-Vail Regional Medical Center, Topeka	4.3	0.0%	1.36	No	0.01	5	0.80	0.057

GASTROENTEROLOGY

Natl. Rank	Hospital	U.S. News index	Reputa-tional score	Gastro-enterology mortality rate	COTH member	Interns and residents to beds	Tech-nology score (of 11)	R.N.'s to beds	Board-certified gastro-enterologists to beds	Pro-cedures to beds
	TIER THREE									
	Providence Medical Center, Kansas City	7.7	0.0%	0.87	No	0.00	6	1.02	0.028	3.36
76	University of Kansas Hospital, Kansas City	13.1	0.0%	0.96	Yes	1.21	9	0.81	0.011	1.42
	TIER FOUR									
	Asbury-Salina Regional Medical Center, Salina	4.2	0.0%	1.34	No	0.04	6	0.62	0.006	3.89
	Bethany Medical Center, Kansas City	6.4	0.0%	0.84	No	0.05	6	0.58	0.012	2.10
	HCA Wesley Medical Center, Wichita	5.1	0.0%	1.47	No	0.15	9	1.10	0.000	2.20
	Mount Carmel Medical Center, Pittsburg	2.8	0.0%	1.53	No	0.00	8	0.28	0.000	3.18
	Overland Park Regional Medical Center, Overland Park	4.9	0.0%	0.85	No	0.00	4	0.41	0.020	1.67
	St. Francis Hospital and Medical Center, Topeka	5.8	0.0%	1.48	No	0.01	8	1.37	0.016	3.49
	St. Francis Regional Medical Center, Wichita	3.3	0.0%	1.76	No	0.20	8	0.65	0.009	2.32
	St. Joseph Medical Center, Wichita	4.4	0.0%	1.58	No	0.08	9	0.91	0.008	2.62
	St. Ormont-Vail Regional Medical Center, Topeka	6.2	0.0%	0.86	No	0.01	5	0.80	0.014	2.03

GERIATRICS

Natl. Rank	Hospital	U.S. News index	Reputa-tional score	Hospital-wide mortality rate	COTH member	Service mix	Interns and residents to beds	Tech-nology score (of 13)	R.N.'s to beds	Discharge planning (of 2)	Geriatric services (of 9)	Board-certified internists to beds
	TIER THREE											
	Bethany Medical Center, Kansas City	17.5	0.0%	0.90	No	5	0.05	8	0.58	2	5	0.032
	Overland Park Regional Medical Center, Overland Park	16.0	0.0%	0.83	No	4	0.00	6	0.41	2	2	0.063
	University of Kansas Hospital, Kansas City	17.4	0.3%	1.19	Yes	8	1.21	11	0.81	2	3	0.043
	TIER FOUR											
	Asbury-Salina Regional Medical Center, Salina	6.2	0.0%	1.36	No	5	0.04	7	0.62	2	3	0.039
	HCA Wesley Medical Center, Wichita	9.6	0.0%	1.34	No	5	0.15	11	1.10	2	3	0.232
	Providence Medical Center, Kansas City	11.4	0.0%	1.13	No	5	0.00	8	1.02	2	3	0.052
	St. Francis Hospital and Medical Center, Topeka	12.5	0.0%	1.13	No	5	0.01	10	1.37	2	2	0.057
	St. Francis Regional Medical Center, Wichita	7.6	0.0%	1.44	No	7	0.20	11	0.65	2	5	0.025
	St. Joseph Medical Center, Wichita	6.7	0.0%	1.43	No	6	0.08	11	0.91	1	6	0.024
	St. Ormont-Vail Regional Medical Center, Topeka	12.8	0.0%	1.07	No	5	0.01	7	0.80	2	5	0.057

GYNECOLOGY

Natl. Rank	Hospital	U.S. News index	Reputational score	Hospital-wide mortality rate	Interns and residents to beds	Technology score (of 10)	R.N.'s to beds	Board-certified OB-GYNs to beds	Procedures to beds
	TIER THREE								
	Bethany Medical Center, Kansas City	15.3	0.0%	0.90	0.05	5	0.58	0.018	0.21
	Overland Park Regional Medical Center, Overland Park	14.7	0.0%	0.83	0.00	4	0.41	0.037	0.35
	St. Francis Hospital and Medical Center, Topeka	14.2	0.0%	1.13	0.01	7	1.37	0.029	0.75
	University of Kansas Hospital, Kansas City	15.9	0.0%	1.19	1.21	7	0.81	0.034	0.41
	TIER FOUR								
	Asbury-Salina Regional Medical Center, Salina	6.1	0.0%	1.36	0.04	6	0.62	0.033	0.74
	HCA Wesley Medical Center, Wichita	10.8	0.0%	1.34	0.15	8	1.10	0.048	0.62
	Providence Medical Center, Kansas City	11.2	0.0%	1.13	0.00	5	1.02	0.038	0.35
	St. Francis Regional Medical Center, Wichita	6.9	0.0%	1.44	0.20	8	0.65	0.017	0.30
	St. Joseph Medical Center, Wichita	7.7	0.0%	1.43	0.08	8	0.91	0.022	0.36
	St. Ormont-Vail Regional Medical Center, Topeka	12.3	0.0%	1.07	0.01	6	0.80	0.031	0.42

NEUROLOGY

Natl. Rank	Hospital	U.S. News index	Reputational score	Neurology mortality rate	COTH member	Interns and residents to beds	Technology score (of 9)	R.N.'s to beds	Board-certified neurologists to beds
	TIER THREE								
	St. Francis Hospital and Medical Center, Topeka	11.0	0.0%	1.01	No	0.01	7	1.37	0.013
	University of Kansas Hospital, Kansas City	12.0	0.0%	1.32	Yes	1.21	7	0.81	0.013
	TIER FOUR								
	Asbury-Salina Regional Medical Center, Salina	1.9	0.0%	1.66	No	0.04	5	0.62	0.006
	Bethany Medical Center, Kansas City	7.2	0.0%	1.05	No	0.05	5	0.58	0.003
	HCA Wesley Medical Center, Wichita	7.6	0.0%	1.25	No	0.15	7	1.10	0.012
	Providence Medical Center, Kansas City	8.2	0.0%	1.06	No	0.00	5	1.02	0.005
	St. Francis Regional Medical Center, Wichita	7.0	0.0%	1.20	No	0.20	7	0.65	0.009
	St. Joseph Medical Center, Wichita	7.7	0.0%	1.14	No	0.08	7	0.91	0.006
	St. Ormont-Vail Regional Medical Center, Topeka	5.8	0.0%	1.29	No	0.01	5	0.80	0.017

ORTHOPEDICS

Natl. Rank	Hospital	U.S. News index	Reputational score	Orthopedics mortality rate	COTH member	Interns and residents to beds	Technology score (of 5)	R.N.'s to beds	Board-certified orthopedists to beds	Procedures to beds
	TIER THREE									
	St. Francis Hospital and Medical Center, Topeka	10.5	0.0%	0.74	No	0.01	3	1.37	0.044	4.42
	St. Ormont-Vail Regional Medical Center, Topeka	8.4	0.0%	0.72	No	0.01	2	0.80	0.037	3.21
95	University of Kansas Hospital, Kansas City	13.2	0.9%	1.29	Yes	1.21	4	0.81	0.022	1.24
	TIER FOUR									
	Asbury-Salina Regional Medical Center, Salina	7.8	0.0%	0.81	No	0.04	3	0.62	0.028	4.80
	Bethany Medical Center, Kansas City	5.8	0.0%	0.85	No	0.05	2	0.58	0.012	1.43
	HCA Wesley Medical Center, Wichita	6.7	0.0%	1.22	No	0.15	4	1.10	0.036	3.12
	Overland Park Regional Medical Center, Overland Park	7.7	0.0%	0.47	No	0.00	2	0.41	0.028	1.44
	Providence Medical Center, Kansas City	7.5	0.0%	0.88	No	0.00	3	1.02	0.019	2.66
	St. Francis Regional Medical Center, Wichita	4.0	0.0%	1.60	No	0.20	4	0.65	0.022	2.42
	St. John's Regional Health Center, Salina	7.9	0.0%	0.85	No	0.01	4	0.71	0.031	3.47
	St. Joseph Medical Center, Wichita	6.9	0.0%	1.01	No	0.08	4	0.91	0.033	1.78

OTOLARYNGOLOGY

Natl. Rank	Hospital	U.S. News index	Reputa-tional score	Hospital-wide mortality rate	COTH member	Interns and residents to beds	Tech-nology score (of 9)	R.N.'s to beds	Board-certified internists to beds	Procedures to beds
	TIER TWO									
	University of Kansas Hospital, Kansas City	13.7	0.3%	1.19	Yes	1.21	7	0.81	0.043	0.205
	TIER THREE									
	HCA Wesley Medical Center, Wichita	7.7	0.0%	1.34	No	0.15	7	1.10	0.232	0.173
	TIER FOUR									
	Asbury-Salina Regional Medical Center, Salina	3.6	0.0%	1.37	No	0.04	5	0.62	0.039	0.304
	Bethany Medical Center, Kansas City	3.8	0.0%	0.90	No	0.05	5	0.58	0.032	0.279
	Mount Carmel Medical Center, Pittsburg	2.7	0.0%	1.14	No	0.00	6	0.28	0.025	0.239
	Overland Park Regional Medical Center, Overland Park	2.9	0.0%	0.82	No	0.00	3	0.41	0.063	0.108
	Providence Medical Center, Kansas City	5.0	0.0%	1.13	No	0.00	5	1.02	0.052	0.384
	St. Francis Hospital and Medical Center, Topeka	6.7	0.0%	1.12	No	0.01	7	1.37	0.057	0.324
	St. Francis Regional Medical Center, Wichita	4.8	0.0%	1.44	No	0.20	7	0.65	0.025	0.135
	St. John's Regional Health Center, Salina	4.6	0.0%	0.99	No	0.01	7	0.71	0.044	0.302
	St. Joseph Medical Center, Wichita	5.1	0.0%	1.43	No	0.08	7	0.91	0.024	0.222
	St. Ormont-Vail Regional Medical Center, Topeka	3.8	0.0%	1.07	No	0.01	3	0.80	0.057	0.209

RHEUMATOLOGY

Natl. Rank	Hospital	U.S. News index	Reputa-tional score	Hospital-wide mortality rate	COTH member	Interns and residents to beds	Tech-nology score (of 5)	R.N.'s to beds	Board-certified internists to beds
	TIER THREE								
	University of Kansas Hospital, Kansas City	14.6	0.5%	1.19	Yes	1.21	4	0.81	0.043
	TIER FOUR								
	Asbury-Salina Regional Medical Center, Salina	5.3	0.0%	1.37	No	0.04	3	0.62	0.039
	Bethany Medical Center, Kansas City	8.2	0.0%	0.90	No	0.05	2	0.58	0.032
	HCA Wesley Medical Center, Wichita	8.9	0.0%	1.34	No	0.15	4	1.10	0.232
	Overland Park Regional Medical Center, Overland Park	8.6	0.0%	0.82	No	0.00	2	0.41	0.063
	Providence Medical Center, Kansas City	7.7	0.0%	1.13	No	0.00	3	1.02	0.052
	St. Francis Hospital and Medical Center, Topeka	8.8	0.0%	1.12	No	0.01	3	1.37	0.057
	St. Francis Regional Medical Center, Wichita	6.7	0.4%	1.44	No	0.20	4	0.65	0.025
	St. Joseph Medical Center, Wichita	5.2	0.0%	1.43	No	0.08	4	0.91	0.024
	St. Ormont-Vail Regional Medical Center, Topeka	7.2	0.0%	1.07	No	0.01	2	0.80	0.057

UROLOGY

Natl. Rank	Hospital	U.S. News index	Reputa-tional score	Urology mortality rate	COTH member	Interns and residents to beds	Tech-nology score (of 11)	R.N.'s to beds	Board-certified internists to beds	Procedures to beds
	TIER TWO									
54	University of Kansas Hospital, Kansas City	17.5	1.0%	0.86	Yes	1.21	9	0.81	0.043	1.94
	TIER THREE									
	Bethany Medical Center, Kansas City	9.9	0.0%	0.71	No	0.05	6	0.58	0.032	1.15
	TIER FOUR									
	Asbury-Salina Regional Medical Center, Salina	4.8	0.0%	1.35	No	0.04	6	0.62	0.039	2.83
	HCA Wesley Medical Center, Wichita	8.1	0.0%	1.25	No	0.15	9	1.10	0.232	1.76
	Mount Carmel Medical Center, Pittsburg	5.1	0.0%	1.16	No	0.00	8	0.28	0.025	2.20
	Overland Park Regional Medical Center, Overland Park	7.0	0.0%	0.86	No	0.00	4	0.41	0.063	0.86
	Providence Medical Center, Kansas City	3.3	0.0%	1.94	No	0.00	6	1.02	0.052	1.51
	St. Francis Hospital and Medical Center, Topeka	7.4	0.0%	1.31	No	0.01	8	1.37	0.057	2.83
	St. Francis Regional Medical Center, Wichita	3.8	0.0%	1.80	No	0.20	8	0.65	0.025	1.71
	St. John's Regional Health Center, Salina	5.5	0.0%	1.32	No	0.01	9	0.71	0.044	1.63
	St. Joseph Medical Center, Wichita	7.7	0.0%	1.08	No	0.08	9	0.91	0.024	1.85
	St. Ormont-Vail Regional Medical Center, Topeka	4.8	0.0%	1.31	No	0.01	5	0.80	0.057	1.59

AIDS

Natl. Rank	Hospital	U.S. News index	Reputa-tional score	Hospital-wide mortality rate	COTH member	Interns and residents to beds	Tech-nology score (of 11)	Discharge planning (of 2)	R.N.'s to beds	Board-certified internists to beds
TIER THREE										
	University of Kentucky Hospital, Lexington	23.6	0.0%	1.04	Yes	0.60	6	2	1.51	0.133
TIER FOUR										
	Central Baptist Hospital, Lexington	19.4	0.0%	1.07	No	0.03	6	2	1.10	0.028
	Humana Hospital-Lexington, Lexington	18.9	0.0%	1.04	No	0.00	5	1	1.19	0.058
	Jennie Stuart Medical Center, Hopkinsville	14.3	0.0%	1.56	No	0.00	6	2	0.97	0.029
	Jewish Hospital, Louisville	17.9	0.0%	1.15	No	0.05	5	2	1.06	0.060
	Lourdes Hospital, Paducah	18.1	0.0%	1.04	No	0.00	5	1	0.79	0.022
	Medical Center-Bowling Green, Bowling Green	18.8	0.0%	1.03	No	0.00	5	2	0.70	0.020
	Norton Hospital of Alliant Health, Louisville	19.2	0.0%	1.08	No	0.16	5	2	1.11	0.052
	Owensboro-Daviess County Hospital, Owensboro	18.4	0.0%	1.15	No	0.00	6	2	1.17	0.030
	Regional Medical Center of Hopkins County, Madisonville	14.6	0.0%	1.53	No	0.04	8	2	0.60	0.005
	St. Anthony Medical Center, Louisville	15.8	0.0%	1.27	No	0.00	7	1	0.60	0.064
	St. Elizabeth Medical Center-North, Covington	15.7	0.0%	1.22	No	0.09	4	1	0.89	0.023
	St. Joseph Hospital, Lexington	18.2	0.0%	1.10	No	0.01	5	2	0.91	0.032
	St. Luke Hospital East, Fort Thomas	17.0	0.0%	1.21	No	0.00	5	2	0.92	0.067

CANCER

Natl. Rank	Hospital	U.S. News index	Reputa-tional score	Cancer mortality rate	COTH member	Interns and residents to beds	Tech-nology score (of 12)	R.N.'s to beds	Board-certified oncologists to beds	Procedures to beds
TIER TWO										
72	University of Kentucky Hospital, Lexington	11.4	0.6%	0.65	Yes	0.60	8	1.51	0.014	1.68
TIER THREE										
	University of Louisville Hospital, Louisville	7.0	0.0%	0.54	Yes	0.53	0	1.16	0.015	0.64
TIER FOUR										
	Central Baptist Hospital, Lexington	4.8	0.0%	0.50	No	0.03	7	1.10	0.012	1.47
	Highlands Regional Medical Center, Prestonsburg	0.7	0.0%	1.32	No	0.00	2	0.52	0.000	0.90
	Humana Hospital-Lexington, Lexington	3.7	0.0%	0.82	No	0.00	4	1.19	0.006	1.20
	Jennie Stuart Medical Center, Hopkinsville	3.5	0.0%	1.68	No	0.00	7	0.97	0.015	1.99
	Jewish Hospital, Louisville	3.3	0.0%	0.94	No	0.05	4	1.06	0.010	1.02
	Lourdes Hospital, Paducah	2.2	0.0%	1.04	No	0.00	3	0.79	0.015	1.49
	Medical Center-Bowling Green, Bowling Green	3.3	0.0%	0.99	No	0.00	8	0.70	0.006	1.25
	Norton Hospital of Alliant Health, Louisville	4.8	0.0%	0.74	No	0.16	6	1.11	0.007	1.65
	Owensboro-Daviess County Hospital, Owensboro	4.7	0.0%	0.91	No	0.00	8	1.17	0.006	1.50
	Regional Medical Center of Hopkins County, Madisonville	3.0	0.0%	1.46	No	0.04	9	0.60	0.002	0.77
	St. Anthony Medical Center, Louisville	2.9	0.0%	1.22	No	0.00	8	0.60	0.023	1.20
	St. Elizabeth Medical Center-North, Covington	4.1	0.0%	0.81	No	0.09	7	0.89	0.008	1.42
	St. Joseph Hospital, Lexington	3.6	0.0%	0.74	No	0.01	5	0.91	0.015	2.20
	St. Luke Hospital East, Fort Thomas	3.4	0.0%	0.99	No	0.00	6	0.92	0.012	1.63
	Western Baptist Hospital, Paducah	3.5	0.0%	1.23	No	0.00	7	0.93	0.006	1.79

CARDIOLOGY

Natl. Rank Hospital	U.S. News index	Reputa- tional score	Cardiology mortality rate	COTH member	Interns and residents to beds	Tech- nology score (of 10)	R.N.'s to beds	Board- certified cardiologists to beds	Procedures to beds
TIER THREE									
University of Kentucky Hospital, Lexington	**14.8**	0.0%	1.32	Yes	0.60	8	1.51	0.025	3.64
University of Louisville Hospital, Louisville	**20.5**	0.0%	0.79	Yes	0.53	0	1.16	0.037	2.31
TIER FOUR									
Central Baptist Hospital, Lexington	**10.1**	0.0%	1.27	No	0.03	8	1.10	0.034	8.93
Highlands Regional Medical Center, Prestonsburg	**6.3**	0.0%	1.30	No	0.00	4	0.52	0.011	8.34
Humana Hospital-Lexington, Lexington	**12.0**	0.0%	1.15	No	0.00	6	1.19	0.069	6.50
Jennie Stuart Medical Center, Hopkinsville	**4.2**	0.0%	1.57	No	0.00	4	0.97	0.007	7.91
Jewish Hospital, Louisville	**12.9**	0.0%	1.11	No	0.05	7	1.06	0.043	14.00
Lourdes Hospital, Paducah	**13.1**	0.0%	1.03	No	0.00	8	0.79	0.018	7.33
Medical Center-Bowling Green, Bowling Green	**10.8**	0.0%	1.10	No	0.00	7	0.70	0.009	4.41
Norton Hospital of Alliant Health, Louisville	**8.1**	0.0%	1.40	No	0.16	7	1.11	0.023	3.88
Owensboro-Daviess County Hospital, Owensboro	**13.0**	0.0%	1.08	No	0.00	7	1.17	0.018	8.72
Regional Medical Center of Hopkins County, Madisonville	**4.1**	0.0%	1.64	No	0.04	9	0.60	0.010	5.30
St. Anthony Medical Center, Louisville	**4.3**	0.0%	1.53	No	0.00	6	0.60	0.027	4.75
St. Elizabeth Medical Center-North, Covington	**7.3**	0.0%	1.33	No	0.09	4	0.89	0.021	7.24
St. Joseph Hospital, Lexington	**9.9**	0.0%	1.24	No	0.01	8	0.91	0.032	8.00
St. Luke Hospital East, Fort Thomas	**10.1**	0.0%	1.18	No	0.00	6	0.92	0.028	7.72
Western Baptist Hospital, Paducah	**12.8**	0.0%	1.04	No	0.00	6	0.93	0.009	11.34

ENDOCRINOLOGY

Natl. Rank Hospital	U.S. News index	Reputa- tional score	Endocrinology mortality rate	COTH member	Interns and residents to beds	Tech- nology score (of 11)	R.N.'s to beds	Board- certified internists to beds
TIER THREE								
Central Baptist Hospital, Lexington	**8.2**	0.0%	0.89	No	0.03	8	1.10	0.028
Norton Hospital of Alliant Health, Louisville	**8.6**	0.0%	0.85	No	0.16	5	1.11	0.052
90 University of Kentucky Hospital, Lexington	**14.1**	0.0%	0.97	Yes	0.60	9	1.51	0.133
94 University of Louisville Hospital, Louisville	**13.9**	0.0%	0.50	Yes	0.53	0	1.16	0.062
TIER FOUR								
Highlands Regional Medical Center, Prestonsburg	**4.2**	0.0%	1.06	No	0.00	3	0.52	0.011
Humana Hospital-Lexington, Lexington	**4.8**	0.0%	1.61	No	0.00	6	1.19	0.058
Jennie Stuart Medical Center, Hopkinsville	**5.2**	0.0%	1.33	No	0.00	8	0.97	0.029
Jewish Hospital, Louisville	**4.4**	0.0%	1.61	No	0.05	5	1.06	0.060
Lourdes Hospital, Paducah	**3.5**	0.0%	1.44	No	0.00	4	0.79	0.022
Medical Center-Bowling Green, Bowling Green	**5.4**	0.0%	1.08	No	0.00	7	0.70	0.020
Owensboro-Daviess County Hospital, Owensboro	**7.8**	0.0%	0.98	No	0.00	9	1.17	0.030
Regional Medical Center of Hopkins County, Madisonville	**3.3**	0.0%	1.70	No	0.04	9	0.60	0.005
St. Anthony Medical Center, Louisville	**6.5**	0.0%	0.98	No	0.00	9	0.60	0.064
St. Elizabeth Medical Center-North, Covington	**4.6**	0.0%	1.45	No	0.09	7	0.89	0.023
St. Joseph Hospital, Lexington	**5.4**	0.0%	1.18	No	0.01	6	0.91	0.032
St. Luke Hospital East, Fort Thomas	**4.3**	0.0%	1.59	No	0.00	7	0.92	0.067
Western Baptist Hospital, Paducah	**6.6**	0.0%	1.02	No	0.00	8	0.93	0.023

GASTROENTEROLOGY

Natl. Rank	Hospital	U.S. News index	Reputa-tional score	Gastro-enterology mortality rate	COTH member	Interns and residents to beds	Tech-nology score (of 11)	R.N.'s to beds	Board-certified gastro-enterologists to beds	Pro-cedures to beds
	TIER THREE									
	Central Baptist Hospital, Lexington	8.3	0.0%	0.83	No	0.03	7	1.10	0.015	2.90
79	University of Kentucky Hospital, Lexington	13.0	0.0%	0.89	Yes	0.60	8	1.51	0.014	1.61
	TIER FOUR									
	Highlands Regional Medical Center, Prestonsburg	5.7	0.0%	0.89	No	0.00	3	0.52	0.005	3.95
	Humana Hospital-Lexington, Lexington	5.3	0.0%	1.26	No	0.00	5	1.19	0.017	3.57
	Jennie Stuart Medical Center, Hopkinsville	4.0	0.0%	2.23	No	0.00	7	0.97	0.007	5.54
	Jewish Hospital, Louisville	4.9	0.0%	1.17	No	0.05	4	1.06	0.002	3.01
	Lourdes Hospital, Paducah	5.8	0.0%	1.08	No	0.00	5	0.79	0.012	4.48
	Medical Center-Bowling Green, Bowling Green	3.8	0.0%	1.24	No	0.00	6	0.70	0.009	2.33
	Norton Hospital of Alliant Health, Louisville	6.7	0.0%	0.90	No	0.16	4	1.11	0.007	1.86
	Owensboro-Daviess County Hospital, Owensboro	6.9	0.0%	1.05	No	0.00	8	1.17	0.000	3.00
	Regional Medical Center of Hopkins County, Madisonville	4.4	0.0%	1.26	No	0.04	8	0.60	0.002	2.67
	St. Anthony Medical Center, Louisville	5.0	0.0%	1.17	No	0.00	8	0.60	0.027	3.00
	St. Elizabeth Medical Center-North, Covington	4.6	0.0%	1.33	No	0.09	6	0.89	0.019	3.01
	St. Joseph Hospital, Lexington	5.1	0.0%	1.09	No	0.01	5	0.91	0.011	2.74
	St. Luke Hospital East, Fort Thomas	4.1	0.0%	1.59	No	0.00	6	0.92	0.020	4.07
	Western Baptist Hospital, Paducah	5.6	0.0%	1.34	No	0.00	7	0.93	0.015	4.70

GERIATRICS

Natl. Rank	Hospital	U.S. News index	Reputa-tional score	Hospital-wide mortality rate	COTH member	Service mix	Interns and residents to beds	Tech-nology score (of 13)	R.N.'s to beds	Discharge planning (of 2)	Geriatric services (of 9)	Board-certified internists to beds
	TIER THREE											
	Medical Center-Bowling Green, Bowling Green	15.7	0.0%	1.03	No	8	0.00	10	0.70	2	6	0.020
	Norton Hospital of Alliant Health, Louisville	14.8	0.0%	1.08	No	7	0.16	7	1.11	2	6	0.052
	University of Kentucky Hospital, Lexington	20.1	0.0%	1.04	Yes	7	0.60	10	1.51	2	4	0.133
	TIER FOUR											
	Central Baptist Hospital, Lexington	13.2	0.0%	1.07	No	5	0.03	10	1.10	2	2	0.028
	Highlands Regional Medical Center, Prestonsburg	6.9	0.0%	1.18	No	4	0.00	4	0.52	1	3	0.011
	Humana Hospital-Lexington, Lexington	11.5	0.0%	1.04	No	3	0.00	7	1.19	1	1	0.058
	Jennie Stuart Medical Center, Hopkinsville	3.6	0.0%	1.56	No	4	0.00	9	0.97	2	1	0.029
	Jewish Hospital, Louisville	10.6	0.0%	1.15	No	4	0.05	6	1.06	2	4	0.060
	Lourdes Hospital, Paducah	11.8	0.0%	1.04	No	6	0.00	6	0.79	1	2	0.022
	Owensboro-Daviess County Hospital, Owensboro	12.2	0.0%	1.15	No	5	0.00	10	1.17	2	5	0.030
	Regional Medical Center of Hopkins County, Madisonville	4.5	0.0%	1.53	No	5	0.04	11	0.60	2	3	0.005
	St. Anthony Medical Center, Louisville	6.1	0.0%	1.27	No	3	0.00	10	0.60	1	2	0.064
	St. Elizabeth Medical Center-North, Covington	8.7	0.0%	1.22	No	7	0.09	7	0.89	1	2	0.023
	St. Joseph Hospital, Lexington	11.7	0.0%	1.10	No	5	0.01	8	0.91	2	2	0.032
	St. Luke Hospital East, Fort Thomas	10.3	0.0%	1.21	No	5	0.00	9	0.92	2	4	0.067

GYNECOLOGY

Natl. Rank	Hospital	U.S. News index	Reputa-tional score	Hospital-wide mortality rate	Interns and residents to beds	Tech-nology score (of 10)	R.N.'s to beds	Board-certified OB-GYNs to beds	Procedures to beds
	TIER THREE								
	Central Baptist Hospital, Lexington	15.8	0.0%	1.07	0.03	7	1.10	0.086	0.73
	Humana Hospital-Lexington, Lexington	15.4	0.0%	1.04	0.00	5	1.19	0.087	0.60
	Norton Hospital of Alliant Health, Louisville	15.3	0.4%	1.08	0.16	5	1.11	0.061	0.54
	Owensboro-Daviess County Hospital, Owensboro	14.4	0.4%	1.15	0.00	8	1.17	0.021	0.32
	University of Kentucky Hospital, Lexington	20.6	0.0%	1.04	0.60	8	1.51	0.047	0.69

Natl. Rank Hospital	U.S. News index	Reputational score	Hospital-wide mortality rate	Interns and residents to beds	Technology score (of 10)	R.N.'s to beds	Board-certified OB-GYNs to beds	Procedures to beds
TIER FOUR								
Highlands Regional Medical Center, Prestonsburg	5.9	0.0%	1.18	0.00	3	0.52	0.005	0.10
Jennie Stuart Medical Center, Hopkinsville	4.6	0.0%	1.56	0.00	6	0.97	0.015	0.79
Jewish Hospital, Louisville	10.0	0.0%	1.15	0.05	4	1.06	0.017	0.18
Lourdes Hospital, Paducah	11.2	0.0%	1.04	0.00	4	0.79	0.012	0.27
Medical Center-Bowling Green, Bowling Green	12.9	0.0%	1.03	0.00	6	0.70	0.031	0.17
Regional Medical Center of Hopkins County, Madisonville	4.8	0.0%	1.53	0.04	8	0.60	0.012	0.25
St. Anthony Medical Center, Louisville	7.6	0.0%	1.27	0.00	7	0.60	0.014	0.35
St. Elizabeth Medical Center-North, Covington	10.3	0.0%	1.22	0.09	6	0.89	0.049	0.33
St. Joseph Hospital, Lexington	10.2	0.0%	1.10	0.01	4	0.91	0.006	0.08
St. Luke Hospital East, Fort Thomas	9.4	0.0%	1.21	0.00	5	0.92	0.039	0.39
Western Baptist Hospital, Paducah	12.0	0.0%	1.11	0.00	6	0.93	0.032	0.48

NEUROLOGY

Natl. Rank Hospital	U.S. News index	Reputational score	Neurology mortality rate	COTH member	Interns and residents to beds	Technology score (of 9)	R.N.'s to beds	Board-certified neurologists to beds
TIER THREE								
Central Baptist Hospital, Lexington	11.4	0.0%	0.93	No	0.03	6	1.10	0.012
96 University of Kentucky Hospital, Lexington	17.3	0.0%	0.95	Yes	0.60	7	1.51	0.025
University of Louisville Hospital, Louisville	12.1	0.6%	1.09	Yes	0.53	0	1.16	0.012
TIER FOUR								
Jewish Hospital, Louisville	7.6	0.0%	1.11	No	0.05	4	1.06	0.005
Lourdes Hospital, Paducah	8.0	0.0%	1.03	No	0.00	4	0.79	0.009
Medical Center-Bowling Green, Bowling Green	9.9	0.0%	0.91	No	0.00	5	0.70	0.006
Norton Hospital of Alliant Health, Louisville	5.9	0.0%	1.35	No	0.16	4	1.11	0.012
Owensboro-Daviess County Hospital, Owensboro	6.4	0.0%	1.29	No	0.00	7	1.17	0.003
Regional Medical Center of Hopkins County, Madisonville	2.2	0.0%	1.66	No	0.04	7	0.60	0.002
St. Anthony Medical Center, Louisville	9.6	0.0%	1.03	No	0.00	7	0.60	0.027
St. Elizabeth Medical Center-North, Covington	9.7	0.0%	0.98	No	0.09	5	0.89	0.011
St. Joseph Hospital, Lexington	10.1	0.0%	0.94	No	0.01	4	0.91	0.013
St. Luke Hospital East, Fort Thomas	8.3	0.0%	1.07	No	0.00	5	0.92	0.012
Western Baptist Hospital, Paducah	7.1	0.0%	1.17	No	0.00	6	0.93	0.009

ORTHOPEDICS

Natl. Rank Hospital	U.S. News index	Reputational score	Orthopedics mortality rate	COTH member	Interns and residents to beds	Technology score (of 5)	R.N.'s to beds	Board-certified orthopedists to beds	Procedures to beds
TIER THREE									
Humana Hospital-Lexington, Lexington	10.6	0.0%	0.68	No	0.00	3	1.19	0.064	2.57
Norton Hospital of Alliant Health, Louisville	12.2	1.4%	0.70	No	0.16	2	1.11	0.031	0.97
St. Joseph Hospital, Lexington	8.2	0.0%	0.78	No	0.01	3	0.91	0.019	2.19
87 University of Kentucky Hospital, Lexington	13.8	0.4%	0.92	Yes	0.60	3	1.51	0.023	1.57
TIER FOUR									
Central Baptist Hospital, Lexington	5.5	0.0%	1.22	No	0.03	3	1.10	0.034	2.44
Jewish Hospital, Louisville	5.7	0.0%	1.16	No	0.05	3	1.06	0.036	2.21
Lourdes Hospital, Paducah	6.7	0.0%	0.90	No	0.00	3	0.79	0.015	2.83
Medical Center-Bowling Green, Bowling Green	5.7	0.0%	0.87	No	0.00	2	0.70	0.020	1.31
Owensboro-Daviess County Hospital, Owensboro	5.6	0.0%	1.18	No	0.00	3	1.17	0.024	2.03
Regional Medical Center of Hopkins County, Madisonville	6.5	0.0%	0.92	No	0.04	4	0.60	0.005	1.96
St. Anthony Medical Center, Louisville	3.5	0.0%	1.45	No	0.00	4	0.60	0.027	1.76
St. Elizabeth Medical Center-North, Covington	4.6	0.0%	1.05	No	0.09	1	0.89	0.026	1.86
St. Luke Hospital East, Fort Thomas	3.1	0.0%	1.68	No	0.00	3	0.92	0.031	1.96
Western Baptist Hospital, Paducah	5.5	0.0%	1.00	No	0.00	2	0.93	0.006	2.69

OTOLARYNGOLOGY

Natl. Rank	Hospital	U.S. News index	Reputa- tional score	Hospital- wide mortality rate	COTH member	Interns and residents to beds	Tech- nology score (of 9)	R.N.'s to beds	Board- certified internists to beds	Procedures to beds
TIER TWO										
84	University of Kentucky Hospital, Lexington	14.4	0.4%	1.04	Yes	0.60	7	1.51	0.133	0.270
TIER THREE										
	Norton Hospital of Alliant Health, Louisville	7.0	0.5%	1.07	No	0.16	3	1.11	0.052	0.140
	University of Louisville Hospital, Louisville	9.5	0.0%	0.91	Yes	0.53	0	1.16	0.062	0.059
TIER FOUR										
	Central Baptist Hospital, Lexington	5.4	0.0%	1.07	No	0.03	6	1.10	0.028	0.225
	Highlands Regional Medical Center, Prestonsburg	1.9	0.0%	1.18	No	0.00	1	0.52	0.011	0.283
	Humana Hospital-Lexington, Lexington	5.3	0.0%	1.04	No	0.00	4	1.19	0.058	0.116
	Jennie Stuart Medical Center, Hopkinsville	4.7	0.0%	1.56	No	0.00	6	0.97	0.029	0.292
	Jewish Hospital, Louisville	4.8	0.0%	1.15	No	0.05	3	1.06	0.060	0.200
	Lourdes Hospital, Paducah	3.2	0.0%	1.04	No	0.00	2	0.79	0.022	0.265
	Medical Center-Bowling Green, Bowling Green	4.0	0.0%	1.03	No	0.00	6	0.70	0.020	0.169
	Owensboro-Daviess County Hospital, Owensboro	5.8	0.0%	1.15	No	0.00	7	1.17	0.030	0.308
	Regional Medical Center of Hopkins County, Madisonville	3.8	0.0%	1.53	No	0.04	7	0.60	0.005	0.285
	St. Anthony Medical Center, Louisville	4.2	0.0%	1.28	No	0.00	7	0.60	0.064	0.205
	St. Elizabeth Medical Center-North, Covington	4.9	0.0%	1.22	No	0.09	6	0.89	0.023	0.257
	St. Joseph Hospital, Lexington	4.2	0.0%	1.10	No	0.01	4	0.91	0.032	0.154
	St. Luke Hospital East, Fort Thomas	4.7	0.0%	1.21	No	0.00	5	0.92	0.067	0.370
	Western Baptist Hospital, Paducah	4.7	0.0%	1.11	No	0.00	6	0.93	0.023	0.319

RHEUMATOLOGY

Natl. Rank	Hospital	U.S. News index	Reputa- tional score	Hospital- wide mortality rate	COTH member	Interns and residents to beds	Tech- nology score (of 5)	R.N.'s to beds	Board- certified internists to beds
TIER THREE									
	University of Kentucky Hospital, Lexington	14.8	0.0%	1.04	Yes	0.60	3	1.51	0.133
	University of Louisville Hospital, Louisville	11.0	0.0%	0.91	Yes	0.53	0	1.16	0.062
TIER FOUR									
	Central Baptist Hospital, Lexington	8.4	0.0%	1.07	No	0.03	3	1.10	0.028
	Highlands Regional Medical Center, Prestonsburg	4.3	0.0%	1.18	No	0.00	2	0.52	0.011
	Humana Hospital-Lexington, Lexington	8.0	0.0%	1.04	No	0.00	3	1.19	0.058
	Jennie Stuart Medical Center, Hopkinsville	5.2	0.0%	1.56	No	0.00	3	0.97	0.029
	Jewish Hospital, Louisville	7.9	0.0%	1.15	No	0.05	3	1.06	0.060
	Lourdes Hospital, Paducah	6.6	0.0%	1.04	No	0.00	3	0.79	0.022
	Medical Center-Bowling Green, Bowling Green	7.0	0.0%	1.03	No	0.00	2	0.70	0.020
	Norton Hospital of Alliant Health, Louisville	8.5	0.0%	1.07	No	0.16	2	1.11	0.052
	Owensboro-Daviess County Hospital, Owensboro	7.9	0.0%	1.15	No	0.00	3	1.17	0.030
	Regional Medical Center of Hopkins County, Madisonville	4.8	0.0%	1.53	No	0.04	4	0.60	0.005
	St. Anthony Medical Center, Louisville	5.2	0.0%	1.28	No	0.00	4	0.60	0.064
	St. Elizabeth Medical Center-North, Covington	4.9	0.0%	1.22	No	0.09	1	0.89	0.023
	St. Joseph Hospital, Lexington	7.6	0.0%	1.10	No	0.01	3	0.91	0.032
	St. Luke Hospital East, Fort Thomas	7.1	0.0%	1.21	No	0.00	3	0.92	0.067
	Western Baptist Hospital, Paducah	6.0	0.0%	1.11	No	0.00	2	0.93	0.023

UROLOGY

Natl. Rank	Hospital	U.S. News index	Reputa-tional score	Urology mortality rate	COTH member	Interns and residents to beds	Tech-nology score (of 11)	R.N.'s to beds	Board-certified internists to beds	Procedures to beds
	TIER THREE									
	University of Kentucky Hospital, Lexington	14.0	0.0%	1.07	Yes	0.60	8	1.51	0.133	1.45
	TIER FOUR									
	Central Baptist Hospital, Lexington	8.2	0.0%	0.99	No	0.03	7	1.10	0.028	1.79
	Highlands Regional Medical Center, Prestonsburg	3.9	0.0%	1.22	No	0.00	3	0.52	0.011	2.06
	Humana Hospital-Lexington, Lexington	6.6	0.0%	1.21	No	0.00	5	1.19	0.058	2.37
	Jennie Stuart Medical Center, Hopkinsville	4.3	0.0%	1.74	No	0.00	7	0.97	0.029	3.07
	Jewish Hospital, Louisville	5.1	0.0%	1.44	No	0.05	4	1.06	0.060	2.77
	Lourdes Hospital, Paducah	3.8	0.0%	1.47	No	0.00	5	0.79	0.022	1.74
	Medical Center-Bowling Green, Bowling Green	3.7	0.0%	1.47	No	0.00	6	0.70	0.020	1.30
	Norton Hospital of Alliant Health, Louisville	5.2	0.0%	1.37	No	0.16	4	1.11	0.052	0.71
	Owensboro-Daviess County Hospital, Owensboro	6.9	0.0%	1.20	No	0.00	8	1.17	0.030	1.33
	Regional Medical Center of Hopkins County, Madisonville	2.9	0.0%	1.78	No	0.04	8	0.60	0.005	1.32
	St. Anthony Medical Center, Louisville	5.3	0.0%	1.30	No	0.00	8	0.60	0.064	2.12
	St. Elizabeth Medical Center-North, Covington	8.0	0.0%	0.94	No	0.09	6	0.89	0.023	1.39
	St. Joseph Hospital, Lexington	3.4	0.0%	1.66	No	0.01	5	0.91	0.032	1.44
	St. Luke Hospital East, Fort Thomas	5.5	0.0%	1.32	No	0.00	6	0.92	0.067	1.89
	Western Baptist Hospital, Paducah	8.0	0.0%	0.97	No	0.00	7	0.93	0.023	2.03

AIDS

Natl. Rank	Hospital	U.S. News index	Reputa- tional score	Hospital- wide mortality rate	COTH member	Interns and residents to beds	Tech- nology score (of 11)	Discharge planning (of 2)	R.N.'s to beds	Board- certified internists to beds
					TIER TWO					
59	Medical Center of Louisiana at New Orleans	26.5	1.3%	1.15	Yes	1.39	8	2	0.91	0.457
79	Ochsner Foundation Hospital, New Orleans	25.4	0.6%	0.83	Yes	0.44	8	1	0.82	0.054
53	Tulane University Hospital and Clinics, New Orleans	26.8	0.0%	0.78	Yes	0.76	8	2	0.88	0.219
					TIER THREE					
	Baton Rouge General Medical Center, Baton Rouge	20.6	0.0%	0.96	No	0.01	7	2	0.55	0.080
	Glenwood Regional Medical Center, Westmonroe	20.4	0.0%	0.93	No	0.00	7	1	0.59	0.026
	LSU Medical Center-University Hospital, Shreveport	22.4	0.0%	1.14	Yes	1.07	7	2	0.90	0.085
	Lake Charles Memorial Hospital, Lake Charles	21.8	0.0%	0.85	No	0.02	6	2	0.59	0.068
	Mercy Hospital of New Orleans	20.3	0.0%	0.97	No	0.00	7	2	0.38	0.075
	Slidell Memorial Hospital and Medical Center, Slidell	20.8	0.0%	0.96	No	0.01	6	2	0.97	0.038
	Touro Infirmary, New Orleans	20.1	0.0%	0.97	No	0.09	6	2	0.31	0.103
	West Jefferson Medical Center, Marrero	21.2	0.0%	0.96	No	0.00	8	2	0.65	0.058
					TIER FOUR					
	E. A. Conway Medical Center, Monroe	11.7	0.0%	1.70	No	0.24	4	1	0.54	0.022
	Earl K. Long Medical Center, Baton Rouge	13.8	0.0%	1.74	No	0.78	5	1	0.59	0.208
	East Jefferson General Hospital, Metairie	15.5	0.0%	1.38	No	0.00	6	2	0.89	0.040
	Huey P. Long Medical Center, Pineville, La.	13.6	0.0%	1.39	No	0.13	3	1	0.75	0.033
	Lafayette General Medical Center, Lafayette	19.1	0.0%	1.10	No	0.00	8	2	0.81	0.035
	Lakeland Medical Center, New Orleans	18.8	0.0%	1.06	No	0.00	6	2	0.67	0.067
	Northshore Regional Medical Center, Slidell	17.4	0.0%	1.14	No	0.00	5	2	0.78	0.033
	Opelousas General Hospital, Opelousas	18.5	0.0%	1.06	No	0.00	7	2	0.33	0.027
	Our Lady of Lake Regional Medical Center, Baton Rouge	18.0	0.0%	1.28	No	0.00	10	2	0.89	0.061
	Our Lady of Lourdes Regional Center, Lafayette	17.6	0.0%	1.16	No	0.00	6	2	0.76	0.056
	Rapides Regional Medical Center, Alexandria	18.4	0.0%	1.17	No	0.00	8	2	0.88	0.040
	Southern Baptist Hospital, New Orleans	14.2	0.0%	1.44	No	0.04	5	2	0.58	0.038
	St. Frances Cabrini Hospital, Alexandria	17.8	0.0%	1.19	No	0.00	7	2	0.94	0.032
	St. Francis Medical Center, Monroe	15.2	0.0%	1.34	No	0.00	6	2	0.59	0.005
	Terrebonne General Medical Center, Houma	18.0	0.0%	1.12	No	0.00	6	2	0.74	0.027
	University Hospital, New Orleans	13.8	0.0%	1.54	No	0.07	6	2	0.57	0.022
	University Medical Center, Lafayette	19.3	0.0%	1.02	No	0.38	6	1	0.52	0.068

CANCER

Natl. Rank	Hospital	U.S. News index	Reputa- tional score	Cancer mortality rate	COTH member	Interns and residents to beds	Tech- nology score (of 12)	R.N.'s to beds	Board- certified oncologists to beds	Procedures to beds
					TIER TWO					
80	Medical Center of Louisiana at New Orleans	11.1	0.0%	0.76	Yes	1.39	8	0.91	0.012	0.36
					TIER THREE					
89	LSU Medical Center-University Hospital, Shreveport	10.6	0.4%	0.76	Yes	1.07	8	0.90	0.017	0.79
	Ochsner Foundation Hospital, New Orleans	8.7	0.0%	0.58	Yes	0.44	10	0.82	0.013	1.54
	Tulane University Hospital and Clinics, New Orleans	8.5	0.0%	0.87	Yes	0.76	6	0.88	0.022	1.50
					TIER FOUR					
	Baton Rouge General Medical Center, Baton Rouge	3.9	0.0%	0.77	No	0.01	10	0.55	0.017	1.61
	East Jefferson General Hospital, Metairie	4.5	0.5%	1.17	No	0.00	8	0.89	0.013	2.39
	Glenwood Regional Medical Center, Westmonroe	3.8	0.0%	0.84	No	0.00	9	0.59	0.010	2.75
	Lafayette General Medical Center, Lafayette	4.4	0.0%	0.87	No	0.00	10	0.81	0.010	1.41
	Mercy Hospital of New Orleans	3.0	0.0%	0.80	No	0.00	9	0.38	0.011	1.48
	Northshore Regional Medical Center, Slidell	2.3	0.0%	1.06	No	0.00	4	0.78	0.008	1.37
	Our Lady of Lake Regional Medical Center, Baton Rouge	3.8	0.0%	1.17	No	0.00	8	0.89	0.009	2.03
	Our Lady of Lourdes Regional Center, Lafayette	3.9	0.0%	0.84	No	0.00	8	0.76	0.015	2.46

Natl. Rank	Hospital	U.S. News index	Reputa- tional score	Cancer mortality rate	COTH member	Interns and residents to beds	Tech- nology score (of 12)	R.N.'s to beds	Board- certified oncologists to beds	Procedures to beds
	Rapides Regional Medical Center, Alexandria	4.2	0.0%	0.97	No	0.00	9	0.88	0.008	1.86
	Schumpert Medical Center, Shreveport	4.0	0.0%	0.97	No	0.01	9	0.82	0.008	1.68
	Southern Baptist Hospital, New Orleans	1.8	0.0%	1.16	No	0.04	4	0.58	0.005	1.33
	St. Frances Cabrini Hospital, Alexandria	4.5	0.0%	0.89	No	0.00	9	0.94	0.012	1.62
	St. Francis Medical Center, Monroe	2.9	0.0%	0.86	No	0.00	7	0.59	0.010	1.52
	Terrebonne General Medical Center, Houma	2.0	0.0%	1.32	No	0.00	4	0.74	0.004	1.12
	Touro Infirmary, New Orleans	2.3	0.0%	1.01	No	0.09	7	0.31	0.027	1.27
	University Hospital, New Orleans	2.8	0.0%	1.16	No	0.07	7	0.57	0.022	0.92
	West Jefferson Medical Center, Marrero	3.2	0.0%	1.30	No	0.00	9	0.65	0.010	1.06
	Willis-Knighton Medical Center, Shreveport	1.0	0.0%	1.00	No	0.06	0	0.63	0.012	1.02
	Woman's Hospital, Baton Rouge	2.0	0.0%	1.73	No	0.00	1	1.07	0.012	1.77

CARDIOLOGY

Natl. Rank	Hospital	U.S. News index	Reputa- tional score	Cardiology mortality rate	COTH member	Interns and residents to beds	Tech- nology score (of 10)	R.N.'s to beds	Board- certified cardiologists to beds	Procedures to beds
	TIER TWO									
80	LSU Medical Center-University Hospital, Shreveport	21.4	0.0%	0.95	Yes	1.07	7	0.90	0.014	3.09
43	Tulane University Hospital and Clinics, New Orleans	23.8	0.0%	0.83	Yes	0.76	9	0.88	0.059	3.40
	TIER THREE									
	Mercy Hospital of New Orleans	15.1	0.0%	0.92	No	0.00	8	0.38	0.023	9.14
	Ochsner Foundation Hospital, New Orleans	19.1	1.4%	1.07	Yes	0.44	8	0.82	0.030	8.77
	Slidell Memorial Hospital and Medical Center, Slidell	14.0	0.0%	1.04	No	0.01	8	0.97	0.044	8.32
	Touro Infirmary, New Orleans	14.4	0.0%	0.97	No	0.09	8	0.31	0.067	5.69
	West Jefferson Medical Center, Marrero	14.7	0.0%	0.98	No	0.00	9	0.65	0.039	8.72
	TIER FOUR									
	Baton Rouge General Medical Center, Baton Rouge	12.8	0.0%	1.03	No	0.01	8	0.55	0.041	6.97
	East Jefferson General Hospital, Metairie	6.5	0.0%	1.52	No	0.00	8	0.89	0.046	8.01
	Glenwood Regional Medical Center, Westmonroe	8.8	0.0%	1.18	No	0.00	6	0.59	0.010	7.11
	Lafayette General Medical Center, Lafayette	7.8	0.0%	1.34	No	0.00	8	0.81	0.016	8.14
	Lakeland Medical Center, New Orleans	9.2	0.0%	1.24	No	0.00	8	0.67	0.027	10.26
	Northshore Regional Medical Center, Slidell	6.7	0.0%	1.41	No	0.00	7	0.78	0.024	8.18
	Our Lady of Lake Regional Medical Center, Baton Rouge	7.8	0.0%	1.42	No	0.00	10	0.89	0.031	6.13
	Our Lady of Lourdes Regional Center, Lafayette	8.2	0.0%	1.32	No	0.00	7	0.76	0.034	10.49
	Rapides Regional Medical Center, Alexandria	8.2	0.0%	1.34	No	0.00	8	0.88	0.024	6.98
	Schumpert Medical Center, Shreveport	8.5	0.0%	1.29	No	0.01	8	0.82	0.018	6.01
	Southern Baptist Hospital, New Orleans	6.8	0.0%	1.39	No	0.04	8	0.58	0.028	6.64
	St. Frances Cabrini Hospital, Alexandria	6.8	0.0%	1.46	No	0.00	8	0.94	0.020	8.11
	St. Francis Medical Center, Monroe	4.0	0.0%	1.61	No	0.00	7	0.59	0.020	8.05
	Terrebonne General Medical Center, Houma	10.4	0.0%	1.21	No	0.00	9	0.74	0.031	13.61
	University Hospital, New Orleans	6.0	0.0%	1.48	No	0.07	8	0.57	0.044	5.14
	Willis-Knighton Medical Center, Shreveport	2.0	0.0%	1.67	No	0.06	0	0.63	0.033	8.96

ENDOCRINOLOGY

Natl. Rank	Hospital	U.S. News index	Reputa- tional score	Endocrinology mortality rate	COTH member	Interns and residents to beds	Tech- nology score (of 11)	R.N.'s to beds	Board- certified internists to beds
	TIER TWO								
77	Tulane University Hospital and Clinics, New Orleans	15.1	0.0%	0.73	Yes	0.76	6	0.88	0.219
	TIER THREE								
	Glenwood Regional Medical Center, Westmonroe	9.6	0.0%	0.39	No	0.00	9	0.59	0.026
	LSU Medical Center-University Hospital, Shreveport	12.0	0.0%	1.26	Yes	1.07	9	0.90	0.085
	Mercy Hospital of New Orleans	9.4	0.0%	0.67	No	0.00	10	0.38	0.075
	Northshore Regional Medical Center, Slidell	8.2	0.0%	0.74	No	0.00	5	0.78	0.033

Natl. Rank	Hospital	U.S. News index	Reputational score	Endocrinology mortality rate	COTH member	Interns and residents to beds	Technology score (of 11)	R.N.'s to beds	Board-certified internists to beds
93	Ochsner Foundation Hospital, New Orleans	13.9	0.5%	0.75	Yes	0.44	10	0.82	0.054
	St. Frances Cabrini Hospital, Alexandria	10.8	0.0%	0.60	No	0.00	10	0.94	0.032
	West Jefferson Medical Center, Marrero	10.0	0.0%	0.63	No	0.00	9	0.65	0.058
	TIER FOUR								
	Baton Rouge General Medical Center, Baton Rouge	7.6	0.0%	0.85	No	0.01	9	0.55	0.080
	East Jefferson General Hospital, Metairie	5.8	0.0%	1.22	No	0.00	9	0.89	0.040
	Lafayette General Medical Center, Lafayette	7.1	0.0%	0.97	No	0.00	10	0.81	0.035
	Lakeland Medical Center, New Orleans	4.6	0.0%	1.42	No	0.00	9	0.67	0.067
	Opelousas General Hospital, Opelousas	3.5	0.0%	1.34	No	0.00	8	0.33	0.027
	Our Lady of Lake Regional Medical Center, Baton Rouge	4.8	0.0%	1.41	No	0.00	7	0.89	0.061
	Our Lady of Lourdes Regional Center, Lafayette	5.8	0.0%	1.16	No	0.00	9	0.76	0.056
	Rapides Regional Medical Center, Alexandria	6.4	0.0%	1.09	No	0.00	9	0.88	0.040
	Schumpert Medical Center, Shreveport	7.7	0.0%	0.88	No	0.01	9	0.82	0.033
	Slidell Memorial Hospital and Medical Center, Slidell	6.2	0.0%	1.06	No	0.01	6	0.97	0.038
	Southern Baptist Hospital, New Orleans	3.4	0.0%	1.44	No	0.04	5	0.58	0.038
	St. Francis Medical Center, Monroe	1.8	0.0%	2.23	No	0.00	7	0.59	0.005
	Terrebonne General Medical Center, Houma	3.4	0.0%	1.52	No	0.00	5	0.74	0.027
	Touro Infirmary, New Orleans	5.6	0.0%	1.06	No	0.09	8	0.31	0.103
	University Hospital, New Orleans	6.2	0.0%	0.98	No	0.07	8	0.57	0.022
	Willis-Knighton Medical Center, Shreveport	6.4	0.0%	0.82	No	0.06	0	0.63	0.073

GASTROENTEROLOGY

Natl. Rank	Hospital	U.S. News index	Reputational score	Gastroenterology mortality rate	COTH member	Interns and residents to beds	Technology score (of 11)	R.N.'s to beds	Board-certified gastroenterologists to beds	Procedures to beds
	TIER THREE									
	Lakeland Medical Center, New Orleans	8.0	0.0%	0.59	No	0.00	8	0.67	0.020	3.31
85	Ochsner Foundation Hospital, New Orleans	12.8	0.8%	0.94	Yes	0.44	10	0.82	0.009	2.78
	Slidell Memorial Hospital and Medical Center, Slidell	7.9	0.0%	0.84	No	0.01	7	0.97	0.016	2.82
	TIER FOUR									
	Baton Rouge General Medical Center, Baton Rouge	7.2	0.0%	0.89	No	0.01	9	0.55	0.024	3.22
	East Jefferson General Hospital, Metairie	5.5	0.0%	1.20	No	0.00	8	0.89	0.029	3.01
	Glenwood Regional Medical Center, Westmonroe	6.9	0.0%	0.96	No	0.00	8	0.59	0.026	4.16
	Lafayette General Medical Center, Lafayette	6.1	0.0%	1.10	No	0.00	10	0.81	0.022	2.43
	Mercy Hospital of New Orleans	5.5	0.0%	1.10	No	0.00	9	0.38	0.026	3.53
	Our Lady of Lake Regional Medical Center, Baton Rouge	4.5	0.0%	1.34	No	0.00	7	0.89	0.016	2.99
	Our Lady of Lourdes Regional Center, Lafayette	6.5	0.0%	1.16	No	0.00	8	0.76	0.030	4.91
	Rapides Regional Medical Center, Alexandria	7.0	0.0%	1.07	No	0.00	9	0.88	0.003	3.92
	Schumpert Medical Center, Shreveport	6.7	0.4%	1.14	No	0.01	9	0.82	0.010	3.23
	Southern Baptist Hospital, New Orleans	2.0	0.0%	1.70	No	0.04	4	0.58	0.018	3.24
	St. Frances Cabrini Hospital, Alexandria	5.0	0.0%	1.51	No	0.00	9	0.94	0.008	3.64
	St. Francis Medical Center, Monroe	4.4	0.0%	1.22	No	0.00	6	0.59	0.015	3.56
	Terrebonne General Medical Center, Houma	5.4	0.0%	1.04	No	0.00	5	0.74	0.008	3.46
	Touro Infirmary, New Orleans	4.7	0.0%	1.05	No	0.09	7	0.31	0.036	2.46
	University Hospital, New Orleans	3.4	0.0%	1.41	No	0.07	7	0.57	0.015	2.31
	West Jefferson Medical Center, Marrero	5.4	0.0%	1.11	No	0.00	9	0.65	0.029	2.43
	Willis-Knighton Medical Center, Shreveport	0.0	0.0%	1.95	No	0.06	0	0.63	0.016	2.41

GERIATRICS

Natl. Rank	Hospital	U.S. News index	Reputa-tional score	Hospital-wide mortality rate	COTH member	Service mix	Interns and residents to beds	Tech-nology score (of 13)	R.N.'s to beds	Discharge planning (of 2)	Geriatric services (of 9)	Board-certified internists to beds
	TIER TWO											
56	Tulane University Hospital and Clinics, New Orleans	23.7	0.0%	0.78	Yes	8	0.76	8	0.88	2	2	0.219
	TIER THREE											
	Baton Rouge General Medical Center, Baton Rouge	17.1	0.0%	0.96	No	6	0.01	11	0.55	2	7	0.080
	LSU Medical Center-University Hospital, Shreveport	15.9	0.0%	1.14	Yes	6	1.07	9	0.90	2	1	0.085
	Mercy Hospital of New Orleans	14.3	0.0%	0.97	No	4	0.00	10	0.38	2	2	0.075
91	Ochsner Foundation Hospital, New Orleans	21.6	0.0%	0.83	Yes	9	0.44	11	0.82	1	1	0.054
	Slidell Memorial Hospital and Medical Center, Slidell	15.3	0.0%	0.96	No	5	0.01	7	0.97	2	2	0.038
	Touro Infirmary, New Orleans	16.0	0.0%	0.97	No	5	0.09	10	0.31	2	6	0.103
	West Jefferson Medical Center, Marrero	15.2	0.0%	0.96	No	3	0.00	11	0.65	2	3	0.058
	TIER FOUR											
	East Jefferson General Hospital, Metairie	6.7	0.0%	1.38	No	5	0.00	10	0.89	2	2	0.040
	Lafayette General Medical Center, Lafayette	12.9	0.0%	1.10	No	6	0.00	10	0.81	2	5	0.035
	Lakeland Medical Center, New Orleans	12.0	0.0%	1.06	No	4	0.00	9	0.67	2	2	0.067
	Our Lady of Lake Regional Medical Center, Baton Rouge	10.2	0.0%	1.28	No	7	0.00	8	0.89	2	7	0.061
	Our Lady of Lourdes Regional Center, Lafayette	10.1	0.0%	1.16	No	4	0.00	9	0.76	2	3	0.056
	Rapides Regional Medical Center, Alexandria	10.9	0.0%	1.17	No	5	0.00	10	0.88	2	4	0.040
	Schumpert Medical Center, Shreveport	13.0	0.0%	1.13	No	6	0.01	10	0.82	2	7	0.033
	Southern Baptist Hospital, New Orleans	5.4	0.0%	1.44	No	6	0.04	7	0.58	2	3	0.038
	St. Frances Cabrini Hospital, Alexandria	11.1	0.0%	1.19	No	5	0.00	10	0.94	2	6	0.032
	St. Francis Medical Center, Monroe	7.7	0.0%	1.34	No	7	0.00	9	0.59	2	4	0.005
	Terrebonne General Medical Center, Houma	9.6	0.0%	1.12	No	3	0.00	7	0.74	2	1	0.027
	University Hospital, New Orleans	3.9	0.0%	1.54	No	5	0.07	8	0.57	2	3	0.022

GYNECOLOGY

Natl. Rank	Hospital	U.S. News index	Reputa-tional score	Hospital-wide mortality rate	Interns and residents to beds	Tech-nology score (of 10)	R.N.'s to beds	Board-certified OB-GYNs to beds	Procedures to beds
	TIER TWO								
69	Ochsner Foundation Hospital, New Orleans	23.7	0.9%	0.83	0.44	9	0.82	0.006	0.38
58	Tulane University Hospital and Clinics, New Orleans	25.2	0.9%	0.78	0.76	6	0.88	0.089	0.27
	TIER THREE								
	Baton Rouge General Medical Center, Baton Rouge	14.1	0.0%	0.96	0.01	7	0.55	0.005	0.08
	Glenwood Regional Medical Center, Westmonroe	16.3	0.0%	0.93	0.00	7	0.59	0.041	0.69
	LSU Medical Center-University Hospital, Shreveport	19.7	1.0%	1.14	1.07	8	0.90	0.028	0.17
	Mercy Hospital of New Orleans	15.5	0.4%	0.97	0.00	8	0.38	0.023	0.32
	Slidell Memorial Hospital and Medical Center, Slidell	16.2	0.0%	0.96	0.01	6	0.97	0.038	0.30
	Touro Infirmary, New Orleans	14.5	0.0%	0.97	0.09	7	0.31	0.052	0.18
	West Jefferson Medical Center, Marrero	15.9	0.0%	0.96	0.00	7	0.65	0.050	0.23
	TIER FOUR								
	East Jefferson General Hospital, Metairie	9.2	0.0%	1.38	0.00	8	0.89	0.073	0.24
	Lafayette General Medical Center, Lafayette	13.4	0.0%	1.10	0.00	9	0.81	0.022	0.27
	Lakeland Medical Center, New Orleans	13.0	0.0%	1.06	0.00	7	0.67	0.047	0.31
	Our Lady of Lake Regional Medical Center, Baton Rouge	8.5	0.0%	1.28	0.00	7	0.89	0.003	0.16
	Our Lady of Lourdes Regional Center, Lafayette	10.5	0.0%	1.16	0.00	7	0.76	0.019	0.16
	Rapides Regional Medical Center, Alexandria	10.7	0.0%	1.17	0.00	7	0.88	0.013	0.38
	Schumpert Medical Center, Shreveport	12.6	0.0%	1.13	0.01	8	0.82	0.033	0.52
	Southern Baptist Hospital, New Orleans	4.8	0.0%	1.44	0.04	5	0.58	0.061	0.40
	St. Frances Cabrini Hospital, Alexandria	12.3	0.0%	1.19	0.00	9	0.94	0.028	0.39
	St. Francis Medical Center, Monroe	5.8	0.0%	1.34	0.00	6	0.59	0.017	0.34
	Terrebonne General Medical Center, Houma	9.8	0.0%	1.12	0.00	5	0.74	0.011	0.42
	University Hospital, New Orleans	3.1	0.0%	1.54	0.07	6	0.57	0.007	0.16

NEUROLOGY

Natl. Rank	Hospital	U.S. News index	Reputa-tional score	Neurology mortality rate	COTH member	Interns and residents to beds	Tech-nology score (of 9)	R.N.'s to beds	Board-certified neurologists to beds
	TIER TWO								
58	**Ochsner Foundation Hospital, New Orleans**	19.0	0.4%	0.71	Yes	0.44	8	0.82	0.009
	TIER THREE								
	Glenwood Regional Medical Center, Westmonroe	13.8	0.0%	0.79	No	0.00	7	0.59	0.021
	LSU Medical Center-University Hospital, Shreveport	15.8	0.0%	0.98	Yes	1.07	7	0.90	0.009
	Lafayette General Medical Center, Lafayette	12.1	0.0%	0.88	No	0.00	8	0.81	0.013
	Our Lady of Lourdes Regional Center, Lafayette	11.1	0.0%	0.92	No	0.00	7	0.76	0.015
	Touro Infirmary, New Orleans	11.4	0.0%	0.88	No	0.09	6	0.31	0.024
	West Jefferson Medical Center, Marrero	11.8	0.0%	0.88	No	0.00	7	0.65	0.018
	TIER FOUR								
	Baton Rouge General Medical Center, Baton Rouge	8.6	0.0%	1.08	No	0.01	7	0.55	0.024
	East Jefferson General Hospital, Metairie	4.8	0.0%	1.50	No	0.00	7	0.89	0.017
	Mercy Hospital of New Orleans	6.5	0.0%	1.12	No	0.00	8	0.38	0.004
	Our Lady of Lake Regional Medical Center, Baton Rouge	8.8	0.0%	1.05	No	0.00	6	0.89	0.013
	Rapides Regional Medical Center, Alexandria	6.8	0.0%	1.18	No	0.00	7	0.88	0.003
	Schumpert Medical Center, Shreveport	7.7	0.0%	1.10	No	0.01	7	0.82	0.004
	Southern Baptist Hospital, New Orleans	4.7	0.0%	1.27	No	0.04	4	0.58	0.010
	St. Frances Cabrini Hospital, Alexandria	10.2	0.0%	0.97	No	0.00	8	0.94	0.004
	St. Francis Medical Center, Monroe	5.4	0.0%	1.19	No	0.00	5	0.59	0.005
	Terrebonne General Medical Center, Houma	7.5	0.0%	1.06	No	0.00	5	0.74	0.004
	University Hospital, New Orleans	7.3	0.0%	1.11	No	0.07	6	0.57	0.011
	Willis-Knighton Medical Center, Shreveport	3.7	0.0%	1.31	No	0.06	0	0.63	0.014

ORTHOPEDICS

Natl. Rank	Hospital	U.S. News index	Reputa-tional score	Orthopedics mortality rate	COTH member	Interns and residents to beds	Tech-nology score (of 5)	R.N.'s to beds	Board-certified orthopedists to beds	Pro-cedures to beds
	TIER TWO									
58	**Tulane University Hospital and Clinics, New Orleans**	15.8	0.0%	0.42	Yes	0.76	4	0.88	0.048	1.99
	TIER THREE									
	Glenwood Regional Medical Center, Westmonroe	8.9	0.0%	0.68	No	0.00	3	0.59	0.041	2.84
82	**Ochsner Foundation Hospital, New Orleans**	14.3	0.0%	0.44	Yes	0.44	4	0.82	0.011	1.70
	Our Lady of Lake Regional Medical Center, Baton Rouge	8.4	0.5%	1.01	No	0.00	5	0.89	0.045	2.64
	West Jefferson Medical Center, Marrero	9.5	0.0%	0.67	No	0.00	4	0.65	0.037	1.36
	TIER FOUR									
	Baton Rouge General Medical Center, Baton Rouge	5.8	0.0%	0.92	No	0.01	3	0.55	0.039	1.64
	East Jefferson General Hospital, Metairie	4.5	0.0%	1.29	No	0.00	3	0.89	0.037	2.40
	Lafayette General Medical Center, Lafayette	6.6	0.0%	0.96	No	0.00	4	0.81	0.029	1.46
	Mercy Hospital of New Orleans	7.0	0.0%	0.81	No	0.00	4	0.38	0.030	2.16
	Northshore Regional Medical Center, Slidell	7.4	0.0%	0.82	No	0.00	3	0.78	0.016	2.73
	Our Lady of Lourdes Regional Center, Lafayette	7.8	0.0%	0.81	No	0.00	3	0.76	0.041	3.40
	Rapides Regional Medical Center, Alexandria	6.1	0.0%	1.09	No	0.00	4	0.88	0.016	2.50
	Schumpert Medical Center, Shreveport	7.7	0.0%	0.87	No	0.01	4	0.82	0.022	2.60
	Southern Baptist Hospital, New Orleans	3.2	0.0%	1.38	No	0.04	3	0.58	0.023	1.87
	St. Frances Cabrini Hospital, Alexandria	7.1	0.0%	0.98	No	0.00	4	0.94	0.028	2.51
	St. Francis Medical Center, Monroe	3.3	0.0%	1.23	No	0.00	2	0.59	0.027	2.61
	Terrebonne General Medical Center, Houma	4.3	0.0%	1.39	No	0.00	4	0.74	0.027	2.48
	Touro Infirmary, New Orleans	7.4	0.0%	0.75	No	0.09	3	0.31	0.061	1.84
	University Hospital, New Orleans	2.3	0.0%	1.98	No	0.07	4	0.57	0.022	1.89

OTOLARYNGOLOGY

Natl. Rank	Hospital	U.S. News index	Reputational score	Hospital-wide mortality rate	COTH member	Interns and residents to beds	Technology score (of 9)	R.N.'s to beds	Board-certified internists to beds	Procedures to beds
	TIER TWO									
44	Medical Center of Louisiana at New Orleans	19.0	0.7%	1.15	Yes	1.39	5	0.91	0.457	0.094
90	Ochsner Foundation Hospital, New Orleans	14.2	1.2%	0.83	Yes	0.44	8	0.82	0.054	0.257
85	Tulane University Hospital and Clinics, New Orleans	14.4	0.7%	0.78	Yes	0.76	4	0.88	0.219	0.178
	TIER THREE									
	LSU Medical Center-University Hospital, Shreveport	12.8	0.0%	1.14	Yes	1.07	7	0.90	0.085	0.101
	TIER FOUR									
	Baton Rouge General Medical Center, Baton Rouge	4.4	0.0%	0.97	No	0.01	7	0.55	0.080	0.165
	E. A. Conway Medical Center, Monroe	3.0	0.0%	1.69	No	0.24	2	0.54	0.022	0.031
	Earl K. Long Medical Center, Baton Rouge	6.6	0.0%	1.72	No	0.78	1	0.59	0.208	0.050
	East Jefferson General Hospital, Metairie	6.0	0.4%	1.38	No	0.00	7	0.89	0.040	0.221
	Eye, Ear, Nose and Throat Hospital, New Orleans	6.5	0.7%	1.00	No	0.33	0	0.77	0.051	0.564
	Glenwood Regional Medical Center, Westmonroe	4.2	0.0%	0.93	No	0.00	7	0.59	0.026	0.500
	Huey P. Long Medical Center, Pineville,La.	2.9	0.0%	1.36	No	0.13	0	0.75	0.033	0.016
	Lafayette General Medical Center, Lafayette	5.0	0.0%	1.10	No	0.00	8	0.81	0.035	0.298
	Lake Charles Memorial Hospital, Lake Charles	4.3	0.0%	0.86	No	0.02	6	0.59	0.068	0.057
	Lakeland Medical Center, New Orleans	4.6	0.0%	1.06	No	0.00	7	0.67	0.067	0.140
	Mercy Hospital of New Orleans	4.1	0.0%	0.97	No	0.00	8	0.38	0.075	0.106
	Northshore Regional Medical Center, Slidell	3.5	0.0%	1.14	No	0.00	3	0.78	0.033	0.220
	Opelousas General Hospital, Opelousas	2.9	0.0%	1.06	No	0.00	6	0.33	0.027	0.201
	Our Lady of Lake Regional Medical Center, Baton Rouge	4.8	0.0%	1.28	No	0.00	6	0.89	0.061	0.212
	Our Lady of Lourdes Regional Center, Lafayette	4.7	0.0%	1.16	No	0.00	7	0.76	0.056	0.321
	Rapides Regional Medical Center, Alexandria	5.0	0.0%	1.17	No	0.00	7	0.88	0.040	0.234
	Schumpert Medical Center, Shreveport	4.8	0.0%	1.13	No	0.01	7	0.82	0.033	0.155
	Slidell Memorial Hospital and Medical Center, Slidell	4.6	0.0%	0.96	No	0.01	4	0.97	0.038	0.275
	Southern Baptist Hospital, New Orleans	2.9	0.0%	1.44	No	0.04	3	0.58	0.038	0.270
	St. Frances Cabrini Hospital, Alexandria	5.3	0.0%	1.19	No	0.00	8	0.94	0.032	0.255
	St. Francis Medical Center, Monroe	3.1	0.0%	1.34	No	0.00	5	0.59	0.005	0.384
	Terrebonne General Medical Center, Houma	3.3	0.0%	1.12	No	0.00	3	0.74	0.027	0.138
	Touro Infirmary, New Orleans	4.0	0.0%	0.97	No	0.09	6	0.31	0.103	0.179
	University Hospital, New Orleans	3.7	0.0%	1.54	No	0.07	6	0.57	0.022	0.294
	University Medical Center, Lafayette	4.3	0.0%	1.02	No	0.38	2	0.52	0.068	0.099
	West Jefferson Medical Center, Marrero	4.6	0.0%	0.96	No	0.00	7	0.65	0.058	0.154
	Willis-Knighton Medical Center, Shreveport	2.6	0.0%	1.45	No	0.06	0	0.63	0.073	0.169

RHEUMATOLOGY

Natl. Rank	Hospital	U.S. News index	Reputational score	Hospital-wide mortality rate	COTH member	Interns and residents to beds	Technology score (of 5)	R.N.'s to beds	Board-certified internists to beds
	TIER TWO								
78	Ochsner Foundation Hospital, New Orleans	16.3	1.3%	0.83	Yes	0.44	4	0.82	0.054
53	Tulane University Hospital and Clinics, New Orleans	17.6	0.4%	0.78	Yes	0.76	4	0.88	0.219
	TIER THREE								
	LSU Medical Center-University Hospital, Shreveport	13.5	0.0%	1.14	Yes	1.07	3	0.90	0.085
	TIER FOUR								
	Baton Rouge General Medical Center, Baton Rouge	8.1	0.0%	0.97	No	0.01	3	0.55	0.080
	East Jefferson General Hospital, Metairie	6.6	0.4%	1.38	No	0.00	3	0.89	0.040
	Glenwood Regional Medical Center, Westmonroe	7.2	0.0%	0.93	No	0.00	3	0.59	0.026
	Lafayette General Medical Center, Lafayette	7.7	0.0%	1.10	No	0.00	4	0.81	0.035
	Lakeland Medical Center, New Orleans	7.9	0.0%	1.06	No	0.00	4	0.67	0.067
	Mercy Hospital of New Orleans	8.1	0.0%	0.97	No	0.00	4	0.38	0.075
	Northshore Regional Medical Center, Slidell	6.9	0.0%	1.14	No	0.00	3	0.78	0.033
	Our Lady of Lake Regional Medical Center, Baton Rouge	7.4	0.0%	1.28	No	0.00	5	0.89	0.061

Natl. Rank	Hospital	U.S. News index	Reputa-tional score	Hospital-wide mortality rate	COTH member	Interns and residents to beds	Tech-nology score (of 5)	R.N.'s to beds	Board-certified internists to beds
	Our Lady of Lourdes Regional Center, Lafayette	6.9	0.0%	1.16	No	0.00	3	0.76	0.056
	Rapides Regional Medical Center, Alexandria	7.5	0.0%	1.17	No	0.00	4	0.88	0.040
	Schumpert Medical Center, Shreveport	7.6	0.0%	1.13	No	0.01	4	0.82	0.033
	Slidell Memorial Hospital and Medical Center, Slidell	9.4	0.0%	0.96	No	0.01	4	0.97	0.038
	Southern Baptist Hospital, New Orleans	4.8	0.0%	1.44	No	0.04	3	0.58	0.038
	St. Frances Cabrini Hospital, Alexandria	7.4	0.0%	1.19	No	0.00	4	0.94	0.032
	St. Francis Medical Center, Monroe	4.5	0.0%	1.34	No	0.00	2	0.59	0.005
	Terrebonne General Medical Center, Houma	7.4	0.0%	1.12	No	0.00	4	0.74	0.027
	Touro Infirmary, New Orleans	7.9	0.0%	0.97	No	0.09	3	0.31	0.103
	University Hospital, New Orleans	4.8	0.0%	1.54	No	0.07	4	0.57	0.022
	West Jefferson Medical Center, Marrero	8.8	0.0%	0.96	No	0.00	4	0.65	0.058
	Willis-Knighton Medical Center, Shreveport	1.9	0.0%	1.45	No	0.06	0	0.63	0.073

UROLOGY

Natl. Rank	Hospital	U.S. News index	Reputa-tional score	Urology mortality rate	COTH member	Interns and residents to beds	Tech-nology score (of 11)	R.N.'s to beds	Board-certified internists to beds	Procedures to beds
	TIER TWO									
48	Ochsner Foundation Hospital, New Orleans	18.5	2.0%	0.74	Yes	0.44	10	0.82	0.054	2.30
56	Tulane University Hospital and Clinics, New Orleans	17.5	0.6%	0.57	Yes	0.76	6	0.88	0.219	1.91
	TIER THREE									
	Glenwood Regional Medical Center, Westmonroe	9.7	0.0%	0.78	No	0.00	8	0.59	0.026	1.97
	LSU Medical Center-University Hospital, Shreveport	11.2	0.0%	1.50	Yes	1.07	8	0.90	0.085	1.46
	Opelousas General Hospital, Opelousas	9.7	0.0%	0.65	No	0.00	7	0.33	0.027	2.33
	St. Francis Medical Center, Monroe	8.7	0.0%	0.80	No	0.00	6	0.59	0.005	1.90
	TIER FOUR									
	Baton Rouge General Medical Center, Baton Rouge	6.1	0.0%	1.20	No	0.01	9	0.55	0.080	1.76
	East Jefferson General Hospital, Metairie	4.5	0.0%	1.60	No	0.00	8	0.89	0.040	1.78
	Lafayette General Medical Center, Lafayette	4.1	0.0%	1.80	No	0.00	10	0.81	0.035	1.73
	Lakeland Medical Center, New Orleans	8.1	0.0%	0.94	No	0.00	8	0.67	0.067	1.72
	Mercy Hospital of New Orleans	4.4	0.0%	1.44	No	0.00	9	0.38	0.075	2.02
	Our Lady of Lake Regional Medical Center, Baton Rouge	5.2	0.0%	1.42	No	0.00	7	0.89	0.061	2.28
	Our Lady of Lourdes Regional Center, Lafayette	4.2	0.0%	1.69	No	0.00	8	0.76	0.056	2.76
	Rapides Regional Medical Center, Alexandria	5.7	0.0%	1.37	No	0.00	9	0.88	0.040	2.04
	Schumpert Medical Center, Shreveport	7.9	0.0%	1.03	No	0.01	9	0.82	0.033	2.23
	Slidell Memorial Hospital and Medical Center, Slidell	5.1	0.0%	1.41	No	0.01	7	0.97	0.038	1.45
	Southern Baptist Hospital, New Orleans	5.3	0.0%	1.10	No	0.04	4	0.58	0.038	1.73
	St. Frances Cabrini Hospital, Alexandria	7.7	0.0%	1.09	No	0.00	9	0.94	0.032	2.24
	Terrebonne General Medical Center, Houma	3.7	0.0%	1.49	No	0.00	5	0.74	0.027	2.12
	Touro Infirmary, New Orleans	5.5	0.0%	1.16	No	0.09	7	0.31	0.103	1.34
	University Hospital, New Orleans	1.9	0.0%	2.30	No	0.07	7	0.57	0.022	2.35
	West Jefferson Medical Center, Marrero	5.6	0.0%	1.29	No	0.00	9	0.65	0.058	1.63
	Willis-Knighton Medical Center, Shreveport	5.6	0.0%	1.01	No	0.06	0	0.63	0.073	2.12

AIDS

Natl. Rank	Hospital	U.S. News index	Reputa-tional score	Hospital-wide mortality rate	COTH member	Interns and residents to beds	Tech-nology score (of 11)	Discharge planning (of 2)	R.N.'s to beds	Board-certified internists to beds
TIER THREE										
	Maine Medical Center, Portland	21.0	0.0%	1.15	Yes	0.49	8	2	0.73	0.067
TIER FOUR										
	Central Maine Medical Center, Lewiston	13.7	0.0%	1.63	No	0.10	7	2	0.57	0.020
	Eastern Maine Medical Center, Bangor	17.6	0.0%	1.20	No	0.12	6	2	0.95	0.039
	Kennebec Valley Medical Center, Augusta	16.3	0.0%	1.14	No	0.07	5	1	0.45	0.024
	Mid-Maine Medical Center, Waterville	19.5	0.0%	1.00	No	0.04	5	2	0.70	0.043

CANCER

Natl. Rank	Hospital	U.S. News index	Reputa-tional score	Cancer mortality rate	COTH member	Interns and residents to beds	Tech-nology score (of 12)	R.N.'s to beds	Board-certified oncologists to beds	Procedures to beds
TIER THREE										
	Maine Medical Center, Portland	7.8	0.0%	1.05	Yes	0.49	8	0.73	0.000	3.45
TIER FOUR										
	Central Maine Medical Center, Lewiston	3.0	0.0%	1.69	No	0.10	7	0.57	0.012	3.17
	Eastern Maine Medical Center, Bangor	3.9	0.0%	1.42	No	0.12	7	0.95	0.012	1.65
	Kennebec Valley Medical Center, Augusta	2.2	0.0%	1.23	No	0.07	6	0.45	0.006	1.81
	Mid-Maine Medical Center, Waterville	2.7	0.0%	1.14	No	0.04	6	0.70	0.004	1.20

CARDIOLOGY

Natl. Rank	Hospital	U.S. News index	Reputa-tional score	Cardiology mortality rate	COTH member	Interns and residents to beds	Tech-nology score (of 10)	R.N.'s to beds	Board-certified cardiologists to beds	Procedures to beds
TIER THREE										
	Maine Medical Center, Portland	15.5	0.0%	1.17	Yes	0.49	9	0.73	0.035	10.32
	Mid-Maine Medical Center, Waterville	13.8	0.0%	0.95	No	0.04	5	0.70	0.004	5.35
TIER FOUR										
	Central Maine Medical Center, Lewiston	2.2	0.0%	1.81	No	0.10	6	0.57	0.016	7.75
	Eastern Maine Medical Center, Bangor	13.3	0.0%	1.07	No	0.12	8	0.95	0.019	8.62
	Kennebec Valley Medical Center, Augusta	10.6	0.0%	1.07	No	0.07	5	0.45	0.018	6.30

ENDOCRINOLOGY

Natl. Rank	Hospital	U.S. News index	Reputa-tional score	Endocrinology mortality rate	COTH member	Interns and residents to beds	Tech-nology score (of 11)	R.N.'s to beds	Board-certified internists to beds
TIER THREE									
	Maine Medical Center, Portland	9.5	0.0%	1.25	Yes	0.49	9	0.73	0.067
	Mid-Maine Medical Center, Waterville	9.7	0.0%	0.59	No	0.04	7	0.70	0.043
TIER FOUR									
	Central Maine Medical Center, Lewiston	3.9	0.0%	1.46	No	0.10	8	0.57	0.020
	Eastern Maine Medical Center, Bangor	4.3	0.0%	1.79	No	0.12	8	0.95	0.039
	Kennebec Valley Medical Center, Augusta	4.4	0.0%	1.19	No	0.07	7	0.45	0.024

GASTROENTEROLOGY

Natl. Rank Hospital	U.S. News index	Reputa-tional score	Gastro-enterology mortality rate	COTH member	Interns and residents to beds	Tech-nology score (of 11)	R.N.'s to beds	Board-certified gastro-enterologists to beds	Pro-cedures to beds
TIER THREE									
Kennebec Valley Medical Center, Augusta	7.5	0.0%	0.83	No	0.07	6	0.45	0.006	4.30
Maine Medical Center, Portland	8.5	0.0%	1.34	Yes	0.49	8	0.73	0.015	2.34
TIER FOUR									
Central Maine Medical Center, Lewiston	4.2	0.0%	1.52	No	0.10	8	0.57	0.016	3.67
Eastern Maine Medical Center, Bangor	5.0	0.0%	1.23	No	0.12	7	0.95	0.010	2.03
Mid-Maine Medical Center, Waterville	6.9	0.0%	0.84	No	0.04	6	0.70	0.008	2.77

GERIATRICS

Natl. Rank Hospital	U.S. News index	Reputa-tional score	Hospital-wide mortality rate	COTH member	Service mix	Interns and residents to beds	Tech-nology score (of 13)	R.N.'s to beds	Discharge planning (of 2)	Geriatric services (of 9)	Board-certified internists to beds
TIER THREE											
Maine Medical Center, Portland	14.7	0.0%	1.15	Yes	7	0.49	11	0.73	2	1	0.067
Mid-Maine Medical Center, Waterville	14.4	0.0%	1.00	No	6	0.04	8	0.70	2	2	0.043
TIER FOUR											
Central Maine Medical Center, Lewiston	2.4	0.0%	1.63	No	4	0.10	9	0.57	2	2	0.020
Eastern Maine Medical Center, Bangor	11.1	0.0%	1.20	No	7	0.12	10	0.95	2	2	0.039
Kennebec Valley Medical Center, Augusta	9.1	0.0%	1.14	No	5	0.07	8	0.45	1	3	0.024

GYNECOLOGY

Natl. Rank Hospital	U.S. News index	Reputa-tional score	Hospital-wide mortality rate	Interns and residents to beds	Tech-nology score (of 10)	R.N.'s to beds	Board-certified OB-GYNs to beds	Procedures to beds
TIER FOUR								
Central Maine Medical Center, Lewiston	3.4	0.0%	1.63	0.10	7	0.57	0.028	0.42
Eastern Maine Medical Center, Bangor	11.0	0.0%	1.20	0.12	7	0.95	0.017	0.24
Kennebec Valley Medical Center, Augusta	8.4	0.0%	1.14	0.07	5	0.45	0.018	0.42
Maine Medical Center, Portland	14.0	0.0%	1.15	0.49	8	0.73	0.043	0.61
Mid-Maine Medical Center, Waterville	12.8	0.0%	1.00	0.04	5	0.70	0.016	0.39

NEUROLOGY

Natl. Rank Hospital	U.S. News index	Reputa-tional score	Neurology mortality rate	COTH member	Interns and residents to beds	Tech-nology score (of 9)	R.N.'s to beds	Board-certified neurologists to beds
TIER FOUR								
Central Maine Medical Center, Lewiston	3.3	0.0%	1.53	No	0.10	7	0.57	0.004
Eastern Maine Medical Center, Bangor	7.4	0.0%	1.20	No	0.12	6	0.95	0.012
Maine Medical Center, Portland	8.4	0.0%	1.44	Yes	0.49	7	0.73	0.012
Mid-Maine Medical Center, Waterville	4.9	0.0%	1.30	No	0.04	5	0.70	0.008

ORTHOPEDICS

Natl. Rank	Hospital	U.S. News index	Reputational score	Orthopedics mortality rate	COTH member	Interns and residents to beds	Technology score (of 5)	R.N.'s to beds	Board-certified orthopedists to beds	Procedures to beds
	TIER THREE									
	Maine Medical Center, Portland	**10.1**	0.0%	1.07	Yes	0.49	4	0.73	0.027	2.17
	TIER FOUR									
	Central Maine Medical Center, Lewiston	**3.7**	0.0%	1.50	No	0.10	4	0.57	0.020	2.18
	Eastern Maine Medical Center, Bangor	**3.7**	0.0%	1.66	No	0.12	3	0.95	0.024	2.58
	Kennebec Valley Medical Center, Augusta	**4.3**	0.0%	1.06	No	0.07	2	0.45	0.024	3.34
	Mid-Maine Medical Center, Waterville	**5.0**	0.0%	1.08	No	0.04	3	0.70	0.016	2.00

OTOLARYNGOLOGY

Natl. Rank	Hospital	U.S. News index	Reputational score	Hospital-wide mortality rate	COTH member	Interns and residents to beds	Technology score (of 9)	R.N.'s to beds	Board-certified internists to beds	Procedures to beds
	TIER THREE									
	Maine Medical Center, Portland	**9.8**	0.0%	1.15	Yes	0.49	7	0.73	0.067	0.239
	TIER FOUR									
	Central Maine Medical Center, Lewiston	**3.7**	0.0%	1.63	No	0.10	6	0.57	0.020	0.300
	Eastern Maine Medical Center, Bangor	**5.3**	0.0%	1.20	No	0.12	6	0.95	0.039	0.329
	Kennebec Valley Medical Center, Augusta	**3.2**	0.0%	1.14	No	0.07	5	0.45	0.024	0.461
	Mid-Maine Medical Center, Waterville	**4.1**	0.0%	1.00	No	0.04	5	0.70	0.043	0.252

RHEUMATOLOGY

Natl. Rank	Hospital	U.S. News index	Reputational score	Hospital-wide mortality rate	COTH member	Interns and residents to beds	Technology score (of 5)	R.N.'s to beds	Board-certified internists to beds
	TIER THREE								
	Maine Medical Center, Portland	**11.4**	0.0%	1.15	Yes	0.49	4	0.73	0.067
	TIER FOUR								
	Central Maine Medical Center, Lewiston	**4.6**	0.0%	1.63	No	0.10	4	0.57	0.020
	Eastern Maine Medical Center, Bangor	**7.4**	0.0%	1.20	No	0.12	3	0.95	0.039
	Kennebec Valley Medical Center, Augusta	**4.7**	0.0%	1.14	No	0.07	2	0.45	0.024
	Mid-Maine Medical Center, Waterville	**8.0**	0.0%	1.00	No	0.04	3	0.70	0.043

UROLOGY

Natl. Rank	Hospital	U.S. News index	Reputational score	Urology mortality rate	COTH member	Interns and residents to beds	Technology score (of 11)	R.N.'s to beds	Board-certified internists to beds	Procedures to beds
	TIER THREE									
	Maine Medical Center, Portland	**10.7**	0.0%	1.16	Yes	0.49	8	0.73	0.067	2.06
	TIER FOUR									
	Central Maine Medical Center, Lewiston	**3.6**	0.0%	1.72	No	0.10	8	0.57	0.020	2.22
	Eastern Maine Medical Center, Bangor	**4.9**	0.0%	1.51	No	0.12	7	0.95	0.039	1.09
	Mid-Maine Medical Center, Waterville	**8.3**	0.0%	0.87	No	0.04	6	0.70	0.043	1.50

AIDS

Natl. Rank	Hospital	U.S. News index	Reputa-tional score	Hospital-wide mortality rate	COTH member	Interns and residents to beds	Tech-nology score (of 11)	Discharge planning (of 2)	R.N.'s to beds	Board-certified internists to beds
	TIER ONE									
2	**Johns Hopkins Hospital, Baltimore**	66.1	31.2%	0.97	Yes	0.73	11	2	1.43	0.084
	TIER TWO									
82	**Sinai Hospital of Baltimore, Baltimore**	25.3	0.0%	0.97	Yes	0.42	9	2	1.43	0.127
33	**University of Maryland Medical System, Baltimore**	29.1	1.4%	0.98	Yes	0.96	9	2	1.67	0.281
	TIER THREE									
	Anne Arundel Medical Center, Annapolis	23.4	0.0%	0.73	No	0.00	8	2	0.96	0.132
	Francis Scott Key Medical Center, Baltimore	19.8	0.0%	1.21	Yes	0.27	7	2	0.61	0.168
	Franklin Square Hospital Center, Baltimore	20.2	0.0%	1.10	Yes	0.34	4	2	0.90	0.063
	Good Samaritan Hospital, Baltimore	20.2	0.0%	1.03	No	0.32	6	2	0.83	0.067
94	**Greater Baltimore Medical Center**	24.7	0.0%	0.89	Yes	0.29	5	2	0.90	0.210
	Harbor Hospital Center, Baltimore	23.0	0.0%	0.77	No	0.34	5	2	0.93	0.150
	Holy Cross Hospital, Silver Spring	23.6	0.0%	0.94	Yes	0.05	6	2	0.64	0.336
	Mercy Medical Center, Baltimore	22.5	0.0%	0.65	No	0.21	6	2	0.50	0.185
	Northwest Hospital Center, Randallstown	20.5	0.0%	1.01	No	0.00	6	2	0.79	0.207
	Washington Adventist Hospital, Takoma Park	19.9	0.0%	1.05	No	0.03	6	2	1.23	0.043
	Washington County Hospital Assn., Hagerstown	21.2	0.0%	0.95	No	0.00	6	2	0.99	0.083
	TIER FOUR									
	Howard County General Hospital, Columbia	18.3	0.0%	1.04	No	0.00	4	2	0.47	0.127
	Maryland General Hospital, Baltimore	19.0	0.0%	1.04	No	0.36	6	1	0.58	0.053
	Memorial Hospital at Easton, Easton	17.8	0.0%	1.20	No	0.00	7	2	1.02	0.030
	Peninsula Regional Medical Center, Salisbury	17.7	0.0%	1.14	No	0.00	6	2	0.67	0.042
	Prince George's Hospital Center, Cheverly	16.5	0.0%	1.29	No	0.32	6	2	0.57	0.056
	St. Agnes Hospital, Baltimore	19.6	0.0%	1.17	No	0.29	8	2	0.82	0.215
	Suburban Hospital, Bethesda	19.0	0.0%	1.02	No	0.02	5	2	0.59	0.094
	Union Memorial Hospital, Baltimore	19.2	0.0%	1.10	No	0.38	6	2	0.56	0.123

CANCER

Natl. Rank	Hospital	U.S. News index	Reputa-tional score	Cancer mortality rate	COTH member	Interns and residents to beds	Tech-nology score (of 12)	R.N.'s to beds	Board-certified oncologists to beds	Procedures to beds
	TIER ONE									
4	**Johns Hopkins Hospital, Baltimore**	47.7	28.7%	0.53	Yes	0.73	11	1.43	0.011	1.57
	TIER TWO									
43	**University of Maryland Medical System, Baltimore**	13.3	0.5%	0.84	Yes	0.96	11	1.67	0.029	0.95
	TIER THREE									
	Francis Scott Key Medical Center, Baltimore	5.3	0.0%	0.82	Yes	0.27	4	0.61	0.003	0.39
	Franklin Square Hospital Center, Baltimore	5.8	0.0%	1.08	Yes	0.34	2	0.90	0.007	2.14
	Greater Baltimore Medical Center	7.1	0.0%	0.76	Yes	0.29	5	0.90	0.016	2.87
	Sinai Hospital of Baltimore, Baltimore	9.8	0.0%	0.77	Yes	0.42	9	1.43	0.012	1.24
	TIER FOUR									
	Anne Arundel Medical Center, Annapolis	4.5	0.0%	1.02	No	0.00	9	0.96	0.010	2.11
	Good Samaritan Hospital, Baltimore	3.3	0.0%	1.01	No	0.32	3	0.83	0.015	1.29
	Harbor Hospital Center, Baltimore	4.4	0.0%	0.64	No	0.34	3	0.93	0.010	2.30
	Holy Cross Hospital, Silver Spring	4.9	0.0%	0.81	Yes	0.05	4	0.64	0.002	1.80
	Howard County General Hospital, Columbia	1.0	0.0%	0.97	No	0.00	2	0.47	0.014	1.23
	Maryland General Hospital, Baltimore	3.6	0.0%	0.92	No	0.36	6	0.58	0.004	1.23
	Memorial Hospital at Easton, Easton	3.9	0.0%	1.25	No	0.00	7	1.02	0.005	2.29
	Mercy Medical Center, Baltimore	3.3	0.0%	0.50	No	0.21	5	0.50	0.007	2.34
	Northwest Hospital Center, Randallstown	3.2	0.0%	0.99	No	0.00	6	0.79	0.013	2.27
	Peninsula Regional Medical Center, Salisbury	3.2	0.0%	0.85	No	0.00	7	0.67	0.007	1.86

Natl. Rank	Hospital	U.S. News index	Reputational score	Cancer mortality rate	COTH member	Interns and residents to beds	Technology score (of 12)	R.N.'s to beds	Board-certified oncologists to beds	Procedures to beds
	Prince George's Hospital Center, Cheverly	2.5	0.0%	1.47	No	0.32	4	0.57	0.022	0.57
	St. Agnes Hospital, Baltimore	4.4	0.0%	0.98	No	0.29	7	0.82	0.008	1.65
	Suburban Hospital, Bethesda	2.5	0.0%	0.88	No	0.02	5	0.59	0.030	1.47
	Union Memorial Hospital, Baltimore	3.4	0.0%	0.90	No	0.38	5	0.56	0.008	1.22
	Washington Adventist Hospital, Takoma Park	4.4	0.0%	1.43	No	0.03	7	1.23	0.027	1.11
	Washington County Hospital Assn., Hagerstown	4.2	0.0%	0.89	No	0.00	8	0.99	0.006	1.44

CARDIOLOGY

Natl. Rank	Hospital	U.S. News index	Reputational score	Cardiology mortality rate	COTH member	Interns and residents to beds	Technology score (of 10)	R.N.'s to beds	Board-certified cardiologists to beds	Procedures to beds
TIER ONE										
9	Johns Hopkins Hospital, Baltimore	40.5	15.6%	1.21	Yes	0.73	10	1.43	0.033	4.66
TIER TWO										
82	Greater Baltimore Medical Center	21.3	0.0%	0.79	Yes	0.29	5	0.90	0.096	7.77
55	Sinai Hospital of Baltimore, Baltimore	22.7	0.0%	0.93	Yes	0.42	8	1.43	0.109	8.58
86	University of Maryland Medical System, Baltimore	21.3	0.0%	1.10	Yes	0.96	9	1.67	0.059	3.85
TIER THREE										
	Anne Arundel Medical Center, Annapolis	17.9	0.0%	0.71	No	0.00	8	0.96	0.026	7.37
	Franklin Square Hospital Center, Baltimore	17.0	0.0%	1.02	Yes	0.34	4	0.90	0.047	9.29
	Good Samaritan Hospital, Baltimore	18.8	0.0%	0.85	No	0.32	7	0.83	0.037	9.91
	Harbor Hospital Center, Baltimore	18.5	0.0%	0.76	No	0.34	5	0.93	0.045	7.71
	Holy Cross Hospital, Silver Spring	18.6	0.0%	0.91	Yes	0.05	6	0.64	0.051	6.03
	Maryland General Hospital, Baltimore	13.7	0.0%	1.03	No	0.36	7	0.58	0.036	4.79
	Mercy Medical Center, Baltimore	16.6	0.0%	0.54	No	0.21	6	0.50	0.026	5.16
	Northwest Hospital Center, Randallstown	14.3	0.0%	1.00	No	0.00	6	0.79	0.057	13.94
	Suburban Hospital, Bethesda	15.9	0.0%	0.91	No	0.02	6	0.59	0.090	6.17
	Union Memorial Hospital, Baltimore	16.4	0.0%	0.93	No	0.38	7	0.56	0.037	7.29
	Washington Adventist Hospital, Takoma Park	19.6	0.0%	0.88	No	0.03	8	1.23	0.133	12.98
	Washington County Hospital Assn., Hagerstown	17.0	0.0%	0.84	No	0.00	5	0.99	0.013	8.99
TIER FOUR										
	Francis Scott Key Medical Center, Baltimore	13.5	0.0%	1.16	Yes	0.27	7	0.61	0.032	3.94
	Howard County General Hospital, Columbia	12.8	0.0%	0.96	No	0.00	3	0.47	0.042	6.87
	Memorial Hospital at Easton, Easton	12.7	0.0%	1.06	No	0.00	6	1.02	0.015	9.16
	Peninsula Regional Medical Center, Salisbury	10.7	0.0%	1.16	No	0.00	8	0.67	0.030	14.32
	Prince George's Hospital Center, Cheverly	11.3	0.0%	1.16	No	0.32	7	0.57	0.062	4.67
	St. Agnes Hospital, Baltimore	12.1	0.0%	1.13	No	0.29	7	0.82	0.013	10.49

ENDOCRINOLOGY

Natl. Rank	Hospital	U.S. News index	Reputational score	Endocrinology mortality rate	COTH member	Interns and residents to beds	Technology score (of 11)	R.N.'s to beds	Board-certified internists to beds
TIER ONE									
4	Johns Hopkins Hospital, Baltimore	41.8	18.4%	0.68	Yes	0.73	11	1.43	0.084
TIER TWO									
57	University of Maryland Medical System, Baltimore	16.5	0.0%	1.03	Yes	0.96	10	1.67	0.281
TIER THREE									
	Anne Arundel Medical Center, Annapolis	11.1	0.0%	0.69	No	0.00	10	0.96	0.132
	Franklin Square Hospital Center, Baltimore	9.4	0.0%	1.03	Yes	0.34	3	0.90	0.063
	Greater Baltimore Medical Center	11.4	0.0%	0.95	Yes	0.29	6	0.90	0.210
	Harbor Hospital Center, Baltimore	10.8	0.0%	0.71	No	0.34	4	0.93	0.150
	Holy Cross Hospital, Silver Spring	12.8	0.0%	0.73	Yes	0.05	5	0.64	0.336
	Sinai Hospital of Baltimore, Baltimore	13.2	0.0%	0.96	Yes	0.42	9	1.43	0.127

Natl. Rank	Hospital	U.S. News index	Reputational score	Endocrinology mortality rate	COTH member	Interns and residents to beds	Technology score (of 11)	R.N.'s to beds	Board-certified internists to beds
	TIER FOUR								
	Francis Scott Key Medical Center, Baltimore	7.8	0.0%	1.40	Yes	0.27	5	0.61	0.168
	Good Samaritan Hospital, Baltimore	5.3	0.0%	1.42	No	0.32	5	0.83	0.067
	Howard County General Hospital, Columbia	4.0	0.0%	1.19	No	0.00	2	0.47	0.127
	Maryland General Hospital, Baltimore	5.1	0.0%	1.38	No	0.36	7	0.58	0.053
	Memorial Hospital at Easton, Easton	4.1	0.0%	1.78	No	0.00	8	1.02	0.030
	Mercy Medical Center, Baltimore	8.1	0.0%	0.86	No	0.21	6	0.50	0.185
	Northwest Hospital Center, Randallstown	7.4	0.0%	0.99	No	0.00	6	0.79	0.207
	Peninsula Regional Medical Center, Salisbury	3.9	0.0%	1.51	No	0.00	8	0.67	0.042
	Prince George's Hospital Center, Cheverly	5.4	0.0%	1.19	No	0.32	5	0.57	0.056
	St. Agnes Hospital, Baltimore	7.1	0.0%	1.28	No	0.29	7	0.82	0.215
	Suburban Hospital, Bethesda	4.1	0.0%	1.35	No	0.02	5	0.59	0.094
	Union Memorial Hospital, Baltimore	6.0	0.0%	1.26	No	0.38	6	0.56	0.123
	Washington Adventist Hospital, Takoma Park	6.5	0.0%	1.23	No	0.03	8	1.23	0.043
	Washington County Hospital Assn., Hagerstown	5.1	0.0%	1.56	No	0.00	9	0.99	0.083

GASTROENTEROLOGY

Natl. Rank	Hospital	U.S. News index	Reputational score	Gastroenterology mortality rate	COTH member	Interns and residents to beds	Technology score (of 11)	R.N.'s to beds	Board-certified gastroenterologists to beds	Procedures to beds
	TIER ONE									
2	Johns Hopkins Hospital, Baltimore	64.8	33.4%	0.81	Yes	0.73	11	1.43	0.015	1.43
	TIER TWO									
69	Sinai Hospital of Baltimore, Baltimore	13.5	0.0%	0.83	Yes	0.42	8	1.43	0.031	2.73
38	University of Maryland Medical System, Baltimore	16.1	0.4%	0.84	Yes	0.96	10	1.67	0.010	1.00
	TIER THREE									
	Anne Arundel Medical Center, Annapolis	9.4	0.0%	0.60	No	0.00	9	0.96	0.020	3.99
	Francis Scott Key Medical Center, Baltimore	8.1	0.4%	1.01	Yes	0.27	5	0.61	0.010	1.15
	Franklin Square Hospital Center, Baltimore	8.6	0.0%	1.26	Yes	0.34	3	0.90	0.028	4.88
	Greater Baltimore Medical Center	11.3	0.0%	0.87	Yes	0.29	5	0.90	0.049	4.06
	Holy Cross Hospital, Silver Spring	8.9	0.0%	0.93	Yes	0.05	5	0.64	0.051	3.35
	Maryland General Hospital, Baltimore	7.7	0.0%	0.84	No	0.36	6	0.58	0.024	2.46
	Mercy Medical Center, Baltimore	7.8	0.0%	0.66	No	0.21	7	0.50	0.030	2.88
	Northwest Hospital Center, Randallstown	8.2	0.0%	0.98	No	0.00	6	0.79	0.044	6.66
	Washington County Hospital Assn., Hagerstown	8.8	0.0%	0.86	No	0.00	8	0.99	0.006	4.30
	TIER FOUR									
	Good Samaritan Hospital, Baltimore	6.0	0.0%	1.26	No	0.32	5	0.83	0.045	4.00
	Harbor Hospital Center, Baltimore	6.6	0.0%	1.05	No	0.34	4	0.93	0.031	3.17
	Howard County General Hospital, Columbia	3.6	0.0%	1.13	No	0.00	2	0.47	0.042	3.75
	Memorial Hospital at Easton, Easton	6.8	0.0%	1.14	No	0.00	8	1.02	0.010	4.28
	Peninsula Regional Medical Center, Salisbury	5.5	0.0%	1.12	No	0.00	7	0.67	0.012	3.79
	Prince George's Hospital Center, Cheverly	3.5	0.0%	1.43	No	0.32	5	0.57	0.056	1.92
	St. Agnes Hospital, Baltimore	7.0	0.0%	1.28	No	0.29	7	0.82	0.018	5.28
	Suburban Hospital, Bethesda	7.2	0.0%	0.75	No	0.02	5	0.59	0.050	3.58
	Union Memorial Hospital, Baltimore	6.7	0.0%	1.02	No	0.38	6	0.56	0.032	3.35
	Washington Adventist Hospital, Takoma Park	6.6	0.0%	1.05	No	0.03	7	1.23	0.053	2.14

GERIATRICS

Natl. Rank	Hospital	U.S. News index	Reputa-tional score	Hospital-wide mortality rate	COTH member	Service mix	Interns and residents to beds	Tech-nology score (of 13)	R.N.'s to beds	Discharge planning (of 2)	Geriatric services (of 9)	Board-certified internists to beds
					TIER ONE							
6	Johns Hopkins Hospital, Baltimore	66.5	16.9%	0.97	Yes	8	0.73	12	1.43	2	1	0.084
					TIER TWO							
66	Francis Scott Key Medical Center, Baltimore	23.0	3.3%	1.21	Yes	7	0.27	7	0.61	2	8	0.168
59	Greater Baltimore Medical Center	23.3	0.5%	0.89	Yes	6	0.29	7	0.90	2	4	0.210
73	Sinai Hospital of Baltimore, Baltimore	22.5	0.0%	0.97	Yes	10	0.42	10	1.43	2	3	0.127
48	University of Maryland Medical System, Baltimore	24.4	0.0%	0.98	Yes	8	0.96	12	1.67	2	3	0.281
					TIER THREE							
	Anne Arundel Medical Center, Annapolis	19.0	0.0%	0.73	No	5	0.00	12	0.96	2	2	0.132
	Franklin Square Hospital Center, Baltimore	15.0	0.0%	1.10	Yes	6	0.34	4	0.90	2	5	0.063
	Harbor Hospital Center, Baltimore	17.8	0.0%	0.77	No	4	0.34	5	0.93	2	1	0.150
	Holy Cross Hospital, Silver Spring	19.9	0.0%	0.94	Yes	6	0.05	7	0.64	2	3	0.336
	Mercy Medical Center, Baltimore	18.5	0.0%	0.65	No	6	0.21	8	0.50	2	2	0.185
	Suburban Hospital, Bethesda	14.6	0.0%	1.02	No	6	0.02	6	0.59	2	7	0.094
	Union Memorial Hospital, Baltimore	13.9	0.0%	1.10	No	8	0.38	8	0.56	2	3	0.123
	Washington County Hospital Assn., Hagerstown	17.3	0.0%	0.95	No	6	0.00	9	0.99	2	4	0.083
					TIER FOUR							
	Good Samaritan Hospital, Baltimore	12.8	0.0%	1.03	No	3	0.32	7	0.83	2	1	0.067
	Howard County General Hospital, Columbia	11.5	0.0%	1.04	No	5	0.00	2	0.47	2	2	0.127
	Maryland General Hospital, Baltimore	12.2	0.0%	1.04	No	5	0.36	9	0.58	1	1	0.053
	Memorial Hospital at Easton, Easton	9.4	0.0%	1.20	No	4	0.00	9	1.02	2	2	0.030
	Northwest Hospital Center, Randallstown	13.4	0.0%	1.01	No	2	0.00	9	0.79	2	1	0.207
	Peninsula Regional Medical Center, Salisbury	10.2	0.0%	1.14	No	3	0.00	10	0.67	2	3	0.042
	Prince George's Hospital Center, Cheverly	6.7	0.0%	1.29	No	3	0.32	6	0.57	2	2	0.056
	Spring Grove Hospital Center, Catonsville	13.8	0.0%	0.77	No	3	0.10	0	0.35	2	1	0.000
	St. Agnes Hospital, Baltimore	12.3	0.0%	1.17	No	7	0.29	9	0.82	2	1	0.215
	Washington Adventist Hospital, Takoma Park	13.8	0.0%	1.05	No	4	0.03	10	1.23	2	3	0.043

GYNECOLOGY

Natl. Rank	Hospital	U.S. News index	Reputa-tional score	Hospital-wide mortality rate	Interns and residents to beds	Tech-nology score (of 10)	R.N.'s to beds	Board-certified OB-GYNs to beds	Procedures to beds
				TIER ONE					
1	Johns Hopkins Hospital, Baltimore	100.0	29.5%	0.97	0.73	10	1.43	0.046	0.46
				TIER TWO					
82	Sinai Hospital of Baltimore, Baltimore	22.4	0.0%	0.97	0.42	8	1.43	0.090	0.34
51	University of Maryland Medical System, Baltimore	26.1	0.4%	0.98	0.96	9	1.67	0.034	0.15
				TIER THREE					
100	Anne Arundel Medical Center, Annapolis	21.0	0.0%	0.73	0.00	8	0.96	0.086	0.44
89	Greater Baltimore Medical Center	22.1	0.4%	0.89	0.29	6	0.90	0.228	0.99
	Harbor Hospital Center, Baltimore	19.9	0.0%	0.77	0.34	4	0.93	0.122	0.43
	Holy Cross Hospital, Silver Spring	16.4	0.0%	0.94	0.05	5	0.64	0.138	0.40
	Mercy Medical Center, Baltimore	18.7	0.0%	0.65	0.21	7	0.50	0.063	0.24
	Northwest Hospital Center, Randallstown	14.2	0.0%	1.01	0.00	5	0.79	0.075	0.34
	St. Agnes Hospital, Baltimore	14.1	0.0%	1.17	0.29	8	0.82	0.088	0.45
	Washington Adventist Hospital, Takoma Park	15.6	0.0%	1.05	0.03	6	1.23	0.063	0.31
	Washington County Hospital Assn., Hagerstown	17.1	0.0%	0.95	0.00	7	0.99	0.032	0.39
				TIER FOUR					
	Francis Scott Key Medical Center, Baltimore	9.7	0.0%	1.21	0.27	6	0.61	0.034	0.10
	Franklin Square Hospital Center, Baltimore	13.2	0.0%	1.10	0.34	4	0.90	0.077	0.36
	Good Samaritan Hospital, Baltimore	14.0	0.0%	1.03	0.32	5	0.83	0.030	0.07
	Maryland General Hospital, Baltimore	13.1	0.0%	1.04	0.36	5	0.58	0.040	0.23
	Memorial Hospital at Easton, Easton	11.5	0.0%	1.20	0.00	7	1.02	0.045	0.38

Natl. Rank	Hospital	U.S. News index	Reputational score	Hospital-wide mortality rate	Interns and residents to beds	Technology score (of 10)	R.N.'s to beds	Board-certified OB-GYNs to beds	Procedures to beds
	Peninsula Regional Medical Center, Salisbury	10.3	0.0%	1.14	0.00	6	0.67	0.035	0.38
	Prince George's Hospital Center, Cheverly	9.1	0.0%	1.29	0.32	6	0.57	0.070	0.25
	Suburban Hospital, Bethesda	12.2	0.0%	1.02	0.02	5	0.59	0.043	0.18
	Union Memorial Hospital, Baltimore	13.6	0.0%	1.10	0.38	6	0.56	0.088	0.33

NEUROLOGY

Natl. Rank	Hospital	U.S. News index	Reputational score	Neurology mortality rate	COTH member	Interns and residents to beds	Technology score (of 9)	R.N.'s to beds	Board-certified neurologists to beds
TIER ONE									
2	Johns Hopkins Hospital, Baltimore	80.7	38.7%	0.84	Yes	0.73	9	1.43	0.014
TIER TWO									
67	Greater Baltimore Medical Center	18.5	0.5%	0.69	Yes	0.29	5	0.90	0.016
40	University of Maryland Medical System, Baltimore	22.2	1.9%	0.97	Yes	0.96	8	1.67	0.031
TIER THREE									
	Anne Arundel Medical Center, Annapolis	12.6	0.0%	0.88	No	0.00	8	0.96	0.013
	Franklin Square Hospital Center, Baltimore	12.1	0.0%	1.00	Yes	0.34	3	0.90	0.012
	Harbor Hospital Center, Baltimore	13.4	0.0%	0.86	No	0.34	4	0.93	0.021
	Holy Cross Hospital, Silver Spring	14.7	0.0%	0.82	Yes	0.05	5	0.64	0.014
	Howard County General Hospital, Columbia	12.4	0.0%	0.66	No	0.00	2	0.47	0.014
	Maryland General Hospital, Baltimore	14.3	0.0%	0.77	No	0.36	5	0.58	0.012
	Mercy Medical Center, Baltimore	14.0	0.0%	0.68	No	0.21	6	0.50	0.010
	Northwest Hospital Center, Randallstown	13.0	0.0%	0.78	No	0.00	5	0.79	0.004
	Sinai Hospital of Baltimore, Baltimore	15.8	0.0%	0.99	Yes	0.42	7	1.43	0.023
	St. Agnes Hospital, Baltimore	12.8	0.0%	0.88	No	0.29	7	0.82	0.013
	Washington Adventist Hospital, Takoma Park	11.7	0.0%	0.96	No	0.03	6	1.23	0.020
TIER FOUR									
	Francis Scott Key Medical Center, Baltimore	9.4	0.0%	1.17	Yes	0.27	5	0.61	0.013
	Good Samaritan Hospital, Baltimore	8.8	0.0%	1.10	No	0.32	5	0.83	0.015
	Memorial Hospital at Easton, Easton	9.1	0.0%	1.04	No	0.00	7	1.02	0.005
	Peninsula Regional Medical Center, Salisbury	8.2	0.0%	1.03	No	0.00	6	0.67	0.007
	Prince George's Hospital Center, Cheverly	7.6	0.0%	1.17	No	0.32	5	0.57	0.020
	Suburban Hospital, Bethesda	9.6	0.0%	0.92	No	0.02	4	0.59	0.010
	Union Memorial Hospital, Baltimore	10.7	0.0%	0.94	No	0.38	5	0.56	0.013
	Washington County Hospital Assn., Hagerstown	10.8	0.0%	0.92	No	0.00	7	0.99	0.003

ORTHOPEDICS

Natl. Rank	Hospital	U.S. News index	Reputational score	Orthopedics mortality rate	COTH member	Interns and residents to beds	Technology score (of 5)	R.N.'s to beds	Board-certified orthopedists to beds	Procedures to beds
TIER ONE										
4	Johns Hopkins Hospital, Baltimore	45.3	14.4%	0.80	Yes	0.73	5	1.43	0.026	1.11
TIER TWO										
71	Sinai Hospital of Baltimore, Baltimore	14.9	0.0%	0.75	Yes	0.42	4	1.43	0.076	1.75
69	University of Maryland Medical System, Baltimore	15.1	0.4%	1.03	Yes	0.96	4	1.67	0.031	0.74
TIER THREE										
	Anne Arundel Medical Center, Annapolis	11.7	0.0%	0.57	No	0.00	5	0.96	0.053	3.23
	Francis Scott Key Medical Center, Baltimore	9.7	0.0%	0.93	Yes	0.27	4	0.61	0.010	0.80
	Good Samaritan Hospital, Baltimore	8.2	0.0%	1.10	No	0.32	4	0.83	0.063	6.55
	Greater Baltimore Medical Center	10.8	0.4%	0.93	Yes	0.29	2	0.90	0.073	2.11
	Harbor Hospital Center, Baltimore	9.4	0.0%	0.78	No	0.34	3	0.93	0.049	1.61
	Holy Cross Hospital, Silver Spring	8.9	0.0%	1.03	Yes	0.05	4	0.64	0.068	2.07
	Mercy Medical Center, Baltimore	9.5	0.0%	0.52	No	0.21	3	0.50	0.056	1.50
	Northwest Hospital Center, Randallstown	8.2	0.0%	0.82	No	0.00	3	0.79	0.132	3.11

Natl. Rank	Hospital	U.S. News index	Reputational score	Orthopedics mortality rate	COTH member	Interns and residents to beds	Technology score (of 5)	R.N.'s to beds	Board-certified orthopedists to beds	Procedures to beds
	St. Agnes Hospital, Baltimore	9.0	0.0%	0.84	No	0.29	4	0.82	0.030	2.87
	Washington County Hospital Assn., Hagerstown	9.0	0.0%	0.75	No	0.00	3	0.99	0.035	2.93
TIER FOUR										
	Franklin Square Hospital Center, Baltimore	6.2	0.0%	1.72	Yes	0.34	2	0.90	0.030	2.25
	Howard County General Hospital, Columbia	2.3	0.0%	1.40	No	0.00	2	0.47	0.056	1.93
	Memorial Hospital at Easton, Easton	5.4	0.0%	1.42	No	0.00	4	1.02	0.030	4.42
	Peninsula Regional Medical Center, Salisbury	3.3	0.0%	1.40	No	0.00	3	0.67	0.015	2.24
	Prince George's Hospital Center, Cheverly	4.1	0.0%	1.54	No	0.32	4	0.57	0.045	1.01
	Suburban Hospital, Bethesda	6.5	0.0%	0.93	No	0.02	3	0.59	0.084	3.32
	Union Memorial Hospital, Baltimore	4.4	0.0%	1.74	No	0.38	4	0.56	0.053	3.26
	Washington Adventist Hospital, Takoma Park	5.6	0.0%	1.18	No	0.03	3	1.23	0.020	1.15

OTOLARYNGOLOGY

Natl. Rank	Hospital	U.S. News index	Reputational score	Hospital-wide mortality rate	COTH member	Interns and residents to beds	Technology score (of 9)	R.N.'s to beds	Board-certified internists to beds	Procedures to beds
TIER ONE										
1	Johns Hopkins Hospital, Baltimore	100.0	27.0%	0.97	Yes	0.73	9	1.43	0.084	0.315
TIER TWO										
37	University of Maryland Medical System, Baltimore	19.9	1.0%	0.98	Yes	0.96	8	1.67	0.281	0.223
TIER THREE										
	Francis Scott Key Medical Center, Baltimore	8.3	0.0%	1.21	Yes	0.27	3	0.61	0.168	0.151
	Franklin Square Hospital Center, Baltimore	8.1	0.0%	1.10	Yes	0.34	1	0.90	0.063	0.363
	Greater Baltimore Medical Center	10.2	0.0%	0.89	Yes	0.29	4	0.90	0.210	0.715
	Holy Cross Hospital, Silver Spring	9.2	0.0%	0.94	Yes	0.05	3	0.64	0.336	0.225
	Sinai Hospital of Baltimore, Baltimore	12.4	0.0%	0.97	Yes	0.42	7	1.43	0.127	0.234
TIER FOUR										
	Anne Arundel Medical Center, Annapolis	6.6	0.0%	0.73	No	0.00	8	0.96	0.132	0.267
	Deaton Hospital and Medical Center, Baltimore	0.0	0.0%	3.80	No	0.00	0	0.14	0.019	0.022
	Good Samaritan Hospital, Baltimore	5.3	0.0%	1.03	No	0.32	3	0.83	0.067	0.271
	Harbor Hospital Center, Baltimore	6.3	0.0%	0.77	No	0.34	2	0.93	0.150	0.195
	Howard County General Hospital, Columbia	2.8	0.0%	1.04	No	0.00	1	0.47	0.127	0.362
	Maryland General Hospital, Baltimore	5.1	0.0%	1.04	No	0.36	5	0.58	0.053	0.211
	Memorial Hospital at Easton, Easton	5.0	0.0%	1.20	No	0.00	6	1.02	0.030	0.323
	Mercy Medical Center, Baltimore	5.3	0.0%	0.66	No	0.21	4	0.50	0.185	0.159
	Northwest Hospital Center, Randallstown	5.4	0.0%	1.01	No	0.00	4	0.79	0.207	0.383
	Peninsula Regional Medical Center, Salisbury	4.1	0.0%	1.14	No	0.00	6	0.67	0.042	0.458
	Prince George's Hospital Center, Cheverly	4.2	0.0%	1.29	No	0.32	3	0.57	0.056	0.154
	St. Agnes Hospital, Baltimore	6.8	0.0%	1.17	No	0.29	5	0.82	0.215	0.331
	Suburban Hospital, Bethesda	3.8	0.0%	1.02	No	0.02	4	0.59	0.094	0.201
	Union Memorial Hospital, Baltimore	5.4	0.0%	1.10	No	0.38	4	0.56	0.123	0.288
	Washington Adventist Hospital, Takoma Park	6.0	0.0%	1.05	No	0.03	6	1.23	0.043	0.133
	Washington County Hospital Assn., Hagerstown	5.8	0.0%	0.95	No	0.00	7	0.99	0.083	0.263

RHEUMATOLOGY

Natl. Rank	Hospital	U.S. News index	Reputational score	Hospital-wide mortality rate	COTH member	Interns and residents to beds	Technology score (of 5)	R.N.'s to beds	Board-certified internists to beds
TIER ONE									
2	Johns Hopkins Hospital, Baltimore	75.3	26.6%	0.97	Yes	0.73	5	1.43	0.084
TIER TWO									
45	University of Maryland Medical System, Baltimore	18.4	0.0%	0.98	Yes	0.96	4	1.67	0.281
TIER THREE									
	Anne Arundel Medical Center, Annapolis	11.9	0.0%	0.73	No	0.00	5	0.96	0.132

Natl. Rank	Hospital	U.S. News index	Reputa- tional score	Hospital- wide mortality rate	COTH member	Interns and residents to beds	Tech- nology score (of 5)	R.N.'s to beds	Board- certified internists to beds
	Francis Scott Key Medical Center, Baltimore	10.8	0.0%	1.21	Yes	0.27	4	0.61	0.168
	Franklin Square Hospital Center, Baltimore	10.8	0.0%	1.10	Yes	0.34	2	0.90	0.063
	Good Samaritan Hospital, Baltimore	10.2	0.3%	1.03	No	0.32	4	0.83	0.067
	Greater Baltimore Medical Center	13.8	0.0%	0.89	Yes	0.29	2	0.90	0.210
	Harbor Hospital Center, Baltimore	12.1	0.0%	0.77	No	0.34	3	0.93	0.150
	Holy Cross Hospital, Silver Spring	13.6	0.0%	0.94	Yes	0.05	4	0.64	0.336
	Mercy Medical Center, Baltimore	10.8	0.0%	0.66	No	0.21	3	0.50	0.185
96	Sinai Hospital of Baltimore, Baltimore	15.0	0.0%	0.97	Yes	0.42	4	1.43	0.127
TIER FOUR									
	Howard County General Hospital, Columbia	7.1	0.0%	1.04	No	0.00	2	0.47	0.127
	Maryland General Hospital, Baltimore	7.9	0.0%	1.04	No	0.36	4	0.58	0.053
	Memorial Hospital at Easton, Easton	7.6	0.0%	1.20	No	0.00	4	1.02	0.030
	Northwest Hospital Center, Randallstown	9.3	0.0%	1.01	No	0.00	3	0.79	0.207
	Peninsula Regional Medical Center, Salisbury	6.7	0.0%	1.14	No	0.00	3	0.67	0.042
	Prince George's Hospital Center, Cheverly	7.0	0.0%	1.29	No	0.32	4	0.57	0.056
	St. Agnes Hospital, Baltimore	9.5	0.0%	1.17	No	0.29	4	0.82	0.215
	Suburban Hospital, Bethesda	7.8	0.0%	1.02	No	0.02	3	0.59	0.094
	Union Memorial Hospital, Baltimore	9.0	0.0%	1.10	No	0.38	4	0.56	0.123
	Washington Adventist Hospital, Takoma Park	9.0	0.0%	1.05	No	0.03	3	1.23	0.043
	Washington County Hospital Assn., Hagerstown	9.5	0.0%	0.95	No	0.00	3	0.99	0.083

UROLOGY

Natl. Rank	Hospital	U.S. News index	Reputa- tional score	Urology mortality rate	COTH member	Interns and residents to beds	Tech- nology score (of 11)	R.N.'s to beds	Board- certified internists to beds	Procedures to beds
TIER ONE										
1	Johns Hopkins Hospital, Baltimore	100.0	63.5%	0.94	Yes	0.73	11	1.43	0.084	1.35
TIER TWO										
59	University of Maryland Medical System, Baltimore	17.3	0.6%	1.04	Yes	0.96	10	1.67	0.281	1.28
TIER THREE										
	Anne Arundel Medical Center, Annapolis	12.5	0.0%	0.67	No	0.00	9	0.96	0.132	2.29
	Francis Scott Key Medical Center, Baltimore	9.7	0.0%	1.09	Yes	0.27	5	0.61	0.168	1.07
	Franklin Square Hospital Center, Baltimore	8.6	0.0%	1.27	Yes	0.34	3	0.90	0.063	2.13
	Greater Baltimore Medical Center	11.8	0.0%	0.98	Yes	0.29	5	0.90	0.210	2.42
	Harbor Hospital Center, Baltimore	10.5	0.0%	0.86	No	0.34	4	0.93	0.150	2.54
	Maryland General Hospital, Baltimore	9.6	0.0%	0.85	No	0.36	6	0.58	0.053	2.29
	Mercy Medical Center, Baltimore	11.6	0.0%	0.63	No	0.21	7	0.50	0.185	2.24
	Sinai Hospital of Baltimore, Baltimore	12.8	0.0%	1.12	Yes	0.42	8	1.43	0.127	1.53
TIER FOUR										
	Good Samaritan Hospital, Baltimore	8.5	0.0%	1.00	No	0.32	5	0.83	0.067	2.56
	Holy Cross Hospital, Silver Spring	8.2	0.0%	1.26	Yes	0.05	5	0.64	0.336	2.20
	Howard County General Hospital, Columbia	2.6	0.0%	1.57	No	0.00	2	0.47	0.127	1.99
	Memorial Hospital at Easton, Easton	5.6	0.0%	1.45	No	0.00	8	1.02	0.030	2.73
	Northwest Hospital Center, Randallstown	8.1	0.0%	1.05	No	0.00	6	0.79	0.207	3.78
	Peninsula Regional Medical Center, Salisbury	4.6	0.0%	1.38	No	0.00	7	0.67	0.042	1.85
	Prince George's Hospital Center, Cheverly	3.2	0.0%	1.76	No	0.32	5	0.57	0.056	0.96
	St. Agnes Hospital, Baltimore	7.1	0.0%	1.38	No	0.29	7	0.82	0.215	3.07
	Suburban Hospital, Bethesda	5.1	0.0%	1.23	No	0.02	5	0.59	0.094	1.71
	Union Memorial Hospital, Baltimore	6.4	0.0%	1.31	No	0.38	6	0.56	0.123	2.44
	Washington Adventist Hospital, Takoma Park	6.3	0.0%	1.32	No	0.03	7	1.23	0.043	1.25
	Washington County Hospital Assn., Hagerstown	8.0	0.0%	1.07	No	0.00	8	0.99	0.083	2.25

AIDS

Natl. Rank	Hospital	U.S. News index	Reputa-tional score	Hospital-wide mortality rate	COTH member	Interns and residents to beds	Tech-nology score (of 11)	Discharge planning (of 2)	R.N.'s to beds	Board-certified internists to beds
TIER ONE										
3	Massachusetts General Hospital, Boston	62.3	26.8%	0.88	Yes	1.00	11	2	1.14	0.085
12	Beth Israel Hospital, Boston	35.2	4.4%	0.85	Yes	0.57	8	2	1.93	0.590
13	New England Deaconess Hospital, Boston	35.2	7.2%	0.99	Yes	1.08	9	2	1.33	0.089
21	Boston City Hospital	31.0	1.8%	0.75	No	1.64	7	2	1.37	0.545
26	Brigham and Women's Hospital, Boston	30.0	2.1%	0.91	Yes	1.49	8	2	0.79	0.179
TIER TWO										
49	Boston University Medical Center-University Hospital	27.4	0.5%	0.82	Yes	0.96	7	2	0.85	0.231
31	New England Medical Center, Boston	29.3	1.0%	0.86	Yes	1.07	8	2	1.66	0.086
57	University of Massachusetts Medical Center, Worcester	26.5	0.8%	0.99	Yes	1.47	8	2	0.96	0.000
TIER THREE										
	Baystate Medical Center, Springfield	20.6	0.5%	1.36	Yes	0.54	9	2	1.07	0.076
	Berkshire Medical Center, Pittsfield	20.1	0.4%	1.25	Yes	0.33	8	2	0.55	0.133
	Brockton Hospital, Brockton	19.9	0.0%	1.04	No	0.06	6	2	1.10	0.060
	Cape Cod Hospital, Hyannis	21.4	0.0%	0.94	No	0.02	5	2	1.28	0.050
	Carney Hospital, Boston	21.1	0.0%	1.02	No	0.51	4	2	1.05	0.237
	Faulkner Hospital, Boston	23.9	0.0%	0.76	Yes	0.35	5	2	0.54	0.137
	Lahey Clinic Hospital, Burlington	22.8	0.0%	0.96	No	0.51	7	2	1.22	0.085
	Medical Center of Central Massachusetts, Worcester	21.6	0.0%	0.92	Yes	0.14	5	1	0.47	0.063
	Metrowest Medical Center, Framingham	21.5	0.0%	0.91	No	0.24	6	2	0.33	0.109
	Mount Auburn Hospital, Cambridge	22.6	0.0%	0.99	Yes	0.50	5	2	0.64	0.185
	New England Baptist Hospital, Boston	20.6	0.0%	0.74	No	0.05	4	1	0.75	0.050
	Newton-Wellesley Hospital, Newton	21.3	0.0%	0.74	No	0.19	4	2	0.40	0.107
100	St. Elizabeth's Hospital of Boston	24.6	0.0%	0.95	Yes	0.77	6	2	0.96	0.154
	St. Vincent Hospital, Worcester	20.8	0.0%	1.24	Yes	0.33	6	2	1.09	0.370
	Walthamweston Hospital and Medical Center, Waltham	21.4	0.0%	0.88	No	0.02	6	2	0.36	0.062
TIER FOUR										
	Atlanticare Medical Center, Lynn	15.2	0.0%	1.46	No	0.01	8	2	0.64	0.045
	Burbank Hospital, Fitchburg	14.1	0.0%	1.34	No	0.03	4	2	0.21	0.038
	Cambridge Hospital, Cambridge	16.9	0.0%	1.34	No	0.60	5	2	0.80	0.118
	Cardinal Cushing General Hospital, Brockton	17.5	0.0%	1.07	No	0.03	4	2	0.32	0.093
	Charlton Memorial Hospital, Fall River	17.3	0.0%	1.12	No	0.00	6	2	0.30	0.045
	Holy Family Hospital and Medical Center, Methuen	12.8	0.0%	1.56	No	0.00	5	2	0.29	0.019
	Jewish Memorial Hospital, Boston	6.0	0.0%	3.92	No	0.00	1	2	0.49	0.184
	Malden Hospital, Malden	16.6	0.0%	1.09	No	0.15	4	1	0.34	0.030
	North Shore Medical Center, Salem	18.4	0.0%	1.12	No	0.12	6	2	0.58	0.115

CANCER

Natl. Rank	Hospital	U.S. News index	Reputa-tional score	Cancer mortality rate	COTH member	Interns and residents to beds	Tech-nology score (of 12)	R.N.'s to beds	Board-certified oncologists to beds	Procedures to beds
TIER ONE										
3	Dana-Farber Cancer Institute, Boston	74.1	46.7%	0.01	No	0.49	4	1.58	0.964	12.91
12	Massachusetts General Hospital, Boston	21.1	7.3%	0.80	Yes	1.00	12	1.14	0.011	2.41
TIER TWO										
67	Beth Israel Hospital, Boston	11.9	0.0%	0.66	Yes	0.57	8	1.93	0.043	1.83
32	Brigham and Women's Hospital, Boston	14.7	1.9%	0.69	Yes	1.49	10	0.79	0.066	1.45
53	New England Deaconess Hospital, Boston	12.8	0.4%	0.70	Yes	1.08	10	1.33	0.034	1.50
48	New England Medical Center, Boston	13.0	0.7%	0.76	Yes	1.07	7	1.66	0.012	1.40
59	University of Massachusetts Medical Center, Worcester	12.4	0.4%	0.78	Yes	1.47	7	0.96	0.054	2.49

Natl. Rank	Hospital	U.S. News index	Reputa- tional score	Cancer mortality rate	COTH member	Interns and residents to beds	Tech- nology score (of 12)	R.N.'s to beds	Board- certified oncologists to beds	Procedures to beds
	TIER THREE									
	Baystate Medical Center, Springfield	8.6	0.0%	1.44	Yes	0.54	9	1.07	0.018	1.29
	Berkshire Medical Center, Pittsfield	6.1	0.0%	1.63	Yes	0.33	8	0.55	0.000	1.91
	Boston City Hospital	10.1	0.0%	0.48	No	1.64	5	1.37	0.000	0.56
99	Boston University Medical Center-University Hospital	10.2	0.0%	0.63	Yes	0.96	8	0.85	0.033	2.15
	Faulkner Hospital, Boston	5.5	0.0%	0.81	Yes	0.35	3	0.54	0.020	2.10
	Lahey Clinic Hospital, Burlington	7.9	0.5%	0.98	No	0.51	9	1.22	0.015	3.83
	Mount Auburn Hospital, Cambridge	5.9	0.0%	1.33	Yes	0.50	4	0.64	0.013	1.29
	St. Elizabeth's Hospital of Boston	8.8	0.0%	0.85	Yes	0.77	6	0.96	0.020	1.72
	St. Vincent Hospital, Worcester	7.5	0.0%	1.28	Yes	0.33	7	1.09	0.005	1.64
	TIER FOUR									
	Atlanticare Medical Center, Lynn	2.9	0.0%	2.03	No	0.01	8	0.64	0.007	2.78
	Brockton Hospital, Brockton	4.1	0.0%	0.97	No	0.06	6	1.10	0.010	1.26
	Burbank Hospital, Fitchburg	0.0	0.0%	1.41	No	0.03	2	0.21	0.005	1.40
	Cape Cod Hospital, Hyannis	4.5	0.0%	0.78	No	0.02	4	1.28	0.008	2.93
	Cardinal Cushing General Hospital, Brockton	0.6	0.0%	1.08	No	0.03	2	0.32	0.017	1.47
	Carney Hospital, Boston	4.5	0.0%	0.81	No	0.51	2	1.05	0.007	1.62
	Charlton Memorial Hospital, Fall River	1.3	0.0%	1.09	No	0.00	5	0.30	0.006	1.40
	Holy Family Hospital and Medical Center, Methuen	1.7	0.0%	1.36	No	0.00	7	0.29	0.006	2.07
	Lawrence Memorial Hospital of Medford, Medford	1.3	0.0%	1.05	No	0.01	2	0.56	0.013	1.84
	Malden Hospital, Malden	1.0	0.0%	1.18	No	0.15	2	0.34	0.010	1.69
	Medical Center of Central Massachusetts, Worcester	4.9	0.0%	1.01	Yes	0.14	6	0.47	0.013	0.60
	Metrowest Medical Center, Framingham	2.0	0.0%	1.03	No	0.24	4	0.33	0.021	1.44
	New England Baptist Hospital, Boston	2.6	0.0%	0.66	No	0.05	2	0.75	0.015	2.19
	Newton-Wellesley Hospital, Newton	1.8	0.0%	0.80	No	0.19	2	0.40	0.009	2.01
	North Shore Medical Center, Salem	2.8	0.0%	1.16	No	0.12	6	0.58	0.013	1.69
	Walthamweston Hospital and Medical Center, Waltham	2.0	0.0%	0.83	No	0.02	6	0.36	0.012	0.98

CARDIOLOGY

Natl. Rank	Hospital	U.S. News index	Reputa- tional score	Cardiology mortality rate	COTH member	Interns and residents to beds	Tech- nology score (of 10)	R.N.'s to beds	Board- certified cardiologists to beds	Procedures to beds
	TIER ONE									
4	Massachusetts General Hospital, Boston	73.3	32.5%	0.71	Yes	1.00	10	1.14	0.034	7.24
6	Brigham and Women's Hospital, Boston	56.3	23.2%	1.03	Yes	1.49	9	0.79	0.071	5.70
14	Beth Israel Hospital, Boston	31.7	3.4%	0.87	Yes	0.57	9	1.93	0.087	10.50
	TIER TWO									
85	Boston University Medical Center-University Hospital	21.3	0.0%	0.99	Yes	0.96	8	0.85	0.087	7.69
27	New England Medical Center, Boston	27.1	0.6%	0.69	Yes	1.07	7	1.66	0.034	6.14
94	University of Massachusetts Medical Center, Worcester	20.9	0.0%	1.10	Yes	1.47	7	0.96	0.075	8.52
	TIER THREE									
	Baystate Medical Center, Springfield	14.9	0.0%	1.28	Yes	0.54	9	1.07	0.045	7.46
	Brockton Hospital, Brockton	17.1	0.0%	0.89	No	0.06	5	1.10	0.017	7.35
	Cape Cod Hospital, Hyannis	16.3	0.0%	0.92	No	0.02	3	1.28	0.023	15.90
	Carney Hospital, Boston	18.9	0.0%	0.80	No	0.51	4	1.05	0.026	8.29
	Faulkner Hospital, Boston	20.1	0.0%	0.72	Yes	0.35	6	0.54	0.020	8.63
	Lahey Clinic Hospital, Burlington	18.6	0.7%	1.01	No	0.51	8	1.22	0.051	12.11
	Lawrence Memorial Hospital of Medford, Medford	15.4	0.0%	0.82	No	0.01	3	0.56	0.020	11.15
	Medical Center of Central Massachusetts, Worcester	18.1	0.0%	0.89	Yes	0.14	5	0.47	0.024	3.31
	Metrowest Medical Center, Framingham	16.5	0.0%	0.85	No	0.24	6	0.33	0.027	8.72
	Mount Auburn Hospital, Cambridge	20.0	0.0%	0.92	Yes	0.50	6	0.64	0.034	10.99
	New England Baptist Hospital, Boston	16.3	0.0%	0.66	No	0.05	3	0.75	0.045	6.87
	New England Deaconess Hospital, Boston	20.6	0.3%	1.17	Yes	1.08	10	1.33	0.066	12.12
	Newton-Wellesley Hospital, Newton	15.4	0.0%	0.86	No	0.19	4	0.40	0.013	5.07
	North Shore Medical Center, Salem	14.7	0.0%	0.94	No	0.12	5	0.58	0.036	6.94

Natl. Rank Hospital	U.S. News index	Reputational score	Cardiology mortality rate	COTH member	Interns and residents to beds	Technology score (of 10)	R.N.'s to beds	Boardcertified cardiologists to beds	Procedures to beds
St. Elizabeth's Hospital of Boston	17.5	0.0%	1.15	Yes	0.77	7	0.96	0.069	9.09
Walthamweston Hospital and Medical Center, Waltham	14.9	0.0%	0.82	No	0.02	4	0.36	0.016	6.79
TIER FOUR									
Atlanticare Medical Center, Lynn	7.2	0.0%	1.31	No	0.01	5	0.64	0.037	7.60
Berkshire Medical Center, Pittsfield	13.4	0.0%	1.13	Yes	0.33	6	0.55	0.000	7.41
Burbank Hospital, Fitchburg	7.9	0.0%	1.13	No	0.03	3	0.21	0.011	6.01
Cambridge Hospital, Cambridge	5.6	0.0%	1.53	No	0.60	2	0.80	0.011	4.85
Cardinal Cushing General Hospital, Brockton	12.3	0.0%	0.98	No	0.03	4	0.32	0.034	9.66
Charlton Memorial Hospital, Fall River	11.3	0.0%	1.04	No	0.00	7	0.30	0.006	11.76
Holy Family Hospital and Medical Center, Methuen	4.1	0.0%	1.43	No	0.00	5	0.29	0.013	5.61
Malden Hospital, Malden	12.5	0.0%	0.97	No	0.15	3	0.34	0.030	5.73
St. Vincent Hospital, Worcester	13.2	0.0%	1.25	Yes	0.33	6	1.09	0.000	12.32

ENDOCRINOLOGY

Natl. Rank Hospital	U.S. News index	Reputational score	Endocrinology mortality rate	COTH member	Interns and residents to beds	Technology score (of 11)	R.N.'s to beds	Boardcertified internists to beds
TIER ONE								
2 Massachusetts General Hospital, Boston	92.0	58.2%	0.93	Yes	1.00	11	1.14	0.085
9 New England Deaconess Hospital, Boston	34.7	13.0%	0.72	Yes	1.08	10	1.33	0.089
11 Brigham and Women's Hospital, Boston	33.5	13.1%	0.89	Yes	1.49	10	0.79	0.179
16 Beth Israel Hospital, Boston	25.9	5.0%	0.86	Yes	0.57	9	1.93	0.590
TIER TWO								
31 Boston City Hospital	20.0	0.0%	0.59	No	1.64	5	1.37	0.545
43 Boston University Medical Center-University Hospital	18.0	0.4%	0.65	Yes	0.96	9	0.85	0.231
42 New England Medical Center, Boston	18.2	0.9%	0.79	Yes	1.07	8	1.66	0.086
66 St. Elizabeth's Hospital of Boston	16.0	0.0%	0.67	Yes	0.77	7	0.96	0.154
37 University of Massachusetts Medical Center, Worcester	18.9	1.0%	0.60	Yes	1.47	8	0.96	0.000
TIER THREE								
Baystate Medical Center, Springfield	8.8	0.0%	1.88	Yes	0.54	9	1.07	0.076
Cape Cod Hospital, Hyannis	8.8	0.0%	0.83	No	0.02	5	1.28	0.050
Carney Hospital, Boston	8.3	0.0%	1.18	No	0.51	3	1.05	0.237
Faulkner Hospital, Boston	10.1	0.0%	0.90	Yes	0.35	4	0.54	0.137
Lahey Clinic Hospital, Burlington	12.9	0.7%	0.79	No	0.51	10	1.22	0.085
Mount Auburn Hospital, Cambridge	9.6	0.0%	1.20	Yes	0.50	5	0.64	0.185
Newton-Wellesley Hospital, Newton	9.1	0.0%	0.45	No	0.19	3	0.40	0.107
St. Vincent Hospital, Worcester	13.0	0.0%	1.04	Yes	0.33	8	1.09	0.370
TIER FOUR								
Atlanticare Medical Center, Lynn	3.7	0.0%	1.65	No	0.01	9	0.64	0.045
Berkshire Medical Center, Pittsfield	7.1	0.0%	1.89	Yes	0.33	9	0.55	0.133
Brockton Hospital, Brockton	5.3	0.0%	1.48	No	0.06	7	1.10	0.060
Burbank Hospital, Fitchburg	1.6	0.0%	1.57	No	0.03	3	0.21	0.038
Cardinal Cushing General Hospital, Brockton	3.8	0.0%	1.15	No	0.03	3	0.32	0.093
Charlton Memorial Hospital, Fall River	2.4	0.0%	1.54	No	0.00	6	0.30	0.045
Holy Family Hospital and Medical Center, Methuen	1.7	0.0%	1.95	No	0.00	8	0.29	0.019
Lawrence Memorial Hospital of Medford, Medford	4.8	0.0%	1.09	No	0.01	3	0.56	0.107
Malden Hospital, Malden	3.2	0.0%	1.29	No	0.15	3	0.34	0.030
Medical Center of Central Massachusetts, Worcester	7.8	0.0%	1.13	Yes	0.14	7	0.47	0.063
Metrowest Medical Center, Framingham	7.5	0.0%	0.81	No	0.24	5	0.33	0.109
North Shore Medical Center, Salem	5.9	0.0%	1.13	No	0.12	7	0.58	0.115
Walthamweston Hospital and Medical Center, Waltham	7.3	0.0%	0.78	No	0.02	7	0.36	0.062

GASTROENTEROLOGY

Natl. Rank	Hospital	U.S. News index	Reputational score	Gastro-enterology mortality rate	COTH member	Interns and residents to beds	Technology score (of 11)	R.N.'s to beds	Board-certified gastro-enterologists to beds	Pro-cedures to beds
TIER ONE										
3	Massachusetts General Hospital, Boston	60.3	29.6%	0.71	Yes	1.00	11	1.14	0.014	2.89
10	Brigham and Women's Hospital, Boston	33.4	12.2%	0.89	Yes	1.49	10	0.79	0.020	1.78
12	Beth Israel Hospital, Boston	26.8	7.1%	0.79	Yes	0.57	9	1.93	0.041	3.48
TIER TWO										
51	Boston University Medical Center-University Hospital	15.1	0.7%	0.86	Yes	0.96	9	0.85	0.024	2.73
43	Lahey Clinic Hospital, Burlington	15.6	2.6%	0.89	No	0.51	10	1.22	0.029	4.77
31	New England Deaconess Hospital, Boston	16.8	0.5%	0.68	Yes	1.08	9	1.33	0.020	2.68
37	New England Medical Center, Boston	16.2	1.3%	0.93	Yes	1.07	7	1.66	0.016	1.47
72	St. Elizabeth's Hospital of Boston	13.4	0.0%	0.84	Yes	0.77	6	0.96	0.029	3.67
48	University of Massachusetts Medical Center, Worcester	15.3	0.0%	0.87	Yes	1.47	8	0.96	0.022	2.10
TIER THREE										
	Baystate Medical Center, Springfield	10.2	0.0%	1.28	Yes	0.54	9	1.07	0.023	2.72
	Berkshire Medical Center, Pittsfield	9.3	0.0%	1.12	Yes	0.33	9	0.55	0.000	3.27
	Cape Cod Hospital, Hyannis	10.2	0.0%	0.93	No	0.02	5	1.28	0.012	8.09
	Faulkner Hospital, Boston	10.4	0.0%	0.88	Yes	0.35	4	0.54	0.015	4.48
	Medical Center of Central Massachusetts, Worcester	9.0	0.0%	0.83	Yes	0.14	6	0.47	0.004	1.98
	Mount Auburn Hospital, Cambridge	9.5	0.0%	1.08	Yes	0.50	5	0.64	0.020	3.67
	St. Vincent Hospital, Worcester	8.7	0.0%	1.61	Yes	0.33	7	1.09	0.000	4.40
TIER FOUR										
	Atlanticare Medical Center, Lynn	4.6	0.0%	1.43	No	0.01	8	0.64	0.015	4.15
	Brockton Hospital, Brockton	5.2	0.0%	1.27	No	0.06	6	1.10	0.010	3.11
	Burbank Hospital, Fitchburg	1.8	0.0%	1.38	No	0.03	3	0.21	0.005	3.30
	Cardinal Cushing General Hospital, Brockton	2.4	0.0%	1.42	No	0.03	3	0.32	0.013	4.18
	Carney Hospital, Boston	6.4	0.0%	1.41	No	0.51	3	1.05	0.015	4.87
	Charlton Memorial Hospital, Fall River	4.4	0.0%	1.31	No	0.00	7	0.30	0.015	4.89
	Holy Family Hospital and Medical Center, Methuen	1.8	0.0%	1.71	No	0.00	7	0.29	0.010	2.71
	Lawrence Memorial Hospital of Medford, Medford	5.8	0.0%	0.98	No	0.01	3	0.56	0.033	5.07
	Malden Hospital, Malden	5.3	0.0%	0.89	No	0.15	3	0.34	0.010	2.98
	Metrowest Medical Center, Framingham	6.0	0.0%	1.02	No	0.24	6	0.33	0.018	3.85
	New England Baptist Hospital, Boston	6.5	0.0%	0.60	No	0.05	3	0.75	0.015	2.69
	Newton-Wellesley Hospital, Newton	6.6	0.0%	0.73	No	0.19	3	0.40	0.019	3.42
	North Shore Medical Center, Salem	5.4	0.0%	1.15	No	0.12	7	0.58	0.026	3.35
	Walthamweston Hospital and Medical Center, Waltham	4.7	0.0%	1.07	No	0.02	7	0.36	0.008	3.01

GERIATRICS

Natl. Rank	Hospital	U.S. News index	Reputational score	Hospital-wide mortality rate	COTH member	Service mix	Interns and residents to beds	Technology score (of 13)	R.N.'s to beds	Discharge planning (of 2)	Geriatric services (of 9)	Board-certified internists to beds
TIER ONE												
2	Massachusetts General Hospital, Boston	86.4	23.1%	0.88	Yes	8	1.00	13	1.14	2	4	0.085
5	Beth Israel Hospital, Boston	69.9	15.7%	0.85	Yes	9	0.57	11	1.93	2	3	0.590
10	Brigham and Women's Hospital, Boston	45.9	7.8%	0.91	Yes	7	1.49	12	0.79	2	4	0.179
TIER TWO												
28	Boston University Medical Center-University Hospital	26.9	1.3%	0.82	Yes	4	0.96	10	0.85	2	5	0.231
53	New England Deaconess Hospital, Boston	24.2	0.9%	0.99	Yes	5	1.08	13	1.33	2	4	0.089
37	New England Medical Center, Boston	26.2	0.3%	0.86	Yes	8	1.07	10	1.66	2	1	0.086
72	St. Elizabeth's Hospital of Boston	22.5	0.0%	0.95	Yes	8	0.77	9	0.96	2	5	0.154
58	University of Massachusetts Medical Center, Worcester	23.4	0.5%	0.99	Yes	9	1.47	9	0.96	2	2	0.000
TIER THREE												
	Cape Cod Hospital, Hyannis	16.8	0.0%	0.94	No	5	0.02	6	1.28	2	3	0.050
	Carney Hospital, Boston	15.9	0.0%	1.02	No	5	0.51	5	1.05	2	3	0.237
	Faulkner Hospital, Boston	20.4	0.0%	0.76	Yes	6	0.35	6	0.54	2	2	0.137

Natl. Rank	Hospital	U.S. News index	Reputa- tional score	Hospital- wide mortality rate	COTH member	Service mix	Interns and residents to beds	Tech- nology score (of 13)	R.N.'s to beds	Discharge planning (of 2)	Geriatric services (of 9)	Board- certified internists to beds
	Lahey Clinic Hospital, Burlington	17.0	0.0%	0.96	No	3	0.51	10	1.22	2	2	0.085
	Medical Center of Central Massachusetts, Worcester	18.7	0.0%	0.92	Yes	8	0.14	9	0.47	1	2	0.063
	Metrowest Medical Center, Framingham	16.6	0.0%	0.91	No	5	0.24	7	0.33	2	2	0.109
	Mount Auburn Hospital, Cambridge	20.0	0.5%	0.99	Yes	6	0.50	7	0.64	2	4	0.185
	New England Baptist Hospital, Boston	14.5	0.0%	0.74	No	3	0.05	4	0.75	1	1	0.050
	Newton-Wellesley Hospital, Newton	17.3	0.0%	0.74	No	6	0.19	4	0.40	2	3	0.107
	St. Vincent Hospital, Worcester	14.9	0.0%	1.24	Yes	5	0.33	9	1.09	2	6	0.370
	Walthamweston Hospital and Medical Center, Waltham	18.6	0.0%	0.88	No	8	0.02	7	0.36	2	5	0.062
TIER FOUR												
	Atlanticare Medical Center, Lynn	6.3	0.0%	1.46	No	7	0.01	9	0.64	2	4	0.045
	Baystate Medical Center, Springfield	12.3	0.0%	1.36	Yes	7	0.54	11	1.07	2	3	0.076
	Berkshire Medical Center, Pittsfield	13.2	0.0%	1.25	Yes	8	0.33	10	0.55	2	3	0.133
	Brockton Hospital, Brockton	13.0	0.0%	1.04	No	4	0.06	8	1.10	2	1	0.060
	Burbank Hospital, Fitchburg	4.5	0.0%	1.34	No	4	0.03	3	0.21	2	3	0.038
	Cardinal Cushing General Hospital, Brockton	10.1	0.0%	1.07	No	3	0.03	4	0.32	2	3	0.093
	Charlton Memorial Hospital, Fall River	9.3	0.0%	1.12	No	3	0.00	8	0.30	2	3	0.045
	Holy Family Hospital and Medical Center, Methuen	2.5	0.0%	1.56	No	4	0.00	9	0.29	2	2	0.019
	Lawrence Memorial Hospital of Medford, Medford	13.3	0.0%	0.92	No	3	0.01	3	0.56	1	1	0.107
	Malden Hospital, Malden	8.8	0.0%	1.09	No	5	0.15	3	0.34	1	1	0.030
	North Shore Medical Center, Salem	12.7	0.0%	1.12	No	7	0.12	9	0.58	2	3	0.115

GYNECOLOGY

Natl. Rank	Hospital	U.S. News index	Reputa- tional score	Hospital- wide mortality rate	Interns and residents to beds	Tech- nology score (of 10)	R.N.'s to beds	Board- certified OB-GYNs to beds	Procedures to beds
TIER ONE									
4	Brigham and Women's Hospital, Boston	80.9	20.9%	0.91	1.49	9	0.79	0.127	0.66
5	Massachusetts General Hospital, Boston	57.7	12.0%	0.88	1.00	10	1.14	0.046	0.53
19	Beth Israel Hospital, Boston	35.3	3.0%	0.85	0.57	7	1.93	0.132	0.55
TIER TWO									
75	Boston University Medical Center-University Hospital	23.1	0.0%	0.82	0.96	7	0.85	0.039	0.37
80	New England Deaconess Hospital, Boston	22.6	0.0%	0.99	1.08	8	1.33	0.009	0.14
76	University of Massachusetts Medical Center, Worcester	23.1	0.0%	0.99	1.47	6	0.96	0.086	0.73
TIER THREE									
	Brockton Hospital, Brockton	14.5	0.0%	1.04	0.06	6	1.10	0.030	0.24
	Cape Cod Hospital, Hyannis	17.5	0.0%	0.94	0.02	5	1.28	0.035	0.88
	Carney Hospital, Boston	14.4	0.0%	1.02	0.51	3	1.05	0.011	0.18
	Faulkner Hospital, Boston	16.7	0.0%	0.76	0.35	4	0.54	0.034	0.29
	Lahey Clinic Hospital, Burlington	20.4	0.0%	0.96	0.51	8	1.22	0.015	0.86
	Medical Center of Central Massachusetts, Worcester	16.8	0.0%	0.92	0.14	6	0.47	0.083	0.11
	Metrowest Medical Center, Framingham	15.8	0.0%	0.91	0.24	5	0.33	0.063	0.46
	Mount Auburn Hospital, Cambridge	14.9	0.0%	0.99	0.50	4	0.64	0.051	0.28
	Newton-Wellesley Hospital, Newton	15.4	0.0%	0.74	0.19	3	0.40	0.066	0.50
	St. Elizabeth's Hospital of Boston	19.5	0.0%	0.95	0.77	5	0.96	0.057	0.37
	Walthamweston Hospital and Medical Center, Waltham	16.2	0.0%	0.88	0.02	6	0.36	0.049	0.23
TIER FOUR									
	Atlanticare Medical Center, Lynn	5.1	0.0%	1.46	0.01	7	0.64	0.019	0.37
	Baystate Medical Center, Springfield	13.1	0.0%	1.36	0.54	8	1.07	0.085	0.53
	Berkshire Medical Center, Pittsfield	9.6	0.0%	1.25	0.33	7	0.55	0.026	0.35
	Burbank Hospital, Fitchburg	2.1	0.0%	1.34	0.03	3	0.21	0.016	0.30
	Cardinal Cushing General Hospital, Brockton	7.8	0.0%	1.07	0.03	3	0.32	0.017	0.17
	Charlton Memorial Hospital, Fall River	7.9	0.0%	1.12	0.00	5	0.30	0.021	0.57
	Holy Family Hospital and Medical Center, Methuen	1.7	0.0%	1.56	0.00	6	0.29	0.019	0.24
	Lawrence Memorial Hospital of Medford, Medford	13.2	0.0%	0.92	0.01	3	0.56	0.020	0.17

Natl. Rank	Hospital	U.S. News index	Reputational score	Hospital-wide mortality rate	Interns and residents to beds	Technology score (of 10)	R.N.'s to beds	Board-certified OB-GYNs to beds	Procedures to beds
	Malden Hospital, Malden	9.0	0.0%	1.09	0.15	3	0.34	0.059	0.47
	North Shore Medical Center, Salem	10.4	0.0%	1.12	0.12	5	0.58	0.044	0.40
	St. Vincent Hospital, Worcester	12.3	0.0%	1.24	0.33	6	1.09	0.065	0.34

NEUROLOGY

Natl. Rank	Hospital	U.S. News index	Reputational score	Neurology mortality rate	COTH member	Interns and residents to beds	Technology score (of 9)	R.N.'s to beds	Board-certified neurologists to beds
	TIER ONE								
4	Massachusetts General Hospital, Boston	61.8	28.6%	1.00	Yes	1.00	9	1.14	0.014
12	Brigham and Women's Hospital, Boston	31.1	5.3%	0.79	Yes	1.49	8	0.79	0.036
18	Beth Israel Hospital, Boston	26.8	1.1%	0.82	Yes	0.57	7	1.93	0.087
	TIER TWO								
32	Boston University Medical Center-University Hospital	23.2	0.0%	0.65	Yes	0.96	7	0.85	0.060
39	New England Deaconess Hospital, Boston	22.3	0.0%	0.70	Yes	1.08	8	1.33	0.017
50	New England Medical Center, Boston	20.3	1.6%	0.98	Yes	1.07	6	1.66	0.014
86	St. Elizabeth's Hospital of Boston	17.9	0.6%	0.88	Yes	0.77	5	0.96	0.020
59	University of Massachusetts Medical Center, Worcester	19.0	0.6%	1.02	Yes	1.47	6	0.96	0.038
	TIER THREE								
	Faulkner Hospital, Boston	15.6	0.0%	0.79	Yes	0.35	4	0.54	0.010
	Lahey Clinic Hospital, Burlington	14.7	0.2%	0.98	No	0.51	8	1.22	0.033
	Medical Center of Central Massachusetts, Worcester	13.9	0.0%	0.84	Yes	0.14	5	0.47	0.013
	Mount Auburn Hospital, Cambridge	15.6	0.0%	0.86	Yes	0.50	4	0.64	0.024
	Newton-Wellesley Hospital, Newton	13.1	0.0%	0.75	No	0.19	3	0.40	0.013
	St. Vincent Hospital, Worcester	14.5	0.0%	1.05	Yes	0.33	6	1.09	0.040
	Walthamweston Hospital and Medical Center, Waltham	11.7	0.0%	0.81	No	0.02	6	0.36	0.008
	TIER FOUR								
	Atlanticare Medical Center, Lynn	5.2	0.0%	1.36	No	0.01	7	0.64	0.015
	Baystate Medical Center, Springfield	10.0	0.0%	1.36	Yes	0.54	7	1.07	0.012
	Berkshire Medical Center, Pittsfield	7.0	0.0%	1.45	Yes	0.33	7	0.55	0.006
	Brockton Hospital, Brockton	7.0	0.0%	1.20	No	0.06	6	1.10	0.003
	Burbank Hospital, Fitchburg	1.3	0.0%	1.49	No	0.03	3	0.21	0.005
	Cardinal Cushing General Hospital, Brockton	8.8	0.0%	0.90	No	0.03	3	0.32	0.008
	Carney Hospital, Boston	10.1	0.0%	1.06	No	0.51	3	1.05	0.015
	Charlton Memorial Hospital, Fall River	5.2	0.0%	1.15	No	0.00	5	0.30	0.006
	Holy Family Hospital and Medical Center, Methuen	3.3	0.0%	1.37	No	0.00	6	0.29	0.006
	Lawrence Memorial Hospital of Medford, Medford	7.3	0.0%	1.07	No	0.01	3	0.56	0.020
	Metrowest Medical Center, Framingham	10.5	0.0%	0.90	No	0.24	5	0.33	0.015
	North Shore Medical Center, Salem	4.9	0.0%	1.37	No	0.12	5	0.58	0.018

ORTHOPEDICS

Natl. Rank	Hospital	U.S. News index	Reputational score	Orthopedics mortality rate	COTH member	Interns and residents to beds	Technology score (of 5)	R.N.'s to beds	Board-certified orthopedists to beds	Procedures to beds
	TIER ONE									
3	Massachusetts General Hospital, Boston	76.5	28.7%	0.72	Yes	1.00	5	1.14	0.026	2.29
15	Brigham and Women's Hospital, Boston	23.7	3.6%	0.79	Yes	1.49	4	0.79	0.034	2.37
	TIER TWO									
35	Beth Israel Hospital, Boston	18.7	0.3%	0.63	Yes	0.57	4	1.93	0.039	2.53
52	Boston University Medical Center-University Hospital	16.3	0.0%	0.63	Yes	0.96	4	0.85	0.039	1.55
56	New England Medical Center, Boston	16.0	0.0%	0.80	Yes	1.07	3	1.66	0.024	1.04
42	University of Massachusetts Medical Center, Worcester	17.4	0.0%	0.68	Yes	1.47	3	0.96	0.059	1.62

Natl. Rank	Hospital	U.S. News index	Reputational score	Orthopedics mortality rate	COTH member	Interns and residents to beds	Technology score (of 5)	R.N.'s to beds	Board-certified orthopedists to beds	Procedures to beds
	TIER THREE									
	Baystate Medical Center, Springfield	8.4	0.0%	1.78	Yes	0.54	4	1.07	0.018	1.95
	Brockton Hospital, Brockton	10.4	0.0%	0.59	No	0.06	3	1.10	0.017	1.81
	Carney Hospital, Boston	8.2	0.0%	0.94	No	0.51	2	1.05	0.026	2.97
	Faulkner Hospital, Boston	12.2	0.0%	0.70	Yes	0.35	3	0.54	0.025	2.46
	Lahey Clinic Hospital, Burlington	10.7	0.4%	0.98	No	0.51	4	1.22	0.029	3.87
	Mount Auburn Hospital, Cambridge	8.3	0.0%	1.13	Yes	0.50	2	0.64	0.034	2.32
	New England Baptist Hospital, Boston	13.0	2.4%	0.94	No	0.05	2	0.75	0.125	9.80
98	New England Deaconess Hospital, Boston	13.1	0.0%	1.26	Yes	1.08	5	1.33	0.023	1.28
	St. Elizabeth's Hospital of Boston	10.7	0.0%	1.02	Yes	0.77	2	0.96	0.023	1.89
	St. Vincent Hospital, Worcester	10.2	0.0%	1.11	Yes	0.33	3	1.09	0.090	2.69
	TIER FOUR									
	Atlanticare Medical Center, Lynn	4.2	0.0%	1.37	No	0.01	4	0.64	0.030	2.78
	Berkshire Medical Center, Pittsfield	7.5	0.0%	1.45	Yes	0.33	4	0.55	0.029	2.83
	Burbank Hospital, Fitchburg	2.7	0.0%	1.19	No	0.03	2	0.21	0.033	2.78
	Cape Cod Hospital, Hyannis	6.7	0.0%	1.04	No	0.02	2	1.28	0.016	4.57
	Cardinal Cushing General Hospital, Brockton	2.2	0.0%	1.31	No	0.03	2	0.32	0.038	2.16
	Charlton Memorial Hospital, Fall River	5.1	0.0%	1.01	No	0.00	4	0.30	0.012	2.70
	Holy Family Hospital and Medical Center, Methuen	1.7	0.0%	1.38	No	0.00	2	0.29	0.032	1.70
	Lawrence Memorial Hospital of Medford, Medford	4.9	0.0%	0.96	No	0.01	2	0.56	0.033	2.24
	Malden Hospital, Malden	5.5	0.0%	0.87	No	0.15	2	0.34	0.035	1.57
	Medical Center of Central Massachusetts, Worcester	7.3	0.0%	0.98	Yes	0.14	2	0.47	0.022	1.27
	Metrowest Medical Center, Framingham	6.6	0.0%	0.86	No	0.24	3	0.33	0.027	2.45
	Newton-Wellesley Hospital, Newton	7.0	0.0%	0.79	No	0.19	2	0.40	0.060	2.87
	North Shore Medical Center, Salem	6.9	0.0%	0.81	No	0.12	2	0.58	0.036	2.58
	Walthamweston Hospital and Medical Center, Waltham	6.6	0.0%	0.74	No	0.02	2	0.36	0.016	1.78

OTOLARYNGOLOGY

Natl. Rank	Hospital	U.S. News index	Reputational score	Hospital-wide mortality rate	COTH member	Interns and residents to beds	Technology score (of 9)	R.N.'s to beds	Board-certified internists to beds	Procedures to beds
	TIER ONE									
2	Massachusetts Eye and Ear Infirmary, Boston	91.3	18.4%	0.04	No	0.86	2	2.18	0.043	4.848
35	Beth Israel Hospital, Boston	20.7	0.7%	0.85	Yes	0.57	7	1.93	0.590	0.245
	TIER TWO									
59	Boston City Hospital	16.4	0.0%	0.75	No	1.64	3	1.37	0.545	0.179
100	Boston University Medical Center-University Hospital	13.8	0.0%	0.82	Yes	0.96	7	0.85	0.231	0.273
48	Brigham and Women's Hospital, Boston	18.5	1.0%	0.91	Yes	1.49	8	0.79	0.179	0.153
72	Lahey Clinic Hospital, Burlington	15.2	2.0%	0.96	No	0.51	8	1.22	0.085	0.456
80	New England Deaconess Hospital, Boston	14.6	0.0%	0.99	Yes	1.08	8	1.33	0.089	0.292
46	New England Medical Center, Boston	18.5	1.1%	0.86	Yes	1.07	6	1.66	0.086	0.151
	University of Massachusetts Medical Center, Worcester	13.6	0.0%	0.99	Yes	1.47	6	0.96	0.000	0.148
	TIER THREE									
	Baystate Medical Center, Springfield	11.0	0.0%	1.35	Yes	0.54	7	1.07	0.076	0.196
	Berkshire Medical Center, Pittsfield	9.2	0.0%	1.25	Yes	0.33	7	0.55	0.133	0.416
	Carney Hospital, Boston	7.6	0.0%	1.02	No	0.51	1	1.05	0.237	0.489
	Dana-Farber Cancer Institute, Boston	7.9	0.0%	0.01	No	0.49	2	1.58	0.018	0.807
	Faulkner Hospital, Boston	8.2	0.0%	0.76	Yes	0.35	2	0.54	0.137	0.201
	Medical Center of Central Massachusetts, Worcester	7.2	0.0%	0.92	Yes	0.14	5	0.47	0.063	0.165
	Mount Auburn Hospital, Cambridge	9.6	0.0%	0.99	Yes	0.50	3	0.64	0.185	0.424
	St. Elizabeth's Hospital of Boston	12.0	0.0%	0.95	Yes	0.77	5	0.96	0.154	0.209
	St. Vincent Hospital, Worcester	12.6	0.0%	1.24	Yes	0.33	6	1.09	0.370	0.430
	TIER FOUR									
	Atlanticare Medical Center, Lynn	4.1	0.0%	1.46	No	0.01	7	0.64	0.045	0.201
	Brockton Hospital, Brockton	5.5	0.0%	1.04	No	0.06	5	1.10	0.060	0.199

Natl. Rank	Hospital	U.S. News index	Reputa-tional score	Hospital-wide mortality rate	COTH member	Interns and residents to beds	Tech-nology score (of 9)	R.N.'s to beds	Board-certified internists to beds	Procedures to beds
	Burbank Hospital, Fitchburg	1.2	0.0%	1.35	No	0.03	1	0.21	0.038	0.179
	Cambridge Hospital, Cambridge	5.9	0.0%	1.34	No	0.60	1	0.80	0.118	0.208
	Cape Cod Hospital, Hyannis	5.5	0.0%	0.94	No	0.02	3	1.28	0.050	0.709
	Cardinal Cushing General Hospital, Brockton	2.2	0.0%	1.07	No	0.03	1	0.32	0.093	0.388
	Charlton Memorial Hospital, Fall River	2.4	0.0%	1.13	No	0.00	4	0.30	0.045	0.265
	Holy Family Hospital and Medical Center, Methuen	2.5	0.0%	1.55	No	0.00	6	0.29	0.019	0.237
	Jewish Memorial Hospital, Boston	2.5	0.0%	3.94	No	0.00	0	0.49	0.184	0.005
	Lawrence Memorial Hospital of Medford, Medford	3.1	0.0%	0.92	No	0.01	1	0.56	0.107	0.480
	Lemuel Shattuck Hospital, Boston	0.2	0.0%	8.00	No	0.04	0	0.20	0.017	0.004
	Malden Hospital, Malden	2.1	0.0%	1.09	No	0.15	1	0.34	0.030	0.149
	Metrowest Medical Center, Framingham	3.9	0.0%	0.91	No	0.24	3	0.33	0.109	0.320
	New England Baptist Hospital, Boston	3.5	0.0%	0.74	No	0.05	1	0.75	0.050	0.180
	Newton-Wellesley Hospital, Newton	3.5	0.0%	0.74	No	0.19	1	0.40	0.107	0.170
	North Shore Medical Center, Salem	4.6	0.0%	1.11	No	0.12	5	0.58	0.115	0.307
	Walthamweston Hospital and Medical Center, Waltham	3.3	0.0%	0.88	No	0.02	5	0.36	0.062	0.416

RHEUMATOLOGY

Natl. Rank	Hospital	U.S. News index	Reputa-tional score	Hospital-wide mortality rate	COTH member	Interns and residents to beds	Tech-nology score (of 5)	R.N.'s to beds	Board-certified internists to beds
	TIER ONE								
3	Brigham and Women's Hospital, Boston	73.3	25.0%	0.91	Yes	1.49	4	0.79	0.179
12	Massachusetts General Hospital, Boston	33.7	7.4%	0.88	Yes	1.00	5	1.14	0.085
16	Beth Israel Hospital, Boston	27.1	2.5%	0.85	Yes	0.57	4	1.93	0.590
	TIER TWO								
57	Boston University Medical Center-University Hospital	17.4	0.0%	0.82	Yes	0.96	4	0.85	0.231
65	New England Deaconess Hospital, Boston	16.9	0.0%	0.99	Yes	1.08	5	1.33	0.089
40	New England Medical Center, Boston	19.3	0.5%	0.86	Yes	1.07	3	1.66	0.086
51	University of Massachusetts Medical Center, Worcester	17.7	1.0%	0.99	Yes	1.47	3	0.96	0.000
	TIER THREE								
	Baystate Medical Center, Springfield	11.4	0.0%	1.35	Yes	0.54	4	1.07	0.076
	Berkshire Medical Center, Pittsfield	10.3	0.0%	1.25	Yes	0.33	4	0.55	0.133
	Cape Cod Hospital, Hyannis	9.7	0.0%	0.94	No	0.02	2	1.28	0.050
	Carney Hospital, Boston	11.3	0.0%	1.02	No	0.51	2	1.05	0.237
	Faulkner Hospital, Boston	13.5	0.0%	0.76	Yes	0.35	3	0.54	0.137
	Lahey Clinic Hospital, Burlington	12.6	0.3%	0.96	No	0.51	4	1.22	0.085
	Medical Center of Central Massachusetts, Worcester	9.7	0.0%	0.92	Yes	0.14	2	0.47	0.063
	Mount Auburn Hospital, Cambridge	12.5	0.0%	0.99	Yes	0.50	2	0.64	0.185
	St. Elizabeth's Hospital of Boston	14.3	0.0%	0.95	Yes	0.77	2	0.96	0.154
	St. Vincent Hospital, Worcester	13.1	0.0%	1.24	Yes	0.33	3	1.09	0.370
	TIER FOUR								
	Atlanticare Medical Center, Lynn	5.3	0.0%	1.46	No	0.01	4	0.64	0.045
	Brockton Hospital, Brockton	8.9	0.0%	1.04	No	0.06	3	1.10	0.060
	Burbank Hospital, Fitchburg	3.9	0.0%	1.35	No	0.03	2	0.21	0.038
	Cardinal Cushing General Hospital, Brockton	6.3	0.0%	1.07	No	0.03	2	0.32	0.093
	Charlton Memorial Hospital, Fall River	6.3	0.0%	1.13	No	0.00	4	0.30	0.045
	Holy Family Hospital and Medical Center, Methuen	2.9	0.0%	1.55	No	0.00	2	0.29	0.019
	Lawrence Memorial Hospital of Medford, Medford	7.4	0.0%	0.92	No	0.01	2	0.56	0.107
	Malden Hospital, Malden	5.1	0.0%	1.09	No	0.15	2	0.34	0.030
	Metrowest Medical Center, Framingham	9.1	0.0%	0.91	No	0.24	3	0.33	0.109
	New England Baptist Hospital, Boston	9.3	0.4%	0.74	No	0.05	2	0.75	0.050
	Newton-Wellesley Hospital, Newton	9.5	0.0%	0.74	No	0.19	2	0.40	0.107
	North Shore Medical Center, Salem	7.1	0.0%	1.11	No	0.12	2	0.58	0.115
	Walthamweston Hospital and Medical Center, Waltham	8.1	0.0%	0.88	No	0.02	2	0.36	0.062

UROLOGY

Natl. Rank	Hospital	U.S. News index	Reputa- tional score	Urology mortality rate	COTH member	Interns and residents to beds	Tech- nology score (of 11)	R.N.'s to beds	Board- certified internists to beds	Procedures to beds
	TIER ONE									
7	Massachusetts General Hospital, Boston	43.2	20.2%	0.92	Yes	1.00	11	1.14	0.085	2.02
22	Brigham and Women's Hospital, Boston	23.4	6.3%	1.16	Yes	1.49	10	0.79	0.179	1.35
	TIER TWO									
39	Beth Israel Hospital, Boston	19.1	0.0%	0.76	Yes	0.57	9	1.93	0.590	2.37
57	Boston City Hospital	17.4	0.0%	0.10	No	1.64	4	1.37	0.545	0.80
61	Boston University Medical Center-University Hospital	17.2	1.3%	0.91	Yes	0.96	9	0.85	0.231	1.98
27	Lahey Clinic Hospital, Burlington	21.1	7.1%	1.04	No	0.51	10	1.22	0.085	4.18
31	New England Deaconess Hospital, Boston	20.0	0.6%	0.69	Yes	1.08	9	1.33	0.089	1.87
42	New England Medical Center, Boston	18.7	0.0%	0.76	Yes	1.07	7	1.66	0.086	1.03
78	St. Elizabeth's Hospital of Boston	16.1	0.0%	0.82	Yes	0.77	6	0.96	0.154	3.70
36	University of Massachusetts Medical Center, Worcester	19.3	0.6%	0.59	Yes	1.47	8	0.96	0.000	1.37
	TIER THREE									
	Baystate Medical Center, Springfield	9.5	0.0%	1.64	Yes	0.54	9	1.07	0.076	1.26
	Berkshire Medical Center, Pittsfield	9.1	0.0%	1.37	Yes	0.33	9	0.55	0.133	1.73
	Cape Cod Hospital, Hyannis	9.0	0.0%	0.99	No	0.02	5	1.28	0.050	3.92
	Faulkner Hospital, Boston	14.0	0.0%	0.70	Yes	0.35	4	0.54	0.137	2.68
	Metrowest Medical Center, Framingham	8.8	0.0%	0.86	No	0.24	6	0.33	0.109	1.99
	Mount Auburn Hospital, Cambridge	13.0	0.0%	0.87	Yes	0.50	5	0.64	0.185	2.31
	New England Baptist Hospital, Boston	9.7	0.0%	0.57	No	0.05	3	0.75	0.050	1.43
	Newton-Wellesley Hospital, Newton	9.9	0.0%	0.68	No	0.19	3	0.40	0.107	1.93
	St. Vincent Hospital, Worcester	9.5	0.0%	1.57	Yes	0.33	7	1.09	0.370	2.54
	Walthamweston Hospital and Medical Center, Waltham	9.9	0.0%	0.50	No	0.02	7	0.36	0.062	1.68
	TIER FOUR									
	Atlanticare Medical Center, Lynn	4.5	0.0%	1.49	No	0.01	8	0.64	0.045	2.29
	Brockton Hospital, Brockton	6.8	0.0%	1.19	No	0.06	6	1.10	0.060	1.84
	Burbank Hospital, Fitchburg	2.1	0.0%	1.45	No	0.03	3	0.21	0.038	1.91
	Cardinal Cushing General Hospital, Brockton	5.6	0.0%	1.00	No	0.03	3	0.32	0.093	1.99
	Carney Hospital, Boston	8.2	0.0%	1.21	No	0.51	3	1.05	0.237	2.89
	Charlton Memorial Hospital, Fall River	3.1	0.0%	1.55	No	0.00	7	0.30	0.045	2.39
	Holy Family Hospital and Medical Center, Methuen	1.1	0.0%	2.08	No	0.00	7	0.29	0.019	1.19
	Lawrence Memorial Hospital of Medford, Medford	6.4	0.0%	1.01	No	0.01	3	0.56	0.107	2.48
	Malden Hospital, Malden	5.2	0.0%	1.05	No	0.15	3	0.34	0.030	1.66
	Medical Center of Central Massachusetts, Worcester	6.9	0.0%	1.34	Yes	0.14	6	0.47	0.063	0.97
	North Shore Medical Center, Salem	5.7	0.0%	1.29	No	0.12	7	0.58	0.115	1.62

AIDS

Natl. Rank Hospital	U.S. News index	Reputa-tional score	Hospital-wide mortality rate	COTH member	Interns and residents to beds	Tech-nology score (of 11)	Discharge planning (of 2)	R.N.'s to beds	Board-certified internists to beds
TIER ONE									
24 Henry Ford Hospital, Detroit	30.2	1.3%	0.96	Yes	1.34	10	2	1.50	0.301
TIER TWO									
37 University of Michigan Medical Center, Ann Arbor	28.6	1.8%	0.98	Yes	1.00	10	2	1.29	0.086
TIER THREE									
Battle Creek Health System, Battle Creek	20.8	0.0%	0.91	No	0.00	7	1	0.65	0.029
Blodgett Memorial Medical Center, Grand Rapids	23.2	0.0%	0.98	Yes	0.33	6	1	1.53	0.093
Bon Secours Hospital, Grosse Pointe	21.1	0.0%	0.96	No	0.23	5	2	0.69	0.163
Butterworth Hospital, Grand Rapids	22.1	0.0%	0.99	No	0.42	8	2	0.97	0.078
Catherine McAuley Health System, Ann Arbor	23.5	0.0%	0.98	Yes	0.36	6	2	1.29	0.080
Detroit Riverview Hospital	20.7	0.0%	0.91	No	0.03	5	1	0.76	0.108
96 Harper Hospital, Detroit	24.6	0.3%	0.99	Yes	0.34	9	2	1.20	0.070
Macomb Hospital Center, Warren	19.9	0.0%	1.00	No	0.01	6	2	0.54	0.151
Mercy Hospital, Port Huron	20.4	0.0%	0.97	No	0.00	6	2	0.73	0.059
Metropolitan Hospital, Grand Rapids	21.3	0.0%	1.00	No	0.47	7	2	0.87	0.029
North Oakland Medical Center, Pontiac	22.6	0.0%	0.89	No	0.25	6	2	0.87	0.048
Providence Hospital, Southfield	20.5	0.0%	1.12	Yes	0.52	5	2	0.85	0.039
Sinai Hospital, Detroit	21.0	0.0%	1.20	Yes	0.70	7	2	0.98	0.072
St. John Hospital and Medical Center, Detroit	21.5	0.0%	1.09	Yes	0.39	7	2	0.95	0.040
St. Joseph Mercy Hospital, Pontiac	21.0	0.0%	0.98	No	0.42	6	2	0.84	0.031
St. Mary's Health Services, Grand Rapids	20.5	0.0%	1.03	No	0.38	8	1	0.86	0.075
William Beaumont Hospital, Royal Oak	24.5	0.0%	1.05	Yes	0.63	9	2	1.46	0.113
TIER FOUR									
Borgess Medical Center, Kalamazoo	17.6	0.0%	1.17	No	0.09	5	2	0.95	0.047
Bronson Methodist Hospital, Kalamazoo	18.0	0.0%	1.21	No	0.09	7	2	0.91	0.078
Detroit Receiving Hospital	19.4	0.0%	1.28	Yes	0.90	4	2	1.00	0.043
Genesys Regional Medical Center-St. Joseph, Flint	15.9	0.0%	1.33	No	0.25	6	2	0.52	0.031
Grace Hospital, Detroit	19.2	0.0%	1.31	Yes	0.23	5	2	1.58	0.096
Hackley Hospital, Muskegon	18.1	0.0%	1.11	No	0.00	6	2	0.60	0.071
Hurley Medical Center, Flint	19.3	0.0%	1.27	Yes	0.31	7	2	0.98	0.030
Hutzel Hospital, Detroit	16.6	0.0%	1.48	Yes	0.28	4	2	0.97	0.099
Marquette General Hospital, Marquette	19.0	0.0%	1.04	No	0.10	7	2	0.35	0.025
McLaren Regional Medical Center, Flint	16.3	0.0%	1.35	No	0.23	7	2	0.65	0.048
Mercy-Memorial Medical Center, St. Joseph	17.1	0.0%	1.25	No	0.00	6	2	0.83	0.151
Michigan Affiliated Health System, Lansing	15.9	0.0%	1.42	No	0.24	6	2	0.83	0.110
Mid Michigan Regional Medical Center, Midland	18.8	0.0%	1.07	No	0.13	6	2	0.65	0.010
Munson Medical Center, Traverse City	17.1	0.0%	1.16	No	0.00	6	2	0.51	0.042
Northern Michigan Hospital, Petoskey	17.0	0.0%	1.24	No	0.00	6	2	0.95	0.061
Oakwood Hospital, Dearborn	18.6	0.0%	1.31	Yes	0.29	7	2	0.80	0.042
Saginaw General Hospital, Saginaw	16.2	0.0%	1.34	No	0.11	5	2	1.26	0.011
Sparrow Hospital, Lansing	15.6	0.0%	1.63	No	0.34	8	2	1.08	0.074
St. Lawrence Hospital and Healthcare, Lansing	19.4	0.0%	0.98	No	0.29	4	2	0.37	0.034
St. Mary Hospital, Livonia	19.3	0.0%	1.03	No	0.00	6	2	0.73	0.063
St. Mary's Medical Center, Saginaw	17.0	0.0%	1.27	No	0.05	7	2	0.97	0.008

CANCER

Natl. Rank	Hospital	U.S. News index	Reputa-tional score	Cancer mortality rate	COTH member	Interns and residents to beds	Tech-nology score (of 12)	R.N.'s to beds	Board-certified oncologists to beds	Procedures to beds
	TIER TWO									
35	**Henry Ford Hospital, Detroit**	**14.1**	0.5%	0.71	Yes	1.34	10	1.50	0.000	1.76
40	**University of Michigan Medical Center, Ann Arbor**	**13.9**	1.6%	0.50	Yes	1.00	10	1.29	0.012	1.68
	TIER THREE									
	Blodgett Memorial Medical Center, Grand Rapids	9.7	0.0%	0.87	Yes	0.33	9	1.53	0.012	1.65
	Butterworth Hospital, Grand Rapids	6.1	0.0%	0.86	No	0.42	9	0.97	0.008	2.15
	Catherine McAuley Health System, Ann Arbor	8.6	0.0%	0.77	Yes	0.36	7	1.29	0.011	1.37
	Grace Hospital, Detroit	8.2	0.0%	0.93	Yes	0.23	5	1.58	0.019	0.94
	Harper Hospital, Detroit	10.0	0.5%	0.81	Yes	0.34	9	1.20	0.057	3.01
	Hurley Medical Center, Flint	7.2	0.0%	1.38	Yes	0.31	8	0.98	0.000	0.82
	Hutzel Hospital, Detroit	6.6	0.0%	0.89	Yes	0.28	4	0.97	0.038	0.85
	Oakwood Hospital, Dearborn	6.9	0.0%	1.35	Yes	0.29	8	0.80	0.007	2.19
	Providence Hospital, Southfield	7.2	0.0%	0.93	Yes	0.52	5	0.85	0.006	1.69
	Sinai Hospital, Detroit	9.0	0.0%	0.96	Yes	0.70	8	0.98	0.010	1.78
	Sparrow Hospital, Lansing	5.8	0.0%	1.32	No	0.34	10	1.08	0.009	1.42
	St. John Hospital and Medical Center, Detroit	8.0	0.0%	0.99	Yes	0.39	8	0.95	0.012	2.33
	St. Mary's Health Services, Grand Rapids	5.5	0.0%	0.96	No	0.38	9	0.86	0.025	1.52
88	William Beaumont Hospital, Royal Oak	10.6	0.0%	1.08	Yes	0.63	10	1.46	0.012	2.03
	TIER FOUR									
	Battle Creek Health System, Battle Creek	3.9	0.0%	0.66	No	0.00	9	0.65	0.003	1.27
	Bon Secours Hospital, Grosse Pointe	3.2	0.0%	0.96	No	0.23	4	0.69	0.031	2.07
	Borgess Medical Center, Kalamazoo	4.5	0.0%	0.71	No	0.09	7	0.95	0.015	1.58
	Bronson Methodist Hospital, Kalamazoo	4.3	0.0%	0.91	No	0.09	8	0.91	0.013	1.22
	Genesys Regional Medical Center-St. Joseph, Flint	3.4	0.0%	1.29	No	0.25	8	0.52	0.005	1.63
	Hackley Hospital, Muskegon	2.9	0.0%	0.98	No	0.00	7	0.60	0.012	1.88
	Macomb Hospital Center, Warren	3.3	0.0%	0.74	No	0.01	8	0.54	0.006	1.60
	Marquette General Hospital, Marquette	3.4	0.0%	0.64	No	0.10	8	0.35	0.009	2.11
	McLaren Regional Medical Center, Flint	3.6	0.0%	1.37	No	0.23	8	0.65	0.002	1.47
	Mercy Hospital, Port Huron	3.3	0.0%	1.01	No	0.00	7	0.73	0.008	2.43
	Mercy-Memorial Medical Center, St. Joseph	3.5	0.0%	1.11	No	0.00	7	0.83	0.007	2.25
	Metropolitan Hospital, Grand Rapids	4.2	0.0%	0.74	No	0.47	3	0.87	0.005	1.06
	Michigan Affiliated Health System, Lansing	3.1	0.0%	1.54	No	0.24	5	0.83	0.016	0.39
	Mid Michigan Regional Medical Center, Midland	3.6	0.0%	1.11	No	0.13	7	0.65	0.007	3.27
	Munson Medical Center, Traverse City	3.1	0.0%	0.98	No	0.00	8	0.51	0.008	2.68
	North Oakland Medical Center, Pontiac	4.1	0.0%	1.12	No	0.25	7	0.87	0.004	0.83
	Northern Michigan Hospital, Petoskey	4.5	0.0%	1.10	No	0.00	8	0.95	0.011	4.45
	Saginaw General Hospital, Saginaw	3.8	0.0%	0.91	No	0.11	3	1.26	0.004	0.94
	St. Joseph Mercy Hospital, Pontiac	4.3	0.0%	0.79	No	0.42	4	0.84	0.011	1.59
	St. Lawrence Hospital and Healthcare, Lansing	1.4	0.0%	1.01	No	0.29	2	0.37	0.007	0.37
	St. Luke's Hospital, Saginaw	2.4	0.0%	1.13	No	0.04	3	0.86	0.011	1.68
	St. Mary Hospital, Livonia	3.7	0.0%	0.74	No	0.00	7	0.73	0.019	1.91
	St. Mary's Medical Center, Saginaw	4.6	0.0%	1.00	No	0.05	9	0.97	0.004	1.94

CARDIOLOGY

Natl. Rank	Hospital	U.S. News index	Reputa-tional score	Cardiology mortality rate	COTH member	Interns and residents to beds	Tech-nology score (of 10)	R.N.'s to beds	Board-certified cardiologists to beds	Procedures to beds
	TIER TWO									
31	**Henry Ford Hospital, Detroit**	**26.0**	1.2%	0.96	Yes	1.34	9	1.50	0.000	7.47
32	**University of Michigan Medical Center, Ann Arbor**	**25.9**	3.9%	1.10	Yes	1.00	10	1.29	0.034	4.25
48	**William Beaumont Hospital, Royal Oak**	**23.1**	1.3%	1.04	Yes	0.63	10	1.46	0.046	10.28
	TIER THREE									
	Battle Creek Health System, Battle Creek	14.9	0.0%	0.91	No	0.00	6	0.65	0.013	5.30

Natl. Rank / Hospital	U.S. News index	Reputational score	Cardiology mortality rate	COTH member	Interns and residents to beds	Technology score (of 10)	R.N.'s to beds	Board-certified cardiologists to beds	Procedures to beds
Blodgett Memorial Medical Center, Grand Rapids	20.5	0.0%	0.99	Yes	0.33	8	1.53	0.029	7.79
Bon Secours Hospital, Grosse Pointe	17.2	0.0%	0.82	No	0.23	5	0.69	0.027	9.00
Butterworth Hospital, Grand Rapids	14.2	0.0%	1.07	No	0.42	8	0.97	0.015	6.71
Catherine McAuley Health System, Ann Arbor	19.1	0.0%	1.02	Yes	0.36	7	1.29	0.041	10.20
Grace Hospital, Detroit	15.8	0.0%	1.17	Yes	0.23	5	1.58	0.048	6.95
Harper Hospital, Detroit	19.4	0.6%	1.07	Yes	0.34	9	1.20	0.065	6.64
Mercy Hospital, Port Huron	15.2	0.0%	0.93	No	0.00	5	0.73	0.042	7.92
North Oakland Medical Center, Pontiac	17.2	0.0%	0.76	No	0.25	5	0.87	0.011	5.19
Providence Hospital, Southfield	16.5	0.0%	1.11	Yes	0.52	8	0.85	0.028	8.76
Sinai Hospital, Detroit	16.1	0.0%	1.23	Yes	0.70	9	0.98	0.054	7.71
St. John Hospital and Medical Center, Detroit	18.2	0.0%	1.05	Yes	0.39	9	0.95	0.038	10.57
St. Joseph Mercy Hospital, Pontiac	14.5	0.0%	1.06	No	0.42	8	0.84	0.040	7.22
St. Mary Hospital, Livonia	14.8	0.0%	0.96	No	0.00	5	0.73	0.059	10.77
St. Mary's Health Services, Grand Rapids	16.4	0.0%	0.94	No	0.38	6	0.86	0.025	4.88
TIER FOUR									
Borgess Medical Center, Kalamazoo	10.2	0.0%	1.29	No	0.09	8	0.95	0.056	12.38
Bronson Methodist Hospital, Kalamazoo	10.1	0.0%	1.22	No	0.09	8	0.91	0.022	5.53
Detroit Riverview Hospital	13.4	0.0%	0.96	No	0.03	3	0.76	0.016	6.75
Genesys Regional Medical Center-St. Joseph, Flint	7.2	0.0%	1.40	No	0.25	8	0.52	0.019	7.08
Hackley Hospital, Muskegon	11.4	0.0%	1.04	No	0.00	5	0.60	0.024	4.44
Hurley Medical Center, Flint	11.8	0.0%	1.32	Yes	0.31	8	0.98	0.006	3.33
Macomb Hospital Center, Warren	9.8	0.0%	1.14	No	0.01	5	0.54	0.036	8.64
Marquette General Hospital, Marquette	11.9	0.0%	1.06	No	0.10	9	0.35	0.019	6.77
McLaren Regional Medical Center, Flint	8.1	0.0%	1.38	No	0.23	9	0.65	0.016	9.06
Mercy-Memorial Medical Center, St. Joseph	7.3	0.0%	1.40	No	0.00	8	0.83	0.029	7.63
Metropolitan Hospital, Grand Rapids	12.6	0.0%	1.13	No	0.47	7	0.87	0.010	6.43
Michigan Affiliated Health System, Lansing	7.5	0.0%	1.46	No	0.24	9	0.83	0.033	1.77
Mid Michigan Regional Medical Center, Midland	12.8	0.0%	1.01	No	0.13	6	0.65	0.010	5.67
Munson Medical Center, Traverse City	8.1	0.0%	1.26	No	0.00	8	0.51	0.017	8.97
Northern Michigan Hospital, Petoskey	6.8	0.0%	1.45	No	0.00	7	0.95	0.023	8.66
Oakwood Hospital, Dearborn	12.7	0.0%	1.28	Yes	0.29	9	0.80	0.015	8.98
Saginaw General Hospital, Saginaw	10.0	0.0%	1.25	No	0.11	6	1.26	0.019	4.83
Sparrow Hospital, Lansing	6.6	0.0%	1.57	No	0.34	7	1.08	0.015	3.99
St. Luke's Hospital, Saginaw	9.9	0.4%	1.25	No	0.04	6	0.86	0.032	9.36
St. Mary's Medical Center, Saginaw	9.4	0.0%	1.31	No	0.05	8	0.97	0.030	15.36

ENDOCRINOLOGY

Natl. Rank / Hospital	U.S. News index	Reputational score	Endocrinology mortality rate	COTH member	Interns and residents to beds	Technology score (of 11)	R.N.'s to beds	Board-certified internists to beds
TIER ONE								
8 University of Michigan Medical Center, Ann Arbor	34.9	12.8%	0.62	Yes	1.00	10	1.29	0.086
TIER TWO								
51 Henry Ford Hospital, Detroit	17.4	0.4%	1.14	Yes	1.34	10	1.50	0.301
TIER THREE								
92 Blodgett Memorial Medical Center, Grand Rapids	14.0	0.0%	0.84	Yes	0.33	9	1.53	0.093
Catherine McAuley Health System, Ann Arbor	10.9	0.0%	1.16	Yes	0.36	8	1.29	0.080
Detroit Receiving Hospital	9.0	0.0%	1.54	Yes	0.90	2	1.00	0.043
Grace Hospital, Detroit	9.3	0.0%	1.63	Yes	0.23	6	1.58	0.096
Harper Hospital, Detroit	11.9	0.4%	1.08	Yes	0.34	10	1.20	0.070
Munson Medical Center, Traverse City	9.5	0.0%	0.64	No	0.00	9	0.51	0.042
Oakwood Hospital, Dearborn	8.3	0.0%	1.40	Yes	0.29	9	0.80	0.042
Sinai Hospital, Detroit	12.0	0.0%	1.04	Yes	0.70	9	0.98	0.072
St. John Hospital and Medical Center, Detroit	10.8	0.0%	1.02	Yes	0.39	9	0.95	0.040
St. Mary's Health Services, Grand Rapids	8.9	0.0%	0.96	No	0.38	10	0.86	0.075

Natl. Rank	Hospital	U.S. News index	Reputa-tional score	Endocrinology mortality rate	COTH member	Interns and residents to beds	Tech-nology score (of 11)	R.N.'s to beds	Board-certified internists to beds
	William Beaumont Hospital, Royal Oak	12.0	0.0%	1.38	Yes	0.63	10	1.46	0.113

TIER FOUR									
	Battle Creek Health System, Battle Creek	5.7	0.0%	1.12	No	0.00	10	0.65	0.029
	Bon Secours Hospital, Grosse Pointe	5.9	0.0%	1.20	No	0.23	4	0.69	0.163
	Borgess Medical Center, Kalamazoo	3.3	0.0%	2.25	No	0.09	7	0.95	0.047
	Bronson Methodist Hospital, Kalamazoo	5.8	0.0%	1.31	No	0.09	8	0.91	0.078
	Butterworth Hospital, Grand Rapids	7.1	0.0%	1.34	No	0.42	9	0.97	0.078
	Detroit Riverview Hospital	8.0	0.0%	0.80	No	0.03	4	0.76	0.108
	Genesys Regional Medical Center-St. Joseph, Flint	3.9	0.0%	1.65	No	0.25	8	0.52	0.031
	Hackley Hospital, Muskegon	2.5	0.0%	2.19	No	0.00	8	0.60	0.071
	Hurley Medical Center, Flint	7.7	0.0%	1.68	Yes	0.31	8	0.98	0.030
	Macomb Hospital Center, Warren	6.3	0.0%	1.03	No	0.01	7	0.54	0.151
	Marquette General Hospital, Marquette	4.8	0.0%	1.16	No	0.10	9	0.35	0.025
	McLaren Regional Medical Center, Flint	5.4	0.0%	1.35	No	0.23	9	0.65	0.048
	Mercy-Memorial Medical Center, St. Joseph	4.9	0.0%	1.59	No	0.00	8	0.83	0.151
	Metropolitan Hospital, Grand Rapids	7.0	0.0%	1.10	No	0.47	5	0.87	0.029
	Mid Michigan Regional Medical Center, Midland	4.5	0.0%	1.39	No	0.13	8	0.65	0.010
	North Oakland Medical Center, Pontiac	7.7	0.0%	0.98	No	0.25	8	0.87	0.048
	Northern Michigan Hospital, Petoskey	5.9	0.0%	1.22	No	0.00	8	0.95	0.061
	Providence Hospital, Southfield	8.1	0.0%	1.53	Yes	0.52	6	0.85	0.039
	Saginaw General Hospital, Saginaw	6.0	0.0%	1.20	No	0.11	4	1.26	0.011
	Sparrow Hospital, Lansing	6.3	0.0%	1.60	No	0.34	9	1.08	0.074
	St. Joseph Mercy Hospital, Pontiac	5.7	0.0%	1.27	No	0.42	4	0.84	0.031
	St. Luke's Hospital, Saginaw	3.9	0.0%	1.38	No	0.04	3	0.86	0.025
	St. Mary Hospital, Livonia	5.7	0.0%	1.13	No	0.00	8	0.73	0.063
	St. Mary's Medical Center, Saginaw	5.1	0.0%	1.45	No	0.05	9	0.97	0.008

GASTROENTEROLOGY

Natl. Rank	Hospital	U.S. News index	Reputa-tional score	Gastro-enterology mortality rate	COTH member	Interns and residents to beds	Tech-nology score (of 11)	R.N.'s to beds	Board-certified gastro-enterologists to beds	Pro-cedures to beds
TIER ONE										
14	University of Michigan Medical Center, Ann Arbor	25.3	6.9%	0.83	Yes	1.00	10	1.29	0.014	1.44
TIER TWO										
70	Blodgett Memorial Medical Center, Grand Rapids	13.4	0.0%	0.83	Yes	0.33	8	1.53	0.009	3.10
32	Henry Ford Hospital, Detroit	16.7	0.0%	0.91	Yes	1.34	10	1.50	0.000	2.81
36	William Beaumont Hospital, Royal Oak	16.3	0.7%	0.82	Yes	0.63	10	1.46	0.019	3.26
TIER THREE										
	Bon Secours Hospital, Grosse Pointe	8.5	0.0%	0.85	No	0.23	4	0.69	0.027	5.37
	Butterworth Hospital, Grand Rapids	8.1	0.0%	1.05	No	0.42	9	0.97	0.009	2.72
	Catherine McAuley Health System, Ann Arbor	11.2	0.0%	1.01	Yes	0.36	7	1.29	0.016	3.15
	Ferguson Hospital, Grand Rapids	8.3	0.0%	0.94	No	0.11	1	0.59	0.000	9.22
	Grace Hospital, Detroit	9.2	0.0%	1.28	Yes	0.23	5	1.58	0.036	2.77
97	Harper Hospital, Detroit	11.9	0.0%	0.93	Yes	0.34	10	1.20	0.020	2.05
	Hurley Medical Center, Flint	8.8	0.0%	1.06	Yes	0.31	7	0.98	0.007	1.11
	Oakwood Hospital, Dearborn	8.1	0.0%	1.41	Yes	0.29	9	0.80	0.002	2.76
	Providence Hospital, Southfield	10.1	0.0%	1.02	Yes	0.52	5	0.85	0.009	3.15
	Sinai Hospital, Detroit	11.2	0.0%	1.10	Yes	0.70	8	0.98	0.020	2.60
	St. John Hospital and Medical Center, Detroit	9.7	0.0%	1.16	Yes	0.39	8	0.95	0.007	2.91
	St. Joseph Mercy Hospital, Pontiac	7.6	0.0%	0.88	No	0.42	4	0.84	0.022	2.57
	St. Mary's Health Services, Grand Rapids	7.7	0.0%	1.09	No	0.38	9	0.86	0.016	3.11
TIER FOUR										
	Battle Creek Health System, Battle Creek	5.1	0.0%	1.24	No	0.00	9	0.65	0.000	3.16
	Borgess Medical Center, Kalamazoo	6.1	0.0%	1.10	No	0.09	6	0.95	0.021	3.32

Natl. Rank	Hospital	U.S. News index	Reputa-tional score	Gastro-enterology mortality rate	COTH member	Interns and residents to beds	Tech-nology score (of 11)	R.N.'s to beds	Board-certified gastro-enterologists to beds	Pro-cedures to beds
	Bronson Methodist Hospital, Kalamazoo	4.4	0.0%	1.42	No	0.09	7	0.91	0.016	2.67
	Genesys Regional Medical Center-St. Joseph, Flint	4.3	0.0%	1.50	No	0.25	8	0.52	0.007	3.02
	Hackley Hospital, Muskegon	5.0	0.0%	1.09	No	0.00	7	0.60	0.016	2.87
	Macomb Hospital Center, Warren	4.4	0.0%	1.14	No	0.01	6	0.54	0.027	3.02
	Marquette General Hospital, Marquette	5.0	0.0%	1.07	No	0.10	8	0.35	0.012	2.43
	McLaren Regional Medical Center, Flint	4.3	0.0%	1.56	No	0.23	8	0.65	0.005	3.01
	Mercy Hospital, Port Huron	6.8	0.0%	0.99	No	0.00	7	0.73	0.017	4.22
	Mercy-Memorial Medical Center, St. Joseph	4.6	0.0%	1.28	No	0.00	7	0.83	0.007	2.96
	Metropolitan Hospital, Grand Rapids	6.3	0.0%	1.19	No	0.47	5	0.87	0.005	3.13
	Michigan Affiliated Health System, Lansing	2.1	0.0%	1.83	No	0.24	5	0.83	0.018	1.05
	Mid Michigan Regional Medical Center, Midland	4.9	0.0%	1.18	No	0.13	7	0.65	0.003	2.64
	Munson Medical Center, Traverse City	5.2	0.0%	1.14	No	0.00	8	0.51	0.008	3.55
	North Oakland Medical Center, Pontiac	6.6	0.0%	1.04	No	0.25	7	0.87	0.000	2.48
	Northern Michigan Hospital, Petoskey	4.7	0.0%	1.38	No	0.00	7	0.95	0.011	3.28
	Saginaw General Hospital, Saginaw	4.0	0.0%	1.54	No	0.11	4	1.26	0.011	2.71
	Sparrow Hospital, Lansing	4.7	0.0%	1.82	No	0.34	9	1.08	0.007	1.88
	St. Luke's Hospital, Saginaw	6.3	0.0%	0.97	No	0.04	3	0.86	0.014	4.45
	St. Mary Hospital, Livonia	6.0	0.0%	1.14	No	0.00	7	0.73	0.026	4.53
	St. Mary's Medical Center, Saginaw	5.2	0.0%	1.19	No	0.05	8	0.97	0.011	1.85

GERIATRICS

Natl. Rank	Hospital	U.S. News index	Reputa-tional score	Hospital-wide mortality rate	COTH member	Service mix	Interns and residents to beds	Tech-nology score (of 13)	R.N.'s to beds	Discharge planning (of 2)	Geriatric services (of 9)	Board-certified internists to beds
	TIER ONE											
8	University of Michigan Medical Center, Ann Arbor	49.6	9.6%	0.98	Yes	9	1.00	12	1.29	2	8	0.086
	TIER TWO											
38	Henry Ford Hospital, Detroit	26.0	0.0%	0.96	Yes	8	1.34	11	1.50	2	6	0.301
62	William Beaumont Hospital, Royal Oak	23.1	1.1%	1.05	Yes	6	0.63	12	1.46	2	6	0.113
	TIER THREE											
	Battle Creek Health System, Battle Creek	15.3	0.0%	0.91	No	3	0.00	10	0.65	1	4	0.029
	Blodgett Memorial Medical Center, Grand Rapids	18.5	0.0%	0.98	Yes	5	0.33	11	1.53	1	1	0.093
	Bon Secours Hospital, Grosse Pointe	16.2	0.0%	0.96	No	5	0.23	6	0.69	2	3	0.163
	Butterworth Hospital, Grand Rapids	16.5	0.0%	0.99	No	6	0.42	10	0.97	2	1	0.078
	Catherine McAuley Health System, Ann Arbor	19.9	0.0%	0.98	Yes	5	0.36	10	1.29	2	5	0.080
	Detroit Riverview Hospital	15.6	0.0%	0.91	No	5	0.03	4	0.76	1	3	0.108
	Harper Hospital, Detroit	19.7	0.0%	0.99	Yes	6	0.34	11	1.20	2	4	0.070
	Macomb Hospital Center, Warren	14.0	0.0%	1.00	No	5	0.01	9	0.54	2	1	0.151
	Mercy Hospital, Port Huron	15.0	0.0%	0.97	No	4	0.00	9	0.73	2	3	0.059
	Metropolitan Hospital, Grand Rapids	15.2	0.0%	1.00	No	5	0.47	6	0.87	2	3	0.029
	North Oakland Medical Center, Pontiac	18.2	0.0%	0.89	No	4	0.25	9	0.87	2	3	0.048
	Oakwood Hospital, Dearborn	14.2	0.5%	1.31	Yes	7	0.29	11	0.80	2	7	0.042
	Providence Hospital, Southfield	15.1	0.0%	1.12	Yes	6	0.52	8	0.85	2	3	0.039
	St. John Hospital and Medical Center, Detroit	15.0	0.0%	1.09	Yes	4	0.39	11	0.95	2	2	0.040
	St. Joseph Mercy Hospital, Pontiac	16.1	0.0%	0.98	No	5	0.42	6	0.84	2	6	0.031
	TIER FOUR											
	Borgess Medical Center, Kalamazoo	10.9	0.0%	1.17	No	4	0.09	10	0.95	2	4	0.047
	Bronson Methodist Hospital, Kalamazoo	11.2	0.0%	1.21	No	5	0.09	10	0.91	2	6	0.078
	Detroit Receiving Hospital	10.5	0.0%	1.28	Yes	3	0.90	4	1.00	2	1	0.043
	Genesys Regional Medical Center-St. Joseph, Flint	7.9	0.0%	1.33	No	5	0.25	11	0.52	2	3	0.031
	Grace Hospital, Detroit	11.2	0.0%	1.31	Yes	4	0.23	8	1.58	2	2	0.096
	Hackley Hospital, Muskegon	11.3	0.0%	1.11	No	4	0.00	9	0.60	2	4	0.071
	Hurley Medical Center, Flint	13.0	0.0%	1.27	Yes	8	0.31	10	0.98	2	3	0.030
	Marquette General Hospital, Marquette	12.8	0.0%	1.04	No	5	0.10	11	0.35	2	2	0.025

Natl. Rank	Hospital	U.S. News index	Reputational score	Hospital-wide mortality rate	COTH member	Service mix	Interns and residents to beds	Technology score (of 13)	R.N.'s to beds	Discharge planning (of 2)	Geriatric services (of 9)	Board-certified internists to beds
	McLaren Regional Medical Center, Flint	7.6	0.0%	1.35	No	5	0.23	11	0.65	2	2	0.048
	Mercy-Memorial Medical Center, St. Joseph	8.9	0.0%	1.25	No	5	0.00	9	0.83	2	1	0.151
	Michigan Affiliated Health System, Lansing	6.9	0.0%	1.42	No	5	0.24	8	0.83	2	3	0.110
	Mid Michigan Regional Medical Center, Midland	12.4	0.0%	1.07	No	3	0.13	10	0.65	2	5	0.010
	Munson Medical Center, Traverse City	11.0	0.0%	1.16	No	6	0.00	10	0.51	2	5	0.042
	Northern Michigan Hospital, Petoskey	8.0	0.0%	1.24	No	3	0.00	9	0.95	2	1	0.061
	Saginaw General Hospital, Saginaw	6.7	0.0%	1.34	No	4	0.11	6	1.26	2	1	0.011
	Sinai Hospital, Detroit	13.8	0.0%	1.20	Yes	5	0.70	11	0.98	2	1	0.072
	Sparrow Hospital, Lansing	5.1	0.0%	1.63	No	5	0.34	12	1.08	2	1	0.074
	St. Luke's Hospital, Saginaw	8.3	0.0%	1.17	No	3	0.04	5	0.86	2	1	0.025
	St. Mary Hospital, Livonia	13.7	0.0%	1.03	No	5	0.00	10	0.73	2	3	0.063
	St. Mary's Health Services, Grand Rapids	13.7	0.0%	1.03	No	5	0.38	10	0.86	1	2	0.075
	St. Mary's Medical Center, Saginaw	7.9	0.0%	1.27	No	3	0.05	12	0.97	2	1	0.008

GYNECOLOGY

Natl. Rank	Hospital	U.S. News index	Reputational score	Hospital-wide mortality rate	Interns and residents to beds	Technology score (of 10)	R.N.'s to beds	Board-certified OB-GYNs to beds	Procedures to beds
	TIER TWO								
49	Henry Ford Hospital, Detroit	26.6	0.0%	0.96	1.34	9	1.50	0.042	0.28
40	University of Michigan Medical Center, Ann Arbor	27.8	1.6%	0.98	1.00	9	1.29	0.046	0.45
	TIER THREE								
	Battle Creek Health System, Battle Creek	17.1	0.0%	0.91	0.00	8	0.65	0.016	0.49
99	Blodgett Memorial Medical Center, Grand Rapids	21.3	0.0%	0.98	0.33	7	1.53	0.081	0.67
	Bon Secours Hospital, Grosse Pointe	15.2	0.0%	0.96	0.23	4	0.69	0.062	0.65
	Butterworth Hospital, Grand Rapids	19.0	0.0%	0.99	0.42	8	0.97	0.055	0.58
	Catherine McAuley Health System, Ann Arbor	18.9	0.0%	0.98	0.36	6	1.29	0.052	0.44
	Detroit Riverview Hospital	16.4	0.0%	0.91	0.03	3	0.76	0.108	0.20
	Harper Hospital, Detroit	18.9	0.0%	0.99	0.34	8	1.20	0.022	0.06
	Macomb Hospital Center, Warren	14.5	0.0%	1.00	0.01	6	0.54	0.139	0.42
	Metropolitan Hospital, Grand Rapids	15.2	0.0%	1.00	0.47	5	0.87	0.005	0.40
	North Oakland Medical Center, Pontiac	20.7	0.0%	0.89	0.25	7	0.87	0.071	0.30
	Providence Hospital, Southfield	14.6	0.0%	1.12	0.52	6	0.85	0.067	0.52
	Sinai Hospital, Detroit	16.4	0.0%	1.20	0.70	8	0.98	0.100	0.41
	St. John Hospital and Medical Center, Detroit	16.4	0.0%	1.09	0.39	8	0.95	0.067	0.46
	St. Joseph Mercy Hospital, Pontiac	15.7	0.0%	0.98	0.42	4	0.84	0.053	0.31
	St. Mary's Health Services, Grand Rapids	17.9	0.0%	1.03	0.38	8	0.86	0.082	0.48
88	William Beaumont Hospital, Royal Oak	22.1	0.0%	1.05	0.63	9	1.46	0.091	0.55
	TIER FOUR								
	Borgess Medical Center, Kalamazoo	10.2	0.0%	1.17	0.09	5	0.95	0.024	0.41
	Bronson Methodist Hospital, Kalamazoo	11.7	0.0%	1.21	0.09	7	0.91	0.065	0.45
	Detroit Receiving Hospital	10.4	0.0%	1.28	0.90	3	1.00	0.013	0.02
	Genesys Regional Medical Center-St. Joseph, Flint	7.9	0.4%	1.33	0.25	6	0.52	0.019	0.38
	Grace Hospital, Detroit	13.5	0.0%	1.31	0.23	6	1.58	0.096	0.30
	Hackley Hospital, Muskegon	10.3	0.0%	1.11	0.00	6	0.60	0.024	0.69
	Hurley Medical Center, Flint	11.1	0.0%	1.27	0.31	7	0.98	0.031	0.23
	Marquette General Hospital, Marquette	12.4	0.0%	1.04	0.10	8	0.35	0.009	0.44
	McLaren Regional Medical Center, Flint	8.0	0.0%	1.35	0.23	7	0.65	0.028	0.46
	Mercy-Memorial Medical Center, St. Joseph	8.3	0.0%	1.25	0.00	6	0.83	0.014	0.41
	Michigan Affiliated Health System, Lansing	6.5	0.0%	1.42	0.24	5	0.83	0.035	0.12
	Mid Michigan Regional Medical Center, Midland	11.9	0.0%	1.07	0.13	6	0.65	0.013	0.41
	Munson Medical Center, Traverse City	9.9	0.0%	1.16	0.00	8	0.51	0.014	0.54
	Northern Michigan Hospital, Petoskey	9.1	0.0%	1.24	0.00	6	0.95	0.019	0.44
	Oakwood Hospital, Dearborn	10.8	0.0%	1.31	0.29	8	0.80	0.057	0.51
	Saginaw General Hospital, Saginaw	9.3	0.0%	1.34	0.11	5	1.26	0.052	0.94

Natl. Rank	Hospital	U.S. News index	Reputa-tional score	Hospital-wide mortality rate	Interns and residents to beds	Tech-nology score (of 10)	R.N.'s to beds	Board-certified OB-GYNs to beds	Procedures to beds
	Sparrow Hospital, Lansing	7.9	0.0%	1.63	0.34	8	1.08	0.046	0.43
	St. Luke's Hospital, Saginaw	7.9	0.0%	1.17	0.04	3	0.86	0.011	0.18
	St. Mary Hospital, Livonia	13.4	0.0%	1.03	0.00	6	0.73	0.052	0.41
	St. Mary's Medical Center, Saginaw	9.3	0.0%	1.27	0.05	7	0.97	0.004	0.08

NEUROLOGY

Natl. Rank	Hospital	U.S. News index	Reputa-tional score	Neurology mortality rate	COTH member	Interns and residents to beds	Tech-nology score (of 9)	R.N.'s to beds	Board-certified neurologists to beds
	TIER ONE								
24	University of Michigan Medical Center, Ann Arbor	24.9	5.3%	1.02	Yes	1.00	8	1.29	0.014
	TIER TWO								
42	Harper Hospital, Detroit	21.5	1.0%	0.70	Yes	0.34	8	1.20	0.022
45	Henry Ford Hospital, Detroit	20.9	0.2%	0.90	Yes	1.34	8	1.50	0.020
61	William Beaumont Hospital, Royal Oak	18.9	0.0%	0.84	Yes	0.63	8	1.46	0.012
	TIER THREE								
	Blodgett Memorial Medical Center, Grand Rapids	15.0	0.0%	0.99	Yes	0.33	7	1.53	0.012
	Bon Secours Hospital, Grosse Pointe	13.5	0.0%	0.78	No	0.23	4	0.69	0.008
	Butterworth Hospital, Grand Rapids	12.8	0.0%	0.92	No	0.42	7	0.97	0.011
	Catherine McAuley Health System, Ann Arbor	13.7	0.0%	0.98	Yes	0.36	6	1.29	0.003
	Detroit Receiving Hospital	11.1	0.0%	1.23	Yes	0.90	2	1.00	0.017
	Grace Hospital, Detroit	12.6	0.0%	1.08	Yes	0.23	5	1.58	0.006
	Hurley Medical Center, Flint	13.6	0.0%	0.95	Yes	0.31	6	0.98	0.007
	Providence Hospital, Southfield	16.2	0.0%	0.82	Yes	0.52	5	0.85	0.006
	Sinai Hospital, Detroit	14.4	0.0%	1.03	Yes	0.70	7	0.98	0.016
	St. John Hospital and Medical Center, Detroit	13.9	0.0%	0.95	Yes	0.39	7	0.95	0.005
	St. Mary's Health Services, Grand Rapids	12.1	0.0%	0.99	No	0.38	8	0.86	0.022
	TIER FOUR								
	Battle Creek Health System, Battle Creek	8.7	0.0%	1.02	No	0.00	8	0.65	0.005
	Borgess Medical Center, Kalamazoo	9.3	0.0%	1.05	No	0.09	5	0.95	0.018
	Bronson Methodist Hospital, Kalamazoo	6.6	0.0%	1.21	No	0.09	6	0.91	0.005
	Genesys Regional Medical Center-St. Joseph, Flint	5.5	0.0%	1.25	No	0.25	6	0.52	0.002
	Hackley Hospital, Muskegon	9.6	0.0%	0.94	No	0.00	6	0.60	0.008
	Macomb Hospital Center, Warren	8.9	0.0%	1.00	No	0.01	5	0.54	0.021
	Marquette General Hospital, Marquette	6.4	0.0%	1.14	No	0.10	7	0.35	0.006
	McLaren Regional Medical Center, Flint	10.3	0.0%	0.98	No	0.23	7	0.65	0.011
	Mercy Hospital, Port Huron	7.6	0.0%	1.09	No	0.00	6	0.73	0.008
	Metropolitan Hospital, Grand Rapids	8.7	0.0%	1.11	No	0.47	5	0.87	0.005
	Mid Michigan Regional Medical Center, Midland	7.7	0.0%	1.09	No	0.13	6	0.65	0.007
	Munson Medical Center, Traverse City	10.4	0.0%	0.89	No	0.00	7	0.51	0.006
	North Oakland Medical Center, Pontiac	7.6	0.0%	1.16	No	0.25	6	0.87	0.004
	Northern Michigan Hospital, Petoskey	10.1	0.0%	0.96	No	0.00	6	0.95	0.008
	Oakwood Hospital, Dearborn	10.6	0.0%	1.11	Yes	0.29	7	0.80	0.003
	Sparrow Hospital, Lansing	5.8	0.0%	1.53	No	0.34	7	1.08	0.011
	St. Joseph Mercy Hospital, Pontiac	9.0	0.0%	1.04	No	0.42	4	0.84	0.004
	St. Luke's Hospital, Saginaw	5.3	0.0%	1.22	No	0.04	3	0.86	0.004
	St. Mary Hospital, Livonia	9.0	0.0%	1.01	No	0.00	6	0.73	0.011
	St. Mary's Medical Center, Saginaw	6.2	0.0%	1.29	No	0.05	7	0.97	0.004

ORTHOPEDICS

Natl. Rank	Hospital	U.S. News index	Reputa-tional score	Orthopedics mortality rate	COTH member	Interns and residents to beds	Tech-nology score (of 5)	R.N.'s to beds	Board-certified orthopedists to beds	Pro-cedures to beds
	TIER ONE									
13	University of Michigan Medical Center, Ann Arbor	25.0	5.7%	1.16	Yes	1.00	5	1.29	0.025	1.21
	TIER TWO									
30	Henry Ford Hospital, Detroit	19.2	1.0%	0.82	Yes	1.34	4	1.50	0.026	1.86
	TIER THREE									
	Blodgett Memorial Medical Center, Grand Rapids	13.0	0.4%	1.03	Yes	0.33	3	1.53	0.035	5.29
	Butterworth Hospital, Grand Rapids	11.1	0.4%	0.81	No	0.42	4	0.97	0.025	2.91
94	Catherine McAuley Health System, Ann Arbor	13.3	0.0%	0.78	Yes	0.36	3	1.29	0.030	3.20
	Detroit Receiving Hospital	11.8	0.0%	0.93	Yes	0.90	2	1.00	0.033	1.05
	Grace Hospital, Detroit	9.7	0.0%	1.24	Yes	0.23	3	1.58	0.025	1.18
	Metropolitan Hospital, Grand Rapids	8.4	0.0%	0.98	No	0.47	4	0.87	0.014	2.78
	Oakwood Hospital, Dearborn	8.6	0.0%	1.24	Yes	0.29	4	0.80	0.011	2.13
	Providence Hospital, Southfield	8.8	0.0%	1.27	Yes	0.52	3	0.85	0.019	2.22
	Sinai Hospital, Detroit	10.4	0.0%	1.27	Yes	0.70	4	0.98	0.040	1.65
	St. John Hospital and Medical Center, Detroit	11.8	0.0%	0.87	Yes	0.39	4	0.95	0.019	1.95
	St. Joseph Mercy Hospital, Pontiac	11.1	0.0%	0.63	No	0.42	3	0.84	0.022	2.11
	St. Mary's Medical Center, Saginaw	10.9	0.0%	0.60	No	0.05	4	0.97	0.011	2.61
	William Beaumont Hospital, Royal Oak	12.5	0.0%	1.23	Yes	0.63	5	1.46	0.022	3.12
	TIER FOUR									
	Battle Creek Health System, Battle Creek	5.9	0.0%	1.00	No	0.00	4	0.65	0.013	1.95
	Bon Secours Hospital, Grosse Pointe	6.5	0.0%	1.05	No	0.23	3	0.69	0.043	4.07
	Borgess Medical Center, Kalamazoo	5.9	0.0%	1.18	No	0.09	3	0.95	0.053	3.85
	Bronson Methodist Hospital, Kalamazoo	7.4	0.0%	0.90	No	0.09	3	0.91	0.048	2.28
	Genesys Regional Medical Center-St. Joseph, Flint	3.9	0.0%	1.32	No	0.25	3	0.52	0.021	1.52
	Hackley Hospital, Muskegon	5.4	0.0%	1.00	No	0.00	3	0.60	0.028	2.81
	Hutzel Hospital, Detroit	6.2	0.0%	1.80	Yes	0.28	2	0.97	0.076	1.79
	Macomb Hospital Center, Warren	5.8	0.0%	0.91	No	0.01	3	0.54	0.036	1.49
	Marquette General Hospital, Marquette	5.7	0.0%	0.99	No	0.10	4	0.35	0.015	2.86
	McLaren Regional Medical Center, Flint	5.3	0.0%	1.28	No	0.23	4	0.65	0.016	2.74
	Mercy Hospital, Port Huron	5.1	0.0%	1.19	No	0.00	3	0.73	0.059	4.17
	Mercy-Memorial Medical Center, St. Joseph	2.4	0.0%	2.23	No	0.00	4	0.83	0.022	2.20
	Michigan Affiliated Health System, Lansing	4.4	0.0%	1.57	No	0.24	4	0.83	0.045	0.67
	Mid Michigan Regional Medical Center, Midland	6.5	0.0%	0.95	No	0.13	3	0.65	0.020	3.62
	Munson Medical Center, Traverse City	4.8	0.0%	1.07	No	0.00	3	0.51	0.017	3.71
	North Oakland Medical Center, Pontiac	8.1	0.0%	0.83	No	0.25	3	0.87	0.030	1.10
	Northern Michigan Hospital, Petoskey	6.6	0.0%	0.96	No	0.00	3	0.95	0.023	2.68
	Saginaw General Hospital, Saginaw	4.0	0.0%	1.71	No	0.11	3	1.26	0.011	1.33
	Sparrow Hospital, Lansing	4.7	0.0%	1.95	No	0.34	4	1.08	0.013	2.21
	St. Luke's Hospital, Saginaw	5.1	0.0%	1.11	No	0.04	2	0.86	0.046	3.19
	St. Mary Hospital, Livonia	4.7	0.0%	1.17	No	0.00	3	0.73	0.026	3.02
	St. Mary's Health Services, Grand Rapids	7.5	0.0%	1.11	No	0.38	4	0.86	0.025	3.58

OTOLARYNGOLOGY

Natl. Rank	Hospital	U.S. News index	Reputa-tional score	Hospital-wide mortality rate	COTH member	Interns and residents to beds	Tech-nology score (of 9)	R.N.'s to beds	Board-certified internists to beds	Procedures to beds
	TIER ONE									
4	University of Michigan Medical Center, Ann Arbor	59.8	14.3%	0.98	Yes	1.00	8	1.29	0.086	0.274
34	Henry Ford Hospital, Detroit	20.8	0.9%	0.96	Yes	1.34	8	1.50	0.301	0.265
	TIER THREE									
	Blodgett Memorial Medical Center, Grand Rapids	12.0	0.0%	0.98	Yes	0.33	7	1.53	0.093	0.157
	Butterworth Hospital, Grand Rapids	7.3	0.0%	0.99	No	0.42	7	0.97	0.078	0.178
	Catherine McAuley Health System, Ann Arbor	11.0	0.0%	0.98	Yes	0.36	6	1.29	0.080	0.207

Natl. Rank Hospital	U.S. News index	Reputa- tional score	Hospital- wide mortality rate	COTH member	Interns and residents to beds	Tech- nology score (of 9)	R.N.'s to beds	Board- certified internists to beds	Procedures to beds
Detroit Receiving Hospital	10.3	0.0%	1.28	Yes	0.90	1	1.00	0.043	0.127
Grace Hospital, Detroit	10.7	0.0%	1.31	Yes	0.23	4	1.58	0.096	0.119
Harper Hospital, Detroit	11.1	0.0%	0.99	Yes	0.34	8	1.20	0.070	0.226
Hurley Medical Center, Flint	9.2	0.0%	1.27	Yes	0.31	6	0.98	0.030	0.054
Hutzel Hospital, Detroit	8.7	0.0%	1.48	Yes	0.28	3	0.97	0.099	0.010
Oakwood Hospital, Dearborn	8.9	0.0%	1.31	Yes	0.29	7	0.80	0.042	0.096
Providence Hospital, Southfield	9.2	0.0%	1.12	Yes	0.52	4	0.85	0.039	0.251
Sinai Hospital, Detroit	11.4	0.0%	1.20	Yes	0.70	7	0.98	0.072	0.177
Sparrow Hospital, Lansing	7.0	0.0%	1.63	No	0.34	7	1.08	0.074	0.116
St. John Hospital and Medical Center, Detroit	9.9	0.0%	1.09	Yes	0.39	7	0.95	0.040	0.138
St. Mary's Health Services, Grand Rapids	7.1	0.0%	1.03	No	0.38	8	0.86	0.075	0.135
William Beaumont Hospital, Royal Oak	13.4	0.0%	1.05	Yes	0.63	8	1.46	0.113	0.194
TIER FOUR									
Battle Creek Health System, Battle Creek	4.6	0.0%	0.91	No	0.00	8	0.65	0.029	0.104
Bon Secours Hospital, Grosse Pointe	5.1	0.0%	0.96	No	0.23	2	0.69	0.163	0.218
Borgess Medical Center, Kalamazoo	5.0	0.0%	1.17	No	0.09	5	0.95	0.047	0.083
Bronson Methodist Hospital, Kalamazoo	5.4	0.0%	1.21	No	0.09	6	0.91	0.078	0.124
Chelsea Community Hospital, Chelsea	3.0	0.0%	0.81	No	0.00	1	0.62	0.067	0.057
Detroit Riverview Hospital	4.1	0.0%	0.91	No	0.03	2	0.76	0.108	0.146
Genesys Regional Medical Center-St. Joseph, Flint	4.4	0.0%	1.33	No	0.25	6	0.52	0.031	0.180
Hackley Hospital, Muskegon	4.1	0.0%	1.11	No	0.00	6	0.60	0.071	0.175
Macomb Hospital Center, Warren	4.7	0.0%	1.01	No	0.01	6	0.54	0.151	0.157
Marquette General Hospital, Marquette	3.7	0.0%	1.04	No	0.10	7	0.35	0.025	0.142
McLaren Regional Medical Center, Flint	5.1	0.0%	1.35	No	0.23	7	0.65	0.048	0.126
Mercy Hospital, Port Huron	4.5	0.0%	0.97	No	0.00	6	0.73	0.059	0.109
Mercy-Memorial Medical Center, St. Joseph	5.4	0.0%	1.25	No	0.00	6	0.83	0.151	0.140
Metropolitan Hospital, Grand Rapids	5.7	0.0%	1.00	No	0.47	3	0.87	0.029	0.116
Michigan Affiliated Health System, Lansing	5.1	0.0%	1.41	No	0.24	3	0.83	0.110	0.039
Mid Michigan Regional Medical Center, Midland	5.5	0.4%	1.07	No	0.13	6	0.65	0.010	0.179
Munson Medical Center, Traverse City	3.8	0.0%	1.16	No	0.00	7	0.51	0.042	0.269
North Oakland Medical Center, Pontiac	5.9	0.0%	0.89	No	0.25	6	0.87	0.048	0.086
Northern Michigan Hospital, Petoskey	5.3	0.0%	1.24	No	0.00	7	0.95	0.061	0.218
Saginaw General Hospital, Saginaw	4.8	0.0%	1.34	No	0.11	2	1.26	0.011	0.153
St. Joseph Mercy Hospital, Pontiac	5.1	0.0%	0.99	No	0.42	2	0.84	0.031	0.122
St. Lawrence Hospital and Healthcare, Lansing	2.9	0.0%	0.98	No	0.29	1	0.37	0.034	0.039
St. Luke's Hospital, Saginaw	3.2	0.0%	1.17	No	0.04	1	0.86	0.025	0.296
St. Mary Hospital, Livonia	4.5	0.0%	1.03	No	0.00	6	0.73	0.063	0.197
St. Mary's Medical Center, Saginaw	5.1	0.0%	1.27	No	0.05	7	0.97	0.008	0.236

RHEUMATOLOGY

Natl. Rank Hospital	U.S. News index	Reputa- tional score	Hospital- wide mortality rate	COTH member	Interns and residents to beds	Tech- nology score (of 5)	R.N.'s to beds	Board- certified internists to beds
TIER ONE								
13 University of Michigan Medical Center, Ann Arbor	32.7	7.2%	0.98	Yes	1.00	5	1.29	0.086
TIER TWO								
27 Henry Ford Hospital, Detroit	21.9	1.1%	0.96	Yes	1.34	4	1.50	0.301
76 William Beaumont Hospital, Royal Oak	16.5	0.5%	1.05	Yes	0.63	5	1.46	0.113
TIER THREE								
Blodgett Memorial Medical Center, Grand Rapids	13.2	0.0%	0.98	Yes	0.33	3	1.53	0.093
Bon Secours Hospital, Grosse Pointe	9.9	0.0%	0.96	No	0.23	3	0.69	0.163
Butterworth Hospital, Grand Rapids	10.8	0.0%	0.99	No	0.42	4	0.97	0.078
Catherine McAuley Health System, Ann Arbor	14.6	0.5%	0.98	Yes	0.36	3	1.29	0.080
Detroit Receiving Hospital	11.6	0.0%	1.28	Yes	0.90	2	1.00	0.043
Grace Hospital, Detroit	11.6	0.0%	1.31	Yes	0.23	3	1.58	0.096

Natl. Rank / Hospital	U.S. News index	Reputational score	Hospital-wide mortality rate	COTH member	Interns and residents to beds	Technology score (of 5)	R.N.'s to beds	Board-certified internists to beds
Harper Hospital, Detroit	13.5	0.0%	0.99	Yes	0.34	4	1.20	0.070
Hurley Medical Center, Flint	10.1	0.0%	1.27	Yes	0.31	3	0.98	0.030
Metropolitan Hospital, Grand Rapids	10.2	0.0%	1.00	No	0.47	4	0.87	0.029
North Oakland Medical Center, Pontiac	10.4	0.0%	0.89	No	0.25	3	0.87	0.048
Oakwood Hospital, Dearborn	9.8	0.0%	1.31	Yes	0.29	4	0.80	0.042
Providence Hospital, Southfield	11.4	0.0%	1.12	Yes	0.52	3	0.85	0.039
Sinai Hospital, Detroit	12.5	0.0%	1.20	Yes	0.70	4	0.98	0.072
St. John Hospital and Medical Center, Detroit	11.9	0.0%	1.09	Yes	0.39	4	0.95	0.040
St. Joseph Mercy Hospital, Pontiac	9.7	0.0%	0.99	No	0.42	3	0.84	0.031
TIER FOUR								
Battle Creek Health System, Battle Creek	8.0	0.0%	0.91	No	0.00	4	0.65	0.029
Borgess Medical Center, Kalamazoo	8.4	0.4%	1.17	No	0.09	3	0.95	0.047
Bronson Methodist Hospital, Kalamazoo	8.3	0.4%	1.21	No	0.09	3	0.91	0.078
Detroit Riverview Hospital	8.6	0.0%	0.91	No	0.03	3	0.76	0.108
Genesys Regional Medical Center-St. Joseph, Flint	5.9	0.0%	1.33	No	0.25	3	0.52	0.031
Hackley Hospital, Muskegon	6.9	0.0%	1.11	No	0.00	3	0.60	0.071
Macomb Hospital Center, Warren	8.3	0.0%	1.01	No	0.01	3	0.54	0.151
Marquette General Hospital, Marquette	7.3	0.0%	1.04	No	0.10	4	0.35	0.025
McLaren Regional Medical Center, Flint	6.6	0.0%	1.35	No	0.23	4	0.65	0.048
Mercy Hospital, Port Huron	8.4	0.0%	0.97	No	0.00	3	0.73	0.059
Mercy-Memorial Medical Center, St. Joseph	7.7	0.0%	1.25	No	0.00	4	0.83	0.151
Michigan Affiliated Health System, Lansing	7.3	0.0%	1.41	No	0.24	4	0.83	0.110
Mid Michigan Regional Medical Center, Midland	7.4	0.0%	1.07	No	0.13	3	0.65	0.010
Munson Medical Center, Traverse City	6.1	0.0%	1.16	No	0.00	3	0.51	0.042
Northern Michigan Hospital, Petoskey	6.9	0.0%	1.24	No	0.00	3	0.95	0.061
Saginaw General Hospital, Saginaw	7.1	0.0%	1.34	No	0.11	3	1.26	0.011
Sparrow Hospital, Lansing	7.1	0.0%	1.63	No	0.34	4	1.08	0.074
St. Luke's Hospital, Saginaw	6.5	0.0%	1.17	No	0.04	2	0.86	0.025
St. Mary Hospital, Livonia	7.8	0.0%	1.03	No	0.00	3	0.73	0.063
St. Mary's Health Services, Grand Rapids	9.0	0.0%	1.03	No	0.38	4	0.86	0.075
St. Mary's Medical Center, Saginaw	7.0	0.0%	1.27	No	0.05	4	0.97	0.008

UROLOGY

Natl. Rank / Hospital	U.S. News index	Reputational score	Urology mortality rate	COTH member	Interns and residents to beds	Technology score (of 11)	R.N.'s to beds	Board-certified internists to beds	Procedures to beds
TIER ONE									
24 University of Michigan Medical Center, Ann Arbor	22.2	3.0%	0.77	Yes	1.00	10	1.29	0.086	1.30
TIER TWO									
70 Harper Hospital, Detroit	16.4	1.0%	0.84	Yes	0.34	10	1.20	0.070	2.58
45 Henry Ford Hospital, Detroit	18.6	0.6%	1.02	Yes	1.34	10	1.50	0.301	2.29
50 William Beaumont Hospital, Royal Oak	18.2	1.4%	0.89	Yes	0.63	10	1.46	0.113	2.42
TIER THREE									
Blodgett Memorial Medical Center, Grand Rapids	12.2	0.0%	1.15	Yes	0.33	8	1.53	0.093	1.32
Butterworth Hospital, Grand Rapids	10.2	0.0%	0.99	No	0.42	9	0.97	0.078	1.97
Catherine McAuley Health System, Ann Arbor	13.7	0.0%	0.91	Yes	0.36	7	1.29	0.080	2.00
Detroit Receiving Hospital	10.0	0.0%	1.27	Yes	0.90	2	1.00	0.043	0.89
Detroit Riverview Hospital	10.4	0.0%	0.73	No	0.03	4	0.76	0.108	1.69
Grace Hospital, Detroit	9.4	0.0%	1.59	Yes	0.23	5	1.58	0.096	2.48
Hurley Medical Center, Flint	13.7	0.0%	0.78	Yes	0.31	7	0.98	0.030	0.89
Metropolitan Hospital, Grand Rapids	9.4	0.0%	0.93	No	0.47	5	0.87	0.029	2.49
Providence Hospital, Southfield	9.5	0.0%	1.26	Yes	0.52	5	0.85	0.039	1.99
Sinai Hospital, Detroit	11.7	0.0%	1.20	Yes	0.70	8	0.98	0.072	1.85
St. John Hospital and Medical Center, Detroit	10.1	0.0%	1.28	Yes	0.39	8	0.95	0.040	2.34
St. Joseph Mercy Hospital, Pontiac	10.0	0.0%	0.82	No	0.42	4	0.84	0.031	1.41

Natl. Rank	Hospital	U.S. News index	Reputational score	Urology mortality rate	COTH member	Interns and residents to beds	Technology score (of 11)	R.N.'s to beds	Board-certified internists to beds	Procedures to beds
	St. Mary's Health Services, Grand Rapids	**9.1**	0.0%	1.10	No	0.38	9	0.86	0.075	2.62
	TIER FOUR									
	Battle Creek Health System, Battle Creek	**5.9**	0.0%	1.21	No	0.00	9	0.65	0.029	1.70
	Bon Secours Hospital, Grosse Pointe	**8.3**	0.0%	0.99	No	0.23	4	0.69	0.163	2.97
	Borgess Medical Center, Kalamazoo	**4.9**	0.0%	1.48	No	0.09	6	0.95	0.047	1.59
	Bronson Methodist Hospital, Kalamazoo	**8.5**	0.0%	0.97	No	0.09	7	0.91	0.078	1.45
	Genesys Regional Medical Center-St. Joseph, Flint	**6.1**	0.0%	1.23	No	0.25	8	0.52	0.031	1.84
	Hackley Hospital, Muskegon	**6.2**	0.0%	1.12	No	0.00	7	0.60	0.071	1.89
	Macomb Hospital Center, Warren	**3.9**	0.0%	1.58	No	0.01	6	0.54	0.151	1.83
	Marquette General Hospital, Marquette	**6.0**	0.0%	1.08	No	0.10	8	0.35	0.025	1.48
	McLaren Regional Medical Center, Flint	**4.2**	0.0%	1.75	No	0.23	8	0.65	0.048	1.93
	Mercy-Memorial Medical Center, St. Joseph	**4.5**	0.0%	1.66	No	0.00	7	0.83	0.151	1.49
	Michigan Affiliated Health System, Lansing	**3.9**	0.0%	1.76	No	0.24	5	0.83	0.110	0.53
	Mid Michigan Regional Medical Center, Midland	**7.3**	0.0%	0.98	No	0.13	7	0.65	0.010	1.21
	Munson Medical Center, Traverse City	**3.5**	0.0%	1.58	No	0.00	8	0.51	0.042	1.53
	Northern Michigan Hospital, Petoskey	**6.3**	0.0%	1.21	No	0.00	7	0.95	0.061	1.71
	Oakwood Hospital, Dearborn	**7.4**	0.0%	1.84	Yes	0.29	9	0.80	0.042	1.88
	Saginaw General Hospital, Saginaw	**4.8**	0.0%	1.48	No	0.11	4	1.26	0.011	1.30
	Sparrow Hospital, Lansing	**8.4**	0.0%	1.17	No	0.34	9	1.08	0.074	1.01
	St. Luke's Hospital, Saginaw	**5.4**	0.0%	1.16	No	0.04	3	0.86	0.025	2.29
	St. Mary Hospital, Livonia	**6.4**	0.0%	1.18	No	0.00	7	0.73	0.063	3.14
	St. Mary's Medical Center, Saginaw	**4.3**	0.0%	1.67	No	0.05	8	0.97	0.008	1.44

AIDS

Natl. Rank	Hospital	U.S. News index	Reputational score	Hospital-wide mortality rate	COTH member	Interns and residents to beds	Technology score (of 11)	Discharge planning (of 2)	R.N.'s to beds	Board-certified internists to beds
	TIER TWO									
67	Hennepin County Medical Center, Minneapolis	26.1	0.0%	0.77	Yes	0.91	8	2	0.78	0.020
43	Mayo Clinic, Rochester	28.0	2.7%	0.72	Yes	0.24	7	2	0.77	0.060
60	St. Paul-Ramsey Medical Center, St. Paul	26.5	1.1%	0.85	Yes	0.57	8	2	0.37	0.112
46	University of Minnesota Hospital and Clinic, Minneapolis	27.6	1.3%	0.81	Yes	0.59	8	2	0.86	0.133
	TIER THREE									
	Abbott Northwestern Hospital, Minneapolis	23.1	0.0%	0.77	No	0.11	9	2	0.48	0.101
	Fairview Riverside Medical Center, Minneapolis	20.5	0.0%	0.92	No	0.03	5	2	0.33	0.085
	Healtheast St. John's Hospital, Maplewood	21.5	0.0%	0.75	No	0.06	6	2	0.37	0.056
	Healtheast St. Joseph's Hospital, St. Paul	22.0	0.0%	0.62	No	0.04	7	2	0.48	0.065
	Healthone Corp, Metro Hospitals, Minneapolis	20.9	0.0%	0.81	No	0.00	4	2	0.60	0.025
	Methodist Hospital, St. Louis Park	21.5	0.0%	0.89	No	0.00	5	2	0.62	0.092
	Miller-Dwan Medical Center, Duluth	21.3	0.0%	0.68	No	0.00	4	2	0.36	0.230
	St. Cloud Hospital, St. Cloud	20.4	0.0%	0.98	No	0.00	6	2	0.87	0.055
	St. Mary's Medical Center, Duluth	21.5	0.0%	0.88	No	0.04	6	2	0.41	0.040
	TIER FOUR									
	Fairview Southdale Hospital, Minneapolis	18.4	0.0%	1.08	No	0.00	6	2	0.57	0.067
	North Memorial Medical Center, Robbinsdale	17.2	0.0%	1.27	No	0.07	7	2	0.87	0.072
	St. Luke's Hospital, Duluth	16.3	0.0%	1.19	No	0.03	5	1	0.34	0.229

CANCER

Natl. Rank	Hospital	U.S. News index	Reputational score	Cancer mortality rate	COTH member	Interns and residents to beds	Technology score (of 12)	R.N.'s to beds	Board-certified oncologists to beds	Procedures to beds
	TIER ONE									
5	Mayo Clinic, Rochester	42.3	27.5%	0.57	Yes	0.24	8	0.77	0.026	3.03
	TIER THREE									
	Hennepin County Medical Center, Minneapolis	9.3	0.0%	0.70	Yes	0.91	8	0.78	0.008	0.49
	St. Paul-Ramsey Medical Center, St. Paul	6.6	0.0%	0.59	Yes	0.57	6	0.37	0.007	0.68
	University of Minnesota Hospital and Clinic, Minneapolis	9.4	0.0%	0.46	Yes	0.59	9	0.86	0.056	2.00
	TIER FOUR									
	Abbott Northwestern Hospital, Minneapolis	3.9	0.0%	0.72	No	0.11	9	0.48	0.010	2.14
	Fairview Riverside Medical Center, Minneapolis	1.1	0.0%	0.80	No	0.03	3	0.33	0.012	0.61
	Fairview Southdale Hospital, Minneapolis	2.4	0.0%	1.16	No	0.00	6	0.57	0.013	2.04
	Healtheast St. John's Hospital, Maplewood	2.2	0.0%	0.18	No	0.06	5	0.37	0.006	1.25
	Healtheast St. Joseph's Hospital, St. Paul	3.7	0.0%	0.30	No	0.04	9	0.48	0.015	1.05
	Healthone Corp. Metro Hospitals, Minneapolis	1.0	0.0%	1.08	No	0.00	2	0.60	0.005	0.21
	Methodist Hospital, St. Louis Park	3.2	0.0%	0.73	No	0.00	6	0.62	0.018	2.51
	North Memorial Medical Center, Robbinsdale	3.8	0.0%	1.25	No	0.07	8	0.87	0.017	1.21
	St. Cloud Hospital, St. Cloud	3.8	0.0%	0.95	No	0.00	8	0.87	0.000	1.43
	St. Luke's Hospital, Duluth	0.8	0.0%	1.40	No	0.03	3	0.34	0.021	1.29
	St. Mary's Medical Center, Duluth	2.4	0.0%	0.98	No	0.04	6	0.41	0.017	2.68

CARDIOLOGY

Natl. Rank	Hospital	U.S. News index	Reputational score	Cardiology mortality rate	COTH member	Interns and residents to beds	Technology score (of 10)	R.N.'s to beds	Board-certified cardiologists to beds	Procedures to beds
	TIER ONE									
2	**Mayo Clinic, Rochester**	**93.4**	49.0%	0.82	Yes	0.24	8	0.77	0.053	6.57
	TIER TWO									
57	**Hennepin County Medical Center, Minneapolis**	**22.7**	0.0%	0.89	Yes	0.91	8	0.78	0.027	4.05
93	**University of Minnesota Hospital and Clinic, Minneapolis**	**21.0**	1.2%	0.99	Yes	0.59	8	0.86	0.041	3.40
	TIER THREE									
	Abbott Northwestern Hospital, Minneapolis	**19.0**	1.0%	0.78	No	0.11	9	0.48	0.029	11.52
	Fairview Riverside Medical Center, Minneapolis	**13.7**	0.0%	0.96	No	0.03	8	0.33	0.033	2.68
	Healtheast St. John's Hospital, Maplewood	**15.5**	0.0%	0.66	No	0.06	5	0.37	0.022	7.64
	Healtheast St. Joseph's Hospital, St. Paul	**16.7**	0.0%	0.71	No	0.04	8	0.48	0.033	5.98
	Healthone Corp. Metro Hospitals, Minneapolis	**14.6**	0.0%	0.90	No	0.00	5	0.60	0.017	1.61
	Methodist Hospital, St. Louis Park	**14.5**	0.0%	0.95	No	0.00	8	0.62	0.015	7.21
	St. Mary's Medical Center, Duluth	**16.7**	0.0%	0.82	No	0.04	8	0.41	0.020	12.49
	St. Paul-Ramsey Medical Center, St. Paul	**18.6**	0.0%	0.96	Yes	0.57	9	0.37	0.020	6.87
	TIER FOUR									
	Fairview Southdale Hospital, Minneapolis	**11.5**	0.0%	1.09	No	0.00	8	0.57	0.031	8.26
	North Memorial Medical Center, Robbinsdale	**10.6**	0.0%	1.22	No	0.07	9	0.87	0.035	6.55
	St. Cloud Hospital, St. Cloud	**13.3**	0.0%	1.03	No	0.00	8	0.87	0.014	8.22
	St. Luke's Hospital, Duluth	**10.7**	0.0%	1.07	No	0.03	8	0.34	0.004	4.37

ENDOCRINOLOGY

Natl. Rank	Hospital	U.S. News index	Reputational score	Endocrinology mortality rate	COTH member	Interns and residents to beds	Technology score (of 11)	R.N.'s to beds	Board-certified internists to beds
	TIER ONE								
1	**Mayo Clinic, Rochester**	**100.0**	65.1%	0.48	Yes	0.24	8	0.77	0.060
	TIER TWO								
73	**Hennepin County Medical Center, Minneapolis**	**15.4**	0.0%	0.24	Yes	0.91	8	0.78	0.020
27	**University of Minnesota Hospital and Clinic, Minneapolis**	**20.5**	4.8%	0.78	Yes	0.59	10	0.86	0.133
	TIER THREE								
	Abbott Northwestern Hospital, Minneapolis	**10.4**	0.0%	0.45	No	0.11	10	0.48	0.101
	Fairview Southdale Hospital, Minneapolis	**8.7**	0.0%	0.72	No	0.00	8	0.57	0.067
	Healtheast St. Joseph's Hospital, St. Paul	**9.9**	0.0%	0.22	No	0.04	10	0.48	0.065
	Healthone Corp. Metro Hospitals, Minneapolis	**8.4**	0.0%	0.39	No	0.00	3	0.60	0.025
	Methodist Hospital, St. Louis Park	**9.8**	0.0%	0.63	No	0.00	7	0.62	0.092
97	St. Paul-Ramsey Medical Center, St. Paul	**13.6**	0.0%	0.46	Yes	0.57	7	0.37	0.112
	TIER FOUR								
	Fairview Riverside Medical Center, Minneapolis	**6.3**	0.0%	0.84	No	0.03	5	0.33	0.085
	Healtheast St. John's Hospital, Maplewood	**7.7**	0.0%	0.73	No	0.06	6	0.37	0.056
	North Memorial Medical Center, Robbinsdale	**6.1**	0.0%	1.24	No	0.07	9	0.87	0.072
	St. Cloud Hospital, St. Cloud	**8.0**	0.0%	0.86	No	0.00	8	0.87	0.055
	St. Mary's Medical Center, Duluth	**4.6**	0.0%	1.10	No	0.04	6	0.41	0.040

GASTROENTEROLOGY

Natl. Rank	Hospital	U.S. News index	Reputa-tional score	Gastro-enterology mortality rate	COTH member	Interns and residents to beds	Tech-nology score (of 11)	R.N.'s to beds	Board-certified gastro-enterologists to beds	Pro-cedures to beds
TIER ONE
1	Mayo Clinic, Rochester	100.0	59.8%	0.05	Yes	0.24	8	0.77	0.029	1.00
TIER TWO
44	University of Minnesota Hospital and Clinic, Minneapolis	15.6	2.0%	0.73	Yes	0.59	10	0.86	0.030	1.29
TIER THREE
	Abbott Northwestern Hospital, Minneapolis	8.7	0.0%	0.80	No	0.11	10	0.48	0.014	3.61
	Healtheast St. John's Hospital, Maplewood	7.4	0.0%	0.71	No	0.06	6	0.37	0.011	4.16
	Healtheast St. Joseph's Hospital, St. Paul	7.9	0.0%	0.60	No	0.04	10	0.48	0.018	2.57
84	Hennepin County Medical Center, Minneapolis	12.8	0.0%	0.75	Yes	0.91	7	0.78	0.008	1.59
	St. Cloud Hospital, St. Cloud	8.4	0.0%	0.68	No	0.00	8	0.87	0.005	3.33
	St. Paul-Ramsey Medical Center, St. Paul	9.9	0.0%	0.92	Yes	0.57	6	0.37	0.010	2.66
TIER FOUR
	Fairview Riverside Medical Center, Minneapolis	5.3	0.0%	0.78	No	0.03	5	0.33	0.014	1.41
	Fairview Southdale Hospital, Minneapolis	5.4	0.0%	1.15	No	0.00	7	0.57	0.018	4.30
	Methodist Hospital, St. Louis Park	7.2	0.0%	0.85	No	0.00	7	0.62	0.010	3.24
	North Memorial Medical Center, Robbinsdale	3.8	0.0%	1.59	No	0.07	8	0.87	0.020	2.42
	St. Luke's Hospital, Duluth	2.4	0.0%	1.39	No	0.03	4	0.34	0.000	3.28
	St. Mary's Medical Center, Duluth	6.3	0.4%	1.03	No	0.04	5	0.41	0.007	4.88

GERIATRICS

Natl. Rank	Hospital	U.S. News index	Reputa-tional score	Hospital-wide mortality rate	COTH member	Service mix	Interns and residents to beds	Tech-nology score (of 13)	R.N.'s to beds	Discharge planning (of 2)	Geriatric services (of 9)	Board-certified internists to beds
TIER ONE
7	Mayo Clinic, Rochester	57.7	14.0%	0.72	Yes	5	0.24	8	0.77	2	5	0.060
21	University of Minnesota Hospital and Clinic, Minneapolis	31.2	2.9%	0.81	Yes	9	0.59	10	0.86	2	2	0.133
TIER TWO
50	Hennepin County Medical Center, Minneapolis	24.2	0.0%	0.77	Yes	8	0.91	10	0.78	2	6	0.020
71	St. Paul-Ramsey Medical Center, St. Paul	22.6	0.0%	0.85	Yes	8	0.57	9	0.37	2	5	0.112
TIER THREE
	Abbott Northwestern Hospital, Minneapolis	19.8	0.0%	0.77	No	8	0.11	11	0.48	2	4	0.101
	Fairview Riverside Medical Center, Minneapolis	17.3	0.0%	0.92	No	6	0.03	7	0.33	2	6	0.085
	Healtheast St. John's Hospital, Maplewood	16.0	0.0%	0.75	No	4	0.06	6	0.37	2	2	0.056
	Healtheast St. Joseph's Hospital, St. Paul	18.5	0.0%	0.62	No	7	0.04	10	0.48	2	3	0.065
	Healthone Corp. Metro Hospitals, Minneapolis	15.9	0.0%	0.81	No	4	0.00	5	0.60	2	2	0.025
	Methodist Hospital, St. Louis Park	17.8	0.0%	0.89	No	5	0.00	9	0.62	2	3	0.092
	St. Cloud Hospital, St. Cloud	16.1	0.0%	0.98	No	7	0.00	11	0.87	2	1	0.055
	St. Mary's Medical Center, Duluth	17.5	0.0%	0.88	No	6	0.04	8	0.41	2	3	0.040
TIER FOUR
	Fairview Southdale Hospital, Minneapolis	12.5	0.0%	1.08	No	6	0.00	9	0.57	2	3	0.067
	North Memorial Medical Center, Robbinsdale	11.3	0.0%	1.27	No	8	0.07	11	0.87	2	6	0.072
	St. Luke's Hospital, Duluth	8.8	0.0%	1.19	No	6	0.03	6	0.34	1	3	0.229

GYNECOLOGY

Natl. Rank	Hospital	U.S. News index	Reputa-tional score	Hospital-wide mortality rate	Interns and residents to beds	Tech-nology score (of 10)	R.N.'s to beds	Board-certified OB-GYNs to beds	Procedures to beds
TIER ONE
2	Mayo Clinic, Rochester	95.4	30.0%	0.72	0.24	6	0.77	0.014	0.35
TIER TWO
81	Hennepin County Medical Center, Minneapolis	22.5	0.0%	0.77	0.91	7	0.78	0.037	0.11
61	University of Minnesota Hospital and Clinic, Minneapolis	24.6	0.8%	0.81	0.59	9	0.86	0.027	0.57

Natl. Rank	Hospital	U.S. News index	Reputational score	Hospital-wide mortality rate	Interns and residents to beds	Technology score (of 10)	R.N.'s to beds	Board-certified OB-GYNs to beds	Procedures to beds
TIER THREE									
	Abbott Northwestern Hospital, Minneapolis	19.9	0.4%	0.77	0.11	8	0.48	0.060	0.42
	Healtheast St. John's Hospital, Maplewood	15.4	0.0%	0.75	0.06	5	0.37	0.034	0.73
	Healtheast St. Joseph's Hospital, St. Paul	18.2	0.0%	0.62	0.04	8	0.48	0.045	0.27
	Methodist Hospital, St. Louis Park	16.7	0.0%	0.89	0.00	5	0.62	0.060	0.49
	St. Cloud Hospital, St. Cloud	16.9	0.4%	0.98	0.00	7	0.87	0.033	0.33
	St. Mary's Medical Center, Duluth	14.8	0.0%	0.88	0.04	4	0.41	0.033	0.68
	St. Paul-Ramsey Medical Center, St. Paul	18.7	0.0%	0.85	0.57	7	0.37	0.020	0.27
TIER FOUR									
	Fairview Riverside Medical Center, Minneapolis	13.0	0.0%	0.92	0.03	3	0.33	0.046	0.23
	Fairview Southdale Hospital, Minneapolis	10.6	0.0%	1.08	0.00	5	0.57	0.044	0.58
	North Memorial Medical Center, Robbinsdale	11.0	0.0%	1.27	0.07	8	0.87	0.064	0.35
	St. Luke's Hospital, Duluth	6.6	0.0%	1.19	0.03	4	0.34	0.042	0.44

NEUROLOGY

Natl. Rank	Hospital	U.S. News index	Reputational score	Neurology mortality rate	COTH member	Interns and residents to beds	Technology score (of 9)	R.N.'s to beds	Board-certified neurologists to beds
TIER ONE									
1	Mayo Clinic, Rochester	100.0	51.5%	0.72	Yes	0.24	6	0.77	0.035
TIER TWO									
27	University of Minnesota Hospital and Clinic, Minneapolis	23.8	1.6%	0.64	Yes	0.59	8	0.86	0.043
TIER THREE									
	Abbott Northwestern Hospital, Minneapolis	15.8	0.0%	0.73	No	0.11	8	0.48	0.033
	Healtheast St. John's Hospital, Maplewood	13.0	0.0%	0.72	No	0.06	5	0.37	0.011
	Healtheast St. Joseph's Hospital, St. Paul	14.2	0.0%	0.60	No	0.04	8	0.48	0.012
	Hennepin County Medical Center, Minneapolis	14.7	0.0%	1.02	Yes	0.91	6	0.78	0.021
	Methodist Hospital, St. Louis Park	11.6	0.0%	0.87	No	0.00	5	0.62	0.020
	Miller-Dwan Medical Center, Duluth	15.1	0.0%	0.30	No	0.00	3	0.36	0.055
	St. Paul-Ramsey Medical Center, St. Paul	15.6	0.0%	0.85	Yes	0.57	6	0.37	0.020
TIER FOUR									
	Fairview Riverside Medical Center, Minneapolis	10.2	0.0%	0.87	No	0.03	4	0.33	0.014
	Fairview Southdale Hospital, Minneapolis	7.7	0.0%	1.07	No	0.00	6	0.57	0.013
	Healthone Corp. Metro Hospitals, Minneapolis	8.8	0.0%	0.94	No	0.00	3	0.60	0.010
	North Memorial Medical Center, Robbinsdale	4.9	0.0%	1.52	No	0.07	7	0.87	0.017
	St. Cloud Hospital, St. Cloud	7.3	0.0%	1.16	No	0.00	6	0.87	0.011
	St. Luke's Hospital, Duluth	7.3	0.0%	1.08	No	0.03	4	0.34	0.025
	St. Mary's Medical Center, Duluth	10.9	0.0%	0.86	No	0.04	4	0.41	0.017

ORTHOPEDICS

Natl. Rank	Hospital	U.S. News index	Reputational score	Orthopedics mortality rate	COTH member	Interns and residents to beds	Technology score (of 5)	R.N.'s to beds	Board-certified orthopedists to beds	Procedures to beds
TIER ONE										
1	Mayo Clinic, Rochester	100.0	41.7%	0.55	Yes	0.24	4	0.77	0.023	1.89
TIER TWO										
51	Hennepin County Medical Center, Minneapolis	16.3	0.5%	0.55	Yes	0.91	3	0.78	0.018	1.87
32	University of Minnesota Hospital and Clinic, Minneapolis	18.8	1.9%	0.35	Yes	0.59	4	0.86	0.016	1.55
TIER THREE										
	St. Mary's Medical Center, Duluth	9.4	0.0%	0.62	No	0.04	3	0.41	0.026	5.43
TIER FOUR										
	Abbott Northwestern Hospital, Minneapolis	7.8	0.0%	0.84	No	0.11	4	0.48	0.039	3.54
	Fairview Riverside Medical Center, Minneapolis	5.2	0.0%	0.92	No	0.03	3	0.33	0.026	1.66
	Fairview Southdale Hospital, Minneapolis	5.0	0.0%	1.11	No	0.00	3	0.57	0.031	4.40

Natl. Rank	Hospital	U.S. News index	Reputational score	Orthopedics mortality rate	COTH member	Interns and residents to beds	Technology score (of 5)	R.N.'s to beds	Board-certified orthopedists to beds	Procedures to beds
	Healtheast St. John's Hospital, Maplewood	3.8	0.0%	1.36	No	0.06	4	0.37	0.028	3.24
	Healtheast St. Joseph's Hospital, St. Paul	6.4	0.0%	0.92	No	0.04	4	0.48	0.033	2.36
	Healthone Corp. Metro Hospitals, Minneapolis	2.3	0.0%	1.35	No	0.00	2	0.60	0.018	0.57
	Methodist Hospital, St. Louis Park	6.9	0.0%	0.85	No	0.00	3	0.62	0.045	3.13
	North Memorial Medical Center, Robbinsdale	6.3	0.0%	1.10	No	0.07	4	0.87	0.040	2.43
	St. Cloud Hospital, St. Cloud	6.5	0.0%	0.96	No	0.00	3	0.87	0.022	3.03
	St. Luke's Hospital, Duluth	2.7	0.0%	1.59	No	0.03	3	0.34	0.050	4.84
	St. Paul-Ramsey Medical Center, St. Paul	8.1	0.0%	1.29	Yes	0.57	4	0.37	0.020	1.55

OTOLARYNGOLOGY

Natl. Rank	Hospital	U.S. News index	Reputational score	Hospital-wide mortality rate	COTH member	Interns and residents to beds	Technology score (of 9)	R.N.'s to beds	Board-certified internists to beds	Procedures to beds
TIER ONE										
6	Mayo Clinic, Rochester	52.8	13.7%	0.72	Yes	0.24	6	0.77	0.089	0.222
30	University of Minnesota Hospital and Clinic, Minneapolis	21.5	3.1%	0.81	Yes	0.59	8	0.86	0.133	0.267
TIER THREE										
	Abbott Northwestern Hospital, Minneapolis	7.5	0.7%	0.77	No	0.11	8	0.48	0.101	0.297
	Hennepin County Medical Center, Minneapolis	11.3	0.0%	0.77	Yes	0.91	6	0.78	0.020	0.170
	St. Paul-Ramsey Medical Center, St. Paul	9.1	0.0%	0.85	Yes	0.57	5	0.37	0.112	0.283
TIER FOUR										
	Fairview Riverside Medical Center, Minneapolis	2.8	0.0%	0.91	No	0.03	3	0.33	0.085	0.200
	Fairview Southdale Hospital, Minneapolis	4.0	0.0%	1.08	No	0.00	6	0.57	0.067	0.451
	Healtheast St. John's Hospital, Maplewood	3.3	0.0%	0.75	No	0.06	4	0.37	0.056	0.218
	Healtheast St. Joseph's Hospital, St. Paul	4.7	0.0%	0.62	No	0.04	8	0.48	0.065	0.262
	Healthone Corp, Metro Hospitals, Minneapolis	2.6	0.0%	0.81	No	0.00	1	0.60	0.025	0.048
	Methodist Hospital, St. Louis Park	4.3	0.0%	0.89	No	0.00	5	0.62	0.092	0.235
	Miller-Dwan Medical Center, Duluth	4.5	0.0%	0.68	No	0.00	4	0.36	0.230	0.212
	North Memorial Medical Center, Robbinsdale	5.4	0.0%	1.27	No	0.07	7	0.87	0.072	0.225
	St. Cloud Hospital, St. Cloud	4.9	0.0%	0.98	No	0.00	6	0.87	0.055	0.373
	St. Luke's Hospital, Duluth	3.6	0.0%	1.19	No	0.03	2	0.34	0.229	0.275
	St. Mary's Medical Center, Duluth	3.1	0.0%	0.88	No	0.04	4	0.41	0.040	0.350

RHEUMATOLOGY

Natl. Rank	Hospital	U.S. News index	Reputational score	Hospital-wide mortality rate	COTH member	Interns and residents to beds	Technology score (of 5)	R.N.'s to beds	Board-certified internists to beds
TIER ONE									
1	Mayo Clinic, Rochester	100.0	38.7%	0.72	Yes	0.24	4	0.77	0.089
TIER TWO									
84	Hennepin County Medical Center, Minneapolis	15.9	0.4%	0.77	Yes	0.91	3	0.78	0.020
43	University of Minnesota Hospital and Clinic, Minneapolis	18.7	1.4%	0.81	Yes	0.59	4	0.86	0.133
TIER THREE									
	Abbott Northwestern Hospital, Minneapolis	11.5	0.5%	0.77	No	0.11	4	0.48	0.101
	Healtheast St. Joseph's Hospital, St. Paul	9.8	0.0%	0.62	No	0.04	4	0.48	0.065
	St. Paul-Ramsey Medical Center, St. Paul	14.0	0.0%	0.85	Yes	0.57	4	0.37	0.112
TIER FOUR									
	Fairview Riverside Medical Center, Minneapolis	8.2	0.0%	0.91	No	0.03	3	0.33	0.085
	Fairview Southdale Hospital, Minneapolis	7.0	0.0%	1.08	No	0.00	3	0.57	0.067
	Healtheast St. John's Hospital, Maplewood	9.5	0.0%	0.75	No	0.06	4	0.37	0.056
	Healthone Corp. Metro Hospitals, Minneapolis	8.8	0.0%	0.81	No	0.00	2	0.60	0.025
	Methodist Hospital, St. Louis Park	9.2	0.0%	0.89	No	0.00	3	0.62	0.092
	North Memorial Medical Center, Robbinsdale	7.3	0.0%	1.27	No	0.07	4	0.87	0.072

Natl. Rank	Hospital	U.S. News index	Reputa-tional score	Hospital-wide mortality rate	COTH member	Interns and residents to beds	Tech-nology score (of 5)	R.N.'s to beds	Board-certified internists to beds
	St. Cloud Hospital, St. Cloud	8.6	0.0%	0.98	No	0.00	3	0.87	0.055
	St. Luke's Hospital, Duluth	5.9	0.0%	1.19	No	0.03	3	0.34	0.229
	St. Mary's Medical Center, Duluth	8.5	0.0%	0.88	No	0.04	3	0.41	0.040

UROLOGY

Natl. Rank	Hospital	U.S. News index	Reputa-tional score	Urology mortality rate	COTH member	Interns and residents to beds	Tech-nology score (of 11)	R.N.'s to beds	Board-certified internists to beds	Procedures to beds
	TIER ONE									
2	Mayo Clinic, Rochester	89.7	56.6%	0.74	Yes	0.24	8	0.77	0.060	2.84
	TIER TWO									
74	Hennepin County Medical Center, Minneapolis	16.2	0.0%	0.58	Yes	0.91	7	0.78	0.020	1.66
40	University of Minnesota Hospital and Clinic, Minneapolis	19.0	1.5%	0.73	Yes	0.59	10	0.86	0.133	2.14
	TIER THREE									
	Abbott Northwestern Hospital, Minneapolis	10.7	0.0%	0.78	No	0.11	10	0.48	0.101	1.91
	Healtheast St. Joseph's Hospital, St. Paul	10.9	0.0%	0.51	No	0.04	10	0.48	0.065	1.23
	Healthone Corp. Metro Hospitals, Minneapolis	8.7	0.0%	0.23	No	0.00	3	0.60	0.025	0.46
	Methodist Hospital, St. Louis Park	9.8	0.6%	0.85	No	0.00	7	0.62	0.092	2.07
	St. Cloud Hospital, St. Cloud	10.2	0.0%	0.80	No	0.00	8	0.87	0.055	1.63
	St. Mary's Medical Center, Duluth	9.7	0.0%	0.45	No	0.04	5	0.41	0.040	2.57
	St. Paul-Ramsey Medical Center, St. Paul	14.3	0.0%	0.23	Yes	0.57	6	0.37	0.112	1.59
	TIER FOUR									
	Fairview Riverside Medical Center, Minneapolis	5.8	0.0%	1.01	No	0.03	5	0.33	0.085	0.82
	Fairview Southdale Hospital, Minneapolis	8.0	0.0%	0.92	No	0.00	7	0.57	0.067	2.46
	Healtheast St. John's Hospital, Maplewood	5.6	0.0%	1.11	No	0.06	6	0.37	0.056	2.32
	North Memorial Medical Center, Robbinsdale	5.7	0.0%	1.36	No	0.07	8	0.87	0.072	1.22
	St. Luke's Hospital, Duluth	5.1	0.0%	1.18	No	0.03	4	0.34	0.229	2.30

AIDS

Natl. Rank Hospital	U.S. News index	Reputa-tional score	Hospital-wide mortality rate	COTH member	Interns and residents to beds	Tech-nology score (of 11)	Discharge planning (of 2)	R.N.'s to beds	Board-certified internists to beds
TIER FOUR									
Memorial Hospital at Gulfport, Gulfport	17.5	0.0%	1.21	No	0.00	5	2	1.36	0.017
Methodist Medical Center, Jackson	15.8	0.0%	1.26	No	0.00	5	2	0.68	0.014
Mississippi Baptist Medical Center, Jackson	17.2	0.0%	1.19	No	0.00	6	2	0.72	0.039
North Mississippi Medical Center, Tupelo	14.7	0.0%	1.42	No	0.00	5	2	0.87	0.012
University Hospitals and Clinics, University Ctr., Jackson	18.6	0.0%	1.54	Yes	1.15	7	2	0.93	0.016

CANCER

Natl. Rank Hospital	U.S. News index	Reputa-tional score	Cancer mortality rate	COTH member	Interns and residents to beds	Tech-nology score (of 12)	R.N.'s to beds	Board-certified oncologists to beds	Procedures to beds
TIER THREE									
University Hospitals and Clinics, University Ctr., Jackson	9.5	0.0%	1.09	Yes	1.15	6	0.93	0.002	1.08
TIER FOUR									
Memorial Hospital at Gulfport, Gulfport	4.5	0.0%	1.09	No	0.00	6	1.36	0.007	1.45
Methodist Medical Center, Jackson	2.8	0.0%	1.43	No	0.00	7	0.68	0.021	1.78
Mississippi Baptist Medical Center, Jackson	3.5	0.0%	1.10	No	0.00	8	0.72	0.010	2.63
North Mississippi Medical Center, Tupelo	2.9	0.0%	1.45	No	0.00	6	0.87	0.003	1.48

CARDIOLOGY

Natl. Rank Hospital	U.S. News index	Reputa-tional score	Cardiology mortality rate	COTH member	Interns and residents to beds	Tech-nology score (of 10)	R.N.'s to beds	Board-certified cardiologists to beds	Procedures to beds
TIER FOUR									
Memorial Hospital at Gulfport, Gulfport	10.6	0.0%	1.23	No	0.00	6	1.36	0.020	9.16
Methodist Medical Center, Jackson	11.7	0.0%	1.03	No	0.00	4	0.68	0.029	6.33
Mississippi Baptist Medical Center, Jackson	9.7	0.0%	1.17	No	0.00	7	0.72	0.013	6.19
North Mississippi Medical Center, Tupelo	4.3	0.0%	1.58	No	0.00	6	0.87	0.006	6.44
University Hospitals and Clinics, University Ctr., Jackson	11.7	0.5%	1.63	Yes	1.15	7	0.93	0.014	2.02

ENDOCRINOLOGY

Natl. Rank Hospital	U.S. News index	Reputa-tional score	Endocrinology mortality rate	COTH member	Interns and residents to beds	Tech-nology score (of 11)	R.N.'s to beds	Board-certified internists to beds
TIER THREE								
University Hospitals and Clinics, University Ctr., Jackson	10.5	0.0%	1.47	Yes	1.15	6	0.93	0.016
TIER FOUR								
Memorial Hospital at Gulfport, Gulfport	5.3	0.0%	1.55	No	0.00	7	1.36	0.017
Methodist Medical Center, Jackson	3.3	0.0%	1.59	No	0.00	7	0.68	0.014
Mississippi Baptist Medical Center, Jackson	3.8	0.0%	1.51	No	0.00	7	0.72	0.039
North Mississippi Medical Center, Tupelo	4.4	0.0%	1.41	No	0.00	7	0.87	0.012

GASTROENTEROLOGY

Natl. Rank	Hospital	U.S. News index	Reputational score	Gastroenterology mortality rate	COTH member	Interns and residents to beds	Technology score (of 11)	R.N.'s to beds	Board-certified gastroenterologists to beds	Procedures to beds
	TIER FOUR									
	Memorial Hospital at Gulfport, Gulfport	5.7	0.0%	1.49	No	0.00	7	1.36	0.007	4.08
	Methodist Medical Center, Jackson	4.6	0.0%	1.33	No	0.00	6	0.68	0.007	4.43
	Mississippi Baptist Medical Center, Jackson	5.4	0.0%	1.10	No	0.00	6	0.72	0.013	3.68
	North Mississippi Medical Center, Tupelo	4.3	0.0%	1.53	No	0.00	7	0.87	0.006	3.90

GERIATRICS

Natl. Rank	Hospital	U.S. News index	Reputational score	Hospital-wide mortality rate	COTH member	Service mix	Interns and residents to beds	Technology score (of 13)	R.N.'s to beds	Discharge planning (of 2)	Geriatric services (of 9)	Board-certified internists to beds
	TIER FOUR											
	Memorial Hospital at Gulfport, Gulfport	9.4	0.0%	1.21	No	4	0.00	8	1.36	2	1	0.017
	Methodist Medical Center, Jackson	7.5	0.0%	1.26	No	4	0.00	9	0.68	2	2	0.014
	Mississippi Baptist Medical Center, Jackson	9.4	0.0%	1.19	No	4	0.00	10	0.72	2	2	0.039
	North Mississippi Medical Center, Tupelo	6.2	0.0%	1.42	No	7	0.00	8	0.87	2	1	0.012
	University Hospitals and Clinics, University Ctr., Jackson	9.9	0.0%	1.54	Yes	7	1.15	8	0.93	2	2	0.016

GYNECOLOGY

Natl. Rank	Hospital	U.S. News index	Reputational score	Hospital-wide mortality rate	Interns and residents to beds	Technology score (of 10)	R.N.'s to beds	Board-certified OB-GYNs to beds	Procedures to beds
	TIER FOUR								
	Memorial Hospital at Gulfport, Gulfport	10.1	0.0%	1.21	0.00	4	1.36	0.020	0.32
	Methodist Medical Center, Jackson	8.1	0.4%	1.26	0.00	5	0.68	0.032	0.52
	Mississippi Baptist Medical Center, Jackson	9.6	0.4%	1.19	0.00	5	0.72	0.026	0.89
	North Mississippi Medical Center, Tupelo	5.0	0.0%	1.42	0.00	5	0.87	0.010	0.34
	University Hospitals and Clinics, University Ctr., Jackson	9.6	0.4%	1.54	1.15	4	0.93	0.022	0.56

NEUROLOGY

Natl. Rank	Hospital	U.S. News index	Reputational score	Neurology mortality rate	COTH member	Interns and residents to beds	Technology score (of 9)	R.N.'s to beds	Board-certified neurologists to beds
	TIER THREE								
	University Hospitals and Clinics, University Ctr., Jackson	11.6	0.0%	1.26	Yes	1.15	4	0.93	0.010
	TIER FOUR								
	Memorial Hospital at Gulfport, Gulfport	7.1	0.0%	1.24	No	0.00	5	1.36	0.007
	Methodist Medical Center, Jackson	5.5	0.0%	1.22	No	0.00	5	0.68	0.007
	Mississippi Baptist Medical Center, Jackson	6.6	0.0%	1.12	No	0.00	5	0.72	0.005
	North Mississippi Medical Center, Tupelo	5.7	0.0%	1.23	No	0.00	5	0.87	0.004

ORTHOPEDICS

Natl. Rank Hospital	U.S. News index	Reputa-tional score	Orthopedics mortality rate	COTH member	Interns and residents to beds	Tech-nology score (of 5)	R.N.'s to beds	Board-certified orthopedists to beds	Pro-cedures to beds
TIER THREE									
University Hospitals and Clinics, University Ctr., Jackson	12.7	0.6%	1.15	Yes	1.15	3	0.93	0.014	1.11
TIER FOUR									
Memorial Hospital at Gulfport, Gulfport	7.5	0.0%	0.96	No	0.00	3	1.36	0.020	2.10
Methodist Medical Center, Jackson	2.4	0.0%	1.66	No	0.00	3	0.68	0.018	1.81
Mississippi Baptist Medical Center, Jackson	4.8	0.0%	1.09	No	0.00	3	0.72	0.018	1.67
North Mississippi Medical Center, Tupelo	4.8	0.0%	1.18	No	0.00	3	0.87	0.006	2.44

OTOLARYNGOLOGY

Natl. Rank Hospital	U.S. News index	Reputa-tional score	Hospital-wide mortality rate	COTH member	Interns and residents to beds	Tech-nology score (of 9)	R.N.'s to beds	Board-certified internists to beds	Procedures to beds
TIER THREE									
University Hospitals and Clinics, University Ctr., Jackson	11.6	0.0%	1.54	Yes	1.15	4	0.93	0.016	0.117
TIER FOUR									
Memorial Hospital at Gulfport, Gulfport	6.8	0.4%	1.21	No	0.00	5	1.36	0.017	0.275
Methodist Medical Center, Jackson	3.5	0.0%	1.26	No	0.00	5	0.68	0.014	0.279
Mississippi Baptist Medical Center, Jackson	3.9	0.0%	1.19	No	0.00	5	0.72	0.039	0.244
North Mississippi Medical Center, Tupelo	4.0	0.0%	1.42	No	0.00	5	0.87	0.012	0.239

RHEUMATOLOGY

Natl. Rank Hospital	U.S. News index	Reputa-tional score	Hospital-wide mortality rate	COTH member	Interns and residents to beds	Tech-nology score (of 5)	R.N.'s to beds	Board-certified internists to beds
TIER THREE								
University Hospitals and Clinics, University Ctr., Jackson	11.2	0.0%	1.54	Yes	1.15	3	0.93	0.016
TIER FOUR								
Memorial Hospital at Gulfport, Gulfport	7.9	0.0%	1.21	No	0.00	3	1.36	0.017
Methodist Medical Center, Jackson	5.7	0.0%	1.26	No	0.00	3	0.68	0.014
Mississippi Baptist Medical Center, Jackson	6.5	0.0%	1.19	No	0.00	3	0.72	0.039
North Mississippi Medical Center, Tupelo	5.4	0.0%	1.42	No	0.00	3	0.87	0.012

UROLOGY

Natl. Rank Hospital	U.S. News index	Reputa-tional score	Urology mortality rate	COTH member	Interns and residents to beds	Tech-nology score (of 11)	R.N.'s to beds	Board-certified internists to beds	Procedures to beds
TIER THREE									
University Hospitals and Clinics, University Ctr., Jackson	11.5	0.0%	1.28	Yes	1.15	6	0.93	0.016	1.09
TIER FOUR									
Memorial Hospital at Gulfport, Gulfport	7.6	0.0%	1.15	No	0.00	7	1.36	0.017	2.08
Methodist Medical Center, Jackson	3.8	0.0%	1.49	No	0.00	6	0.68	0.014	2.36
Mississippi Baptist Medical Center, Jackson	6.0	0.0%	1.12	No	0.00	6	0.72	0.039	1.85
North Mississippi Medical Center, Tupelo	3.4	0.0%	1.79	No	0.00	7	0.87	0.012	2.01

AIDS

Natl. Rank	Hospital	U.S. News index	Reputa-tional score	Hospital-wide mortality rate	COTH member	Interns and residents to beds	Tech-nology score (of 11)	Discharge planning (of 2)	R.N.'s to beds	Board-certified internists to beds
		TIER ONE								
22	Barnes Hospital, St. Louis	30.8	4.0%	0.98	Yes	0.89	9	2	0.82	0.273
		TIER THREE								
	AMI Lucy Lee Hospital, Poplar Bluff	20.8	0.0%	0.92	No	0.00	7	2	0.34	0.017
	Boone Hospital Center, Columbia	20.0	0.0%	1.02	No	0.00	7	2	0.82	0.039
98	Jewish Hospital of St. Louis	24.6	0.0%	0.97	Yes	0.63	7	2	1.22	0.100
	Missouri Baptist Medical Ctr., Town and Country, St. Louis	20.6	0.0%	1.00	No	0.00	8	2	0.84	0.039
	St. John's Mercy Medical Center, St. Louis	24.6	0.0%	0.82	Yes	0.19	8	2	0.66	0.052
	St. John's Regional Health Center, Springfield	22.6	0.0%	0.89	No	0.00	7	2	0.87	0.097
	St. Joseph Health Center, St. Charles	22.0	0.0%	0.68	No	0.00	6	2	0.77	0.061
	St. Louis University Hospital	23.9	0.0%	1.24	Yes	1.89	8	2	1.33	0.057
	St. Luke's Hospital, Chesterfield	20.3	0.0%	1.01	No	0.17	6	2	0.83	0.077
	St. Luke's Hospital, Kansas City	22.4	0.0%	1.00	Yes	0.25	7	2	0.81	0.034
	Truman Medical Center-West, Kansas City	19.8	0.0%	1.37	Yes	0.54	7	2	1.52	0.056
	University Hospitals and Clinics, Columbia	21.7	0.0%	1.25	Yes	1.10	8	2	1.19	0.015
		TIER FOUR								
	Baptist Medical Center, Kansas City	16.6	0.0%	1.18	No	0.11	6	1	0.64	0.048
	Bethesda General Hospital, St. Louis	13.9	0.0%	1.28	No	0.10	4	1	0.22	0.000
	De Paul Health Center, St. Louis	19.3	0.0%	1.04	No	0.00	7	2	0.55	0.058
	Deaconess Hospital, St. Louis	17.9	0.0%	1.26	No	0.37	5	2	0.99	0.227
	Independence Regional Health Center, Independence	17.8	0.0%	1.07	No	0.00	5	2	0.40	0.012
	Kirksville Osteo Medical Center, Kirksville	18.0	0.0%	1.07	No	0.13	5	2	0.41	0.017
	Lester E. Cox Medical Centers, Springfield	18.8	0.0%	1.10	No	0.04	6	2	0.96	0.033
	Lutheran Medical Center, St. Louis	17.6	0.0%	1.13	No	0.00	7	2	0.39	0.020
	Menorah Medical Center, Kansas City	18.8	0.0%	1.07	No	0.03	6	2	0.58	0.126
	North Kansas City Hospital, North Kansas City	16.6	0.0%	1.26	No	0.00	7	1	1.07	0.037
	Phelps County Regional Medical Center, Rolla	17.2	0.0%	1.15	No	0.02	6	2	0.46	0.032
	Research Medical Center, Kansas City	19.2	0.0%	1.09	No	0.02	6	2	1.02	0.113
	Southeast Missouri Hospital, Cape Girardeau	16.4	0.0%	1.35	No	0.00	8	2	0.88	0.015
	St. Anthony's Medical Center, St. Louis	18.0	0.0%	1.12	No	0.00	7	2	0.56	0.028
	St. Francis Medical Center, Cape Girardeau	15.1	0.0%	1.41	No	0.00	6	2	0.83	0.027
	St. John's Regional Medical Center, Joplin	15.7	0.0%	1.38	No	0.00	6	2	1.00	0.030
	St. Joseph Health Center, Kansas City	19.2	0.0%	1.05	No	0.00	6	2	0.80	0.048
	St. Joseph Hospital, St. Louis	17.1	0.0%	1.20	No	0.00	6	2	0.74	0.050
	St. Louis Regional Medical Center	18.7	0.0%	1.09	No	0.19	5	2	0.92	0.048
	St. Mary's Health Center, Jefferson City	17.2	0.0%	1.17	No	0.00	6	2	0.74	0.013
	St. Mary's Health Center, St. Louis	18.7	0.0%	1.06	No	0.15	5	2	0.62	0.055
	Trinity Lutheran Hospital, Kansas City	19.4	0.4%	1.07	No	0.09	7	2	0.56	0.036
	Truman Medical Center-East, Kansas City	19.4	0.0%	0.91	No	0.09	2	2	0.25	0.040

CANCER

Natl. Rank	Hospital	U.S. News index	Reputa-tional score	Cancer mortality rate	COTH member	Interns and residents to beds	Tech-nology score (of 12)	R.N.'s to beds	Board-certified oncologists to beds	Procedures to beds
		TIER TWO								
39	Barnes Hospital, St. Louis	13.9	2.7%	0.65	Yes	0.89	11	0.82	0.000	1.66
33	St. Louis University Hospital	14.7	0.0%	0.82	Yes	1.89	10	1.33	0.016	1.61
		TIER THREE								
94	Jewish Hospital of St. Louis	10.4	0.0%	0.88	Yes	0.63	10	1.22	0.045	1.90
	St. John's Mercy Medical Center, St. Louis	7.0	0.0%	0.71	Yes	0.19	9	0.66	0.007	1.48
	St. Luke's Hospital, Kansas City	7.3	0.0%	0.94	Yes	0.25	9	0.81	0.011	1.55

STATE RANKINGS ■ MISSOURI

Natl. Rank	Hospital	U.S. News index	Reputa-tional score	Cancer mortality rate	COTH member	Interns and residents to beds	Tech-nology score (of 12)	R.N.'s to beds	Board-certified oncologists to beds	Procedures to beds
	Truman Medical Center-West, Kansas City	8.5	0.0%	1.22	Yes	0.54	4	1.52	0.019	0.81
92	University Hospitals and Clinics, Columbia	10.4	0.0%	0.76	Yes	1.10	6	1.19	0.020	0.46
TIER FOUR										
	AMI Lucy Lee Hospital, Poplar Bluff	2.3	0.0%	0.97	No	0.00	8	0.34	0.006	1.08
	Baptist Medical Center, Kansas City	2.6	0.0%	0.93	No	0.11	5	0.64	0.006	0.94
	Boone Hospital Center, Columbia	4.6	0.0%	0.72	No	0.00	9	0.82	0.026	1.95
	De Paul Health Center, St. Louis	2.7	0.0%	1.04	No	0.00	8	0.55	0.008	0.84
	Deaconess Hospital, St. Louis	4.8	0.0%	1.12	No	0.37	6	0.99	0.008	2.29
	Independence Regional Health Center, Independence	1.9	0.0%	0.72	No	0.00	5	0.40	0.006	1.07
	Lester E. Cox Medical Centers, Springfield	4.0	0.0%	0.87	No	0.04	7	0.96	0.006	1.10
	Menorah Medical Center, Kansas City	3.5	0.0%	0.65	No	0.03	8	0.58	0.014	0.88
	Missouri Baptist Medical Ctr., Town and Country, St. Louis	4.8	0.0%	0.70	No	0.00	10	0.84	0.013	1.73
	North Kansas City Hospital, North Kansas City	4.3	0.0%	1.07	No	0.00	8	1.07	0.012	1.58
	Phelps County Regional Medical Center, Rolla	2.6	0.0%	1.06	No	0.02	8	0.46	0.014	1.08
	Research Medical Center, Kansas City	4.2	0.0%	0.93	No	0.02	7	1.02	0.023	1.66
	Southeast Missouri Hospital, Cape Girardeau	3.8	0.0%	1.37	No	0.00	9	0.88	0.008	1.08
	St. Anthony's Medical Center, St. Louis	3.5	0.0%	0.90	No	0.00	10	0.56	0.005	0.96
	St. Francis Medical Center, Cape Girardeau	2.3	0.0%	1.22	No	0.00	4	0.83	0.004	1.15
	St. John's Regional Health Center, Springfield	4.7	0.0%	0.66	No	0.00	9	0.87	0.010	1.77
	St. John's Regional Medical Center, Joplin	4.0	0.0%	1.42	No	0.00	8	1.00	0.015	1.95
	St. Joseph Health Center, Kansas City	3.1	0.0%	0.77	No	0.00	5	0.80	0.012	1.65
	St. Joseph Health Center, St. Charles	3.7	0.0%	0.62	No	0.00	7	0.77	0.014	1.00
	St. Joseph Hospital, St. Louis	2.9	0.0%	1.28	No	0.00	7	0.74	0.013	1.26
	St. Luke's Hospital, Chesterfield	4.4	0.0%	0.86	No	0.17	8	0.83	0.014	1.31
	St. Mary's Health Center, Jefferson City	3.2	0.0%	0.76	No	0.00	6	0.74	0.007	1.73
	St. Mary's Health Center, St. Louis	3.3	0.0%	0.80	No	0.15	6	0.62	0.007	1.33
	Trinity Lutheran Hospital, Kansas City	2.8	0.0%	1.18	No	0.09	7	0.56	0.011	1.18

CARDIOLOGY

Natl. Rank	Hospital	U.S. News index	Reputa-tional score	Cardiology mortality rate	COTH member	Interns and residents to beds	Tech-nology score (of 10)	R.N.'s to beds	Board-certified cardiologists to beds	Procedures to beds
TIER ONE										
20	Barnes Hospital, St. Louis	28.8	6.9%	1.06	Yes	0.89	10	0.82	0.000	5.45
TIER TWO										
52	Jewish Hospital of St. Louis	22.9	0.4%	0.94	Yes	0.63	8	1.22	0.045	9.90
45	St. Louis University Hospital	23.6	0.9%	1.22	Yes	1.89	10	1.33	0.092	10.57
TIER THREE										
	Missouri Baptist Medical Ctr., Town and Country, St. Louis	14.1	0.0%	1.03	No	0.00	10	0.84	0.024	8.45
	St. John's Mercy Medical Center, St. Louis	20.4	0.0%	0.76	Yes	0.19	9	0.66	0.022	3.22
	St. John's Regional Health Center, Springfield	13.9	0.0%	1.01	No	0.00	8	0.87	0.014	8.92
	St. Joseph Health Center, Kansas City	14.2	0.0%	1.01	No	0.00	8	0.80	0.040	7.33
	St. Joseph Health Center, St. Charles	16.9	0.0%	0.82	No	0.00	7	0.77	0.025	4.81
	St. Luke's Hospital, Kansas City	20.3	0.0%	0.94	Yes	0.25	9	0.81	0.052	10.62
	Truman Medical Center-West, Kansas City	16.0	0.0%	1.18	Yes	0.54	6	1.52	0.014	3.92
	University Hospitals and Clinics, Columbia	14.1	0.0%	1.50	Yes	1.10	9	1.19	0.033	5.74
TIER FOUR										
	Baptist Medical Center, Kansas City	10.5	0.0%	1.15	No	0.11	8	0.64	0.019	4.08
	Boone Hospital Center, Columbia	10.4	0.0%	1.19	No	0.00	8	0.82	0.026	10.11
	De Paul Health Center, St. Louis	11.0	0.0%	1.11	No	0.00	8	0.55	0.041	4.59
	Deaconess Hospital, St. Louis	10.9	0.0%	1.22	No	0.37	6	0.99	0.019	7.43
	Independence Regional Health Center, Independence	6.6	0.0%	1.30	No	0.00	7	0.40	0.012	5.36
	Lester E. Cox Medical Centers, Springfield	9.2	0.0%	1.28	No	0.04	8	0.96	0.016	6.33
	Menorah Medical Center, Kansas City	12.6	0.0%	1.04	No	0.03	8	0.58	0.032	4.64
	North Kansas City Hospital, North Kansas City	9.3	0.0%	1.31	No	0.00	9	1.07	0.019	7.29

Natl. Rank Hospital	U.S. News index	Reputa- tional score	Cardiology mortality rate	COTH member	Interns and residents to beds	Tech- nology score (of 10)	R.N.'s to beds	Board- certified cardiologists to beds	Procedures to beds
Phelps County Regional Medical Center, Rolla	9.5	0.0%	1.12	No	0.02	4	0.46	0.041	5.57
Research Medical Center, Kansas City	10.6	0.0%	1.16	No	0.02	6	1.02	0.019	6.64
Southeast Missouri Hospital, Cape Girardeau	6.2	0.0%	1.53	No	0.00	9	0.88	0.019	8.36
St. Anthony's Medical Center, St. Louis	9.9	0.0%	1.17	No	0.00	9	0.56	0.018	4.83
St. Francis Medical Center, Cape Girardeau	3.4	0.0%	1.78	No	0.00	8	0.83	0.019	6.28
St. John's Regional Medical Center, Joplin	8.7	0.0%	1.34	No	0.00	8	1.00	0.024	11.30
St. Joseph Hospital, St. Louis	9.6	0.0%	1.26	No	0.00	8	0.74	0.059	8.09
St. Luke's Hospital, Chesterfield	10.6	0.0%	1.24	No	0.17	8	0.83	0.057	6.01
St. Mary's Health Center, Jefferson City	10.8	0.0%	1.17	No	0.00	8	0.74	0.034	10.51
St. Mary's Health Center, St. Louis	11.8	0.0%	1.10	No	0.15	8	0.62	0.018	6.51
Trinity Lutheran Hospital, Kansas City	8.7	0.0%	1.20	No	0.09	6	0.56	0.017	4.58

ENDOCRINOLOGY

Natl. Rank Hospital	U.S. News index	Reputa- tional score	Endocrinology mortality rate	COTH member	Interns and residents to beds	Tech- nology score (of 11)	R.N.'s to beds	Board- certified internists to beds
TIER ONE								
5 Barnes Hospital, St. Louis	39.1	17.8%	0.86	Yes	0.89	11	0.82	0.273
TIER TWO								
75 Jewish Hospital of St. Louis	15.2	0.3%	0.80	Yes	0.63	10	1.22	0.100
45 St. Louis University Hospital	17.9	0.0%	0.94	Yes	1.89	11	1.33	0.057
TIER THREE								
AMI Lucy Lee Hospital, Poplar Bluff	8.9	0.0%	0.51	No	0.00	9	0.34	0.017
Deaconess Hospital, St. Louis	9.3	0.0%	1.01	No	0.37	7	0.99	0.227
Menorah Medical Center, Kansas City	10.2	0.0%	0.67	No	0.03	9	0.58	0.126
St. John's Mercy Medical Center, St. Louis	13.1	0.0%	0.60	Yes	0.19	9	0.66	0.052
St. John's Regional Health Center, Springfield	9.0	0.0%	0.80	No	0.00	9	0.87	0.097
St. Luke's Hospital, Kansas City	9.0	0.0%	1.22	Yes	0.25	10	0.81	0.034
Truman Medical Center-West, Kansas City	9.6	0.0%	1.67	Yes	0.54	5	1.52	0.056
University Hospitals and Clinics, Columbia	12.0	0.0%	1.15	Yes	1.10	5	1.19	0.015
TIER FOUR								
Baptist Medical Center, Kansas City	4.5	0.0%	1.27	No	0.11	5	0.64	0.048
Boone Hospital Center, Columbia	7.7	0.0%	0.89	No	0.00	9	0.82	0.039
De Paul Health Center, St. Louis	5.3	0.0%	1.15	No	0.00	9	0.55	0.058
Independence Regional Health Center, Independence	4.9	0.0%	0.99	No	0.00	6	0.40	0.012
Lester E. Cox Medical Centers, Springfield	7.9	0.0%	0.90	No	0.04	8	0.96	0.033
Missouri Baptist Medical Ctr., Town and Country, St. Louis	7.7	0.0%	0.94	No	0.00	11	0.84	0.039
North Kansas City Hospital, North Kansas City	6.6	0.0%	1.15	No	0.00	9	1.07	0.037
Phelps County Regional Medical Center, Rolla	3.9	0.0%	1.38	No	0.02	9	0.46	0.032
Research Medical Center, Kansas City	8.0	0.0%	0.95	No	0.02	8	1.02	0.113
Southeast Missouri Hospital, Cape Girardeau	4.6	0.0%	1.48	No	0.00	9	0.88	0.015
St. Anthony's Medical Center, St. Louis	6.5	0.0%	0.96	No	0.00	10	0.56	0.028
St. Francis Medical Center, Cape Girardeau	6.9	0.0%	0.88	No	0.00	5	0.83	0.027
St. John's Regional Medical Center, Joplin	4.3	0.0%	1.76	No	0.00	9	1.00	0.030
St. Joseph Health Center, Kansas City	3.7	0.0%	1.58	No	0.00	6	0.80	0.048
St. Joseph Health Center, St. Charles	7.9	0.0%	0.84	No	0.00	8	0.77	0.061
St. Joseph Hospital, St. Louis	5.1	0.0%	1.24	No	0.00	8	0.74	0.050
St. Louis Regional Medical Center	3.0	0.0%	2.07	No	0.19	3	0.92	0.048
St. Luke's Hospital, Chesterfield	7.8	0.0%	0.95	No	0.17	8	0.83	0.077
St. Mary's Health Center, St. Louis	3.6	0.0%	1.72	No	0.15	7	0.62	0.055
Trinity Lutheran Hospital, Kansas City	7.3	0.0%	0.86	No	0.09	8	0.56	0.036

GASTROENTEROLOGY

Natl. Rank	Hospital	U.S. News index	Reputational score	Gastroenterology mortality rate	COTH member	Interns and residents to beds	Technology score (of 11)	R.N.'s to beds	Board-certified gastroenterologists to beds	Procedures to beds
	TIER ONE									
18	**Barnes Hospital, St. Louis**	21.4	6.1%	1.01	Yes	0.89	11	0.82	0.000	1.71
	TIER TWO									
62	Jewish Hospital of St. Louis	14.1	0.0%	0.90	Yes	0.63	9	1.22	0.022	4.02
40	St. Louis University Hospital	15.9	0.0%	1.28	Yes	1.89	10	1.33	0.032	2.50
	TIER THREE									
	Menorah Medical Center, Kansas City	7.5	0.0%	0.79	No	0.03	8	0.58	0.029	2.49
	St. John's Mercy Medical Center, St. Louis	10.3	0.0%	0.77	Yes	0.19	8	0.66	0.012	1.59
	St. John's Regional Health Center, Springfield	8.6	0.0%	0.74	No	0.00	9	0.87	0.008	3.16
	St. Luke's Hospital, Chesterfield	7.7	0.0%	0.86	No	0.17	7	0.83	0.018	2.62
	St. Luke's Hospital, Kansas City	8.4	0.0%	1.26	Yes	0.25	9	0.81	0.011	2.37
	University Hospitals and Clinics, Columbia	10.6	0.0%	1.32	Yes	1.10	6	1.19	0.013	1.41
	TIER FOUR									
	AMI Lucy Lee Hospital, Poplar Bluff	4.6	0.0%	1.08	No	0.00	8	0.34	0.000	2.78
	Baptist Medical Center, Kansas City	4.6	0.0%	1.15	No	0.11	5	0.64	0.016	3.00
	Boone Hospital Center, Columbia	5.1	0.0%	1.19	No	0.00	8	0.82	0.013	2.67
	De Paul Health Center, St. Louis	4.8	0.0%	1.08	No	0.00	8	0.55	0.023	2.10
	Deaconess Hospital, St. Louis	6.5	0.0%	1.28	No	0.37	6	0.99	0.006	3.91
	Independence Regional Health Center, Independence	3.9	0.0%	1.07	No	0.00	5	0.40	0.012	2.53
	Lester E. Cox Medical Centers, Springfield	4.7	0.0%	1.37	No	0.04	8	0.96	0.007	2.46
	Missouri Baptist Medical Ctr., Town and Country, St. Louis	6.0	0.0%	1.19	No	0.00	10	0.84	0.018	2.93
	North Kansas City Hospital, North Kansas City	4.9	0.0%	1.49	No	0.00	8	1.07	0.012	3.32
	Phelps County Regional Medical Center, Rolla	5.0	0.0%	1.21	No	0.02	9	0.46	0.000	3.46
	Research Medical Center, Kansas City	7.2	0.0%	0.95	No	0.02	7	1.02	0.010	3.21
	Southeast Missouri Hospital, Cape Girardeau	4.8	0.0%	1.30	No	0.00	8	0.88	0.019	2.67
	St. Anthony's Medical Center, St. Louis	5.1	0.0%	1.06	No	0.00	9	0.56	0.005	1.99
	St. Francis Medical Center, Cape Girardeau	4.0	0.0%	1.41	No	0.00	6	0.83	0.023	3.24
	St. John's Regional Medical Center, Joplin	4.9	0.0%	1.65	No	0.00	9	1.00	0.012	3.95
	St. Joseph Health Center, Kansas City	5.1	0.0%	1.18	No	0.00	6	0.80	0.024	3.53
	St. Joseph Health Center, St. Charles	7.1	0.0%	0.81	No	0.00	7	0.77	0.022	1.87
	St. Joseph Hospital, St. Louis	4.8	0.0%	1.26	No	0.00	7	0.74	0.029	3.41
	St. Mary's Health Center, Jefferson City	3.4	0.0%	1.63	No	0.00	6	0.74	0.020	3.70
	St. Mary's Health Center, St. Louis	5.4	0.0%	1.09	No	0.15	6	0.62	0.018	3.07
	Trinity Lutheran Hospital, Kansas City	5.1	0.0%	1.06	No	0.09	7	0.56	0.020	2.34

GERIATRICS

Natl. Rank	Hospital	U.S. News index	Reputational score	Hospital-wide mortality rate	COTH member	Service mix	Interns and residents to beds	Technology score (of 13)	R.N.'s to beds	Discharge planning (of 2)	Geriatric services (of 9)	Board-certified internists to beds
	TIER ONE											
17	**Barnes Hospital, St. Louis**	32.5	3.4%	0.98	Yes	10	0.89	13	0.82	2	4	0.273
	TIER TWO											
40	Jewish Hospital of St. Louis	26.0	1.0%	0.97	Yes	9	0.63	11	1.22	2	7	0.100
63	St. John's Mercy Medical Center, St. Louis	23.1	0.0%	0.82	Yes	9	0.19	11	0.66	2	6	0.052
35	St. Louis University Hospital	26.5	3.2%	1.24	Yes	6	1.89	12	1.33	2	5	0.057
	TIER THREE											
	Boone Hospital Center, Columbia	14.7	0.0%	1.02	No	5	0.00	11	0.82	2	4	0.039
	De Paul Health Center, St. Louis	13.9	0.0%	1.04	No	6	0.00	10	0.55	2	4	0.058
	Lester E. Cox Medical Centers, Springfield	15.1	0.0%	1.10	No	9	0.04	10	0.96	2	6	0.033
	Missouri Baptist Medical Ctr., Town and Country, St. Louis	15.8	0.0%	1.00	No	8	0.00	12	0.84	2	1	0.039
	St. John's Regional Health Center, Springfield	19.7	0.0%	0.89	No	6	0.00	10	0.87	2	6	0.097
	St. Joseph Health Center, St. Charles	19.6	0.0%	0.68	No	7	0.00	9	0.77	2	6	0.061
	St. Luke's Hospital, Chesterfield	17.5	0.0%	1.01	No	9	0.17	11	0.83	2	5	0.077

Natl. Rank	Hospital	U.S. News index	Reputa-tional score	Hospital-wide mortality rate	COTH member	Service mix	Interns and residents to beds	Technology score (of 13)	R.N.'s to beds	Discharge planning (of 2)	Geriatric services (of 9)	Board-certified internists to beds
	St. Luke's Hospital, Kansas City	18.4	0.0%	1.00	Yes	7	0.25	11	0.81	2	3	0.034
	St. Mary's Health Center, St. Louis	14.9	0.0%	1.06	No	9	0.15	9	0.62	2	4	0.055
	University Hospitals and Clinics, Columbia	15.1	0.0%	1.25	Yes	8	1.10	8	1.19	2	3	0.015
	TIER FOUR											
	Baptist Medical Center, Kansas City	10.2	0.0%	1.18	No	7	0.11	7	0.64	1	6	0.048
	Deaconess Hospital, St. Louis	12.1	0.0%	1.26	No	7	0.37	9	0.99	2	5	0.227
	Independence Regional Health Center, Independence	12.8	0.0%	1.07	No	7	0.00	7	0.40	2	5	0.012
	Menorah Medical Center, Kansas City	12.6	0.0%	1.07	No	4	0.03	10	0.58	2	4	0.126
	Phelps County Regional Medical Center, Rolla	9.7	0.0%	1.15	No	5	0.02	8	0.46	2	2	0.032
	Research Medical Center, Kansas City	13.6	0.0%	1.09	No	6	0.02	8	1.02	2	5	0.113
	Southeast Missouri Hospital, Cape Girardeau	7.4	0.0%	1.35	No	6	0.00	11	0.88	2	1	0.015
	St. Anthony's Medical Center, St. Louis	13.1	0.0%	1.12	No	7	0.00	12	0.56	2	6	0.028
	St. Francis Medical Center, Cape Girardeau	4.9	0.0%	1.41	No	4	0.00	6	0.83	2	2	0.027
	St. John's Regional Medical Center, Joplin	8.4	0.0%	1.38	No	6	0.00	10	1.00	2	6	0.030
	St. Joseph Health Center, Kansas City	11.8	0.0%	1.05	No	3	0.00	7	0.80	2	2	0.048
	St. Joseph Hospital, St. Louis	9.8	0.0%	1.20	No	6	0.00	9	0.74	2	2	0.050
	St. Mary's Health Center, Jefferson City	9.5	0.0%	1.17	No	5	0.00	8	0.74	2	2	0.013
	Trinity Lutheran Hospital, Kansas City	12.7	0.0%	1.07	No	7	0.09	8	0.56	2	2	0.036

GYNECOLOGY

Natl. Rank	Hospital	U.S. News index	Reputa-tional score	Hospital-wide mortality rate	Interns and residents to beds	Technology score (of 10)	R.N.'s to beds	Board-certified OB-GYNs to beds	Procedures to beds
	TIER ONE								
26	Barnes Hospital, St. Louis	32.1	4.0%	0.98	0.89	9	0.82	0.071	0.56
	TIER TWO								
78	Jewish Hospital of St. Louis	22.7	0.0%	0.97	0.63	8	1.22	0.118	0.23
	TIER THREE								
	Missouri Baptist Medical Ctr., Town and Country, St. Louis	16.8	0.0%	1.00	0.00	9	0.84	0.055	0.28
94	St. John's Mercy Medical Center, St. Louis	21.5	0.5%	0.82	0.19	8	0.66	0.075	0.36
	St. John's Regional Health Center, Springfield	19.0	0.0%	0.89	0.00	8	0.87	0.021	0.57
	St. Joseph Health Center, St. Charles	17.7	0.0%	0.68	0.00	6	0.77	0.039	0.17
96	St. Louis University Hospital	21.3	0.0%	1.24	1.89	9	1.33	0.019	0.29
	St. Luke's Hospital, Chesterfield	16.4	0.0%	1.01	0.17	6	0.83	0.147	0.43
	St. Luke's Hospital, Kansas City	17.7	0.0%	1.00	0.25	9	0.81	0.041	0.59
	University Hospitals and Clinics, Columbia	15.3	0.0%	1.25	1.10	6	1.19	0.041	0.19
	TIER FOUR								
	Baptist Medical Center, Kansas City	8.9	0.0%	1.18	0.11	5	0.64	0.032	0.24
	Boone Hospital Center, Columbia	14.0	0.0%	1.02	0.00	7	0.82	0.016	0.59
	De Paul Health Center, St. Louis	13.6	0.0%	1.04	0.00	7	0.55	0.071	0.24
	Deaconess Hospital, St. Louis	11.1	0.0%	1.26	0.37	5	0.99	0.075	0.43
	Independence Regional Health Center, Independence	9.2	0.0%	1.07	0.00	4	0.40	0.030	0.43
	Lester E. Cox Medical Centers, Springfield	13.3	0.0%	1.10	0.04	7	0.96	0.034	0.34
	Menorah Medical Center, Kansas City	12.5	0.0%	1.07	0.03	7	0.58	0.051	0.34
	North Kansas City Hospital, North Kansas City	10.3	0.0%	1.26	0.00	7	1.07	0.034	0.25
	Phelps County Regional Medical Center, Rolla	9.5	0.0%	1.15	0.02	7	0.46	0.018	0.51
	Research Medical Center, Kansas City	13.8	0.0%	1.09	0.02	7	1.02	0.046	0.40
	Southeast Missouri Hospital, Cape Girardeau	8.4	0.0%	1.35	0.00	8	0.88	0.023	0.62
	St. Anthony's Medical Center, St. Louis	11.3	0.0%	1.12	0.00	8	0.56	0.025	0.28
	St. Francis Medical Center, Cape Girardeau	5.2	0.0%	1.41	0.00	5	0.83	0.019	0.16
	St. John's Regional Medical Center, Joplin	7.5	0.0%	1.38	0.00	7	1.00	0.009	0.62
	St. Joseph Health Center, Kansas City	13.5	0.0%	1.05	0.00	5	0.80	0.088	0.46
	St. Joseph Hospital, St. Louis	10.7	0.0%	1.20	0.00	6	0.74	0.101	0.52

Natl. Rank	Hospital	U.S. News index	Reputa- tional score	Hospital- wide mortality rate	Interns and residents to beds	Tech- nology score (of 10)	R.N.'s to beds	Board- certified OB-GYNs to beds	Procedures to beds
	St. Mary's Health Center, Jefferson City	9.1	0.0%	1.17	0.00	5	0.74	0.034	0.29
	St. Mary's Health Center, St. Louis	11.8	0.0%	1.06	0.15	5	0.62	0.035	0.60
	Trinity Lutheran Hospital, Kansas City	10.9	0.0%	1.07	0.09	6	0.56	0.003	0.14

NEUROLOGY

Natl. Rank	Hospital	U.S. News index	Reputa- tional score	Neurology mortality rate	COTH member	Interns and residents to beds	Tech- nology score (of 9)	R.N.'s to beds	Board- certified neurologists to beds
TIER ONE									
9	Barnes Hospital, St. Louis	39.6	12.5%	0.87	Yes	0.89	9	0.82	0.042
TIER TWO									
52	St. Louis University Hospital	19.8	0.5%	1.25	Yes	1.89	9	1.33	0.047
73	University Hospitals and Clinics, Columbia	18.3	0.0%	0.86	Yes	1.10	5	1.19	0.010
TIER THREE									
	Baptist Medical Center, Kansas City	12.2	0.0%	0.83	No	0.11	5	0.64	0.010
	Boone Hospital Center, Columbia	11.2	0.0%	0.93	No	0.00	7	0.82	0.016
	Deaconess Hospital, St. Louis	12.1	0.0%	0.94	No	0.37	5	0.99	0.019
	Independence Regional Health Center, Independence	12.4	0.0%	0.77	No	0.00	4	0.40	0.012
	Jewish Hospital of St. Louis	15.1	0.0%	1.04	Yes	0.63	8	1.22	0.018
	Lester E. Cox Medical Centers, Springfield	14.2	0.0%	0.77	No	0.04	6	0.96	0.007
	Missouri Baptist Medical Ctr., Town and Country, St. Louis	12.8	0.0%	0.86	No	0.00	9	0.84	0.011
	North Kansas City Hospital, North Kansas City	12.1	0.0%	0.90	No	0.00	7	1.07	0.012
92	St. John's Mercy Medical Center, St. Louis	17.6	0.5%	0.74	Yes	0.19	7	0.66	0.008
	St. John's Regional Health Center, Springfield	12.6	0.0%	0.84	No	0.00	7	0.87	0.008
	St. Joseph Health Center, St. Charles	14.2	0.0%	0.47	No	0.00	6	0.77	0.011
	St. Joseph Hospital, St. Louis	12.0	0.0%	0.85	No	0.00	6	0.74	0.013
	St. Luke's Hospital, Chesterfield	12.3	0.0%	0.89	No	0.17	6	0.83	0.018
95	St. Luke's Hospital, Kansas City	17.4	0.0%	0.78	Yes	0.25	8	0.81	0.009
	Trinity Lutheran Hospital, Kansas City	14.1	0.0%	0.68	No	0.09	6	0.56	0.014
TIER FOUR									
	De Paul Health Center, St. Louis	10.1	0.0%	0.96	No	0.00	7	0.55	0.019
	Menorah Medical Center, Kansas City	8.0	0.0%	1.07	No	0.03	7	0.58	0.011
	Phelps County Regional Medical Center, Rolla	6.9	0.0%	1.10	No	0.02	7	0.46	0.005
	Research Medical Center, Kansas City	7.0	0.0%	1.21	No	0.02	6	1.02	0.010
	Southeast Missouri Hospital, Cape Girardeau	10.1	0.0%	1.00	No	0.00	7	0.88	0.015
	St. Anthony's Medical Center, St. Louis	7.6	0.0%	1.08	No	0.00	8	0.56	0.005
	St. Francis Medical Center, Cape Girardeau	7.9	0.0%	1.10	No	0.00	5	0.83	0.015
	St. John's Regional Medical Center, Joplin	7.2	0.0%	1.21	No	0.00	7	1.00	0.009
	St. Joseph Health Center, Kansas City	8.1	0.0%	1.06	No	0.00	5	0.80	0.012
	St. Mary's Health Center, St. Louis	9.7	0.0%	0.97	No	0.15	5	0.62	0.015

ORTHOPEDICS

Natl. Rank	Hospital	U.S. News index	Reputa- tional score	Orthopedics mortality rate	COTH member	Interns and residents to beds	Tech- nology score (of 5)	R.N.'s to beds	Board- certified orthopedists to beds	Pro- cedures to beds
TIER TWO										
41	Barnes Hospital, St. Louis	17.5	1.9%	0.90	Yes	0.89	5	0.82	0.017	1.34
54	Jewish Hospital of St. Louis	16.2	0.0%	0.62	Yes	0.63	4	1.22	0.025	2.15
53	St. Louis University Hospital	16.2	0.0%	1.29	Yes	1.89	5	1.33	0.035	3.20
33	University Hospitals and Clinics, Columbia	18.8	0.8%	0.67	Yes	1.10	4	1.19	0.015	1.18
TIER THREE										
	AMI Lucy Lee Hospital, Poplar Bluff	8.8	0.0%	0.65	No	0.00	4	0.34	0.017	1.56
	Boone Hospital Center, Columbia	10.4	0.0%	0.61	No	0.00	4	0.82	0.039	2.26
	De Paul Health Center, St. Louis	8.5	0.0%	0.76	No	0.00	4	0.55	0.035	3.53

Natl. Rank	Hospital	U.S. News index	Reputa-tional score	Orthopedics mortality rate	COTH member	Interns and residents to beds	Tech-nology score (of 5)	R.N.'s to beds	Board-certified orthopedists to beds	Pro-cedures to beds
	Independence Regional Health Center, Independence	8.4	0.0%	0.38	No	0.00	3	0.40	0.015	1.98
99	St. John's Mercy Medical Center, St. Louis	13.1	0.0%	0.47	Yes	0.19	4	0.66	0.027	1.60
	St. Joseph Health Center, St. Charles	9.4	0.0%	0.44	No	0.00	3	0.77	0.025	1.68
	St. Luke's Hospital, Chesterfield	8.2	0.0%	0.83	No	0.17	3	0.83	0.047	2.67
	St. Luke's Hospital, Kansas City	8.5	0.0%	1.29	Yes	0.25	4	0.81	0.027	2.51
	Trinity Lutheran Hospital, Kansas City	8.5	0.0%	0.62	No	0.09	2	0.56	0.011	2.13
	TIER FOUR									
	Baptist Medical Center, Kansas City	4.2	0.0%	1.43	No	0.11	4	0.64	0.032	2.12
	Deaconess Hospital, St. Louis	6.2	0.0%	1.09	No	0.37	2	0.99	0.028	1.87
	Lester E. Cox Medical Centers, Springfield	5.2	0.0%	1.18	No	0.04	3	0.96	0.023	2.31
	Menorah Medical Center, Kansas City	5.9	0.0%	0.91	No	0.03	3	0.58	0.040	1.22
	Missouri Baptist Medical Ctr., Town and Country, St. Louis	5.9	0.0%	1.25	No	0.00	5	0.84	0.039	2.71
	North Kansas City Hospital, North Kansas City	5.7	0.0%	1.27	No	0.00	4	1.07	0.034	2.37
	Phelps County Regional Medical Center, Rolla	3.1	0.0%	1.33	No	0.02	3	0.46	0.009	2.35
	Research Medical Center, Kansas City	6.6	0.4%	1.06	No	0.02	2	1.02	0.027	3.73
	Southeast Missouri Hospital, Cape Girardeau	3.7	0.0%	1.57	No	0.00	4	0.88	0.019	1.38
	St. Anthony's Medical Center, St. Louis	4.3	0.0%	1.24	No	0.00	4	0.56	0.019	2.19
	St. Francis Medical Center, Cape Girardeau	4.3	0.0%	1.57	No	0.00	4	0.83	0.019	4.55
	St. John's Regional Health Center, Springfield	6.3	0.0%	0.99	No	0.00	3	0.87	0.022	3.35
	St. John's Regional Medical Center, Joplin	6.2	0.0%	1.04	No	0.00	3	1.00	0.021	3.05
	St. Joseph Health Center, Kansas City	7.5	0.0%	0.90	No	0.00	4	0.80	0.036	2.84
	St. Joseph Hospital, St. Louis	6.6	0.0%	1.03	No	0.00	4	0.74	0.084	2.94
	St. Mary's Health Center, Jefferson City	2.3	0.0%	2.14	No	0.00	4	0.74	0.034	2.05
	St. Mary's Health Center, St. Louis	4.5	0.0%	1.25	No	0.15	3	0.62	0.024	2.95

OTOLARYNGOLOGY

Natl. Rank	Hospital	U.S. News index	Reputa-tional score	Hospital-wide mortality rate	COTH member	Interns and residents to beds	Tech-nology score (of 9)	R.N.'s to beds	Board-certified internists to beds	Procedures to beds
	TIER ONE									
7	Barnes Hospital, St. Louis	50.7	11.5%	0.98	Yes	0.89	9	0.82	0.273	0.261
	TIER TWO									
54	St. Louis University Hospital	17.6	0.0%	1.24	Yes	1.89	9	1.33	0.057	0.282
	TIER THREE									
	Deaconess Hospital, St. Louis	7.7	0.0%	1.26	No	0.37	5	0.99	0.227	0.210
	Jewish Hospital of St. Louis	12.6	0.0%	0.97	Yes	0.63	8	1.22	0.100	0.219
	St. John's Mercy Medical Center, St. Louis	8.6	0.0%	0.82	Yes	0.19	7	0.66	0.052	0.140
	St. Luke's Hospital, Kansas City	9.2	0.0%	1.00	Yes	0.25	8	0.81	0.034	0.135
	Truman Medical Center-West, Kansas City	11.1	0.0%	1.37	Yes	0.54	3	1.52	0.056	0.158
	University Hospitals and Clinics, Columbia	13.2	0.4%	1.25	Yes	1.10	3	1.19	0.015	0.268
	TIER FOUR									
	AMI Lucy Lee Hospital, Poplar Bluff	3.3	0.0%	0.92	No	0.00	7	0.34	0.017	0.193
	Baptist Medical Center, Kansas City	3.6	0.0%	1.18	No	0.11	3	0.64	0.048	0.200
	Bethesda General Hospital, St. Louis	1.5	0.0%	1.29	No	0.10	2	0.22	0.000	0.033
	Boone Hospital Center, Columbia	4.9	0.0%	1.02	No	0.00	7	0.82	0.039	0.186
	De Paul Health Center, St. Louis	4.2	0.0%	1.04	No	0.00	7	0.55	0.058	0.108
	Independence Regional Health Center, Independence	2.5	0.0%	1.06	No	0.00	4	0.40	0.012	0.129
	Kirksville Osteo Medical Center, Kirksville	3.6	0.0%	1.07	No	0.13	6	0.41	0.017	0.130
	Lester E. Cox Medical Centers, Springfield	5.1	0.0%	1.10	No	0.04	6	0.96	0.033	0.189
	Lutheran Medical Center, St. Louis	3.6	0.0%	1.13	No	0.00	8	0.39	0.020	0.034
	Menorah Medical Center, Kansas City	4.9	0.0%	1.07	No	0.03	7	0.58	0.126	0.141
	Missouri Baptist Medical Ctr., Town and Country, St. Louis	5.5	0.0%	1.00	No	0.00	9	0.84	0.039	0.179
	North Kansas City Hospital, North Kansas City	5.5	0.0%	1.26	No	0.00	7	1.07	0.037	0.176
	Phelps County Regional Medical Center, Rolla	3.7	0.0%	1.15	No	0.02	7	0.46	0.032	0.192
	Research Medical Center, Kansas City	5.8	0.0%	1.09	No	0.02	6	1.02	0.113	0.215

Natl. Rank	Hospital	U.S. News index	Reputational score	Hospital-wide mortality rate	COTH member	Interns and residents to beds	Technology score (of 9)	R.N.'s to beds	Board-certified internists to beds	Procedures to beds
	Southeast Missouri Hospital, Cape Girardeau	4.6	0.0%	1.35	No	0.00	7	0.88	0.015	0.153
	St. Anthony's Medical Center, St. Louis	4.2	0.0%	1.12	No	0.00	8	0.56	0.028	0.130
	St. Francis Medical Center, Cape Girardeau	3.4	0.0%	1.41	No	0.00	3	0.83	0.027	0.163
	St. John's Regional Health Center, Springfield	5.6	0.0%	0.89	No	0.00	7	0.87	0.097	0.181
	St. John's Regional Medical Center, Joplin	5.1	0.0%	1.38	No	0.00	7	1.00	0.030	0.334
	St. Joseph Health Center, Kansas City	4.0	0.0%	1.04	No	0.00	4	0.80	0.048	0.219
	St. Joseph Health Center, St. Charles	4.9	0.0%	0.68	No	0.00	6	0.77	0.061	0.091
	St. Joseph Hospital, St. Louis	4.3	0.0%	1.20	No	0.00	6	0.74	0.050	0.147
	St. Louis Regional Medical Center	4.2	0.0%	1.09	No	0.19	1	0.92	0.048	0.117
	St. Luke's Hospital, Chesterfield	5.6	0.0%	1.01	No	0.17	6	0.83	0.077	0.169
	St. Mary's Health Center, Jefferson City	3.7	0.0%	1.17	No	0.00	5	0.74	0.013	0.295
	St. Mary's Health Center, St. Louis	4.4	0.0%	1.06	No	0.15	5	0.62	0.055	0.176
	Trinity Lutheran Hospital, Kansas City	4.1	0.0%	1.07	No	0.09	6	0.56	0.036	0.288
	Truman Medical Center-East, Kansas City	1.6	0.0%	0.91	No	0.09	0	0.25	0.040	0.003

RHEUMATOLOGY

Natl. Rank	Hospital	U.S. News index	Reputational score	Hospital-wide mortality rate	COTH member	Interns and residents to beds	Technology score (of 5)	R.N.'s to beds	Board-certified internists to beds
TIER ONE									
18	Barnes Hospital, St. Louis	26.0	4.4%	0.98	Yes	0.89	5	0.82	0.273
TIER TWO									
60	St. Louis University Hospital	17.3	0.0%	1.24	Yes	1.89	5	1.33	0.057
TIER THREE									
99	Jewish Hospital of St. Louis	15.0	0.0%	0.97	Yes	0.63	4	1.22	0.100
	St. John's Mercy Medical Center, St. Louis	13.2	0.0%	0.82	Yes	0.19	4	0.66	0.052
	St. John's Regional Health Center, Springfield	9.9	0.0%	0.89	No	0.00	3	0.87	0.097
	St. Joseph Health Center, St. Charles	10.0	0.0%	0.68	No	0.00	3	0.77	0.061
	St. Luke's Hospital, Kansas City	11.9	0.0%	1.00	Yes	0.25	4	0.81	0.034
	University Hospitals and Clinics, Columbia	13.6	0.0%	1.25	Yes	1.10	4	1.19	0.015
TIER FOUR									
	Baptist Medical Center, Kansas City	6.1	0.0%	1.18	No	0.11	4	0.64	0.048
	Boone Hospital Center, Columbia	8.5	0.0%	1.02	No	0.00	4	0.82	0.039
	De Paul Health Center, St. Louis	7.7	0.0%	1.04	No	0.00	4	0.55	0.058
	Deaconess Hospital, St. Louis	8.8	0.0%	1.26	No	0.37	2	0.99	0.227
	Independence Regional Health Center, Independence	6.3	0.0%	1.06	No	0.00	3	0.40	0.012
	Lester E. Cox Medical Centers, Springfield	7.8	0.0%	1.10	No	0.04	3	0.96	0.033
	Menorah Medical Center, Kansas City	7.6	0.0%	1.07	No	0.03	3	0.58	0.126
	Missouri Baptist Medical Ctr., Town and Country, St. Louis	9.1	0.0%	1.00	No	0.00	5	0.84	0.039
	North Kansas City Hospital, North Kansas City	6.4	0.0%	1.26	No	0.00	4	1.07	0.037
	Phelps County Regional Medical Center, Rolla	6.1	0.0%	1.15	No	0.02	3	0.46	0.032
	Research Medical Center, Kansas City	8.1	0.0%	1.09	No	0.02	2	1.02	0.113
	Southeast Missouri Hospital, Cape Girardeau	6.2	0.0%	1.35	No	0.00	4	0.88	0.015
	St. Anthony's Medical Center, St. Louis	6.9	0.0%	1.12	No	0.00	4	0.56	0.028
	St. Francis Medical Center, Cape Girardeau	5.9	0.0%	1.41	No	0.00	4	0.83	0.027
	St. John's Regional Medical Center, Joplin	6.1	0.0%	1.38	No	0.00	3	1.00	0.030
	St. Joseph Health Center, Kansas City	8.3	0.0%	1.04	No	0.00	4	0.80	0.048
	St. Joseph Hospital, St. Louis	7.0	0.0%	1.20	No	0.00	4	0.74	0.050
	St. Luke's Hospital, Chesterfield	9.0	0.0%	1.01	No	0.17	3	0.83	0.077
	St. Mary's Health Center, Jefferson City	6.9	0.0%	1.17	No	0.00	4	0.74	0.013
	St. Mary's Health Center, St. Louis	7.7	0.0%	1.06	No	0.15	3	0.62	0.055
	Trinity Lutheran Hospital, Kansas City	6.7	0.0%	1.07	No	0.09	2	0.56	0.036

UROLOGY

Natl. Rank	Hospital	U.S. News index	Reputa- tional score	Urology mortality rate	COTH member	Interns and residents to beds	Tech- nology score (of 11)	R.N.'s to beds	Board- certified internists to beds	Procedures to beds
	TIER ONE									
8	**Barnes Hospital, St. Louis**	**42.3**	21.3%	1.08	Yes	0.89	11	0.82	0.273	1.52
	TIER TWO									
69	**Jewish Hospital of St. Louis**	**16.6**	0.0%	0.80	Yes	0.63	9	1.22	0.100	2.13
73	**St. Louis University Hospital**	**16.2**	0.0%	1.36	Yes	1.89	10	1.33	0.057	2.10
	TIER THREE									
	Missouri Baptist Medical Ctr., Town and Country, St. Louis	11.4	0.0%	0.74	No	0.00	10	0.84	0.039	1.41
	St. John's Mercy Medical Center, St. Louis	10.4	0.0%	0.99	Yes	0.19	8	0.66	0.052	0.86
	St. John's Regional Health Center, Springfield	9.6	0.6%	0.99	No	0.00	9	0.87	0.097	2.33
	St. Joseph Health Center, St. Charles	10.6	0.0%	0.36	No	0.00	7	0.77	0.061	1.00
	St. Luke's Hospital, Kansas City	11.5	0.0%	0.99	Yes	0.25	9	0.81	0.034	2.01
	University Hospitals and Clinics, Columbia	13.2	0.0%	1.11	Yes	1.10	6	1.19	0.015	1.27
	TIER FOUR									
	Baptist Medical Center, Kansas City	7.1	0.0%	0.98	No	0.11	5	0.64	0.048	1.72
	Boone Hospital Center, Columbia	8.3	0.0%	0.95	No	0.00	8	0.82	0.039	2.21
	De Paul Health Center, St. Louis	7.8	0.0%	0.92	No	0.00	8	0.55	0.058	1.30
	Deaconess Hospital, St. Louis	7.1	0.0%	1.41	No	0.37	6	0.99	0.227	2.44
	Independence Regional Health Center, Independence	3.6	0.0%	1.28	No	0.00	5	0.40	0.012	1.39
	Lester E. Cox Medical Centers, Springfield	4.9	0.0%	1.51	No	0.04	8	0.96	0.033	1.20
	Menorah Medical Center, Kansas City	5.6	0.0%	1.28	No	0.03	8	0.58	0.126	1.31
	North Kansas City Hospital, North Kansas City	5.3	0.0%	1.50	No	0.00	8	1.07	0.037	1.72
	Phelps County Regional Medical Center, Rolla	8.1	0.0%	0.91	No	0.02	9	0.46	0.032	2.26
	Research Medical Center, Kansas City	8.3	0.0%	1.02	No	0.02	7	1.02	0.113	1.69
	Southeast Missouri Hospital, Cape Girardeau	4.2	0.0%	1.61	No	0.00	8	0.88	0.015	1.73
	St. Anthony's Medical Center, St. Louis	4.8	0.0%	1.33	No	0.00	9	0.56	0.028	1.31
	St. Francis Medical Center, Cape Girardeau	5.4	0.0%	1.22	No	0.00	6	0.83	0.027	1.47
	St. John's Regional Medical Center, Joplin	3.6	0.0%	2.14	No	0.00	9	1.00	0.030	2.15
	St. Joseph Health Center, Kansas City	4.4	0.0%	1.49	No	0.00	6	0.80	0.048	2.29
	St. Joseph Hospital, St. Louis	4.9	0.0%	1.35	No	0.00	7	0.74	0.050	1.58
	St. Luke's Hospital, Chesterfield	7.1	0.0%	1.14	No	0.17	7	0.83	0.077	1.45
	St. Mary's Health Center, Jefferson City	2.2	0.0%	2.00	No	0.00	6	0.74	0.013	1.69
	St. Mary's Health Center, St. Louis	8.3	0.0%	0.89	No	0.15	6	0.62	0.055	1.52
	Trinity Lutheran Hospital, Kansas City	4.4	0.0%	1.39	No	0.09	7	0.56	0.036	1.48

STATE RANKINGS ■ MISSOURI

AIDS

Natl. Rank	Hospital	U.S. News index	Reputa-tional score	Hospital-wide mortality rate	COTH member	Interns and residents to beds	Tech-nology score (of 11)	Discharge planning (of 2)	R.N.'s to beds	Board-certified internists to beds
	TIER THREE									
	Kalispell Regional Hospital, Kalispell	22.7	0.0%	0.73	No	0.00	7	2	0.87	0.082
	Montana Deaconess Medical Center, Great Falls	20.1	0.0%	0.99	No	0.00	7	2	0.65	0.040
	St. Patrick Hospital, Missoula	20.9	0.0%	0.90	No	0.00	6	1	0.76	0.052
	St. Vincent Hospital, Billings	19.9	0.0%	0.97	No	0.00	4	2	0.86	0.062
	TIER FOUR									
	Columbus Hospital, Great Falls	18.2	0.0%	1.04	No	0.00	5	1	0.69	0.099
	St. James Community Hospital, Butte	18.5	0.0%	1.15	No	0.00	7	2	0.93	0.079

CANCER

Natl. Rank	Hospital	U.S. News index	Reputa-tional score	Cancer mortality rate	COTH member	Interns and residents to beds	Tech-nology score (of 12)	R.N.'s to beds	Board-certified oncologists to beds	Procedures to beds
	TIER FOUR									
	Columbus Hospital, Great Falls	3.6	0.0%	0.74	No	0.00	7	0.69	0.006	2.58
	Kalispell Regional Hospital, Kalispell	4.1	0.0%	0.77	No	0.00	7	0.87	0.000	3.03
	Montana Deaconess Medical Center, Great Falls	2.7	0.0%	0.64	No	0.00	5	0.65	0.007	0.78
	St. James Community Hospital, Butte	4.1	0.0%	0.98	No	0.00	8	0.93	0.010	1.83
	St. Patrick Hospital, Missoula	4.0	0.0%	0.60	No	0.00	7	0.76	0.033	2.05
	St. Vincent Hospital, Billings	3.2	0.0%	0.96	No	0.00	5	0.86	0.022	2.17

CARDIOLOGY

Natl. Rank	Hospital	U.S. News index	Reputa-tional score	Cardiology mortality rate	COTH member	Interns and residents to beds	Tech-nology score (of 10)	R.N.'s to beds	Board-certified cardiologists to beds	Procedures to beds
	TIER THREE									
	Kalispell Regional Hospital, Kalispell	17.4	0.0%	0.79	No	0.00	7	0.87	0.018	9.83
	St. Patrick Hospital, Missoula	13.9	0.0%	1.04	No	0.00	8	0.76	0.052	11.44
	St. Vincent Hospital, Billings	14.1	0.0%	0.98	No	0.00	5	0.86	0.043	7.51
	TIER FOUR									
	Montana Deaconess Medical Center, Great Falls	10.8	0.0%	1.12	No	0.00	9	0.65	0.009	3.62

ENDOCRINOLOGY

Natl. Rank	Hospital	U.S. News index	Reputa-tional score	Endocrinology mortality rate	COTH member	Interns and residents to beds	Tech-nology score (of 11)	R.N.'s to beds	Board-certified internists to beds
	TIER FOUR								
	St. Vincent Hospital, Billings	6.8	0.0%	0.92	No	0.00	5	0.86	0.062

GASTROENTEROLOGY

Natl. Rank	Hospital	U.S. News index	Reputa-tional score	Gastro-enterology mortality rate	COTH member	Interns and residents to beds	Tech-nology score (of 11)	R.N.'s to beds	Board-certified gastro-enterologists to beds	Pro-cedures to beds
	TIER THREE									
	Kalispell Regional Hospital, Kalispell	10.1	0.0%	0.62	No	0.00	8	0.87	0.018	6.15
	St. James Community Hospital, Butte	7.7	0.0%	1.33	No	0.00	9	0.93	0.000	7.25
	TIER FOUR									
	Columbus Hospital, Great Falls	5.3	0.0%	1.24	No	0.00	8	0.69	0.012	3.99

Natl. Rank	Hospital	U.S. News index	Reputational score	Gastroenterology mortality rate	COTH member	Interns and residents to beds	Technology score (of 11)	R.N.'s to beds	Board-certified gastroenterologists to beds	Procedures to beds
	Montana Deaconess Medical Center, Great Falls	2.9	0.0%	1.34	No	0.00	6	0.65	0.005	1.73
	St. Patrick Hospital, Missoula	6.2	0.0%	1.07	No	0.00	7	0.76	0.019	3.98
	St. Vincent Hospital, Billings	5.5	0.0%	1.08	No	0.00	5	0.86	0.014	3.68

GERIATRICS

Natl. Rank	Hospital	U.S. News index	Reputational score	Hospital-wide mortality rate	COTH member	Service mix	Interns and residents to beds	Technology score (of 13)	R.N.'s to beds	Discharge planning (of 2)	Geriatric services (of 9)	Board-certified internists to beds
TIER THREE												
	Kalispell Regional Hospital, Kalispell	17.7	0.0%	0.73	No	5	0.00	9	0.87	2	1	0.082
	Montana Deaconess Medical Center, Great Falls	15.4	0.0%	0.99	No	6	0.00	7	0.65	2	7	0.040
	St. Patrick Hospital, Missoula	15.9	0.0%	0.90	No	5	0.00	9	0.76	1	1	0.052
	St. Vincent Hospital, Billings	15.1	0.0%	0.97	No	4	0.00	6	0.86	2	5	0.062
TIER FOUR												
	Columbus Hospital, Great Falls	12.1	0.0%	1.04	No	5	0.00	8	0.69	1	3	0.099

GYNECOLOGY

Natl. Rank	Hospital	U.S. News index	Reputational score	Hospital-wide mortality rate	Interns and residents to beds	Technology score (of 10)	R.N.'s to beds	Board-certified OB-GYNs to beds	Procedures to beds
TIER THREE									
	Kalispell Regional Hospital, Kalispell	18.8	0.0%	0.73	0.00	7	0.87	0.036	1.25
	St. Patrick Hospital, Missoula	17.2	0.0%	0.90	0.00	6	0.76	0.042	0.35
	St. Vincent Hospital, Billings	14.1	0.0%	0.97	0.00	4	0.86	0.043	0.49
TIER FOUR									
	Columbus Hospital, Great Falls	12.9	0.0%	1.04	0.00	6	0.69	0.050	0.43
	Montana Deaconess Medical Center, Great Falls	13.3	0.0%	0.99	0.00	6	0.65	0.019	0.23

NEUROLOGY

Natl. Rank	Hospital	U.S. News index	Reputational score	Neurology mortality rate	COTH member	Interns and residents to beds	Technology score (of 9)	R.N.'s to beds	Board-certified neurologists to beds
TIER THREE									
	Columbus Hospital, Great Falls	14.5	0.0%	0.54	No	0.00	6	0.69	0.019
	Kalispell Regional Hospital, Kalispell	13.1	0.0%	0.84	No	0.00	7	0.87	0.018
TIER FOUR									
	Montana Deaconess Medical Center, Great Falls	8.9	0.0%	0.96	No	0.00	5	0.65	0.005
	St. Patrick Hospital, Missoula	9.0	0.0%	1.02	No	0.00	6	0.76	0.014
	St. Vincent Hospital, Billings	10.2	0.0%	0.91	No	0.00	3	0.86	0.014

ORTHOPEDICS

Natl. Rank	Hospital	U.S. News index	Reputa-tional score	Orthopedics mortality rate	COTH member	Interns and residents to beds	Tech-nology score (of 5)	R.N.'s to beds	Board-certified orthopedists to beds	Pro-cedures to beds
	TIER THREE									
	Columbus Hospital, Great Falls	9.3	0.0%	0.69	No	0.00	3	0.69	0.062	3.52
	Kalispell Regional Hospital, Kalispell	10.9	0.0%	0.67	No	0.00	4	0.87	0.036	4.63
	Montana Deaconess Medical Center, Great Falls	9.7	0.0%	0.40	No	0.00	4	0.65	0.023	1.59
	St. Patrick Hospital, Missoula	9.6	0.0%	0.76	No	0.00	4	0.76	0.075	4.73
	TIER FOUR									
	St. James Community Hospital, Butte	7.5	0.0%	0.96	No	0.00	4	0.93	0.030	3.83
	St. Vincent Hospital, Billings	6.0	0.3%	1.03	No	0.00	1	0.86	0.054	5.27

OTOLARYNGOLOGY

Natl. Rank	Hospital	U.S. News index	Reputa-tional score	Hospital-wide mortality rate	COTH member	Interns and residents to beds	Tech-nology score (of 9)	R.N.'s to beds	Board-certified internists to beds	Procedures to beds
	TIER FOUR									
	Columbus Hospital, Great Falls	4.7	0.0%	1.04	No	0.00	6	0.69	0.099	0.298
	Kalispell Regional Hospital, Kalispell	5.4	0.0%	0.73	No	0.00	6	0.87	0.082	0.627
	Montana Deaconess Medical Center, Great Falls	3.2	0.0%	0.99	No	0.00	3	0.65	0.040	0.176
	St. James Community Hospital, Butte	5.5	0.0%	1.15	No	0.00	7	0.93	0.079	0.673
	St. Patrick Hospital, Missoula	4.6	0.0%	0.90	No	0.00	6	0.76	0.052	0.357
	St. Vincent Hospital, Billings	4.4	0.0%	0.97	No	0.00	4	0.86	0.062	0.239

RHEUMATOLOGY

Natl. Rank	Hospital	U.S. News index	Reputa-tional score	Hospital-wide mortality rate	COTH member	Interns and residents to beds	Tech-nology score (of 5)	R.N.'s to beds	Board-certified internists to beds
	TIER THREE								
	Kalispell Regional Hospital, Kalispell	10.8	0.0%	0.73	No	0.00	4	0.87	0.082
	TIER FOUR								
	Columbus Hospital, Great Falls	6.9	0.0%	1.04	No	0.00	3	0.69	0.099
	Montana Deaconess Medical Center, Great Falls	8.3	0.0%	0.99	No	0.00	4	0.65	0.040
	St. Patrick Hospital, Missoula	8.6	0.0%	0.90	No	0.00	4	0.76	0.052
	St. Vincent Hospital, Billings	7.9	0.0%	0.97	No	0.00	1	0.86	0.062

UROLOGY

Natl. Rank	Hospital	U.S. News index	Reputa-tional score	Urology mortality rate	COTH member	Interns and residents to beds	Tech-nology score (of 11)	R.N.'s to beds	Board-certified internists to beds	Procedures to beds
	TIER THREE									
	Kalispell Regional Hospital, Kalispell	11.8	0.0%	0.68	No	0.00	8	0.87	0.082	2.79
	St. James Community Hospital, Butte	10.5	0.0%	0.86	No	0.00	9	0.93	0.079	3.52
	TIER FOUR									
	Columbus Hospital, Great Falls	7.2	0.0%	1.08	No	0.00	8	0.69	0.099	2.03
	Montana Deaconess Medical Center, Great Falls	7.3	0.0%	0.91	No	0.00	6	0.65	0.040	0.64
	St. Patrick Hospital, Missoula	7.5	0.0%	1.01	No	0.00	7	0.76	0.052	2.46
	St. Vincent Hospital, Billings	7.5	0.0%	0.97	No	0.00	5	0.86	0.062	1.84

AIDS

Natl. Rank	Hospital	U.S. News index	Reputa-tional score	Hospital-wide mortality rate	COTH member	Interns and residents to beds	Tech-nology score (of 11)	Discharge planning (of 2)	R.N.'s to beds	Board-certified internists to beds
	TIER TWO									
62	University of Nebraska Medical Center, Omaha	26.4	0.2%	1.04	Yes	1.37	9	2	1.23	0.205
	TIER THREE									
	AMI St. Joseph Hospital, Omaha	20.3	0.0%	1.19	Yes	0.43	7	2	0.90	0.044
	TIER FOUR									
	Archbishop Bergan Mercy Center, Omaha	19.2	0.0%	1.04	No	0.01	7	2	0.57	0.032
	Bishop Clarkson Memorial Hospital, Omaha	15.4	0.0%	1.48	No	0.07	6	1	1.57	0.076
	Bryan Memorial Hospital, Lincoln	15.9	0.0%	1.29	No	0.01	6	1	1.04	0.058
	Good Samaritan Hospital, Kearney	17.1	0.0%	1.20	No	0.00	7	2	0.58	0.019
	Immanuel Medical Center, Omaha	15.8	0.0%	1.19	No	0.00	6	1	0.40	0.019
	Lincoln General Hospital, Lincoln	14.3	0.0%	1.38	No	0.01	5	2	0.41	0.028
	Lincoln Regional Center, Lincoln	0.4	0.0%	3.43	No	0.00	1	1	0.22	0.000
	Methodist Hospital, Omaha	15.6	0.0%	1.46	No	0.04	7	2	0.94	0.085
	Regional West Medical Center, Scottsbluff	15.8	0.0%	1.27	No	0.00	6	2	0.45	0.023
	St. Elizabeth Community Health Center, Lincoln	17.6	0.0%	1.13	No	0.02	4	2	0.84	0.092

CANCER

Natl. Rank	Hospital	U.S. News index	Reputa-tional score	Cancer mortality rate	COTH member	Interns and residents to beds	Tech-nology score (of 12)	R.N.'s to beds	Board-certified oncologists to beds	Procedures to beds
	TIER TWO									
21	University of Nebraska Medical Center, Omaha	15.9	2.8%	0.89	Yes	1.37	10	1.23	0.000	0.99
	TIER THREE									
	AMI St. Joseph Hospital, Omaha	8.0	0.0%	0.78	Yes	0.43	8	0.90	0.013	1.04
	Bishop Clarkson Memorial Hospital, Omaha	6.9	0.0%	0.87	No	0.07	10	1.57	0.004	2.82
	TIER FOUR									
	Archbishop Bergan Mercy Center, Omaha	3.7	0.0%	0.60	No	0.01	9	0.57	0.003	0.96
	Bryan Memorial Hospital, Lincoln	3.3	0.0%	0.93	No	0.01	4	1.04	0.015	1.27
	Good Samaritan Hospital, Kearney	2.6	0.0%	0.99	No	0.00	7	0.58	0.004	1.09
	Immanuel Medical Center, Omaha	2.2	0.0%	0.91	No	0.00	7	0.40	0.010	0.63
	Lincoln General Hospital, Lincoln	2.0	0.0%	1.61	No	0.01	7	0.41	0.020	1.44
	Methodist Hospital, Omaha	4.3	0.0%	1.14	No	0.04	9	0.94	0.020	1.34
	Regional West Medical Center, Scottsbluff	3.0	0.0%	0.62	No	0.00	8	0.45	0.000	1.06
	St. Elizabeth Community Health Center, Lincoln	2.2	0.0%	0.91	No	0.02	2	0.84	0.023	1.08

CARDIOLOGY

Natl. Rank	Hospital	U.S. News index	Reputa-tional score	Cardiology mortality rate	COTH member	Interns and residents to beds	Tech-nology score (of 10)	R.N.'s to beds	Board-certified cardiologists to beds	Procedures to beds
	TIER THREE									
	AMI St. Joseph Hospital, Omaha	16.3	0.0%	1.15	Yes	0.43	8	0.90	0.064	9.23
	University of Nebraska Medical Center, Omaha	16.7	0.0%	1.30	Yes	1.37	8	1.23	0.000	4.43
	TIER FOUR									
	Archbishop Bergan Mercy Center, Omaha	11.1	0.0%	1.09	No	0.01	9	0.57	0.008	3.67
	Bishop Clarkson Memorial Hospital, Omaha	7.7	0.0%	1.63	No	0.07	9	1.57	0.033	9.22
	Bryan Memorial Hospital, Lincoln	8.9	0.0%	1.34	No	0.01	8	1.04	0.026	11.70
	Good Samaritan Hospital, Kearney	10.9	0.0%	1.07	No	0.00	7	0.58	0.004	3.62
	Immanuel Medical Center, Omaha	5.1	0.0%	1.44	No	0.00	8	0.40	0.015	2.92
	Methodist Hospital, Omaha	6.7	0.0%	1.49	No	0.04	9	0.94	0.017	5.54
	Regional West Medical Center, Scottsbluff	8.0	0.0%	1.21	No	0.00	6	0.45	0.023	3.91

ENDOCRINOLOGY

Natl. Rank Hospital	U.S. News index	Reputational score	Endocrinology mortality rate	COTH member	Interns and residents to beds	Technology score (of 11)	R.N.'s to beds	Board-certified internists to beds
TIER THREE								
AMI St. Joseph Hospital, Omaha	12.9	0.0%	0.76	Yes	0.43	8	0.90	0.044
Methodist Hospital, Omaha	8.5	0.0%	0.90	No	0.04	10	0.94	0.085
TIER FOUR								
Archbishop Bergan Mercy Center, Omaha	5.2	0.0%	1.18	No	0.01	10	0.57	0.032
Bishop Clarkson Memorial Hospital, Omaha	7.7	0.0%	1.36	No	0.07	10	1.57	0.076
Bryan Memorial Hospital, Lincoln	4.3	0.4%	1.90	No	0.01	6	1.04	0.058
Immanuel Medical Center, Omaha	6.8	0.0%	0.82	No	0.00	8	0.40	0.019

GASTROENTEROLOGY

Natl. Rank Hospital	U.S. News index	Reputational score	Gastro-enterology mortality rate	COTH member	Interns and residents to beds	Technology score (of 11)	R.N.'s to beds	Board-certified gastro-enterologists to beds	Pro-cedures to beds
TIER THREE									
AMI St. Joseph Hospital, Omaha	7.7	0.0%	1.49	Yes	0.43	7	0.90	0.013	2.13
TIER FOUR									
Archbishop Bergan Mercy Center, Omaha	6.1	0.0%	0.92	No	0.01	9	0.57	0.007	1.78
Bishop Clarkson Memorial Hospital, Omaha	6.8	0.0%	1.66	No	0.07	10	1.57	0.011	4.04
Bryan Memorial Hospital, Lincoln	5.6	0.0%	1.23	No	0.01	6	1.04	0.017	3.74
Good Samaritan Hospital, Kearney	3.2	0.0%	1.38	No	0.00	7	0.58	0.000	2.23
Immanuel Medical Center, Omaha	4.4	0.0%	0.98	No	0.00	7	0.40	0.010	1.24
Lincoln General Hospital, Lincoln	3.4	0.0%	1.25	No	0.01	7	0.41	0.020	2.27
Methodist Hospital, Omaha	4.4	0.0%	1.74	No	0.04	10	0.94	0.011	2.98
Regional West Medical Center, Scottsbluff	3.3	0.0%	1.40	No	0.00	8	0.45	0.000	2.66
St. Elizabeth Community Health Center, Lincoln	4.4	0.0%	1.13	No	0.02	4	0.84	0.037	2.61

GERIATRICS

Natl. Rank Hospital	U.S. News index	Reputational score	Hospital-wide mortality rate	COTH member	Service mix	Interns and residents to beds	Technology score (of 13)	R.N.'s to beds	Discharge planning (of 2)	Geriatric services (of 9)	Board-certified internists to beds
TIER TWO											
65 University of Nebraska Medical Center, Omaha	23.0	0.0%	1.04	Yes	9	1.37	10	1.23	2	6	0.205
TIER FOUR											
AMI St. Joseph Hospital, Omaha	12.0	0.0%	1.19	Yes	3	0.43	10	0.90	2	1	0.044
Archbishop Bergan Mercy Center, Omaha	13.6	0.0%	1.04	No	5	0.01	11	0.57	2	4	0.032
Bishop Clarkson Memorial Hospital, Omaha	6.3	0.0%	1.48	No	5	0.07	12	1.57	1	2	0.076
Bryan Memorial Hospital, Lincoln	6.4	0.0%	1.29	No	4	0.01	7	1.04	1	2	0.058
Good Samaritan Hospital, Kearney	10.9	0.0%	1.20	No	8	0.00	9	0.58	2	5	0.019
Immanuel Medical Center, Omaha	8.3	0.0%	1.19	No	5	0.00	10	0.40	1	4	0.019
Methodist Hospital, Omaha	5.9	0.0%	1.46	No	5	0.04	11	0.94	2	1	0.085
Regional West Medical Center, Scottsbluff	9.4	0.0%	1.27	No	9	0.00	9	0.45	2	3	0.023

GYNECOLOGY

Natl. Rank	Hospital	U.S. News index	Reputa- tional score	Hospital- wide mortality rate	Interns and residents to beds	Tech- nology score (of 10)	R.N.'s to beds	Board- certified OB-GYNs to beds	Procedures to beds
	TIER TWO								
57	University of Nebraska Medical Center, Omaha	25.3	1.0%	1.04	1.37	9	1.23	0.015	0.37
	TIER THREE								
	Archbishop Bergan Mercy Center, Omaha	14.3	0.0%	1.04	0.01	9	0.57	0.035	0.29
	TIER FOUR								
	AMI St. Joseph Hospital, Omaha	13.0	0.0%	1.19	0.43	7	0.90	0.044	0.26
	Bishop Clarkson Memorial Hospital, Omaha	10.0	0.0%	1.48	0.07	8	1.57	0.022	0.54
	Bryan Memorial Hospital, Lincoln	7.9	0.0%	1.29	0.01	5	1.04	0.020	0.43
	Good Samaritan Hospital, Kearney	9.4	0.0%	1.20	0.00	8	0.58	0.011	0.49
	Immanuel Medical Center, Omaha	7.3	0.0%	1.19	0.00	6	0.40	0.008	0.17
	Methodist Hospital, Omaha	8.0	0.0%	1.46	0.04	8	0.94	0.054	0.43
	Regional West Medical Center, Scottsbluff	7.6	0.0%	1.27	0.00	8	0.45	0.011	0.43

NEUROLOGY

Natl. Rank	Hospital	U.S. News index	Reputa- tional score	Neurology mortality rate	COTH member	Interns and residents to beds	Tech- nology score (of 9)	R.N.'s to beds	Board- certified neurologists to beds
	TIER THREE								
	AMI St. Joseph Hospital, Omaha	12.5	0.0%	1.07	Yes	0.43	6	0.90	0.017
	Archbishop Bergan Mercy Center, Omaha	14.0	0.0%	0.69	No	0.01	8	0.57	0.007
	TIER FOUR								
	Bishop Clarkson Memorial Hospital, Omaha	9.3	0.0%	1.23	No	0.07	8	1.57	0.015
	Bryan Memorial Hospital, Lincoln	6.3	0.0%	1.30	No	0.01	5	1.04	0.017
	Good Samaritan Hospital, Kearney	7.1	0.0%	1.10	No	0.00	7	0.58	0.004
	Immanuel Medical Center, Omaha	4.6	0.0%	1.31	No	0.00	6	0.40	0.013
	Methodist Hospital, Omaha	7.1	0.0%	1.31	No	0.04	8	0.94	0.020
	Regional West Medical Center, Scottsbluff	4.9	0.0%	1.26	No	0.00	7	0.45	0.004

ORTHOPEDICS

Natl. Rank	Hospital	U.S. News index	Reputa- tional score	Orthopedics mortality rate	COTH member	Interns and residents to beds	Tech- nology score (of 5)	R.N.'s to beds	Board- certified orthopedists to beds	Pro- cedures to beds
	TIER TWO									
78	University of Nebraska Medical Center, Omaha	14.7	0.0%	1.00	Yes	1.37	4	1.23	0.012	1.29
	TIER THREE									
	AMI St. Joseph Hospital, Omaha	8.2	0.0%	1.32	Yes	0.43	3	0.90	0.017	1.56
	TIER FOUR									
	Archbishop Bergan Mercy Center, Omaha	4.9	0.0%	1.15	No	0.01	4	0.57	0.023	2.47
	Bishop Clarkson Memorial Hospital, Omaha	6.4	0.0%	1.55	No	0.07	4	1.57	0.022	3.60
	Bryan Memorial Hospital, Lincoln	4.0	0.0%	2.06	No	0.01	4	1.04	0.032	5.06
	Good Samaritan Hospital, Kearney	7.0	0.0%	0.94	No	0.00	4	0.58	0.030	4.97
	Immanuel Medical Center, Omaha	6.8	0.0%	0.76	No	0.00	3	0.40	0.017	1.14
	Lincoln General Hospital, Lincoln	4.9	0.0%	1.00	No	0.01	3	0.41	0.024	2.74
	Methodist Hospital, Omaha	5.1	0.0%	1.41	No	0.04	4	0.94	0.023	3.32
	Regional West Medical Center, Scottsbluff	2.3	0.0%	1.59	No	0.00	3	0.45	0.019	3.02
	St. Elizabeth Community Health Center, Lincoln	4.5	0.0%	1.18	No	0.02	2	0.84	0.032	3.49

OTOLARYNGOLOGY

Natl. Rank	Hospital	U.S. News index	Reputational score	Hospital-wide mortality rate	COTH member	Interns and residents to beds	Technology score (of 9)	R.N.'s to beds	Board-certified internists to beds	Procedures to beds
	TIER TWO									
42	**University of Nebraska Medical Center, Omaha**	**19.3**	0.9%	1.05	Yes	1.37	8	1.23	0.205	0.145
	TIER THREE									
	AMI St. Joseph Hospital, Omaha	**9.6**	0.0%	1.19	Yes	0.43	6	0.90	0.044	0.121
	Bishop Clarkson Memorial Hospital, Omaha	**7.8**	0.0%	1.48	No	0.07	8	1.57	0.076	0.360
	TIER FOUR									
	Archbishop Bergan Mercy Center, Omaha	**4.3**	0.0%	1.04	No	0.01	8	0.57	0.032	0.102
	Bryan Memorial Hospital, Lincoln	**4.7**	0.0%	1.30	No	0.01	4	1.04	0.058	0.209
	Good Samaritan Hospital, Kearney	**3.5**	0.0%	1.20	No	0.00	6	0.58	0.019	0.143
	Immanuel Medical Center, Omaha	**3.0**	0.0%	1.19	No	0.00	6	0.40	0.019	0.092
	Lincoln General Hospital, Lincoln	**3.0**	0.0%	1.38	No	0.01	6	0.41	0.028	0.167
	Methodist Hospital, Omaha	**5.8**	0.0%	1.46	No	0.04	8	0.94	0.085	0.242
	Regional West Medical Center, Scottsbluff	**3.4**	0.0%	1.27	No	0.00	7	0.45	0.023	0.164
	St. Elizabeth Community Health Center, Lincoln	**3.7**	0.0%	1.13	No	0.02	1	0.84	0.092	0.165

RHEUMATOLOGY

Natl. Rank	Hospital	U.S. News index	Reputational score	Hospital-wide mortality rate	COTH member	Interns and residents to beds	Technology score (of 5)	R.N.'s to beds	Board-certified internists to beds
	TIER TWO								
59	**University of Nebraska Medical Center, Omaha**	**17.4**	0.0%	1.05	Yes	1.37	4	1.23	0.205
	TIER THREE								
	AMI St. Joseph Hospital, Omaha	**10.8**	0.0%	1.19	Yes	0.43	3	0.90	0.044
	TIER FOUR								
	Archbishop Bergan Mercy Center, Omaha	**7.6**	0.0%	1.04	No	0.01	4	0.57	0.032
	Bishop Clarkson Memorial Hospital, Omaha	**8.1**	0.5%	1.48	No	0.07	4	1.57	0.076
	Bryan Memorial Hospital, Lincoln	**6.3**	0.0%	1.30	No	0.01	4	1.04	0.058
	Good Samaritan Hospital, Kearney	**6.3**	0.0%	1.20	No	0.00	4	0.58	0.019
	Immanuel Medical Center, Omaha	**4.4**	0.0%	1.19	No	0.00	3	0.40	0.019
	Methodist Hospital, Omaha	**6.5**	0.0%	1.46	No	0.04	4	0.94	0.085
	Regional West Medical Center, Scottsbluff	**5.1**	0.0%	1.27	No	0.00	3	0.45	0.023

UROLOGY

Natl. Rank	Hospital	U.S. News index	Reputational score	Urology mortality rate	COTH member	Interns and residents to beds	Technology score (of 11)	R.N.'s to beds	Board-certified internists to beds	Procedures to beds
	TIER THREE									
	AMI St. Joseph Hospital, Omaha	**9.5**	0.0%	1.28	Yes	0.43	7	0.90	0.044	1.01
	Lincoln General Hospital, Lincoln	**9.6**	0.0%	0.72	No	0.01	7	0.41	0.028	1.31
	TIER FOUR									
	Archbishop Bergan Mercy Center, Omaha	**7.5**	0.0%	0.96	No	0.01	9	0.57	0.032	1.09
	Bishop Clarkson Memorial Hospital, Omaha	**6.1**	0.0%	2.05	No	0.07	10	1.57	0.076	2.48
	Bryan Memorial Hospital, Lincoln	**5.4**	0.0%	1.36	No	0.01	6	1.04	0.058	1.38
	Good Samaritan Hospital, Kearney	**2.7**	0.0%	1.81	No	0.00	7	0.58	0.019	2.10
	Immanuel Medical Center, Omaha	**5.3**	0.0%	1.08	No	0.00	7	0.40	0.019	0.67
	Methodist Hospital, Omaha	**7.8**	0.0%	1.13	No	0.04	10	0.94	0.085	1.37
	Regional West Medical Center, Scottsbluff	**3.3**	0.0%	1.55	No	0.00	8	0.45	0.023	1.53
	St. Elizabeth Community Health Center, Lincoln	**4.9**	0.0%	1.29	No	0.02	4	0.84	0.092	1.39

AIDS

Natl. Rank	Hospital	U.S. News index	Reputa- tional score	Hospital- wide mortality rate	COTH member	Interns and residents to beds	Tech- nology score (of 11)	Discharge planning (of 2)	R.N.'s to beds	Board- certified internists to beds
	TIER THREE									
	St. Mary's Regional Medical Center, Reno	20.0	0.0%	1.00	No	0.00	5	2	0.92	0.104
	TIER FOUR									
	University Medical Center, Las Vegas	19.1	0.0%	1.21	No	0.15	9	2	1.23	0.032
	Valley Hospital Medical Center, Las Vegas	16.9	0.0%	1.21	No	0.00	7	1	0.89	0.048
	Washoe Medical Center, Reno	17.6	0.0%	1.25	No	0.03	8	2	0.89	0.055

CANCER

Natl. Rank	Hospital	U.S. News index	Reputa- tional score	Cancer mortality rate	COTH member	Interns and residents to beds	Tech- nology score (of 12)	R.N.'s to beds	Board- certified oncologists to beds	Procedures to beds
	TIER FOUR									
	St. Mary's Regional Medical Center, Reno	2.4	0.0%	1.12	No	0.00	3	0.92	0.016	1.17
	University Medical Center, Las Vegas	4.6	0.0%	1.32	No	0.15	7	1.23	0.010	0.70
	Valley Hospital Medical Center, Las Vegas	3.2	0.0%	0.98	No	0.00	5	0.89	0.032	1.33
	Washoe Medical Center, Reno	4.2	0.0%	1.09	No	0.03	9	0.89	0.020	1.16

CARDIOLOGY

Natl. Rank	Hospital	U.S. News index	Reputa- tional score	Cardiology mortality rate	COTH member	Interns and residents to beds	Tech- nology score (of 10)	R.N.'s to beds	Board- certified cardiologists to beds	Procedures to beds
	TIER THREE									
	St. Mary's Regional Medical Center, Reno	15.2	0.0%	0.97	No	0.00	7	0.92	0.052	5.75
	Washoe Medical Center, Reno	13.8	0.0%	1.06	No	0.03	9	0.89	0.051	6.22
	TIER FOUR									
	University Medical Center, Las Vegas	11.6	0.0%	1.23	No	0.15	9	1.23	0.046	2.89
	Valley Hospital Medical Center, Las Vegas	11.4	0.0%	1.21	No	0.00	9	0.89	0.074	9.80

ENDOCRINOLOGY

Natl. Rank	Hospital	U.S. News index	Reputa- tional score	Endocrinology mortality rate	COTH member	Interns and residents to beds	Tech- nology score (of 11)	R.N.'s to beds	Board- certified internists to beds
	TIER FOUR								
	St. Mary's Regional Medical Center, Reno	4.7	0.0%	1.31	No	0.00	3	0.92	0.104
	University Medical Center, Las Vegas	5.8	0.0%	1.47	No	0.15	7	1.23	0.032
	Valley Hospital Medical Center, Las Vegas	5.2	0.0%	1.23	No	0.00	6	0.89	0.048
	Washoe Medical Center, Reno	6.1	0.0%	1.19	No	0.03	9	0.89	0.055

GASTROENTEROLOGY

Natl. Rank	Hospital	U.S. News index	Reputa- tional score	Gastro- enterology mortality rate	COTH member	Interns and residents to beds	Tech- nology score (of 11)	R.N.'s to beds	Board- certified gastro- enterologists to beds	Pro- cedures to beds
	TIER FOUR									
	St. Mary's Regional Medical Center, Reno	5.4	0.0%	1.02	No	0.00	4	0.92	0.019	3.05
	University Medical Center, Las Vegas	4.6	0.0%	1.39	No	0.15	7	1.23	0.018	1.19
	Valley Hospital Medical Center, Las Vegas	5.0	0.0%	1.36	No	0.00	6	0.89	0.029	4.39
	Washoe Medical Center, Reno	5.0	0.0%	1.23	No	0.03	8	0.89	0.018	2.21

GERIATRICS

Natl. Rank	Hospital	U.S. News index	Reputa-tional score	Hospital-wide mortality rate	COTH member	Service mix	Interns and residents to beds	Tech-nology score (of 13)	R.N.'s to beds	Discharge planning (of 2)	Geriatric services (of 9)	Board-certified internists to beds
TIER THREE												
	St. Mary's Regional Medical Center, Reno	14.7	0.0%	1.00	No	7	0.00	5	0.92	2	1	0.104
TIER FOUR												
	University Medical Center, Las Vegas	10.4	0.0%	1.21	No	5	0.15	9	1.23	2	2	0.032
	Valley Hospital Medical Center, Las Vegas	7.0	0.0%	1.21	No	3	0.00	7	0.89	1	1	0.048
	Washoe Medical Center, Reno	10.9	0.0%	1.25	No	7	0.03	11	0.89	2	5	0.055

GYNECOLOGY

Natl. Rank	Hospital	U.S. News index	Reputa-tional score	Hospital-wide mortality rate	Interns and residents to beds	Tech-nology score (of 10)	R.N.'s to beds	Board-certified OB-GYNs to beds	Procedures to beds
TIER FOUR									
	St. Mary's Regional Medical Center, Reno	13.9	0.0%	1.00	0.00	4	0.92	0.057	0.50
	University Medical Center, Las Vegas	11.7	0.0%	1.21	0.15	6	1.23	0.026	0.21
	Valley Hospital Medical Center, Las Vegas	9.8	0.0%	1.21	0.00	6	0.89	0.035	0.59
	Washoe Medical Center, Reno	10.9	0.0%	1.25	0.03	8	0.89	0.046	0.19

NEUROLOGY

Natl. Rank	Hospital	U.S. News index	Reputa-tional score	Neurology mortality rate	COTH member	Interns and residents to beds	Tech-nology score (of 9)	R.N.'s to beds	Board-certified neurologists to beds
TIER FOUR									
	St. Mary's Regional Medical Center, Reno	8.0	0.0%	1.09	No	0.00	3	0.92	0.022
	University Medical Center, Las Vegas	9.3	0.0%	1.04	No	0.15	5	1.23	0.002
	Valley Hospital Medical Center, Las Vegas	6.0	0.0%	1.27	No	0.00	6	0.89	0.010
	Washoe Medical Center, Reno	6.7	0.0%	1.33	No	0.03	7	0.89	0.022

ORTHOPEDICS

Natl. Rank	Hospital	U.S. News index	Reputa-tional score	Orthopedics mortality rate	COTH member	Interns and residents to beds	Tech-nology score (of 5)	R.N.'s to beds	Board-certified orthopedists to beds	Pro-cedures to beds
TIER FOUR										
	St. Mary's Regional Medical Center, Reno	6.7	0.0%	0.90	No	0.00	2	0.92	0.065	2.70
	University Medical Center, Las Vegas	6.2	0.0%	1.26	No	0.15	4	1.23	0.022	0.82
	Valley Hospital Medical Center, Las Vegas	7.8	0.0%	0.97	No	0.00	5	0.89	0.061	2.50
	Washoe Medical Center, Reno	5.2	0.0%	1.27	No	0.03	4	0.89	0.046	1.74

OTOLARYNGOLOGY

Natl. Rank	Hospital	U.S. News index	Reputa-tional score	Hospital-wide mortality rate	COTH member	Interns and residents to beds	Tech-nology score (of 9)	R.N.'s to beds	Board-certified internists to beds	Procedures to beds
TIER FOUR										
	St. Mary's Regional Medical Center, Reno	4.1	0.0%	1.00	No	0.00	1	0.92	0.104	0.294
	University Medical Center, Las Vegas	6.0	0.0%	1.21	No	0.15	5	1.23	0.032	0.038
	Valley Hospital Medical Center, Las Vegas	4.2	0.0%	1.21	No	0.00	4	0.89	0.048	0.281
	Washoe Medical Center, Reno	5.2	0.0%	1.25	No	0.03	7	0.89	0.055	0.216

RHEUMATOLOGY

Natl. Rank	Hospital	U.S. News index	Reputa- tional score	Hospital- wide mortality rate	COTH member	Interns and residents to beds	Tech- nology score (of 5)	R.N.'s to beds	Board- certified internists to beds
	TIER FOUR								
	St. Mary's Regional Medical Center, Reno	8.5	0.0%	1.00	No	0.00	2	0.92	0.104
	University Medical Center, Las Vegas	8.6	0.0%	1.21	No	0.15	4	1.23	0.032
	Valley Hospital Medical Center, Las Vegas	6.8	0.0%	1.21	No	0.00	5	0.89	0.048
	Washoe Medical Center, Reno	7.2	0.0%	1.25	No	0.03	4	0.89	0.055

UROLOGY

Natl. Rank	Hospital	U.S. News index	Reputa- tional score	Urology mortality rate	COTH member	Interns and residents to beds	Tech- nology score (of 11)	R.N.'s to beds	Board- certified internists to beds	Procedures to beds
	TIER FOUR									
	St. Mary's Regional Medical Center, Reno	4.6	0.0%	1.41	No	0.00	4	0.92	0.104	1.42
	University Medical Center, Las Vegas	6.7	0.0%	1.27	No	0.15	7	1.23	0.032	0.89
	Valley Hospital Medical Center, Las Vegas	4.9	0.0%	1.44	No	0.00	6	0.89	0.048	2.73
	Washoe Medical Center, Reno	4.6	0.0%	1.57	No	0.03	8	0.89	0.055	1.07

AIDS

Natl. Rank	Hospital	U.S. News index	Reputa-tional score	Hospital-wide mortality rate	COTH member	Interns and residents to beds	Tech-nology score (of 11)	Discharge planning (of 2)	R.N.'s to beds	Board-certified internists to beds
	TIER THREE									
95	Mary Hitchcock Memorial Hospital, Lebanon	24.7	0.0%	1.04	Yes	1.04	8	2	1.35	0.045
	TIER FOUR									
	Elliot Hospital, Manchester	16.1	0.0%	1.33	No	0.00	7	2	0.64	0.077
	St. Joseph Hospital and Trauma Center, Nashua	15.2	0.0%	1.36	No	0.00	7	1	0.79	0.044

CANCER

Natl. Rank	Hospital	U.S. News index	Reputa-tional score	Cancer mortality rate	COTH member	Interns and residents to beds	Tech-nology score (of 12)	R.N.'s to beds	Board-certified oncologists to beds	Procedures to beds
	TIER TWO									
61	Mary Hitchcock Memorial Hospital, Lebanon	12.3	0.0%	0.74	Yes	1.04	10	1.35	0.034	2.18
	TIER FOUR									
	Elliot Hospital, Manchester	3.0	0.0%	1.63	No	0.00	9	0.64	0.003	1.54
	St. Joseph Hospital and Trauma Center, Nashua	2.6	0.0%	1.57	No	0.00	6	0.79	0.006	1.15

CARDIOLOGY

Natl. Rank	Hospital	U.S. News index	Reputa-tional score	Cardiology mortality rate	COTH member	Interns and residents to beds	Tech-nology score (of 10)	R.N.'s to beds	Board-certified cardiologists to beds	Procedures to beds
	TIER TWO									
95	Mary Hitchcock Memorial Hospital, Lebanon	20.9	0.0%	1.09	Yes	1.04	9	1.35	0.050	6.98
	TIER FOUR									
	Elliot Hospital, Manchester	8.7	0.0%	1.22	No	0.00	6	0.64	0.035	5.65
	St. Joseph Hospital and Trauma Center, Nashua	12.5	0.0%	1.04	No	0.00	6	0.79	0.033	5.72

ENDOCRINOLOGY

Natl. Rank	Hospital	U.S. News index	Reputa-tional score	Endocrinology mortality rate	COTH member	Interns and residents to beds	Tech-nology score (of 11)	R.N.'s to beds	Board-certified internists to beds
	TIER TWO								
79	Mary Hitchcock Memorial Hospital, Lebanon	15.0	0.0%	0.91	Yes	1.04	10	1.35	0.045
	TIER FOUR								
	Elliot Hospital, Manchester	5.4	0.0%	1.21	No	0.00	9	0.64	0.077

GASTROENTEROLOGY

Natl. Rank	Hospital	U.S. News index	Reputa-tional score	Gastro-enterology mortality rate	COTH member	Interns and residents to beds	Tech-nology score (of 11)	R.N.'s to beds	Board-certified gastro-enterologists to beds	Pro-cedures to beds
	TIER TWO									
64	Mary Hitchcock Memorial Hospital, Lebanon	14.0	0.0%	1.03	Yes	1.04	10	1.35	0.013	2.17
	TIER FOUR									
	Elliot Hospital, Manchester	4.2	0.0%	1.39	No	0.00	9	0.64	0.017	2.61
	St. Joseph Hospital and Trauma Center, Nashua	3.8	0.0%	1.58	No	0.00	8	0.79	0.017	2.94

GERIATRICS

Natl. Rank	Hospital	U.S. News index	Reputational score	Hospital-wide mortality rate	COTH member	Service mix	Interns and residents to beds	Technology score (of 13)	R.N.'s to beds	Discharge planning (of 2)	Geriatric services (of 9)	Board-certified internists to beds
	TIER THREE											
	Mary Hitchcock Memorial Hospital, Lebanon	**19.0**	0.0%	1.04	Yes	5	1.04	11	1.35	2	1	0.045
	TIER FOUR											
	Elliot Hospital, Manchester	**9.1**	0.0%	1.33	No	7	0.00	11	0.64	2	5	0.077
	St. Joseph Hospital and Trauma Center, Nashua	**5.5**	0.0%	1.36	No	6	0.00	8	0.79	1	1	0.044

GYNECOLOGY

Natl. Rank	Hospital	U.S. News index	Reputational score	Hospital-wide mortality rate	Interns and residents to beds	Technology score (of 10)	R.N.'s to beds	Board-certified OB-GYNs to beds	Procedures to beds
	TIER TWO								
83	Mary Hitchcock Memorial Hospital, Lebanon	**22.4**	0.0%	1.04	1.04	9	1.35	0.034	0.37
	TIER FOUR								
	Elliot Hospital, Manchester	**8.3**	0.0%	1.33	0.00	8	0.64	0.045	0.49

NEUROLOGY

Natl. Rank	Hospital	U.S. News index	Reputational score	Neurology mortality rate	COTH member	Interns and residents to beds	Technology score (of 9)	R.N.'s to beds	Board-certified neurologists to beds
	TIER THREE								
94	Mary Hitchcock Memorial Hospital, Lebanon	**17.5**	0.0%	1.00	Yes	1.04	8	1.35	0.021
	TIER FOUR								
	Elliot Hospital, Manchester	**6.1**	0.0%	1.32	No	0.00	7	0.64	0.024

ORTHOPEDICS

Natl. Rank	Hospital	U.S. News index	Reputational score	Orthopedics mortality rate	COTH member	Interns and residents to beds	Technology score (of 5)	R.N.'s to beds	Board-certified orthopedists to beds	Procedures to beds
	TIER TWO									
74	Mary Hitchcock Memorial Hospital, Lebanon	**14.8**	0.0%	0.93	Yes	1.04	4	1.35	0.019	2.78
	TIER FOUR									
	Elliot Hospital, Manchester	**4.0**	0.0%	1.36	No	0.00	4	0.64	0.028	1.93
	St. Joseph Hospital and Trauma Center, Nashua	**4.5**	0.0%	1.35	No	0.00	4	0.79	0.033	2.08

OTOLARYNGOLOGY

Natl. Rank	Hospital	U.S. News index	Reputational score	Hospital-wide mortality rate	COTH member	Interns and residents to beds	Technology score (of 9)	R.N.'s to beds	Board-certified internists to beds	Procedures to beds
	TIER TWO									
92	Mary Hitchcock Memorial Hospital, Lebanon	**14.1**	0.0%	1.04	Yes	1.04	8	1.35	0.045	0.246
	TIER FOUR									
	Elliot Hospital, Manchester	**4.4**	0.0%	1.32	No	0.00	7	0.64	0.077	0.189
	St. Joseph Hospital and Trauma Center, Nashua	**4.0**	0.0%	1.36	No	0.00	5	0.79	0.044	0.239

RHEUMATOLOGY

Natl. Rank	Hospital	U.S. News index	Reputa- tional score	Hospital- wide mortality rate	COTH member	Interns and residents to beds	Tech- nology score (of 5)	R.N.'s to beds	Board- certified internists to beds
	TIER TWO								
69	**Mary Hitchcock Memorial Hospital, Lebanon**	**16.6**	0.5%	1.04	Yes	1.04	4	1.35	0.045
	TIER FOUR								
	Elliot Hospital, Manchester	**6.2**	0.0%	1.32	No	0.00	4	0.64	0.077
	St. Joseph Hospital and Trauma Center, Nashua	**5.1**	0.0%	1.36	No	0.00	4	0.79	0.044

UROLOGY

Natl. Rank	Hospital	U.S. News index	Reputa- tional score	Urology mortality rate	COTH member	Interns and residents to beds	Tech- nology score (of 11)	R.N.'s to beds	Board- certified internists to beds	Procedures to beds
	TIER TWO									
86	**Mary Hitchcock Memorial Hospital, Lebanon**	**15.2**	0.0%	1.04	Yes	1.04	10	1.35	0.045	1.50
	TIER FOUR									
	Elliot Hospital, Manchester	**4.4**	0.0%	1.55	No	0.00	9	0.64	0.077	1.38

AIDS

Natl. Rank	Hospital	U.S. News index	Reputa-tional score	Hospital-wide mortality rate	COTH member	Interns and residents to beds	Tech-nology score (of 11)	Discharge planning (of 2)	R.N.'s to beds	Board-certified internists to beds
TIER THREE										
	Atlantic City Medical Center, Atlantic City	20.9	0.0%	1.00	No	0.15	7	2	0.98	0.064
	Cooper Hospital-University Medical Center, Camden	20.2	0.0%	1.34	Yes	0.55	9	2	1.10	0.056
	Hackensack Medical Center, Hackensack	23.7	0.0%	1.10	Yes	0.40	8	2	1.54	0.281
	Medical Center at Princeton, Princeton	19.7	0.4%	1.01	No	0.09	6	1	0.61	0.095
	Overlook Hospital, Summit	21.9	0.0%	1.08	Yes	0.39	7	2	0.96	0.114
	Robert Wood Johnson University Hospital, New Brunswick	20.4	0.0%	1.22	Yes	0.43	5	2	1.51	0.090
	St. Barnabas Medical Center, Livingston	19.8	0.0%	1.22	Yes	0.40	8	2	0.62	0.046
	University Hospital, Newark	21.6	0.3%	1.33	Yes	0.94	9	2	1.28	0.019
TIER FOUR										
	Bergen Pines County Hospital, Paramus	13.0	0.0%	1.48	No	0.06	6	1	0.24	0.009
	Christ Hospital, Jersey City	15.3	0.0%	1.41	No	0.00	8	2	0.53	0.022
	Community Medical Center, Toms River	17.5	0.0%	1.19	No	0.00	6	2	0.98	0.025
	Elizabeth General Medical Center, Elizabeth	16.8	0.0%	1.18	No	0.02	6	1	0.60	0.127
	Englewood Hospital, Englewood	16.7	0.4%	1.25	No	0.18	6	1	0.63	0.075
	Helene Fuld Medical Center, Trenton	16.3	0.0%	1.28	No	0.19	5	2	0.84	0.024
	Hunterdon Medical Center, Flemington	19.1	0.0%	1.00	No	0.20	4	2	0.60	0.006
	JFK Medical Center, Edison	16.5	0.0%	1.25	No	0.16	5	2	0.66	0.086
	Jersey City Medical Center, Jersey City	15.5	0.0%	1.55	No	0.40	7	2	0.88	0.046
	Jersey Shore Medical Center, Neptune	17.9	0.0%	1.42	Yes	0.30	8	2	0.71	0.051
	Kennedy Memorial Hosp.-University Med. Ctr., Cherry Hill	18.4	0.0%	1.18	No	0.27	7	2	0.92	0.028
	Memorial Hospital of Burlington County, Mount Holly	15.4	0.0%	1.42	No	0.25	6	2	0.68	0.041
	Mercer Medical Center, Trenton	15.0	0.0%	1.47	No	0.00	6	2	1.04	0.039
	Monmouth Medical Center, Long Branch	17.9	0.0%	1.36	Yes	0.50	5	2	0.78	0.061
	Morristown Memorial Hospital, Morristown	18.2	0.0%	1.30	Yes	0.35	6	2	0.55	0.068
	Mountainside Hospital, Montclair	16.8	0.0%	1.27	No	0.24	6	2	0.62	0.086
	Muhlenberg Regional Medical Center, Plainfield	16.3	0.0%	1.36	No	0.18	7	2	0.73	0.066
	Our Lady of Lourdes Medical Center, Camden	15.8	0.0%	1.38	No	0.09	5	2	1.23	0.015
	Raritan Bay Medical Center, Perth Amboy	14.6	0.0%	1.40	No	0.12	6	1	0.72	0.033
	Riverview Medical Center, Red Bank	14.5	0.0%	1.50	No	0.00	6	2	0.63	0.108
	Somerset Medical Center, Somerville	16.0	0.0%	1.25	No	0.11	5	2	0.49	0.040
	St. Elizabeth Hospital, Elizabeth	19.6	0.0%	1.02	No	0.18	7	1	0.68	0.076
	St. Francis Medical Center, Trenton	17.7	0.0%	1.19	No	0.21	7	2	0.65	0.021
	St. Joseph's Hospital and Medical Center, Paterson	18.7	0.0%	1.39	Yes	0.38	9	2	0.76	0.042
	St. Michael's Medical Center, Newark	16.7	0.0%	1.58	Yes	0.48	7	2	0.71	0.029
	St. Peter's Medical Center, New Brunswick	17.0	0.0%	1.32	No	0.51	6	2	0.75	0.056
	United Hospital Medical Center, Newark	18.4	0.0%	1.23	No	0.38	8	2	0.94	0.014
	Valley Hospital, Ridgewood	17.5	0.0%	1.20	No	0.00	6	2	1.01	0.044
	Warren Hospital, Phillipsburg	15.5	0.0%	1.28	No	0.17	4	2	0.61	0.023
	West Jersey Hospital-Voorhees, Voorhees	18.3	0.0%	1.15	No	0.09	4	2	1.13	0.179

CANCER

Natl. Rank	Hospital	U.S. News index	Reputa-tional score	Cancer mortality rate	COTH member	Interns and residents to beds	Tech-nology score (of 12)	R.N.'s to beds	Board-certified oncologists to beds	Procedures to beds
TIER THREE										
	Cooper Hospital-University Medical Center, Camden	9.5	0.0%	1.06	Yes	0.55	10	1.10	0.025	2.09
	Hackensack Medical Center, Hackensack	9.6	0.0%	1.13	Yes	0.40	8	1.54	0.013	2.46
	Jersey Shore Medical Center, Neptune	6.6	0.0%	1.36	Yes	0.30	8	0.71	0.006	1.66
	Monmouth Medical Center, Long Branch	7.1	0.0%	1.20	Yes	0.50	6	0.78	0.004	2.30
	Morristown Memorial Hospital, Morristown	6.3	0.0%	1.30	Yes	0.35	8	0.55	0.010	1.65

STATE RANKINGS ■ NEW JERSEY

Natl. Rank	Hospital	U.S. News index	Reputa- tional score	Cancer mortality rate	COTH member	Interns and residents to beds	Tech- nology score (of 12)	R.N.'s to beds	Board- certified oncologists to beds	Procedures to beds
	Newark Beth Israel Medical Center, Newark	5.5	0.0%	1.14	Yes	0.40	0	1.02	0.011	0.79
	Overlook Hospital, Summit	7.9	0.0%	1.22	Yes	0.39	8	0.96	0.014	2.79
	Robert Wood Johnson University Hospital, New Brunswick	8.0	0.0%	1.25	Yes	0.43	3	1.51	0.033	1.68
	St. Barnabas Medical Center, Livingston	7.3	0.0%	1.12	Yes	0.40	9	0.62	0.007	2.40
	St. Joseph's Hospital and Medical Center, Paterson	7.2	0.0%	1.17	Yes	0.38	9	0.76	0.008	0.69
	St. Michael's Medical Center, Newark	5.5	0.0%	1.46	Yes	0.48	3	0.71	0.007	0.50
84	University Hospital, Newark	10.8	0.0%	1.09	Yes	0.94	10	1.28	0.008	0.62
	TIER FOUR									
	Atlantic City Medical Center, Atlantic City	4.2	0.0%	1.24	No	0.15	7	0.98	0.008	1.84
	Christ Hospital, Jersey City	2.6	0.0%	1.42	No	0.00	8	0.53	0.002	1.80
	Community Medical Center, Toms River	4.3	0.0%	1.07	No	0.00	7	0.98	0.007	4.51
	Elizabeth General Medical Center, Elizabeth	2.5	0.0%	0.92	No	0.02	6	0.60	0.002	0.99
	Englewood Hospital, Englewood	3.4	0.0%	1.39	No	0.18	7	0.63	0.015	2.25
	Helene Fuld Medical Center, Trenton	3.3	0.0%	1.21	No	0.19	5	0.84	0.003	1.52
	Hospital Center at Orange, Orange	1.3	0.0%	1.46	No	0.07	0	0.80	0.012	1.78
	Hunterdon Medical Center, Flemington	2.7	0.0%	1.01	No	0.20	4	0.60	0.011	2.10
	JFK Medical Center, Edison	2.7	0.0%	1.49	No	0.16	5	0.66	0.012	1.84
	Kennedy Memorial Hosp.-University Med. Ctr., Cherry Hill	4.3	0.0%	0.94	No	0.27	6	0.92	0.009	1.30
	Medical Center at Princeton, Princeton	3.5	0.0%	0.83	No	0.09	7	0.61	0.012	2.16
	Memorial Hospital of Burlington County, Mount Holly	3.7	0.0%	1.36	No	0.25	7	0.68	0.016	2.24
	Mercer Medical Center, Trenton	3.7	0.0%	1.26	No	0.00	7	1.04	0.006	1.29
	Mountainside Hospital, Montclair	3.8	0.0%	1.08	No	0.24	7	0.62	0.022	2.47
	Muhlenberg Regional Medical Center, Plainfield	3.7	0.0%	1.62	No	0.18	8	0.73	0.008	1.77
	Our Lady of Lourdes Medical Center, Camden	3.7	0.0%	1.16	No	0.09	4	1.23	0.018	0.71
	Raritan Bay Medical Center, Perth Amboy	1.6	0.0%	1.61	No	0.12	2	0.72	0.015	0.94
	Riverview Medical Center, Red Bank	2.8	0.0%	1.51	No	0.00	8	0.63	0.006	1.78
	Somerset Medical Center, Somerville	1.8	0.0%	1.40	No	0.11	4	0.49	0.013	1.79
	St. Elizabeth Hospital, Elizabeth	4.0	0.0%	1.01	No	0.18	8	0.68	0.009	1.91
	St. Francis Medical Center, Trenton	3.4	0.0%	1.38	No	0.21	7	0.65	0.005	2.21
	St. Peter's Medical Center, New Brunswick	4.9	0.0%	1.46	No	0.51	7	0.75	0.029	2.49
	Underwood-Memorial Hospital, Woodbury	2.0	0.0%	0.97	No	0.06	3	0.59	0.009	2.21
	United Hospital Medical Center, Newark	5.0	0.0%	1.12	No	0.38	8	0.94	0.012	0.54
	Valley Hospital, Ridgewood	4.1	0.0%	1.21	No	0.00	7	1.01	0.019	2.75
	Warren Hospital, Phillipsburg	2.1	0.0%	1.11	No	0.17	3	0.61	0.000	1.63
	West Jersey Hospital-Voorhees, Voorhees	3.8	0.0%	1.12	No	0.09	2	1.13	0.042	4.46

CARDIOLOGY

Natl. Rank	Hospital	U.S. News index	Reputa- tional score	Cardiology mortality rate	COTH member	Interns and residents to beds	Tech- nology score (of 10)	R.N.'s to beds	Board- certified cardiologists to beds	Procedures to beds
	TIER TWO									
64	Hackensack Medical Center, Hackensack	21.9	0.0%	0.98	Yes	0.40	9	1.54	0.106	10.82
	TIER THREE									
	Atlantic City Medical Center, Atlantic City	17.8	0.0%	0.81	No	0.15	6	0.98	0.016	8.58
	Deborah Heart and Lung Center, Browns Mills	18.4	0.0%	0.48	No	0.48	6	0.81	0.000	26.37
	Englewood Hospital, Englewood	15.4	0.0%	0.95	No	0.18	7	0.63	0.048	6.26
	Helene Fuld Medical Center, Trenton	14.4	0.0%	0.97	No	0.19	5	0.84	0.015	6.02
	Hunterdon Medical Center, Flemington	16.0	0.0%	0.76	No	0.20	3	0.60	0.022	6.49
	Medical Center at Princeton, Princeton	13.8	0.0%	0.96	No	0.09	5	0.61	0.031	5.19
	Monmouth Medical Center, Long Branch	14.2	0.0%	1.11	Yes	0.50	3	0.78	0.011	4.63
	Morristown Memorial Hospital, Morristown	14.9	0.6%	1.16	Yes	0.35	7	0.55	0.037	9.10
	Overlook Hospital, Summit	20.1	0.0%	0.96	Yes	0.39	7	0.96	0.062	7.22
	Robert Wood Johnson University Hospital, New Brunswick	17.8	0.0%	1.15	Yes	0.43	7	1.51	0.152	12.50
	St. Barnabas Medical Center, Livingston	17.1	0.0%	1.02	Yes	0.40	7	0.62	0.038	6.01
	St. Elizabeth Hospital, Elizabeth	17.8	0.0%	0.82	No	0.18	5	0.68	0.094	10.43

Natl. Rank Hospital	U.S. News index	Reputational score	Cardiology mortality rate	COTH member	Interns and residents to beds	Technology score (of 10)	R.N.'s to beds	Board-certified cardiologists to beds	Procedures to beds
St. Francis Medical Center, Trenton	15.0	0.0%	0.96	No	0.21	7	0.65	0.033	5.45
St. Peter's Medical Center, New Brunswick	14.7	0.0%	1.04	No	0.51	5	0.75	0.086	6.99
Underwood-Memorial Hospital, Woodbury	15.1	0.0%	0.91	No	0.06	5	0.59	0.022	8.12
TIER FOUR									
Christ Hospital, Jersey City	8.2	0.0%	1.22	No	0.00	6	0.53	0.035	4.37
Community Medical Center, Toms River	11.4	0.0%	1.12	No	0.00	6	0.98	0.015	11.33
Cooper Hospital-University Medical Center, Camden	13.2	0.0%	1.38	Yes	0.55	8	1.10	0.043	6.10
Elizabeth General Medical Center, Elizabeth	4.2	0.0%	1.43	No	0.02	3	0.60	0.011	2.79
Hospital Center at Orange, Orange	5.5	0.0%	1.36	No	0.07	0	0.80	0.034	4.21
JFK Medical Center, Edison	6.1	0.0%	1.36	No	0.16	2	0.66	0.035	6.07
Jersey Shore Medical Center, Neptune	12.3	0.0%	1.30	Yes	0.30	8	0.71	0.028	10.18
Kennedy Memorial Hosp.-University Med. Ctr., Cherry Hill	13.5	0.0%	1.07	No	0.27	6	0.92	0.042	8.43
Memorial Hospital of Burlington County, Mount Holly	8.4	0.0%	1.30	No	0.25	5	0.68	0.025	13.72
Mercer Medical Center, Trenton	7.5	0.0%	1.33	No	0.00	5	1.04	0.016	5.37
Mountainside Hospital, Montclair	12.6	0.0%	1.09	No	0.24	6	0.62	0.078	8.46
Muhlenberg Regional Medical Center, Plainfield	9.1	0.0%	1.27	No	0.18	6	0.73	0.047	7.41
Newark Beth Israel Medical Center, Newark	8.2	0.0%	1.55	Yes	0.40	0	1.02	0.035	9.31
Our Lady of Lourdes Medical Center, Camden	10.8	0.0%	1.29	No	0.09	7	1.23	0.113	11.47
Raritan Bay Medical Center, Perth Amboy	7.1	0.0%	1.37	No	0.12	5	0.72	0.046	5.93
Riverview Medical Center, Red Bank	6.4	0.0%	1.33	No	0.00	5	0.63	0.024	4.60
Somerset Medical Center, Somerville	12.3	0.0%	1.03	No	0.11	6	0.49	0.029	7.27
St. Joseph's Hospital and Medical Center, Paterson	12.8	0.0%	1.31	Yes	0.38	8	0.76	0.049	6.89
St. Michael's Medical Center, Newark	10.4	0.0%	1.52	Yes	0.48	7	0.71	0.119	8.12
University Hospital, Newark	13.3	0.0%	1.43	Yes	0.94	7	1.28	0.010	1.93
Valley Hospital, Ridgewood	12.6	0.0%	1.13	No	0.00	7	1.01	0.063	11.81
Warren Hospital, Phillipsburg	7.7	0.0%	1.26	No	0.17	3	0.61	0.028	7.99
West Jersey Hospital-Voorhees, Voorhees	13.3	0.0%	1.05	No	0.09	2	1.13	0.103	22.52

ENDOCRINOLOGY

Natl. Rank Hospital	U.S. News index	Reputational score	Endocrinology mortality rate	COTH member	Interns and residents to beds	Technology score (of 11)	R.N.'s to beds	Board-certified internists to beds
TIER THREE								
Atlantic City Medical Center, Atlantic City	8.9	0.0%	0.85	No	0.15	8	0.98	0.064
Cooper Hospital-University Medical Center, Camden	10.3	0.0%	1.34	Yes	0.55	9	1.10	0.056
Hackensack Medical Center, Hackensack	11.8	0.0%	1.58	Yes	0.40	9	1.54	0.281
Morristown Memorial Hospital, Morristown	9.1	0.0%	1.13	Yes	0.35	9	0.55	0.068
Newark Beth Israel Medical Center, Newark	12.7	0.4%	0.73	Yes	0.40	0	1.02	0.086
Overlook Hospital, Summit	10.4	0.0%	1.18	Yes	0.39	9	0.96	0.114
Robert Wood Johnson University Hospital, New Brunswick	9.2	0.4%	1.81	Yes	0.43	3	1.51	0.090
TIER FOUR								
Bergen Pines County Hospital, Paramus	1.8	0.0%	1.82	No	0.06	7	0.24	0.009
Christ Hospital, Jersey City	2.3	0.0%	2.09	No	0.00	9	0.53	0.022
Community Medical Center, Toms River	3.6	0.0%	1.94	No	0.00	8	0.98	0.025
Elizabeth General Medical Center, Elizabeth	6.3	0.0%	1.03	No	0.02	7	0.60	0.127
Englewood Hospital, Englewood	4.1	0.0%	1.69	No	0.18	8	0.63	0.075
Helene Fuld Medical Center, Trenton	4.2	0.0%	1.60	No	0.19	6	0.84	0.024
Hospital Center at Orange, Orange	3.0	0.0%	1.53	No	0.07	0	0.80	0.068
JFK Medical Center, Edison	4.6	0.0%	1.48	No	0.16	7	0.66	0.086
Jersey Shore Medical Center, Neptune	6.4	0.0%	2.01	Yes	0.30	8	0.71	0.051
Kennedy Memorial Hosp.-University Med. Ctr., Cherry Hill	5.8	0.0%	1.34	No	0.27	7	0.92	0.028
Medical Center at Princeton, Princeton	4.4	0.0%	1.50	No	0.09	8	0.61	0.095
Memorial Hospital of Burlington County, Mount Holly	3.6	0.0%	2.01	No	0.25	8	0.68	0.041
Mercer Medical Center, Trenton	3.7	0.0%	2.05	No	0.00	8	1.04	0.039
Monmouth Medical Center, Long Branch	6.8	0.0%	2.27	Yes	0.50	7	0.78	0.061

Natl. Rank	Hospital	U.S. News index	Reputational score	Endocrinology mortality rate	COTH member	Interns and residents to beds	Technology score (of 11)	R.N.'s to beds	Board-certified internists to beds
	Mountainside Hospital, Montclair	3.7	0.0%	2.03	No	0.24	8	0.62	0.086
	Muhlenberg Regional Medical Center, Plainfield	3.8	0.0%	1.98	No	0.18	8	0.73	0.066
	Our Lady of Lourdes Medical Center, Camden	4.9	0.0%	1.47	No	0.09	4	1.23	0.015
	Raritan Bay Medical Center, Perth Amboy	3.6	0.5%	1.75	No	0.12	4	0.72	0.033
	Riverview Medical Center, Red Bank	2.5	0.0%	2.68	No	0.00	9	0.63	0.108
	Somerset Medical Center, Somerville	4.2	0.0%	1.24	No	0.11	5	0.49	0.040
	St. Barnabas Medical Center, Livingston	7.4	0.0%	1.68	Yes	0.40	9	0.62	0.046
	St. Elizabeth Hospital, Elizabeth	5.5	0.0%	1.30	No	0.18	8	0.68	0.076
	St. Francis Medical Center, Trenton	4.7	0.0%	1.42	No	0.21	8	0.65	0.021
	St. Joseph's Hospital and Medical Center, Paterson	7.8	0.0%	1.63	Yes	0.38	9	0.76	0.042
	St. Michael's Medical Center, Newark	6.4	0.0%	1.83	Yes	0.48	4	0.71	0.029
	St. Peter's Medical Center, New Brunswick	4.9	0.0%	1.97	No	0.51	8	0.75	0.056
	Underwood-Memorial Hospital, Woodbury	4.0	0.0%	1.28	No	0.06	5	0.59	0.031
	United Hospital Medical Center, Newark	5.5	0.0%	1.52	No	0.38	7	0.94	0.014
	Valley Hospital, Ridgewood	4.2	0.0%	1.78	No	0.00	8	1.01	0.044
	Warren Hospital, Phillipsburg	2.7	0.0%	1.75	No	0.17	4	0.61	0.023
	West Jersey Hospital-Voorhees, Voorhees	6.0	0.0%	1.41	No	0.09	4	1.13	0.179

GASTROENTEROLOGY

Natl. Rank	Hospital	U.S. News index	Reputational score	Gastro-enterology mortality rate	COTH member	Interns and residents to beds	Technology score (of 11)	R.N.'s to beds	Board-certified gastro-enterologists to beds	Procedures to beds
	TIER THREE									
	Community Medical Center, Toms River	8.6	0.6%	1.05	No	0.00	7	0.98	0.018	5.62
	Cooper Hospital-University Medical Center, Camden	10.3	0.5%	1.24	Yes	0.55	8	1.10	0.032	1.57
87	Hackensack Medical Center, Hackensack	12.7	0.0%	0.99	Yes	0.40	8	1.54	0.023	3.68
	Medical Center at Princeton, Princeton	8.4	0.5%	0.77	No	0.09	7	0.61	0.031	2.95
	Monmouth Medical Center, Long Branch	8.0	0.0%	1.40	Yes	0.50	6	0.78	0.009	2.79
	Overlook Hospital, Summit	10.8	0.0%	1.09	Yes	0.39	8	0.96	0.025	3.84
	Robert Wood Johnson University Hospital, New Brunswick	9.5	0.0%	1.14	Yes	0.43	3	1.51	0.069	2.00
	St. Barnabas Medical Center, Livingston	8.8	0.0%	1.23	Yes	0.40	8	0.62	0.031	3.03
	St. Joseph's Hospital and Medical Center, Paterson	7.7	0.0%	1.32	Yes	0.38	8	0.76	0.015	1.43
	Valley Hospital, Ridgewood	7.5	0.0%	1.02	No	0.00	7	1.01	0.030	4.68
89	West Jersey Hospital-Voorhees, Voorhees	12.7	0.0%	1.02	No	0.09	4	1.13	0.095	13.65
	TIER FOUR									
	Atlantic City Medical Center, Atlantic City	6.2	0.0%	1.16	No	0.15	7	0.98	0.010	3.10
	Christ Hospital, Jersey City	2.9	0.0%	1.61	No	0.00	8	0.53	0.030	2.60
	Elizabeth General Medical Center, Elizabeth	4.3	0.0%	1.03	No	0.02	6	0.60	0.016	1.40
	Englewood Hospital, Englewood	6.0	0.0%	1.12	No	0.18	7	0.63	0.027	3.52
	Helene Fuld Medical Center, Trenton	5.2	0.0%	1.22	No	0.19	6	0.84	0.018	2.72
	Hospital Center at Orange, Orange	2.3	0.0%	1.30	No	0.07	0	0.80	0.015	2.32
	Hunterdon Medical Center, Flemington	5.4	0.0%	1.08	No	0.20	4	0.60	0.017	3.87
	JFK Medical Center, Edison	4.6	0.0%	1.26	No	0.16	6	0.66	0.016	3.03
	Jersey Shore Medical Center, Neptune	6.8	0.0%	1.61	Yes	0.30	7	0.71	0.014	2.83
	Kennedy Memorial Hosp.-University Med. Ctr., Cherry Hill	7.2	0.0%	1.06	No	0.27	6	0.92	0.028	3.91
	Memorial Hospital of Burlington County, Mount Holly	4.6	0.0%	1.61	No	0.25	7	0.68	0.038	3.82
	Mercer Medical Center, Trenton	4.1	0.0%	1.58	No	0.00	7	1.04	0.010	3.08
	Morristown Memorial Hospital, Morristown	7.3	0.0%	1.40	Yes	0.35	8	0.55	0.013	2.40
	Mountainside Hospital, Montclair	5.2	0.0%	1.44	No	0.24	7	0.62	0.042	4.33
	Muhlenberg Regional Medical Center, Plainfield	5.1	0.0%	1.33	No	0.18	7	0.73	0.014	3.54
	Newark Beth Israel Medical Center, Newark	4.4	0.0%	1.79	Yes	0.40	0	1.02	0.015	1.24
	Our Lady of Lourdes Medical Center, Camden	4.5	0.5%	1.50	No	0.09	4	1.23	0.036	2.20
	Raritan Bay Medical Center, Perth Amboy	4.2	0.0%	1.19	No	0.12	4	0.72	0.039	2.62
	Riverview Medical Center, Red Bank	4.2	0.0%	1.31	No	0.00	8	0.63	0.004	2.86

Natl. Rank	Hospital	U.S. News index	Reputational score	Gastro-enterology mortality rate	COTH member	Interns and residents to beds	Technology score (of 11)	R.N.'s to beds	Board-certified gastro-enterologists to beds	Pro-cedures to beds
	Somerset Medical Center, Somerville	3.1	0.0%	1.37	No	0.11	4	0.49	0.019	3.11
	St. Elizabeth Hospital, Elizabeth	7.2	0.0%	0.93	No	0.18	7	0.68	0.030	3.16
	St. Francis Medical Center, Trenton	4.4	0.0%	1.35	No	0.21	7	0.65	0.013	2.62
	St. Peter's Medical Center, New Brunswick	5.5	0.0%	1.47	No	0.51	7	0.75	0.027	2.85
	Underwood-Memorial Hospital, Woodbury	4.5	0.5%	1.40	No	0.06	5	0.59	0.025	4.09
	Warren Hospital, Phillipsburg	5.0	0.0%	1.21	No	0.17	4	0.61	0.009	4.52

GERIATRICS

Natl. Rank	Hospital	U.S. News index	Reputational score	Hospital-wide mortality rate	COTH member	Service mix	Interns and residents to beds	Technology score (of 13)	R.N.'s to beds	Discharge planning (of 2)	Geriatric services (of 9)	Board-certified internists to beds
	TIER THREE											
	Atlantic City Medical Center, Atlantic City	17.5	0.0%	1.00	No	8	0.15	10	0.98	2	6	0.064
98	Hackensack Medical Center, Hackensack	20.6	0.0%	1.10	Yes	10	0.40	11	1.54	2	5	0.281
	Hunterdon Medical Center, Flemington	14.5	0.0%	1.00	No	7	0.20	5	0.60	2	3	0.006
	Medical Center at Princeton, Princeton	13.9	0.0%	1.01	No	7	0.09	9	0.61	1	2	0.095
	Overlook Hospital, Summit	19.1	0.0%	1.08	Yes	9	0.39	11	0.96	2	7	0.114
	TIER FOUR											
	Christ Hospital, Jersey City	6.9	0.0%	1.41	No	9	0.00	10	0.53	2	1	0.022
	Community Medical Center, Toms River	11.3	0.0%	1.19	No	6	0.00	10	0.98	2	5	0.025
	Cooper Hospital-University Medical Center, Camden	12.6	0.0%	1.34	Yes	7	0.55	12	1.10	2	2	0.056
	Elizabeth General Medical Center, Elizabeth	9.3	0.0%	1.18	No	7	0.02	7	0.60	1	2	0.127
	Helene Fuld Medical Center, Trenton	8.6	0.0%	1.28	No	7	0.19	6	0.84	2	2	0.024
	JFK Medical Center, Edison	9.0	0.0%	1.25	No	7	0.16	7	0.66	2	1	0.086
	Jersey Shore Medical Center, Neptune	10.3	0.0%	1.42	Yes	9	0.30	10	0.71	2	2	0.051
	Kennedy Memorial Hosp.-University Med. Ctr., Cherry Hill	12.9	0.0%	1.18	No	8	0.27	9	0.92	2	6	0.028
	Memorial Hospital of Burlington County, Mount Holly	7.6	0.0%	1.42	No	6	0.25	9	0.68	2	6	0.041
	Mercer Medical Center, Trenton	6.3	0.0%	1.47	No	5	0.00	9	1.04	2	5	0.039
	Monmouth Medical Center, Long Branch	12.6	0.0%	1.36	Yes	8	0.50	8	0.78	2	8	0.061
	Morristown Memorial Hospital, Morristown	12.6	0.0%	1.30	Yes	7	0.35	10	0.55	2	7	0.068
	Mountainside Hospital, Montclair	9.2	0.0%	1.27	No	5	0.24	10	0.62	2	3	0.086
	Muhlenberg Regional Medical Center, Plainfield	8.2	0.0%	1.36	No	7	0.18	9	0.73	2	3	0.066
	Our Lady of Lourdes Medical Center, Camden	7.4	0.0%	1.38	No	6	0.09	6	1.23	2	3	0.015
	Raritan Bay Medical Center, Perth Amboy	4.9	0.0%	1.40	No	7	0.12	5	0.72	1	1	0.033
	Riverview Medical Center, Red Bank	6.6	0.0%	1.50	No	8	0.00	9	0.63	2	4	0.108
	Robert Wood Johnson University Hospital, New Brunswick	13.0	0.0%	1.22	Yes	5	0.43	5	1.51	2	2	0.090
	Somerset Medical Center, Somerville	7.6	0.0%	1.25	No	5	0.11	6	0.49	2	2	0.040
	St. Barnabas Medical Center, Livingston	13.2	0.0%	1.22	Yes	7	0.40	12	0.62	2	2	0.046
	St. Elizabeth Hospital, Elizabeth	13.8	0.0%	1.02	No	6	0.18	9	0.68	1	3	0.076
	St. Francis Medical Center, Trenton	9.9	0.0%	1.19	No	5	0.21	10	0.65	2	2	0.021
	St. Joseph's Hospital and Medical Center, Paterson	12.4	0.0%	1.39	Yes	8	0.38	10	0.76	2	9	0.042
	St. Michael's Medical Center, Newark	5.3	0.0%	1.58	Yes	4	0.48	5	0.71	2	1	0.029
	St. Peter's Medical Center, New Brunswick	9.8	0.0%	1.32	No	6	0.51	9	0.75	2	5	0.056
	Underwood-Memorial Hospital, Woodbury	9.5	0.0%	1.05	No	2	0.06	6	0.59	1	2	0.031
	Valley Hospital, Ridgewood	10.1	0.0%	1.20	No	5	0.00	10	1.01	2	2	0.044
	Warren Hospital, Phillipsburg	7.9	0.0%	1.28	No	5	0.17	4	0.61	2	6	0.023
	West Jersey Hospital-Voorhees, Voorhees	10.8	0.0%	1.15	No	5	0.09	4	1.13	2	1	0.179

GYNECOLOGY

Natl. Rank / Hospital	U.S. News index	Reputational score	Hospital-wide mortality rate	Interns and residents to beds	Technology score (of 10)	R.N.'s to beds	Board-certified OB-GYNs to beds	Procedures to beds
TIER THREE								
Atlantic City Medical Center, Atlantic City	16.2	0.0%	1.00	0.15	7	0.98	0.034	0.35
Hackensack Medical Center, Hackensack	18.7	0.0%	1.10	0.40	8	1.54	0.064	0.45
Medical Center at Princeton, Princeton	14.3	0.0%	1.01	0.09	7	0.61	0.036	0.27
Overlook Hospital, Summit	16.4	0.0%	1.08	0.39	8	0.96	0.058	0.35
St. Barnabas Medical Center, Livingston	15.1	1.0%	1.22	0.40	8	0.62	0.081	0.70
St. Elizabeth Hospital, Elizabeth	15.0	0.0%	1.02	0.18	7	0.68	0.045	0.22
TIER FOUR								
Christ Hospital, Jersey City	5.1	0.0%	1.41	0.00	7	0.53	0.012	0.16
Community Medical Center, Toms River	10.9	0.0%	1.19	0.00	7	0.98	0.020	0.43
Cooper Hospital-University Medical Center, Camden	12.8	0.0%	1.34	0.55	8	1.10	0.051	0.44
Elizabeth General Medical Center, Elizabeth	8.2	0.0%	1.18	0.02	5	0.60	0.023	0.13
Englewood Hospital, Englewood	9.2	0.0%	1.25	0.18	6	0.63	0.058	0.32
Helene Fuld Medical Center, Trenton	8.6	0.0%	1.28	0.19	6	0.84	0.015	0.21
Hunterdon Medical Center, Flemington	12.2	0.0%	1.00	0.20	3	0.60	0.039	0.34
JFK Medical Center, Edison	8.2	0.0%	1.25	0.16	5	0.66	0.045	0.25
Jersey Shore Medical Center, Neptune	6.4	0.0%	1.42	0.30	6	0.71	0.016	0.28
Kennedy Memorial Hosp.-University Med. Ctr., Cherry Hill	11.4	0.0%	1.18	0.27	5	0.92	0.055	0.24
Memorial Hospital of Burlington County, Mount Holly	7.8	0.0%	1.42	0.25	6	0.68	0.090	0.38
Mercer Medical Center, Trenton	7.6	0.0%	1.47	0.00	7	1.04	0.058	0.40
Monmouth Medical Center, Long Branch	9.3	0.0%	1.36	0.50	6	0.78	0.050	0.25
Morristown Memorial Hospital, Morristown	9.9	0.0%	1.30	0.35	8	0.55	0.045	0.29
Muhlenberg Regional Medical Center, Plainfield	8.1	0.0%	1.36	0.18	7	0.73	0.041	0.38
Our Lady of Lourdes Medical Center, Camden	8.5	0.0%	1.38	0.09	5	1.23	0.049	0.17
Raritan Bay Medical Center, Perth Amboy	4.7	0.0%	1.40	0.12	4	0.72	0.022	0.18
Riverview Medical Center, Red Bank	4.5	0.0%	1.50	0.00	6	0.63	0.047	0.31
Robert Wood Johnson University Hospital, New Brunswick	13.6	0.0%	1.22	0.43	3	1.51	0.157	0.37
Somerset Medical Center, Somerville	6.1	0.0%	1.25	0.11	4	0.49	0.024	0.25
St. Francis Medical Center, Trenton	9.6	0.0%	1.19	0.21	6	0.65	0.018	0.23
St. Joseph's Hospital and Medical Center, Paterson	9.1	0.0%	1.39	0.38	8	0.76	0.025	0.22
St. Michael's Medical Center, Newark	3.9	0.0%	1.58	0.48	4	0.71	0.015	0.15
St. Peter's Medical Center, New Brunswick	11.7	0.0%	1.32	0.51	7	0.75	0.097	0.64
Underwood-Memorial Hospital, Woodbury	11.8	0.0%	1.05	0.06	5	0.59	0.050	0.30
Valley Hospital, Ridgewood	11.1	0.0%	1.20	0.00	6	1.01	0.065	0.37
Warren Hospital, Phillipsburg	5.2	0.0%	1.28	0.17	3	0.61	0.009	0.36
West Jersey Hospital-Voorhees, Voorhees	12.5	0.0%	1.15	0.09	4	1.13	0.240	0.81

NEUROLOGY

Natl. Rank / Hospital	U.S. News index	Reputational score	Neurology mortality rate	COTH member	Interns and residents to beds	Technology score (of 9)	R.N.'s to beds	Board-certified neurologists to beds
TIER THREE								
Hackensack Medical Center, Hackensack	16.0	0.0%	0.94	Yes	0.40	7	1.54	0.011
JFK Medical Center, Edison	13.5	0.0%	0.79	No	0.16	5	0.66	0.014
99 Robert Wood Johnson University Hospital, New Brunswick	17.0	0.0%	0.94	Yes	0.43	3	1.51	0.044
United Hospital Medical Center, Newark	11.7	0.0%	0.91	No	0.38	5	0.94	0.005
University Hospital, Newark	13.0	0.0%	1.35	Yes	0.94	7	1.28	0.027
Valley Hospital, Ridgewood	11.4	0.0%	0.95	No	0.00	6	1.01	0.021
West Jersey Hospital-Voorhees, Voorhees	12.1	0.0%	1.06	No	0.09	3	1.13	0.065
TIER FOUR								
Atlantic City Medical Center, Atlantic City	9.6	0.0%	1.01	No	0.15	6	0.98	0.004
Christ Hospital, Jersey City	5.8	0.0%	1.20	No	0.00	7	0.53	0.005
Community Medical Center, Toms River	7.6	0.0%	1.12	No	0.00	6	0.98	0.005

Natl. Rank	Hospital	U.S. News index	Reputational score	Neurology mortality rate	COTH member	Interns and residents to beds	Technology score (of 9)	R.N.'s to beds	Board-certified neurologists to beds
	Cooper Hospital-University Medical Center, Camden	10.2	0.0%	1.39	Yes	0.55	7	1.10	0.016
	Elizabeth General Medical Center, Elizabeth	6.4	0.0%	1.12	No	0.02	5	0.60	0.005
	Englewood Hospital, Englewood	5.9	0.0%	1.29	No	0.18	6	0.63	0.013
	Helene Fuld Medical Center, Trenton	4.1	0.0%	1.51	No	0.19	5	0.84	0.009
	Hospital Center at Orange, Orange	3.3	0.0%	1.39	No	0.07	0	0.80	0.012
	Jersey Shore Medical Center, Neptune	9.5	0.0%	1.24	Yes	0.30	6	0.71	0.016
	Kennedy Memorial Hosp.-University Med. Ctr., Cherry Hill	7.6	0.0%	1.26	No	0.27	5	0.92	0.023
	Medical Center at Princeton, Princeton	8.7	0.0%	1.05	No	0.09	6	0.61	0.017
	Memorial Hospital of Burlington County, Mount Holly	7.9	0.0%	1.24	No	0.25	6	0.68	0.030
	Mercer Medical Center, Trenton	7.5	0.0%	1.20	No	0.00	6	1.04	0.016
	Monmouth Medical Center, Long Branch	7.6	0.0%	1.49	Yes	0.50	5	0.78	0.011
	Morristown Memorial Hospital, Morristown	10.5	0.0%	1.13	Yes	0.35	7	0.55	0.013
	Mountainside Hospital, Montclair	6.8	0.0%	1.25	No	0.24	6	0.62	0.017
	Muhlenberg Regional Medical Center, Plainfield	5.0	0.0%	1.36	No	0.18	6	0.73	0.005
	Newark Beth Israel Medical Center, Newark	9.2	0.0%	1.20	Yes	0.40	0	1.02	0.015
	Our Lady of Lourdes Medical Center, Camden	6.7	0.0%	1.28	No	0.09	4	1.23	0.013
	Overlook Hospital, Summit	10.1	0.0%	1.29	Yes	0.39	7	0.96	0.014
	Raritan Bay Medical Center, Perth Amboy	6.7	0.0%	1.15	No	0.12	4	0.72	0.009
	Riverview Medical Center, Red Bank	5.2	0.0%	1.34	No	0.00	7	0.63	0.014
	Somerset Medical Center, Somerville	3.4	0.0%	1.43	No	0.11	4	0.49	0.011
	St. Barnabas Medical Center, Livingston	8.1	0.0%	1.38	Yes	0.40	7	0.62	0.009
	St. Elizabeth Hospital, Elizabeth	8.9	0.0%	1.05	No	0.18	6	0.68	0.012
	St. Francis Medical Center, Trenton	6.6	0.0%	1.21	No	0.21	6	0.65	0.008
	St. Joseph's Hospital and Medical Center, Paterson	8.4	0.0%	1.39	Yes	0.38	7	0.76	0.010
	St. Peter's Medical Center, New Brunswick	7.5	0.0%	1.24	No	0.51	6	0.75	0.009
	Underwood-Memorial Hospital, Woodbury	6.9	0.0%	1.09	No	0.06	5	0.59	0.006
	Warren Hospital, Phillipsburg	5.5	0.0%	1.21	No	0.17	3	0.61	0.009

ORTHOPEDICS

Natl. Rank	Hospital	U.S. News index	Reputational score	Orthopedics mortality rate	COTH member	Interns and residents to beds	Technology score (of 5)	R.N.'s to beds	Board-certified orthopedists to beds	Procedures to beds
	TIER THREE									
	Cooper Hospital-University Medical Center, Camden	9.8	0.0%	1.30	Yes	0.55	4	1.10	0.022	0.86
89	Hackensack Medical Center, Hackensack	13.6	0.0%	0.90	Yes	0.40	4	1.54	0.060	2.36
	Overlook Hospital, Summit	12.5	0.0%	0.84	Yes	0.39	4	0.96	0.043	2.31
	Robert Wood Johnson University Hospital, New Brunswick	10.8	0.0%	1.09	Yes	0.43	2	1.51	0.059	1.97
	St. Barnabas Medical Center, Livingston	8.8	0.5%	1.45	Yes	0.40	4	0.62	0.057	1.75
	West Jersey Hospital-Voorhees, Voorhees	8.4	0.0%	0.94	No	0.09	2	1.13	0.141	6.02
	TIER FOUR									
	Atlantic City Medical Center, Atlantic City	6.5	0.0%	1.03	No	0.15	3	0.98	0.018	1.93
	Christ Hospital, Jersey City	3.7	0.0%	1.31	No	0.00	4	0.53	0.017	1.27
	Community Medical Center, Toms River	7.4	0.5%	1.00	No	0.00	3	0.98	0.022	2.73
	Elizabeth General Medical Center, Elizabeth	0.5	0.0%	2.05	No	0.02	2	0.60	0.023	0.68
	Englewood Hospital, Englewood	4.7	0.0%	1.32	No	0.18	4	0.63	0.027	1.82
	Helene Fuld Medical Center, Trenton	3.3	0.0%	1.62	No	0.19	3	0.84	0.006	0.91
	Hunterdon Medical Center, Flemington	5.5	0.0%	0.98	No	0.20	2	0.60	0.028	2.38
	JFK Medical Center, Edison	5.1	0.0%	1.05	No	0.16	2	0.66	0.025	2.54
	Jersey Shore Medical Center, Neptune	6.7	0.0%	1.52	Yes	0.30	3	0.71	0.024	1.94
	Kennedy Memorial Hosp.-University Med. Ctr., Cherry Hill	7.3	0.0%	1.06	No	0.27	4	0.92	0.028	2.25
	Medical Center at Princeton, Princeton	6.8	0.0%	0.87	No	0.09	3	0.61	0.043	2.06
	Memorial Hospital of Burlington County, Mount Holly	3.9	0.0%	1.52	No	0.25	3	0.68	0.036	2.62
	Mercer Medical Center, Trenton	3.3	0.0%	1.70	No	0.00	3	1.04	0.016	1.95
	Monmouth Medical Center, Long Branch	6.7	0.0%	1.59	Yes	0.50	2	0.78	0.037	1.73
	Morristown Memorial Hospital, Morristown	6.8	0.0%	1.44	Yes	0.35	3	0.55	0.028	2.53

Natl. Rank	Hospital	U.S. News index	Reputational score	Orthopedics mortality rate	COTH member	Interns and residents to beds	Technology score (of 5)	R.N.'s to beds	Board-certified orthopedists to beds	Procedures to beds
	Mountainside Hospital, Montclair	3.1	0.0%	1.79	No	0.24	3	0.62	0.042	2.88
	Muhlenberg Regional Medical Center, Plainfield	5.7	0.0%	1.17	No	0.18	4	0.73	0.022	1.75
	Our Lady of Lourdes Medical Center, Camden	4.1	0.0%	1.60	No	0.09	3	1.23	0.013	0.87
	Raritan Bay Medical Center, Perth Amboy	4.0	0.0%	1.32	No	0.12	3	0.72	0.035	1.18
	Riverview Medical Center, Red Bank	2.4	0.0%	1.64	No	0.00	3	0.63	0.035	1.73
	Somerset Medical Center, Somerville	6.7	0.0%	0.84	No	0.11	3	0.49	0.027	1.77
	St. Elizabeth Hospital, Elizabeth	5.3	0.0%	1.09	No	0.18	3	0.68	0.036	1.34
	St. Francis Medical Center, Trenton	5.1	0.0%	1.11	No	0.21	3	0.65	0.018	1.37
	St. Joseph's Hospital and Medical Center, Paterson	4.8	0.0%	2.50	Yes	0.38	3	0.76	0.014	0.64
	St. Peter's Medical Center, New Brunswick	7.4	0.0%	1.01	No	0.51	3	0.75	0.050	1.74
	Underwood-Memorial Hospital, Woodbury	5.1	0.0%	1.16	No	0.06	4	0.59	0.028	2.27
	Valley Hospital, Ridgewood	4.7	0.0%	1.39	No	0.00	3	1.01	0.053	3.34
	Warren Hospital, Phillipsburg	3.0	0.0%	1.38	No	0.17	2	0.61	0.028	1.61

OTOLARYNGOLOGY

Natl. Rank	Hospital	U.S. News index	Reputational score	Hospital-wide mortality rate	COTH member	Interns and residents to beds	Technology score (of 9)	R.N.'s to beds	Board-certified internists to beds	Procedures to beds
	TIER TWO									
97	Hackensack Medical Center, Hackensack	13.8	0.0%	1.10	Yes	0.40	7	1.54	0.281	0.232
69	University Hospital, Newark	15.4	0.8%	1.33	Yes	0.94	7	1.28	0.019	0.091
	TIER THREE									
	Cooper Hospital-University Medical Center, Camden	11.0	0.0%	1.33	Yes	0.55	7	1.10	0.056	0.179
	Jersey Shore Medical Center, Neptune	8.4	0.0%	1.42	Yes	0.30	6	0.71	0.051	0.274
	Monmouth Medical Center, Long Branch	9.3	0.0%	1.36	Yes	0.50	5	0.78	0.061	0.232
	Morristown Memorial Hospital, Morristown	8.6	0.0%	1.30	Yes	0.35	7	0.55	0.068	0.230
	Newark Beth Israel Medical Center, Newark	8.4	0.0%	1.47	Yes	0.40	0	1.02	0.086	0.139
	Overlook Hospital, Summit	10.6	0.0%	1.08	Yes	0.39	7	0.96	0.114	0.227
	Robert Wood Johnson University Hospital, New Brunswick	10.4	0.0%	1.22	Yes	0.43	1	1.51	0.090	0.075
	St. Barnabas Medical Center, Livingston	8.9	0.0%	1.22	Yes	0.40	7	0.62	0.046	0.242
	St. Joseph's Hospital and Medical Center, Paterson	9.1	0.0%	1.39	Yes	0.38	7	0.76	0.042	0.107
	St. Michael's Medical Center, Newark	7.8	0.0%	1.57	Yes	0.48	2	0.71	0.029	0.066
	United Hospital Medical Center, Newark	8.4	0.8%	1.23	No	0.38	5	0.94	0.014	0.116
	TIER FOUR									
	Atlantic City Medical Center, Atlantic City	5.9	0.0%	1.00	No	0.15	6	0.98	0.064	0.210
	Bergen Pines County Hospital, Paramus	2.2	0.0%	1.48	No	0.06	5	0.24	0.009	0.015
	Christ Hospital, Jersey City	3.6	0.0%	1.41	No	0.00	7	0.53	0.022	0.254
	Community Medical Center, Toms River	4.9	0.0%	1.19	No	0.00	6	0.98	0.025	0.371
	Deborah Heart and Lung Center, Browns Mills	5.2	0.0%	0.52	No	0.48	2	0.81	0.000	0.039
	Elizabeth General Medical Center, Elizabeth	4.3	0.0%	1.18	No	0.02	5	0.60	0.127	0.130
	Englewood Hospital, Englewood	4.9	0.0%	1.25	No	0.18	6	0.63	0.075	0.242
	Helene Fuld Medical Center, Trenton	4.5	0.0%	1.28	No	0.19	4	0.84	0.024	0.165
	Hospital Center at Orange, Orange	3.1	0.0%	1.38	No	0.07	0	0.80	0.068	0.212
	Hunterdon Medical Center, Flemington	3.6	0.0%	1.00	No	0.20	3	0.60	0.006	0.315
	JFK Medical Center, Edison	4.7	0.0%	1.25	No	0.16	5	0.66	0.086	0.327
	Jersey City Medical Center, Jersey City	5.0	0.0%	1.54	No	0.40	2	0.88	0.046	0.085
	Kennedy Memorial Hosp.-University Med. Ctr., Cherry Hill	5.5	0.0%	1.18	No	0.27	5	0.92	0.028	0.277
	Medical Center at Princeton, Princeton	4.8	0.0%	1.01	No	0.09	6	0.61	0.095	0.322
	Memorial Hospital of Burlington County, Mount Holly	4.9	0.0%	1.42	No	0.25	6	0.68	0.041	0.370
	Mercer Medical Center, Trenton	5.0	0.0%	1.47	No	0.00	6	1.04	0.039	0.321
	Mountainside Hospital, Montclair	5.2	0.0%	1.27	No	0.24	6	0.62	0.086	0.344
	Muhlenberg Regional Medical Center, Plainfield	5.3	0.0%	1.36	No	0.18	7	0.73	0.066	0.247
	Our Lady of Lourdes Medical Center, Camden	4.7	0.0%	1.38	No	0.09	2	1.23	0.015	0.126
	Raritan Bay Medical Center, Perth Amboy	3.4	0.0%	1.40	No	0.12	2	0.72	0.033	0.360
	Riverview Medical Center, Red Bank	4.6	0.0%	1.50	No	0.00	7	0.63	0.108	0.306

Natl. Rank	Hospital	U.S. News index	Reputational score	Hospital-wide mortality rate	COTH member	Interns and residents to beds	Technology score (of 9)	R.N.'s to beds	Board-certified internists to beds	Procedures to beds
	Somerset Medical Center, Somerville	3.0	0.0%	1.25	No	0.11	3	0.49	0.040	0.316
	St. Elizabeth Hospital, Elizabeth	5.5	0.0%	1.02	No	0.18	7	0.68	0.076	0.208
	St. Francis Medical Center, Trenton	4.6	0.0%	1.19	No	0.21	6	0.65	0.021	0.192
	St. Peter's Medical Center, New Brunswick	6.3	0.0%	1.32	No	0.51	6	0.75	0.056	0.330
	Underwood-Memorial Hospital, Woodbury	3.2	0.0%	1.05	No	0.06	3	0.59	0.031	0.368
	Valley Hospital, Ridgewood	5.1	0.0%	1.20	No	0.00	6	1.01	0.044	0.391
	Warren Hospital, Phillipsburg	3.2	0.0%	1.28	No	0.17	2	0.61	0.023	0.350
	West Jersey Hospital-Voorhees, Voorhees	6.0	0.0%	1.15	No	0.09	2	1.13	0.179	0.996

RHEUMATOLOGY

Natl. Rank	Hospital	U.S. News index	Reputational score	Hospital-wide mortality rate	COTH member	Interns and residents to beds	Technology score (of 5)	R.N.'s to beds	Board-certified internists to beds
	TIER THREE								
	Cooper Hospital-University Medical Center, Camden	11.4	0.0%	1.33	Yes	0.55	4	1.10	0.056
	Deborah Heart and Lung Center, Browns Mills	10.1	0.0%	0.52	No	0.48	3	0.81	0.000
94	Hackensack Medical Center, Hackensack	15.2	0.0%	1.10	Yes	0.40	4	1.54	0.281
	Overlook Hospital, Summit	12.6	0.0%	1.08	Yes	0.39	4	0.96	0.114
	Robert Wood Johnson University Hospital, New Brunswick	12.1	0.0%	1.22	Yes	0.43	2	1.51	0.090
	St. Barnabas Medical Center, Livingston	11.2	0.4%	1.22	Yes	0.40	4	0.62	0.046
	TIER FOUR								
	Atlantic City Medical Center, Atlantic City	9.2	0.0%	1.00	No	0.15	3	0.98	0.064
	Christ Hospital, Jersey City	5.1	0.0%	1.41	No	0.00	4	0.53	0.022
	Community Medical Center, Toms River	7.0	0.0%	1.19	No	0.00	3	0.98	0.025
	Elizabeth General Medical Center, Elizabeth	5.4	0.0%	1.18	No	0.02	2	0.60	0.127
	Englewood Hospital, Englewood	6.1	0.0%	1.25	No	0.18	4	0.63	0.075
	Helene Fuld Medical Center, Trenton	6.7	0.0%	1.28	No	0.19	3	0.84	0.024
	Hospital Center at Orange, Orange	2.6	0.0%	1.38	No	0.07	0	0.80	0.068
	Hunterdon Medical Center, Flemington	7.6	0.0%	1.00	No	0.20	2	0.60	0.006
	JFK Medical Center, Edison	6.3	0.0%	1.25	No	0.16	2	0.66	0.086
	Jersey Shore Medical Center, Neptune	8.7	0.0%	1.42	Yes	0.30	3	0.71	0.051
	Kennedy Memorial Hosp.-University Med. Ctr., Cherry Hill	8.3	0.0%	1.18	No	0.27	4	0.92	0.028
	Medical Center at Princeton, Princeton	7.2	0.0%	1.01	No	0.09	3	0.61	0.095
	Memorial Hospital of Burlington County, Mount Holly	5.9	0.0%	1.42	No	0.25	3	0.68	0.041
	Mercer Medical Center, Trenton	5.8	0.0%	1.47	No	0.00	3	1.04	0.039
	Monmouth Medical Center, Long Branch	9.4	0.0%	1.36	Yes	0.50	2	0.78	0.061
	Morristown Memorial Hospital, Morristown	9.2	0.0%	1.30	Yes	0.35	3	0.55	0.068
	Mountainside Hospital, Montclair	6.8	0.0%	1.27	No	0.24	3	0.62	0.086
	Muhlenberg Regional Medical Center, Plainfield	6.7	0.0%	1.36	No	0.18	4	0.73	0.066
	Newark Beth Israel Medical Center, Newark	6.5	0.0%	1.47	Yes	0.40	0	1.02	0.086
	Our Lady of Lourdes Medical Center, Camden	6.9	0.0%	1.38	No	0.09	3	1.23	0.015
	Raritan Bay Medical Center, Perth Amboy	4.6	0.0%	1.40	No	0.12	3	0.72	0.033
	Riverview Medical Center, Red Bank	5.1	0.0%	1.50	No	0.00	3	0.63	0.108
	Somerset Medical Center, Somerville	5.9	0.0%	1.25	No	0.11	3	0.49	0.040
	St. Elizabeth Hospital, Elizabeth	7.5	0.0%	1.02	No	0.18	3	0.68	0.076
	St. Francis Medical Center, Trenton	6.8	0.0%	1.19	No	0.21	3	0.65	0.021
	St. Joseph's Hospital and Medical Center, Paterson	9.2	0.0%	1.39	Yes	0.38	3	0.76	0.042
	St. Michael's Medical Center, Newark	8.5	0.0%	1.57	Yes	0.48	3	0.71	0.029
	St. Peter's Medical Center, New Brunswick	7.5	0.0%	1.32	No	0.51	3	0.75	0.056
	Underwood-Memorial Hospital, Woodbury	6.7	0.0%	1.05	No	0.06	4	0.59	0.031
	Valley Hospital, Ridgewood	7.2	0.0%	1.20	No	0.00	3	1.01	0.044
	Warren Hospital, Phillipsburg	5.6	0.0%	1.28	No	0.17	2	0.61	0.023
	West Jersey Hospital-Voorhees, Voorhees	8.7	0.0%	1.15	No	0.09	2	1.13	0.179

UROLOGY

Natl. Rank	Hospital	U.S. News index	Reputa-tional score	Urology mortality rate	COTH member	Interns and residents to beds	Tech-nology score (of 11)	R.N.'s to beds	Board-certified internists to beds	Procedures to beds
	TIER THREE									
	Hackensack Medical Center, Hackensack	12.0	0.0%	1.36	Yes	0.40	8	1.54	0.281	2.55
	Hunterdon Medical Center, Flemington	10.0	0.0%	0.58	No	0.20	4	0.60	0.006	1.93
	Overlook Hospital, Summit	11.5	0.0%	1.17	Yes	0.39	8	0.96	0.114	2.89
	Robert Wood Johnson University Hospital, New Brunswick	11.0	0.0%	1.19	Yes	0.43	3	1.51	0.090	1.71
	TIER FOUR									
	Atlantic City Medical Center, Atlantic City	7.9	0.0%	1.08	No	0.15	7	0.98	0.064	1.93
	Bergen Pines County Hospital, Paramus	3.1	0.0%	1.31	No	0.06	6	0.24	0.009	0.35
	Christ Hospital, Jersey City	3.8	0.0%	1.52	No	0.00	8	0.53	0.022	1.82
	Community Medical Center, Toms River	7.2	0.0%	1.15	No	0.00	7	0.98	0.025	3.91
	Cooper Hospital-University Medical Center, Camden	8.4	0.0%	1.90	Yes	0.55	8	1.10	0.056	1.00
	Elizabeth General Medical Center, Elizabeth	4.8	0.0%	1.31	No	0.02	6	0.60	0.127	0.82
	Englewood Hospital, Englewood	4.4	0.0%	1.61	No	0.18	7	0.63	0.075	1.88
	Helene Fuld Medical Center, Trenton	3.8	0.0%	1.76	No	0.19	6	0.84	0.024	1.73
	Hospital Center at Orange, Orange	3.7	0.0%	1.30	No	0.07	0	0.80	0.068	1.42
	JFK Medical Center, Edison	4.3	0.0%	1.57	No	0.16	6	0.66	0.086	1.67
	Jersey Shore Medical Center, Neptune	7.2	0.0%	1.61	Yes	0.30	7	0.71	0.051	1.44
	Kennedy Memorial Hosp.-University Med. Ctr., Cherry Hill	5.5	0.0%	1.50	No	0.27	6	0.92	0.028	2.83
	Medical Center at Princeton, Princeton	7.3	0.0%	1.03	No	0.09	7	0.61	0.095	1.90
	Memorial Hospital of Burlington County, Mount Holly	4.5	0.0%	1.61	No	0.25	7	0.68	0.041	1.95
	Mercer Medical Center, Trenton	5.6	0.0%	1.35	No	0.00	7	1.04	0.039	1.62
	Monmouth Medical Center, Long Branch	7.7	0.0%	1.66	Yes	0.50	6	0.78	0.061	1.42
	Morristown Memorial Hospital, Morristown	8.2	0.0%	1.42	Yes	0.35	8	0.55	0.068	1.62
	Mountainside Hospital, Montclair	4.7	0.0%	1.71	No	0.24	7	0.62	0.086	3.13
	Muhlenberg Regional Medical Center, Plainfield	4.6	0.0%	1.58	No	0.18	7	0.73	0.066	1.70
	Newark Beth Israel Medical Center, Newark	6.3	0.0%	1.69	Yes	0.40	0	1.02	0.086	0.92
	Our Lady of Lourdes Medical Center, Camden	3.5	0.0%	1.93	No	0.09	4	1.23	0.015	1.81
	Raritan Bay Medical Center, Perth Amboy	3.3	0.0%	1.59	No	0.12	4	0.72	0.033	1.59
	Riverview Medical Center, Red Bank	4.0	0.0%	1.63	No	0.00	8	0.63	0.108	1.33
	Somerset Medical Center, Somerville	3.1	0.0%	1.50	No	0.11	4	0.49	0.040	1.52
	St. Barnabas Medical Center, Livingston	8.3	0.0%	1.50	Yes	0.40	8	0.62	0.046	2.42
	St. Elizabeth Hospital, Elizabeth	7.8	0.0%	1.02	No	0.18	7	0.68	0.076	1.92
	St. Francis Medical Center, Trenton	6.5	0.0%	1.14	No	0.21	7	0.65	0.021	1.87
	St. Joseph's Hospital and Medical Center, Paterson	7.9	0.0%	1.57	Yes	0.38	8	0.76	0.042	1.08
	St. Michael's Medical Center, Newark	6.2	0.0%	1.79	Yes	0.48	4	0.71	0.029	0.81
	St. Peter's Medical Center, New Brunswick	6.9	0.0%	1.30	No	0.51	7	0.75	0.056	1.45
	Underwood-Memorial Hospital, Woodbury	4.2	0.0%	1.35	No	0.06	5	0.59	0.031	2.09
	Valley Hospital, Ridgewood	5.7	0.0%	1.37	No	0.00	7	1.01	0.044	2.41
	Warren Hospital, Phillipsburg	3.9	0.0%	1.48	No	0.17	4	0.61	0.023	2.85
	West Jersey Hospital-Voorhees, Voorhees	7.6	0.0%	1.33	No	0.09	4	1.13	0.179	6.23

AIDS

Natl. Rank	Hospital	U.S. News index	Reputational score	Hospital-wide mortality rate	COTH member	Interns and residents to beds	Technology score (of 11)	Discharge planning (of 2)	R.N.'s to beds	Board-certified internists to beds
	TIER THREE									
	Lovelace Medical Center, Albuquerque	**23.7**	0.0%	0.94	No	0.06	5	2	2.67	0.063
	St. Joseph Medical Center, Albuquerque	**20.3**	0.0%	1.01	No	0.00	6	2	0.83	0.175
	University Hospital, Albuquerque	**24.4**	0.5%	1.31	Yes	1.20	8	2	1.82	0.373
	TIER FOUR									
	Memorial Medical Center, Las Cruces	**17.6**	0.0%	1.12	No	0.00	7	1	0.73	0.020
	Presbyterian Hospital, Albuquerque	**18.8**	0.0%	1.09	No	0.00	6	2	0.91	0.062

CANCER

Natl. Rank	Hospital	U.S. News index	Reputational score	Cancer mortality rate	COTH member	Interns and residents to beds	Technology score (of 12)	R.N.'s to beds	Board-certified oncologists to beds	Procedures to beds
	TIER TWO									
56	University Hospital, Albuquerque	**12.5**	0.5%	1.34	Yes	1.20	6	1.82	0.022	0.62
	TIER THREE									
	Lovelace Medical Center, Albuquerque	**7.7**	0.0%	0.90	No	0.06	3	2.67	0.015	1.16
	TIER FOUR									
	Memorial Medical Center, Las Cruces	**3.3**	0.0%	1.02	No	0.00	8	0.73	0.004	1.32
	Presbyterian Hospital, Albuquerque	**3.4**	0.0%	0.95	No	0.00	6	0.91	0.017	1.24
	St. Joseph Medical Center, Albuquerque	**4.2**	0.0%	0.86	No	0.00	8	0.83	0.025	2.74

CARDIOLOGY

Natl. Rank	Hospital	U.S. News index	Reputational score	Cardiology mortality rate	COTH member	Interns and residents to beds	Technology score (of 10)	R.N.'s to beds	Board-certified cardiologists to beds	Procedures to beds
	TIER TWO									
90	Lovelace Medical Center, Albuquerque	**21.1**	0.0%	0.93	No	0.06	6	2.67	0.034	8.09
	TIER THREE									
	Presbyterian Hospital, Albuquerque	**15.6**	0.0%	0.98	No	0.00	8	0.91	0.059	10.77
	TIER FOUR									
	Memorial Medical Center, Las Cruces	**11.2**	0.0%	1.10	No	0.00	8	0.73	0.012	5.97
	St. Joseph Medical Center, Albuquerque	**11.1**	0.0%	1.13	No	0.00	8	0.83	0.018	6.23

ENDOCRINOLOGY

Natl. Rank	Hospital	U.S. News index	Reputational score	Endocrinology mortality rate	COTH member	Interns and residents to beds	Technology score (of 11)	R.N.'s to beds	Board-certified internists to beds
	TIER TWO								
49	University Hospital, Albuquerque	**17.6**	0.0%	1.01	Yes	1.20	6	1.82	0.373
	TIER THREE								
	Lovelace Medical Center, Albuquerque	**10.3**	0.0%	1.12	No	0.06	3	2.67	0.063
	TIER FOUR								
	Memorial Medical Center, Las Cruces	**5.8**	0.0%	1.09	No	0.00	9	0.73	0.020
	Presbyterian Hospital, Albuquerque	**5.0**	0.0%	1.26	No	0.00	5	0.91	0.062
	St. Joseph Medical Center, Albuquerque	**7.7**	0.0%	1.01	No	0.00	9	0.83	0.175

GASTROENTEROLOGY

Natl. Rank	Hospital	U.S. News index	Reputa-tional score	Gastro-enterology mortality rate	COTH member	Interns and residents to beds	Tech-nology score (of 11)	R.N.'s to beds	Board-certified gastro-enterologists to beds	Pro-cedures to beds
	TIER THREE									
	Lovelace Medical Center, Albuquerque	10.1	0.0%	1.06	No	0.06	3	2.67	0.024	4.54
	St. Joseph Medical Center, Albuquerque	8.6	0.0%	0.82	No	0.00	8	0.83	0.022	3.80
	TIER FOUR									
	Memorial Medical Center, Las Cruces	6.6	0.0%	1.02	No	0.00	8	0.73	0.004	3.77
	Presbyterian Hospital, Albuquerque	4.5	0.0%	1.26	No	0.00	4	0.91	0.025	3.74

GERIATRICS

Natl. Rank	Hospital	U.S. News index	Reputa-tional score	Hospital-wide mortality rate	COTH member	Service mix	Interns and residents to beds	Tech-nology score (of 13)	R.N.'s to beds	Discharge planning (of 2)	Geriatric services (of 9)	Board-certified internists to beds
	TIER THREE											
94	Lovelace Medical Center, Albuquerque	20.9	0.0%	0.94	No	8	0.06	4	2.67	2	5	0.063
	St. Joseph Medical Center, Albuquerque	14.2	0.0%	1.01	No	3	0.00	10	0.83	2	3	0.175
	University Hospital, Albuquerque	17.6	0.0%	1.31	Yes	8	1.20	6	1.82	2	5	0.373
	TIER FOUR											
	Memorial Medical Center, Las Cruces	9.3	0.0%	1.12	No	4	0.00	10	0.73	1	1	0.020
	Presbyterian Hospital, Albuquerque	11.4	0.0%	1.09	No	4	0.00	8	0.91	2	1	0.062

GYNECOLOGY

Natl. Rank	Hospital	U.S. News index	Reputa-tional score	Hospital-wide mortality rate	Interns and residents to beds	Tech-nology score (of 10)	R.N.'s to beds	Board-certified OB-GYNs to beds	Procedures to beds
	TIER TWO								
86	Lovelace Medical Center, Albuquerque	22.3	0.0%	0.94	0.06	3	2.67	0.039	0.69
	TIER THREE								
	St. Joseph Medical Center, Albuquerque	15.3	0.0%	1.01	0.00	7	0.83	0.065	0.62
	TIER FOUR								
	Memorial Medical Center, Las Cruces	12.0	0.0%	1.12	0.00	7	0.73	0.052	0.46
	Presbyterian Hospital, Albuquerque	13.0	0.0%	1.09	0.00	5	0.91	0.091	0.45

NEUROLOGY

Natl. Rank	Hospital	U.S. News index	Reputa-tional score	Neurology mortality rate	COTH member	Interns and residents to beds	Tech-nology score (of 9)	R.N.'s to beds	Board-certified neurologists to beds
	TIER THREE								
	Lovelace Medical Center, Albuquerque	13.7	0.0%	1.00	No	0.06	3	2.67	0.015
	St. Joseph Medical Center, Albuquerque	11.0	0.0%	0.99	No	0.00	7	0.83	0.029
	TIER FOUR								
	Memorial Medical Center, Las Cruces	10.4	0.0%	0.94	No	0.00	7	0.73	0.012
	Presbyterian Hospital, Albuquerque	5.7	0.0%	1.23	No	0.00	4	0.91	0.007

ORTHOPEDICS

Natl. Rank	Hospital	U.S. News index	Reputa-tional score	Orthopedics mortality rate	COTH member	Interns and residents to beds	Tech-nology score (of 5)	R.N.'s to beds	Board-certified orthopedists to beds	Pro-cedures to beds
	TIER TWO									
66	University Hospital, Albuquerque	15.3	0.0%	1.06	Yes	1.20	4	1.82	0.038	1.00
	TIER THREE									
	Lovelace Medical Center, Albuquerque	10.7	0.0%	1.00	No	0.06	2	2.67	0.024	3.83
	St. Joseph Medical Center, Albuquerque	10.6	0.0%	0.60	No	0.00	3	0.83	0.084	4.76
	TIER FOUR									
	Memorial Medical Center, Las Cruces	4.1	0.0%	1.41	No	0.00	4	0.73	0.020	2.43
	Presbyterian Hospital, Albuquerque	5.2	0.0%	1.22	No	0.00	3	0.91	0.079	2.70

OTOLARYNGOLOGY

Natl. Rank	Hospital	U.S. News index	Reputa-tional score	Hospital-wide mortality rate	COTH member	Interns and residents to beds	Tech-nology score (of 9)	R.N.'s to beds	Board-certified internists to beds	Procedures to beds
	TIER TWO									
53	University Hospital, Albuquerque	17.6	0.0%	1.31	Yes	1.20	4	1.82	0.373	0.168
	TIER THREE									
	Lovelace Medical Center, Albuquerque	9.7	0.0%	0.94	No	0.06	2	2.67	0.063	0.170
	TIER FOUR									
	Memorial Medical Center, Las Cruces	4.4	0.0%	1.12	No	0.00	7	0.73	0.020	0.333
	Presbyterian Hospital, Albuquerque	4.2	0.0%	1.09	No	0.00	3	0.91	0.062	0.227
	St. Joseph Medical Center, Albuquerque	6.1	0.0%	1.01	No	0.00	7	0.83	0.175	0.353

RHEUMATOLOGY

Natl. Rank	Hospital	U.S. News index	Reputa-tional score	Hospital-wide mortality rate	COTH member	Interns and residents to beds	Tech-nology score (of 5)	R.N.'s to beds	Board-certified internists to beds
	TIER TWO								
50	University Hospital, Albuquerque	17.8	0.0%	1.31	Yes	1.20	4	1.82	0.373
	TIER THREE								
	Lovelace Medical Center, Albuquerque	13.5	0.0%	0.94	No	0.06	2	2.67	0.063
	TIER FOUR								
	Memorial Medical Center, Las Cruces	6.3	0.0%	1.12	No	0.00	4	0.73	0.020
	Presbyterian Hospital, Albuquerque	7.9	0.0%	1.09	No	0.00	3	0.91	0.062
	St. Joseph Medical Center, Albuquerque	9.1	0.0%	1.01	No	0.00	3	0.83	0.175

UROLOGY

Natl. Rank	Hospital	U.S. News index	Reputa-tional score	Urology mortality rate	COTH member	Interns and residents to beds	Tech-nology score (of 11)	R.N.'s to beds	Board-certified internists to beds	Procedures to beds
	TIER TWO									
38	University Hospital, Albuquerque	19.2	0.0%	0.80	Yes	1.20	6	1.82	0.373	1.38
	TIER THREE									
	Lovelace Medical Center, Albuquerque	14.1	0.0%	0.78	No	0.06	3	2.67	0.063	1.73
	St. Joseph Medical Center, Albuquerque	12.1	0.0%	0.46	No	0.00	8	0.83	0.175	2.35
	TIER FOUR									
	Memorial Medical Center, Las Cruces	3.8	0.0%	1.71	No	0.00	8	0.73	0.020	2.51
	Presbyterian Hospital, Albuquerque	6.5	0.0%	1.06	No	0.00	4	0.91	0.062	1.92

AIDS

Natl. Rank	Hospital	U.S. News index	Reputational score	Hospital-wide mortality rate	COTH member	Interns and residents to beds	Technology score (of 11)	Discharge planning (of 2)	R.N.'s to beds	Board-certified internists to beds
	TIER ONE									
7	Memorial Sloan-Kettering Cancer Center, New York	41.4	12.6%	0.91	Yes	0.38	7	2	1.37	0.074
8	New York University Medical Center	39.5	9.7%	0.98	Yes	1.30	8	2	1.15	0.360
9	New York Hospital-Cornell Medical Center	37.9	10.9%	1.07	Yes	0.79	10	2	1.00	0.113
16	Columbia-Presbyterian Medical Center, New York	33.0	8.3%	1.25	Yes	0.85	11	2	1.05	0.111
19	Mount Sinai Medical Center, New York	31.6	4.9%	1.09	Yes	0.99	9	2	1.50	0.253
23	Montefiore Medical Center, Bronx	30.3	6.2%	1.19	Yes	0.53	10	2	1.28	0.095
	TIER TWO									
65	Beth Israel Medical Center, New York	26.3	1.9%	1.09	Yes	0.65	10	2	1.27	0.085
88	Methodist Hospital, Brooklyn	25.1	0.0%	0.94	Yes	0.57	8	2	0.77	0.229
80	North Shore University Hospital, Manhasset	25.4	1.0%	1.12	Yes	0.58	10	2	1.10	0.327
73	St. Vincent's Hospital and Medical Center, New York	25.8	3.4%	1.36	Yes	0.88	9	2	1.08	0.255
	TIER THREE									
	Albany Medical Center Hospital, Albany	23.7	0.4%	1.12	Yes	0.76	8	2	1.33	0.103
	Bellevue Hospital Center, New York	22.8	1.5%	1.10	Yes	0.34	5	2	0.89	0.137
	Bronx-Lebanon Hospital Center, Bronx	19.9	0.3%	1.37	Yes	0.79	7	2	1.00	0.075
	Brooklyn Hospital Center, Brooklyn	19.9	0.0%	1.32	Yes	0.75	8	2	0.67	0.107
	Cabrini Medical Center, New York	20.7	0.0%	1.20	Yes	0.53	8	2	0.69	0.120
	Lenox Hill Hospital, New York	21.7	0.8%	1.25	Yes	0.57	7	2	1.18	0.104
	Lincoln Medical and Mental Health Center, Bronx	21.4	0.5%	1.18	No	1.07	7	2	1.36	0.045
	Long Island College Hospital, Brooklyn	20.8	0.0%	1.21	Yes	0.62	5	2	1.23	0.156
	Long Island Jewish Medical Center, New York	21.7	0.0%	1.34	Yes	1.17	9	2	1.20	0.097
	Maimonides Medical Center, Brooklyn	21.3	0.6%	1.21	Yes	0.78	6	2	0.93	0.070
	Mary Imogene Bassett Hospital, Cooperstown	23.7	0.0%	1.03	Yes	0.22	8	2	1.69	0.066
	Northern Westchester Hospital Center, Mount Kisco	20.5	0.0%	1.05	No	0.00	6	2	1.32	0.170
	St. Luke's-Roosevelt Hospital Center, New York	21.2	0.6%	1.29	Yes	0.69	7	2	1.07	0.142
	Strong Memorial Hospital-Rochester University	23.6	0.5%	1.26	Yes	1.00	10	2	1.45	0.111
	University Hosp.-SUNY Health Science Ctr., Syracuse	23.9	0.3%	1.28	Yes	1.30	9	2	1.61	0.160
	University Hospital, Stony Brook	22.7	0.3%	1.31	Yes	1.12	10	2	1.22	0.108
	Winthrop-University Hospital, Mineola	19.7	0.0%	1.23	Yes	0.21	7	2	0.95	0.085
	TIER FOUR									
	Arnot Ogden Medical Center, Elmira	16.4	0.0%	1.40	No	0.00	7	2	1.18	0.093
	Auburn Memorial Hospital, Auburn	14.5	0.0%	1.39	No	0.00	5	2	0.52	0.044
	Bayley Seton Hospital, Staten Island	16.2	0.0%	1.29	No	0.06	5	2	0.78	0.106
	Benedictine Hospital, Kingston	15.4	0.0%	1.29	No	0.08	4	2	0.59	0.068
	Bronx Municipal Hospital Center, Bronx	18.3	0.7%	1.59	Yes	1.07	4	2	1.07	0.072
	Brookdale Hospital Medical Center, Brooklyn	16.8	0.0%	1.59	Yes	0.45	7	2	0.79	0.085
	Buffalo General Hospital, Buffalo	16.1	0.0%	1.54	Yes	0.04	5	2	0.96	0.133
	Catholic Medical Center, Jamaica	17.2	0.0%	1.53	Yes	0.29	6	2	0.80	0.220
	Central General Hospital, Plainview	18.5	0.0%	1.10	No	0.00	5	2	0.59	0.246
	Community-General Hospital, Syracuse	16.1	0.0%	1.16	No	0.03	4	1	0.63	0.065
	Coney Island Hospital, Brooklyn	15.7	0.0%	1.46	No	0.56	4	2	1.06	0.070
	Crouse Irving Memorial Hospital, Syracuse	15.2	0.0%	1.33	No	0.12	4	1	1.06	0.061
	Ellis Hospital, Schenectady	16.8	0.0%	1.23	No	0.02	6	2	0.78	0.042
	Elmhurst Hospital Center, Elmhurst	17.2	0.0%	1.56	Yes	0.60	6	2	1.02	0.050
	Erie County Medical Center, Buffalo	16.1	0.0%	1.54	Yes	0.20	6	2	0.72	0.068
	Flushing Hospital Medical Center, Flushing	16.8	0.0%	1.37	No	0.45	6	2	1.05	0.056
	Franklin Hospital Medical Center, Valley Stream	13.3	0.0%	1.62	No	0.04	7	2	0.29	0.052
	Genesee Hospital, Rochester	17.5	0.0%	1.35	Yes	0.28	4	2	0.78	0.146
	Goldwater Memorial Hospital, New York	5.5	0.0%	4.91	No	0.01	5	2	0.25	0.018
	Good Samaritan Hospital, Suffern	16.8	0.0%	1.24	No	0.00	6	2	0.92	0.022
	Good Samaritan Hospital, West Islip	14.3	0.0%	1.57	No	0.00	7	2	0.74	0.055

Natl. Rank	Hospital	U.S. News index	Reputa-tional score	Hospital-wide mortality rate	COTH member	Interns and residents to beds	Tech-nology score (of 11)	Discharge planning (of 2)	R.N.'s to beds	Board-certified internists to beds
	Harlem Hospital Center, New York	15.6	0.5%	2.25	Yes	0.83	8	2	0.91	0.041
	Highland Hospital of Rochester, Rochester	16.6	0.0%	1.35	No	0.51	5	2	0.54	0.184
	House of the Good Samaritan, Watertown	16.0	0.0%	1.35	No	0.00	6	2	1.06	0.034
	Huntington Hospital, Huntington	17.2	0.0%	1.12	No	0.02	6	1	0.59	0.065
	Interfaith Medical Center, Brooklyn	14.6	0.0%	1.73	No	0.53	8	2	0.73	0.010
	Jamaica Hospital, Jamaica	15.7	0.0%	1.37	No	0.50	4	1	1.17	0.066
	John T. Mather Memorial Hospital, Port Jefferson	14.6	0.0%	1.56	No	0.00	6	2	1.15	0.059
	Kings County Hospital Center, Brooklyn	18.5	0.3%	1.61	Yes	0.54	10	2	0.86	0.076
	Kingsboro Psychiatric Center, Brooklyn	14.0	0.0%	1.22	No	0.02	1	2	0.20	0.002
	Kingsbrook Jewish Medical Center, Brooklyn	12.9	0.0%	1.57	No	0.17	5	2	0.23	0.012
	Kingston Hospital, Kingston	13.3	0.0%	1.41	No	0.14	2	1	0.85	0.057
	La Guardia Hospital, Flushing	13.7	0.0%	1.58	No	0.28	3	2	0.78	0.132
	Lutheran Medical Center, Brooklyn	18.7	0.0%	1.21	No	0.38	8	2	0.79	0.073
	Mercy Hospital, Buffalo	14.4	0.0%	1.34	No	0.12	3	2	0.48	0.045
	Mercy Medical Center, Rockville Centre	17.2	0.0%	1.22	No	0.01	6	2	0.77	0.101
	Metropolitan Hospital Center, New York	17.6	0.0%	1.65	Yes	0.97	7	2	0.84	0.059
	Mount Vernon Hospital, Mount Vernon	18.9	0.0%	1.12	No	0.30	5	2	0.93	0.090
	Nassau County Medical Center, East Meadow	19.3	0.0%	1.69	Yes	1.01	10	2	1.17	0.121
	Nathan Littauer Hospital, Gloversville	14.0	0.0%	1.37	No	0.00	4	2	0.37	0.024
	New Rochelle Hospital Medical Center, New Rochelle	18.5	0.0%	1.14	No	0.20	6	2	0.89	0.073
	New York Downtown Hospital	18.1	0.0%	1.26	No	0.67	6	2	1.06	0.000
	New York Hospital Medical Center, Flushing	18.3	0.9%	1.43	Yes	0.27	7	2	0.52	0.084
	North Central Bronx Hospital, Bronx	17.8	0.0%	1.29	No	0.71	5	2	1.07	0.056
	North General Hospital, New York	16.3	0.0%	1.29	No	0.23	4	2	0.95	0.070
	North Shore University Hospital-Glen Cove, Glen Cove	18.1	0.0%	1.29	No	0.09	6	2	0.66	0.506
	Nyack Hospital, Nyack	16.6	0.0%	1.14	No	0.06	4	1	0.74	0.067
	Our Lady of Mercy Medical Center, Bronx	17.2	0.0%	1.44	Yes	0.42	7	1	0.62	0.158
	Queens Hospital Center, Jamaica	18.3	0.0%	1.25	No	0.60	6	2	1.09	0.033
	Rochester General Hospital, Rochester	19.6	0.0%	1.26	Yes	0.22	7	2	0.96	0.135
	Saratoga Hospital, Saratoga Springs	16.2	0.0%	1.22	No	0.00	4	2	0.86	0.027
	Sisters of Charity Hospital, Buffalo	14.1	0.0%	1.47	No	0.07	4	2	0.60	0.120
	South Nassau Community Hospital, Oceanside	16.5	0.0%	1.22	No	0.07	5	1	0.85	0.147
	Southampton Hospital, Southampton	14.4	0.0%	1.39	No	0.00	7	1	0.44	0.036
	Southside Hospital, Bay Shore	11.7	0.0%	1.75	No	0.13	5	1	0.60	0.017
	St. Charles Hospital and Rehab. Ctr., Port Jefferson	16.4	0.0%	1.39	No	0.04	5	2	0.90	0.332
	St. Clare's Hospital of Schenectady, Schenectady	16.0	0.0%	1.40	No	0.20	5	2	1.05	0.122
	St. Elizabeth Hospital, Utica	17.9	0.0%	1.13	No	0.20	5	2	0.82	0.009
	St. John's Episcopal Hospital, Smithtown	12.6	0.0%	1.70	No	0.00	6	2	0.34	0.087
	St. Joseph's Medical Center, Yonkers	16.5	0.0%	1.24	No	0.26	4	2	0.79	0.046
	St. Mary's Hospital of Troy, Troy	14.5	0.0%	1.38	No	0.00	4	2	0.66	0.060
	St. Mary's Hospital, Rochester	16.5	0.0%	1.30	No	0.37	4	2	0.84	0.110
	St. Vincent's Medical Center, Staten Island	16.7	0.0%	1.41	No	0.46	7	2	0.92	0.075
	Staten Island University Hospital, Staten Island	17.6	0.0%	1.26	No	0.46	7	2	0.53	0.071
	United Health Services Hospitals, Binghamton	18.0	0.0%	1.25	Yes	0.20	5	2	0.61	0.050
	University Hospital of Brooklyn-SUNY Center, Brooklyn	19.6	0.0%	1.48	Yes	0.70	9	2	1.12	0.128
	Vassar Brothers Hospital, Poughkeepsie	15.0	0.0%	1.50	No	0.01	7	2	0.69	0.120
	Westchester County Medical Center, Valhalla	19.4	0.0%	1.50	Yes	0.81	7	2	1.59	0.052

CANCER

Natl. Rank	Hospital	U.S. News index	Reputational score	Cancer mortality rate	COTH member	Interns and residents to beds	Technology score (of 12)	R.N.'s to beds	Board-certified oncologists to beds	Procedures to beds
	TIER ONE									
1	Memorial Sloan-Kettering Cancer Center, New York	100.0	70.8%	0.97	Yes	0.38	9	1.37	0.083	7.93
10	Roswell Park Cancer Institute, Buffalo	24.7	8.5%	0.52	No	0.68	9	2.58	0.000	14.09
	TIER TWO									
76	Columbia-Presbyterian Medical Center, New York	11.3	1.0%	1.07	Yes	0.85	10	1.05	0.010	1.39
69	Long Island Jewish Medical Center, New York	11.6	0.0%	1.21	Yes	1.17	10	1.20	0.035	1.32
73	Montefiore Medical Center, Bronx	11.3	1.0%	0.90	Yes	0.53	10	1.28	0.020	2.21
29	Mount Sinai Medical Center, New York	14.9	2.6%	1.05	Yes	0.99	9	1.50	0.010	2.45
64	New York University Medical Center	12.1	0.0%	0.92	Yes	1.30	9	1.15	0.000	3.46
57	Strong Memorial Hospital-Rochester University	12.5	0.4%	1.09	Yes	1.00	11	1.45	0.030	1.20
52	University Hosp.-SUNY Health Science Ctr., Syracuse	12.9	0.0%	1.08	Yes	1.30	9	1.61	0.016	1.42
78	University Hospital, Stony Brook	11.2	0.0%	1.06	Yes	1.12	9	1.22	0.010	1.48
	TIER THREE									
93	Albany Medical Center Hospital, Albany	10.4	0.0%	0.95	Yes	0.76	9	1.33	0.021	0.99
	Bellevue Hospital Center, New York	6.1	0.0%	1.03	Yes	0.34	4	0.89	0.013	0.20
	Beth Israel Medical Center, New York	9.8	0.0%	1.09	Yes	0.65	9	1.27	0.011	1.70
	Bronx Municipal Hospital Center, Bronx	8.2	0.0%	1.22	Yes	1.07	2	1.07	0.008	0.24
	Brookdale Hospital Medical Center, Brooklyn	6.3	0.0%	1.29	Yes	0.45	5	0.79	0.011	0.44
	Brooklyn Hospital Center, Brooklyn	8.1	0.0%	1.24	Yes	0.75	9	0.67	0.003	0.84
	Buffalo General Hospital, Buffalo	5.7	0.0%	1.28	Yes	0.04	6	0.96	0.000	1.03
	Cabrini Medical Center, New York	7.1	0.0%	1.25	Yes	0.53	7	0.69	0.016	1.47
	Catholic Medical Center, Jamaica	6.1	0.0%	1.23	Yes	0.29	6	0.80	0.000	0.90
	Flushing Hospital Medical Center, Flushing	5.3	0.0%	1.25	No	0.45	7	1.05	0.011	1.24
	Genesee Hospital, Rochester	6.1	0.0%	1.37	Yes	0.28	6	0.78	0.019	1.29
	Harlem Hospital Center, New York	8.1	0.0%	2.01	Yes	0.83	7	0.91	0.003	0.25
	Kings County Hospital Center, Brooklyn	8.3	0.0%	1.00	Yes	0.54	10	0.86	0.000	0.16
	Lenox Hill Hospital, New York	8.1	0.0%	1.34	Yes	0.57	5	1.18	0.011	2.33
	Lincoln Medical and Mental Health Center, Bronx	8.1	0.0%	1.10	No	1.07	7	1.36	0.004	0.34
	Long Island College Hospital, Brooklyn	8.7	0.0%	1.31	Yes	0.62	7	1.23	0.000	1.18
	Maimonides Medical Center, Brooklyn	8.4	0.0%	1.09	Yes	0.78	6	0.93	0.014	1.45
	Mary Imogene Bassett Hospital, Cooperstown	9.5	0.0%	0.81	Yes	0.22	8	1.69	0.013	1.47
	Methodist Hospital, Brooklyn	9.4	0.0%	0.47	Yes	0.57	11	0.77	0.000	2.47
	Millard Fillmore Hospitals, Buffalo	5.3	0.0%	1.35	Yes	0.15	4	0.82	0.010	1.56
	New York Downtown Hospital	5.3	0.0%	1.25	No	0.67	4	1.06	0.023	1.44
	New York Hospital Medical Center, Flushing	5.9	0.0%	1.02	Yes	0.27	7	0.52	0.011	1.61
83	New York Hospital-Cornell Medical Center	10.8	0.9%	0.90	Yes	0.79	9	1.00	0.015	1.48
95	North Shore University Hospital, Manhasset	10.3	0.5%	0.98	Yes	0.58	10	1.10	0.031	2.10
	Our Lady of Mercy Medical Center, Bronx	5.9	0.0%	1.03	Yes	0.42	5	0.62	0.004	0.92
	Rochester General Hospital, Rochester	7.3	0.0%	1.15	Yes	0.22	9	0.96	0.006	1.00
	St. Luke's-Roosevelt Hospital Center, New York	7.3	0.0%	1.38	Yes	0.69	3	1.07	0.014	0.94
	St. Vincent's Hospital and Medical Center, New York	9.7	0.0%	1.31	Yes	0.88	9	1.08	0.000	1.10
	University Hospital of Brooklyn-SUNY Center, Brooklyn	9.6	0.0%	1.28	Yes	0.70	10	1.12	0.021	0.77
91	Westchester County Medical Center, Valhalla	10.4	0.0%	1.30	Yes	0.81	7	1.59	0.019	1.17
	Winthrop-University Hospital, Mineola	7.2	0.0%	1.10	Yes	0.21	8	0.95	0.010	2.10
	TIER FOUR									
	Arnot Ogden Medical Center, Elmira	4.5	0.0%	1.62	No	0.00	9	1.18	0.014	1.12
	Auburn Memorial Hospital, Auburn	1.3	0.0%	1.65	No	0.00	4	0.52	0.004	1.41
	Bayley Seton Hospital, Staten Island	1.9	0.0%	1.18	No	0.06	2	0.78	0.025	0.89
	Benedictine Hospital, Kingston	1.7	0.0%	1.20	No	0.08	2	0.59	0.014	2.65
	Central General Hospital, Plainview	2.7	0.0%	1.23	No	0.00	6	0.59	0.038	2.65
	Community-General Hospital, Syracuse	1.4	0.0%	1.33	No	0.03	2	0.63	0.014	2.02
	Coney Island Hospital, Brooklyn	4.1	0.0%	1.25	No	0.56	2	1.06	0.011	0.48
	Crouse Irving Memorial Hospital, Syracuse	2.9	0.0%	1.30	No	0.12	2	1.06	0.009	1.90
	Ellis Hospital, Schenectady	2.7	0.0%	1.52	No	0.02	6	0.78	0.016	1.24

Natl. Rank	Hospital	U.S. News index	Reputa-tional score	Cancer mortality rate	COTH member	Interns and residents to beds	Tech-nology score (of 12)	R.N.'s to beds	Board-certified oncologists to beds	Procedures to beds
	Erie County Medical Center, Buffalo	4.5	0.0%	1.32	Yes	0.20	3	0.72	0.001	0.23
	Franklin Hospital Medical Center, Valley Stream	1.8	0.0%	1.66	No	0.04	8	0.29	0.002	1.01
	Good Samaritan Hospital, Suffern	4.0	0.0%	1.20	No	0.00	8	0.92	0.030	1.66
	Good Samaritan Hospital, West Islip	3.4	0.0%	1.61	No	0.00	9	0.74	0.013	1.47
	Highland Hospital of Rochester, Rochester	4.0	0.0%	1.38	No	0.51	7	0.54	0.011	1.32
	House of the Good Samaritan, Watertown	3.8	0.0%	1.21	No	0.00	7	1.06	0.009	1.35
	Huntington Hospital, Huntington	2.9	0.0%	1.14	No	0.02	7	0.59	0.012	2.57
	Interfaith Medical Center, Brooklyn	4.4	0.0%	1.28	No	0.53	7	0.73	0.000	0.36
	Jamaica Hospital, Jamaica	4.4	0.0%	1.21	No	0.50	2	1.17	0.028	0.77
	John T. Mather Memorial Hospital, Port Jefferson	4.0	0.0%	1.60	No	0.00	6	1.15	0.025	2.58
	Kingsboro Psychiatric Center, Brooklyn	0.0	0.0%	0.81	No	0.02	1	0.20	0.000	0.55
	Kingsbrook Jewish Medical Center, Brooklyn	1.3	0.0%	1.23	No	0.17	5	0.23	0.005	0.21
	Kingston Hospital, Kingston	2.6	0.0%	1.12	No	0.14	2	0.85	0.007	2.67
	La Guardia Hospital, Flushing	2.5	0.0%	1.11	No	0.28	1	0.78	0.007	1.91
	Lutheran Medical Center, Brooklyn	4.3	0.0%	1.17	No	0.38	7	0.79	0.004	1.10
	Mercy Hospital, Buffalo	1.6	0.0%	1.26	No	0.12	3	0.48	0.007	1.92
	Mercy Medical Center, Rockville Centre	3.6	0.0%	1.18	No	0.01	8	0.77	0.026	2.04
	Mount Vernon Hospital, Mount Vernon	3.2	0.0%	0.78	No	0.30	1	0.93	0.008	1.39
	Nathan Littauer Hospital, Gloversville	0.2	0.0%	1.61	No	0.00	2	0.37	0.005	0.94
	New Rochelle Hospital Medical Center, New Rochelle	4.6	0.0%	1.10	No	0.20	8	0.89	0.007	2.42
	North Shore University Hospital-Glen Cove, Glen Cove	3.2	0.0%	1.04	No	0.09	5	0.66	0.023	3.91
	Northern Westchester Hospital Center, Mount Kisco	4.7	0.0%	1.29	No	0.00	7	1.32	0.015	1.86
	Nyack Hospital, Nyack	2.5	0.0%	1.06	No	0.06	4	0.74	0.015	1.43
	Samaritan Hospital, Troy	3.3	0.0%	1.06	No	0.00	8	0.66	0.022	1.48
	Sisters of Charity Hospital, Buffalo	1.9	0.0%	1.24	No	0.07	4	0.60	0.000	1.59
	South Nassau Community Hospital, Oceanside	3.3	0.0%	1.35	No	0.07	6	0.85	0.016	1.84
	Southampton Hospital, Southampton	2.1	0.0%	1.84	No	0.00	8	0.44	0.005	1.36
	Southside Hospital, Bay Shore	2.5	0.0%	1.60	No	0.13	6	0.60	0.015	1.14
	St. Barnabas Hospital, Bronx	2.6	0.0%	1.14	No	0.41	0	0.86	0.013	0.43
	St. Charles Hospital and Rehab. Ctr., Port Jefferson	2.5	0.0%	1.47	No	0.04	3	0.90	0.026	1.86
	St. Clare's Hospital of Schenectady, Schenectady	3.1	0.0%	1.32	No	0.20	2	1.05	0.027	1.36
	St. Elizabeth Hospital, Utica	3.5	0.0%	0.99	No	0.20	5	0.82	0.009	1.33
	St. John's Episcopal Hospital, Far Rockaway	1.5	0.0%	1.76	No	0.24	0	0.74	0.013	1.41
	St. Joseph's Medical Center, Yonkers	3.0	0.0%	0.89	No	0.26	2	0.79	0.026	1.40
	St. Mary's Hospital of Troy, Troy	1.9	0.0%	0.79	No	0.00	2	0.66	0.025	1.48
	St. Mary's Hospital, Rochester	3.4	0.0%	1.17	No	0.37	3	0.84	0.018	1.15
	St. Peter's Hospital, Albany	5.0	0.0%	0.92	No	0.09	9	0.98	0.020	2.02
	St. Vincent's Medical Center, Staten Island	4.4	0.0%	1.19	No	0.46	5	0.92	0.018	1.20
	Staten Island University Hospital, Staten Island	4.6	0.0%	0.90	No	0.46	8	0.53	0.011	1.68
	United Health Services Hospitals, Binghamton	5.1	0.0%	0.93	Yes	0.20	4	0.61	0.011	0.92
	Vassar Brothers Hospital, Poughkeepsie	3.3	0.0%	1.44	No	0.01	8	0.69	0.010	2.63

CARDIOLOGY

Natl. Rank	Hospital	U.S. News index	Reputa-tional score	Cardiology mortality rate	COTH member	Interns and residents to beds	Tech-nology score (of 10)	R.N.'s to beds	Board-certified cardiologists to beds	Procedures to beds
	TIER ONE									
11	Columbia-Presbyterian Medical Center, New York	33.7	10.8%	1.16	Yes	0.85	10	1.05	0.044	3.76
19	Mount Sinai Medical Center, New York	29.1	2.0%	0.84	Yes	0.99	8	1.50	0.068	3.94
23	New York Hospital-Cornell Medical Center	28.3	4.7%	0.96	Yes	0.79	9	1.00	0.034	3.80
	TIER TWO									
88	Albany Medical Center Hospital, Albany	21.2	0.0%	1.00	Yes	0.76	9	1.33	0.031	6.76
70	Beth Israel Medical Center, New York	21.8	0.0%	0.96	Yes	0.65	10	1.27	0.034	3.90
50	Mary Imogene Bassett Hospital, Cooperstown	23.0	0.0%	0.84	Yes	0.22	6	1.69	0.026	8.04
28	New York University Medical Center	26.7	3.7%	1.02	Yes	1.30	8	1.15	0.000	4.84

Natl. Rank Hospital	U.S. News index	Reputa- tional score	Cardiology mortality rate	COTH member	Interns and residents to beds	Tech- nology score (of 10)	R.N.'s to beds	Board- certified cardiologists to beds	Procedures to beds
TIER THREE									
Bronx Municipal Hospital Center, Bronx	15.0	0.0%	1.21	Yes	1.07	2	1.07	0.022	3.12
Bronx-Lebanon Hospital Center, Bronx	13.7	0.0%	1.22	Yes	0.79	4	1.00	0.001	2.34
Brooklyn Hospital Center, Brooklyn	14.2	0.0%	1.18	Yes	0.75	6	0.67	0.003	4.28
Cabrini Medical Center, New York	18.8	0.0%	0.92	Yes	0.53	4	0.69	0.018	3.63
Huntington Hospital, Huntington	14.4	0.0%	0.94	No	0.02	4	0.59	0.051	7.37
Lenox Hill Hospital, New York	16.5	0.0%	1.15	Yes	0.57	6	1.18	0.043	7.10
Lincoln Medical and Mental Health Center, Bronx	18.5	0.0%	0.94	No	1.07	2	1.36	0.009	2.41
Long Island College Hospital, Brooklyn	14.9	0.0%	1.16	Yes	0.62	4	1.23	0.000	4.30
Long Island Jewish Medical Center, New York	17.6	0.0%	1.27	Yes	1.17	8	1.20	0.100	5.64
Maimonides Medical Center, Brooklyn	20.2	0.7%	1.06	Yes	0.78	9	0.93	0.044	8.18
Mercy Medical Center, Rockville Centre	14.2	0.0%	0.95	No	0.01	5	0.77	0.026	5.37
Methodist Hospital, Brooklyn	18.6	0.0%	0.96	Yes	0.57	6	0.77	0.000	5.75
Montefiore Medical Center, Bronx	18.0	0.6%	1.18	Yes	0.53	9	1.28	0.053	6.31
Mount Vernon Hospital, Mount Vernon	14.1	0.0%	0.99	No	0.30	4	0.93	0.016	6.10
North Shore University Hospital, Manhasset	18.6	0.0%	1.09	Yes	0.58	9	1.10	0.073	5.65
Northern Westchester Hospital Center, Mount Kisco	17.1	0.0%	0.88	No	0.00	3	1.32	0.015	6.33
Rochester General Hospital, Rochester	16.2	0.0%	1.10	Yes	0.22	8	0.96	0.038	8.65
St. Elizabeth Hospital, Utica	14.0	0.0%	1.01	No	0.20	5	0.82	0.032	10.82
St. Luke's-Roosevelt Hospital Center, New York	16.2	0.0%	1.15	Yes	0.69	7	1.07	0.024	3.36
St. Vincent's Hospital and Medical Center, New York	15.2	0.0%	1.25	Yes	0.88	8	1.08	0.000	3.96
Strong Memorial Hospital-Rochester University	18.0	0.0%	1.24	Yes	1.00	8	1.45	0.057	4.84
United Health Services Hospitals, Binghamton	13.6	0.0%	1.17	Yes	0.20	8	0.61	0.030	8.59
University Hosp.-SUNY Health Science Ctr., Syracuse	19.1	0.0%	1.26	Yes	1.30	7	1.61	0.083	5.26
University Hospital of Brooklyn-SUNY Center, Brooklyn	15.0	0.0%	1.32	Yes	0.70	9	1.12	0.053	4.30
University Hospital, Stony Brook	15.5	0.0%	1.34	Yes	1.12	7	1.22	0.032	5.32
Westchester County Medical Center, Valhalla	16.8	0.0%	1.25	Yes	0.81	5	1.59	0.091	5.82
Winthrop-University Hospital, Mineola	16.9	0.0%	1.04	Yes	0.21	7	0.95	0.033	9.09
TIER FOUR									
Arnot Ogden Medical Center, Elmira	10.2	0.0%	1.24	No	0.00	8	1.18	0.017	7.17
Auburn Memorial Hospital, Auburn	5.4	0.0%	1.35	No	0.00	4	0.52	0.000	7.70
Bayley Seton Hospital, Staten Island	8.8	0.0%	1.23	No	0.06	4	0.78	0.051	4.47
Bellevue Hospital Center, New York	10.6	0.0%	1.38	Yes	0.34	6	0.89	0.030	0.77
Benedictine Hospital, Kingston	6.8	0.0%	1.29	No	0.08	3	0.59	0.027	5.55
Brookdale Hospital Medical Center, Brooklyn	9.4	0.0%	1.46	Yes	0.45	4	0.79	0.034	2.14
Buffalo General Hospital, Buffalo	11.0	0.0%	1.29	Yes	0.04	7	0.96	0.000	6.67
Catholic Medical Center, Jamaica	9.3	0.0%	1.38	Yes	0.29	4	0.80	0.000	4.88
Central General Hospital, Plainview	10.8	0.0%	1.06	No	0.00	3	0.59	0.038	7.09
Community-General Hospital, Syracuse	11.3	0.0%	1.04	No	0.03	4	0.63	0.017	5.63
Coney Island Hospital, Brooklyn	11.1	0.0%	1.25	No	0.56	6	1.06	0.018	5.54
Crouse Irving Memorial Hospital, Syracuse	11.6	0.0%	1.12	No	0.12	5	1.06	0.029	5.57
Ellis Hospital, Schenectady	11.9	0.0%	1.10	No	0.02	7	0.78	0.042	8.03
Elmhurst Hospital Center, Elmhurst	12.9	0.0%	1.26	Yes	0.60	5	1.02	0.005	1.57
Erie County Medical Center, Buffalo	8.0	0.0%	1.52	Yes	0.20	7	0.72	0.007	2.27
Flushing Hospital Medical Center, Flushing	9.5	0.0%	1.29	No	0.45	4	1.05	0.020	5.74
Franklin Hospital Medical Center, Valley Stream	4.4	0.0%	1.44	No	0.04	5	0.29	0.026	5.92
Genesee Hospital, Rochester	11.7	0.0%	1.24	Yes	0.28	5	0.78	0.009	5.37
Good Samaritan Hospital, Suffern	12.1	0.0%	1.10	No	0.00	6	0.92	0.062	6.41
Good Samaritan Hospital, West Islip	8.7	0.0%	1.24	No	0.00	6	0.74	0.032	6.36
Harlem Hospital Center, New York	4.7	0.0%	2.24	Yes	0.83	4	0.91	0.006	1.53
Highland Hospital of Rochester, Rochester	12.0	0.0%	1.07	No	0.51	4	0.54	0.018	4.52
House of the Good Samaritan, Watertown	5.5	0.0%	1.47	No	0.00	4	1.06	0.009	5.45
Jamaica Hospital, Jamaica	13.0	0.0%	1.10	No	0.50	3	1.17	0.019	5.83
John T. Mather Memorial Hospital, Port Jefferson	8.5	0.0%	1.32	No	0.00	5	1.15	0.029	8.85
Kingsbrook Jewish Medical Center, Brooklyn	0.0	0.0%	1.81	No	0.17	3	0.23	0.007	1.46
Kingston Hospital, Kingston	6.5	0.0%	1.34	No	0.14	1	0.85	0.021	9.01

Natl. Rank	Hospital	U.S. News index	Reputational score	Cardiology mortality rate	COTH member	Interns and residents to beds	Technology score (of 10)	R.N.'s to beds	Board-certified cardiologists to beds	Procedures to beds
	La Guardia Hospital, Flushing	3.8	0.0%	1.54	No	0.28	0	0.78	0.015	5.17
	Lutheran Medical Center, Brooklyn	12.8	0.0%	1.04	No	0.38	4	0.79	0.010	4.52
	Mercy Hospital, Buffalo	5.8	0.0%	1.40	No	0.12	5	0.48	0.026	7.21
	Millard Fillmore Hospitals, Buffalo	11.5	0.0%	1.36	Yes	0.15	9	0.82	0.035	7.61
	Nassau County Medical Center, East Meadow	13.2	0.0%	1.39	Yes	1.01	6	1.17	0.000	2.61
	Nathan Littauer Hospital, Gloversville	6.9	0.0%	1.19	No	0.00	3	0.37	0.000	5.54
	New Rochelle Hospital Medical Center, New Rochelle	12.4	0.0%	1.09	No	0.20	5	0.89	0.031	8.17
	New York Downtown Hospital	10.6	0.0%	1.31	No	0.67	4	1.06	0.055	4.63
	New York Hospital Medical Center, Flushing	9.1	0.0%	1.37	Yes	0.27	4	0.52	0.034	4.73
	North Shore University Hospital-Glen Cove, Glen Cove	9.4	0.0%	1.18	No	0.09	4	0.66	0.049	6.17
	Nyack Hospital, Nyack	10.4	0.0%	1.10	No	0.06	3	0.74	0.032	6.22
	Our Lady of Mercy Medical Center, Bronx	9.7	0.0%	1.34	Yes	0.42	3	0.62	0.013	4.24
	Queens Hospital Center, Jamaica	9.6	0.0%	1.31	No	0.60	5	1.09	0.000	1.79
	Samaritan Hospital, Troy	6.7	0.0%	1.30	No	0.00	4	0.66	0.022	5.15
	Sisters of Charity Hospital, Buffalo	3.6	0.0%	1.52	No	0.07	4	0.60	0.000	4.29
	South Nassau Community Hospital, Oceanside	12.7	0.0%	1.07	No	0.07	5	0.85	0.072	7.39
	Southampton Hospital, Southampton	7.9	0.0%	1.21	No	0.00	6	0.44	0.015	5.41
	Southside Hospital, Bay Shore	3.0	0.0%	1.69	No	0.13	4	0.60	0.035	5.18
	St. Barnabas Hospital, Bronx	9.2	0.0%	1.20	No	0.41	0	0.86	0.033	3.86
	St. Charles Hospital and Rehab. Ctr., Port Jefferson	9.3	0.0%	1.23	No	0.04	4	0.90	0.087	5.00
	St. Clare's Hospital of Schenectady, Schenectady	10.0	0.0%	1.27	No	0.20	4	1.05	0.072	9.33
	St. John's Episcopal Hospital, Far Rockaway	0.6	0.0%	1.92	No	0.24	0	0.74	0.032	3.77
	St. John's Episcopal Hospital, Smithtown	3.2	0.0%	1.60	No	0.00	6	0.34	0.043	3.61
	St. Joseph's Medical Center, Yonkers	9.0	0.0%	1.23	No	0.26	3	0.79	0.036	6.64
	St. Mary's Hospital of Troy, Troy	4.6	0.0%	1.53	No	0.00	3	0.66	0.070	8.28
	St. Mary's Hospital, Rochester	8.7	0.0%	1.28	No	0.37	4	0.84	0.018	5.65
	St. Peter's Hospital, Albany	12.4	0.0%	1.18	No	0.09	9	0.98	0.063	9.94
	St. Vincent's Medical Center, Staten Island	9.9	0.0%	1.31	No	0.46	6	0.92	0.043	5.54
	Staten Island University Hospital, Staten Island	8.7	0.0%	1.27	No	0.46	5	0.53	0.019	6.23
	Vassar Brothers Hospital, Poughkeepsie	4.1	0.0%	1.53	No	0.01	5	0.69	0.013	6.16

ENDOCRINOLOGY

Natl. Rank	Hospital	U.S. News index	Reputational score	Endocrinology mortality rate	COTH member	Interns and residents to beds	Technology score (of 11)	R.N.'s to beds	Board-certified internists to beds
TIER ONE									
21	Columbia-Presbyterian Medical Center, New York	22.6	8.2%	1.35	Yes	0.85	10	1.05	0.111
TIER TWO									
48	Mount Sinai Medical Center, New York	17.7	2.7%	1.35	Yes	0.99	9	1.50	0.253
52	New York Hospital-Cornell Medical Center	17.4	1.4%	0.72	Yes	0.79	9	1.00	0.113
53	New York University Medical Center	17.3	1.0%	1.12	Yes	1.30	9	1.15	0.360
80	University Hosp.-SUNY Health Science Ctr., Syracuse	15.0	0.0%	1.31	Yes	1.30	9	1.61	0.160
TIER THREE									
	Albany Medical Center Hospital, Albany	10.6	0.0%	1.82	Yes	0.76	9	1.33	0.103
	Beth Israel Medical Center, New York	11.3	0.0%	1.39	Yes	0.65	10	1.27	0.085
	Bronx Municipal Hospital Center, Bronx	10.1	0.0%	1.44	Yes	1.07	1	1.07	0.072
	Bronx-Lebanon Hospital Center, Bronx	9.7	0.0%	1.61	Yes	0.79	7	1.00	0.075
	Brooklyn Hospital Center, Brooklyn	9.4	0.0%	1.56	Yes	0.75	9	0.67	0.107
	Cabrini Medical Center, New York	9.0	0.0%	1.44	Yes	0.53	8	0.69	0.120
	Lenox Hill Hospital, New York	10.9	0.0%	1.20	Yes	0.57	6	1.18	0.104
	Lincoln Medical and Mental Health Center, Bronx	9.8	0.0%	1.31	No	1.07	7	1.36	0.045
	Long Island College Hospital, Brooklyn	11.1	0.0%	1.41	Yes	0.62	8	1.23	0.156
	Long Island Jewish Medical Center, New York	11.6	0.0%	1.86	Yes	1.17	10	1.20	0.097
	Maimonides Medical Center, Brooklyn	10.2	0.0%	1.35	Yes	0.78	7	0.93	0.070
	Mary Imogene Bassett Hospital, Cooperstown	10.9	0.0%	1.32	Yes	0.22	9	1.69	0.066

Natl. Rank	Hospital	U.S. News index	Reputa-tional score	Endocrinology mortality rate	COTH member	Interns and residents to beds	Tech-nology score (of 11)	R.N.'s to beds	Board-certified internists to beds
	Memorial Sloan-Kettering Cancer Center, New York	10.6	0.0%	1.33	Yes	0.38	9	1.37	0.074
	Methodist Hospital, Brooklyn	12.5	0.0%	1.01	Yes	0.57	10	0.77	0.229
	Metropolitan Hospital Center, New York	8.9	0.0%	1.78	Yes	0.97	5	0.84	0.059
	Montefiore Medical Center, Bronx	12.9	0.9%	1.22	Yes	0.53	10	1.28	0.095
	Nassau County Medical Center, East Meadow	12.1	0.0%	1.42	Yes	1.01	9	1.17	0.121
	North Shore University Hospital, Manhasset	11.4	0.0%	1.72	Yes	0.58	10	1.10	0.327
	Northern Westchester Hospital Center, Mount Kisco	11.1	0.0%	0.75	No	0.00	8	1.32	0.170
	Rochester General Hospital, Rochester	8.9	0.0%	1.53	Yes	0.22	10	0.96	0.135
	St. Luke's-Roosevelt Hospital Center, New York	9.4	0.0%	1.62	Yes	0.69	4	1.07	0.142
	St. Vincent's Hospital and Medical Center, New York	12.4	0.0%	1.49	Yes	0.88	10	1.08	0.255
95	Strong Memorial Hospital-Rochester University	13.8	0.9%	1.53	Yes	1.00	10	1.45	0.111
	University Hospital, Stony Brook	12.1	0.0%	1.56	Yes	1.12	9	1.22	0.108
	Westchester County Medical Center, Valhalla	12.7	0.0%	1.14	Yes	0.81	6	1.59	0.052

TIER FOUR

Natl. Rank	Hospital	U.S. News index	Reputa-tional score	Endocrinology mortality rate	COTH member	Interns and residents to beds	Tech-nology score (of 11)	R.N.'s to beds	Board-certified internists to beds
	Auburn Memorial Hospital, Auburn	2.3	0.0%	1.74	No	0.00	5	0.52	0.044
	Bayley Seton Hospital, Staten Island	3.1	0.0%	1.80	No	0.06	3	0.78	0.106
	Benedictine Hospital, Kingston	4.4	0.0%	1.21	No	0.08	4	0.59	0.068
	Brookdale Hospital Medical Center, Brooklyn	6.9	0.0%	2.21	Yes	0.45	7	0.79	0.085
	Buffalo General Hospital, Buffalo	6.3	0.0%	2.24	Yes	0.04	7	0.96	0.133
	Catholic Medical Center, Jamaica	7.9	0.0%	1.88	Yes	0.29	7	0.80	0.220
	Central General Hospital, Plainview	5.3	0.0%	1.34	No	0.00	6	0.59	0.246
	Community-General Hospital, Syracuse	5.1	0.0%	1.04	No	0.03	3	0.63	0.065
	Coney Island Hospital, Brooklyn	5.0	0.0%	1.94	No	0.56	3	1.06	0.070
	Crouse Irving Memorial Hospital, Syracuse	3.5	0.0%	1.84	No	0.12	2	1.06	0.061
	Ellis Hospital, Schenectady	3.0	0.0%	1.97	No	0.02	7	0.78	0.042
	Erie County Medical Center, Buffalo	6.8	0.0%	1.44	Yes	0.20	4	0.72	0.068
	Flushing Hospital Medical Center, Flushing	5.3	0.0%	2.09	No	0.45	8	1.05	0.056
	Franklin Hospital Medical Center, Valley Stream	2.0	0.0%	2.07	No	0.04	9	0.29	0.052
	Genesee Hospital, Rochester	7.8	0.0%	1.65	Yes	0.28	7	0.78	0.146
	Good Samaritan Hospital, Suffern	3.9	0.0%	1.81	No	0.00	9	0.92	0.022
	Good Samaritan Hospital, West Islip	2.8	0.0%	2.51	No	0.00	10	0.74	0.055
	Harlem Hospital Center, New York	8.0	0.0%	2.35	Yes	0.83	7	0.91	0.041
	Highland Hospital of Rochester, Rochester	7.4	0.0%	1.21	No	0.51	8	0.54	0.184
	Huntington Hospital, Huntington	4.6	0.0%	1.32	No	0.02	8	0.59	0.065
	Interfaith Medical Center, Brooklyn	4.1	0.0%	2.14	No	0.53	7	0.73	0.010
	Jamaica Hospital, Jamaica	5.6	0.0%	1.69	No	0.50	3	1.17	0.066
	John T. Mather Memorial Hospital, Port Jefferson	5.6	0.0%	1.38	No	0.00	7	1.15	0.059
	Kingsbrook Jewish Medical Center, Brooklyn	1.4	0.0%	2.09	No	0.17	6	0.23	0.012
	Kingston Hospital, Kingston	5.0	0.0%	1.19	No	0.14	2	0.85	0.057
	La Guardia Hospital, Flushing	2.3	0.0%	2.56	No	0.28	0	0.78	0.132
	Lutheran Medical Center, Brooklyn	5.4	0.0%	1.62	No	0.38	8	0.79	0.073
	Mercy Hospital, Buffalo	3.1	0.0%	1.44	No	0.12	3	0.48	0.045
	Mercy Medical Center, Rockville Centre	3.1	0.0%	2.24	No	0.01	8	0.77	0.101
	Millard Fillmore Hospitals, Buffalo	5.5	0.0%	1.92	Yes	0.15	4	0.82	0.031
	Mount Vernon Hospital, Mount Vernon	6.1	0.0%	1.19	No	0.30	3	0.93	0.090
	New Rochelle Hospital Medical Center, New Rochelle	5.8	0.0%	1.45	No	0.20	9	0.89	0.073
	New York Downtown Hospital	5.6	0.0%	1.76	No	0.67	5	1.06	0.000
	New York Hospital Medical Center, Flushing	5.6	0.0%	2.17	Yes	0.27	7	0.52	0.084
	North Shore University Hospital-Glen Cove, Glen Cove	6.6	0.4%	1.91	No	0.09	6	0.66	0.506
	Nyack Hospital, Nyack	3.9	0.0%	1.52	No	0.06	5	0.74	0.067
	Our Lady of Mercy Medical Center, Bronx	7.2	0.0%	1.86	Yes	0.42	6	0.62	0.158
	Queens Hospital Center, Jamaica	6.9	0.0%	1.29	No	0.60	4	1.09	0.033
	Samaritan Hospital, Troy	4.4	0.0%	1.42	No	0.00	9	0.66	0.044
	Saratoga Hospital, Saratoga Springs	1.9	0.0%	2.19	No	0.00	3	0.86	0.027
	Sisters of Charity Hospital, Buffalo	3.4	0.0%	1.71	No	0.07	5	0.60	0.120
	South Nassau Community Hospital, Oceanside	5.0	0.0%	1.59	No	0.07	7	0.85	0.147

Natl. Rank	Hospital	U.S. News index	Reputational score	Endocrinology mortality rate	COTH member	Interns and residents to beds	Technology score (of 11)	R.N.'s to beds	Board-certified internists to beds
	Southampton Hospital, Southampton	1.5	0.0%	2.67	No	0.00	9	0.44	0.036
	Southside Hospital, Bay Shore	2.0	0.0%	2.51	No	0.13	7	0.60	0.017
	St. Barnabas Hospital, Bronx	4.5	0.0%	1.47	No	0.41	0	0.86	0.072
	St. Charles Hospital and Rehab. Ctr., Port Jefferson	4.9	0.0%	1.95	No	0.04	4	0.90	0.332
	St. Clare's Hospital of Schenectady, Schenectady	5.5	0.0%	1.46	No	0.20	4	1.05	0.122
	St. Elizabeth Hospital, Utica	8.0	0.0%	0.84	No	0.20	6	0.82	0.009
	St. John's Episcopal Hospital, Far Rockaway	1.7	0.0%	2.45	No	0.24	0	0.74	0.068
	St. John's Episcopal Hospital, Smithtown	1.6	0.0%	2.43	No	0.00	8	0.34	0.087
	St. Joseph's Medical Center, Yonkers	5.1	0.0%	1.24	No	0.26	3	0.79	0.046
	St. Mary's Hospital of Troy, Troy	3.3	0.0%	1.42	No	0.00	3	0.66	0.060
	St. Mary's Hospital, Rochester	5.4	0.0%	1.47	No	0.37	4	0.84	0.110
	St. Peter's Hospital, Albany	6.1	0.0%	1.32	No	0.09	9	0.98	0.065
	St. Vincent's Medical Center, Staten Island	5.0	0.0%	1.81	No	0.46	5	0.92	0.075
	Staten Island University Hospital, Staten Island	4.4	0.0%	1.97	No	0.46	9	0.53	0.071
	United Health Services Hospitals, Binghamton	6.2	0.0%	1.56	Yes	0.20	5	0.61	0.050
	Vassar Brothers Hospital, Poughkeepsie	3.8	0.0%	1.88	No	0.01	9	0.69	0.120
	Winthrop-University Hospital, Mineola	7.7	0.0%	1.76	Yes	0.21	9	0.95	0.085

GASTROENTEROLOGY

Natl. Rank	Hospital	U.S. News index	Reputational score	Gastroenterology mortality rate	COTH member	Interns and residents to beds	Technology score (of 11)	R.N.'s to beds	Board-certified gastroenterologists to beds	Procedures to beds
TIER ONE										
7	Mount Sinai Medical Center, New York	51.3	24.3%	0.91	Yes	0.99	9	1.50	0.037	2.23
20	Memorial Sloan-Kettering Cancer Center, New York	19.5	4.3%	0.83	Yes	0.38	8	1.37	0.011	2.58
TIER TWO										
67	Beth Israel Medical Center, New York	13.5	0.9%	1.03	Yes	0.65	9	1.27	0.014	2.16
50	Columbia-Presbyterian Medical Center, New York	15.1	2.4%	1.13	Yes	0.85	10	1.05	0.014	1.29
54	Montefiore Medical Center, Bronx	14.8	2.0%	1.09	Yes	0.53	10	1.28	0.043	2.44
41	New York Hospital-Cornell Medical Center	15.9	2.3%	0.92	Yes	0.79	9	1.00	0.015	1.37
30	New York University Medical Center	16.8	1.6%	0.94	Yes	1.30	8	1.15	0.000	2.01
42	Roswell Park Cancer Institute, Buffalo	15.8	0.0%	0.21	No	0.68	9	2.58	0.000	4.46
TIER THREE										
	Albany Medical Center Hospital, Albany	9.8	0.0%	1.47	Yes	0.76	8	1.33	0.019	1.33
	Bronx Municipal Hospital Center, Bronx	8.2	0.0%	1.38	Yes	1.07	1	1.07	0.011	0.83
	Bronx-Lebanon Hospital Center, Bronx	8.7	0.0%	1.32	Yes	0.79	6	1.00	0.003	0.75
	Brooklyn Hospital Center, Brooklyn	8.0	0.0%	1.64	Yes	0.75	8	0.67	0.012	1.89
	Cabrini Medical Center, New York	8.4	0.0%	1.32	Yes	0.53	7	0.69	0.010	2.49
	Genesee Hospital, Rochester	8.5	0.0%	1.08	Yes	0.28	6	0.78	0.012	2.37
	Huntington Hospital, Huntington	7.6	0.0%	0.84	No	0.02	7	0.59	0.033	3.86
	Lenox Hill Hospital, New York	11.2	1.5%	1.35	Yes	0.57	5	1.18	0.017	2.42
100	Long Island College Hospital, Brooklyn	11.7	0.0%	0.98	Yes	0.62	8	1.23	0.000	1.78
81	Long Island Jewish Medical Center, New York	12.9	0.0%	1.25	Yes	1.17	10	1.20	0.046	2.03
	Maimonides Medical Center, Brooklyn	10.4	0.0%	1.14	Yes	0.78	6	0.93	0.018	2.43
99	Mary Imogene Bassett Hospital, Cooperstown	11.7	0.0%	1.14	Yes	0.22	8	1.69	0.018	4.13
	Methodist Hospital, Brooklyn	11.0	0.0%	1.07	Yes	0.57	9	0.77	0.000	3.19
93	North Shore University Hospital, Manhasset	12.3	0.0%	1.01	Yes	0.58	10	1.10	0.034	2.76
	Northern Westchester Hospital Center, Mount Kisco	8.6	0.0%	0.93	No	0.00	8	1.32	0.019	3.69
	Our Lady of Mercy Medical Center, Bronx	7.7	0.6%	1.41	Yes	0.42	5	0.62	0.026	2.18
	Rochester General Hospital, Rochester	9.5	0.0%	1.19	Yes	0.22	9	0.96	0.017	3.15
	St. Joseph's Medical Center, Yonkers	7.6	0.0%	0.78	No	0.26	3	0.79	0.036	2.96
	St. Luke's-Roosevelt Hospital Center, New York	10.3	0.5%	1.06	Yes	0.69	4	1.07	0.017	1.28
	St. Peter's Hospital, Albany	7.7	0.0%	1.03	No	0.09	9	0.98	0.022	3.66
	St. Vincent's Hospital and Medical Center, New York	11.0	0.0%	1.21	Yes	0.88	9	1.08	0.000	1.45

Natl. Rank	Hospital	U.S. News index	Reputational score	Gastroenterology mortality rate	COTH member	Interns and residents to beds	Technology score (of 11)	R.N.'s to beds	Board-certified gastroenterologists to beds	Procedures to beds
94	Strong Memorial Hospital-Rochester University	12.1	0.0%	1.36	Yes	1.00	10	1.45	0.021	1.71
91	University Hosp.-SUNY Health Science Ctr., Syracuse	12.4	0.0%	1.65	Yes	1.30	9	1.61	0.042	1.58
95	University Hospital, Stony Brook	12.1	0.0%	1.23	Yes	1.12	9	1.22	0.016	1.35
	Westchester County Medical Center, Valhalla	10.1	0.0%	1.30	Yes	0.81	5	1.59	0.014	1.02
	Winthrop-University Hospital, Mineola	10.3	0.0%	1.05	Yes	0.21	8	0.95	0.013	3.85
TIER FOUR										
	Arnot Ogden Medical Center, Elmira	5.6	0.0%	1.27	No	0.00	9	1.18	0.014	2.10
	Auburn Memorial Hospital, Auburn	3.2	0.0%	1.34	No	0.00	4	0.52	0.007	3.75
	Benedictine Hospital, Kingston	3.5	0.0%	1.29	No	0.08	4	0.59	0.018	3.02
	Brookdale Hospital Medical Center, Brooklyn	5.5	0.0%	1.86	Yes	0.45	6	0.79	0.014	0.95
	Buffalo General Hospital, Buffalo	6.8	0.0%	1.32	Yes	0.04	7	0.96	0.000	1.71
	Catholic Medical Center, Jamaica	6.6	0.0%	1.48	Yes	0.29	6	0.80	0.000	2.14
	Central General Hospital, Plainview	4.7	0.0%	1.18	No	0.00	5	0.59	0.030	4.08
	Community-General Hospital, Syracuse	4.3	0.0%	1.14	No	0.03	3	0.63	0.014	3.87
	Crouse Irving Memorial Hospital, Syracuse	4.2	0.0%	1.23	No	0.12	2	1.06	0.005	2.76
	Ellis Hospital, Schenectady	5.3	0.0%	1.10	No	0.02	7	0.78	0.013	2.58
	Erie County Medical Center, Buffalo	4.7	0.0%	1.50	Yes	0.20	4	0.72	0.007	0.75
	Flushing Hospital Medical Center, Flushing	6.6	0.0%	1.29	No	0.45	7	1.05	0.028	2.75
	Franklin Hospital Medical Center, Valley Stream	3.1	0.0%	1.48	No	0.04	9	0.29	0.028	2.58
	Good Samaritan Hospital, Suffern	6.2	0.0%	1.08	No	0.00	8	0.92	0.022	3.01
	Good Samaritan Hospital, West Islip	4.2	0.0%	1.59	No	0.00	9	0.74	0.023	3.34
	Highland Hospital of Rochester, Rochester	5.8	0.0%	1.23	No	0.51	7	0.54	0.011	2.69
	House of the Good Samaritan, Watertown	4.3	0.0%	1.74	No	0.00	7	1.06	0.004	4.06
	Jamaica Hospital, Jamaica	4.0	0.0%	1.65	No	0.50	3	1.17	0.016	1.78
	John T. Mather Memorial Hospital, Port Jefferson	4.8	0.0%	1.59	No	0.00	6	1.15	0.008	4.52
	Kingsbrook Jewish Medical Center, Brooklyn	1.9	0.0%	1.38	No	0.17	6	0.23	0.006	0.98
	Kingston Hospital, Kingston	5.3	0.0%	1.17	No	0.14	2	0.85	0.014	4.99
	La Guardia Hospital, Flushing	2.3	0.0%	1.59	No	0.28	0	0.78	0.007	2.99
	Lutheran Medical Center, Brooklyn	5.2	0.0%	1.35	No	0.38	7	0.79	0.010	2.28
	Mercy Hospital, Buffalo	3.2	0.0%	1.30	No	0.12	3	0.48	0.012	3.41
	Mercy Medical Center, Rockville Centre	5.5	0.0%	1.19	No	0.01	8	0.77	0.031	3.36
	Millard Fillmore Hospitals, Buffalo	6.5	0.0%	1.37	Yes	0.15	4	0.82	0.012	2.94
	Mount Vernon Hospital, Mount Vernon	5.5	0.0%	1.09	No	0.30	3	0.93	0.016	2.48
	Nathan Littauer Hospital, Gloversville	2.1	0.0%	1.32	No	0.00	3	0.37	0.005	2.90
	New Rochelle Hospital Medical Center, New Rochelle	6.0	0.0%	1.30	No	0.20	8	0.89	0.021	3.54
	New York Downtown Hospital	7.2	0.0%	1.15	No	0.67	4	1.06	0.023	2.80
	New York Hospital Medical Center, Flushing	6.8	0.0%	1.29	Yes	0.27	6	0.52	0.014	2.30
	North Shore University Hospital-Glen Cove, Glen Cove	4.1	0.0%	1.47	No	0.09	6	0.66	0.064	3.71
	Nyack Hospital, Nyack	5.3	0.0%	1.09	No	0.06	5	0.74	0.017	3.44
	Samaritan Hospital, Troy	3.9	0.0%	1.43	No	0.00	8	0.66	0.018	2.78
	Saratoga Hospital, Saratoga Springs	4.6	0.0%	1.07	No	0.00	3	0.86	0.013	2.88
	Sisters of Charity Hospital, Buffalo	2.8	0.0%	1.38	No	0.07	4	0.60	0.000	2.63
	South Nassau Community Hospital, Oceanside	5.5	0.0%	1.16	No	0.07	6	0.85	0.047	3.22
	Southampton Hospital, Southampton	5.9	0.0%	1.00	No	0.00	8	0.44	0.015	3.47
	Southside Hospital, Bay Shore	2.9	0.0%	1.62	No	0.13	6	0.60	0.020	2.68
	St. Barnabas Hospital, Bronx	3.1	0.0%	1.36	No	0.41	0	0.86	0.017	1.99
	St. Charles Hospital and Rehab. Ctr., Port Jefferson	2.7	0.0%	1.59	No	0.04	4	0.90	0.026	2.44
	St. Clare's Hospital of Schenectady, Schenectady	5.2	0.0%	1.58	No	0.20	4	1.05	0.027	5.16
	St. Elizabeth Hospital, Utica	4.1	0.0%	1.56	No	0.20	5	0.82	0.014	3.74
	St. John's Episcopal Hospital, Far Rockaway	1.3	0.0%	1.74	No	0.24	0	0.74	0.016	2.32
	St. John's Episcopal Hospital, Smithtown	0.9	0.0%	2.01	No	0.00	7	0.34	0.017	1.97
	St. Mary's Hospital of Troy, Troy	4.2	0.0%	1.23	No	0.00	3	0.66	0.035	4.44
	St. Mary's Hospital, Rochester	4.3	0.0%	1.43	No	0.37	4	0.84	0.013	2.57
	St. Vincent's Medical Center, Staten Island	5.1	0.0%	1.31	No	0.46	4	0.92	0.020	2.32

Natl. Rank	Hospital	U.S. News index	Reputational score	Gastro-enterology mortality rate	COTH member	Interns and residents to beds	Technology score (of 11)	R.N.'s to beds	Board-certified gastro-enterologists to beds	Procedures to beds
	Staten Island University Hospital, Staten Island	6.5	0.0%	1.13	No	0.46	8	0.53	0.010	2.86
	United Health Services Hospitals, Binghamton	6.9	0.0%	1.32	Yes	0.20	5	0.61	0.019	3.30
	Vassar Brothers Hospital, Poughkeepsie	3.7	0.0%	1.60	No	0.01	8	0.69	0.010	3.34

GERIATRICS

Natl. Rank	Hospital	U.S. News index	Reputational score	Hospital-wide mortality rate	COTH member	Service mix	Interns and residents to beds	Technology score (of 13)	R.N.'s to beds	Discharge planning (of 2)	Geriatric services (of 9)	Board-certified internists to beds
TIER ONE
3	Mount Sinai Medical Center, New York	85.9	24.3%	1.09	Yes	9	0.99	10	1.50	2	6	0.253
15	New York University Medical Center	33.7	4.4%	0.98	Yes	4	1.30	10	1.15	2	1	0.360
25	New York Hospital-Cornell Medical Center	29.5	3.5%	1.07	Yes	9	0.79	11	1.00	2	6	0.113
TIER TWO
26	Columbia-Presbyterian Medical Center, New York	29.1	5.3%	1.25	Yes	7	0.85	11	1.05	2	4	0.111
31	Montefiore Medical Center, Bronx	26.8	4.0%	1.19	Yes	7	0.53	11	1.28	2	5	0.095
TIER THREE
	Albany Medical Center Hospital, Albany	18.9	0.4%	1.12	Yes	7	0.76	11	1.33	2	2	0.103
	Bellevue Hospital Center, New York	16.4	0.3%	1.10	Yes	7	0.34	6	0.89	2	3	0.137
	Beth Israel Medical Center, New York	20.1	0.0%	1.09	Yes	9	0.65	12	1.27	2	6	0.085
	Long Island College Hospital, Brooklyn	15.2	0.0%	1.21	Yes	8	0.62	8	1.23	2	1	0.156
93	Long Island Jewish Medical Center, New York	21.3	2.1%	1.34	Yes	9	1.17	11	1.20	2	5	0.097
	Maimonides Medical Center, Brooklyn	14.1	0.0%	1.21	Yes	5	0.78	9	0.93	2	4	0.070
	Mary Imogene Bassett Hospital, Cooperstown	20.3	0.7%	1.03	Yes	6	0.22	10	1.69	2	2	0.066
92	Methodist Hospital, Brooklyn	21.4	0.0%	0.94	Yes	6	0.57	12	0.77	2	2	0.229
	North Shore University Hospital, Manhasset	19.0	0.0%	1.12	Yes	8	0.58	12	1.10	2	3	0.327
	Northern Westchester Hospital Center, Mount Kisco	15.4	0.0%	1.05	No	6	0.00	8	1.32	2	4	0.170
	St. Vincent's Hospital and Medical Center, New York	15.3	0.0%	1.36	Yes	9	0.88	10	1.08	2	5	0.255
	Strong Memorial Hospital-Rochester University	19.5	1.3%	1.26	Yes	8	1.00	11	1.45	2	2	0.111
	University Hosp.-SUNY Health Science Ctr., Syracuse	16.6	0.0%	1.28	Yes	7	1.30	10	1.61	2	3	0.160
	University Hospital, Stony Brook	15.7	0.3%	1.31	Yes	7	1.12	10	1.22	2	4	0.108
	Winthrop-University Hospital, Mineola	15.3	0.9%	1.23	Yes	6	0.21	10	0.95	2	3	0.085
TIER FOUR
	Arnot Ogden Medical Center, Elmira	6.9	0.0%	1.40	No	3	0.00	10	1.18	2	4	0.093
	Auburn Memorial Hospital, Auburn	3.9	0.0%	1.39	No	3	0.00	6	0.52	2	1	0.044
	Benedictine Hospital, Kingston	5.8	0.0%	1.29	No	3	0.08	5	0.59	2	1	0.068
	Bronx Municipal Hospital Center, Bronx	8.6	0.0%	1.59	Yes	8	1.07	2	1.07	2	1	0.072
	Bronx-Lebanon Hospital Center, Bronx	13.2	0.0%	1.37	Yes	8	0.79	8	1.00	2	6	0.075
	Brookdale Hospital Medical Center, Brooklyn	8.0	0.0%	1.59	Yes	8	0.45	9	0.79	2	1	0.085
	Brooklyn Hospital Center, Brooklyn	13.0	0.0%	1.32	Yes	7	0.75	11	0.67	2	4	0.107
	Buffalo General Hospital, Buffalo	11.2	1.0%	1.54	Yes	8	0.04	9	0.96	2	3	0.133
	Cabrini Medical Center, New York	13.5	0.0%	1.20	Yes	7	0.53	9	0.69	2	1	0.120
	Catholic Medical Center, Jamaica	9.2	0.0%	1.53	Yes	7	0.29	8	0.80	2	4	0.220
	Central General Hospital, Plainview	11.7	0.0%	1.10	No	3	0.00	8	0.59	2	4	0.246
	Community-General Hospital, Syracuse	7.2	0.0%	1.16	No	4	0.03	3	0.63	1	1	0.065
	Coney Island Hospital, Brooklyn	8.2	0.0%	1.46	No	6	0.56	5	1.06	2	7	0.070
	Crouse Irving Memorial Hospital, Syracuse	5.1	0.0%	1.33	No	4	0.12	3	1.06	1	1	0.061
	Ellis Hospital, Schenectady	9.4	0.0%	1.23	No	5	0.02	9	0.78	2	4	0.042
	Erie County Medical Center, Buffalo	7.4	0.0%	1.54	Yes	6	0.20	5	0.72	2	6	0.068
	Flushing Hospital Medical Center, Flushing	8.3	0.0%	1.37	No	6	0.45	9	1.05	2	1	0.056
	Franklin Hospital Medical Center, Valley Stream	3.0	0.0%	1.62	No	4	0.04	10	0.29	2	5	0.052
	Genesee Hospital, Rochester	9.6	0.0%	1.35	Yes	5	0.28	8	0.78	2	1	0.146
	Good Samaritan Hospital, Suffern	9.4	0.0%	1.24	No	6	0.00	10	0.92	2	2	0.022
	Good Samaritan Hospital, West Islip	4.6	0.0%	1.57	No	5	0.00	10	0.74	2	4	0.055
	Harlem Hospital Center, New York	4.2	0.0%	2.25	Yes	8	0.83	8	0.91	2	4	0.041

Natl. Rank	Hospital	U.S. News index	Reputa-tional score	Hospital-wide mortality rate	COTH member	Service mix	Interns and residents to beds	Tech-nology score (of 13)	R.N.'s to beds	Discharge planning (of 2)	Geriatric services (of 9)	Board-certified internists to beds
	Highland Hospital of Rochester, Rochester	7.4	0.0%	1.35	No	3	0.51	7	0.54	2	3	0.184
	House of the Good Samaritan, Watertown	6.9	0.0%	1.35	No	4	0.00	8	1.06	2	3	0.034
	Jamaica Hospital, Jamaica	5.8	0.0%	1.37	No	4	0.50	4	1.17	1	1	0.066
	John T. Mather Memorial Hospital, Port Jefferson	5.4	0.0%	1.56	No	6	0.00	8	1.15	2	4	0.059
	Kingsboro Psychiatric Center, Brooklyn	6.0	0.0%	1.22	No	4	0.02	0	0.20	2	4	0.002
	Kingsbrook Jewish Medical Center, Brooklyn	3.7	0.0%	1.57	No	6	0.17	6	0.23	2	5	0.012
	Kingston Hospital, Kingston	3.0	0.0%	1.41	No	3	0.14	3	0.85	1	1	0.057
	La Guardia Hospital, Flushing	1.5	0.0%	1.58	No	2	0.28	0	0.78	2	1	0.132
	Lenox Hill Hospital, New York	13.8	0.0%	1.25	Yes	8	0.57	8	1.18	2	1	0.104
	Lutheran Medical Center, Brooklyn	12.7	0.0%	1.21	No	8	0.38	9	0.79	2	6	0.073
	Mercy Hospital, Buffalo	6.6	0.0%	1.34	No	5	0.12	6	0.48	2	4	0.045
	Mercy Medical Center, Rockville Centre	9.8	0.0%	1.22	No	5	0.01	10	0.77	2	3	0.101
	Millard Fillmore Hospitals, Buffalo	7.5	0.0%	1.45	Yes	4	0.15	6	0.82	2	5	0.031
	Mount Vernon Hospital, Mount Vernon	12.1	0.0%	1.12	No	7	0.30	4	0.93	2	1	0.090
	Nassau County Medical Center, East Meadow	9.6	0.0%	1.69	Yes	8	1.01	11	1.17	2	1	0.121
	New Rochelle Hospital Medical Center, New Rochelle	13.4	0.0%	1.14	No	7	0.20	9	0.89	2	6	0.073
	New York Downtown Hospital	10.5	0.0%	1.26	No	7	0.67	6	1.06	2	2	0.000
	New York Hospital Medical Center, Flushing	9.8	0.3%	1.43	Yes	8	0.27	9	0.52	2	1	0.084
	North Shore University Hospital-Glen Cove, Glen Cove	9.9	0.0%	1.29	No	5	0.09	7	0.66	2	2	0.506
	Our Lady of Mercy Medical Center, Bronx	8.3	0.0%	1.44	Yes	7	0.42	7	0.62	1	2	0.158
	Richard H. Hutchings Psychiatric Center, Syracuse	4.7	0.0%	1.33	No	5	0.42	0	0.48	1	3	0.000
	Rochester General Hospital, Rochester	12.1	0.0%	1.26	Yes	4	0.22	10	0.96	2	4	0.135
	Samaritan Hospital, Troy	9.0	0.0%	1.24	No	6	0.00	9	0.66	2	2	0.044
	Saratoga Hospital, Saratoga Springs	6.6	0.0%	1.22	No	2	0.00	3	0.86	2	2	0.027
	Sisters of Charity Hospital, Buffalo	6.3	0.0%	1.47	No	7	0.07	6	0.60	2	5	0.120
	South Nassau Community Hospital, Oceanside	9.0	0.0%	1.22	No	6	0.07	9	0.85	1	1	0.147
	Southside Hospital, Bay Shore	0.0	0.0%	1.75	No	4	0.13	9	0.60	1	1	0.017
	St. Charles Hospital and Rehab. Ctr., Port Jefferson	7.0	0.0%	1.39	No	5	0.04	4	0.90	2	2	0.332
	St. Clare's Hospital of Schenectady, Schenectady	6.4	0.0%	1.40	No	3	0.20	4	1.05	2	5	0.122
	St. Elizabeth Hospital, Utica	10.2	0.0%	1.13	No	4	0.20	7	0.82	2	1	0.009
	St. John's Episcopal Hospital, Smithtown	1.9	0.0%	1.70	No	4	0.00	10	0.34	2	3	0.087
	St. Joseph's Medical Center, Yonkers	9.1	0.0%	1.24	No	5	0.26	3	0.79	2	6	0.046
	St. Luke's-Roosevelt Hospital Center, New York	12.8	0.0%	1.29	Yes	8	0.69	5	1.07	2	1	0.142
	St. Mary's Hospital of Troy, Troy	4.3	0.0%	1.38	No	3	0.00	3	0.66	2	3	0.060
	St. Mary's Hospital, Rochester	7.6	0.0%	1.30	No	3	0.37	5	0.84	2	3	0.110
	St. Peter's Hospital, Albany	12.3	0.0%	1.15	No	6	0.09	11	0.98	2	3	0.065
	St. Vincent's Medical Center, Staten Island	9.8	0.0%	1.41	No	8	0.46	7	0.92	2	8	0.075
	Staten Island University Hospital, Staten Island	11.8	0.0%	1.26	No	9	0.46	10	0.53	2	5	0.071
	United Health Services Hospitals, Binghamton	11.4	0.0%	1.25	Yes	7	0.20	6	0.61	2	4	0.050
	University Hospital of Brooklyn-SUNY Center, Brooklyn	10.3	0.3%	1.48	Yes	4	0.70	11	1.12	2	1	0.128
	Vassar Brothers Hospital, Poughkeepsie	4.3	0.0%	1.50	No	3	0.01	10	0.69	2	2	0.120
	Westchester County Medical Center, Valhalla	11.7	0.0%	1.50	Yes	8	0.81	8	1.59	2	3	0.052

GYNECOLOGY

Natl. Rank	Hospital	U.S. News index	Reputa-tional score	Hospital-wide mortality rate	Interns and residents to beds	Tech-nology score (of 10)	R.N.'s to beds	Board-certified OB-GYNs to beds	Procedures to beds
	TIER ONE								
11	Memorial Sloan-Kettering Cancer Center, New York	45.6	9.4%	0.91	0.38	7	1.37	0.007	0.50
18	Roswell Park Cancer Institute, Buffalo	36.1	2.5%	0.56	0.68	8	2.58	0.023	0.91
29	New York Hospital-Cornell Medical Center	31.5	5.0%	1.07	0.79	8	1.00	0.055	0.23
31	New York University Medical Center	30.5	2.3%	0.98	1.30	8	1.15	0.074	0.36
	TIER TWO								
33	Columbia-Presbyterian Medical Center, New York	29.9	5.2%	1.25	0.85	10	1.05	0.036	0.22
36	Mount Sinai Medical Center, New York	28.2	2.9%	1.09	0.99	7	1.50	0.061	0.28

Natl. Rank Hospital	U.S. News index	Reputa- tional score	Hospital- wide mortality rate	Interns and residents to beds	Tech- nology score (of 10)	R.N.'s to beds	Board- certified OB-GYNs to beds	Procedures to beds
TIER THREE								
Albany Medical Center Hospital, Albany	19.3	0.0%	1.12	0.76	8	1.33	0.074	0.57
Beth Israel Medical Center, New York	19.3	0.0%	1.09	0.65	9	1.27	0.046	0.19
Lenox Hill Hospital, New York	18.7	2.1%	1.25	0.57	5	1.18	0.091	0.29
Long Island College Hospital, Brooklyn	15.2	0.0%	1.21	0.62	7	1.23	0.050	0.20
Long Island Jewish Medical Center, New York	17.7	0.0%	1.34	1.17	9	1.20	0.104	0.29
Mary Imogene Bassett Hospital, Cooperstown	19.0	0.0%	1.03	0.22	7	1.69	0.039	0.28
Methodist Hospital, Brooklyn	20.8	0.0%	0.94	0.57	9	0.77	0.051	0.26
Montefiore Medical Center, Bronx	17.2	0.0%	1.19	0.53	9	1.28	0.071	0.25
North Shore University Hospital, Manhasset	20.3	0.6%	1.12	0.58	9	1.10	0.116	0.57
Northern Westchester Hospital Center, Mount Kisco	16.2	0.0%	1.05	0.00	6	1.32	0.077	0.37
St. Peter's Hospital, Albany	14.4	0.0%	1.15	0.09	9	0.98	0.058	0.31
St. Vincent's Hospital and Medical Center, New York	14.7	0.0%	1.36	0.88	9	1.08	0.058	0.15
Strong Memorial Hospital-Rochester University	19.4	0.0%	1.26	1.00	9	1.45	0.118	0.51
University Hosp.-SUNY Health Science Ctr., Syracuse	19.7	0.0%	1.28	1.30	7	1.61	0.134	0.08
University Hospital, Stony Brook	18.4	0.4%	1.31	1.12	8	1.22	0.112	0.57
TIER FOUR								
Arnot Ogden Medical Center, Elmira	9.9	0.0%	1.40	0.00	9	1.18	0.027	0.42
Auburn Memorial Hospital, Auburn	3.3	0.0%	1.39	0.00	4	0.52	0.018	0.40
Bellevue Hospital Center, New York	13.3	0.5%	1.10	0.34	4	0.89	0.028	0.07
Bronx Municipal Hospital Center, Bronx	9.0	0.5%	1.59	1.07	3	1.07	0.034	0.09
Bronx-Lebanon Hospital Center, Bronx	10.8	0.0%	1.37	0.79	6	1.00	0.017	0.08
Brookdale Hospital Medical Center, Brooklyn	6.5	0.5%	1.59	0.45	5	0.79	0.046	0.12
Brooklyn Hospital Center, Brooklyn	12.1	0.0%	1.32	0.75	8	0.67	0.053	0.21
Buffalo General Hospital, Buffalo	5.8	0.4%	1.54	0.04	5	0.96	0.042	0.25
Cabrini Medical Center, New York	11.0	0.0%	1.20	0.53	6	0.69	0.020	0.12
Catholic Medical Center, Jamaica	5.5	0.0%	1.53	0.29	6	0.80	0.022	0.15
Central General Hospital, Plainview	10.0	0.0%	1.10	0.00	4	0.59	0.064	0.28
Community-General Hospital, Syracuse	8.2	0.0%	1.16	0.03	3	0.63	0.056	0.49
Coney Island Hospital, Brooklyn	6.4	0.0%	1.46	0.56	3	1.06	0.009	0.07
Crouse Irving Memorial Hospital, Syracuse	8.7	0.0%	1.33	0.12	4	1.06	0.080	0.62
Ellis Hospital, Schenectady	8.5	0.0%	1.23	0.02	6	0.78	0.016	0.11
Erie County Medical Center, Buffalo	3.5	0.0%	1.54	0.20	4	0.72	0.033	0.03
Flushing Hospital Medical Center, Flushing	11.9	0.0%	1.37	0.45	7	1.05	0.098	0.20
Franklin Hospital Medical Center, Valley Stream	2.6	0.0%	1.62	0.04	7	0.29	0.049	0.15
Genesee Hospital, Rochester	7.8	0.0%	1.35	0.28	5	0.78	0.052	0.32
Good Samaritan Hospital, Suffern	9.8	0.0%	1.24	0.00	7	0.92	0.027	0.17
Good Samaritan Hospital, West Islip	6.3	0.0%	1.57	0.00	9	0.74	0.050	0.38
Highland Hospital of Rochester, Rochester	9.4	0.0%	1.35	0.51	6	0.54	0.088	0.36
House of the Good Samaritan, Watertown	9.0	0.0%	1.35	0.00	7	1.06	0.043	0.45
Huntington Hospital, Huntington	10.8	0.0%	1.12	0.02	6	0.59	0.054	0.39
Jamaica Hospital, Jamaica	8.8	0.0%	1.37	0.50	3	1.17	0.054	0.16
John T. Mather Memorial Hospital, Port Jefferson	6.1	0.0%	1.56	0.00	5	1.15	0.084	0.18
Kingsbrook Jewish Medical Center, Brooklyn	1.0	0.0%	1.57	0.17	5	0.23	0.006	0.03
La Guardia Hospital, Flushing	1.5	0.0%	1.58	0.28	1	0.78	0.033	0.17
Lutheran Medical Center, Brooklyn	11.2	0.0%	1.21	0.38	6	0.79	0.038	0.18
Maimonides Medical Center, Brooklyn	13.8	0.0%	1.21	0.78	6	0.93	0.052	0.27
Mercy Hospital, Buffalo	4.2	0.0%	1.34	0.12	3	0.48	0.033	0.37
Mercy Medical Center, Rockville Centre	10.2	0.0%	1.22	0.01	7	0.77	0.052	0.32
Millard Fillmore Hospitals, Buffalo	7.6	0.4%	1.45	0.15	5	0.82	0.073	0.43
Nassau County Medical Center, East Meadow	10.4	0.0%	1.69	1.01	8	1.17	0.039	0.12
New Rochelle Hospital Medical Center, New Rochelle	12.8	0.0%	1.14	0.20	7	0.89	0.038	0.22
New York Downtown Hospital	12.2	0.0%	1.26	0.67	4	1.06	0.082	0.10
New York Hospital Medical Center, Flushing	5.3	0.0%	1.43	0.27	5	0.52	0.046	0.19
North Shore University Hospital-Glen Cove, Glen Cove	8.6	0.0%	1.29	0.09	5	0.66	0.136	0.22
Our Lady of Mercy Medical Center, Bronx	7.2	0.0%	1.44	0.42	6	0.62	0.051	0.22

Natl. Rank	Hospital	U.S. News index	Reputa-tional score	Hospital-wide mortality rate	Interns and residents to beds	Tech-nology score (of 10)	R.N.'s to beds	Board-certified OB-GYNs to beds	Procedures to beds
	Rochester General Hospital, Rochester	12.1	0.0%	1.26	0.22	9	0.96	0.027	0.33
	Samaritan Hospital, Troy	8.9	0.0%	1.24	0.00	7	0.66	0.033	0.43
	Saratoga Hospital, Saratoga Springs	6.7	0.0%	1.22	0.00	3	0.86	0.009	0.21
	Sisters of Charity Hospital, Buffalo	2.9	0.0%	1.47	0.07	3	0.60	0.045	0.45
	South Nassau Community Hospital, Oceanside	9.0	0.0%	1.22	0.07	5	0.85	0.037	0.27
	Southside Hospital, Bay Shore	1.6	0.0%	1.75	0.13	5	0.60	0.049	0.16
	St. Charles Hospital and Rehab. Ctr., Port Jefferson	6.9	0.0%	1.39	0.04	4	0.90	0.092	0.41
	St. Clare's Hospital of Schenectady, Schenectady	7.5	0.0%	1.40	0.20	4	1.05	0.063	0.44
	St. Elizabeth Hospital, Utica	9.2	0.0%	1.13	0.20	3	0.82	0.009	0.30
	St. John's Episcopal Hospital, Smithtown	0.4	0.0%	1.70	0.00	5	0.34	0.050	0.14
	St. Joseph's Medical Center, Yonkers	7.2	0.0%	1.24	0.26	3	0.79	0.010	0.26
	St. Luke's-Roosevelt Hospital Center, New York	13.1	0.6%	1.29	0.69	5	1.07	0.042	0.14
	St. Vincent's Medical Center, Staten Island	8.1	0.0%	1.41	0.46	5	0.92	0.045	0.22
	Staten Island University Hospital, Staten Island	10.8	0.0%	1.26	0.46	8	0.53	0.037	0.22
	United Health Services Hospitals, Binghamton	8.4	0.0%	1.25	0.20	6	0.61	0.026	0.30
	Vassar Brothers Hospital, Poughkeepsie	6.8	0.0%	1.50	0.01	8	0.69	0.073	0.66
	Westchester County Medical Center, Valhalla	12.5	0.0%	1.50	0.81	5	1.59	0.083	0.24
	Winthrop-University Hospital, Mineola	12.4	0.0%	1.23	0.21	8	0.95	0.047	0.36

NEUROLOGY

Natl. Rank	Hospital	U.S. News index	Reputa-tional score	Neurology mortality rate	COTH member	Interns and residents to beds	Tech-nology score (of 9)	R.N.'s to beds	Board-certified neurologists to beds
	TIER ONE								
5	Columbia-Presbyterian Medical Center, New York	54.8	23.7%	1.02	Yes	0.85	9	1.05	0.040
8	New York Hospital-Cornell Medical Center	40.2	12.8%	0.78	Yes	0.79	7	1.00	0.024
13	New York University Medical Center	28.6	3.7%	0.73	Yes	1.30	7	1.15	0.024
22	Mount Sinai Medical Center, New York	25.4	1.9%	0.78	Yes	0.99	7	1.50	0.026
	TIER TWO								
75	Montefiore Medical Center, Bronx	18.2	0.4%	0.96	Yes	0.53	8	1.28	0.040
80	North Shore University Hospital, Manhasset	18.0	0.0%	0.91	Yes	0.58	8	1.10	0.036
43	Strong Memorial Hospital-Rochester University	21.5	1.8%	1.09	Yes	1.00	8	1.45	0.057
	TIER THREE								
	Albany Medical Center Hospital, Albany	15.1	0.0%	1.01	Yes	0.76	7	1.33	0.005
	Beth Israel Medical Center, New York	16.5	0.0%	0.94	Yes	0.65	8	1.27	0.013
	Bronx-Lebanon Hospital Center, Bronx	12.1	0.0%	1.12	Yes	0.79	5	1.00	0.004
	Cabrini Medical Center, New York	12.7	0.0%	1.07	Yes	0.53	6	0.69	0.024
	Lenox Hill Hospital, New York	11.9	0.0%	1.14	Yes	0.57	4	1.18	0.012
	Long Island College Hospital, Brooklyn	13.6	0.0%	1.09	Yes	0.62	6	1.23	0.016
	Long Island Jewish Medical Center, New York	14.1	0.0%	1.33	Yes	1.17	8	1.20	0.029
	Maimonides Medical Center, Brooklyn	12.0	0.0%	1.18	Yes	0.78	5	0.93	0.016
	Mary Imogene Bassett Hospital, Cooperstown	12.4	0.0%	1.19	Yes	0.22	7	1.69	0.013
	Memorial Sloan-Kettering Cancer Center, New York	16.0	0.3%	0.94	Yes	0.38	7	1.37	0.011
	Northern Westchester Hospital Center, Mount Kisco	12.0	0.0%	0.96	No	0.00	6	1.32	0.023
	St. Luke's-Roosevelt Hospital Center, New York	11.6	0.0%	1.14	Yes	0.69	4	1.07	0.008
	St. Vincent's Hospital and Medical Center, New York	15.3	0.0%	1.23	Yes	0.88	8	1.08	0.051
91	University Hosp.-SUNY Health Science Ctr., Syracuse	17.6	0.0%	1.19	Yes	1.30	7	1.61	0.042
	University Hospital, Stony Brook	14.2	0.0%	1.31	Yes	1.12	7	1.22	0.034
	Winthrop-University Hospital, Mineola	12.6	0.0%	1.03	Yes	0.21	7	0.95	0.013
	TIER FOUR								
	Arnot Ogden Medical Center, Elmira	5.9	0.0%	1.54	No	0.00	8	1.18	0.021
	Auburn Memorial Hospital, Auburn	2.7	0.0%	1.43	No	0.00	4	0.52	0.004
	Benedictine Hospital, Kingston	3.6	0.0%	1.45	No	0.08	4	0.59	0.014
	Bronx Municipal Hospital Center, Bronx	7.8	0.0%	1.70	Yes	1.07	1	1.07	0.014
	Brookdale Hospital Medical Center, Brooklyn	7.6	0.0%	1.48	Yes	0.45	5	0.79	0.013

Natl. Rank	Hospital	U.S. News index	Reputa-tional score	Neurology mortality rate	COTH member	Interns and residents to beds	Tech-nology score (of 9)	R.N.'s to beds	Board-certified neurologists to beds
	Brooklyn Hospital Center, Brooklyn	10.7	0.0%	1.25	Yes	0.75	7	0.67	0.011
	Buffalo General Hospital, Buffalo	5.4	0.0%	1.67	Yes	0.04	5	0.96	0.011
	Central General Hospital, Plainview	8.4	0.0%	1.02	No	0.00	4	0.59	0.021
	Community-General Hospital, Syracuse	5.1	0.0%	1.20	No	0.03	3	0.63	0.006
	Coney Island Hospital, Brooklyn	3.4	0.0%	1.76	No	0.56	3	1.06	0.004
	Crouse Irving Memorial Hospital, Syracuse	5.6	0.0%	1.33	No	0.12	2	1.06	0.018
	Ellis Hospital, Schenectady	6.7	0.0%	1.20	No	0.02	6	0.78	0.013
	Erie County Medical Center, Buffalo	6.6	0.0%	1.44	Yes	0.20	4	0.72	0.013
	Flushing Hospital Medical Center, Flushing	7.8	0.0%	1.28	No	0.45	6	1.05	0.011
	Franklin Hospital Medical Center, Valley Stream	5.6	0.0%	1.21	No	0.04	7	0.29	0.012
	Genesee Hospital, Rochester	7.1	0.0%	1.44	Yes	0.28	5	0.78	0.009
	Good Samaritan Hospital, Suffern	8.9	0.0%	1.07	No	0.00	7	0.92	0.011
	Good Samaritan Hospital, West Islip	4.3	0.0%	1.55	No	0.00	8	0.74	0.015
	Harlem Hospital Center, New York	6.4	0.0%	1.93	Yes	0.83	6	0.91	0.006
	Highland Hospital of Rochester, Rochester	6.9	0.0%	1.23	No	0.51	6	0.54	0.007
	Huntington Hospital, Huntington	5.3	0.0%	1.37	No	0.02	6	0.59	0.024
	Jamaica Hospital, Jamaica	8.6	0.0%	1.27	No	0.50	3	1.17	0.028
	John T. Mather Memorial Hospital, Port Jefferson	2.5	0.0%	1.94	No	0.00	5	1.15	0.017
	Kings County Hospital Center, Brooklyn	10.1	0.0%	1.32	Yes	0.54	7	0.86	0.016
	Kingsbrook Jewish Medical Center, Brooklyn	0.0	0.0%	1.88	No	0.17	5	0.23	0.003
	Kingston Hospital, Kingston	2.4	0.0%	1.60	No	0.14	2	0.85	0.007
	La Guardia Hospital, Flushing	4.3	0.0%	1.37	No	0.28	0	0.78	0.015
	Mercy Hospital, Buffalo	2.7	0.0%	1.44	No	0.12	3	0.48	0.005
	Mercy Medical Center, Rockville Centre	6.1	0.0%	1.22	No	0.01	6	0.77	0.008
	Millard Fillmore Hospitals, Buffalo	6.0	0.0%	1.54	Yes	0.15	4	0.82	0.012
	Mount Vernon Hospital, Mount Vernon	6.7	0.0%	1.21	No	0.30	3	0.93	0.008
	Nassau County Medical Center, East Meadow	9.4	0.0%	1.77	Yes	1.01	7	1.17	0.017
	New Rochelle Hospital Medical Center, New Rochelle	9.3	0.0%	1.09	No	0.20	7	0.89	0.014
	New York Downtown Hospital	10.4	0.0%	1.02	No	0.67	3	1.06	0.005
	New York Hospital Medical Center, Flushing	7.3	0.0%	1.36	Yes	0.27	5	0.52	0.014
	North Shore University Hospital-Glen Cove, Glen Cove	10.7	0.0%	1.10	No	0.09	5	0.66	0.060
	Nyack Hospital, Nyack	6.4	0.0%	1.18	No	0.06	4	0.74	0.012
	Our Lady of Mercy Medical Center, Bronx	9.1	0.0%	1.21	Yes	0.42	5	0.62	0.007
	Rochester General Hospital, Rochester	9.4	0.0%	1.33	Yes	0.22	8	0.96	0.013
	Samaritan Hospital, Troy	8.3	0.0%	1.08	No	0.00	7	0.66	0.015
	Sisters of Charity Hospital, Buffalo	1.2	0.0%	1.70	No	0.07	3	0.60	0.006
	South Nassau Community Hospital, Oceanside	6.8	0.0%	1.17	No	0.07	5	0.85	0.007
	Southside Hospital, Bay Shore	3.4	0.0%	1.51	No	0.13	5	0.60	0.010
	St. Barnabas Hospital, Bronx	6.8	0.0%	1.17	No	0.41	0	0.86	0.013
	St. Charles Hospital and Rehab. Ctr., Port Jefferson	7.4	0.0%	1.15	No	0.04	4	0.90	0.017
	St. Clare's Hospital of Schenectady, Schenectady	5.5	0.0%	1.48	No	0.20	4	1.05	0.023
	St. John's Episcopal Hospital, Far Rockaway	4.8	0.0%	1.27	No	0.24	0	0.74	0.013
	St. John's Episcopal Hospital, Smithtown	2.1	0.0%	1.66	No	0.00	6	0.34	0.017
	St. Joseph's Medical Center, Yonkers	7.2	0.0%	1.19	No	0.26	3	0.79	0.021
	St. Mary's Hospital of Troy, Troy	4.7	0.0%	1.44	No	0.00	3	0.66	0.035
	St. Mary's Hospital, Rochester	7.8	0.3%	1.18	No	0.37	3	0.84	0.013
	St. Peter's Hospital, Albany	7.3	0.0%	1.29	No	0.09	8	0.98	0.016
	St. Vincent's Medical Center, Staten Island	6.4	0.0%	1.37	No	0.46	4	0.92	0.016
	Staten Island University Hospital, Staten Island	7.9	0.0%	1.15	No	0.46	7	0.53	0.006
	United Health Services Hospitals, Binghamton	5.5	0.0%	1.52	Yes	0.20	5	0.61	0.004
	Vassar Brothers Hospital, Poughkeepsie	3.1	0.0%	1.58	No	0.01	7	0.69	0.007
	Westchester County Medical Center, Valhalla	9.3	0.0%	1.82	Yes	0.81	4	1.59	0.025

ORTHOPEDICS

Natl. Rank	Hospital	U.S. News index	Reputational score	Orthopedics mortality rate	COTH member	Interns and residents to beds	Technology score (of 5)	R.N.'s to beds	Board-certified orthopedists to beds	Procedures to beds
	TIER ONE									
2	Hospital for Special Surgery, New York	95.9	36.6%	0.24	Yes	0.68	4	0.78	0.271	17.09
8	Hospital for Joint Diseases-Orthopedic Institute, New York	33.9	7.6%	0.11	Yes	0.27	4	1.26	0.277	9.68
	TIER TWO									
43	Columbia-Presbyterian Medical Center, New York	17.3	3.5%	1.68	Yes	0.85	5	1.05	0.035	1.23
68	Mount Sinai Medical Center, New York	15.1	0.9%	1.02	Yes	0.99	3	1.50	0.021	1.23
27	New York University Medical Center	19.9	1.6%	0.78	Yes	1.30	4	1.15	0.032	1.28
77	North Shore University Hospital, Manhasset	14.7	0.0%	0.78	Yes	0.58	5	1.10	0.031	1.99
62	Strong Memorial Hospital-Rochester University	15.6	1.8%	1.47	Yes	1.00	4	1.45	0.060	1.67
40	University Hosp.-SUNY Health Science Ctr., Syracuse	17.6	0.0%	0.78	Yes	1.30	3	1.61	0.086	2.50
	TIER THREE									
93	Albany Medical Center Hospital, Albany	13.4	0.5%	1.09	Yes	0.76	4	1.33	0.036	1.38
	Beth Israel Medical Center, New York	12.8	0.0%	1.03	Yes	0.65	5	1.27	0.025	1.27
	Brooklyn Hospital Center, Brooklyn	8.7	0.0%	1.28	Yes	0.75	3	0.67	0.020	0.66
	Lenox Hill Hospital, New York	9.8	0.4%	1.33	Yes	0.57	2	1.18	0.026	1.94
	Long Island College Hospital, Brooklyn	8.7	0.0%	1.39	Yes	0.62	2	1.23	0.024	0.85
91	Long Island Jewish Medical Center, New York	13.5	0.0%	1.09	Yes	1.17	4	1.20	0.064	1.08
	Maimonides Medical Center, Brooklyn	10.4	0.0%	1.26	Yes	0.78	4	0.93	0.028	1.28
	Mary Imogene Bassett Hospital, Cooperstown	10.2	0.0%	1.41	Yes	0.22	4	1.69	0.026	2.43
81	Memorial Sloan-Kettering Cancer Center, New York	14.3	0.3%	0.84	Yes	0.38	5	1.37	0.009	0.98
	Montefiore Medical Center, Bronx	10.2	0.0%	1.32	Yes	0.53	4	1.28	0.020	1.42
	St. Luke's-Roosevelt Hospital Center, New York	8.6	0.0%	1.55	Yes	0.69	3	1.07	0.021	0.99
	St. Vincent's Hospital and Medical Center, New York	9.6	0.0%	1.73	Yes	0.88	4	1.08	0.032	1.19
	University Hospital, Stony Brook	12.5	0.0%	1.19	Yes	1.12	4	1.22	0.012	1.04
	Westchester County Medical Center, Valhalla	8.8	0.0%	1.66	Yes	0.81	1	1.59	0.033	0.58
	Winthrop-University Hospital, Mineola	9.2	0.0%	1.16	Yes	0.21	4	0.95	0.025	2.03
	TIER FOUR									
	Arnot Ogden Medical Center, Elmira	3.4	0.0%	2.22	No	0.00	4	1.18	0.027	2.15
	Auburn Memorial Hospital, Auburn	3.0	0.0%	1.35	No	0.00	3	0.52	0.015	2.17
	Brookdale Hospital Medical Center, Brooklyn	8.0	0.0%	1.15	Yes	0.45	2	0.79	0.026	0.31
	Buffalo General Hospital, Buffalo	4.7	0.0%	1.88	Yes	0.04	2	0.96	0.020	1.29
	Cabrini Medical Center, New York	7.4	0.0%	1.49	Yes	0.53	3	0.69	0.043	1.27
	Central General Hospital, Plainview	5.2	0.0%	0.94	No	0.00	2	0.59	0.059	1.85
	Community-General Hospital, Syracuse	6.5	0.0%	0.83	No	0.03	2	0.63	0.028	2.82
	Coney Island Hospital, Brooklyn	5.0	0.0%	1.45	No	0.56	2	1.06	0.007	0.71
	Crouse Irving Memorial Hospital, Syracuse	4.6	0.0%	1.34	No	0.12	2	1.06	0.043	2.59
	Ellis Hospital, Schenectady	4.1	0.0%	1.31	No	0.02	3	0.78	0.023	2.25
	Erie County Medical Center, Buffalo	6.9	0.5%	1.58	Yes	0.20	3	0.72	0.007	0.75
	Flushing Hospital Medical Center, Flushing	5.1	0.0%	1.54	No	0.45	3	1.05	0.011	1.37
	Franklin Hospital Medical Center, Valley Stream	1.5	0.0%	1.91	No	0.04	4	0.29	0.035	1.38
	Genesee Hospital, Rochester	4.9	0.0%	1.76	Yes	0.28	1	0.78	0.028	2.32
	Good Samaritan Hospital, Suffern	2.5	0.0%	1.86	No	0.00	3	0.92	0.016	1.65
	Good Samaritan Hospital, West Islip	3.0	0.0%	1.73	No	0.00	4	0.74	0.036	1.37
	Highland Hospital of Rochester, Rochester	2.7	0.0%	1.98	No	0.51	2	0.54	0.026	2.85
	House of the Good Samaritan, Watertown	5.7	0.0%	1.15	No	0.00	3	1.06	0.030	2.89
	Huntington Hospital, Huntington	3.0	0.0%	1.55	No	0.02	3	0.59	0.051	2.71
	Jamaica Hospital, Jamaica	4.7	0.0%	1.63	No	0.50	2	1.17	0.022	1.05
	John T. Mather Memorial Hospital, Port Jefferson	4.1	0.0%	1.56	No	0.00	3	1.15	0.038	1.95
	Kingsbrook Jewish Medical Center, Brooklyn	0.8	0.0%	1.62	No	0.17	2	0.23	0.010	0.33
	La Guardia Hospital, Flushing	1.1	0.0%	1.85	No	0.28	0	0.78	0.026	1.09
	Lutheran Medical Center, Brooklyn	5.8	0.0%	1.15	No	0.38	3	0.79	0.013	1.27
	Mercy Hospital, Buffalo	1.9	0.0%	1.59	No	0.12	2	0.48	0.019	1.97
	Mercy Medical Center, Rockville Centre	5.6	0.0%	1.03	No	0.01	3	0.77	0.039	2.18
	Millard Fillmore Hospitals, Buffalo	7.2	0.0%	1.52	Yes	0.15	4	0.82	0.020	2.31

Natl. Rank	Hospital	U.S. News index	Reputational score	Orthopedics mortality rate	COTH member	Interns and residents to beds	Technology score (of 5)	R.N.'s to beds	Board-certified orthopedists to beds	Procedures to beds
	Nathan Littauer Hospital, Gloversville	0.0	0.0%	2.06	No	0.00	2	0.37	0.010	1.83
	New Rochelle Hospital Medical Center, New Rochelle	7.0	0.0%	0.96	No	0.20	3	0.89	0.017	2.04
	New York Hospital Medical Center, Flushing	5.2	0.0%	1.54	Yes	0.27	2	0.52	0.026	1.21
	North Shore University Hospital-Glen Cove, Glen Cove	4.8	0.0%	1.18	No	0.09	3	0.66	0.087	1.74
	Northern Westchester Hospital Center, Mount Kisco	7.8	0.0%	0.92	No	0.00	3	1.32	0.023	2.07
	Nyack Hospital, Nyack	5.5	0.0%	0.96	No	0.06	2	0.74	0.032	2.00
	Our Lady of Mercy Medical Center, Bronx	5.3	0.0%	1.76	Yes	0.42	2	0.62	0.027	0.93
	Rochester General Hospital, Rochester	7.7	0.0%	1.54	Yes	0.22	4	0.96	0.021	2.28
	Samaritan Hospital, Troy	3.6	0.0%	1.29	No	0.00	3	0.66	0.026	1.69
	Saratoga Hospital, Saratoga Springs	4.8	0.0%	1.04	No	0.00	2	0.86	0.022	1.51
	Sisters of Charity Hospital, Buffalo	1.7	0.0%	1.63	No	0.07	2	0.60	0.010	1.37
	South Nassau Community Hospital, Oceanside	4.7	0.0%	1.27	No	0.07	3	0.85	0.058	2.12
	Southampton Hospital, Southampton	2.6	0.0%	1.59	No	0.00	4	0.44	0.010	2.01
	Southside Hospital, Bay Shore	1.0	0.0%	2.10	No	0.13	2	0.60	0.030	1.15
	St. Charles Hospital and Rehab. Ctr., Port Jefferson	3.5	0.0%	1.61	No	0.04	3	0.90	0.044	2.03
	St. Clare's Hospital of Schenectady, Schenectady	3.7	0.0%	1.99	No	0.20	3	1.05	0.050	2.53
	St. Elizabeth Hospital, Utica	6.0	0.0%	1.05	No	0.20	3	0.82	0.014	1.61
	St. John's Episcopal Hospital, Smithtown	1.4	0.0%	1.65	No	0.00	3	0.34	0.040	0.96
	St. Joseph's Medical Center, Yonkers	4.1	0.0%	1.31	No	0.26	2	0.79	0.021	1.66
	St. Mary's Hospital of Troy, Troy	3.8	0.0%	1.20	No	0.00	2	0.66	0.030	2.95
	St. Mary's Hospital, Rochester	4.7	0.0%	1.27	No	0.37	2	0.84	0.018	1.48
	St. Peter's Hospital, Albany	7.2	0.0%	1.07	No	0.09	4	0.98	0.051	3.17
	St. Vincent's Medical Center, Staten Island	4.0	0.0%	1.79	No	0.46	3	0.92	0.009	1.04
	Staten Island University Hospital, Staten Island	4.1	0.0%	1.45	No	0.46	3	0.53	0.013	1.54
	United Health Services Hospitals, Binghamton	6.9	0.0%	1.35	Yes	0.20	3	0.61	0.030	2.49
	Vassar Brothers Hospital, Poughkeepsie	1.8	0.0%	2.35	No	0.01	4	0.69	0.027	1.75

OTOLARYNGOLOGY

Natl. Rank	Hospital	U.S. News index	Reputational score	Hospital-wide mortality rate	COTH member	Interns and residents to beds	Technology score (of 9)	R.N.'s to beds	Board-certified internists to beds	Procedures to beds
TIER ONE										
13	Mount Sinai Medical Center, New York	37.5	6.8%	1.09	Yes	0.99	7	1.50	0.253	0.216
15	New York University Medical Center	33.2	5.1%	0.98	Yes	1.30	7	1.15	0.360	0.271
21	Manhattan Eye, Ear and Throat Hospital, New York	24.6	5.4%	0.01	No	0.86	1	0.53	0.181	1.833
TIER TWO										
83	Albany Medical Center Hospital, Albany	14.5	0.5%	1.12	Yes	0.76	7	1.33	0.103	0.226
38	Columbia-Presbyterian Medical Center, New York	19.7	2.2%	1.25	Yes	0.85	8	1.05	0.111	0.130
86	Long Island Jewish Medical Center, New York	14.4	0.0%	1.34	Yes	1.17	8	1.20	0.097	0.345
61	Memorial Sloan-Kettering Cancer Center, New York	16.2	1.4%	0.91	Yes	0.38	7	1.37	0.074	0.568
65	Montefiore Medical Center, Bronx	15.9	1.2%	1.19	Yes	0.53	8	1.28	0.095	0.223
50	New York Eye and Ear Infirmary	18.1	3.3%	0.38	No	0.64	2	0.84	0.194	1.039
70	New York Hospital-Cornell Medical Center	15.3	1.0%	1.07	Yes	0.79	7	1.00	0.113	0.095
95	North Shore University Hospital, Manhasset	13.8	0.0%	1.12	Yes	0.58	8	1.10	0.327	0.148
91	Roswell Park Cancer Institute, Buffalo	14.1	0.0%	0.56	No	0.68	8	2.58	0.109	0.438
55	St. Vincent's Hospital and Medical Center, New York	17.3	1.0%	1.36	Yes	0.88	8	1.08	0.255	0.204
78	Strong Memorial Hospital-Rochester University	14.6	0.0%	1.26	Yes	1.00	8	1.45	0.111	0.209
41	University Hosp.-SUNY Health Science Ctr., Syracuse	19.4	0.9%	1.28	Yes	1.30	7	1.61	0.160	0.550
93	University Hospital, Stony Brook	14.1	0.0%	1.31	Yes	1.12	7	1.22	0.108	0.299
TIER THREE										
	Bellevue Hospital Center, New York	9.2	0.0%	1.10	Yes	0.34	3	0.89	0.137	0.076
	Beth Israel Medical Center, New York	12.6	0.0%	1.09	Yes	0.65	8	1.27	0.085	0.245
	Bronx Municipal Hospital Center, Bronx	11.3	0.0%	1.59	Yes	1.07	1	1.07	0.072	0.139
	Bronx-Lebanon Hospital Center, Bronx	11.2	0.0%	1.37	Yes	0.79	5	1.00	0.075	0.042
	Brookdale Hospital Medical Center, Brooklyn	9.2	0.0%	1.59	Yes	0.45	5	0.79	0.085	0.053

Natl. Rank Hospital	U.S. News index	Reputational score	Hospital-wide mortality rate	COTH member	Interns and residents to beds	Technology score (of 9)	R.N.'s to beds	Board-certified internists to beds	Procedures to beds
Brooklyn Hospital Center, Brooklyn	10.9	0.0%	1.32	Yes	0.75	7	0.67	0.107	0.145
Buffalo General Hospital, Buffalo	8.6	0.0%	1.54	Yes	0.04	5	0.96	0.133	0.149
Cabrini Medical Center, New York	10.0	0.0%	1.20	Yes	0.53	6	0.69	0.120	0.144
Catholic Medical Center, Jamaica	9.8	0.0%	1.53	Yes	0.29	5	0.80	0.220	0.128
Elmhurst Hospital Center, Elmhurst	9.7	0.0%	1.56	Yes	0.60	3	1.02	0.050	0.048
Erie County Medical Center, Buffalo	7.0	0.0%	1.54	Yes	0.20	2	0.72	0.068	0.058
Flushing Hospital Medical Center, Flushing	7.0	0.0%	1.37	No	0.45	6	1.05	0.056	0.134
Genesee Hospital, Rochester	9.1	0.0%	1.35	Yes	0.28	5	0.78	0.146	0.233
Harlem Hospital Center, New York	10.5	0.0%	2.26	Yes	0.83	5	0.91	0.041	0.065
Hospital for Joint Diseases-Orthopedic Institute, New York	11.1	0.0%	0.10	Yes	0.27	3	1.26	0.227	0.009
Hospital for Special Surgery, New York	11.0	0.5%	0.36	Yes	0.68	3	0.78	0.000	0.021
Kings County Hospital Center, Brooklyn	10.3	0.0%	1.61	Yes	0.54	7	0.86	0.076	0.045
Lenox Hill Hospital, New York	12.2	0.4%	1.25	Yes	0.57	4	1.18	0.104	0.254
Lincoln Medical and Mental Health Center, Bronx	10.1	0.0%	1.19	No	1.07	5	1.36	0.045	0.060
Long Island College Hospital, Brooklyn	12.3	0.0%	1.20	Yes	0.62	6	1.23	0.156	0.167
Maimonides Medical Center, Brooklyn	12.7	0.5%	1.21	Yes	0.78	5	0.93	0.070	0.091
Mary Imogene Bassett Hospital, Cooperstown	11.8	0.0%	1.03	Yes	0.22	7	1.69	0.066	0.456
Methodist Hospital, Brooklyn	12.1	0.0%	0.94	Yes	0.57	8	0.77	0.229	0.147
Metropolitan Hospital Center, New York	10.6	0.0%	1.64	Yes	0.97	3	0.84	0.059	0.059
Millard Fillmore Hospitals, Buffalo	7.2	0.0%	1.45	Yes	0.15	3	0.82	0.031	0.279
Nassau County Medical Center, East Meadow	13.4	0.0%	1.69	Yes	1.01	7	1.17	0.121	0.093
New York Hospital Medical Center, Flushing	7.7	0.0%	1.43	Yes	0.27	5	0.52	0.084	0.206
North Shore University Hospital-Glen Cove, Glen Cove	7.7	0.0%	1.29	No	0.09	4	0.66	0.506	0.140
Northern Westchester Hospital Center, Mount Kisco	7.2	0.0%	1.05	No	0.00	6	1.32	0.170	0.239
Our Lady of Mercy Medical Center, Bronx	9.0	0.0%	1.44	Yes	0.42	4	0.62	0.158	0.177
Rochester General Hospital, Rochester	10.3	0.0%	1.26	Yes	0.22	8	0.96	0.135	0.283
St. Luke's-Roosevelt Hospital Center, New York	10.8	0.0%	1.29	Yes	0.69	2	1.07	0.142	0.135
United Health Services Hospitals, Binghamton	7.0	0.0%	1.25	Yes	0.20	3	0.61	0.050	0.458
University Hospital of Brooklyn-SUNY Center, Brooklyn	12.5	0.0%	1.48	Yes	0.70	8	1.12	0.128	0.098
Westchester County Medical Center, Valhalla	12.8	0.0%	1.50	Yes	0.81	5	1.59	0.052	0.113
Winthrop-University Hospital, Mineola	9.5	0.0%	1.23	Yes	0.21	7	0.95	0.085	0.161
TIER FOUR									
Arnot Ogden Medical Center, Elmira	6.5	0.0%	1.40	No	0.00	8	1.18	0.093	0.162
Auburn Memorial Hospital, Auburn	2.7	0.0%	1.40	No	0.00	3	0.52	0.044	0.495
Bayley Seton Hospital, Staten Island	3.7	0.0%	1.29	No	0.06	1	0.78	0.106	0.111
Benedictine Hospital, Kingston	3.1	0.0%	1.29	No	0.08	2	0.59	0.068	0.176
Central General Hospital, Plainview	5.0	0.0%	1.10	No	0.00	4	0.59	0.246	0.347
Community-General Hospital, Syracuse	2.9	0.0%	1.16	No	0.03	1	0.63	0.065	0.216
Coney Island Hospital, Brooklyn	6.1	0.0%	1.46	No	0.56	1	1.06	0.070	0.200
Crouse Irving Memorial Hospital, Syracuse	4.4	0.0%	1.33	No	0.12	1	1.06	0.061	0.285
Ellis Hospital, Schenectady	4.1	0.0%	1.23	No	0.02	5	0.78	0.042	0.224
Franklin Hospital Medical Center, Valley Stream	3.2	0.0%	1.62	No	0.04	7	0.29	0.052	0.188
Goldwater Memorial Hospital, New York	0.6	0.0%	4.86	No	0.01	1	0.25	0.018	0.006
Good Samaritan Hospital, Suffern	4.9	0.0%	1.24	No	0.00	7	0.92	0.022	0.214
Good Samaritan Hospital, West Islip	4.7	0.0%	1.57	No	0.00	8	0.74	0.055	0.190
Highland Hospital of Rochester, Rochester	6.7	0.0%	1.35	No	0.51	6	0.54	0.184	0.143
House of the Good Samaritan, Watertown	5.1	0.0%	1.35	No	0.00	6	1.06	0.034	0.333
Huntington Hospital, Huntington	4.1	0.0%	1.12	No	0.02	6	0.59	0.065	0.188
Interfaith Medical Center, Brooklyn	5.5	0.0%	1.73	No	0.53	5	0.73	0.010	0.036
Jamaica Hospital, Jamaica	6.2	0.0%	1.37	No	0.50	1	1.17	0.066	0.091
John T. Mather Memorial Hospital, Port Jefferson	5.2	0.0%	1.57	No	0.00	5	1.15	0.059	0.370
Kingsbrook Jewish Medical Center, Brooklyn	2.3	0.0%	1.56	No	0.17	4	0.23	0.012	0.031
Kingston Hospital, Kingston	3.8	0.0%	1.41	No	0.14	1	0.85	0.057	0.407
La Guardia Hospital, Flushing	4.4	0.0%	1.58	No	0.28	0	0.78	0.132	0.173
Lutheran Medical Center, Brooklyn	6.1	0.0%	1.21	No	0.38	6	0.79	0.073	0.092
Mercy Hospital, Buffalo	2.5	0.0%	1.34	No	0.12	1	0.48	0.045	0.331

Natl. Rank	Hospital	U.S. News index	Reputa-tional score	Hospital-wide mortality rate	COTH member	Interns and residents to beds	Tech-nology score (of 9)	R.N.'s to beds	Board-certified internists to beds	Procedures to beds
	Mercy Medical Center, Rockville Centre	4.9	0.0%	1.22	No	0.01	6	0.77	0.101	0.305
	Monroe Community Hospital, Rochester	1.4	0.0%	2.32	No	0.10	0	0.26	0.073	0.010
	Mount Vernon Hospital, Mount Vernon	5.1	0.0%	1.12	No	0.30	1	0.93	0.090	0.302
	Nathan Littauer Hospital, Gloversville	1.5	0.0%	1.37	No	0.00	1	0.37	0.024	0.207
	New Rochelle Hospital Medical Center, New Rochelle	6.1	0.0%	1.14	No	0.20	7	0.89	0.073	0.263
	New York Downtown Hospital	6.6	0.0%	1.26	No	0.67	3	1.06	0.000	0.182
	North Central Bronx Hospital, Bronx	6.7	0.0%	1.28	No	0.71	1	1.07	0.056	0.048
	North General Hospital, New York	4.8	0.0%	1.30	No	0.23	2	0.95	0.070	0.112
	Nyack Hospital, Nyack	3.9	0.0%	1.14	No	0.06	3	0.74	0.067	0.358
	Queens Hospital Center, Jamaica	6.4	0.0%	1.25	No	0.60	2	1.09	0.033	0.073
	Samaritan Hospital, Troy	4.3	0.0%	1.24	No	0.00	7	0.66	0.044	0.250
	Saratoga Hospital, Saratoga Springs	3.1	0.0%	1.22	No	0.00	1	0.86	0.027	0.211
	Sisters of Charity Hospital, Buffalo	3.8	0.0%	1.47	No	0.07	3	0.60	0.120	0.227
	South Nassau Community Hospital, Oceanside	5.5	0.0%	1.22	No	0.07	5	0.85	0.147	0.200
	Southampton Hospital, Southampton	3.5	0.0%	1.39	No	0.00	7	0.44	0.036	0.366
	Southside Hospital, Bay Shore	3.6	0.0%	1.75	No	0.13	5	0.60	0.017	0.422
	St. Barnabas Hospital, Bronx	4.7	0.0%	1.47	No	0.41	0	0.86	0.072	0.207
	St. Charles Hospital and Rehab. Ctr., Port Jefferson	6.1	0.0%	1.39	No	0.04	2	0.90	0.332	0.197
	St. Clare's Hospital of Schenectady, Schenectady	5.4	0.0%	1.40	No	0.20	2	1.05	0.122	0.312
	St. Elizabeth Hospital, Utica	4.5	0.0%	1.13	No	0.20	4	0.82	0.009	0.212
	St. John's Episcopal Hospital, Far Rockaway	3.5	0.0%	1.66	No	0.24	0	0.74	0.068	0.113
	St. John's Episcopal Hospital, Smithtown	3.2	0.0%	1.70	No	0.00	6	0.34	0.087	0.123
	St. Joseph's Medical Center, Yonkers	4.0	0.0%	1.24	No	0.26	1	0.79	0.046	0.149
	St. Mary's Hospital of Troy, Troy	2.7	0.0%	1.38	No	0.00	1	0.66	0.060	0.313
	St. Mary's Hospital, Rochester	5.4	0.0%	1.30	No	0.37	2	0.84	0.110	0.172
	St. Peter's Hospital, Albany	5.9	0.0%	1.15	No	0.09	7	0.98	0.065	0.324
	St. Vincent's Medical Center, Staten Island	5.9	0.0%	1.42	No	0.46	3	0.92	0.075	0.145
	Staten Island University Hospital, Staten Island	5.9	0.0%	1.26	No	0.46	7	0.53	0.071	0.204
	Vassar Brothers Hospital, Poughkeepsie	4.9	0.0%	1.50	No	0.01	7	0.69	0.120	0.400

RHEUMATOLOGY

Natl. Rank	Hospital	U.S. News index	Reputa-tional score	Hospital-wide mortality rate	COTH member	Interns and residents to beds	Tech-nology score (of 5)	R.N.'s to beds	Board-certified internists to beds
	TIER ONE								
5	Hospital for Special Surgery, New York	53.3	17.4%	0.36	Yes	0.68	4	0.78	0.000
9	New York University Medical Center	36.0	7.7%	0.98	Yes	1.30	4	1.15	0.360
22	Hospital for Joint Diseases-Orthopedic Institute, New York	24.2	3.6%	0.10	Yes	0.27	4	1.26	0.227
25	Mount Sinai Medical Center, New York	22.3	2.6%	1.09	Yes	0.99	3	1.50	0.253
	TIER TWO								
83	Albany Medical Center Hospital, Albany	16.1	0.7%	1.12	Yes	0.76	4	1.33	0.103
67	Columbia-Presbyterian Medical Center, New York	16.8	1.4%	1.25	Yes	0.85	5	1.05	0.111
68	Long Island Jewish Medical Center, New York	16.7	1.2%	1.34	Yes	1.17	4	1.20	0.097
75	Memorial Sloan-Kettering Cancer Center, New York	16.5	0.4%	0.91	Yes	0.38	5	1.37	0.074
80	Montefiore Medical Center, Bronx	16.2	1.4%	1.19	Yes	0.53	4	1.28	0.095
63	New York Hospital-Cornell Medical Center	17.0	1.4%	1.07	Yes	0.79	4	1.00	0.113
66	Strong Memorial Hospital-Rochester University	16.9	1.0%	1.26	Yes	1.00	4	1.45	0.111
73	University Hosp.-SUNY Health Science Ctr., Syracuse	16.5	0.3%	1.28	Yes	1.30	3	1.61	0.160
	TIER THREE								
	Bellevue Hospital Center, New York	11.4	0.0%	1.10	Yes	0.34	2	0.89	0.137
91	Beth Israel Medical Center, New York	15.4	0.4%	1.09	Yes	0.65	5	1.27	0.085
	Bronx Municipal Hospital Center, Bronx	12.1	0.7%	1.59	Yes	1.07	1	1.07	0.072
	Bronx-Lebanon Hospital Center, Bronx	11.5	0.0%	1.37	Yes	0.79	3	1.00	0.075
	Brooklyn Hospital Center, Brooklyn	10.9	0.0%	1.32	Yes	0.75	3	0.67	0.107
	Cabrini Medical Center, New York	11.0	0.0%	1.20	Yes	0.53	3	0.69	0.120

Natl. Rank	Hospital	U.S. News index	Reputa-tional score	Hospital-wide mortality rate	COTH member	Interns and residents to beds	Tech-nology score (of 5)	R.N.'s to beds	Board-certified internists to beds
	Lenox Hill Hospital, New York	11.6	0.0%	1.25	Yes	0.57	2	1.18	0.104
	Long Island College Hospital, Brooklyn	12.6	0.0%	1.20	Yes	0.62	2	1.23	0.156
	Maimonides Medical Center, Brooklyn	12.5	0.0%	1.21	Yes	0.78	4	0.93	0.070
	Mary Imogene Bassett Hospital, Cooperstown	14.0	0.0%	1.03	Yes	0.22	4	1.69	0.066
	Methodist Hospital, Brooklyn	14.8	0.0%	0.94	Yes	0.57	4	0.77	0.229
	Nassau County Medical Center, East Meadow	12.1	0.0%	1.69	Yes	1.01	4	1.17	0.121
	New York Eye and Ear Infirmary	11.7	0.0%	0.38	No	0.64	2	0.84	0.194
92	North Shore University Hospital, Manhasset	15.3	0.0%	1.12	Yes	0.58	5	1.10	0.327
	Northern Westchester Hospital Center, Mount Kisco	10.1	0.0%	1.05	No	0.00	3	1.32	0.170
	Rochester General Hospital, Rochester	11.0	0.0%	1.26	Yes	0.22	4	0.96	0.135
	St. Luke's-Roosevelt Hospital Center, New York	12.2	0.0%	1.29	Yes	0.69	3	1.07	0.142
	St. Vincent's Hospital and Medical Center, New York	14.8	0.4%	1.36	Yes	0.88	4	1.08	0.255
	University Hospital of Brooklyn-SUNY Center, Brooklyn	11.8	0.0%	1.48	Yes	0.70	4	1.12	0.128
	University Hospital, Stony Brook	14.1	0.0%	1.31	Yes	1.12	4	1.22	0.108
	Westchester County Medical Center, Valhalla	11.4	0.0%	1.50	Yes	0.81	1	1.59	0.052
	Winthrop-University Hospital, Mineola	10.8	0.0%	1.23	Yes	0.21	4	0.95	0.085
TIER FOUR									
	Arnot Ogden Medical Center, Elmira	7.3	0.0%	1.40	No	0.00	4	1.18	0.093
	Auburn Memorial Hospital, Auburn	4.8	0.0%	1.40	No	0.00	3	0.52	0.044
	Benedictine Hospital, Kingston	5.5	0.0%	1.29	No	0.08	2	0.59	0.068
	Brookdale Hospital Medical Center, Brooklyn	8.5	0.0%	1.59	Yes	0.45	2	0.79	0.085
	Buffalo General Hospital, Buffalo	8.9	0.3%	1.54	Yes	0.04	2	0.96	0.133
	Catholic Medical Center, Jamaica	9.2	0.0%	1.53	Yes	0.29	2	0.80	0.220
	Central General Hospital, Plainview	7.8	0.0%	1.10	No	0.00	2	0.59	0.246
	Community-General Hospital, Syracuse	5.3	0.0%	1.16	No	0.03	2	0.63	0.065
	Coney Island Hospital, Brooklyn	7.5	0.0%	1.46	No	0.56	2	1.06	0.070
	Crouse Irving Memorial Hospital, Syracuse	5.6	0.0%	1.33	No	0.12	2	1.06	0.061
	Ellis Hospital, Schenectady	6.4	0.0%	1.23	No	0.02	3	0.78	0.042
	Erie County Medical Center, Buffalo	8.0	0.0%	1.54	Yes	0.20	3	0.72	0.068
	Flushing Hospital Medical Center, Flushing	7.9	0.0%	1.37	No	0.45	3	1.05	0.056
	Franklin Hospital Medical Center, Valley Stream	3.9	0.0%	1.62	No	0.04	4	0.29	0.052
	Genesee Hospital, Rochester	8.9	0.0%	1.35	Yes	0.28	1	0.78	0.146
	Good Samaritan Hospital, Suffern	6.5	0.0%	1.24	No	0.00	3	0.92	0.022
	Good Samaritan Hospital, West Islip	5.2	0.0%	1.57	No	0.00	4	0.74	0.055
	Harlem Hospital Center, New York	8.0	0.0%	2.26	Yes	0.83	2	0.91	0.041
	Highland Hospital of Rochester, Rochester	7.3	0.0%	1.35	No	0.51	2	0.54	0.184
	House of the Good Samaritan, Watertown	6.4	0.0%	1.35	No	0.00	3	1.06	0.034
	Huntington Hospital, Huntington	5.8	0.0%	1.12	No	0.02	3	0.59	0.065
	Jamaica Hospital, Jamaica	6.9	0.0%	1.37	No	0.50	2	1.17	0.066
	John T. Mather Memorial Hospital, Port Jefferson	5.9	0.0%	1.57	No	0.00	3	1.15	0.059
	Kingsbrook Jewish Medical Center, Brooklyn	3.2	0.0%	1.56	No	0.17	2	0.23	0.012
	Kingston Hospital, Kingston	4.2	0.0%	1.41	No	0.14	1	0.85	0.057
	La Guardia Hospital, Flushing	4.9	0.0%	1.58	No	0.28	0	0.78	0.132
	Lutheran Medical Center, Brooklyn	8.0	0.0%	1.21	No	0.38	3	0.79	0.073
	Mercy Hospital, Buffalo	4.9	0.0%	1.34	No	0.12	2	0.48	0.045
	Mercy Medical Center, Rockville Centre	6.9	0.0%	1.22	No	0.01	3	0.77	0.101
	Millard Fillmore Hospitals, Buffalo	9.4	0.3%	1.45	Yes	0.15	4	0.82	0.031
	Mount Vernon Hospital, Mount Vernon	8.4	0.0%	1.12	No	0.30	2	0.93	0.090
	New Rochelle Hospital Medical Center, New Rochelle	8.1	0.0%	1.14	No	0.20	3	0.89	0.073
	New York Downtown Hospital	8.3	0.0%	1.26	No	0.67	2	1.06	0.000
	New York Hospital Medical Center, Flushing	7.8	0.0%	1.43	Yes	0.27	2	0.52	0.084
	North Shore University Hospital-Glen Cove, Glen Cove	9.4	0.0%	1.29	No	0.09	3	0.66	0.506
	Nyack Hospital, Nyack	5.8	0.0%	1.14	No	0.06	2	0.74	0.067
	Our Lady of Mercy Medical Center, Bronx	8.1	0.0%	1.44	Yes	0.42	2	0.62	0.158
	Samaritan Hospital, Troy	6.0	0.0%	1.24	No	0.00	3	0.66	0.044
	Saratoga Hospital, Saratoga Springs	6.1	0.0%	1.22	No	0.00	2	0.86	0.027

Natl. Rank	Hospital	U.S. News index	Reputational score	Hospital-wide mortality rate	COTH member	Interns and residents to beds	Technology score (of 5)	R.N.'s to beds	Board-certified internists to beds
	Sisters of Charity Hospital, Buffalo	5.0	0.0%	1.47	No	0.07	2	0.60	0.120
	South Nassau Community Hospital, Oceanside	6.6	0.0%	1.22	No	0.07	3	0.85	0.147
	Southampton Hospital, Southampton	4.0	0.0%	1.39	No	0.00	4	0.44	0.036
	Southside Hospital, Bay Shore	2.4	0.0%	1.75	No	0.13	2	0.60	0.017
	St. Barnabas Hospital, Bronx	3.5	0.0%	1.47	No	0.41	0	0.86	0.072
	St. Charles Hospital and Rehab. Ctr., Port Jefferson	8.1	0.0%	1.39	No	0.04	3	0.90	0.332
	St. Clare's Hospital of Schenectady, Schenectady	7.4	0.0%	1.40	No	0.20	3	1.05	0.122
	St. Elizabeth Hospital, Utica	7.5	0.0%	1.13	No	0.20	3	0.82	0.009
	St. John's Episcopal Hospital, Far Rockaway	1.9	0.0%	1.66	No	0.24	0	0.74	0.068
	St. John's Episcopal Hospital, Smithtown	3.5	0.0%	1.70	No	0.00	3	0.34	0.087
	St. Joseph's Medical Center, Yonkers	6.7	0.0%	1.24	No	0.26	2	0.79	0.046
	St. Mary's Hospital of Troy, Troy	4.9	0.0%	1.38	No	0.00	2	0.66	0.060
	St. Mary's Hospital, Rochester	7.4	0.0%	1.30	No	0.37	2	0.84	0.110
	St. Peter's Hospital, Albany	8.3	0.0%	1.15	No	0.09	4	0.98	0.065
	St. Vincent's Medical Center, Staten Island	7.5	0.0%	1.42	No	0.46	3	0.92	0.075
	Staten Island University Hospital, Staten Island	7.2	0.0%	1.26	No	0.46	3	0.53	0.071
	United Health Services Hospitals, Binghamton	9.0	0.0%	1.25	Yes	0.20	3	0.61	0.050
	Vassar Brothers Hospital, Poughkeepsie	5.9	0.0%	1.50	No	0.01	4	0.69	0.120

UROLOGY

Natl. Rank	Hospital	U.S. News index	Reputational score	Urology mortality rate	COTH member	Interns and residents to beds	Technology score (of 11)	R.N.'s to beds	Board-certified internists to beds	Procedures to beds
	TIER ONE									
10	Memorial Sloan-Kettering Cancer Center, New York	34.8	16.0%	0.98	Yes	0.38	8	1.37	0.074	2.26
12	New York Hospital-Cornell Medical Center	28.6	10.3%	0.90	Yes	0.79	9	1.00	0.113	1.43
20	Columbia-Presbyterian Medical Center, New York	23.9	7.4%	1.07	Yes	0.85	10	1.05	0.111	1.45
	TIER TWO									
72	Albany Medical Center Hospital, Albany	16.3	0.7%	0.91	Yes	0.76	8	1.33	0.103	1.64
80	Mount Sinai Medical Center, New York	15.9	2.1%	1.49	Yes	0.99	9	1.50	0.253	1.30
49	New York University Medical Center	18.4	2.5%	1.17	Yes	1.30	8	1.15	0.360	1.93
37	Roswell Park Cancer Institute, Buffalo	19.3	0.5%	0.26	No	0.68	9	2.58	0.109	2.05
87	University Hosp.-SUNY Health Science Ctr., Syracuse	15.2	0.8%	1.61	Yes	1.30	9	1.61	0.160	1.63
	TIER THREE									
	Bellevue Hospital Center, New York	11.1	2.1%	1.43	Yes	0.34	5	0.89	0.137	0.28
	Beth Israel Medical Center, New York	11.3	0.0%	1.44	Yes	0.65	9	1.27	0.085	1.62
	Brooklyn Hospital Center, Brooklyn	11.4	0.0%	1.17	Yes	0.75	8	0.67	0.107	1.35
	Cabrini Medical Center, New York	11.8	0.6%	1.18	Yes	0.53	7	0.69	0.120	2.71
	Crouse Irving Memorial Hospital, Syracuse	8.6	0.0%	0.87	No	0.12	2	1.06	0.061	1.44
	Genesee Hospital, Rochester	8.6	0.0%	1.38	Yes	0.28	6	0.78	0.146	1.13
	Huntington Hospital, Huntington	9.8	0.0%	0.77	No	0.02	7	0.59	0.065	1.70
	Lenox Hill Hospital, New York	9.6	0.0%	1.49	Yes	0.57	5	1.18	0.104	1.19
	Lincoln Medical and Mental Health Center, Bronx	10.9	0.0%	1.11	No	1.07	6	1.36	0.045	0.50
	Long Island College Hospital, Brooklyn	12.7	0.0%	1.19	Yes	0.62	8	1.23	0.156	1.80
	Long Island Jewish Medical Center, New York	13.2	0.0%	1.44	Yes	1.17	10	1.20	0.097	1.65
	Maimonides Medical Center, Brooklyn	10.8	0.0%	1.30	Yes	0.78	6	0.93	0.070	2.10
	Mary Imogene Bassett Hospital, Cooperstown	12.2	0.0%	1.17	Yes	0.22	8	1.69	0.066	2.03
	Methodist Hospital, Brooklyn	13.4	0.0%	0.98	Yes	0.57	9	0.77	0.229	1.91
	Metropolitan Hospital Center, New York	8.9	0.0%	1.64	Yes	0.97	5	0.84	0.059	0.44
	Montefiore Medical Center, Bronx	11.5	0.0%	1.43	Yes	0.53	10	1.28	0.095	2.29
	Nassau County Medical Center, East Meadow	11.7	0.0%	1.51	Yes	1.01	8	1.17	0.121	0.60
	North Shore University Hospital, Manhasset	14.2	0.0%	0.99	Yes	0.58	10	1.10	0.327	1.46
	Rochester General Hospital, Rochester	10.3	0.6%	1.43	Yes	0.22	9	0.96	0.135	1.70
	St. Luke's-Roosevelt Hospital Center, New York	9.7	0.0%	1.46	Yes	0.69	4	1.07	0.142	1.01
	St. Vincent's Hospital and Medical Center, New York	12.2	0.0%	1.36	Yes	0.88	9	1.08	0.255	0.88

Natl. Rank	Hospital	U.S. News index	Reputational score	Urology mortality rate	COTH member	Interns and residents to beds	Technology score (of 11)	R.N.'s to beds	Board-certified internists to beds	Procedures to beds
	Strong Memorial Hospital-Rochester University	13.8	0.0%	1.37	Yes	1.00	10	1.45	0.111	1.76
	University Hospital of Brooklyn-SUNY Center, Brooklyn	11.3	0.0%	1.50	Yes	0.70	10	1.12	0.128	1.17
92	University Hospital, Stony Brook	14.9	0.0%	1.09	Yes	1.12	9	1.22	0.108	1.33
	Westchester County Medical Center, Valhalla	10.5	0.0%	1.63	Yes	0.81	5	1.59	0.052	1.25
TIER FOUR										
	Arnot Ogden Medical Center, Elmira	5.9	0.0%	1.53	No	0.00	9	1.18	0.093	1.19
	Auburn Memorial Hospital, Auburn	2.4	0.0%	1.60	No	0.00	4	0.52	0.044	1.44
	Bronx Municipal Hospital Center, Bronx	6.7	0.0%	2.74	Yes	1.07	1	1.07	0.072	0.61
	Bronx-Lebanon Hospital Center, Bronx	7.9	0.0%	2.11	Yes	0.79	6	1.00	0.075	0.57
	Brookdale Hospital Medical Center, Brooklyn	6.4	0.0%	2.10	Yes	0.45	6	0.79	0.085	0.96
	Buffalo General Hospital, Buffalo	7.3	0.0%	1.68	Yes	0.04	7	0.96	0.133	1.54
	Catholic Medical Center, Jamaica	6.6	0.0%	2.11	Yes	0.29	6	0.80	0.220	1.59
	Central General Hospital, Plainview	3.9	0.0%	1.59	No	0.00	5	0.59	0.246	2.53
	Community-General Hospital, Syracuse	3.3	0.0%	1.46	No	0.03	3	0.63	0.065	1.84
	Coney Island Hospital, Brooklyn	3.8	0.0%	2.16	No	0.56	3	1.06	0.070	0.59
	Ellis Hospital, Schenectady	5.9	0.0%	1.17	No	0.02	7	0.78	0.042	1.27
	Erie County Medical Center, Buffalo	6.0	0.0%	1.62	Yes	0.20	4	0.72	0.068	0.83
	Flushing Hospital Medical Center, Flushing	6.2	0.0%	1.62	No	0.45	7	1.05	0.056	1.94
	Franklin Hospital Medical Center, Valley Stream	1.0	0.0%	2.69	No	0.04	9	0.29	0.052	1.58
	Good Samaritan Hospital, Suffern	7.5	0.0%	1.02	No	0.00	8	0.92	0.022	1.35
	Good Samaritan Hospital, West Islip	6.5	0.0%	1.16	No	0.00	9	0.74	0.055	1.49
	Highland Hospital of Rochester, Rochester	5.8	0.0%	1.55	No	0.51	7	0.54	0.184	1.40
	House of the Good Samaritan, Watertown	5.6	0.0%	1.38	No	0.00	7	1.06	0.034	2.29
	Jamaica Hospital, Jamaica	3.9	0.0%	2.21	No	0.50	3	1.17	0.066	1.00
	John T. Mather Memorial Hospital, Port Jefferson	2.8	0.0%	2.43	No	0.00	6	1.15	0.059	1.99
	Kingsbrook Jewish Medical Center, Brooklyn	2.1	0.0%	1.68	No	0.17	6	0.23	0.012	0.99
	Kingston Hospital, Kingston	3.9	0.0%	1.61	No	0.14	2	0.85	0.057	3.86
	La Guardia Hospital, Flushing	3.0	0.0%	1.82	No	0.28	0	0.78	0.132	2.04
	Lutheran Medical Center, Brooklyn	5.9	0.0%	1.45	No	0.38	7	0.79	0.073	1.33
	Mercy Hospital, Buffalo	3.7	0.0%	1.34	No	0.12	3	0.48	0.045	1.73
	Mercy Medical Center, Rockville Centre	5.8	0.0%	1.33	No	0.01	8	0.77	0.101	1.80
	Millard Fillmore Hospitals, Buffalo	4.8	0.0%	2.08	Yes	0.15	4	0.82	0.031	1.44
	Mount Vernon Hospital, Mount Vernon	7.0	0.0%	1.11	No	0.30	3	0.93	0.090	1.50
	Nathan Littauer Hospital, Gloversville	1.2	0.0%	1.69	No	0.00	3	0.37	0.024	1.25
	New Rochelle Hospital Medical Center, New Rochelle	8.5	0.0%	1.08	No	0.20	8	0.89	0.073	3.01
	New York Downtown Hospital	5.9	0.0%	1.64	No	0.67	4	1.06	0.000	2.54
	New York Hospital Medical Center, Flushing	8.2	0.7%	1.46	Yes	0.27	6	0.52	0.084	1.85
	North Shore University Hospital-Glen Cove, Glen Cove	3.2	0.0%	2.04	No	0.09	6	0.66	0.506	1.85
	Northern Westchester Hospital Center, Mount Kisco	6.0	0.0%	1.75	No	0.00	8	1.32	0.170	2.33
	Nyack Hospital, Nyack	5.4	0.0%	1.23	No	0.06	5	0.74	0.067	1.84
	Our Lady of Mercy Medical Center, Bronx	7.1	0.0%	1.74	Yes	0.42	5	0.62	0.158	1.18
	Samaritan Hospital, Troy	3.2	0.0%	1.79	No	0.00	8	0.66	0.044	1.58
	Sisters of Charity Hospital, Buffalo	3.2	0.0%	1.60	No	0.07	4	0.60	0.120	0.87
	South Nassau Community Hospital, Oceanside	6.6	0.0%	1.23	No	0.07	6	0.85	0.147	2.04
	Southside Hospital, Bay Shore	2.1	0.0%	2.03	No	0.13	6	0.60	0.017	1.19
	St. Barnabas Hospital, Bronx	2.8	0.0%	1.90	No	0.41	0	0.86	0.072	1.25
	St. Charles Hospital and Rehab. Ctr., Port Jefferson	5.5	0.0%	1.30	No	0.04	4	0.90	0.332	1.34
	St. Clare's Hospital of Schenectady, Schenectady	6.1	0.0%	1.37	No	0.20	4	1.05	0.122	2.07
	St. Elizabeth Hospital, Utica	4.6	0.0%	1.46	No	0.20	5	0.82	0.009	1.97
	St. John's Episcopal Hospital, Far Rockaway	1.8	0.0%	1.92	No	0.24	0	0.74	0.068	1.25
	St. John's Episcopal Hospital, Smithtown	2.1	0.0%	1.86	No	0.00	7	0.34	0.087	1.12
	St. Joseph's Medical Center, Yonkers	5.7	0.0%	1.27	No	0.26	3	0.79	0.046	3.08
	St. Mary's Hospital of Troy, Troy	1.9	0.0%	1.96	No	0.00	3	0.66	0.060	2.78
	St. Mary's Hospital, Rochester	5.6	0.0%	1.42	No	0.37	4	0.84	0.110	1.42
	St. Peter's Hospital, Albany	6.8	0.0%	1.29	No	0.09	9	0.98	0.065	1.85
	St. Vincent's Medical Center, Staten Island	3.8	0.0%	2.05	No	0.46	4	0.92	0.075	1.30

AMERICA'S BEST HOSPITALS

Natl. Rank	Hospital	U.S. News index	Reputa-tional score	Urology mortality rate	COTH member	Interns and residents to beds	Tech-nology score (of 11)	R.N.'s to beds	Board-certified internists to beds	Procedures to beds
	Staten Island University Hospital, Staten Island	7.7	0.0%	1.14	No	0.46	8	0.53	0.071	1.99
	United Health Services Hospitals, Binghamton	6.7	0.0%	1.48	Yes	0.20	5	0.61	0.050	1.76
	Vassar Brothers Hospital, Poughkeepsie	5.7	0.0%	1.36	No	0.01	8	0.69	0.120	2.20
	Winthrop-University Hospital, Mineola	8.1	0.0%	1.67	Yes	0.21	8	0.95	0.085	2.27

AIDS

Natl. Rank	Hospital	U.S. News index	Reputa-tional score	Hospital-wide mortality rate	COTH member	Interns and residents to beds	Tech-nology score (of 11)	Discharge planning (of 2)	R.N.'s to beds	Board-certified internists to beds
	TIER ONE									
14	Duke University Medical Center, Durham	34.5	5.0%	0.90	Yes	0.91	10	2	1.61	0.081
	TIER TWO									
68	North Carolina Baptist Hospital, Winston-Salem	26.0	1.0%	1.07	Yes	1.06	10	2	1.24	0.042
44	University of North Carolina Hospitals, Chapel Hill	27.8	2.4%	1.23	Yes	1.41	9	2	1.71	0.246
	TIER THREE									
	Memorial Mission Medical Center, Asheville	19.7	0.0%	1.09	No	0.06	8	1	1.44	0.052
	Moore Regional Hospital, Pinehurst	21.1	0.0%	0.97	No	0.00	7	2	1.06	0.041
	Moses H. Cone Memorial Hospital, Greensboro	20.9	0.0%	1.12	Yes	0.10	8	2	0.98	0.020
	Pitt County Memorial Hospital, Greenville	20.5	0.0%	1.24	Yes	0.62	6	2	1.34	0.048
	TIER FOUR									
	Cape Fear Valley Medical Center, Fayetteville	13.4	0.0%	1.68	No	0.04	6	2	0.91	0.026
	Carolinas Medical Center, Charlotte	18.0	0.0%	1.72	Yes	0.41	9	2	1.26	0.218
	Catawba Memorial Hospital, Hickory	19.5	0.0%	1.09	No	0.00	6	2	1.47	0.011
	Craven Regional Medical Center, New Bern	16.8	0.0%	1.21	No	0.00	7	1	0.79	0.065
	Dorothea Dix Hospital, Raleigh	12.5	0.0%	1.48	No	0.01	3	2	0.26	0.003
	Durham Regional Hospital, Durham	17.4	0.0%	1.22	No	0.08	6	2	0.91	0.060
	Forsyth Memorial Hospital, Winston-Salem	15.3	0.0%	1.49	No	0.04	7	2	1.03	0.037
	Gaston Memorial Hospital, Gastonia	13.9	0.0%	1.59	No	0.00	6	2	0.85	0.043
	Halifax Memorial Hospital, Roanoke Rapids	13.8	0.0%	1.47	No	0.00	6	1	0.78	0.012
	High Point Regional Hospital, High Point	13.3	0.0%	1.59	No	0.00	5	2	0.66	0.046
	Iredell Memorial Hospital, Statesville	16.1	0.0%	1.48	No	0.00	7	2	1.51	0.034
	Lenoir Memorial Hospital, Kinston	17.9	0.0%	1.14	No	0.00	6	2	0.81	0.018
	Mercy Hospital, Charlotte	15.2	0.0%	1.34	No	0.00	6	1	0.76	0.088
	Nash General Hospital, Rocky Mount	17.9	0.0%	1.16	No	0.00	7	2	0.69	0.060
	New Hanover Regional Medical Center, Wilmington	15.5	0.0%	1.58	No	0.15	7	2	1.44	0.035
	Presbyterian Hospital, Charlotte	16.8	0.0%	1.32	No	0.00	7	1	1.27	0.142
	Rex Hospital, Raleigh	19.3	0.0%	1.14	No	0.00	7	2	1.30	0.090
	Wake Medical Center, Raleigh	18.0	0.0%	1.24	No	0.06	8	2	1.11	0.025
	Wesley Long Community Hospital, Greensboro	18.5	0.0%	1.15	No	0.00	5	2	1.36	0.088

CANCER

Natl. Rank	Hospital	U.S. News index	Reputa-tional score	Cancer mortality rate	COTH member	Interns and residents to beds	Tech-nology score (of 12)	R.N.'s to beds	Board-certified oncologists to beds	Procedures to beds
	TIER ONE									
8	Duke University Medical Center, Durham	28.7	12.3%	0.71	Yes	0.91	12	1.61	0.028	2.76
	TIER TWO									
44	North Carolina Baptist Hospital, Winston-Salem	13.3	0.6%	0.76	Yes	1.06	12	1.24	0.014	2.57
31	University of North Carolina Hospitals, Chapel Hill	14.8	0.6%	0.90	Yes	1.41	10	1.71	0.013	1.28
	TIER THREE									
	Carolinas Medical Center, Charlotte	9.3	0.0%	1.69	Yes	0.41	12	1.26	0.000	0.88
	Memorial Mission Medical Center, Asheville	6.6	0.0%	0.78	No	0.06	10	1.44	0.016	1.97
	Moses H. Cone Memorial Hospital, Greensboro	7.1	0.0%	1.02	Yes	0.10	9	0.98	0.012	1.25
	New Hanover Regional Medical Center, Wilmington	5.6	0.0%	1.40	No	0.15	8	1.44	0.010	1.51
	Pitt County Memorial Hospital, Greenville	8.2	0.0%	1.30	Yes	0.62	4	1.34	0.007	1.52
	TIER FOUR									
	AMI Frye Regional Medical Center, Hickory	2.3	0.0%	1.50	No	0.00	4	0.93	0.008	0.72
	Cape Fear Valley Medical Center, Fayetteville	3.3	0.0%	1.37	No	0.04	7	0.91	0.004	0.73
	Catawba Memorial Hospital, Hickory	4.7	0.0%	1.78	No	0.00	7	1.47	0.011	1.03
	Craven Regional Medical Center, New Bern	3.6	0.0%	1.35	No	0.00	9	0.79	0.007	1.50

STATE RANKINGS ■ NORTH CAROLINA

Natl. Rank	Hospital	U.S. News index	Reputa- tional score	Cancer mortality rate	COTH member	Interns and residents to beds	Tech- nology score (of 12)	R.N.'s to beds	Board- certified oncologists to beds	Procedures to beds
	Durham Regional Hospital, Durham	3.1	0.0%	1.47	No	0.08	5	0.91	0.003	1.95
	Forsyth Memorial Hospital, Winston-Salem	4.1	0.0%	1.43	No	0.04	8	1.03	0.010	1.42
	Gaston Memorial Hospital, Gastonia	2.9	0.0%	1.67	No	0.00	7	0.85	0.003	1.11
	Halifax Memorial Hospital, Roanoke Rapids	2.2	0.0%	1.22	No	0.00	4	0.78	0.006	1.22
	High Point Regional Hospital, High Point	2.3	0.0%	1.72	No	0.00	6	0.66	0.003	1.91
	Iredell Memorial Hospital, Statesville	5.0	0.0%	1.42	No	0.00	7	1.51	0.010	1.64
	Lenoir Memorial Hospital, Kinston	3.1	0.0%	1.27	No	0.00	7	0.81	0.004	1.49
	Mercy Hospital, Charlotte	1.8	0.0%	1.32	No	0.00	3	0.76	0.011	1.03
	Moore Regional Hospital, Pinehurst	3.9	0.0%	0.90	No	0.00	6	1.06	0.006	1.56
	Nash General Hospital, Rocky Mount	3.0	0.0%	1.15	No	0.00	7	0.69	0.011	2.13
	Presbyterian Hospital, Charlotte	5.1	0.0%	1.33	No	0.00	9	1.27	0.017	2.09
	Rex Hospital, Raleigh	5.0	0.0%	1.58	No	0.00	9	1.30	0.021	1.73
	Wesley Long Community Hospital, Greensboro	4.6	0.0%	1.07	No	0.00	6	1.36	0.000	2.09

CARDIOLOGY

Natl. Rank	Hospital	U.S. News index	Reputa- tional score	Cardiology mortality rate	COTH member	Interns and residents to beds	Tech- nology score (of 10)	R.N.'s to beds	Board- certified cardiologists to beds	Procedures to beds
	TIER ONE									
5	Duke University Medical Center, Durham	63.7	25.1%	0.85	Yes	0.91	10	1.61	0.054	6.30
	TIER TWO									
41	North Carolina Baptist Hospital, Winston-Salem	23.8	1.1%	0.99	Yes	1.06	9	1.24	0.024	6.83
60	University of North Carolina Hospitals, Chapel Hill	22.2	0.0%	1.12	Yes	1.41	9	1.71	0.042	3.83
	TIER THREE									
	Catawba Memorial Hospital, Hickory	14.0	0.0%	1.03	No	0.00	5	1.47	0.021	4.58
	Durham Regional Hospital, Durham	13.9	0.0%	1.03	No	0.08	9	0.91	0.017	6.50
	Lenoir Memorial Hospital, Kinston	16.5	0.0%	0.85	No	0.00	6	0.81	0.000	8.19
	Memorial Mission Medical Center, Asheville	15.1	0.5%	1.10	No	0.06	9	1.44	0.031	10.35
	Moore Regional Hospital, Pinehurst	16.9	0.0%	0.92	No	0.00	9	1.06	0.006	8.00
	Moses H. Cone Memorial Hospital, Greensboro	17.7	0.0%	1.01	Yes	0.10	9	0.98	0.028	7.02
	Pitt County Memorial Hospital, Greenville	17.4	0.0%	1.15	Yes	0.62	8	1.34	0.031	7.61
	TIER FOUR									
	AMI Frye Regional Medical Center, Hickory	9.6	0.0%	1.24	No	0.00	8	0.93	0.020	6.14
	Cape Fear Valley Medical Center, Fayetteville	5.3	0.0%	1.50	No	0.04	6	0.91	0.007	3.41
	Carolinas Medical Center, Charlotte	10.8	0.5%	1.66	Yes	0.41	10	1.26	0.000	7.54
	Craven Regional Medical Center, New Bern	12.7	0.0%	1.05	No	0.00	8	0.79	0.014	8.04
	Forsyth Memorial Hospital, Winston-Salem	7.2	0.0%	1.47	No	0.04	9	1.03	0.020	6.23
	Gaston Memorial Hospital, Gastonia	5.5	0.0%	1.42	No	0.00	4	0.85	0.005	6.88
	Halifax Memorial Hospital, Roanoke Rapids	6.5	0.0%	1.35	No	0.00	4	0.78	0.012	9.99
	High Point Regional Hospital, High Point	7.7	0.0%	1.31	No	0.00	8	0.66	0.012	7.31
	Iredell Memorial Hospital, Statesville	12.7	0.0%	1.14	No	0.00	7	1.51	0.020	8.14
	Mercy Hospital, Charlotte	11.0	0.0%	1.18	No	0.00	8	0.76	0.088	8.24
	Nash General Hospital, Rocky Mount	10.4	0.0%	1.13	No	0.00	7	0.69	0.011	7.60
	New Hanover Regional Medical Center, Wilmington	9.4	0.0%	1.41	No	0.15	8	1.44	0.022	8.19
	Presbyterian Hospital, Charlotte	12.8	0.0%	1.15	No	0.00	8	1.27	0.047	8.90
	Rex Hospital, Raleigh	13.4	0.0%	1.12	No	0.00	9	1.30	0.045	5.13
	Wake Medical Center, Raleigh	10.8	0.0%	1.25	No	0.06	9	1.11	0.029	9.10
	Wesley Long Community Hospital, Greensboro	13.0	0.0%	1.09	No	0.00	7	1.36	0.000	8.24

ENDOCRINOLOGY

Natl. Rank	Hospital	U.S. News index	Reputa-tional score	Endocrinology mortality rate	COTH member	Interns and residents to beds	Tech-nology score (of 11)	R.N.'s to beds	Board-certified internists to beds
	TIER ONE								
13	**Duke University Medical Center, Durham**	**27.1**	6.7%	0.69	Yes	0.91	11	1.61	0.081
	TIER TWO								
35	**University of North Carolina Hospitals, Chapel Hill**	**19.1**	1.2%	1.08	Yes	1.41	10	1.71	0.246
	TIER THREE								
	Carolinas Medical Center, Charlotte	12.5	0.0%	1.17	Yes	0.41	11	1.26	0.218
	Memorial Mission Medical Center, Asheville	12.5	0.0%	0.66	No	0.06	10	1.44	0.052
	Moses H. Cone Memorial Hospital, Greensboro	9.1	0.0%	1.13	Yes	0.10	9	0.98	0.020
	North Carolina Baptist Hospital, Winston-Salem	13.1	0.0%	1.21	Yes	1.06	11	1.24	0.042
	Pitt County Memorial Hospital, Greenville	10.1	0.0%	1.28	Yes	0.62	3	1.34	0.048
	Rex Hospital, Raleigh	9.2	0.0%	0.90	No	0.00	9	1.30	0.090
	TIER FOUR								
	AMI Frye Regional Medical Center, Hickory	4.4	0.0%	1.30	No	0.00	4	0.93	0.020
	Cape Fear Valley Medical Center, Fayetteville	3.9	0.0%	1.79	No	0.04	8	0.91	0.026
	Craven Regional Medical Center, New Bern	3.9	0.0%	1.87	No	0.00	10	0.79	0.065
	Durham Regional Hospital, Durham	3.5	0.0%	1.88	No	0.08	5	0.91	0.060
	Forsyth Memorial Hospital, Winston-Salem	5.0	0.0%	1.50	No	0.04	8	1.03	0.037
	Gaston Memorial Hospital, Gastonia	3.1	0.0%	2.13	No	0.00	8	0.85	0.043
	Halifax Memorial Hospital, Roanoke Rapids	1.6	0.0%	2.55	No	0.00	5	0.78	0.012
	High Point Regional Hospital, High Point	2.8	0.0%	1.81	No	0.00	6	0.66	0.046
	Iredell Memorial Hospital, Statesville	7.1	0.0%	1.24	No	0.00	8	1.51	0.034
	Lenoir Memorial Hospital, Kinston	3.9	0.0%	1.58	No	0.00	8	0.81	0.018
	Mercy Hospital, Charlotte	2.6	0.0%	2.14	No	0.00	5	0.76	0.088
	Moore Regional Hospital, Pinehurst	5.8	0.0%	1.18	No	0.00	6	1.06	0.041
	Nash General Hospital, Rocky Mount	4.4	0.0%	1.42	No	0.00	8	0.69	0.060
	New Hanover Regional Medical Center, Wilmington	5.5	0.0%	1.81	No	0.15	7	1.44	0.035
	North Carolina Eye and Ear Hospital, Durham	0.0	0.0%	2.13	No	0.00	0	0.41	0.000
	Presbyterian Hospital, Charlotte	7.5	0.6%	1.35	No	0.00	8	1.27	0.142
	Wake Medical Center, Raleigh	5.2	0.0%	1.45	No	0.06	7	1.11	0.025
	Wesley Long Community Hospital, Greensboro	5.1	0.0%	1.74	No	0.00	6	1.36	0.088

GASTROENTEROLOGY

Natl. Rank	Hospital	U.S. News index	Reputa-tional score	Gastro-enterology mortality rate	COTH member	Interns and residents to beds	Tech-nology score (of 11)	R.N.'s to beds	Board-certified gastro-enterologists to beds	Pro-cedures to beds
	TIER ONE									
6	**Duke University Medical Center, Durham**	**51.5**	24.2%	0.88	Yes	0.91	11	1.61	0.017	1.55
	TIER TWO									
58	**North Carolina Baptist Hospital, Winston-Salem**	**14.3**	0.4%	1.05	Yes	1.06	11	1.24	0.008	1.66
46	**University of North Carolina Hospitals, Chapel Hill**	**15.6**	0.8%	1.29	Yes	1.41	9	1.71	0.037	1.80
	TIER THREE									
	Carolinas Medical Center, Charlotte	8.0	0.0%	1.88	Yes	0.41	10	1.26	0.000	1.63
	Memorial Mission Medical Center, Asheville	7.7	0.0%	1.18	No	0.06	10	1.44	0.029	3.07
	Moore Regional Hospital, Pinehurst	7.4	0.0%	0.95	No	0.00	6	1.06	0.006	4.08
	Moses H. Cone Memorial Hospital, Greensboro	8.8	0.0%	1.14	Yes	0.10	9	0.98	0.016	2.26
	Pitt County Memorial Hospital, Greenville	9.3	0.0%	1.34	Yes	0.62	4	1.34	0.010	2.62
	Rex Hospital, Raleigh	8.5	0.0%	0.95	No	0.00	9	1.30	0.015	3.30
	Wesley Long Community Hospital, Greensboro	8.4	0.0%	0.99	No	0.00	6	1.36	0.000	5.07
	TIER FOUR									
	AMI Frye Regional Medical Center, Hickory	3.8	0.0%	1.32	No	0.00	4	0.93	0.008	2.97
	Cape Fear Valley Medical Center, Fayetteville	1.4	0.0%	2.45	No	0.04	7	0.91	0.011	1.53
	Catawba Memorial Hospital, Hickory	6.9	0.0%	1.14	No	0.00	7	1.47	0.000	3.19
	Craven Regional Medical Center, New Bern	5.5	0.0%	1.37	No	0.00	10	0.79	0.007	3.83

Natl. Rank	Hospital	U.S. News index	Reputa-tional score	Gastro-enterology mortality rate	COTH member	Interns and residents to beds	Tech-nology score (of 11)	R.N.'s to beds	Board-certified gastro-enterologists to beds	Pro-cedures to beds
	Durham Regional Hospital, Durham	6.5	0.0%	1.01	No	0.08	6	0.91	0.017	3.17
	Forsyth Memorial Hospital, Winston-Salem	5.1	0.0%	1.42	No	0.04	8	1.03	0.018	3.09
	Gaston Memorial Hospital, Gastonia	3.6	0.0%	1.68	No	0.00	8	0.85	0.000	3.06
	Halifax Memorial Hospital, Roanoke Rapids	4.1	0.0%	1.45	No	0.00	6	0.78	0.012	4.04
	High Point Regional Hospital, High Point	3.0	0.0%	1.68	No	0.00	5	0.66	0.009	4.33
	Iredell Memorial Hospital, Statesville	5.9	0.0%	1.58	No	0.00	8	1.51	0.020	3.80
	Lenoir Memorial Hospital, Kinston	4.3	0.0%	1.37	No	0.00	7	0.81	0.007	3.09
	Mercy Hospital, Charlotte	3.0	0.0%	1.49	No	0.00	5	0.76	0.032	2.70
	Nash General Hospital, Rocky Mount	5.9	0.0%	1.11	No	0.00	9	0.69	0.000	3.37
	New Hanover Regional Medical Center, Wilmington	5.6	0.0%	1.50	No	0.15	6	1.44	0.000	3.36
	Presbyterian Hospital, Charlotte	6.2	0.0%	1.32	No	0.00	7	1.27	0.025	4.21
	Wake Medical Center, Raleigh	5.7	0.0%	1.18	No	0.06	8	1.11	0.008	1.96

GERIATRICS

Natl. Rank	Hospital	U.S. News index	Reputa-tional score	Hospital-wide mortality rate	COTH member	Service mix	Interns and residents to beds	Tech-nology score (of 13)	R.N.'s to beds	Discharge planning (of 2)	Geriatric services (of 9)	Board-certified internists to beds
TIER ONE
4	Duke University Medical Center, Durham	77.0	19.5%	0.90	Yes	7	0.91	13	1.61	2	4	0.081
24	North Carolina Baptist Hospital, Winston-Salem	29.7	3.4%	1.07	Yes	8	1.06	13	1.24	2	5	0.042
TIER TWO
52	University of North Carolina Hospitals, Chapel Hill	24.2	1.9%	1.23	Yes	7	1.41	11	1.71	2	5	0.246
TIER THREE
	Moore Regional Hospital, Pinehurst	14.5	0.0%	0.97	No	3	0.00	8	1.06	2	2	0.041
	Moses H. Cone Memorial Hospital, Greensboro	16.2	0.0%	1.12	Yes	7	0.10	12	0.98	2	6	0.020
TIER FOUR
	AMI Frye Regional Medical Center, Hickory	6.7	0.0%	1.33	No	5	0.00	7	0.93	2	1	0.020
	Cape Fear Valley Medical Center, Fayetteville	3.5	0.0%	1.68	No	6	0.04	10	0.91	2	2	0.026
	Carolinas Medical Center, Charlotte	8.1	0.0%	1.72	Yes	6	0.41	13	1.26	2	1	0.218
	Craven Regional Medical Center, New Bern	9.3	0.0%	1.21	No	5	0.00	11	0.79	1	4	0.065
	Durham Regional Hospital, Durham	9.7	0.0%	1.22	No	5	0.08	8	0.91	2	3	0.060
	Forsyth Memorial Hospital, Winston-Salem	4.7	0.0%	1.49	No	3	0.04	11	1.03	2	1	0.037
	Gaston Memorial Hospital, Gastonia	3.6	0.0%	1.59	No	4	0.00	9	0.85	2	3	0.043
	High Point Regional Hospital, High Point	4.2	0.0%	1.59	No	5	0.00	9	0.66	2	5	0.046
	Iredell Memorial Hospital, Statesville	5.9	0.0%	1.48	No	3	0.00	10	1.51	2	3	0.034
	Lenoir Memorial Hospital, Kinston	10.1	0.0%	1.14	No	3	0.00	10	0.81	2	2	0.018
	Mercy Hospital, Charlotte	5.5	0.0%	1.34	No	5	0.00	6	0.76	1	2	0.088
	Nash General Hospital, Rocky Mount	10.2	0.0%	1.16	No	4	0.00	10	0.69	2	3	0.060
	New Hanover Regional Medical Center, Wilmington	6.6	0.0%	1.58	No	7	0.15	9	1.44	2	4	0.035
	Pitt County Memorial Hospital, Greenville	11.7	0.0%	1.24	Yes	3	0.62	5	1.34	2	2	0.048
	Presbyterian Hospital, Charlotte	7.8	0.0%	1.32	No	5	0.00	11	1.27	1	1	0.142
	Rex Hospital, Raleigh	11.5	0.0%	1.14	No	3	0.00	12	1.30	2	1	0.090
	Wake Medical Center, Raleigh	8.9	0.0%	1.24	No	4	0.06	9	1.11	2	2	0.025
	Wesley Long Community Hospital, Greensboro	11.3	0.0%	1.15	No	3	0.00	9	1.36	2	3	0.088

GYNECOLOGY

Natl. Rank	Hospital	U.S. News index	Reputa-tional score	Hospital-wide mortality rate	Interns and residents to beds	Tech-nology score (of 10)	R.N.'s to beds	Board-certified OB-GYNs to beds	Procedures to beds
TIER ONE
7	Duke University Medical Center, Durham	53.9	10.2%	0.90	0.91	10	1.61	0.028	0.45
21	University of North Carolina Hospitals, Chapel Hill	33.8	4.5%	1.23	1.41	9	1.71	0.064	0.50
TIER TWO
66	North Carolina Baptist Hospital, Winston-Salem	24.0	1.0%	1.07	1.06	10	1.24	0.017	0.46
TIER THREE
	Memorial Mission Medical Center, Asheville	17.4	0.0%	1.09	0.06	9	1.44	0.050	0.59
	Moore Regional Hospital, Pinehurst	15.8	0.0%	0.97	0.00	6	1.06	0.022	0.60
	Moses H. Cone Memorial Hospital, Greensboro	14.2	0.0%	1.12	0.10	8	0.98	0.049	0.31
	Rex Hospital, Raleigh	15.0	0.0%	1.14	0.00	7	1.30	0.088	0.42
	Wesley Long Community Hospital, Greensboro	14.6	0.0%	1.15	0.00	6	1.36	0.118	0.67
TIER FOUR
	AMI Frye Regional Medical Center, Hickory	7.1	0.0%	1.33	0.00	5	0.93	0.031	0.28
	Cape Fear Valley Medical Center, Fayetteville	4.4	0.0%	1.68	0.04	7	0.91	0.039	0.39
	Carolinas Medical Center, Charlotte	11.7	0.4%	1.72	0.41	10	1.26	0.098	0.36
	Craven Regional Medical Center, New Bern	10.7	0.0%	1.21	0.00	8	0.79	0.029	0.50
	Durham Regional Hospital, Durham	10.4	0.0%	1.22	0.08	5	0.91	0.077	0.54
	Forsyth Memorial Hospital, Winston-Salem	7.2	0.0%	1.49	0.04	7	1.03	0.045	0.34
	Gaston Memorial Hospital, Gastonia	4.1	0.0%	1.59	0.00	6	0.85	0.036	0.38
	Halifax Memorial Hospital, Roanoke Rapids	4.0	0.0%	1.47	0.00	5	0.78	0.012	0.32
	High Point Regional Hospital, High Point	2.8	0.0%	1.59	0.00	5	0.66	0.043	0.48
	Iredell Memorial Hospital, Statesville	9.0	0.0%	1.48	0.00	7	1.51	0.034	0.25
	Mercy Hospital, Charlotte	7.6	0.0%	1.34	0.00	6	0.76	0.060	0.34
	Nash General Hospital, Rocky Mount	10.5	0.0%	1.16	0.00	7	0.69	0.032	0.41
	New Hanover Regional Medical Center, Wilmington	8.4	0.0%	1.58	0.15	7	1.44	0.045	0.50
	Pitt County Memorial Hospital, Greenville	13.2	0.0%	1.24	0.62	5	1.34	0.035	0.60
	Presbyterian Hospital, Charlotte	11.7	0.0%	1.32	0.00	7	1.27	0.097	0.69
	Wake Medical Center, Raleigh	11.1	0.0%	1.24	0.06	7	1.11	0.037	0.20

NEUROLOGY

Natl. Rank	Hospital	U.S. News index	Reputa-tional score	Neurology mortality rate	COTH member	Interns and residents to beds	Tech-nology score (of 9)	R.N.'s to beds	Board-certified neurologists to beds
TIER ONE
11	Duke University Medical Center, Durham	33.2	8.6%	0.89	Yes	0.91	9	1.61	0.017
TIER TWO
71	North Carolina Baptist Hospital, Winston-Salem	18.4	1.3%	1.07	Yes	1.06	9	1.24	0.017
66	University of North Carolina Hospitals, Chapel Hill	18.5	0.0%	1.05	Yes	1.41	8	1.71	0.014
TIER THREE
	Catawba Memorial Hospital, Hickory	12.4	0.0%	0.92	No	0.00	6	1.47	0.011
	Memorial Mission Medical Center, Asheville	12.6	0.0%	0.97	No	0.06	8	1.44	0.016
	Moore Regional Hospital, Pinehurst	11.5	0.0%	0.92	No	0.00	6	1.06	0.013
	Pitt County Memorial Hospital, Greenville	12.1	0.5%	1.18	Yes	0.62	3	1.34	0.007
TIER FOUR
	AMI Frye Regional Medical Center, Hickory	6.0	0.0%	1.26	No	0.00	4	0.93	0.016
	Cape Fear Valley Medical Center, Fayetteville	3.2	0.0%	1.60	No	0.04	6	0.91	0.004
	Carolinas Medical Center, Charlotte	8.9	0.0%	1.70	Yes	0.41	9	1.26	0.020
	Craven Regional Medical Center, New Bern	9.5	0.0%	1.03	No	0.00	8	0.79	0.014
	Durham Regional Hospital, Durham	5.0	0.0%	1.35	No	0.08	5	0.91	0.006
	Forsyth Memorial Hospital, Winston-Salem	4.7	0.0%	1.49	No	0.04	7	1.03	0.006
	Gaston Memorial Hospital, Gastonia	3.6	0.0%	1.51	No	0.00	6	0.85	0.005
	High Point Regional Hospital, High Point	2.4	0.0%	1.72	No	0.00	5	0.66	0.018
	Mercy Hospital, Charlotte	2.1	0.0%	1.93	No	0.00	5	0.76	0.025

Natl. Rank	Hospital	U.S. News index	Reputa-tional score	Neurology mortality rate	COTH member	Interns and residents to beds	Tech-nology score (of 9)	R.N.'s to beds	Board-certified neurologists to beds
	Moses H. Cone Memorial Hospital, Greensboro	10.3	0.0%	1.15	Yes	0.10	7	0.98	0.008
	Nash General Hospital, Rocky Mount	7.1	0.0%	1.13	No	0.00	7	0.69	0.007
	New Hanover Regional Medical Center, Wilmington	5.7	0.0%	1.51	No	0.15	5	1.44	0.012
	Presbyterian Hospital, Charlotte	9.1	0.0%	1.16	No	0.00	6	1.27	0.024
	Rex Hospital, Raleigh	9.5	0.0%	1.13	No	0.00	7	1.30	0.019
	Wake Medical Center, Raleigh	6.4	0.0%	1.26	No	0.06	6	1.11	0.003

ORTHOPEDICS

Natl. Rank	Hospital	U.S. News index	Reputa-tional score	Orthopedics mortality rate	COTH member	Interns and residents to beds	Tech-nology score (of 5)	R.N.'s to beds	Board-certified orthopedists to beds	Pro-cedures to beds
	TIER ONE									
5	Duke University Medical Center, Durham	41.0	11.4%	0.75	Yes	0.91	5	1.61	0.016	1.54
23	University of North Carolina Hospitals, Chapel Hill	20.8	0.6%	0.68	Yes	1.41	4	1.71	0.018	1.21
	TIER TWO									
64	North Carolina Baptist Hospital, Winston-Salem	15.5	0.5%	0.98	Yes	1.06	5	1.24	0.009	1.79
	TIER THREE									
	Carolinas Medical Center, Charlotte	11.3	0.5%	1.47	Yes	0.41	5	1.26	0.061	2.19
	Catawba Memorial Hospital, Hickory	9.0	0.0%	0.84	No	0.00	3	1.47	0.042	1.83
	Moore Regional Hospital, Pinehurst	11.5	0.0%	0.38	No	0.00	4	1.06	0.022	4.88
	Moses H. Cone Memorial Hospital, Greensboro	9.5	0.0%	1.06	Yes	0.10	4	0.98	0.031	1.60
	Pitt County Memorial Hospital, Greenville	9.0	0.0%	1.67	Yes	0.62	3	1.34	0.018	2.30
	TIER FOUR									
	AMI Frye Regional Medical Center, Hickory	4.9	0.0%	1.22	No	0.00	3	0.93	0.031	2.56
	Cape Fear Valley Medical Center, Fayetteville	3.8	0.0%	1.38	No	0.04	3	0.91	0.013	1.06
	Craven Regional Medical Center, New Bern	4.1	0.0%	1.50	No	0.00	4	0.79	0.025	3.09
	Durham Regional Hospital, Durham	7.9	0.0%	0.95	No	0.08	4	0.91	0.040	3.97
	Forsyth Memorial Hospital, Winston-Salem	5.8	0.0%	1.22	No	0.04	4	1.03	0.015	2.41
	Gaston Memorial Hospital, Gastonia	1.9	0.0%	2.10	No	0.00	3	0.85	0.018	1.68
	High Point Regional Hospital, High Point	2.6	0.0%	1.64	No	0.00	3	0.66	0.018	2.56
	Iredell Memorial Hospital, Statesville	5.9	0.0%	1.54	No	0.00	4	1.51	0.020	3.10
	Lenoir Memorial Hospital, Kinston	4.3	0.0%	1.22	No	0.00	3	0.81	0.015	1.54
	Memorial Mission Medical Center, Asheville	6.2	0.0%	1.46	No	0.06	4	1.44	0.055	2.38
	Mercy Hospital, Charlotte	4.0	0.0%	1.53	No	0.00	4	0.76	0.070	2.06
	Nash General Hospital, Rocky Mount	6.0	0.0%	1.00	No	0.00	4	0.69	0.014	2.14
	New Hanover Regional Medical Center, Wilmington	5.1	0.0%	1.60	No	0.15	3	1.44	0.025	1.91
	Presbyterian Hospital, Charlotte	5.1	0.0%	1.40	No	0.00	3	1.27	0.069	1.82
	Rex Hospital, Raleigh	6.7	0.0%	1.18	No	0.00	4	1.30	0.054	1.87
	Wake Medical Center, Raleigh	7.7	0.0%	0.96	No	0.06	4	1.11	0.020	1.99

OTOLARYNGOLOGY

Natl. Rank	Hospital	U.S. News index	Reputa-tional score	Hospital-wide mortality rate	COTH member	Interns and residents to beds	Tech-nology score (of 9)	R.N.'s to beds	Board-certified internists to beds	Procedures to beds
	TIER ONE									
18	Duke University Medical Center, Durham	26.9	3.7%	0.90	Yes	0.91	9	1.61	0.081	0.126
22	University of North Carolina Hospitals, Chapel Hill	24.5	2.0%	1.23	Yes	1.41	8	1.71	0.246	0.235
	TIER TWO									
49	North Carolina Baptist Hospital, Winston-Salem	18.4	1.4%	1.07	Yes	1.06	9	1.24	0.042	0.210
	TIER THREE									
	Carolinas Medical Center, Charlotte	12.7	0.0%	1.72	Yes	0.41	9	1.26	0.218	0.118
	Memorial Mission Medical Center, Asheville	7.3	0.0%	1.09	No	0.06	8	1.44	0.052	0.210
	Moses H. Cone Memorial Hospital, Greensboro	8.6	0.0%	1.12	Yes	0.10	7	0.98	0.020	0.091
	Pitt County Memorial Hospital, Greenville	10.6	0.0%	1.24	Yes	0.62	2	1.34	0.048	0.145

Natl. Rank	Hospital	U.S. News index	Reputa-tional score	Hospital-wide mortality rate	COTH member	Interns and residents to beds	Tech-nology score (of 9)	R.N.'s to beds	Board-certified internists to beds	Procedures to beds
	Presbyterian Hospital, Charlotte	8.3	0.5%	1.32	No	0.00	6	1.27	0.142	0.176
	TIER FOUR									
	AMI Frye Regional Medical Center, Hickory	3.4	0.0%	1.33	No	0.00	2	0.93	0.020	0.039
	Cape Fear Valley Medical Center, Fayetteville	4.6	0.0%	1.68	No	0.04	6	0.91	0.026	0.083
	Catawba Memorial Hospital, Hickory	6.3	0.0%	1.09	No	0.00	6	1.47	0.011	0.095
	Craven Regional Medical Center, New Bern	5.1	0.0%	1.21	No	0.00	8	0.79	0.065	0.261
	Durham Regional Hospital, Durham	4.4	0.0%	1.22	No	0.08	3	0.91	0.060	0.151
	Forsyth Memorial Hospital, Winston-Salem	5.1	0.0%	1.49	No	0.04	6	1.03	0.037	0.140
	Gaston Memorial Hospital, Gastonia	4.4	0.0%	1.59	No	0.00	6	0.85	0.043	0.119
	Halifax Memorial Hospital, Roanoke Rapids	3.1	0.0%	1.47	No	0.00	3	0.78	0.012	0.226
	High Point Regional Hospital, High Point	3.3	0.0%	1.59	No	0.00	4	0.66	0.046	0.149
	Iredell Memorial Hospital, Statesville	6.4	0.0%	1.48	No	0.00	6	1.51	0.034	0.250
	Lenoir Memorial Hospital, Kinston	4.3	0.0%	1.14	No	0.00	6	0.81	0.018	0.225
	Mercy Hospital, Charlotte	3.8	0.0%	1.34	No	0.00	3	0.76	0.088	0.102
	Moore Regional Hospital, Pinehurst	4.8	0.0%	0.97	No	0.00	4	1.06	0.041	0.363
	Nash General Hospital, Rocky Mount	4.3	0.0%	1.16	No	0.00	6	0.69	0.060	0.223
	New Hanover Regional Medical Center, Wilmington	6.7	0.0%	1.58	No	0.15	6	1.44	0.035	0.215
	North Carolina Eye and Ear Hospital, Durham	1.1	0.0%	1.59	No	0.00	0	0.41	0.000	1.270
	Rex Hospital, Raleigh	6.7	0.0%	1.14	No	0.00	7	1.30	0.090	0.195
	Wake Medical Center, Raleigh	5.1	0.0%	1.24	No	0.06	5	1.11	0.025	0.113
	Wesley Long Community Hospital, Greensboro	6.0	0.0%	1.15	No	0.00	4	1.36	0.088	0.154

RHEUMATOLOGY

Natl. Rank	Hospital	U.S. News index	Reputa-tional score	Hospital-wide mortality rate	COTH member	Interns and residents to beds	Tech-nology score (of 5)	R.N.'s to beds	Board-certified internists to beds
	TIER ONE								
6	Duke University Medical Center, Durham	48.0	13.5%	0.90	Yes	0.91	5	1.61	0.081
	TIER TWO								
58	North Carolina Baptist Hospital, Winston-Salem	17.4	0.9%	1.07	Yes	1.06	5	1.24	0.042
33	University of North Carolina Hospitals, Chapel Hill	20.7	1.3%	1.23	Yes	1.41	4	1.71	0.246
	TIER THREE								
	Carolinas Medical Center, Charlotte	11.5	0.0%	1.72	Yes	0.41	5	1.26	0.218
	Moore Regional Hospital, Pinehurst	9.6	0.0%	0.97	No	0.00	4	1.06	0.041
	Moses H. Cone Memorial Hospital, Greensboro	10.7	0.0%	1.12	Yes	0.10	4	0.98	0.020
	Pitt County Memorial Hospital, Greenville	12.3	0.0%	1.24	Yes	0.62	3	1.34	0.048
	TIER FOUR								
	AMI Frye Regional Medical Center, Hickory	6.1	0.0%	1.33	No	0.00	3	0.93	0.020
	Cape Fear Valley Medical Center, Fayetteville	4.7	0.0%	1.68	No	0.04	3	0.91	0.026
	Craven Regional Medical Center, New Bern	6.2	0.0%	1.21	No	0.00	4	0.79	0.065
	Durham Regional Hospital, Durham	7.7	0.0%	1.22	No	0.08	4	0.91	0.060
	Forsyth Memorial Hospital, Winston-Salem	6.3	0.0%	1.49	No	0.04	4	1.03	0.037
	Gaston Memorial Hospital, Gastonia	4.9	0.0%	1.59	No	0.00	3	0.85	0.043
	Halifax Memorial Hospital, Roanoke Rapids	4.4	0.0%	1.47	No	0.00	4	0.78	0.012
	High Point Regional Hospital, High Point	4.4	0.0%	1.59	No	0.00	3	0.66	0.046
	Iredell Memorial Hospital, Statesville	7.4	0.0%	1.48	No	0.00	4	1.51	0.034
	Lenoir Memorial Hospital, Kinston	6.9	0.0%	1.14	No	0.00	3	0.81	0.018
	Memorial Mission Medical Center, Asheville	8.8	0.0%	1.09	No	0.06	4	1.44	0.052
	Mercy Hospital, Charlotte	5.5	0.0%	1.34	No	0.00	4	0.76	0.088
	Nash General Hospital, Rocky Mount	7.2	0.0%	1.16	No	0.00	4	0.69	0.060
	New Hanover Regional Medical Center, Wilmington	6.9	0.0%	1.58	No	0.15	3	1.44	0.035
	North Carolina Eye and Ear Hospital, Durham	0.0	0.0%	1.59	No	0.00	0	0.41	0.000
	Presbyterian Hospital, Charlotte	6.9	0.0%	1.32	No	0.00	3	1.27	0.142

Natl. Rank	Hospital	U.S. News index	Reputational score	Hospital-wide mortality rate	COTH member	Interns and residents to beds	Technology score (of 5)	R.N.'s to beds	Board-certified internists to beds
	Rex Hospital, Raleigh	9.2	0.0%	1.14	No	0.00	4	1.30	0.090
	Wake Medical Center, Raleigh	7.7	0.0%	1.24	No	0.06	4	1.11	0.025
	Wesley Long Community Hospital, Greensboro	8.8	0.0%	1.15	No	0.00	3	1.36	0.088

UROLOGY

Natl. Rank	Hospital	U.S. News index	Reputational score	Urology mortality rate	COTH member	Interns and residents to beds	Technology score (of 11)	R.N.'s to beds	Board-certified internists to beds	Procedures to beds
	TIER ONE									
6	Duke University Medical Center, Durham	44.1	19.8%	0.86	Yes	0.91	11	1.61	0.081	1.68
	TIER TWO									
53	North Carolina Baptist Hospital, Winston-Salem	17.6	1.9%	1.05	Yes	1.06	11	1.24	0.042	1.16
83	University of North Carolina Hospitals, Chapel Hill	15.6	0.0%	1.38	Yes	1.41	9	1.71	0.246	1.16
	TIER THREE									
	Carolinas Medical Center, Charlotte	9.4	0.0%	1.93	Yes	0.41	10	1.26	0.218	1.06
	Pitt County Memorial Hospital, Greenville	9.5	0.0%	1.53	Yes	0.62	4	1.34	0.048	1.68
	Rex Hospital, Raleigh	10.0	0.0%	0.94	No	0.00	9	1.30	0.090	1.47
	TIER FOUR									
	AMI Frye Regional Medical Center, Hickory	5.2	0.0%	1.20	No	0.00	4	0.93	0.020	1.57
	Cape Fear Valley Medical Center, Fayetteville	2.6	0.0%	2.13	No	0.04	7	0.91	0.026	1.09
	Craven Regional Medical Center, New Bern	5.4	0.0%	1.46	No	0.00	10	0.79	0.065	1.40
	Durham Regional Hospital, Durham	4.9	0.0%	1.52	No	0.08	6	0.91	0.060	2.55
	Forsyth Memorial Hospital, Winston-Salem	4.3	0.0%	1.74	No	0.04	8	1.03	0.037	1.08
	Gaston Memorial Hospital, Gastonia	4.4	0.0%	1.56	No	0.00	8	0.85	0.043	1.35
	Halifax Memorial Hospital, Roanoke Rapids	3.9	0.0%	1.55	No	0.00	6	0.78	0.012	2.52
	High Point Regional Hospital, High Point	2.3	0.0%	1.93	No	0.00	5	0.66	0.046	2.09
	Iredell Memorial Hospital, Statesville	5.6	0.0%	1.86	No	0.00	8	1.51	0.034	2.97
	Lenoir Memorial Hospital, Kinston	3.6	0.0%	1.63	No	0.00	7	0.81	0.018	1.37
	Memorial Mission Medical Center, Asheville	8.1	0.0%	1.25	No	0.06	10	1.44	0.052	1.07
	Mercy Hospital, Charlotte	4.9	0.0%	1.28	No	0.00	5	0.76	0.088	1.30
	Moore Regional Hospital, Pinehurst	7.6	0.0%	1.06	No	0.00	6	1.06	0.041	2.58
	Moses H. Cone Memorial Hospital, Greensboro	8.2	0.0%	1.44	Yes	0.10	9	0.98	0.020	1.18
	Nash General Hospital, Rocky Mount	4.1	0.0%	1.68	No	0.00	9	0.69	0.060	1.78
	New Hanover Regional Medical Center, Wilmington	4.6	0.0%	2.01	No	0.15	6	1.44	0.035	1.77
	Presbyterian Hospital, Charlotte	6.8	0.6%	1.63	No	0.00	7	1.27	0.142	2.50
	Wake Medical Center, Raleigh	4.9	0.0%	1.63	No	0.06	8	1.11	0.025	1.32
	Wesley Long Community Hospital, Greensboro	6.2	0.0%	1.44	No	0.00	6	1.36	0.088	2.19

AIDS

Natl. Rank	Hospital	U.S. News index	Reputational score	Hospital-wide mortality rate	COTH member	Interns and residents to beds	Technology score (of 11)	Discharge planning (of 2)	R.N.'s to beds	Board-certified internists to beds
TIER THREE										
	St. Alexius Medical Center, Bismarck	20.6	0.0%	0.92	No	0.03	5	1	1.11	0.014
	St. Joseph's Hospital, Minot	21.1	0.0%	0.88	No	0.02	5	2	0.40	0.064
TIER FOUR										
	Dakota Hospital, Fargo	18.1	0.0%	1.11	No	0.05	2	2	1.55	0.036
	MedCenter One, Bismarck	16.2	0.0%	1.23	No	0.03	4	2	0.86	0.025
	St. Luke's Hospitals Meritcare, Fargo	17.9	0.0%	1.18	No	0.04	8	2	0.55	0.068
	Trinity Medical Center, Minot	16.1	0.0%	1.14	No	0.01	6	1	0.17	0.019
	United Health Services, Grand Forks	18.4	0.0%	1.11	No	0.06	7	2	0.58	0.020

CANCER

Natl. Rank	Hospital	U.S. News index	Reputational score	Cancer mortality rate	COTH member	Interns and residents to beds	Technology score (of 12)	R.N.'s to beds	Board-certified oncologists to beds	Procedures to beds
TIER FOUR										
	Dakota Hospital, Fargo	4.0	0.0%	0.88	No	0.05	1	1.55	0.005	1.65
	MedCenter One, Bismarck	3.6	0.0%	0.97	No	0.03	7	0.86	0.013	1.40
	St. Alexius Medical Center, Bismarck	3.9	0.0%	0.66	No	0.03	4	1.11	0.011	1.25
	St. Joseph's Hospital, Minot	2.7	0.0%	0.45	No	0.02	7	0.40	0.006	0.96
	St. Luke's Hospitals Meritcare, Fargo	3.5	0.0%	0.98	No	0.04	9	0.55	0.013	1.94
	Trinity Medical Center, Minot	0.8	0.0%	0.66	No	0.01	3	0.17	0.004	0.40
	United Health Services, Grand Forks	3.6	0.0%	0.95	No	0.06	9	0.58	0.008	1.56

CARDIOLOGY

Natl. Rank	Hospital	U.S. News index	Reputational score	Cardiology mortality rate	COTH member	Interns and residents to beds	Technology score (of 10)	R.N.'s to beds	Board-certified cardiologists to beds	Procedures to beds
TIER THREE										
	St. Alexius Medical Center, Bismarck	17.6	0.0%	0.85	No	0.03	6	1.11	0.018	5.72
TIER FOUR										
	Dakota Hospital, Fargo	9.7	0.0%	1.26	No	0.05	3	1.55	0.016	7.66
	MedCenter One, Bismarck	9.8	0.0%	1.17	No	0.03	6	0.86	0.013	5.99
	St. Luke's Hospitals Meritcare, Fargo	9.0	0.0%	1.24	No	0.04	9	0.55	0.018	6.32
	Trinity Medical Center, Minot	4.3	0.0%	1.42	No	0.01	8	0.17	0.002	2.25
	United Health Services, Grand Forks	8.7	0.0%	1.23	No	0.06	8	0.58	0.004	6.97

ENDOCRINOLOGY

Natl. Rank	Hospital	U.S. News index	Reputational score	Endocrinology mortality rate	COTH member	Interns and residents to beds	Technology score (of 11)	R.N.'s to beds	Board-certified internists to beds
TIER THREE									
	Dakota Hospital, Fargo	8.3	0.0%	0.86	No	0.05	0	1.55	0.036
	St. Alexius Medical Center, Bismarck	10.0	0.0%	0.36	No	0.03	4	1.11	0.014
	United Health Services, Grand Forks	10.0	0.0%	0.60	No	0.06	10	0.58	0.020
TIER FOUR									
	MedCenter One, Bismarck	5.3	0.0%	1.22	No	0.03	7	0.86	0.025
	St. Luke's Hospitals Meritcare, Fargo	6.1	0.0%	1.04	No	0.04	9	0.55	0.068

GASTROENTEROLOGY

Natl. Rank	Hospital	U.S. News index	Reputa-tional score	Gastro-enterology mortality rate	COTH member	Interns and residents to beds	Tech-nology score (of 11)	R.N.'s to beds	Board-certified gastro-enterologists to beds	Pro-cedures to beds
		TIER FOUR								
	Dakota Hospital, Fargo	6.6	0.0%	0.92	No	0.05	0	1.55	0.010	3.12
	MedCenter One, Bismarck	4.4	0.0%	1.25	No	0.03	6	0.86	0.004	2.67
	St. Alexius Medical Center, Bismarck	3.6	0.0%	1.30	No	0.03	3	1.11	0.004	2.30
	St. Luke's Hospitals Meritcare, Fargo	5.0	0.0%	1.20	No	0.04	9	0.55	0.008	2.94
	Trinity Medical Center, Minot	3.6	0.0%	0.93	No	0.01	5	0.17	0.002	1.17
	United Health Services, Grand Forks	5.3	0.0%	1.24	No	0.06	9	0.58	0.004	3.50

GERIATRICS

Natl. Rank	Hospital	U.S. News index	Reputa-tional score	Hospital-wide mortality rate	COTH member	Service mix	Interns and residents to beds	Tech-nology score (of 13)	R.N.'s to beds	Discharge planning (of 2)	Geriatric services (of 9)	Board-certified internists to beds
		TIER THREE										
	St. Alexius Medical Center, Bismarck	16.2	0.0%	0.92	No	6	0.03	5	1.11	1	4	0.014
		TIER FOUR										
	Dakota Hospital, Fargo	10.9	0.0%	1.11	No	4	0.05	1	1.55	2	2	0.036
	MedCenter One, Bismarck	9.1	0.0%	1.23	No	4	0.03	8	0.86	2	5	0.025
	St. Luke's Hospitals Meritcare, Fargo	10.1	0.0%	1.18	No	4	0.04	11	0.55	2	4	0.068
	Trinity Medical Center, Minot	7.8	0.0%	1.14	No	5	0.01	6	0.17	1	2	0.019
	United Health Services, Grand Forks	12.2	0.0%	1.11	No	7	0.06	10	0.58	2	2	0.020

GYNECOLOGY

Natl. Rank	Hospital	U.S. News index	Reputa-tional score	Hospital-wide mortality rate	Interns and residents to beds	Tech-nology score (of 10)	R.N.'s to beds	Board-certified OB-GYNs to beds	Procedures to beds
		TIER THREE							
	St. Alexius Medical Center, Bismarck	16.1	0.0%	0.92	0.03	4	1.11	0.014	0.54
		TIER FOUR							
	Dakota Hospital, Fargo	10.9	0.0%	1.11	0.05	1	1.55	0.016	0.31
	MedCenter One, Bismarck	8.3	0.0%	1.23	0.03	5	0.86	0.021	0.34
	St. Luke's Hospitals Meritcare, Fargo	9.6	0.0%	1.18	0.04	7	0.55	0.029	0.39
	Trinity Medical Center, Minot	7.5	0.0%	1.14	0.01	6	0.17	0.006	0.14
	United Health Services, Grand Forks	11.9	0.0%	1.11	0.06	8	0.58	0.020	0.51

NEUROLOGY

Natl. Rank	Hospital	U.S. News index	Reputa-tional score	Neurology mortality rate	COTH member	Interns and residents to beds	Tech-nology score (of 9)	R.N.'s to beds	Board-certified neurologists to beds
		TIER FOUR							
	St. Alexius Medical Center, Bismarck	8.4	0.0%	1.07	No	0.03	3	1.11	0.014
	St. Luke's Hospitals Meritcare, Fargo	6.5	0.0%	1.22	No	0.04	7	0.55	0.016
	United Health Services, Grand Forks	9.0	0.0%	1.04	No	0.06	8	0.58	0.012

ORTHOPEDICS

Natl. Rank	Hospital	U.S. News index	Reputa-tional score	Orthopedics mortality rate	COTH member	Interns and residents to beds	Tech-nology score (of 5)	R.N.'s to beds	Board-certified orthopedists to beds	Pro-cedures to beds
	TIER FOUR									
	Dakota Hospital, Fargo	6.0	0.0%	1.16	No	0.05	0	1.55	0.026	6.33
	MedCenter One, Bismarck	3.1	0.0%	1.31	No	0.03	1	0.86	0.017	2.87
	St. Alexius Medical Center, Bismarck	6.1	0.3%	1.13	No	0.03	2	1.11	0.018	3.41
	St. Joseph's Hospital, Minot	6.1	0.0%	0.79	No	0.02	2	0.40	0.017	2.36
	St. Luke's Hospitals Meritcare, Fargo	7.0	0.0%	0.90	No	0.04	4	0.55	0.018	3.41
	Trinity Medical Center, Minot	7.1	0.0%	0.74	No	0.01	4	0.17	0.006	1.18
	United Health Services, Grand Forks	4.4	0.0%	1.47	No	0.06	4	0.58	0.024	5.15

OTOLARYNGOLOGY

Natl. Rank	Hospital	U.S. News index	Reputa-tional score	Hospital-wide mortality rate	COTH member	Interns and residents to beds	Tech-nology score (of 9)	R.N.'s to beds	Board-certified internists to beds	Procedures to beds
	TIER FOUR									
	Dakota Hospital, Fargo	5.2	0.0%	1.11	No	0.05	0	1.55	0.036	0.151
	MedCenter One, Bismarck	4.3	0.0%	1.23	No	0.03	5	0.86	0.025	0.222
	St. Alexius Medical Center, Bismarck	4.3	0.0%	0.92	No	0.03	2	1.11	0.014	0.149
	St. Joseph's Hospital, Minot	3.7	0.0%	0.87	No	0.02	6	0.40	0.064	0.249
	St. Luke's Hospitals Meritcare, Fargo	4.3	0.0%	1.18	No	0.04	7	0.55	0.068	0.260
	Trinity Medical Center, Minot	1.5	0.0%	1.14	No	0.01	3	0.17	0.019	0.113
	United Health Services, Grand Forks	4.4	0.0%	1.11	No	0.06	8	0.58	0.020	0.249

RHEUMATOLOGY

Natl. Rank	Hospital	U.S. News index	Reputa-tional score	Hospital-wide mortality rate	COTH member	Interns and residents to beds	Tech-nology score (of 5)	R.N.'s to beds	Board-certified internists to beds
	TIER FOUR								
	Dakota Hospital, Fargo	8.0	0.0%	1.11	No	0.05	0	1.55	0.036
	MedCenter One, Bismarck	5.6	0.0%	1.23	No	0.03	1	0.86	0.025
	St. Alexius Medical Center, Bismarck	8.2	0.0%	0.92	No	0.03	2	1.11	0.014
	St. Luke's Hospitals Meritcare, Fargo	6.8	0.0%	1.18	No	0.04	4	0.55	0.068
	Trinity Medical Center, Minot	4.7	0.0%	1.14	No	0.01	4	0.17	0.019
	United Health Services, Grand Forks	7.2	0.0%	1.11	No	0.06	4	0.58	0.020

UROLOGY

Natl. Rank	Hospital	U.S. News index	Reputa-tional score	Urology mortality rate	COTH member	Interns and residents to beds	Tech-nology score (of 11)	R.N.'s to beds	Board-certified internists to beds	Procedures to beds
	TIER THREE									
	MedCenter One, Bismarck	10.7	0.0%	0.49	No	0.03	6	0.86	0.025	1.68
	St. Alexius Medical Center, Bismarck	9.4	0.0%	0.79	No	0.03	3	1.11	0.014	1.45
	TIER FOUR									
	Dakota Hospital, Fargo	4.1	0.0%	1.65	No	0.05	0	1.55	0.036	2.19
	St. Luke's Hospitals Meritcare, Fargo	7.0	0.0%	1.07	No	0.04	9	0.55	0.068	1.82
	Trinity Medical Center, Minot	2.7	0.0%	1.34	No	0.01	5	0.17	0.019	1.15
	United Health Services, Grand Forks	7.5	0.0%	1.01	No	0.06	9	0.58	0.020	2.10

AIDS

Natl. Rank	Hospital	U.S. News index	Reputa- tional score	Hospital- wide mortality rate	COTH member	Interns and residents to beds	Tech- nology score (of 11)	Discharge planning (of 2)	R.N.'s to beds	Board- certified internists to beds
	TIER ONE									
25	**Cleveland Clinic**	**30.1**	1.2%	0.87	Yes	1.22	10	2	1.47	0.015
	TIER TWO									
64	**Medical College of Ohio Hospital, Toledo**	**26.3**	0.8%	1.11	Yes	1.42	10	2	1.23	0.132
75	**Mount Sinai Medical Center, Cleveland**	**25.7**	0.0%	0.87	Yes	0.76	6	2	0.86	0.144
55	**Ohio State University Medical Center, Columbus**	**26.7**	1.0%	0.94	Yes	0.81	8	2	1.11	0.029
47	**University Hospitals of Cleveland**	**27.6**	0.3%	1.07	Yes	1.60	11	2	1.73	0.080
	TIER THREE									
	Aultman Hospital, Canton	21.5	0.0%	0.92	No	0.19	6	2	0.67	0.054
	Deaconess Hospital, Cincinnati	20.2	0.0%	0.97	No	0.00	6	2	0.52	0.094
	Jewish Hospital of Cincinnati	21.9	0.0%	0.90	No	0.15	7	2	0.48	0.074
	Lakewood Hospital, Lakewood	21.8	0.0%	0.90	No	0.01	6	2	0.80	0.037
	Lorain Community Hospital, Lorain	21.6	0.0%	0.87	No	0.00	6	2	0.58	0.021
	Mercy Medical Center, Springfield	19.9	0.0%	1.04	No	0.00	7	2	1.04	0.022
	MetroHealth Medical Center, Cleveland	20.8	0.0%	1.20	Yes	0.54	9	2	0.69	0.038
	Middletown Regional Hospital, Middletown	20.7	0.0%	0.96	No	0.00	6	2	0.93	0.014
	Park Medical Center, Columbus	20.8	0.0%	0.86	No	0.02	5	1	0.77	0.011
	Riverside Methodist Hospitals, Columbus	21.0	0.0%	1.23	Yes	0.28	8	2	1.50	0.063
	St. Ann's Hospital of Columbus, Westerville	22.2	0.0%	0.95	No	0.02	6	2	1.26	0.181
	St. Luke's Medical Center, Cleveland	20.0	0.0%	1.25	Yes	0.42	7	2	1.01	0.105
	St. Rita's Medical Center, Lima	21.7	0.0%	0.94	No	0.00	7	2	1.11	0.019
	St. Vincent Medical Center, Toledo	22.9	0.0%	1.04	No	0.34	7	2	2.26	0.081
	Summa Health System, Akron	21.3	0.0%	1.17	Yes	0.39	7	2	1.39	0.039
	The Toledo Hospital, Toledo	22.5	0.8%	1.14	Yes	0.14	9	2	1.14	0.037
	TIER FOUR									
	Akron General Medical Center, Akron	18.8	0.0%	1.21	No	0.44	7	2	1.04	0.054
	Barberton Citizens Hospital, Barberton	16.8	0.0%	1.18	No	0.12	5	2	0.57	0.018
	Bethesda Hospital, Zanesville	16.9	0.0%	1.22	No	0.00	4	2	1.23	0.042
	Bethesda Oak Hospital, Cincinnati	19.5	0.0%	1.07	No	0.16	7	2	0.63	0.109
	Doctor's Hospital, Columbus	17.4	0.0%	1.24	No	0.35	7	1	0.90	0.071
	Elyria Memorial Hospital and Medical Center, Elyria	18.5	0.0%	1.08	No	0.01	6	2	0.78	0.021
	Fairview General Hospital, Cleveland	19.3	0.0%	1.01	No	0.17	4	2	0.84	0.024
	Flower Hospital, Sylvania	18.8	0.0%	1.04	No	0.11	6	2	0.46	0.016
	Good Samaritan Hospital and Health Center, Dayton	17.1	0.0%	1.20	No	0.20	5	2	0.79	0.018
	Good Samaritan Hospital, Cincinnati	19.2	0.0%	1.25	Yes	0.23	6	2	1.03	0.075
	Grant Medical Center, Columbus	19.5	0.0%	1.17	Yes	0.20	5	2	1.09	0.011
	Greene Memorial Hospital, Xenia	16.5	0.0%	1.22	No	0.01	5	2	0.80	0.024
	Kettering Medical Center, Kettering	19.0	0.0%	1.31	Yes	0.18	8	2	0.97	0.039
	Licking Memorial Hospital, Newark	18.0	0.0%	1.22	No	0.00	6	2	1.53	0.016
	Lima Memorial Hospital, Lima	18.7	0.0%	1.05	No	0.00	6	1	0.94	0.040
	Mansfield General Hospital, Mansfield	16.4	0.0%	1.28	No	0.00	7	2	0.60	0.038
	Mercy Hospital, Hamilton	17.9	0.0%	1.15	No	0.20	6	2	0.56	0.077
	Mercy Hospital, Toledo	18.4	0.0%	1.20	No	0.29	6	2	1.22	0.040
	Meridia Huron Hospital, Cleveland	15.3	0.0%	1.35	No	0.35	4	2	0.62	0.042
	Miami Valley Hospital, Dayton	19.4	0.0%	1.29	Yes	0.27	8	2	0.95	0.036
	Mount Carmel Health, Columbus	16.8	0.0%	1.34	No	0.17	8	2	0.78	0.039
	Providence Hospital, Sandusky	16.0	0.0%	1.17	No	0.00	6	1	0.32	0.027
	Robinson Memorial Hospital, Ravenna	19.2	0.0%	1.04	No	0.04	6	2	0.73	0.021
	St. Elizabeth Hospital Medical Center, Youngstown	17.5	0.0%	1.37	Yes	0.21	6	2	0.87	0.028
	St. Elizabeth Medical Center, Dayton	17.5	0.0%	1.15	No	0.15	5	1	1.11	0.041
	St. John Medical Center, Steubenville	16.0	0.0%	1.27	No	0.00	6	2	0.61	0.025
	St. Vincent Charity Hospital, Cleveland	17.7	0.0%	1.13	No	0.06	5	2	0.73	0.067

Natl. Rank	Hospital	U.S. News index	Reputational score	Hospital-wide mortality rate	COTH member	Interns and residents to beds	Technology score (of 11)	Discharge planning (of 2)	R.N.'s to beds	Board-certified internists to beds
	Stouder Memorial Hospital, Troy	18.2	0.0%	1.16	No	0.00	7	2	0.88	0.043
	Timken Mercy Medical Center, Canton	15.7	0.0%	1.28	No	0.04	7	1	0.58	0.040
	Western Reserve System-Southside, Youngstown	19.1	0.0%	1.17	No	0.65	5	2	1.12	0.059

CANCER

Natl. Rank	Hospital	U.S. News index	Reputational score	Cancer mortality rate	COTH member	Interns and residents to beds	Technology score (of 12)	R.N.'s to beds	Board-certified oncologists to beds	Procedures to beds
TIER TWO										
23	Cleveland Clinic	15.8	1.9%	0.64	Yes	1.22	11	1.47	0.009	1.80
47	Medical College of Ohio Hospital, Toledo	13.1	0.5%	0.76	Yes	1.42	9	1.23	0.022	0.92
25	University Hospitals of Cleveland	15.5	0.0%	0.79	Yes	1.60	12	1.73	0.032	1.54
TIER THREE										
	Akron General Medical Center, Akron	5.7	0.0%	1.13	No	0.44	8	1.04	0.013	1.99
	Good Samaritan Hospital, Cincinnati	7.6	0.0%	1.05	Yes	0.23	9	1.03	0.015	0.80
	Grant Medical Center, Columbus	7.2	0.0%	0.81	Yes	0.20	6	1.09	0.018	1.20
	Kettering Medical Center, Kettering	7.4	0.0%	1.01	Yes	0.18	9	0.97	0.014	0.98
	MetroHealth Medical Center, Cleveland	8.2	0.0%	1.02	Yes	0.54	11	0.69	0.008	0.61
	Miami Valley Hospital, Dayton	7.6	0.0%	0.99	Yes	0.27	9	0.95	0.006	1.34
82	Mount Sinai Medical Center, Cleveland	10.9	1.5%	0.87	Yes	0.76	8	0.86	0.016	1.36
100	Ohio State University Medical Center, Columbus	10.2	1.1%	0.44	Yes	0.81	4	1.11	0.014	0.41
	Riverside Methodist Hospitals, Columbus	10.0	0.0%	0.90	Yes	0.28	11	1.50	0.008	2.01
	St. Elizabeth Hospital Medical Center, Youngstown	6.7	0.0%	1.26	Yes	0.21	8	0.87	0.007	1.16
	St. Luke's Medical Center, Cleveland	7.2	0.0%	1.18	Yes	0.42	6	1.01	0.000	0.96
	St. Vincent Medical Center, Toledo	9.7	0.0%	0.50	No	0.34	9	2.26	0.032	0.99
	Summa Health System, Akron	8.2	0.0%	1.17	Yes	0.39	6	1.39	0.009	1.02
	The Toledo Hospital, Toledo	8.2	0.0%	0.85	Yes	0.14	10	1.14	0.009	1.13
	University of Cincinnati Hospital	7.7	0.0%	0.47	Yes	0.78	0	1.10	0.008	0.92
	Western Reserve System-Southside, Youngstown	6.5	0.0%	0.90	No	0.65	6	1.12	0.010	3.12
TIER FOUR										
	Aultman Hospital, Canton	4.3	0.0%	0.69	No	0.19	8	0.67	0.007	1.50
	Barberton Citizens Hospital, Barberton	2.8	0.0%	1.03	No	0.12	6	0.57	0.007	1.88
	Bethesda Hospital, Zanesville	3.5	0.0%	1.14	No	0.00	4	1.23	0.004	1.29
	Bethesda Oak Hospital, Cincinnati	4.1	0.0%	0.85	No	0.16	8	0.63	0.030	1.99
	Christ Hospital, Cincinnati	3.7	0.0%	0.85	No	0.12	9	0.54	0.011	1.17
	Deaconess Hospital, Cincinnati	2.8	0.0%	0.63	No	0.00	6	0.52	0.015	1.25
	Doctor's Hospital, Columbus	4.6	0.0%	1.18	No	0.35	7	0.90	0.012	1.30
	Elyria Memorial Hospital and Medical Center, Elyria	3.1	0.0%	0.69	No	0.01	5	0.78	0.007	1.21
	Fairview General Hospital, Cleveland	2.9	0.0%	0.89	No	0.17	3	0.84	0.004	1.21
	Firelands Community Hospital, Sandusky	4.5	0.0%	0.59	No	0.08	10	0.59	0.011	1.69
	Flower Hospital, Sylvania	3.1	0.0%	0.70	No	0.11	7	0.46	0.016	0.79
	Good Samaritan Hospital and Health Center, Dayton	3.6	0.0%	0.95	No	0.20	6	0.79	0.000	1.09
	Greene Memorial Hospital, Xenia	2.3	0.0%	1.06	No	0.01	4	0.80	0.005	0.94
	Jewish Hospital of Cincinnati	3.7	0.0%	0.84	No	0.15	9	0.48	0.008	1.38
	Lakewood Hospital, Lakewood	3.0	0.0%	0.98	No	0.01	6	0.80	0.003	1.40
	Licking Memorial Hospital, Newark	5.2	0.0%	1.04	No	0.00	7	1.53	0.000	1.10
	Lima Memorial Hospital, Lima	4.5	0.0%	0.67	No	0.00	8	0.94	0.015	1.24
	Lorain Community Hospital, Lorain	2.6	0.0%	0.80	No	0.00	6	0.58	0.008	0.87
	Mansfield General Hospital, Mansfield	3.1	0.0%	1.30	No	0.00	9	0.60	0.006	1.40
	Mercy Hospital, Hamilton	3.5	0.0%	0.69	No	0.20	6	0.56	0.022	1.02
	Mercy Hospital, Toledo	5.0	0.0%	0.97	No	0.29	5	1.22	0.017	1.53
	Mercy Medical Center, Springfield	4.4	0.0%	0.88	No	0.00	8	1.04	0.004	1.42
	Meridia Huron Hospital, Cleveland	2.4	0.0%	1.36	No	0.35	3	0.62	0.007	0.63
	Middletown Regional Hospital, Middletown	3.9	0.0%	0.65	No	0.00	6	0.93	0.011	1.04
	Mount Carmel Health, Columbus	4.5	0.0%	0.94	No	0.17	9	0.78	0.007	1.88

Natl. Rank	Hospital	U.S. News index	Reputational score	Cancer mortality rate	COTH member	Interns and residents to beds	Technology score (of 12)	R.N.'s to beds	Board-certified oncologists to beds	Procedures to beds
	Park Medical Center, Columbus	2.9	0.0%	0.72	No	0.02	4	0.77	0.022	1.24
	Providence Hospital, Sandusky	2.4	0.0%	0.46	No	0.00	7	0.32	0.008	0.84
	Robinson Memorial Hospital, Ravenna	3.1	0.0%	0.61	No	0.04	5	0.73	0.011	0.71
	St. Ann's Hospital of Columbus, Westerville	4.4	0.0%	0.67	No	0.02	4	1.26	0.030	1.22
	St. Elizabeth Medical Center, Dayton	4.8	0.0%	0.65	No	0.15	6	1.11	0.000	0.96
	St. Rita's Medical Center, Lima	4.6	0.0%	0.84	No	0.00	8	1.11	0.009	1.33
	St. Vincent Charity Hospital, Cleveland	3.4	0.0%	0.78	No	0.06	7	0.73	0.012	0.53
	Timken Mercy Medical Center, Canton	3.5	0.0%	0.92	No	0.04	9	0.58	0.010	1.26
	Trumbull Memorial Hospital, Warren	3.6	0.0%	1.01	No	0.00	8	0.84	0.000	1.03

CARDIOLOGY

Natl. Rank	Hospital	U.S. News index	Reputational score	Cardiology mortality rate	COTH member	Interns and residents to beds	Technology score (of 10)	R.N.'s to beds	Board-certified cardiologists to beds	Procedures to beds
TIER ONE										
1	Cleveland Clinic	100.0	49.9%	0.90	Yes	1.22	10	1.47	0.035	9.03
TIER TWO										
37	Mount Sinai Medical Center, Cleveland	24.6	1.0%	0.81	Yes	0.76	8	0.86	0.024	8.29
78	Ohio State University Medical Center, Columbus	21.4	1.0%	1.04	Yes	0.81	9	1.11	0.041	6.01
35	University Hospitals of Cleveland	25.0	0.0%	1.03	Yes	1.60	10	1.73	0.037	4.70
TIER THREE										
	Aultman Hospital, Canton	16.3	0.0%	0.93	No	0.19	9	0.67	0.018	6.52
	Christ Hospital, Cincinnati	14.4	0.0%	0.99	No	0.12	8	0.54	0.042	6.97
	Elyria Memorial Hospital and Medical Center, Elyria	13.8	0.0%	1.05	No	0.01	9	0.78	0.046	10.99
	Lakewood Hospital, Lakewood	15.9	0.0%	0.94	No	0.01	9	0.80	0.019	9.75
	Lima Memorial Hospital, Lima	14.0	0.0%	0.98	No	0.00	6	0.94	0.000	8.62
	Lorain Community Hospital, Lorain	14.0	0.0%	0.97	No	0.00	7	0.58	0.041	5.58
	Medical College of Ohio Hospital, Toledo	17.4	0.0%	1.31	Yes	1.42	8	1.23	0.040	5.15
	Park Medical Center, Columbus	16.6	0.0%	0.86	No	0.02	5	0.77	0.033	5.96
	Riverside Methodist Hospitals, Columbus	15.1	0.0%	1.29	Yes	0.28	10	1.50	0.024	9.99
	Robinson Memorial Hospital, Ravenna	15.5	0.0%	0.91	No	0.04	6	0.73	0.018	6.83
	St. Ann's Hospital of Columbus, Westerville	15.6	0.0%	1.00	No	0.02	6	1.26	0.120	8.61
	St. Luke's Medical Center, Cleveland	15.2	0.0%	1.18	Yes	0.42	8	1.01	0.031	5.55
	St. Rita's Medical Center, Lima	17.6	0.0%	0.85	No	0.00	7	1.11	0.003	6.36
	St. Vincent Medical Center, Toledo	17.6	0.0%	1.12	No	0.34	8	2.26	0.063	8.83
	Summa Health System, Akron	15.4	0.0%	1.21	Yes	0.39	8	1.39	0.021	3.85
	The Toledo Hospital, Toledo	16.4	0.0%	1.11	Yes	0.14	10	1.14	0.024	6.42
TIER FOUR										
	Akron General Medical Center, Akron	12.1	0.0%	1.24	No	0.44	9	1.04	0.017	11.29
	Barberton Citizens Hospital, Barberton	6.2	0.0%	1.36	No	0.12	5	0.57	0.004	8.67
	Bethesda Hospital, Zanesville	9.1	0.0%	1.25	No	0.00	4	1.23	0.021	7.09
	Bethesda Oak Hospital, Cincinnati	9.2	0.0%	1.23	No	0.16	5	0.63	0.047	9.66
	Deaconess Hospital, Cincinnati	10.2	0.0%	1.17	No	0.00	9	0.52	0.030	8.28
	Doctor's Hospital, Columbus	10.8	0.0%	1.27	No	0.35	9	0.90	0.033	5.79
	Fairview General Hospital, Cleveland	10.9	0.0%	1.18	No	0.17	7	0.84	0.026	8.87
	Firelands Community Hospital, Sandusky	7.4	0.0%	1.28	No	0.08	6	0.59	0.016	4.70
	Flower Hospital, Sylvania	12.4	0.0%	0.99	No	0.11	6	0.46	0.005	3.09
	Good Samaritan Hospital and Health Center, Dayton	9.9	0.4%	1.30	No	0.20	7	0.79	0.036	9.53
	Good Samaritan Hospital, Cincinnati	12.4	0.0%	1.32	Yes	0.23	8	1.03	0.024	7.07
	Grant Medical Center, Columbus	11.3	0.0%	1.38	Yes	0.20	7	1.09	0.024	6.43
	Greene Memorial Hospital, Xenia	5.9	0.0%	1.36	No	0.01	4	0.80	0.005	4.41
	Jewish Hospital of Cincinnati	12.5	0.0%	1.06	No	0.15	9	0.48	0.032	5.38
	Kettering Medical Center, Kettering	11.1	0.0%	1.42	Yes	0.18	10	0.97	0.019	6.39
	Licking Memorial Hospital, Newark	10.6	0.0%	1.25	No	0.00	6	1.53	0.010	8.50
	Mansfield General Hospital, Mansfield	9.9	0.0%	1.14	No	0.00	7	0.60	0.013	6.47

Natl. Rank	Hospital	U.S. News index	Reputa-tional score	Cardiology mortality rate	COTH member	Interns and residents to beds	Tech-nology score (of 10)	R.N.'s to beds	Board-certified cardiologists to beds	Procedures to beds
	Mercy Hospital, Hamilton	8.3	0.0%	1.33	No	0.20	7	0.56	0.047	7.30
	Mercy Hospital, Toledo	8.4	0.0%	1.39	No	0.29	5	1.22	0.017	6.57
	Mercy Medical Center, Springfield	13.3	0.0%	1.05	No	0.00	6	1.04	0.031	9.06
	Meridia Huron Hospital, Cleveland	10.5	0.0%	1.19	No	0.35	6	0.62	0.035	8.09
	MetroHealth Medical Center, Cleveland	11.9	0.0%	1.36	Yes	0.54	9	0.69	0.026	2.05
	Miami Valley Hospital, Dayton	11.9	0.0%	1.37	Yes	0.27	9	0.95	0.030	6.08
	Middletown Regional Hospital, Middletown	11.5	0.0%	1.11	No	0.00	7	0.93	0.022	6.39
	Mount Carmel Health, Columbus	7.3	0.0%	1.46	No	0.17	8	0.78	0.025	10.87
	Providence Hospital, Sandusky	4.9	0.0%	1.41	No	0.00	6	0.32	0.027	4.03
	St. Elizabeth Hospital Medical Center, Youngstown	11.1	0.0%	1.37	Yes	0.21	8	0.87	0.015	8.70
	St. Elizabeth Medical Center, Dayton	8.6	0.0%	1.33	No	0.15	7	1.11	0.000	6.38
	St. John Medical Center, Steubenville	6.9	0.0%	1.33	No	0.00	6	0.61	0.025	7.55
	St. Vincent Charity Hospital, Cleveland	8.1	0.0%	1.32	No	0.06	7	0.73	0.034	8.35
	Stouder Memorial Hospital, Troy	11.1	0.0%	1.11	No	0.00	6	0.88	0.022	7.49
	Timken Mercy Medical Center, Canton	6.3	0.0%	1.45	No	0.04	9	0.58	0.020	7.16
	Trumbull Memorial Hospital, Warren	11.2	0.0%	1.12	No	0.00	7	0.84	0.026	6.52
	University of Cincinnati Hospital	10.0	0.0%	1.47	Yes	0.78	0	1.10	0.021	4.12
	Western Reserve System-Southside, Youngstown	11.3	0.0%	1.22	No	0.65	2	1.12	0.021	14.91

ENDOCRINOLOGY

Natl. Rank	Hospital	U.S. News index	Reputa-tional score	Endocrinology mortality rate	COTH member	Interns and residents to beds	Tech-nology score (of 11)	R.N.'s to beds	Board-certified internists to beds
	TIER ONE								
22	Cleveland Clinic	22.5	5.5%	1.02	Yes	1.22	11	1.47	0.015
	TIER TWO								
34	Medical College of Ohio Hospital, Toledo	19.3	0.0%	0.55	Yes	1.42	9	1.23	0.132
32	Ohio State University Medical Center, Columbus	19.9	3.2%	0.44	Yes	0.81	6	1.11	0.029
38	University Hospitals of Cleveland	18.7	0.0%	0.88	Yes	1.60	11	1.73	0.080
	TIER THREE								
	Akron General Medical Center, Akron	9.6	0.0%	0.91	No	0.44	9	1.04	0.054
	Aultman Hospital, Canton	9.4	0.0%	0.73	No	0.19	8	0.67	0.054
	Bethesda Hospital, Zanesville	9.0	0.0%	0.78	No	0.00	5	1.23	0.042
	Flower Hospital, Sylvania	9.3	0.0%	0.36	No	0.11	8	0.46	0.016
	Good Samaritan Hospital and Health Center, Dayton	8.5	0.0%	0.80	No	0.20	7	0.79	0.018
	Good Samaritan Hospital, Cincinnati	8.6	0.0%	1.51	Yes	0.23	9	1.03	0.075
	Grant Medical Center, Columbus	9.2	0.0%	1.16	Yes	0.20	7	1.09	0.011
	Jewish Hospital of Cincinnati	8.9	0.0%	0.74	No	0.15	9	0.48	0.074
	Kettering Medical Center, Kettering	8.6	0.0%	1.39	Yes	0.18	10	0.97	0.039
	MetroHealth Medical Center, Cleveland	12.8	0.0%	0.78	Yes	0.54	10	0.69	0.038
	Mount Sinai Medical Center, Cleveland	12.1	0.0%	1.08	Yes	0.76	9	0.86	0.144
	Riverside Methodist Hospitals, Columbus	10.7	0.0%	1.39	Yes	0.28	11	1.50	0.063
	St. Luke's Medical Center, Cleveland	9.0	0.0%	1.49	Yes	0.42	7	1.01	0.105
	St. Rita's Medical Center, Lima	9.7	0.0%	0.75	No	0.00	9	1.11	0.019
	St. Vincent Medical Center, Toledo	10.2	0.0%	1.34	No	0.34	8	2.26	0.081
	Summa Health System, Akron	12.5	0.0%	0.92	Yes	0.39	8	1.39	0.039
	The Toledo Hospital, Toledo	9.1	0.0%	1.33	Yes	0.14	10	1.14	0.037
	University of Cincinnati Hospital	13.0	0.3%	0.82	Yes	0.78	0	1.10	0.074
	TIER FOUR								
	Barberton Citizens Hospital, Barberton	4.5	0.0%	1.27	No	0.12	7	0.57	0.018
	Bethesda Oak Hospital, Cincinnati	7.8	0.0%	0.94	No	0.16	9	0.63	0.109
	Christ Hospital, Cincinnati	7.0	0.0%	0.96	No	0.12	10	0.54	0.052
	Deaconess Hospital, Cincinnati	4.8	0.0%	1.22	No	0.00	7	0.52	0.094
	Doctor's Hospital, Columbus	7.1	0.0%	1.24	No	0.35	9	0.90	0.071
	Elyria Memorial Hospital and Medical Center, Elyria	6.7	0.0%	0.90	No	0.01	6	0.78	0.021

Natl. Rank	Hospital	U.S. News index	Reputa- tional score	Endocrinology mortality rate	COTH member	Interns and residents to beds	Tech- nology score (of 11)	R.N.'s to beds	Board- certified internists to beds
	Fairview General Hospital, Cleveland	7.3	0.0%	0.87	No	0.17	4	0.84	0.024
	Firelands Community Hospital, Sandusky	4.5	0.0%	1.50	No	0.08	11	0.59	0.027
	Lakewood Hospital, Lakewood	6.7	0.0%	0.92	No	0.01	6	0.80	0.037
	Licking Memorial Hospital, Newark	6.7	0.0%	1.32	No	0.00	8	1.53	0.016
	Lima Memorial Hospital, Lima	7.4	0.0%	0.96	No	0.00	9	0.94	0.040
	Lorain Community Hospital, Lorain	5.5	0.0%	1.02	No	0.00	7	0.58	0.021
	Mansfield General Hospital, Mansfield	3.9	0.0%	1.59	No	0.00	10	0.60	0.038
	Mercy Hospital, Hamilton	5.6	0.0%	1.16	No	0.20	7	0.56	0.077
	Mercy Hospital, Toledo	5.0	0.0%	1.93	No	0.29	6	1.22	0.040
	Mercy Medical Center, Springfield	5.2	0.0%	1.39	No	0.00	8	1.04	0.022
	Meridia Huron Hospital, Cleveland	4.2	0.0%	1.42	No	0.35	3	0.62	0.042
	Miami Valley Hospital, Dayton	7.7	0.0%	1.79	Yes	0.27	10	0.95	0.036
	Middletown Regional Hospital, Middletown	8.0	0.0%	0.82	No	0.00	7	0.93	0.014
	Mount Carmel Health, Columbus	5.1	0.0%	1.47	No	0.17	9	0.78	0.039
	Park Medical Center, Columbus	7.2	0.0%	0.82	No	0.02	5	0.77	0.011
	Providence Hospital, Sandusky	2.9	0.0%	1.49	No	0.00	8	0.32	0.027
	Robinson Memorial Hospital, Ravenna	4.0	0.0%	1.41	No	0.04	6	0.73	0.021
	St. Ann's Hospital of Columbus, Westerville	6.9	0.0%	1.24	No	0.02	5	1.26	0.181
	St. Elizabeth Hospital Medical Center, Youngstown	7.6	0.0%	1.56	Yes	0.21	9	0.87	0.028
	St. Elizabeth Medical Center, Dayton	5.7	0.0%	1.40	No	0.15	7	1.11	0.041
	St. John Medical Center, Steubenville	5.3	0.0%	1.07	No	0.00	7	0.61	0.025
	St. Vincent Charity Hospital, Cleveland	6.0	0.4%	1.20	No	0.06	7	0.73	0.067
	Timken Mercy Medical Center, Canton	3.5	0.0%	1.71	No	0.04	9	0.58	0.040
	Trumbull Memorial Hospital, Warren	5.9	0.0%	1.16	No	0.00	9	0.84	0.034
	Western Reserve System-Southside, Youngstown	7.9	0.0%	1.31	No	0.65	7	1.12	0.059

GASTROENTEROLOGY

Natl. Rank	Hospital	U.S. News index	Reputa- tional score	Gastro- enterology mortality rate	COTH member	Interns and residents to beds	Tech- nology score (of 11)	R.N.'s to beds	Board- certified gastro- enterologists to beds	Pro- cedures to beds
TIER ONE										
4	**Cleveland Clinic**	53.0	24.1%	0.71	Yes	1.22	10	1.47	0.012	2.31
TIER TWO										
59	**Mount Sinai Medical Center, Cleveland**	14.3	1.1%	0.95	Yes	0.76	8	0.86	0.035	3.25
26	**University Hospitals of Cleveland**	17.7	0.0%	0.97	Yes	1.60	11	1.73	0.027	2.15
TIER THREE										
	Christ Hospital, Cincinnati	7.4	0.0%	0.77	No	0.12	9	0.54	0.012	1.58
	Elyria Memorial Hospital and Medical Center, Elyria	7.4	0.0%	0.73	No	0.01	6	0.78	0.007	2.95
	Fairview General Hospital, Cleveland	7.4	0.0%	0.83	No	0.17	4	0.84	0.009	3.07
	Good Samaritan Hospital, Cincinnati	8.3	0.0%	1.31	Yes	0.23	8	1.03	0.011	2.26
	Grant Medical Center, Columbus	9.9	0.0%	0.93	Yes	0.20	6	1.09	0.015	2.08
	Jewish Hospital of Cincinnati	7.6	0.0%	0.79	No	0.15	8	0.48	0.020	2.51
	Kettering Medical Center, Kettering	8.2	0.0%	1.38	Yes	0.18	9	0.97	0.014	2.58
	Mercy Hospital, Toledo	8.1	0.0%	1.04	No	0.29	6	1.22	0.017	3.98
	Mercy Medical Center, Springfield	8.2	0.0%	0.87	No	0.00	7	1.04	0.013	3.81
	MetroHealth Medical Center, Cleveland	8.7	0.0%	1.15	Yes	0.54	9	0.69	0.010	0.72
	Miami Valley Hospital, Dayton	8.4	0.0%	1.40	Yes	0.27	9	0.95	0.016	2.58
	Ohio State University Medical Center, Columbus	10.8	0.4%	1.19	Yes	0.81	6	1.11	0.011	1.58
	Park Medical Center, Columbus	7.6	0.0%	0.63	No	0.02	5	0.77	0.027	3.58
98	Riverside Methodist Hospitals, Columbus	11.8	0.0%	1.10	Yes	0.28	10	1.50	0.015	3.29
	St. Luke's Medical Center, Cleveland	8.4	0.0%	1.35	Yes	0.42	7	1.01	0.008	2.20
	St. Vincent Medical Center, Toledo	9.8	0.0%	1.09	No	0.34	7	2.26	0.021	2.24
	Summa Health System, Akron	10.0	0.0%	1.14	Yes	0.39	7	1.39	0.010	1.81
	The Toledo Hospital, Toledo	9.4	0.0%	1.16	Yes	0.14	9	1.14	0.016	2.52

Natl. Rank	Hospital	U.S. News index	Reputa-tional score	Gastro-enterology mortality rate	COTH member	Interns and residents to beds	Tech-nology score (of 11)	R.N.'s to beds	Board-certified gastro-enterologists to beds	Pro-cedures to beds
	University of Cincinnati Hospital	10.3	0.4%	0.94	Yes	0.78	0	1.10	0.011	1.45
	Western Reserve System-Southside, Youngstown	10.8	0.0%	1.07	No	0.65	6	1.12	0.003	7.14
TIER FOUR										
	Akron General Medical Center, Akron	6.9	0.0%	1.37	No	0.44	8	1.04	0.010	3.44
	Aultman Hospital, Canton	5.3	0.0%	1.16	No	0.19	7	0.67	0.010	2.63
	Barberton Citizens Hospital, Barberton	6.0	0.0%	1.03	No	0.12	6	0.57	0.004	3.81
	Bethesda Hospital, Zanesville	3.9	0.0%	1.49	No	0.00	4	1.23	0.000	3.22
	Bethesda Oak Hospital, Cincinnati	7.0	0.0%	1.18	No	0.16	9	0.63	0.017	5.01
	Deaconess Hospital, Cincinnati	5.8	0.0%	0.95	No	0.00	6	0.52	0.023	3.34
	Doctor's Hospital, Columbus	5.3	0.0%	1.44	No	0.35	8	0.90	0.017	2.33
	Firelands Community Hospital, Sandusky	6.2	0.0%	1.09	No	0.08	10	0.59	0.011	2.85
	Flower Hospital, Sylvania	4.2	0.0%	1.12	No	0.11	7	0.46	0.005	1.78
	Good Samaritan Hospital and Health Center, Dayton	4.9	0.0%	1.24	No	0.20	6	0.79	0.009	2.63
	Lakewood Hospital, Lakewood	5.8	0.0%	1.10	No	0.01	6	0.80	0.006	4.03
	Licking Memorial Hospital, Newark	6.7	0.0%	1.38	No	0.00	7	1.53	0.010	4.54
	Lima Memorial Hospital, Lima	4.2	0.0%	1.66	No	0.00	8	0.94	0.015	3.56
	Lorain Community Hospital, Lorain	5.3	0.0%	0.94	No	0.00	6	0.58	0.012	2.28
	Mansfield General Hospital, Mansfield	3.9	0.0%	1.42	No	0.00	9	0.60	0.006	2.69
	Mercy Hospital, Hamilton	6.3	0.0%	1.00	No	0.20	6	0.56	0.018	3.40
	Meridia Huron Hospital, Cleveland	1.8	0.0%	1.94	No	0.35	3	0.62	0.024	2.09
	Middletown Regional Hospital, Middletown	6.8	0.0%	0.93	No	0.00	6	0.93	0.018	3.11
	Mount Carmel Health, Columbus	5.7	0.0%	1.29	No	0.17	8	0.78	0.013	3.58
	Robinson Memorial Hospital, Ravenna	5.0	0.0%	1.08	No	0.04	6	0.73	0.004	2.63
	St. Ann's Hospital of Columbus, Westerville	7.3	0.0%	1.01	No	0.02	5	1.26	0.072	3.83
	St. Elizabeth Hospital Medical Center, Youngstown	7.2	0.0%	1.67	Yes	0.21	8	0.87	0.003	3.24
	St. Elizabeth Medical Center, Dayton	5.6	0.0%	1.20	No	0.15	6	1.11	0.000	2.53
	St. John Medical Center, Steubenville	4.5	0.0%	1.20	No	0.00	7	0.61	0.012	3.02
	St. Rita's Medical Center, Lima	6.6	0.0%	1.05	No	0.00	8	1.11	0.009	2.75
	St. Vincent Charity Hospital, Cleveland	6.8	0.0%	0.77	No	0.06	6	0.73	0.018	1.59
	Stouder Memorial Hospital, Troy	4.9	0.0%	1.39	No	0.00	8	0.88	0.007	3.58
	Timken Mercy Medical Center, Canton	4.8	0.0%	1.16	No	0.04	8	0.58	0.018	2.45
	Trumbull Memorial Hospital, Warren	6.5	0.0%	1.00	No	0.00	8	0.84	0.006	2.88

GERIATRICS

Natl. Rank	Hospital	U.S. News index	Reputa-tional score	Hospital-wide mortality rate	COTH member	Service mix	Interns and residents to beds	Tech-nology score (of 13)	R.N.'s to beds	Discharge planning (of 2)	Geriatric services (of 9)	Board-certified internists to beds
TIER ONE												
12	Cleveland Clinic	42.0	5.8%	0.87	Yes	9	1.22	12	1.47	2	4	0.015
TIER TWO												
41	Mount Sinai Medical Center, Cleveland	25.7	0.4%	0.87	Yes	8	0.76	10	0.86	2	6	0.144
78	Ohio State University Medical Center, Columbus	22.3	0.0%	0.94	Yes	8	0.81	7	1.11	2	5	0.029
30	University Hospitals of Cleveland	26.9	1.4%	1.07	Yes	8	1.60	13	1.73	2	5	0.080
TIER THREE												
	Aultman Hospital, Canton	18.5	0.0%	0.92	No	7	0.19	11	0.67	2	3	0.054
	Christ Hospital, Cincinnati	14.9	0.0%	0.92	No	4	0.12	10	0.54	1	1	0.052
	Deaconess Hospital, Cincinnati	15.8	0.0%	0.97	No	6	0.00	9	0.52	2	4	0.094
	Fairview General Hospital, Cleveland	14.1	0.0%	1.01	No	5	0.17	6	0.84	2	4	0.024
	Jewish Hospital of Cincinnati	19.5	0.0%	0.90	No	6	0.15	12	0.48	2	7	0.074
	Lakewood Hospital, Lakewood	18.5	0.0%	0.90	No	6	0.01	9	0.80	2	4	0.037
	Lorain Community Hospital, Lorain	16.9	0.0%	0.87	No	6	0.00	7	0.58	2	1	0.021
	Medical College of Ohio Hospital, Toledo	19.7	0.0%	1.11	Yes	7	1.42	10	1.23	2	4	0.132
	MetroHealth Medical Center, Cleveland	15.5	0.0%	1.20	Yes	8	0.54	12	0.69	2	6	0.038
	Miami Valley Hospital, Dayton	14.8	0.0%	1.29	Yes	9	0.27	11	0.95	2	9	0.036

Natl. Rank	Hospital	U.S. News index	Reputational score	Hospital-wide mortality rate	COTH member	Service mix	Interns and residents to beds	Technology score (of 13)	R.N.'s to beds	Discharge planning (of 2)	Geriatric services (of 9)	Board-certified internists to beds
	Middletown Regional Hospital, Middletown	16.8	0.0%	0.96	No	7	0.00	9	0.93	2	3	0.014
	Park Medical Center, Columbus	15.5	0.0%	0.86	No	5	0.02	6	0.77	1	1	0.011
	Riverside Methodist Hospitals, Columbus	16.3	0.0%	1.23	Yes	8	0.28	13	1.50	2	6	0.063
	St. Ann's Hospital of Columbus, Westerville	16.2	0.0%	0.95	No	4	0.02	6	1.26	2	1	0.181
	St. Luke's Medical Center, Cleveland	13.9	0.0%	1.25	Yes	7	0.42	9	1.01	2	5	0.105
	St. Rita's Medical Center, Lima	18.1	0.0%	0.94	No	7	0.00	11	1.11	2	3	0.019
	St. Vincent Medical Center, Toledo	18.7	0.0%	1.04	No	8	0.34	11	2.26	2	2	0.081
	Summa Health System, Akron	15.6	0.0%	1.17	Yes	7	0.39	10	1.39	2	3	0.039
	The Toledo Hospital, Toledo	15.3	0.0%	1.14	Yes	7	0.14	12	1.14	2	2	0.037
TIER FOUR												
	Akron General Medical Center, Akron	11.6	0.0%	1.21	No	5	0.44	11	1.04	2	3	0.054
	Barberton Citizens Hospital, Barberton	9.6	0.0%	1.18	No	5	0.12	7	0.57	2	4	0.018
	Bethesda Hospital, Zanesville	9.7	0.0%	1.22	No	6	0.00	6	1.23	2	2	0.042
	Bethesda Oak Hospital, Cincinnati	13.5	0.0%	1.07	No	7	0.16	10	0.63	2	1	0.109
	Doctor's Hospital, Columbus	10.1	0.0%	1.24	No	7	0.35	11	0.90	1	2	0.071
	Elyria Memorial Hospital and Medical Center, Elyria	10.9	0.0%	1.08	No	3	0.01	8	0.78	2	2	0.021
	Firelands Community Hospital, Sandusky	11.4	0.0%	1.11	No	5	0.08	10	0.59	2	2	0.027
	Flower Hospital, Sylvania	12.3	0.0%	1.04	No	3	0.11	10	0.46	2	4	0.016
	Good Samaritan Hospital and Health Center, Dayton	9.5	0.0%	1.20	No	5	0.20	9	0.79	2	1	0.018
	Good Samaritan Hospital, Cincinnati	12.8	0.0%	1.25	Yes	6	0.23	11	1.03	2	3	0.075
	Grant Medical Center, Columbus	13.0	0.0%	1.17	Yes	5	0.20	9	1.09	2	2	0.011
	Kettering Medical Center, Kettering	11.8	0.0%	1.31	Yes	6	0.18	12	0.97	2	4	0.039
	Licking Memorial Hospital, Newark	10.2	0.0%	1.22	No	4	0.00	10	1.53	2	2	0.016
	Lima Memorial Hospital, Lima	11.9	0.0%	1.05	No	4	0.00	10	0.94	1	2	0.040
	Mansfield General Hospital, Mansfield	8.5	0.0%	1.28	No	6	0.00	11	0.60	2	2	0.038
	Mercy Hospital, Hamilton	10.4	0.0%	1.15	No	3	0.20	8	0.56	2	5	0.077
	Mercy Hospital, Toledo	10.5	0.0%	1.20	No	5	0.29	7	1.22	2	2	0.040
	Mercy Medical Center, Springfield	13.0	0.0%	1.04	No	3	0.00	10	1.04	2	3	0.022
	Meridia Huron Hospital, Cleveland	7.7	0.0%	1.35	No	5	0.35	5	0.62	2	7	0.042
	Mount Carmel Health, Columbus	10.7	0.0%	1.34	No	8	0.17	12	0.78	2	8	0.039
	Robinson Memorial Hospital, Ravenna	12.3	0.0%	1.04	No	4	0.04	7	0.73	2	2	0.021
	St. Elizabeth Hospital Medical Center, Youngstown	10.7	0.0%	1.37	Yes	6	0.21	10	0.87	2	6	0.028
	St. Elizabeth Medical Center, Dayton	10.6	0.0%	1.15	No	6	0.15	9	1.11	1	1	0.041
	St. John Medical Center, Steubenville	8.6	0.0%	1.27	No	6	0.00	9	0.61	2	4	0.025
	St. Vincent Charity Hospital, Cleveland	11.2	0.0%	1.13	No	5	0.06	10	0.73	2	2	0.067
	Timken Mercy Medical Center, Canton	7.8	0.0%	1.28	No	6	0.04	12	0.58	1	3	0.040
	Trumbull Memorial Hospital, Warren	10.6	0.0%	1.07	No	3	0.00	11	0.84	1	1	0.034
	Western Reserve System-Southside, Youngstown	10.9	0.0%	1.17	No	3	0.65	7	1.12	2	1	0.059

GYNECOLOGY

Natl. Rank	Hospital	U.S. News index	Reputational score	Hospital-wide mortality rate	Interns and residents to beds	Technology score (of 10)	R.N.'s to beds	Board-certified OB-GYNs to beds	Procedures to beds
TIER ONE									
8	Cleveland Clinic	50.3	8.8%	0.87	1.22	9	1.47	0.009	0.48
TIER TWO									
62	Mount Sinai Medical Center, Cleveland	24.5	0.4%	0.87	0.76	7	0.86	0.093	0.38
43	Ohio State University Medical Center, Columbus	27.5	2.2%	0.94	0.81	7	1.11	0.041	0.12
42	University Hospitals of Cleveland	27.6	0.0%	1.07	1.60	10	1.73	0.083	0.42
TIER THREE									
	Aultman Hospital, Canton	17.8	0.0%	0.92	0.19	7	0.67	0.045	0.41
	Bethesda Oak Hospital, Cincinnati	14.5	0.0%	1.07	0.16	7	0.63	0.114	0.61
	Christ Hospital, Cincinnati	19.3	0.5%	0.92	0.12	8	0.54	0.065	0.46
	Jewish Hospital of Cincinnati	17.5	0.0%	0.90	0.15	7	0.48	0.054	0.29
	Lakewood Hospital, Lakewood	16.0	0.0%	0.90	0.01	5	0.80	0.006	0.19

Natl. Rank	Hospital	U.S. News index	Reputa- tional score	Hospital- wide mortality rate	Interns and residents to beds	Tech- nology score (of 10)	R.N.'s to beds	Board- certified OB-GYNs to beds	Procedures to beds
	Lorain Community Hospital, Lorain	16.4	0.0%	0.87	0.00	6	0.58	0.017	0.37
	Medical College of Ohio Hospital, Toledo	19.8	0.0%	1.11	1.42	7	1.23	0.015	0.15
	MetroHealth Medical Center, Cleveland	14.4	0.5%	1.20	0.54	9	0.69	0.021	0.23
	Middletown Regional Hospital, Middletown	14.9	0.0%	0.96	0.00	5	0.93	0.018	0.31
	Park Medical Center, Columbus	15.6	0.0%	0.86	0.02	4	0.77	0.005	0.12
	Riverside Methodist Hospitals, Columbus	16.4	0.0%	1.23	0.28	10	1.50	0.044	0.45
	St. Rita's Medical Center, Lima	17.6	0.0%	0.94	0.00	7	1.11	0.013	0.40
91	St. Vincent Medical Center, Toledo	21.9	0.0%	1.04	0.34	7	2.26	0.039	0.23
	The Toledo Hospital, Toledo	15.3	0.0%	1.14	0.14	9	1.14	0.043	0.58
	TIER FOUR								
	Akron General Medical Center, Akron	13.2	0.0%	1.21	0.44	7	1.04	0.038	0.45
	Barberton Citizens Hospital, Barberton	8.0	0.0%	1.18	0.12	5	0.57	0.007	0.31
	Bethesda Hospital, Zanesville	8.8	0.0%	1.22	0.00	3	1.23	0.029	0.31
	Deaconess Hospital, Cincinnati	12.9	0.0%	0.97	0.00	5	0.52	0.026	0.20
	Doctor's Hospital, Columbus	11.8	0.0%	1.24	0.35	7	0.90	0.045	0.30
	Elyria Memorial Hospital and Medical Center, Elyria	10.9	0.0%	1.08	0.01	5	0.78	0.018	0.39
	Fairview General Hospital, Cleveland	13.8	0.0%	1.01	0.17	4	0.84	0.057	0.33
	Firelands Community Hospital, Sandusky	13.0	0.0%	1.11	0.08	9	0.59	0.033	0.43
	Flower Hospital, Sylvania	11.8	0.0%	1.04	0.11	6	0.46	0.026	0.17
	Good Samaritan Hospital and Health Center, Dayton	10.2	0.0%	1.20	0.20	6	0.79	0.029	0.25
	Good Samaritan Hospital, Cincinnati	13.1	0.0%	1.25	0.23	8	1.03	0.080	0.42
	Grant Medical Center, Columbus	12.9	0.0%	1.17	0.20	6	1.09	0.061	0.22
	Kettering Medical Center, Kettering	11.8	0.0%	1.31	0.18	9	0.97	0.058	0.33
	Licking Memorial Hospital, Newark	12.1	0.0%	1.22	0.00	6	1.53	0.021	0.55
	Lima Memorial Hospital, Lima	13.8	0.0%	1.05	0.00	7	0.94	0.015	0.28
	Mansfield General Hospital, Mansfield	8.4	0.0%	1.28	0.00	8	0.60	0.019	0.33
	Mercy Hospital, Hamilton	10.3	0.0%	1.15	0.20	5	0.56	0.062	0.22
	Mercy Hospital, Toledo	12.3	0.0%	1.20	0.29	5	1.22	0.051	0.24
	Mercy Medical Center, Springfield	13.8	0.0%	1.04	0.00	6	1.04	0.022	0.31
	Meridia Huron Hospital, Cleveland	5.1	0.0%	1.35	0.35	3	0.62	0.014	0.08
	Miami Valley Hospital, Dayton	12.6	0.0%	1.29	0.27	9	0.95	0.061	0.59
	Mount Carmel Health, Columbus	8.5	0.0%	1.34	0.17	7	0.78	0.034	0.53
	Robinson Memorial Hospital, Ravenna	11.9	0.0%	1.04	0.04	5	0.73	0.014	0.21
	St. Elizabeth Hospital Medical Center, Youngstown	9.2	0.0%	1.37	0.21	8	0.87	0.028	0.48
	St. Elizabeth Medical Center, Dayton	11.7	0.0%	1.15	0.15	5	1.11	0.025	0.21
	St. Luke's Medical Center, Cleveland	11.7	0.0%	1.25	0.42	7	1.01	0.018	0.19
	St. Vincent Charity Hospital, Cleveland	10.3	0.0%	1.13	0.06	5	0.73	0.043	0.11
	Summa Health System, Akron	13.9	0.0%	1.17	0.39	5	1.39	0.037	0.34
	Timken Mercy Medical Center, Canton	8.6	0.0%	1.28	0.04	8	0.58	0.030	0.31
	Trumbull Memorial Hospital, Warren	12.8	0.0%	1.07	0.00	7	0.84	0.013	0.20
	Western Reserve System-Southside, Youngstown	13.4	0.0%	1.17	0.65	5	1.12	0.017	0.67

NEUROLOGY

Natl. Rank	Hospital	U.S. News index	Reputa- tional score	Neurology mortality rate	COTH member	Interns and residents to beds	Tech- nology score (of 9)	R.N.'s to beds	Board- certified neurologists to beds
	TIER ONE								
7	Cleveland Clinic	40.6	10.6%	0.62	Yes	1.22	9	1.47	0.023
	TIER TWO								
53	Mount Sinai Medical Center, Cleveland	19.7	0.0%	0.63	Yes	0.76	7	0.86	0.016
60	Ohio State University Medical Center, Columbus	18.9	0.0%	0.82	Yes	0.81	6	1.11	0.017
79	St. Vincent Medical Center, Toledo	18.0	0.0%	0.84	No	0.34	6	2.26	0.025
77	Summa Health System, Akron	18.1	0.0%	0.80	Yes	0.39	6	1.39	0.008
28	University Hospitals of Cleveland	23.7	0.0%	0.93	Yes	1.60	9	1.73	0.050

Natl. Rank	Hospital	U.S. News index	Reputa-tional score	Neurology mortality rate	COTH member	Interns and residents to beds	Tech-nology score (of 9)	R.N.'s to beds	Board-certified neurologists to beds
	TIER THREE								
	Akron General Medical Center, Akron	13.4	0.0%	0.91	No	0.44	7	1.04	0.013
	Aultman Hospital, Canton	14.4	0.0%	0.69	No	0.19	6	0.67	0.010
	Bethesda Oak Hospital, Cincinnati	11.1	0.0%	0.91	No	0.16	7	0.63	0.010
	Christ Hospital, Cincinnati	14.8	0.0%	0.75	No	0.12	8	0.54	0.015
	Deaconess Hospital, Cincinnati	13.5	0.0%	0.60	No	0.00	5	0.52	0.015
	Doctor's Hospital, Columbus	13.0	0.0%	0.89	No	0.35	7	0.90	0.012
	Good Samaritan Hospital, Cincinnati	11.1	0.0%	1.16	Yes	0.23	7	1.03	0.013
	Grant Medical Center, Columbus	12.9	0.0%	0.95	Yes	0.20	5	1.09	0.002
	Jewish Hospital of Cincinnati	14.0	0.0%	0.69	No	0.15	7	0.48	0.008
	Lorain Community Hospital, Lorain	12.1	0.0%	0.84	No	0.00	6	0.58	0.017
	Medical College of Ohio Hospital, Toledo	16.0	0.3%	1.23	Yes	1.42	7	1.23	0.026
	Mercy Hospital, Toledo	16.3	0.0%	0.76	No	0.29	5	1.22	0.017
	MetroHealth Medical Center, Cleveland	11.8	0.3%	1.21	Yes	0.54	8	0.69	0.018
	Miami Valley Hospital, Dayton	12.1	0.0%	1.08	Yes	0.27	8	0.95	0.011
	Middletown Regional Hospital, Middletown	11.3	0.0%	0.87	No	0.00	5	0.93	0.004
	Park Medical Center, Columbus	11.1	0.0%	0.86	No	0.02	4	0.77	0.011
	Riverside Methodist Hospitals, Columbus	14.7	0.0%	1.01	Yes	0.28	9	1.50	0.006
	St. Ann's Hospital of Columbus, Westerville	16.1	0.0%	0.73	No	0.02	5	1.26	0.024
	The Toledo Hospital, Toledo	12.4	0.0%	1.07	Yes	0.14	8	1.14	0.010
	University of Cincinnati Hospital	11.3	0.0%	1.13	Yes	0.78	0	1.10	0.013
	Western Reserve System-Southside, Youngstown	12.7	0.0%	0.93	No	0.65	5	1.12	0.007
	TIER FOUR								
	Barberton Citizens Hospital, Barberton	5.7	0.0%	1.28	No	0.12	5	0.57	0.018
	Bethesda Hospital, Zanesville	9.3	0.0%	1.00	No	0.00	3	1.23	0.008
	Elyria Memorial Hospital and Medical Center, Elyria	3.3	0.0%	1.51	No	0.01	5	0.78	0.007
	Fairview General Hospital, Cleveland	7.0	0.0%	1.11	No	0.17	3	0.84	0.004
	Flower Hospital, Sylvania	5.6	0.0%	1.19	No	0.11	6	0.46	0.002
	Good Samaritan Hospital and Health Center, Dayton	7.4	0.0%	1.16	No	0.20	5	0.79	0.011
	Kettering Medical Center, Kettering	10.5	0.0%	1.18	Yes	0.18	8	0.97	0.008
	Lakewood Hospital, Lakewood	9.7	0.0%	0.92	No	0.01	5	0.80	0.003
	Lima Memorial Hospital, Lima	8.1	0.0%	1.10	No	0.00	7	0.94	0.005
	Mansfield General Hospital, Mansfield	6.9	0.0%	1.17	No	0.00	8	0.60	0.009
	Mercy Hospital, Hamilton	9.5	0.0%	0.98	No	0.20	5	0.56	0.015
	Mercy Medical Center, Springfield	10.2	0.0%	0.97	No	0.00	6	1.04	0.009
	Meridia Huron Hospital, Cleveland	7.6	0.0%	1.09	No	0.35	3	0.62	0.010
	Mount Carmel Health, Columbus	6.2	0.0%	1.27	No	0.17	7	0.78	0.005
	Robinson Memorial Hospital, Ravenna	10.2	0.0%	0.91	No	0.04	5	0.73	0.007
	St. Elizabeth Hospital Medical Center, Youngstown	8.3	0.0%	1.37	Yes	0.21	7	0.87	0.009
	St. Elizabeth Medical Center, Dayton	7.7	0.0%	1.15	No	0.15	5	1.11	0.004
	St. Luke's Medical Center, Cleveland	10.7	0.0%	1.17	Yes	0.42	6	1.01	0.005
	St. Rita's Medical Center, Lima	10.4	0.0%	0.97	No	0.00	7	1.11	0.003
	St. Vincent Charity Hospital, Cleveland	7.3	0.0%	1.12	No	0.06	5	0.73	0.012
	Timken Mercy Medical Center, Canton	7.2	0.0%	1.17	No	0.04	7	0.58	0.018
	Trumbull Memorial Hospital, Warren	9.0	0.0%	1.01	No	0.00	7	0.84	0.004

ORTHOPEDICS

Natl. Rank	Hospital	U.S. News index	Reputa-tional score	Orthopedics mortality rate	COTH member	Interns and residents to beds	Tech-nology score (of 5)	R.N.'s to beds	Board-certified orthopedists to beds	Pro-cedures to beds
	TIER ONE									
7	Cleveland Clinic	37.7	8.8%	0.65	Yes	1.22	5	1.47	0.020	2.33
	TIER TWO									
34	Medical College of Ohio Hospital, Toledo	18.8	0.0%	0.67	Yes	1.42	4	1.23	0.051	1.81
29	Ohio State University Medical Center, Columbus	19.3	1.5%	0.62	Yes	0.81	4	1.11	0.018	0.90

Natl. Rank	Hospital	U.S. News index	Reputational score	Orthopedics mortality rate	COTH member	Interns and residents to beds	Technology score (of 5)	R.N.'s to beds	Board-certified orthopedists to beds	Procedures to beds
46	University Hospitals of Cleveland	17.2	0.0%	1.09	Yes	1.60	5	1.73	0.033	2.50
	TIER THREE									
	Akron General Medical Center, Akron	8.2	0.0%	1.09	No	0.44	4	1.04	0.050	2.75
	Christ Hospital, Cincinnati	9.9	0.0%	0.49	No	0.12	4	0.54	0.026	1.96
	Deaconess Hospital, Cincinnati	8.2	0.0%	0.77	No	0.00	4	0.52	0.042	3.16
	Fairview General Hospital, Cleveland	8.4	0.0%	0.73	No	0.17	2	0.84	0.020	1.69
	Firelands Community Hospital, Sandusky	10.5	0.0%	0.13	No	0.08	5	0.59	0.027	1.75
	Good Samaritan Hospital, Cincinnati	12.6	0.0%	0.74	Yes	0.23	3	1.03	0.047	2.11
	Grant Medical Center, Columbus	8.5	0.5%	1.47	Yes	0.20	2	1.09	0.022	4.02
	Greene Memorial Hospital, Xenia	9.0	0.0%	0.69	No	0.01	3	0.80	0.010	1.40
	Jewish Hospital of Cincinnati	8.8	0.0%	0.72	No	0.15	4	0.48	0.030	1.60
	Kettering Medical Center, Kettering	10.1	0.0%	1.11	Yes	0.18	5	0.97	0.023	2.16
	Lakewood Hospital, Lakewood	10.4	0.0%	0.53	No	0.01	4	0.80	0.041	2.58
	Lima Memorial Hospital, Lima	8.7	0.0%	0.78	No	0.00	3	0.94	0.045	3.48
	Lorain Community Hospital, Lorain	8.6	0.0%	0.74	No	0.00	4	0.58	0.033	2.73
	Mercy Medical Center, Springfield	9.1	0.0%	0.74	No	0.00	3	1.04	0.022	2.54
	MetroHealth Medical Center, Cleveland	9.7	0.0%	1.09	Yes	0.54	4	0.69	0.028	0.49
	Miami Valley Hospital, Dayton	9.1	0.0%	1.23	Yes	0.27	4	0.95	0.031	2.14
84	Mount Sinai Medical Center, Cleveland	14.1	0.0%	0.73	Yes	0.76	3	0.86	0.059	2.10
	Park Medical Center, Columbus	9.6	0.0%	0.49	No	0.02	3	0.77	0.033	2.04
	Riverside Methodist Hospitals, Columbus	13.0	0.5%	1.14	Yes	0.28	5	1.50	0.030	3.16
	St. Ann's Hospital of Columbus, Westerville	9.3	0.0%	0.97	No	0.02	4	1.26	0.241	2.69
	St. Rita's Medical Center, Lima	11.2	0.0%	0.53	No	0.00	4	1.11	0.028	2.63
	St. Vincent Charity Hospital, Cleveland	8.8	0.0%	0.61	No	0.06	2	0.73	0.034	1.61
90	St. Vincent Medical Center, Toledo	13.5	0.0%	0.75	No	0.34	3	2.26	0.039	2.63
	Summa Health System, Akron	9.6	0.0%	1.31	Yes	0.39	3	1.39	0.041	1.78
	The Toledo Hospital, Toledo	9.6	0.0%	1.29	Yes	0.14	5	1.14	0.021	2.48
	Western Reserve System-Southside, Youngstown	9.5	0.0%	0.88	No	0.65	2	1.12	0.003	3.89
	TIER FOUR									
	Aultman Hospital, Canton	8.1	0.0%	0.84	No	0.19	4	0.67	0.016	2.09
	Barberton Citizens Hospital, Barberton	4.8	0.0%	1.10	No	0.12	3	0.57	0.021	1.83
	Bethesda Hospital, Zanesville	5.0	0.0%	1.19	No	0.00	2	1.23	0.025	1.78
	Bethesda Oak Hospital, Cincinnati	7.1	0.0%	1.00	No	0.16	4	0.63	0.062	3.66
	Doctor's Hospital, Columbus	4.5	0.0%	1.74	No	0.35	4	0.90	0.026	1.35
	Elyria Memorial Hospital and Medical Center, Elyria	6.7	0.0%	0.95	No	0.01	4	0.78	0.018	1.95
	Flower Hospital, Sylvania	7.4	0.0%	0.76	No	0.11	3	0.46	0.012	1.52
	Good Samaritan Hospital and Health Center, Dayton	3.9	0.0%	1.32	No	0.20	2	0.79	0.014	1.87
	Licking Memorial Hospital, Newark	5.5	0.0%	1.46	No	0.00	3	1.53	0.026	2.70
	Mansfield General Hospital, Mansfield	4.9	0.0%	1.13	No	0.00	4	0.60	0.006	1.81
	Mercy Hospital, Hamilton	5.0	0.0%	1.33	No	0.20	4	0.56	0.084	2.03
	Mercy Hospital, Toledo	4.7	0.0%	1.71	No	0.29	3	1.22	0.017	2.05
	Middletown Regional Hospital, Middletown	6.4	0.0%	1.05	No	0.00	4	0.93	0.014	2.38
	Mount Carmel Health, Columbus	5.9	0.0%	1.22	No	0.17	4	0.78	0.039	2.82
	Providence Hospital, Sandusky	5.2	0.0%	0.88	No	0.00	3	0.32	0.015	1.28
	Robinson Memorial Hospital, Ravenna	4.6	0.0%	1.26	No	0.04	4	0.73	0.018	1.37
	St. Elizabeth Hospital Medical Center, Youngstown	7.6	0.0%	1.28	Yes	0.21	3	0.87	0.009	1.78
	St. Elizabeth Medical Center, Dayton	4.9	0.0%	1.21	No	0.15	2	1.11	0.014	1.52
	St. Luke's Medical Center, Cleveland	7.9	0.0%	1.54	Yes	0.42	3	1.01	0.039	1.68
	Timken Mercy Medical Center, Canton	3.4	0.0%	1.52	No	0.04	4	0.58	0.018	2.32
	Trumbull Memorial Hospital, Warren	4.2	0.0%	1.43	No	0.00	4	0.84	0.017	1.66

OTOLARYNGOLOGY

Natl. Rank	Hospital	U.S. News index	Reputational score	Hospital-wide mortality rate	COTH member	Interns and residents to beds	Technology score (of 9)	R.N.'s to beds	Board-certified internists to beds	Procedures to beds
	TIER ONE									
10	**Cleveland Clinic**	**41.1**	8.1%	0.87	Yes	1.22	9	1.47	0.015	0.231
19	**University of Cincinnati Hospital**	**26.9**	5.2%	1.11	Yes	0.78	0	1.10	0.074	0.246
29	**University Hospitals of Cleveland**	**21.9**	1.2%	1.07	Yes	1.60	9	1.73	0.080	0.284
	TIER TWO									
66	**Medical College of Ohio Hospital, Toledo**	**15.6**	0.0%	1.11	Yes	1.42	7	1.23	0.132	0.154
98	**Mount Sinai Medical Center, Cleveland**	**13.8**	0.5%	0.87	Yes	0.76	7	0.86	0.144	0.304
64	**Ohio State University Medical Center, Columbus**	**16.0**	1.5%	0.94	Yes	0.81	4	1.11	0.029	0.253
	TIER THREE									
	Akron General Medical Center, Akron	**7.3**	0.0%	1.21	No	0.44	7	1.04	0.054	0.326
	Good Samaritan Hospital, Cincinnati	**9.7**	0.0%	1.25	Yes	0.23	7	1.03	0.075	0.146
	Grant Medical Center, Columbus	**8.7**	0.0%	1.17	Yes	0.20	5	1.09	0.011	0.096
	Kettering Medical Center, Kettering	**9.3**	0.0%	1.31	Yes	0.18	8	0.97	0.039	0.148
	MetroHealth Medical Center, Cleveland	**9.9**	0.0%	1.20	Yes	0.54	8	0.69	0.038	0.127
	Miami Valley Hospital, Dayton	**9.5**	0.0%	1.29	Yes	0.27	8	0.95	0.036	0.164
	Riverside Methodist Hospitals, Columbus	**11.9**	0.0%	1.23	Yes	0.28	9	1.50	0.063	0.252
	St. Elizabeth Hospital Medical Center, Youngstown	**8.7**	0.0%	1.37	Yes	0.21	7	0.87	0.028	0.250
	St. Luke's Medical Center, Cleveland	**11.4**	0.4%	1.25	Yes	0.42	5	1.01	0.105	0.150
	St. Vincent Medical Center, Toledo	**10.7**	0.0%	1.04	No	0.34	6	2.26	0.081	0.167
	Summa Health System, Akron	**10.9**	0.0%	1.17	Yes	0.39	6	1.39	0.039	0.201
	The Toledo Hospital, Toledo	**9.7**	0.0%	1.14	Yes	0.14	8	1.14	0.037	0.155
	Western Reserve System-Southside, Youngstown	**7.9**	0.0%	1.17	No	0.65	5	1.12	0.059	0.537
	TIER FOUR									
	Aultman Hospital, Canton	**5.1**	0.0%	0.92	No	0.19	6	0.67	0.054	0.164
	Barberton Citizens Hospital, Barberton	**3.7**	0.0%	1.18	No	0.12	5	0.57	0.018	0.298
	Bethesda Hospital, Zanesville	**4.9**	0.0%	1.22	No	0.00	3	1.23	0.042	0.250
	Bethesda Oak Hospital, Cincinnati	**5.5**	0.0%	1.07	No	0.16	7	0.63	0.109	0.431
	Christ Hospital, Cincinnati	**5.0**	0.0%	0.92	No	0.12	8	0.54	0.052	0.141
	Deaconess Hospital, Cincinnati	**3.9**	0.0%	0.97	No	0.00	5	0.52	0.094	0.204
	Doctor's Hospital, Columbus	**6.6**	0.0%	1.24	No	0.35	7	0.90	0.071	0.181
	Elyria Memorial Hospital and Medical Center, Elyria	**3.7**	0.0%	1.08	No	0.01	4	0.78	0.021	0.314
	Fairview General Hospital, Cleveland	**4.1**	0.0%	1.01	No	0.17	2	0.84	0.024	0.225
	Firelands Community Hospital, Sandusky	**4.8**	0.0%	1.11	No	0.08	9	0.59	0.027	0.180
	Flower Hospital, Sylvania	**3.7**	0.0%	1.04	No	0.11	6	0.46	0.016	0.112
	Good Samaritan Hospital and Health Center, Dayton	**4.7**	0.0%	1.20	No	0.20	5	0.79	0.018	0.218
	Greene Memorial Hospital, Xenia	**3.5**	0.0%	1.22	No	0.01	3	0.80	0.024	0.148
	Jewish Hospital of Cincinnati	**4.8**	0.0%	0.90	No	0.15	7	0.48	0.074	0.142
	Lakewood Hospital, Lakewood	**4.1**	0.0%	0.90	No	0.01	4	0.80	0.037	0.344
	Licking Memorial Hospital, Newark	**6.4**	0.0%	1.22	No	0.00	6	1.53	0.016	0.250
	Lima Memorial Hospital, Lima	**5.2**	0.0%	1.04	No	0.00	7	0.94	0.040	0.210
	Lorain Community Hospital, Lorain	**3.5**	0.0%	0.87	No	0.00	5	0.58	0.021	0.129
	Mansfield General Hospital, Mansfield	**4.3**	0.0%	1.28	No	0.00	8	0.60	0.038	0.138
	Mercy Hospital, Hamilton	**4.5**	0.0%	1.15	No	0.20	5	0.56	0.077	0.150
	Mercy Hospital, Toledo	**6.3**	0.0%	1.20	No	0.29	4	1.22	0.040	0.211
	Mercy Medical Center, Springfield	**5.1**	0.0%	1.04	No	0.00	6	1.04	0.022	0.205
	Meridia Huron Hospital, Cleveland	**3.7**	0.0%	1.35	No	0.35	1	0.62	0.042	0.121
	Middletown Regional Hospital, Middletown	**4.5**	0.0%	0.96	No	0.00	5	0.93	0.014	0.240
	Mount Carmel Health, Columbus	**5.2**	0.0%	1.34	No	0.17	7	0.78	0.039	0.340
	Park Medical Center, Columbus	**3.6**	0.0%	0.86	No	0.02	3	0.77	0.011	0.120
	Providence Hospital, Sandusky	**2.8**	0.0%	1.16	No	0.00	6	0.32	0.027	0.138
	Robinson Memorial Hospital, Ravenna	**3.7**	0.0%	1.03	No	0.04	4	0.73	0.021	0.126
	St. Ann's Hospital of Columbus, Westerville	**6.5**	0.0%	0.95	No	0.02	3	1.26	0.181	0.331
	St. Elizabeth Medical Center, Dayton	**5.7**	0.0%	1.15	No	0.15	5	1.11	0.041	0.275
	St. John Medical Center, Steubenville	**3.4**	0.0%	1.28	No	0.00	5	0.61	0.025	0.153

Natl. Rank	Hospital	U.S. News index	Reputational score	Hospital-wide mortality rate	COTH member	Interns and residents to beds	Technology score (of 9)	R.N.'s to beds	Board-certified internists to beds	Procedures to beds
	St. Rita's Medical Center, Lima	5.7	0.0%	0.94	No	0.00	7	1.11	0.019	0.238
	St. Vincent Charity Hospital, Cleveland	4.4	0.0%	1.13	No	0.06	5	0.73	0.067	0.116
	Stouder Memorial Hospital, Troy	5.0	0.0%	1.16	No	0.00	7	0.88	0.043	0.297
	Timken Mercy Medical Center, Canton	4.1	0.0%	1.28	No	0.04	7	0.58	0.040	0.241
	Trumbull Memorial Hospital, Warren	4.9	0.0%	1.07	No	0.00	7	0.84	0.034	0.480

RHEUMATOLOGY

Natl. Rank	Hospital	U.S. News index	Reputational score	Hospital-wide mortality rate	COTH member	Interns and residents to beds	Technology score (of 5)	R.N.'s to beds	Board-certified internists to beds
	TIER ONE								
8	Cleveland Clinic	41.5	10.4%	0.87	Yes	1.22	5	1.47	0.015
26	University Hospitals of Cleveland	22.0	1.5%	1.07	Yes	1.60	5	1.73	0.080
	TIER TWO								
55	Medical College of Ohio Hospital, Toledo	17.5	0.5%	1.11	Yes	1.42	4	1.23	0.132
70	Ohio State University Medical Center, Columbus	16.6	0.7%	0.94	Yes	0.81	4	1.11	0.029
	TIER THREE								
	Aultman Hospital, Canton	9.8	0.0%	0.92	No	0.19	4	0.67	0.054
	Good Samaritan Hospital, Cincinnati	10.4	0.0%	1.25	Yes	0.23	3	1.03	0.075
	Grant Medical Center, Columbus	10.0	0.0%	1.17	Yes	0.20	2	1.09	0.011
	Kettering Medical Center, Kettering	10.3	0.0%	1.31	Yes	0.18	5	0.97	0.039
	Lakewood Hospital, Lakewood	9.7	0.0%	0.90	No	0.01	4	0.80	0.037
	MetroHealth Medical Center, Cleveland	10.9	0.0%	1.20	Yes	0.54	4	0.69	0.038
	Miami Valley Hospital, Dayton	10.3	0.0%	1.29	Yes	0.27	4	0.95	0.036
90	Mount Sinai Medical Center, Cleveland	15.4	0.0%	0.87	Yes	0.76	3	0.86	0.144
	Riverside Methodist Hospitals, Columbus	12.7	0.0%	1.23	Yes	0.28	5	1.50	0.063
	St. Ann's Hospital of Columbus, Westerville	11.4	0.0%	0.95	No	0.02	4	1.26	0.181
	St. Luke's Medical Center, Cleveland	11.1	0.0%	1.25	Yes	0.42	3	1.01	0.105
	St. Rita's Medical Center, Lima	9.9	0.0%	0.94	No	0.00	4	1.11	0.019
	St. Vincent Medical Center, Toledo	13.0	0.0%	1.04	No	0.34	3	2.26	0.081
	Summa Health System, Akron	12.1	0.0%	1.17	Yes	0.39	3	1.39	0.039
	The Toledo Hospital, Toledo	11.8	0.0%	1.14	Yes	0.14	5	1.14	0.037
	University of Cincinnati Hospital	11.4	0.7%	1.11	Yes	0.78	0	1.10	0.074
	TIER FOUR								
	Akron General Medical Center, Akron	9.2	0.0%	1.21	No	0.44	4	1.04	0.054
	Barberton Citizens Hospital, Barberton	6.3	0.0%	1.18	No	0.12	3	0.57	0.018
	Bethesda Hospital, Zanesville	7.2	0.0%	1.22	No	0.00	2	1.23	0.042
	Bethesda Oak Hospital, Cincinnati	8.5	0.0%	1.07	No	0.16	4	0.63	0.109
	Christ Hospital, Cincinnati	8.2	0.0%	0.92	No	0.12	4	0.54	0.052
	Deaconess Hospital, Cincinnati	8.6	0.0%	0.97	No	0.00	4	0.52	0.094
	Doctor's Hospital, Columbus	7.4	0.0%	1.24	No	0.35	4	0.90	0.071
	Elyria Memorial Hospital and Medical Center, Elyria	7.7	0.0%	1.08	No	0.01	4	0.78	0.021
	Fairview General Hospital, Cleveland	8.1	0.0%	1.01	No	0.17	2	0.84	0.024
	Firelands Community Hospital, Sandusky	7.8	0.0%	1.11	No	0.08	5	0.59	0.027
	Flower Hospital, Sylvania	7.0	0.0%	1.04	No	0.11	3	0.46	0.016
	Good Samaritan Hospital and Health Center, Dayton	6.6	0.0%	1.20	No	0.20	2	0.79	0.018
	Jewish Hospital of Cincinnati	9.5	0.0%	0.90	No	0.15	4	0.48	0.074
	Licking Memorial Hospital, Newark	8.2	0.0%	1.22	No	0.00	3	1.53	0.016
	Lima Memorial Hospital, Lima	7.1	0.0%	1.04	No	0.00	3	0.94	0.040
	Lorain Community Hospital, Lorain	9.2	0.0%	0.87	No	0.00	4	0.58	0.021
	Mansfield General Hospital, Mansfield	6.1	0.0%	1.28	No	0.00	4	0.60	0.038
	Mercy Hospital, Hamilton	7.7	0.0%	1.15	No	0.20	4	0.56	0.077
	Mercy Hospital, Toledo	8.6	0.0%	1.20	No	0.29	3	1.22	0.040
	Mercy Medical Center, Springfield	8.3	0.0%	1.04	No	0.00	3	1.04	0.022
	Meridia Huron Hospital, Cleveland	5.9	0.0%	1.35	No	0.35	2	0.62	0.042

Natl. Rank Hospital	U.S. News index	Reputa-tional score	Hospital-wide mortality rate	COTH member	Interns and residents to beds	Tech-nology score (of 5)	R.N.'s to beds	Board-certified internists to beds
Middletown Regional Hospital, Middletown	9.2	0.0%	0.96	No	0.00	4	0.93	0.014
Mount Carmel Health, Columbus	6.7	0.0%	1.34	No	0.17	4	0.78	0.039
Park Medical Center, Columbus	8.4	0.0%	0.86	No	0.02	3	0.77	0.011
Robinson Memorial Hospital, Ravenna	8.1	0.0%	1.03	No	0.04	4	0.73	0.021
St. Elizabeth Hospital Medical Center, Youngstown	8.9	0.0%	1.37	Yes	0.21	3	0.87	0.028
St. Elizabeth Medical Center, Dayton	6.8	0.0%	1.15	No	0.15	2	1.11	0.041
St. John Medical Center, Steubenville	5.5	0.0%	1.28	No	0.00	3	0.61	0.025
St. Vincent Charity Hospital, Cleveland	6.8	0.0%	1.13	No	0.06	2	0.73	0.067
Timken Mercy Medical Center, Canton	5.1	0.0%	1.28	No	0.04	4	0.58	0.040
Trumbull Memorial Hospital, Warren	7.1	0.0%	1.07	No	0.00	4	0.84	0.034
Western Reserve System-Southside, Youngstown	9.4	0.0%	1.17	No	0.65	2	1.12	0.059

UROLOGY

Natl. Rank Hospital	U.S. News index	Reputa-tional score	Urology mortality rate	COTH member	Interns and residents to beds	Tech-nology score (of 11)	R.N.'s to beds	Board-certified internists to beds	Procedures to beds
TIER ONE									
3 **Cleveland Clinic**	65.0	34.2%	0.62	Yes	1.22	10	1.47	0.015	1.59
TIER TWO									
51 **Mount Sinai Medical Center, Cleveland**	18.0	0.6%	0.68	Yes	0.76	8	0.86	0.144	2.30
58 **University Hospitals of Cleveland**	17.4	0.5%	1.32	Yes	1.60	11	1.73	0.080	1.50
TIER THREE									
Aultman Hospital, Canton	10.0	0.6%	0.86	No	0.19	7	0.67	0.054	1.34
Christ Hospital, Cincinnati	10.7	0.0%	0.76	No	0.12	9	0.54	0.052	1.57
Doctor's Hospital, Columbus	8.6	0.0%	1.08	No	0.35	8	0.90	0.071	1.48
Good Samaritan Hospital, Cincinnati	9.4	0.8%	1.59	Yes	0.23	8	1.03	0.075	1.51
Grant Medical Center, Columbus	12.0	0.0%	0.87	Yes	0.20	6	1.09	0.011	0.90
Jewish Hospital of Cincinnati	9.0	0.0%	0.86	No	0.15	8	0.48	0.074	1.62
Kettering Medical Center, Kettering	10.0	0.0%	1.18	Yes	0.18	9	0.97	0.039	1.43
Lakewood Hospital, Lakewood	10.0	0.0%	0.76	No	0.01	6	0.80	0.037	1.75
100 Medical College of Ohio Hospital, Toledo	14.4	0.0%	1.32	Yes	1.42	8	1.23	0.132	1.38
MetroHealth Medical Center, Cleveland	9.8	0.0%	1.26	Yes	0.54	9	0.69	0.038	0.50
91 Ohio State University Medical Center, Columbus	15.0	1.3%	1.00	Yes	0.81	6	1.11	0.029	2.22
Park Medical Center, Columbus	10.2	0.0%	0.63	No	0.02	5	0.77	0.011	2.14
Riverside Methodist Hospitals, Columbus	9.4	0.0%	1.92	Yes	0.28	10	1.50	0.063	2.12
St. Ann's Hospital of Columbus, Westerville	12.2	0.0%	0.74	No	0.02	5	1.26	0.181	2.12
St. Luke's Medical Center, Cleveland	10.8	0.0%	1.18	Yes	0.42	7	1.01	0.105	1.33
St. Rita's Medical Center, Lima	8.9	0.0%	0.93	No	0.00	8	1.11	0.019	1.41
St. Vincent Medical Center, Toledo	12.0	0.0%	1.08	No	0.34	7	2.26	0.081	2.31
Summa Health System, Akron	9.3	0.0%	1.57	Yes	0.39	7	1.39	0.039	1.17
The Toledo Hospital, Toledo	10.7	0.0%	1.15	Yes	0.14	9	1.14	0.037	1.78
University of Cincinnati Hospital	11.3	0.0%	1.03	Yes	0.78	0	1.10	0.074	1.22
Western Reserve System-Southside, Youngstown	9.9	0.0%	1.13	No	0.65	6	1.12	0.059	4.12
TIER FOUR									
Akron General Medical Center, Akron	7.5	0.6%	1.54	No	0.44	8	1.04	0.054	1.98
Barberton Citizens Hospital, Barberton	4.5	0.0%	1.34	No	0.12	6	0.57	0.018	1.62
Bethesda Hospital, Zanesville	6.4	0.0%	1.17	No	0.00	4	1.23	0.042	1.65
Bethesda Oak Hospital, Cincinnati	6.5	0.0%	1.36	No	0.16	9	0.63	0.109	2.99
Deaconess Hospital, Cincinnati	8.0	0.0%	0.89	No	0.00	6	0.52	0.094	2.06
Elyria Memorial Hospital and Medical Center, Elyria	3.6	0.0%	1.58	No	0.01	6	0.78	0.021	1.54
Fairview General Hospital, Cleveland	6.8	0.0%	1.04	No	0.17	4	0.84	0.024	1.77
Firelands Community Hospital, Sandusky	4.8	0.0%	1.51	No	0.08	10	0.59	0.027	2.00
Flower Hospital, Sylvania	4.7	0.0%	1.25	No	0.11	7	0.46	0.016	0.96
Good Samaritan Hospital and Health Center, Dayton	4.8	0.0%	1.42	No	0.20	6	0.79	0.018	1.20
Greene Memorial Hospital, Xenia	4.9	0.0%	1.25	No	0.01	5	0.80	0.024	1.53

Natl. Rank	Hospital	U.S. News index	Reputa- tional score	Urology mortality rate	COTH member	Interns and residents to beds	Tech- nology score (of 11)	R.N.'s to beds	Board- certified internists to beds	Procedures to beds
	Licking Memorial Hospital, Newark	8.0	0.0%	1.15	No	0.00	7	1.53	0.016	2.16
	Lima Memorial Hospital, Lima	4.3	0.0%	1.70	No	0.00	8	0.94	0.040	1.90
	Lorain Community Hospital, Lorain	7.0	0.0%	0.93	No	0.00	6	0.58	0.021	1.11
	Mansfield General Hospital, Mansfield	7.2	0.0%	1.01	No	0.00	9	0.60	0.038	1.45
	Mercy Hospital, Hamilton	6.0	0.0%	1.22	No	0.20	6	0.56	0.077	2.50
	Mercy Hospital, Toledo	6.5	0.0%	1.46	No	0.29	6	1.22	0.040	2.50
	Mercy Medical Center, Springfield	6.2	0.0%	1.22	No	0.00	7	1.04	0.022	1.55
	Meridia Huron Hospital, Cleveland	3.7	0.0%	1.57	No	0.35	3	0.62	0.042	1.56
	Miami Valley Hospital, Dayton	8.3	0.0%	1.58	Yes	0.27	9	0.95	0.036	1.42
	Middletown Regional Hospital, Middletown	6.5	0.0%	1.10	No	0.00	6	0.93	0.014	2.03
	Mount Carmel Health, Columbus	5.1	0.0%	1.59	No	0.17	8	0.78	0.039	2.60
	Providence Hospital, Sandusky	2.6	0.0%	1.58	No	0.00	7	0.32	0.027	1.22
	Robinson Memorial Hospital, Ravenna	4.4	0.0%	1.36	No	0.04	6	0.73	0.021	1.26
	St. Elizabeth Hospital Medical Center, Youngstown	8.5	0.0%	1.41	Yes	0.21	8	0.87	0.028	2.22
	St. Elizabeth Medical Center, Dayton	4.9	0.0%	1.57	No	0.15	6	1.11	0.041	1.29
	St. John Medical Center, Steubenville	2.5	0.0%	1.93	No	0.00	7	0.61	0.025	2.10
	Stouder Memorial Hospital, Troy	5.8	0.0%	1.31	No	0.00	8	0.88	0.043	2.18
	Timken Mercy Medical Center, Canton	4.4	0.0%	1.42	No	0.04	8	0.58	0.040	1.42
	Trumbull Memorial Hospital, Warren	6.9	0.0%	1.09	No	0.00	8	0.84	0.034	1.39

AIDS

Natl. Rank	Hospital	U.S. News index	Reputa- tional score	Hospital- wide mortality rate	COTH member	Interns and residents to beds	Tech- nology score (of 11)	Discharge planning (of 2)	R.N.'s to beds	Board- certified internists to beds
	TIER TWO									
48	**University Hospitals, Oklahoma City**	27.5	0.0%	0.98	Yes	1.60	9	2	1.56	0.040
	TIER THREE									
	St. Francis Hospital, Tulsa	22.6	0.3%	1.04	Yes	0.13	8	2	0.93	0.076
	Tulsa Regional Medical Center, Tulsa	20.0	0.0%	1.08	No	0.51	8	2	0.53	0.015
	TIER FOUR									
	Baptist Medical Center of Oklahoma, Oklahoma City	17.0	0.0%	1.24	No	0.04	8	1	0.95	0.036
	Bass Memorial Baptist Hospital, Enid	17.8	0.0%	1.07	No	0.00	5	1	0.72	0.083
	Comanche County Memorial Hospital, Lawton	15.5	0.0%	1.35	No	0.00	7	2	0.45	0.028
	Deaconess Hospital, Oklahoma City	16.7	0.0%	1.33	No	0.00	7	2	1.14	0.042
	Griffin Memorial Hospital, Norman	6.2	0.0%	3.20	No	0.17	1	2	0.26	0.008
	Hillcrest Medical Center, Tulsa	19.1	0.0%	1.07	No	0.09	6	2	0.84	0.028
	Memorial Hospital of Southern Oklahoma, Ardmore	15.7	0.0%	1.30	No	0.00	5	2	0.84	0.024
	Mercy Health Center, Oklahoma City	18.3	0.0%	1.08	No	0.00	7	1	0.79	0.027
	Norman Regional Hospital, Norman	15.4	0.0%	1.32	No	0.00	6	1	0.92	0.038
	Presbyterian Hospital, Oklahoma City	18.9	0.0%	1.10	No	0.06	7	2	0.82	0.037
	Southwest Medical Center of Oklahoma, Oklahoma City	17.2	0.0%	1.18	No	0.00	6	2	0.72	0.021
	St. Anthony Hospital, Oklahoma City	14.7	0.0%	1.37	No	0.04	6	1	0.62	0.067
	St. John Medical Center, Tulsa	15.6	0.0%	1.37	No	0.06	7	2	0.51	0.068
	St. Mary's Hospital, Enid	15.8	0.0%	1.18	No	0.00	5	1	0.49	0.051

CANCER

Natl. Rank	Hospital	U.S. News index	Reputa- tional score	Cancer mortality rate	COTH member	Interns and residents to beds	Tech- nology score (of 12)	R.N.'s to beds	Board- certified oncologists to beds	Procedures to beds
	TIER TWO									
30	**University Hospitals, Oklahoma City**	14.9	0.0%	0.65	Yes	1.60	11	1.56	0.029	0.86
	TIER THREE									
	St. Francis Hospital, Tulsa	7.1	0.0%	1.11	Yes	0.13	9	0.93	0.013	1.66
	TIER FOUR									
	Baptist Medical Center of Oklahoma, Oklahoma City	5.0	0.0%	1.16	No	0.04	11	0.95	0.011	1.86
	Bass Memorial Baptist Hospital, Enid	3.1	0.0%	0.75	No	0.00	6	0.72	0.000	1.48
	Comanche County Memorial Hospital, Lawton	3.1	0.0%	0.68	No	0.00	8	0.45	0.008	1.44
	Deaconess Hospital, Oklahoma City	4.2	0.0%	1.25	No	0.00	7	1.14	0.019	1.89
	Hillcrest Medical Center, Tulsa	4.2	0.0%	0.73	No	0.09	8	0.84	0.000	0.77
	Jane Phillips-Memorial Medical Center, Bartlesville	1.7	0.0%	1.33	No	0.01	5	0.52	0.000	1.39
	Memorial Hospital of Southern Oklahoma, Ardmore	3.4	0.0%	1.04	No	0.00	7	0.84	0.012	1.56
	Mercy Health Center, Oklahoma City	3.7	0.0%	1.08	No	0.00	8	0.79	0.021	2.10
	Norman Regional Hospital, Norman	3.2	0.0%	1.20	No	0.00	6	0.92	0.008	1.68
	Presbyterian Hospital, Oklahoma City	4.2	0.0%	0.89	No	0.06	8	0.82	0.017	2.14
	Southwest Medical Center of Oklahoma, Oklahoma City	3.1	0.0%	1.27	No	0.00	7	0.72	0.010	2.28
	St. Anthony Hospital, Oklahoma City	2.9	0.0%	1.25	No	0.04	8	0.62	0.002	0.78
	St. John Medical Center, Tulsa	3.1	0.0%	1.15	No	0.06	9	0.51	0.009	1.34
	St. Mary's Hospital, Enid	1.7	0.0%	0.46	No	0.00	3	0.49	0.000	1.08
	Tulsa Regional Medical Center, Tulsa	4.9	0.0%	0.90	No	0.51	9	0.53	0.009	1.07

CARDIOLOGY

Natl. Rank	Hospital	U.S. News index	Reputational score	Cardiology mortality rate	COTH member	Interns and residents to beds	Technology score (of 10)	R.N.'s to beds	Board-certified cardiologists to beds	Procedures to beds
	TIER TWO									
68	University Hospitals, Oklahoma City	21.9	0.0%	1.13	Yes	1.60	9	1.56	0.032	1.95
	TIER THREE									
	Presbyterian Hospital, Oklahoma City	15.2	0.0%	0.98	No	0.06	9	0.82	0.028	8.31
	St. Francis Hospital, Tulsa	19.1	0.6%	0.98	Yes	0.13	9	0.93	0.022	7.18
	TIER FOUR									
	Baptist Medical Center of Oklahoma, Oklahoma City	9.9	0.0%	1.29	No	0.04	9	0.95	0.034	9.79
	Comanche County Memorial Hospital, Lawton	2.2	0.0%	1.83	No	0.00	9	0.45	0.012	7.39
	Deaconess Hospital, Oklahoma City	11.5	0.0%	1.19	No	0.00	8	1.14	0.047	7.24
	Hillcrest Medical Center, Tulsa	13.1	0.0%	1.06	No	0.09	8	0.84	0.031	5.92
	Jane Phillips-Memorial Medical Center, Bartlesville	4.6	0.0%	1.44	No	0.01	5	0.52	0.004	6.31
	Memorial Hospital of Southern Oklahoma, Ardmore	6.6	0.0%	1.31	No	0.00	3	0.84	0.000	7.79
	Mercy Health Center, Oklahoma City	12.7	0.0%	1.07	No	0.00	9	0.79	0.039	4.80
	Norman Regional Hospital, Norman	9.3	0.0%	1.27	No	0.00	9	0.92	0.013	7.79
	Southwest Medical Center of Oklahoma, Oklahoma City	8.9	0.0%	1.24	No	0.00	7	0.72	0.021	8.77
	St. Anthony Hospital, Oklahoma City	7.4	0.0%	1.36	No	0.04	8	0.62	0.036	5.16
	St. John Medical Center, Tulsa	6.6	0.0%	1.40	No	0.06	8	0.51	0.036	6.28
	Tulsa Regional Medical Center, Tulsa	9.4	0.0%	1.31	No	0.51	9	0.53	0.015	5.80

ENDOCRINOLOGY

Natl. Rank	Hospital	U.S. News index	Reputational score	Endocrinology mortality rate	COTH member	Interns and residents to beds	Technology score (of 11)	R.N.'s to beds	Board-certified internists to beds
	TIER TWO								
29	University Hospitals, Oklahoma City	20.3	0.0%	0.64	Yes	1.60	10	1.56	0.040
	TIER THREE								
	St. Francis Hospital, Tulsa	11.3	0.0%	0.86	Yes	0.13	9	0.93	0.076
	TIER FOUR								
	Baptist Medical Center of Oklahoma, Oklahoma City	7.0	0.0%	1.03	No	0.04	9	0.95	0.036
	Comanche County Memorial Hospital, Lawton	3.1	0.0%	1.64	No	0.00	9	0.45	0.028
	Deaconess Hospital, Oklahoma City	4.8	0.0%	1.58	No	0.00	7	1.14	0.042
	Hillcrest Medical Center, Tulsa	7.9	0.0%	0.87	No	0.09	8	0.84	0.028
	Jane Phillips-Memorial Medical Center, Bartlesville	4.8	0.0%	1.10	No	0.01	6	0.52	0.036
	Memorial Hospital of Southern Oklahoma, Ardmore	5.2	0.0%	1.25	No	0.00	8	0.84	0.024
	Mercy Health Center, Oklahoma City	7.5	0.0%	0.88	No	0.00	9	0.79	0.027
	Norman Regional Hospital, Norman	4.9	0.0%	1.30	No	0.00	6	0.92	0.038
	Presbyterian Hospital, Oklahoma City	4.3	0.0%	1.65	No	0.06	9	0.82	0.037
	Southwest Medical Center of Oklahoma, Oklahoma City	5.8	0.0%	1.10	No	0.00	9	0.72	0.021
	St. Anthony Hospital, Oklahoma City	5.3	0.0%	1.23	No	0.04	9	0.62	0.067
	St. John Medical Center, Tulsa	4.7	0.0%	1.32	No	0.06	9	0.51	0.068
	Tulsa Regional Medical Center, Tulsa	7.9	0.0%	0.98	No	0.51	10	0.53	0.015

GASTROENTEROLOGY

Natl. Rank	Hospital	U.S. News index	Reputational score	Gastroenterology mortality rate	COTH member	Interns and residents to beds	Technology score (of 11)	R.N.'s to beds	Board-certified gastroenterologists to beds	Procedures to beds
	TIER TWO									
56	University Hospitals, Oklahoma City	14.6	0.0%	1.22	Yes	1.60	9	1.56	0.025	1.14
	TIER THREE									
	St. Francis Hospital, Tulsa	9.8	0.0%	1.04	Yes	0.13	9	0.93	0.017	2.96
	TIER FOUR									
	Baptist Medical Center of Oklahoma, Oklahoma City	6.0	0.0%	1.25	No	0.04	8	0.95	0.011	3.86

Natl. Rank	Hospital	U.S. News index	Reputational score	Gastro-enterology mortality rate	COTH member	Interns and residents to beds	Technology score (of 11)	R.N.'s to beds	Board-certified gastro-enterologists to beds	Procedures to beds
	Comanche County Memorial Hospital, Lawton	3.4	0.0%	1.41	No	0.00	8	0.45	0.008	2.78
	Deaconess Hospital, Oklahoma City	5.7	0.0%	1.58	No	0.00	8	1.14	0.028	4.80
	Hillcrest Medical Center, Tulsa	4.0	0.0%	1.41	No	0.09	8	0.84	0.004	1.83
	Jane Phillips-Memorial Medical Center, Bartlesville	1.3	0.0%	2.32	No	0.01	6	0.52	0.004	3.39
	Memorial Hospital of Southern Oklahoma, Ardmore	4.8	0.0%	1.54	No	0.00	8	0.84	0.006	4.48
	Mercy Health Center, Oklahoma City	6.2	0.0%	1.03	No	0.00	8	0.79	0.009	2.99
	Norman Regional Hospital, Norman	4.8	0.0%	1.32	No	0.00	5	0.92	0.008	4.32
	Presbyterian Hospital, Oklahoma City	6.7	0.0%	0.97	No	0.06	8	0.82	0.026	2.44
	Southwest Medical Center of Oklahoma, Oklahoma City	6.2	0.0%	1.15	No	0.00	8	0.72	0.014	4.46
	St. Anthony Hospital, Oklahoma City	3.4	0.0%	1.43	No	0.04	8	0.62	0.006	1.95
	St. John Medical Center, Tulsa	4.0	0.0%	1.37	No	0.06	9	0.51	0.006	2.56
	St. Mary's Hospital, Enid	2.8	0.0%	1.36	No	0.00	4	0.49	0.006	3.40
	Tulsa Regional Medical Center, Tulsa	6.2	0.0%	1.32	No	0.51	10	0.53	0.009	2.56

GERIATRICS

Natl. Rank	Hospital	U.S. News index	Reputational score	Hospital-wide mortality rate	COTH member	Service mix	Interns and residents to beds	Technology score (of 13)	R.N.'s to beds	Discharge planning (of 2)	Geriatric services (of 9)	Board-certified internists to beds
	TIER TWO											
51	University Hospitals, Oklahoma City	24.2	0.0%	0.98	Yes	7	1.60	12	1.56	2	4	0.040
	TIER THREE											
	St. Francis Hospital, Tulsa	16.2	0.0%	1.04	Yes	5	0.13	11	0.93	2	1	0.076
	TIER FOUR											
	Baptist Medical Center of Oklahoma, Oklahoma City	8.9	0.0%	1.24	No	7	0.04	11	0.95	1	1	0.036
	Comanche County Memorial Hospital, Lawton	7.5	0.0%	1.35	No	6	0.00	11	0.45	2	4	0.028
	Deaconess Hospital, Oklahoma City	7.4	0.0%	1.33	No	4	0.00	8	1.14	2	3	0.042
	Hillcrest Medical Center, Tulsa	13.1	0.0%	1.07	No	5	0.09	11	0.84	2	2	0.028
	Jane Phillips-Memorial Medical Center, Bartlesville	3.3	0.0%	1.44	No	4	0.01	8	0.52	1	2	0.036
	Memorial Hospital of Southern Oklahoma, Ardmore	7.2	0.0%	1.30	No	5	0.00	7	0.84	2	2	0.024
	Mercy Health Center, Oklahoma City	11.6	0.0%	1.08	No	6	0.00	11	0.79	1	1	0.027
	Presbyterian Hospital, Oklahoma City	11.9	0.0%	1.10	No	5	0.06	11	0.82	2	1	0.037
	Southwest Medical Center of Oklahoma, Oklahoma City	9.0	0.0%	1.18	No	3	0.00	9	0.72	2	3	0.021
	St. Anthony Hospital, Oklahoma City	6.1	0.0%	1.37	No	5	0.04	10	0.62	1	4	0.067
	St. John Medical Center, Tulsa	7.3	0.0%	1.37	No	7	0.06	10	0.51	2	2	0.068
	St. Mary's Hospital, Enid	6.5	0.0%	1.18	No	3	0.00	5	0.49	1	2	0.051
	Tulsa Regional Medical Center, Tulsa	13.2	0.0%	1.08	No	5	0.51	11	0.53	2	2	0.015

GYNECOLOGY

Natl. Rank	Hospital	U.S. News index	Reputational score	Hospital-wide mortality rate	Interns and residents to beds	Technology score (of 10)	R.N.'s to beds	Board-certified OB-GYNs to beds	Procedures to beds
	TIER TWO								
37	University Hospitals, Oklahoma City	28.1	0.0%	0.98	1.60	8	1.56	0.095	0.19
	TIER THREE								
	Mercy Health Center, Oklahoma City	14.2	0.0%	1.08	0.00	8	0.79	0.060	0.46
	St. Francis Hospital, Tulsa	15.9	0.0%	1.04	0.13	8	0.93	0.039	0.36
	Tulsa Regional Medical Center, Tulsa	14.9	0.0%	1.08	0.51	9	0.53	0.012	0.36
	TIER FOUR								
	Baptist Medical Center of Oklahoma, Oklahoma City	11.9	0.0%	1.24	0.04	9	0.95	0.044	0.55
	Comanche County Memorial Hospital, Lawton	6.0	0.0%	1.35	0.00	7	0.45	0.024	0.34
	Deaconess Hospital, Oklahoma City	11.2	0.0%	1.33	0.00	8	1.14	0.079	1.02
	Hillcrest Medical Center, Tulsa	13.7	0.0%	1.07	0.09	7	0.84	0.031	0.33
	Jane Phillips-Memorial Medical Center, Bartlesville	3.4	0.0%	1.44	0.01	5	0.52	0.013	0.50

Natl. Rank	Hospital	U.S. News index	Reputational score	Hospital-wide mortality rate	Interns and residents to beds	Technology score (of 10)	R.N.'s to beds	Board-certified OB-GYNs to beds	Procedures to beds
	Memorial Hospital of Southern Oklahoma, Ardmore	7.5	0.0%	1.30	0.00	6	0.84	0.018	0.55
	Norman Regional Hospital, Norman	7.6	0.0%	1.32	0.00	6	0.92	0.021	0.95
	Presbyterian Hospital, Oklahoma City	13.9	0.0%	1.10	0.06	8	0.82	0.054	0.58
	Southwest Medical Center of Oklahoma, Oklahoma City	10.2	0.0%	1.18	0.00	7	0.72	0.028	0.46
	St. Anthony Hospital, Oklahoma City	6.3	0.0%	1.37	0.04	7	0.62	0.010	0.18
	St. John Medical Center, Tulsa	7.2	0.0%	1.37	0.06	8	0.51	0.038	0.36
	St. Mary's Hospital, Enid	7.7	0.0%	1.18	0.00	5	0.49	0.028	0.48

NEUROLOGY

Natl. Rank	Hospital	U.S. News index	Reputational score	Neurology mortality rate	COTH member	Interns and residents to beds	Technology score (of 9)	R.N.'s to beds	Board-certified neurologists to beds
	TIER TWO								
30	University Hospitals, Oklahoma City	23.6	0.0%	0.80	Yes	1.60	8	1.56	0.017
	TIER THREE								
	Presbyterian Hospital, Oklahoma City	12.0	0.0%	0.90	No	0.06	7	0.82	0.017
	St. Francis Hospital, Tulsa	11.9	0.0%	1.03	Yes	0.13	7	0.93	0.009
	TIER FOUR								
	Baptist Medical Center of Oklahoma, Oklahoma City	7.9	0.0%	1.15	No	0.04	7	0.95	0.010
	Comanche County Memorial Hospital, Lawton	10.9	0.0%	0.87	No	0.00	7	0.45	0.008
	Deaconess Hospital, Oklahoma City	6.6	0.0%	1.28	No	0.00	6	1.14	0.009
	Jane Phillips-Memorial Medical Center, Bartlesville	5.3	0.0%	1.18	No	0.01	5	0.52	0.004
	Mercy Health Center, Oklahoma City	8.7	0.0%	1.10	No	0.00	7	0.79	0.021
	Norman Regional Hospital, Norman	7.8	0.0%	1.11	No	0.00	5	0.92	0.013
	Southwest Medical Center of Oklahoma, Oklahoma City	8.5	0.0%	1.02	No	0.00	7	0.72	0.003
	St. Anthony Hospital, Oklahoma City	9.7	0.0%	0.98	No	0.04	7	0.62	0.012
	St. John Medical Center, Tulsa	5.0	0.0%	1.32	No	0.06	7	0.51	0.010
	St. Mary's Hospital, Enid	4.5	0.0%	1.31	No	0.00	4	0.49	0.017
	Tulsa Regional Medical Center, Tulsa	8.8	0.0%	1.11	No	0.51	8	0.53	0.006

ORTHOPEDICS

Natl. Rank	Hospital	U.S. News index	Reputational score	Orthopedics mortality rate	COTH member	Interns and residents to beds	Technology score (of 5)	R.N.'s to beds	Board-certified orthopedists to beds	Procedures to beds
	TIER TWO									
36	Bone and Joint Hospital, Oklahoma City	18.6	0.4%	0.49	No	0.04	0	0.63	0.157	43.45
25	University Hospitals, Oklahoma City	20.1	0.0%	0.53	Yes	1.60	4	1.56	0.023	0.90
	TIER THREE									
	Comanche County Memorial Hospital, Lawton	9.2	0.0%	0.58	No	0.00	4	0.45	0.008	2.25
	St. Francis Hospital, Tulsa	12.3	0.0%	0.79	Yes	0.13	4	0.93	0.032	3.63
	TIER FOUR									
	Baptist Medical Center of Oklahoma, Oklahoma City	5.5	0.0%	1.27	No	0.04	4	0.95	0.029	2.39
	Bass Memorial Baptist Hospital, Enid	2.4	0.0%	1.70	No	0.00	2	0.72	0.042	3.89
	Deaconess Hospital, Oklahoma City	5.2	0.0%	1.40	No	0.00	4	1.14	0.014	2.43
	Hillcrest Medical Center, Tulsa	5.8	0.0%	1.02	No	0.09	3	0.84	0.007	1.42
	Jane Phillips-Memorial Medical Center, Bartlesville	4.2	0.0%	1.15	No	0.01	3	0.52	0.009	2.75
	Memorial Hospital of Southern Oklahoma, Ardmore	4.1	0.0%	1.27	No	0.00	2	0.84	0.018	3.93
	Mercy Health Center, Oklahoma City	8.0	0.0%	0.82	No	0.00	4	0.79	0.024	1.95
	Norman Regional Hospital, Norman	5.0	0.0%	1.38	No	0.00	4	0.92	0.021	3.59
	Presbyterian Hospital, Oklahoma City	6.9	0.0%	0.94	No	0.06	4	0.82	0.026	1.07
	Southwest Medical Center of Oklahoma, Oklahoma City	2.4	0.0%	1.75	No	0.00	3	0.72	0.017	2.41
	St. Anthony Hospital, Oklahoma City	2.6	0.0%	1.56	No	0.04	3	0.62	0.016	1.44

Natl. Rank	Hospital	U.S. News index	Reputational score	Orthopedics mortality rate	COTH member	Interns and residents to beds	Technology score (of 5)	R.N.'s to beds	Board-certified orthopedists to beds	Procedures to beds
	St. John Medical Center, Tulsa	3.2	0.0%	1.37	No	0.06	3	0.51	0.014	2.62
	St. Mary's Hospital, Enid	3.9	0.0%	1.26	No	0.00	3	0.49	0.028	3.99
	Tulsa Regional Medical Center, Tulsa	6.3	0.0%	1.31	No	0.51	5	0.53	0.015	2.49

OTOLARYNGOLOGY

Natl. Rank	Hospital	U.S. News index	Reputational score	Hospital-wide mortality rate	COTH member	Interns and residents to beds	Technology score (of 9)	R.N.'s to beds	Board-certified internists to beds	Procedures to beds
	TIER TWO									
56	University Hospitals, Oklahoma City	16.9	0.0%	0.98	Yes	1.60	8	1.56	0.040	0.263
	TIER THREE									
	St. Francis Hospital, Tulsa	9.2	0.0%	1.04	Yes	0.13	7	0.93	0.076	0.228
	TIER FOUR									
	Baptist Medical Center of Oklahoma, Oklahoma City	5.6	0.0%	1.24	No	0.04	8	0.95	0.036	0.418
	Bass Memorial Baptist Hospital, Enid	4.3	0.0%	1.07	No	0.00	5	0.72	0.083	0.267
	Comanche County Memorial Hospital, Lawton	3.4	0.0%	1.35	No	0.00	7	0.45	0.028	0.127
	Deaconess Hospital, Oklahoma City	5.4	0.0%	1.33	No	0.00	6	1.14	0.042	0.377
	Hillcrest Medical Center, Tulsa	4.8	0.0%	1.07	No	0.09	6	0.84	0.028	0.072
	Jane Phillips-Memorial Medical Center, Bartlesville	2.9	0.0%	1.43	No	0.01	4	0.52	0.036	0.228
	Memorial Hospital of Southern Oklahoma, Ardmore	4.4	0.0%	1.30	No	0.00	6	0.84	0.024	0.401
	Mercy Health Center, Oklahoma City	4.6	0.0%	1.08	No	0.00	7	0.79	0.027	0.389
	Norman Regional Hospital, Norman	4.4	0.0%	1.32	No	0.00	5	0.92	0.038	0.213
	Presbyterian Hospital, Oklahoma City	5.0	0.0%	1.10	No	0.06	7	0.82	0.037	0.154
	Southwest Medical Center of Oklahoma, Oklahoma City	4.3	0.0%	1.18	No	0.00	7	0.72	0.021	0.219
	St. Anthony Hospital, Oklahoma City	4.4	0.0%	1.37	No	0.04	7	0.62	0.067	0.116
	St. John Medical Center, Tulsa	4.2	0.0%	1.37	No	0.06	7	0.51	0.068	0.139
	St. Mary's Hospital, Enid	2.4	0.0%	1.18	No	0.00	2	0.49	0.051	0.271
	Tulsa Regional Medical Center, Tulsa	6.0	0.0%	1.08	No	0.51	8	0.53	0.015	0.136

RHEUMATOLOGY

Natl. Rank	Hospital	U.S. News index	Reputational score	Hospital-wide mortality rate	COTH member	Interns and residents to beds	Technology score (of 5)	R.N.'s to beds	Board-certified internists to beds
	TIER TWO								
46	University Hospitals, Oklahoma City	18.4	0.0%	0.98	Yes	1.60	4	1.56	0.040
	TIER THREE								
	St. Francis Hospital, Tulsa	11.8	0.0%	1.04	Yes	0.13	4	0.93	0.076
	TIER FOUR								
	Baptist Medical Center of Oklahoma, Oklahoma City	6.3	0.0%	1.24	No	0.04	4	0.95	0.036
	Comanche County Memorial Hospital, Lawton	5.2	0.0%	1.35	No	0.00	4	0.45	0.028
	Deaconess Hospital, Oklahoma City	7.2	0.0%	1.33	No	0.00	4	1.14	0.042
	Hillcrest Medical Center, Tulsa	7.9	0.0%	1.07	No	0.09	3	0.84	0.028
	Jane Phillips-Memorial Medical Center, Bartlesville	3.6	0.0%	1.43	No	0.01	3	0.52	0.036
	Memorial Hospital of Southern Oklahoma, Ardmore	5.5	0.0%	1.30	No	0.00	2	0.84	0.024
	Mercy Health Center, Oklahoma City	6.8	0.0%	1.08	No	0.00	4	0.79	0.027
	Norman Regional Hospital, Norman	5.6	0.0%	1.32	No	0.00	4	0.92	0.038
	Presbyterian Hospital, Oklahoma City	8.0	0.0%	1.10	No	0.06	4	0.82	0.037
	Southwest Medical Center of Oklahoma, Oklahoma City	6.4	0.0%	1.18	No	0.00	3	0.72	0.021
	St. Anthony Hospital, Oklahoma City	4.5	0.0%	1.37	No	0.04	3	0.62	0.067
	St. John Medical Center, Tulsa	5.3	0.0%	1.37	No	0.06	3	0.51	0.068
	St. Mary's Hospital, Enid	5.0	0.0%	1.18	No	0.00	3	0.49	0.051
	Tulsa Regional Medical Center, Tulsa	9.1	0.0%	1.08	No	0.51	5	0.53	0.015

UROLOGY

Natl. Rank	Hospital	U.S. News index	Reputa- tional score	Urology mortality rate	COTH member	Interns and residents to beds	Tech- nology score (of 11)	R.N.'s to beds	Board- certified internists to beds	Procedures to beds
TIER TWO										
81	**University Hospitals, Oklahoma City**	**15.9**	0.0%	1.22	Yes	1.60	9	1.56	0.040	1.04
TIER THREE										
	Bass Memorial Baptist Hospital, Enid	**10.8**	0.0%	0.42	No	0.00	6	0.72	0.083	2.28
	St. Francis Hospital, Tulsa	**9.4**	0.0%	1.30	Yes	0.13	9	0.93	0.076	1.77
	Tulsa Regional Medical Center, Tulsa	**11.3**	0.0%	0.80	No	0.51	10	0.53	0.015	1.67
TIER FOUR										
	Baptist Medical Center of Oklahoma, Oklahoma City	**7.7**	0.0%	1.09	No	0.04	8	0.95	0.036	2.73
	Comanche County Memorial Hospital, Lawton	**2.6**	0.0%	1.84	No	0.00	8	0.45	0.028	1.85
	Deaconess Hospital, Oklahoma City	**5.4**	0.0%	1.74	No	0.00	8	1.14	0.042	4.17
	Hillcrest Medical Center, Tulsa	**6.3**	0.0%	1.20	No	0.09	8	0.84	0.028	1.39
	Jane Phillips-Memorial Medical Center, Bartlesville	**2.6**	0.0%	1.71	No	0.01	6	0.52	0.036	1.67
	Memorial Hospital of Southern Oklahoma, Ardmore	**7.1**	0.0%	1.13	No	0.00	8	0.84	0.024	3.43
	Mercy Health Center, Oklahoma City	**5.3**	0.0%	1.32	No	0.00	8	0.79	0.027	1.53
	Norman Regional Hospital, Norman	**3.7**	0.0%	1.71	No	0.00	5	0.92	0.038	2.82
	Presbyterian Hospital, Oklahoma City	**5.5**	0.0%	1.33	No	0.06	8	0.82	0.037	1.19
	Southwest Medical Center of Oklahoma, Oklahoma City	**6.8**	0.0%	1.11	No	0.00	8	0.72	0.021	2.88
	St. Anthony Hospital, Oklahoma City	**4.2**	0.0%	1.55	No	0.04	8	0.62	0.067	1.62
	St. John Medical Center, Tulsa	**5.0**	0.0%	1.37	No	0.06	9	0.51	0.068	1.47
	St. Mary's Hospital, Enid	**8.1**	0.0%	0.83	No	0.00	4	0.49	0.051	3.07

AIDS

Natl. Rank	Hospital	U.S. News index	Reputa-tional score	Hospital-wide mortality rate	COTH member	Interns and residents to beds	Tech-nology score (of 11)	Discharge planning (of 2)	R.N.'s to beds	Board-certified internists to beds
	TIER ONE									
20	University Hospital, Portland	31.1	0.3%	0.80	Yes	1.54	9	2	2.31	0.164
	TIER THREE									
	Bess Kaiser Medical Center, Portland	21.6	0.0%	0.91	No	0.02	4	2	0.78	0.236
	Emanuel Hospital and Health Center, Portland	21.0	0.0%	1.02	No	0.22	8	2	0.94	0.048
	Good Samaritan Hospital Corvallis, Corvallis	20.8	0.0%	0.92	No	0.00	5	1	0.76	0.190
	Good Samaritan Hospital and Medical Center, Portland	22.7	0.0%	0.87	No	0.23	6	2	0.69	0.141
	Mercy Medical Center, Roseburg	22.3	0.0%	0.76	No	0.00	5	2	1.25	0.029
	Portland Adventist Medical Center, Portland	22.2	0.0%	0.80	No	0.01	6	2	0.97	0.015
	Providence Medical Center, Portland	21.9	0.0%	0.84	No	0.15	6	1	0.81	0.104
	Rogue Valley Medical Center, Medford	20.4	0.0%	1.01	No	0.00	7	2	0.77	0.121
	Sacred Heart General Hospital, Eugene	22.9	0.0%	0.91	No	0.00	6	2	1.44	0.143
	St. Charles Medical Center, Bend	21.3	0.0%	1.02	No	0.00	7	2	1.61	0.039
	TIER FOUR									
	Oregon State Hospital, Salem	0.0	0.0%	4.20	No	0.00	1	1	0.10	0.000
	Salem Hospital, Salem	17.8	0.0%	1.13	No	0.00	6	1	1.09	0.045
	St. Vincent Hospital and Medical Center, Portland	18.7	0.0%	1.07	No	0.14	6	1	0.75	0.129

CANCER

Natl. Rank	Hospital	U.S. News index	Reputa-tional score	Cancer mortality rate	COTH member	Interns and residents to beds	Tech-nology score (of 12)	R.N.'s to beds	Board-certified oncologists to beds	Procedures to beds
	TIER TWO									
18	University Hospital, Portland	16.2	0.0%	0.40	Yes	1.54	9	2.31	0.017	1.45
	TIER THREE									
	Emanuel Hospital and Health Center, Portland	5.5	0.0%	0.58	No	0.22	9	0.94	0.018	0.59
	Sacred Heart General Hospital, Eugene	5.6	0.0%	0.59	No	0.00	7	1.44	0.000	1.50
	St. Charles Medical Center, Bend	5.9	0.0%	0.93	No	0.00	8	1.61	0.006	1.68
	TIER FOUR									
	Bess Kaiser Medical Center, Portland	2.7	0.0%	1.03	No	0.02	4	0.78	0.037	1.79
	Good Samaritan Hospital Corvallis, Corvallis	3.8	0.0%	0.67	No	0.00	6	0.76	0.029	2.87
	Good Samaritan Hospital and Medical Center, Portland	4.4	0.0%	0.78	No	0.23	8	0.69	0.016	1.57
	Providence Medical Center, Portland	4.0	0.0%	0.91	No	0.15	7	0.81	0.018	1.39
	Rogue Valley Medical Center, Medford	4.1	0.0%	0.76	No	0.00	9	0.77	0.013	1.25
	Salem Hospital, Salem	4.5	0.0%	0.97	No	0.00	8	1.09	0.010	1.88
	St. Vincent Hospital and Medical Center, Portland	3.7	0.0%	0.93	No	0.14	7	0.75	0.004	1.37

CARDIOLOGY

Natl. Rank	Hospital	U.S. News index	Reputa-tional score	Cardiology mortality rate	COTH member	Interns and residents to beds	Tech-nology score (of 10)	R.N.'s to beds	Board-certified cardiologists to beds	Procedures to beds
	TIER ONE									
21	University Hospital, Portland	28.6	0.0%	0.93	Yes	1.54	9	2.31	0.043	2.76
	TIER THREE									
	Bess Kaiser Medical Center, Portland	15.6	0.0%	0.88	No	0.02	3	0.78	0.000	10.05
	Good Samaritan Hospital and Medical Center, Portland	17.0	0.0%	0.90	No	0.23	7	0.69	0.031	7.35
	Mercy Medical Center, Roseburg	18.1	0.0%	0.87	No	0.00	5	1.25	0.029	9.28
	Providence Medical Center, Portland	16.0	0.0%	0.94	No	0.15	7	0.81	0.038	6.85
	Sacred Heart General Hospital, Eugene	16.4	0.0%	0.95	No	0.00	7	1.44	0.002	9.27
	St. Charles Medical Center, Bend	18.0	0.0%	0.93	No	0.00	8	1.61	0.017	7.71

STATE RANKINGS ■ OREGON

Natl. Rank	Hospital	U.S. News index	Reputational score	Cardiology mortality rate	COTH member	Interns and residents to beds	Technology score (of 10)	R.N.'s to beds	Board-certified cardiologists to beds	Procedures to beds
	St. Vincent Hospital and Medical Center, Portland	14.5	1.4%	1.09	No	0.14	7	0.75	0.033	10.90
TIER FOUR										
	Emanuel Hospital and Health Center, Portland	13.2	0.0%	1.07	No	0.22	7	0.94	0.033	2.73
	Good Samaritan Hospital Corvallis, Corvallis	11.9	0.0%	1.05	No	0.00	5	0.76	0.019	8.48
	Rogue Valley Medical Center, Medford	11.1	0.0%	1.12	No	0.00	7	0.77	0.023	7.45
	Salem Hospital, Salem	11.5	0.0%	1.14	No	0.00	8	1.09	0.007	7.72

ENDOCRINOLOGY

Natl. Rank	Hospital	U.S. News index	Reputational score	Endocrinology mortality rate	COTH member	Interns and residents to beds	Technology score (of 11)	R.N.'s to beds	Board-certified internists to beds
TIER ONE									
18	University Hospital, Portland	24.9	2.3%	0.73	Yes	1.54	9	2.31	0.164
TIER THREE									
	Good Samaritan Hospital and Medical Center, Portland	8.4	0.0%	0.93	No	0.23	9	0.69	0.141
	Providence Medical Center, Portland	9.6	0.0%	0.76	No	0.15	8	0.81	0.104
	Sacred Heart General Hospital, Eugene	12.4	0.0%	0.67	No	0.00	8	1.44	0.143
	St. Vincent Hospital and Medical Center, Portland	11.0	0.0%	0.65	No	0.14	8	0.75	0.129
TIER FOUR									
	Bess Kaiser Medical Center, Portland	7.8	0.3%	0.97	No	0.02	4	0.78	0.236
	Emanuel Hospital and Health Center, Portland	8.1	0.0%	0.95	No	0.22	8	0.94	0.048
	Rogue Valley Medical Center, Medford	6.2	0.0%	1.15	No	0.00	8	0.77	0.121
	Salem Hospital, Salem	6.0	0.0%	1.24	No	0.00	8	1.09	0.045

GASTROENTEROLOGY

Natl. Rank	Hospital	U.S. News index	Reputational score	Gastro-enterology mortality rate	COTH member	Interns and residents to beds	Technology score (of 11)	R.N.'s to beds	Board-certified gastro-enterologists to beds	Pro-cedures to beds
TIER THREE										
	Bess Kaiser Medical Center, Portland	7.9	0.0%	0.74	No	0.02	3	0.78	0.000	5.33
	Emanuel Hospital and Health Center, Portland	8.0	0.0%	0.82	No	0.22	7	0.94	0.013	1.44
	Good Samaritan Hospital Corvallis, Corvallis	7.5	0.0%	0.94	No	0.00	6	0.76	0.029	5.19
	Good Samaritan Hospital and Medical Center, Portland	8.2	0.0%	0.75	No	0.23	8	0.69	0.018	2.19
	Mercy Medical Center, Roseburg	10.0	0.0%	0.86	No	0.00	6	1.25	0.020	6.34
	Providence Medical Center, Portland	9.1	0.0%	0.70	No	0.15	8	0.81	0.035	3.59
	Sacred Heart General Hospital, Eugene	8.2	0.0%	0.96	No	0.00	7	1.44	0.000	3.53
	Salem Hospital, Salem	8.0	0.0%	0.98	No	0.00	7	1.09	0.005	4.91
	St. Charles Medical Center, Bend	9.8	0.0%	0.88	No	0.00	8	1.61	0.011	3.90
	St. Vincent Hospital and Medical Center, Portland	8.2	0.0%	0.85	No	0.14	7	0.75	0.018	3.59
TIER FOUR										
	Rogue Valley Medical Center, Medford	6.4	0.4%	0.99	No	0.00	7	0.77	0.020	2.59

GERIATRICS

Natl. Rank	Hospital	U.S. News index	Reputational score	Hospital-wide mortality rate	COTH member	Service mix	Interns and residents to beds	Technology score (of 13)	R.N.'s to beds	Discharge planning (of 2)	Geriatric services (of 9)	Board-certified internists to beds
TIER ONE												
22	University Hospital, Portland	31.2	1.1%	0.80	Yes	7	1.54	11	2.31	2	2	0.164
TIER THREE												
	Bess Kaiser Medical Center, Portland	17.6	0.0%	0.91	No	5	0.02	6	0.78	2	2	0.236
	Emanuel Hospital and Health Center, Portland	15.5	0.0%	1.02	No	7	0.22	10	0.94	2	2	0.048
	Good Samaritan Hospital Corvallis, Corvallis	15.9	0.0%	0.92	No	5	0.00	8	0.76	1	1	0.190

Natl. Rank	Hospital	U.S. News index	Reputational score	Hospital-wide mortality rate	COTH member	Service mix	Interns and residents to beds	Technology score (of 13)	R.N.'s to beds	Discharge planning (of 2)	Geriatric services (of 9)	Board-certified internists to beds
	Good Samaritan Hospital and Medical Center, Portland	19.3	0.3%	0.87	No	3	0.23	9	0.69	2	6	0.141
	Providence Medical Center, Portland	20.5	0.4%	0.84	No	7	0.15	9	0.81	1	7	0.104
	Rogue Valley Medical Center, Medford	15.7	0.0%	1.01	No	6	0.00	11	0.77	2	4	0.121
	Sacred Heart General Hospital, Eugene	20.3	0.0%	0.91	No	8	0.00	9	1.44	2	3	0.143
	St. Charles Medical Center, Bend	14.7	0.0%	1.02	No	3	0.00	10	1.61	2	2	0.039
TIER FOUR												
	Salem Hospital, Salem	10.4	0.0%	1.13	No	4	0.00	11	1.09	1	2	0.045
	St. Vincent Hospital and Medical Center, Portland	13.2	0.0%	1.07	No	8	0.14	9	0.75	1	2	0.129

GYNECOLOGY

Natl. Rank	Hospital	U.S. News index	Reputational score	Hospital-wide mortality rate	Interns and residents to beds	Technology score (of 10)	R.N.'s to beds	Board-certified OB-GYNs to beds	Procedures to beds
TIER ONE									
23	University Hospital, Portland	33.1	0.0%	0.80	1.54	8	2.31	0.055	0.38
TIER THREE									
	Bess Kaiser Medical Center, Portland	17.9	0.4%	0.91	0.02	4	0.78	0.088	0.71
	Emanuel Hospital and Health Center, Portland	17.4	0.0%	1.02	0.22	7	0.94	0.127	0.22
	Good Samaritan Hospital and Medical Center, Portland	20.5	0.0%	0.87	0.23	7	0.69	0.099	0.59
	Providence Medical Center, Portland	18.6	0.0%	0.84	0.15	6	0.81	0.042	0.53
	Rogue Valley Medical Center, Medford	14.5	0.0%	1.01	0.00	7	0.77	0.036	0.56
	Sacred Heart General Hospital, Eugene	20.0	0.0%	0.91	0.00	6	1.44	0.048	0.76
	St. Charles Medical Center, Bend	17.5	0.0%	1.02	0.00	6	1.61	0.044	0.98
TIER FOUR									
	Salem Hospital, Salem	12.5	0.0%	1.13	0.00	6	1.09	0.043	0.55
	St. Vincent Hospital and Medical Center, Portland	13.3	0.0%	1.07	0.14	6	0.75	0.060	0.82

NEUROLOGY

Natl. Rank	Hospital	U.S. News index	Reputational score	Neurology mortality rate	COTH member	Interns and residents to beds	Technology score (of 9)	R.N.'s to beds	Board-certified neurologists to beds
TIER ONE									
21	University Hospital, Portland	25.8	0.6%	0.95	Yes	1.54	7	2.31	0.063
TIER THREE									
	Good Samaritan Hospital and Medical Center, Portland	12.7	0.0%	0.96	No	0.23	7	0.69	0.042
	Providence Medical Center, Portland	13.5	0.0%	0.80	No	0.15	6	0.81	0.009
	Rogue Valley Medical Center, Medford	11.6	0.0%	0.86	No	0.00	6	0.77	0.010
	Sacred Heart General Hospital, Eugene	11.1	0.0%	1.02	No	0.00	6	1.44	0.018
TIER FOUR									
	Emanuel Hospital and Health Center, Portland	9.0	0.0%	1.10	No	0.22	6	0.94	0.013
	Good Samaritan Hospital Corvallis, Corvallis	10.2	0.0%	0.99	No	0.00	5	0.76	0.029
	Salem Hospital, Salem	7.6	0.0%	1.16	No	0.00	6	1.09	0.007
	St. Charles Medical Center, Bend	8.2	0.0%	1.36	No	0.00	7	1.61	0.022
	St. Vincent Hospital and Medical Center, Portland	8.6	0.0%	1.06	No	0.14	6	0.75	0.009

ORTHOPEDICS

Natl. Rank	Hospital	U.S. News index	Reputational score	Orthopedics mortality rate	COTH member	Interns and residents to beds	Technology score (of 5)	R.N.'s to beds	Board-certified orthopedists to beds	Procedures to beds
TIER TWO										
45	**University Hospital, Portland**	**17.2**	0.0%	1.14	Yes	1.54	4	2.31	0.017	1.36
TIER THREE										
	Emanuel Hospital and Health Center, Portland	10.4	0.0%	0.69	No	0.22	3	0.94	0.043	2.01
	Good Samaritan Hospital Corvallis, Corvallis	10.9	0.0%	0.24	No	0.00	3	0.76	0.067	7.16
	Good Samaritan Hospital and Medical Center, Portland	10.2	0.0%	0.64	No	0.23	3	0.69	0.036	2.41
	Mercy Medical Center, Roseburg	11.2	0.0%	0.62	No	0.00	3	1.25	0.039	3.61
	Providence Medical Center, Portland	10.1	0.0%	0.70	No	0.15	3	0.81	0.060	3.88
	Sacred Heart General Hospital, Eugene	9.9	0.0%	0.81	No	0.00	3	1.44	0.040	4.38
	St. Charles Medical Center, Bend	10.5	0.0%	0.91	No	0.00	4	1.61	0.050	6.49
TIER FOUR										
	Bess Kaiser Medical Center, Portland	5.5	0.0%	1.01	No	0.02	2	0.78	0.037	3.66
	Portland Adventist Medical Center, Portland	4.5	0.0%	1.30	No	0.01	3	0.97	0.026	1.87
	Rogue Valley Medical Center, Medford	7.7	0.0%	0.79	No	0.00	3	0.77	0.030	2.19
	Salem Hospital, Salem	7.4	0.3%	1.10	No	0.00	3	1.09	0.048	4.84
	St. Vincent Hospital and Medical Center, Portland	5.0	0.0%	1.25	No	0.14	3	0.75	0.053	3.19

OTOLARYNGOLOGY

Natl. Rank	Hospital	U.S. News index	Reputational score	Hospital-wide mortality rate	COTH member	Interns and residents to beds	Technology score (of 9)	R.N.'s to beds	Board-certified internists to beds	Procedures to beds
TIER ONE										
24	**University Hospital, Portland**	**23.8**	1.2%	0.80	Yes	1.54	7	2.31	0.164	0.374
TIER THREE										
	Sacred Heart General Hospital, Eugene	7.5	0.0%	0.91	No	0.00	6	1.44	0.143	0.251
	St. Charles Medical Center, Bend	7.3	0.0%	1.02	No	0.00	7	1.61	0.039	0.260
TIER FOUR										
	Bess Kaiser Medical Center, Portland	5.2	0.0%	0.91	No	0.02	2	0.78	0.236	0.458
	Emanuel Hospital and Health Center, Portland	5.9	0.0%	1.02	No	0.22	6	0.94	0.048	0.132
	Good Samaritan Hospital Corvallis, Corvallis	5.5	0.0%	0.92	No	0.00	5	0.76	0.190	0.257
	Good Samaritan Hospital and Medical Center, Portland	6.4	0.0%	0.87	No	0.23	7	0.69	0.141	0.234
	Mercy Medical Center, Roseburg	5.5	0.0%	0.76	No	0.00	4	1.25	0.029	0.441
	Portland Adventist Medical Center, Portland	5.1	0.0%	0.80	No	0.01	6	0.97	0.015	0.052
	Providence Medical Center, Portland	5.9	0.0%	0.84	No	0.15	6	0.81	0.104	0.162
	Rogue Valley Medical Center, Medford	6.8	0.5%	1.01	No	0.00	6	0.77	0.121	0.125
	Salem Hospital, Salem	5.4	0.0%	1.13	No	0.00	6	1.09	0.045	0.133
	St. Vincent Hospital and Medical Center, Portland	5.6	0.0%	1.07	No	0.14	6	0.75	0.129	0.175

RHEUMATOLOGY

Natl. Rank	Hospital	U.S. News index	Reputational score	Hospital-wide mortality rate	COTH member	Interns and residents to beds	Technology score (of 5)	R.N.'s to beds	Board-certified internists to beds
TIER ONE									
24	**University Hospital, Portland**	**22.6**	0.0%	0.80	Yes	1.54	4	2.31	0.164
TIER THREE									
	Bess Kaiser Medical Center, Portland	10.1	0.0%	0.91	No	0.02	2	0.78	0.236
	Good Samaritan Hospital and Medical Center, Portland	10.7	0.0%	0.87	No	0.23	3	0.69	0.141
	Mercy Medical Center, Roseburg	11.0	0.0%	0.76	No	0.00	3	1.25	0.029
	Providence Medical Center, Portland	9.9	0.0%	0.84	No	0.15	3	0.81	0.104
	Sacred Heart General Hospital, Eugene	11.5	0.0%	0.91	No	0.00	3	1.44	0.143
	St. Charles Medical Center, Bend	10.6	0.0%	1.02	No	0.00	4	1.61	0.039

Natl. Rank Hospital	U.S. News index	Reputa-tional score	Hospital-wide mortality rate	COTH member	Interns and residents to beds	Tech-nology score (of 5)	R.N.'s to beds	Board-certified internists to beds
TIER FOUR								
Emanuel Hospital and Health Center, Portland	9.1	0.0%	1.02	No	0.22	3	0.94	0.048
Good Samaritan Hospital Corvallis, Corvallis	8.9	0.0%	0.92	No	0.00	3	0.76	0.190
Rogue Valley Medical Center, Medford	8.6	0.0%	1.01	No	0.00	3	0.77	0.121
Salem Hospital, Salem	6.9	0.0%	1.13	No	0.00	3	1.09	0.045
St. Vincent Hospital and Medical Center, Portland	7.5	0.0%	1.07	No	0.14	3	0.75	0.129

UROLOGY

Natl. Rank Hospital	U.S. News index	Reputa-tional score	Urology mortality rate	COTH member	Interns and residents to beds	Tech-nology score (of 11)	R.N.'s to beds	Board-certified internists to beds	Procedures to beds
TIER ONE									
18 University Hospital, Portland	25.0	1.0%	0.53	Yes	1.54	9	2.31	0.164	2.08
TIER THREE									
Good Samaritan Hospital Corvallis, Corvallis	11.8	0.0%	0.59	No	0.00	6	0.76	0.190	3.76
Good Samaritan Hospital and Medical Center, Portland	12.3	0.0%	0.67	No	0.23	8	0.69	0.141	1.88
Providence Medical Center, Portland	9.0	0.0%	0.98	No	0.15	8	0.81	0.104	2.15
Sacred Heart General Hospital, Eugene	13.2	0.0%	0.73	No	0.00	7	1.44	0.143	2.13
Salem Hospital, Salem	8.9	0.0%	0.95	No	0.00	7	1.09	0.045	2.39
St. Charles Medical Center, Bend	11.2	0.0%	0.93	No	0.00	8	1.61	0.039	4.24
TIER FOUR									
Bess Kaiser Medical Center, Portland	6.5	0.0%	1.11	No	0.02	3	0.78	0.236	2.46
Emanuel Hospital and Health Center, Portland	7.5	0.0%	1.10	No	0.22	7	0.94	0.048	1.00
Mercy Medical Center, Roseburg	6.4	0.0%	1.29	No	0.00	6	1.25	0.029	2.67
St. Vincent Hospital and Medical Center, Portland	6.8	0.0%	1.21	No	0.14	7	0.75	0.129	1.84

AIDS

Natl. Rank	Hospital	U.S. News index	Reputa-tional score	Hospital-wide mortality rate	COTH member	Interns and residents to beds	Tech-nology score (of 11)	Discharge planning (of 2)	R.N.'s to beds	Board-certified internists to beds
TIER ONE										
27	Hospital of the University of Pennsylvania, Philadelphia	30.0	2.0%	0.97	Yes	1.72	9	2	1.33	0.007
TIER TWO										
83	Graduate Hospital, Philadelphia	25.3	0.9%	1.04	Yes	0.74	9	2	1.07	0.109
93	Mercy Hospital of Pittsburgh, Pittsburgh	24.8	0.0%	0.90	Yes	0.37	7	2	0.94	0.053
61	Penn State's Milton S. Hershey Medical Ctr., Hershey	26.4	0.0%	1.03	Yes	1.55	9	2	1.57	0.023
91	Temple University Hospital, Philadelphia	24.9	0.5%	1.05	Yes	1.25	7	2	1.15	0.055
40	Thomas Jefferson University Hospital, Philadelphia	28.3	0.5%	0.85	Yes	0.96	9	2	1.44	0.042
56	University of Pittsburgh-Presbyterian University Hospital	26.6	0.0%	1.10	Yes	1.48	7	2	2.10	0.291
92	Western Pennsylvania Hospital, Pittsburgh	24.8	0.0%	0.95	Yes	0.43	7	2	1.44	0.091
TIER THREE										
	Abington Memorial Hospital, Abington	21.8	0.0%	0.93	No	0.36	5	2	0.84	0.088
	Albert Einstein Medical Center, Philadelphia	23.8	0.6%	1.07	Yes	0.75	8	2	0.89	0.098
	Allegheny General Hospital, Pittsburgh	22.8	0.0%	1.04	Yes	0.52	6	2	1.36	0.025
	Bryn Mawr Hospital, Bryn Mawr	24.6	0.0%	0.80	Yes	0.14	5	2	1.35	0.083
	Chester County Hospital, Westchester	21.4	0.0%	0.91	No	0.00	6	2	0.69	0.074
	Chestnut Hill Hospital, Philadelphia	20.2	0.0%	1.03	No	0.26	5	2	0.99	0.121
	Conemaugh Memorial Hospital, Johnstown	23.1	0.0%	0.79	No	0.43	5	2	1.14	0.043
	Easton Hospital, Easton	20.4	0.0%	1.01	No	0.20	5	2	0.99	0.106
	Forbes Regional Hospital, Monroeville	21.3	0.0%	0.94	No	0.11	6	2	0.85	0.068
	Frankford Hospital, Philadelphia	21.2	0.0%	1.06	Yes	0.17	5	2	1.07	0.077
	Geisinger Medical Center, Danville	23.5	0.0%	1.06	Yes	0.68	7	2	1.23	0.140
	Hahnemann University Hospital, Philadelphia	21.5	0.0%	1.22	Yes	1.19	6	2	1.11	0.045
	Lehigh Valley Hospital, Allentown	22.2	0.4%	1.08	Yes	0.19	7	2	1.19	0.044
	McKeesport Hospital, McKeesport	20.0	0.0%	1.03	No	0.28	6	2	0.78	0.064
	Medical College Hospital, Philadelphia	22.6	0.0%	1.13	Yes	1.39	5	2	0.81	0.138
	Paoli Memorial Hospital, Paoli	21.0	0.0%	0.94	No	0.00	5	2	0.82	0.113
	Presbyterian Medical Center of Philadelphia	19.8	0.0%	1.08	No	0.64	5	2	0.72	0.114
	Shadyside Hospital, Pittsburgh	22.4	0.0%	1.02	Yes	0.23	7	2	0.88	0.103
	University of Pittsburgh-Montefiore Hospital	23.2	0.5%	1.08	No	0.93	5	2	1.43	0.388
	Westmoreland Hospital, Greensburg	20.5	0.0%	1.01	No	0.00	7	2	1.09	0.022
	York Hospital, York	20.5	0.0%	1.13	Yes	0.33	6	2	0.92	0.063
TIER FOUR										
	Allegheny Valley Hospital, Natrona Heights	19.1	0.0%	1.04	No	0.00	7	1	0.85	0.061
	Altoona Hospital, Altoona	15.8	0.0%	1.36	No	0.12	4	2	1.15	0.069
	Crozer-Chester Medical Center, Upland	19.5	0.0%	1.22	Yes	0.12	8	2	0.72	0.058
	Delaware County Memorial Hospital, Drexel Hill	18.7	0.0%	1.05	No	0.09	6	1	0.81	0.083
	Delaware Valley Medical Center, Langhorne	19.2	0.0%	1.19	No	0.47	6	2	0.45	0.393
	Divine Providence Hospital, Williamsport	17.2	0.0%	1.11	No	0.00	5	1	0.85	0.017
	Dubois Regional Medical Center, Dubois	18.2	0.0%	1.13	No	0.00	7	2	0.77	0.014
	Episcopal Hospital, Philadelphia	18.2	0.0%	1.22	Yes	0.40	4	2	0.54	0.033
	Germantown Hospital and Medical Center, Philadelphia	18.9	0.0%	1.24	Yes	0.21	5	2	0.99	0.097
	Good Samaritan Hospital, Lebanon	16.2	0.0%	1.21	No	0.06	4	2	0.72	0.021
	Hamot Medical Center, Erie	17.1	0.0%	1.29	Yes	0.10	5	1	0.95	0.016
	Harrisburg Hospital, Harrisburg	16.1	0.0%	1.34	No	0.17	5	2	0.96	0.065
	Lancaster General Hospital, Lancaster	18.4	0.0%	1.12	No	0.14	6	2	0.85	0.009
	Lankenau Hospital, Wynnewood	19.5	0.0%	1.18	No	0.47	7	2	1.21	0.072
	Latrobe Area Hospital, Latrobe	19.4	0.0%	0.97	No	0.10	3	2	0.80	0.030
	Lee Hospital, Johnstown	19.2	0.0%	1.09	No	0.00	5	2	1.20	0.138
	Lewistown Hospital, Lewistown	18.4	0.0%	1.07	No	0.00	7	1	0.68	0.070
	Lower Bucks Hospital, Bristol	16.9	0.0%	1.25	No	0.01	6	2	0.87	0.070
	Mercy Health Corporation, Bala Cynwyd	16.2	0.0%	1.47	Yes	0.32	5	2	0.54	0.051

Natl. Rank	Hospital	U.S. News index	Reputational score	Hospital-wide mortality rate	COTH member	Interns and residents to beds	Technology score (of 11)	Discharge planning (of 2)	R.N.'s to beds	Board-certified internists to beds
	Mercy Hospital of Scranton, Scranton	16.9	0.0%	1.29	No	0.02	7	2	0.91	0.044
	Methodist Hospital, Philadelphia	19.3	0.0%	1.15	No	0.06	4	2	1.57	0.254
	Monongahela Valley Hospital, Monongahela	15.8	0.0%	1.27	No	0.00	5	2	0.72	0.032
	Montgomery Hospital, Norristown	18.0	0.0%	1.11	No	0.12	5	2	0.61	0.076
	Moses Taylor Hospital, Scranton	18.1	0.4%	1.11	No	0.04	4	2	0.73	0.056
	Nazareth Hospital, Philadelphia	18.3	0.0%	1.10	No	0.00	6	2	0.76	0.037
	Northeastern Hospital of Philadelphia	17.2	0.0%	1.16	No	0.02	5	2	0.71	0.046
	Northwest Medical Center, Franklin	19.5	0.0%	1.03	No	0.00	7	2	0.64	0.022
	Polyclinic Medical Center, Harrisburg	15.9	0.0%	1.35	No	0.20	6	2	0.66	0.041
	Reading Hospital and Medical Center, Reading	17.1	0.0%	1.29	No	0.20	7	2	0.84	0.057
	Robert Packer Hospital, Sayre	19.3	0.0%	1.06	No	0.27	7	1	0.97	0.022
	Sacred Heart Hospital, Allentown	18.4	0.0%	1.20	No	0.15	6	2	0.85	0.231
	St. Agnes Medical Center, Philadelphia	16.9	0.0%	1.20	No	0.13	5	2	0.58	0.085
	St. Francis Medical Center, Pittsburgh	18.0	0.0%	1.33	Yes	0.14	6	2	0.69	0.130
	St. Joseph Hospital, Reading	16.4	0.0%	1.25	No	0.11	5	2	0.77	0.047
	St. Luke's Hospital, Bethlehem	16.5	0.0%	1.27	No	0.14	7	1	0.85	0.053
	St. Margaret Memorial Hospital, Pittsburgh	17.8	0.0%	1.11	No	0.27	5	1	0.64	0.109
	St. Vincent Health System, Erie	18.1	0.0%	1.14	No	0.08	5	2	1.11	0.026
	The Medical Center, Beaver	17.2	0.0%	1.24	No	0.08	7	2	0.80	0.040
	Thomas Jefferson University Hospital, Philadelphia	15.5	0.0%	1.29	No	0.01	4	2	0.55	0.140
	Washington Hospital, Washington	19.5	0.0%	0.98	No	0.12	5	1	0.78	0.074
	Wilkes-Barre General Hospital, Wilkes-Barre	15.7	0.0%	1.32	No	0.01	6	2	0.75	0.009
	Williamsport Hospital and Medical Center, Williamsport	17.4	0.0%	1.17	No	0.13	5	2	0.73	0.055

CANCER

Natl. Rank	Hospital	U.S. News index	Reputational score	Cancer mortality rate	COTH member	Interns and residents to beds	Technology score (of 12)	R.N.'s to beds	Board-certified oncologists to beds	Procedures to beds
TIER ONE										
14	Hospital of the University of Pennsylvania, Philadelphia	19.2	4.0%	0.86	Yes	1.72	10	1.33	0.033	1.87
TIER TWO										
19	Fox Chase Cancer Center, Philadelphia	16.1	3.7%	0.14	No	0.36	7	1.42	0.290	15.49
38	Penn State's Milton S. Hershey Medical Ctr., Hershey	14.0	0.0%	0.81	Yes	1.55	9	1.57	0.007	2.15
62	Temple University Hospital, Philadelphia	12.1	0.0%	0.90	Yes	1.25	10	1.15	0.059	1.13
66	Thomas Jefferson University Hospital, Philadelphia	12.0	0.0%	0.87	Yes	0.96	10	1.44	0.020	2.38
26	University of Pittsburgh-Presbyterian University Hospital	15.5	0.0%	0.58	Yes	1.48	8	2.10	0.062	1.71
TIER THREE										
96	Albert Einstein Medical Center, Philadelphia	10.3	0.5%	0.99	Yes	0.75	11	0.89	0.008	1.30
97	Allegheny General Hospital, Pittsburgh	10.3	0.0%	0.64	Yes	0.52	9	1.36	0.019	1.54
	Bryn Mawr Hospital, Bryn Mawr	8.1	0.0%	0.73	Yes	0.14	6	1.35	0.019	2.40
	Conemaugh Memorial Hospital, Johnstown	5.7	0.0%	0.75	No	0.43	6	1.14	0.006	1.39
	Crozer-Chester Medical Center, Upland	6.4	0.0%	1.20	Yes	0.12	9	0.72	0.016	1.05
	Frankford Hospital, Philadelphia	6.4	0.0%	0.95	Yes	0.17	4	1.07	0.019	1.67
	Geisinger Medical Center, Danville	9.6	0.0%	0.93	Yes	0.68	8	1.23	0.014	1.30
	Germantown Hospital and Medical Center, Philadelphia	6.9	0.0%	0.84	Yes	0.21	6	0.99	0.009	1.12
	Graduate Hospital, Philadelphia	9.8	0.0%	1.02	Yes	0.74	9	1.07	0.022	2.16
85	Hahnemann University Hospital, Philadelphia	10.8	0.0%	0.83	Yes	1.19	7	1.11	0.014	1.35
	Hamot Medical Center, Erie	6.6	0.0%	0.86	Yes	0.10	7	0.95	0.006	1.11
	Lankenau Hospital, Wynnewood	6.5	0.0%	1.43	No	0.47	9	1.21	0.012	2.56
	Lehigh Valley Hospital, Allentown	7.8	0.0%	0.99	Yes	0.19	8	1.19	0.006	1.28
	Magee-Womens Hospital, Pittsburgh	6.0	0.0%	0.44	Yes	0.00	3	1.05	0.000	2.30
98	Medical College Hospital, Philadelphia	10.3	0.0%	0.87	Yes	1.39	6	0.81	0.016	1.08
	Mercy Health Corporation, Bala Cynwyd	5.8	0.0%	1.36	Yes	0.32	6	0.54	0.010	2.49
	Mercy Hospital of Pittsburgh, Pittsburgh	8.1	0.0%	0.86	Yes	0.37	9	0.94	0.002	1.62
	Shadyside Hospital, Pittsburgh	7.4	0.0%	0.85	Yes	0.23	8	0.88	0.017	1.88

Natl. Rank Hospital	U.S. News index	Reputational score	Cancer mortality rate	COTH member	Interns and residents to beds	Technology score (of 12)	R.N.'s to beds	Board-certified oncologists to beds	Procedures to beds
St. Francis Medical Center, Pittsburgh	5.8	0.0%	1.26	Yes	0.14	8	0.69	0.003	0.57
University of Pittsburgh-Montefiore Hospital	8.1	0.0%	0.87	No	0.93	3	1.43	0.091	3.37
Western Pennsylvania Hospital, Pittsburgh	9.7	0.0%	1.02	Yes	0.43	9	1.44	0.026	1.67
York Hospital, York	7.2	0.0%	1.05	Yes	0.33	7	0.92	0.004	1.86
TIER FOUR									
Abington Memorial Hospital, Abington	4.2	0.0%	0.90	No	0.36	5	0.84	0.000	2.20
Allegheny Valley Hospital, Natrona Heights	4.1	0.0%	0.96	No	0.00	9	0.85	0.007	1.62
Altoona Hospital, Altoona	3.8	0.0%	1.39	No	0.12	5	1.15	0.003	1.56
Chester County Hospital, Westchester	3.1	0.0%	1.16	No	0.00	7	0.69	0.013	2.19
Chestnut Hill Hospital, Philadelphia	4.2	0.0%	0.76	No	0.26	3	0.99	0.016	2.72
Delaware County Memorial Hospital, Drexel Hill	3.9	0.0%	1.00	No	0.09	7	0.81	0.011	2.67
Delaware Valley Medical Center, Langhorne	3.8	0.0%	0.94	No	0.47	6	0.45	0.037	1.09
Divine Providence Hospital, Williamsport	4.3	0.0%	0.77	No	0.00	7	0.85	0.028	3.52
Dubois Regional Medical Center, Dubois	3.7	0.0%	0.95	No	0.00	8	0.77	0.009	2.03
Easton Hospital, Easton	3.9	0.0%	0.98	No	0.20	4	0.99	0.003	2.66
Forbes Regional Hospital, Monroeville	4.6	0.0%	0.60	No	0.11	6	0.85	0.048	2.68
Good Samaritan Hospital, Lebanon	1.8	0.0%	1.26	No	0.06	2	0.72	0.000	2.27
Harrisburg Hospital, Harrisburg	3.0	0.0%	1.09	No	0.17	3	0.96	0.005	0.97
Lancaster General Hospital, Lancaster	4.3	0.0%	0.88	No	0.14	8	0.85	0.005	1.55
Latrobe Area Hospital, Latrobe	2.8	0.0%	1.04	No	0.10	3	0.80	0.004	3.14
Lee Hospital, Johnstown	4.1	0.0%	1.00	No	0.00	6	1.20	0.004	1.39
Lewistown Hospital, Lewistown	3.1	0.0%	1.15	No	0.00	8	0.68	0.005	1.51
Lower Bucks Hospital, Bristol	2.5	0.0%	1.21	No	0.01	4	0.87	0.008	1.42
McKeesport Hospital, McKeesport	4.4	0.0%	0.95	No	0.28	7	0.78	0.009	2.26
Mercy Hospital of Scranton, Scranton	3.7	0.0%	1.43	No	0.02	7	0.91	0.014	2.62
Methodist Hospital, Philadelphia	3.8	0.0%	1.27	No	0.06	1	1.57	0.013	1.80
Monongahela Valley Hospital, Monongahela	3.1	0.0%	1.33	No	0.00	7	0.72	0.007	2.81
Montgomery Hospital, Norristown	2.8	0.0%	1.13	No	0.12	6	0.61	0.023	1.26
Moses Taylor Hospital, Scranton	2.2	0.0%	0.77	No	0.04	2	0.73	0.019	1.67
Nazareth Hospital, Philadelphia	3.5	0.0%	1.22	No	0.00	8	0.76	0.031	1.63
Northeastern Hospital of Philadelphia	1.9	0.0%	1.16	No	0.02	3	0.71	0.015	1.37
Northwest Medical Center, Franklin	3.2	0.0%	1.01	No	0.00	8	0.64	0.005	1.88
Paoli Memorial Hospital, Paoli	3.6	0.0%	0.93	No	0.00	6	0.82	0.012	3.34
Polyclinic Medical Center, Harrisburg	3.4	0.0%	1.15	No	0.20	7	0.66	0.010	0.94
Presbyterian Medical Center of Philadelphia	4.4	0.0%	0.90	No	0.64	3	0.72	0.009	2.67
Reading Hospital and Medical Center, Reading	4.3	0.0%	1.29	No	0.20	8	0.84	0.010	2.22
Robert Packer Hospital, Sayre	5.2	0.0%	1.23	No	0.27	9	0.97	0.008	2.10
Sacred Heart Hospital, Allentown	3.8	0.0%	1.24	No	0.15	7	0.85	0.020	1.55
St. Agnes Medical Center, Philadelphia	1.9	0.0%	1.16	No	0.13	3	0.58	0.017	1.40
St. Joseph Hospital, Reading	3.3	0.0%	1.21	No	0.11	7	0.77	0.004	1.10
St. Luke's Hospital, Bethlehem	3.6	0.0%	1.55	No	0.14	7	0.85	0.007	1.86
St. Margaret Memorial Hospital, Pittsburgh	3.4	0.0%	0.87	No	0.27	4	0.64	0.030	2.51
St. Vincent Health System, Erie	3.8	0.0%	1.08	No	0.08	5	1.11	0.007	1.75
The Medical Center, Beaver	4.0	0.0%	0.89	No	0.08	8	0.80	0.000	1.75
Washington Hospital, Washington	4.0	0.0%	0.84	No	0.12	7	0.78	0.023	1.52
Westmoreland Hospital, Greensburg	4.5	0.0%	0.88	No	0.00	7	1.09	0.006	2.65
Wilkes-Barre General Hospital, Wilkes-Barre	3.2	0.0%	1.35	No	0.01	8	0.75	0.000	1.67
Williamsport Hospital and Medical Center, Williamsport	4.0	0.0%	0.64	No	0.13	6	0.73	0.022	1.98

CARDIOLOGY

Natl. Rank	Hospital	U.S. News index	Reputa-tional score	Cardiology mortality rate	COTH member	Interns and residents to beds	Tech-nology score (of 10)	R.N.'s to beds	Board-certified cardiologists to beds	Procedures to beds
TIER ONE
22	Hospital of the University of Pennsylvania, Philadelphia	28.4	0.8%	0.91	Yes	1.72	9	1.33	0.035	4.88
TIER TWO
79	Albert Einstein Medical Center, Philadelphia	21.4	0.0%	0.98	Yes	0.75	9	0.89	0.116	9.34
61	Bryn Mawr Hospital, Bryn Mawr	22.1	0.0%	0.88	Yes	0.14	7	1.35	0.025	11.24
92	Graduate Hospital, Philadelphia	21.0	0.0%	1.01	Yes	0.74	9	1.07	0.066	8.68
56	Mercy Hospital of Pittsburgh, Pittsburgh	22.7	0.0%	0.70	Yes	0.37	8	0.94	0.055	11.55
38	Penn State's Milton S. Hershey Medical Ctr., Hershey	24.2	0.0%	1.02	Yes	1.55	8	1.57	0.034	6.51
47	Temple University Hospital, Philadelphia	23.2	0.6%	1.03	Yes	1.25	9	1.15	0.092	5.62
33	Thomas Jefferson University Hospital, Philadelphia	25.7	0.6%	0.91	Yes	0.96	9	1.44	0.047	5.18
40	University of Pittsburgh-Presbyterian University Hospital	24.1	1.1%	1.19	Yes	1.48	8	2.10	0.056	6.32
39	Western Pennsylvania Hospital, Pittsburgh	24.2	0.0%	0.90	Yes	0.43	9	1.44	0.083	10.97
TIER THREE
	Abington Memorial Hospital, Abington	18.0	0.0%	0.81	No	0.36	5	0.84	0.026	8.02
96	Allegheny General Hospital, Pittsburgh	20.8	0.6%	1.06	Yes	0.52	9	1.36	0.058	9.63
	Chester County Hospital, Westchester	16.6	0.0%	0.77	No	0.00	6	0.69	0.026	8.44
	Chestnut Hill Hospital, Philadelphia	18.5	0.0%	0.88	No	0.26	5	0.99	0.042	11.24
	Conemaugh Memorial Hospital, Johnstown	20.4	0.0%	0.74	No	0.43	8	1.14	0.037	11.26
	Crozer-Chester Medical Center, Upland	17.6	0.0%	0.99	Yes	0.12	9	0.72	0.031	6.25
	Delaware County Memorial Hospital, Drexel Hill	14.5	0.0%	0.98	No	0.09	5	0.81	0.045	9.08
	Forbes Regional Hospital, Monroeville	14.7	0.0%	1.00	No	0.11	7	0.85	0.042	9.50
	Frankford Hospital, Philadelphia	19.3	0.0%	0.94	Yes	0.17	5	1.07	0.041	10.41
	Geisinger Medical Center, Danville	18.0	0.0%	1.11	Yes	0.68	8	1.23	0.031	7.09
	Hahnemann University Hospital, Philadelphia	17.9	0.0%	1.23	Yes	1.19	7	1.11	0.090	8.24
	Lankenau Hospital, Wynnewood	17.1	0.0%	1.03	No	0.47	8	1.21	0.096	14.52
	Lee Hospital, Johnstown	16.0	0.0%	0.92	No	0.00	5	1.20	0.000	12.86
	Lehigh Valley Hospital, Allentown	15.8	0.0%	1.14	Yes	0.19	8	1.19	0.036	6.32
	McKeesport Hospital, McKeesport	14.5	0.0%	1.00	No	0.28	6	0.78	0.017	10.13
	Medical College Hospital, Philadelphia	20.5	0.0%	1.08	Yes	1.39	8	0.81	0.086	6.05
	Methodist Hospital, Philadelphia	17.6	0.0%	0.94	No	0.06	4	1.57	0.080	10.35
	Montgomery Hospital, Norristown	14.5	0.0%	0.97	No	0.12	5	0.61	0.065	6.75
	Nazareth Hospital, Philadelphia	14.5	0.0%	0.98	No	0.00	6	0.76	0.056	11.68
	Northeastern Hospital of Philadelphia	15.6	0.0%	0.91	No	0.02	3	0.71	0.061	9.03
	Northwest Medical Center, Franklin	14.1	0.0%	0.93	No	0.00	6	0.64	0.003	4.83
	Paoli Memorial Hospital, Paoli	15.7	0.0%	0.91	No	0.00	5	0.82	0.036	8.21
	Presbyterian Medical Center of Philadelphia	19.5	0.0%	0.91	No	0.64	8	0.72	0.075	12.73
	Robert Packer Hospital, Sayre	18.1	0.0%	0.91	No	0.27	8	0.97	0.025	9.81
	Sacred Heart Hospital, Allentown	13.9	0.0%	1.04	No	0.15	6	0.85	0.069	7.19
	Shadyside Hospital, Pittsburgh	17.3	0.0%	1.07	Yes	0.23	9	0.88	0.052	13.77
	St. Agnes Medical Center, Philadelphia	14.5	0.0%	0.97	No	0.13	5	0.58	0.089	7.94
	St. Vincent Health System, Erie	15.0	0.0%	1.01	No	0.08	8	1.11	0.019	9.61
	University of Pittsburgh-Montefiore Hospital	18.9	0.0%	1.03	No	0.93	8	1.43	0.072	4.39
	Washington Hospital, Washington	16.1	0.0%	0.92	No	0.12	6	0.78	0.023	10.66
	Westmoreland Hospital, Greensburg	13.8	0.0%	1.04	No	0.00	7	1.09	0.025	9.38
	York Hospital, York	15.1	0.0%	1.13	Yes	0.33	7	0.92	0.010	9.27
TIER FOUR
	Allegheny Valley Hospital, Natrona Heights	13.2	0.0%	1.02	No	0.00	6	0.85	0.022	9.21
	Altoona Hospital, Altoona	10.4	0.0%	1.26	No	0.12	7	1.15	0.026	11.86
	Delaware Valley Medical Center, Langhorne	13.0	0.0%	1.09	No	0.47	6	0.45	0.110	8.99
	Divine Providence Hospital, Williamsport	9.1	0.0%	1.18	No	0.00	4	0.85	0.017	6.48
	Dubois Regional Medical Center, Dubois	5.5	0.0%	1.38	No	0.00	4	0.77	0.000	5.55
	Easton Hospital, Easton	12.7	0.0%	1.07	No	0.20	4	0.99	0.026	11.70
	Episcopal Hospital, Philadelphia	11.4	0.0%	1.33	Yes	0.40	6	0.54	0.057	7.68
	Germantown Hospital and Medical Center, Philadelphia	13.0	0.0%	1.20	Yes	0.21	4	0.99	0.032	6.54

Natl. Rank Hospital	U.S. News index	Reputational score	Cardiology mortality rate	COTH member	Interns and residents to beds	Technology score (of 10)	R.N.'s to beds	Board-certified cardiologists to beds	Procedures to beds
Good Samaritan Hospital, Lebanon	10.5	0.0%	1.11	No	0.06	3	0.72	0.036	12.59
Hamot Medical Center, Erie	9.4	0.0%	1.45	Yes	0.10	6	0.95	0.016	8.08
Harrisburg Hospital, Harrisburg	7.6	0.0%	1.45	No	0.17	7	0.96	0.025	10.59
Lancaster General Hospital, Lancaster	11.2	0.0%	1.17	No	0.14	7	0.85	0.027	10.87
Latrobe Area Hospital, Latrobe	11.4	0.0%	1.08	No	0.10	4	0.80	0.011	12.67
Lewistown Hospital, Lewistown	12.1	0.0%	1.03	No	0.00	5	0.68	0.009	10.16
Lower Bucks Hospital, Bristol	10.0	0.0%	1.25	No	0.01	7	0.87	0.066	9.12
Mercy Health Corporation, Bala Cynwyd	9.3	0.0%	1.41	Yes	0.32	6	0.54	0.013	6.52
Mercy Hospital of Scranton, Scranton	9.8	0.0%	1.23	No	0.02	7	0.91	0.025	11.64
Monongahela Valley Hospital, Monongahela	9.0	0.0%	1.18	No	0.00	3	0.72	0.028	11.81
Moses Taylor Hospital, Scranton	9.6	0.0%	1.16	No	0.04	3	0.73	0.037	10.00
Polyclinic Medical Center, Harrisburg	7.7	0.0%	1.39	No	0.20	8	0.66	0.031	7.84
Reading Hospital and Medical Center, Reading	9.8	0.0%	1.31	No	0.20	9	0.84	0.029	10.90
St. Francis Medical Center, Pittsburgh	9.0	0.0%	1.44	Yes	0.14	8	0.69	0.000	4.63
St. Joseph Hospital, Reading	9.6	0.0%	1.21	No	0.11	6	0.77	0.023	8.16
St. Luke's Hospital, Bethlehem	11.1	0.0%	1.22	No	0.14	8	0.85	0.057	11.60
St. Margaret Memorial Hospital, Pittsburgh	11.5	0.0%	1.11	No	0.27	4	0.64	0.052	9.26
The Medical Center, Beaver	8.7	0.0%	1.28	No	0.08	7	0.80	0.017	8.11
Wilkes-Barre General Hospital, Wilkes-Barre	7.7	0.0%	1.34	No	0.01	8	0.75	0.013	9.24
Williamsport Hospital and Medical Center, Williamsport	11.4	0.0%	1.14	No	0.13	8	0.73	0.029	6.63

ENDOCRINOLOGY

Natl. Rank Hospital	U.S. News index	Reputational score	Endocrinology mortality rate	COTH member	Interns and residents to beds	Technology score (of 11)	R.N.'s to beds	Board-certified internists to beds
TIER ONE								
19 University of Pittsburgh-Presbyterian University Hospital	24.3	3.1%	0.91	Yes	1.48	9	2.10	0.291
23 Hospital of the University of Pennsylvania, Philadelphia	22.5	2.4%	0.71	Yes	1.72	11	1.33	0.007
TIER TWO								
84 Bryn Mawr Hospital, Bryn Mawr	14.6	0.0%	0.36	Yes	0.14	7	1.35	0.083
63 Geisinger Medical Center, Danville	16.2	0.0%	0.69	Yes	0.68	8	1.23	0.140
83 Penn State's Milton S. Hershey Medical Ctr., Hershey	14.8	0.0%	1.30	Yes	1.55	9	1.57	0.023
70 Temple University Hospital, Philadelphia	15.8	0.0%	0.85	Yes	1.25	10	1.15	0.055
50 Thomas Jefferson University Hospital, Philadelphia	17.5	0.5%	0.74	Yes	0.96	10	1.44	0.042
TIER THREE								
Abington Memorial Hospital, Abington	8.6	0.0%	0.89	No	0.36	6	0.84	0.088
Albert Einstein Medical Center, Philadelphia	12.1	0.0%	1.07	Yes	0.75	10	0.89	0.098
Allegheny General Hospital, Pittsburgh	11.4	0.0%	1.17	Yes	0.52	9	1.36	0.025
Chester County Hospital, Westchester	10.0	0.0%	0.25	No	0.00	8	0.69	0.074
Conemaugh Memorial Hospital, Johnstown	10.0	0.0%	0.84	No	0.43	7	1.14	0.043
Crozer-Chester Medical Center, Upland	8.7	0.0%	1.19	Yes	0.12	10	0.72	0.058
Frankford Hospital, Philadelphia	8.4	0.0%	1.30	Yes	0.17	5	1.07	0.077
Graduate Hospital, Philadelphia	11.9	0.0%	1.17	Yes	0.74	9	1.07	0.109
88 Hahnemann University Hospital, Philadelphia	14.1	0.3%	1.01	Yes	1.19	8	1.11	0.045
Hamot Medical Center, Erie	8.7	0.0%	1.12	Yes	0.10	7	0.95	0.016
Latrobe Area Hospital, Latrobe	9.3	0.0%	0.52	No	0.10	3	0.80	0.030
Lehigh Valley Hospital, Allentown	11.1	0.0%	0.98	Yes	0.19	9	1.19	0.044
Medical College Hospital, Philadelphia	11.6	0.0%	1.59	Yes	1.39	7	0.81	0.138
Mercy Hospital of Pittsburgh, Pittsburgh	10.9	0.3%	1.02	Yes	0.37	8	0.94	0.053
Methodist Hospital, Philadelphia	8.6	0.0%	1.09	No	0.06	2	1.57	0.254
Montgomery Hospital, Norristown	10.0	0.0%	0.66	No	0.12	7	0.61	0.076
Robert Packer Hospital, Sayre	10.2	0.0%	0.77	No	0.27	10	0.97	0.022
Shadyside Hospital, Pittsburgh	10.1	0.0%	1.10	Yes	0.23	9	0.88	0.103
St. Francis Medical Center, Pittsburgh	8.2	0.0%	1.33	Yes	0.14	8	0.69	0.130
University of Pittsburgh-Montefiore Hospital	12.7	0.0%	1.01	No	0.93	3	1.43	0.388

Natl. Rank	Hospital	U.S. News index	Reputa-tional score	Endocrinology mortality rate	COTH member	Interns and residents to beds	Tech-nology score (of 11)	R.N.'s to beds	Board-certified internists to beds
	Western Pennsylvania Hospital, Pittsburgh	13.1	0.0%	0.95	Yes	0.43	9	1.44	0.091
	York Hospital, York	10.9	0.0%	0.95	Yes	0.33	8	0.92	0.063
TIER FOUR									
	Allegheny Valley Hospital, Natrona Heights	5.8	0.0%	1.23	No	0.00	9	0.85	0.061
	Altoona Hospital, Altoona	6.6	0.0%	1.15	No	0.12	5	1.15	0.069
	Chestnut Hill Hospital, Philadelphia	5.9	0.0%	1.36	No	0.26	4	0.99	0.121
	Delaware County Memorial Hospital, Drexel Hill	6.1	0.0%	1.20	No	0.09	8	0.81	0.083
	Delaware Valley Medical Center, Langhorne	7.9	0.0%	1.30	No	0.47	7	0.45	0.393
	Easton Hospital, Easton	6.4	0.0%	1.16	No	0.20	4	0.99	0.106
	Episcopal Hospital, Philadelphia	6.7	0.0%	1.50	Yes	0.40	5	0.54	0.033
	Forbes Regional Hospital, Monroeville	7.4	0.0%	0.95	No	0.11	7	0.85	0.068
	Germantown Hospital and Medical Center, Philadelphia	7.6	0.0%	1.71	Yes	0.21	7	0.99	0.097
	Good Samaritan Hospital, Lebanon	3.7	0.0%	1.32	No	0.06	3	0.72	0.021
	Harrisburg Hospital, Harrisburg	3.8	0.0%	1.85	No	0.17	4	0.96	0.065
	Lancaster General Hospital, Lancaster	5.6	0.0%	1.24	No	0.14	8	0.85	0.009
	Lankenau Hospital, Wynnewood	7.7	0.0%	1.44	No	0.47	10	1.21	0.072
	Lee Hospital, Johnstown	5.6	0.0%	1.60	No	0.00	7	1.20	0.138
	Lewistown Hospital, Lewistown	6.3	0.0%	1.02	No	0.00	8	0.68	0.070
	Lower Bucks Hospital, Bristol	3.7	0.0%	1.63	No	0.01	5	0.87	0.070
	McKeesport Hospital, McKeesport	6.2	0.0%	1.27	No	0.28	8	0.78	0.064
	Mercy Health Corporation, Bala Cynwyd	6.9	0.0%	1.52	Yes	0.32	7	0.54	0.051
	Mercy Hospital of Scranton, Scranton	3.8	0.0%	1.89	No	0.02	8	0.91	0.044
	Monongahela Valley Hospital, Monongahela	4.2	0.0%	1.39	No	0.00	7	0.72	0.032
	Moses Taylor Hospital, Scranton	3.1	0.0%	1.60	No	0.04	3	0.73	0.056
	Nazareth Hospital, Philadelphia	5.9	0.0%	1.08	No	0.00	8	0.76	0.037
	Northeastern Hospital of Philadelphia	3.9	0.0%	1.34	No	0.02	4	0.71	0.046
	Northwest Medical Center, Franklin	6.2	0.0%	1.00	No	0.00	9	0.64	0.022
	Paoli Memorial Hospital, Paoli	7.8	0.0%	0.89	No	0.00	7	0.82	0.113
	Polyclinic Medical Center, Harrisburg	5.7	0.0%	1.19	No	0.20	8	0.66	0.041
	Presbyterian Medical Center of Philadelphia	7.0	0.0%	1.20	No	0.64	4	0.72	0.114
	Reading Hospital and Medical Center, Reading	6.3	0.0%	1.25	No	0.20	9	0.84	0.057
	Sacred Heart Hospital, Allentown	6.8	0.0%	1.33	No	0.15	8	0.85	0.231
	St. Agnes Medical Center, Philadelphia	3.8	0.0%	1.44	No	0.13	4	0.58	0.085
	St. Joseph Hospital, Reading	4.7	0.0%	1.47	No	0.11	8	0.77	0.047
	St. Luke's Hospital, Bethlehem	5.0	0.0%	1.48	No	0.14	8	0.85	0.053
	St. Margaret Memorial Hospital, Pittsburgh	4.6	0.0%	1.50	No	0.27	5	0.64	0.109
	St. Vincent Health System, Erie	5.3	0.0%	1.37	No	0.08	6	1.11	0.026
	The Medical Center, Beaver	5.3	0.0%	1.33	No	0.08	9	0.80	0.040
	Washington Hospital, Washington	5.8	0.0%	1.24	No	0.12	8	0.78	0.074
	Westmoreland Hospital, Greensburg	7.7	0.0%	0.93	No	0.00	8	1.09	0.022
	Wilkes-Barre General Hospital, Wilkes-Barre	4.2	0.0%	1.42	No	0.01	8	0.75	0.009
	Williamsport Hospital and Medical Center, Williamsport	4.8	0.0%	1.34	No	0.13	6	0.73	0.055

GASTROENTEROLOGY

Natl. Rank	Hospital	U.S. News index	Reputa-tional score	Gastro-enterology mortality rate	COTH member	Interns and residents to beds	Tech-nology score (of 11)	R.N.'s to beds	Board-certified gastro-enterologists to beds	Pro-cedures to beds
TIER ONE										
11	University of Pittsburgh-Presbyterian University Hospital	31.6	9.5%	0.97	Yes	1.48	8	2.10	0.056	2.18
13	Hospital of the University of Pennsylvania, Philadelphia	26.5	5.6%	0.84	Yes	1.72	11	1.33	0.017	1.82
TIER TWO										
71	Graduate Hospital, Philadelphia	13.4	0.3%	0.92	Yes	0.74	9	1.07	0.000	2.51
39	Penn State's Milton S. Hershey Medical Ctr., Hershey	16.0	0.0%	1.00	Yes	1.55	9	1.57	0.011	1.80
73	Temple University Hospital, Philadelphia	13.3	0.5%	1.24	Yes	1.25	9	1.15	0.027	1.69

Natl. Rank	Hospital	U.S. News index	Reputa- tional score	Gastro- enterology mortality rate	COTH member	Interns and residents to beds	Tech- nology score (of 11)	R.N.'s to beds	Board- certified gastro- enterologists to beds	Pro- cedures to beds
35	Thomas Jefferson University Hospital, Philadelphia	16.5	0.5%	0.65	Yes	0.96	10	1.44	0.024	2.09
	TIER THREE									
	Abington Memorial Hospital, Abington	9.0	0.0%	0.80	No	0.36	5	0.84	0.019	3.63
	Albert Einstein Medical Center, Philadelphia	11.1	0.4%	1.20	Yes	0.75	9	0.89	0.019	2.18
88	Allegheny General Hospital, Pittsburgh	12.7	0.0%	0.91	Yes	0.52	9	1.36	0.012	2.13
	Allegheny Valley Hospital, Natrona Heights	9.0	0.0%	0.71	No	0.00	8	0.85	0.011	4.27
	Bryn Mawr Hospital, Bryn Mawr	11.2	0.0%	0.98	Yes	0.14	6	1.35	0.017	4.28
	Chester County Hospital, Westchester	8.1	0.0%	0.76	No	0.00	7	0.69	0.013	3.93
	Chestnut Hill Hospital, Philadelphia	9.8	0.0%	0.78	No	0.26	4	0.99	0.021	5.66
	Conemaugh Memorial Hospital, Johnstown	10.2	0.0%	0.82	No	0.43	6	1.14	0.014	3.85
	Crozer-Chester Medical Center, Upland	8.4	0.0%	1.17	Yes	0.12	10	0.72	0.018	2.17
	Easton Hospital, Easton	7.5	0.0%	1.02	No	0.20	4	0.99	0.007	5.18
	Forbes Regional Hospital, Monroeville	8.4	0.0%	0.95	No	0.11	6	0.85	0.042	5.71
	Frankford Hospital, Philadelphia	9.0	0.0%	1.23	Yes	0.17	5	1.07	0.041	4.43
	Geisinger Medical Center, Danville	11.3	0.0%	1.12	Yes	0.68	8	1.23	0.014	2.21
	Hahnemann University Hospital, Philadelphia	11.6	0.0%	1.20	Yes	1.19	7	1.11	0.022	1.25
	Lankenau Hospital, Wynnewood	7.7	0.0%	1.41	No	0.47	9	1.21	0.017	3.68
	Lehigh Valley Hospital, Allentown	10.5	0.0%	0.98	Yes	0.19	8	1.19	0.014	2.42
	Medical College Hospital, Philadelphia	11.3	0.0%	1.25	Yes	1.39	6	0.81	0.026	1.60
	Mercy Hospital of Pittsburgh, Pittsburgh	9.8	0.0%	1.11	Yes	0.37	7	0.94	0.014	3.15
	Paoli Memorial Hospital, Paoli	7.7	0.0%	0.90	No	0.00	6	0.82	0.024	4.67
	Shadyside Hospital, Pittsburgh	9.5	0.0%	1.09	Yes	0.23	8	0.88	0.014	3.04
	St. Margaret Memorial Hospital, Pittsburgh	8.9	0.0%	0.81	No	0.27	5	0.64	0.026	4.85
	University of Pittsburgh-Montefiore Hospital	9.7	0.0%	1.05	No	0.93	4	1.43	0.088	2.50
82	Western Pennsylvania Hospital, Pittsburgh	12.9	0.0%	0.91	Yes	0.43	8	1.44	0.020	3.13
	Westmoreland Hospital, Greensburg	7.7	0.0%	1.02	No	0.00	7	1.09	0.017	4.66
	York Hospital, York	10.7	0.0%	1.05	Yes	0.33	7	0.92	0.008	4.37
	TIER FOUR									
	Altoona Hospital, Altoona	5.4	0.0%	1.39	No	0.12	4	1.15	0.003	4.71
	Delaware County Memorial Hospital, Drexel Hill	7.2	0.0%	1.03	No	0.09	7	0.81	0.023	4.54
	Divine Providence Hospital, Williamsport	4.8	0.0%	1.27	No	0.00	7	0.85	0.017	3.15
	Dubois Regional Medical Center, Dubois	6.6	0.0%	1.02	No	0.00	8	0.77	0.005	3.70
	Germantown Hospital and Medical Center, Philadelphia	7.3	0.0%	1.50	Yes	0.21	6	0.99	0.014	3.11
	Good Samaritan Hospital, Lebanon	3.6	0.0%	1.61	No	0.06	3	0.72	0.005	5.37
	Hamot Medical Center, Erie	6.8	0.0%	1.33	Yes	0.10	6	0.95	0.006	2.02
	Harrisburg Hospital, Harrisburg	3.9	0.0%	1.44	No	0.17	4	0.96	0.010	2.86
	Lancaster General Hospital, Lancaster	4.7	0.0%	1.44	No	0.14	7	0.85	0.013	3.26
	Latrobe Area Hospital, Latrobe	6.4	0.0%	1.03	No	0.10	3	0.80	0.000	5.41
	Lee Hospital, Johnstown	7.3	0.0%	1.06	No	0.00	6	1.20	0.000	4.57
	Lewistown Hospital, Lewistown	4.8	0.0%	1.38	No	0.00	7	0.68	0.005	4.73
	Lower Bucks Hospital, Bristol	3.7	0.0%	1.47	No	0.01	5	0.87	0.029	3.31
	McKeesport Hospital, McKeesport	6.5	0.0%	1.34	No	0.28	7	0.78	0.012	5.08
	Mercy Health Corporation, Bala Cynwyd	7.2	0.0%	1.40	Yes	0.32	7	0.54	0.013	2.88
	Mercy Hospital of Scranton, Scranton	5.4	0.0%	1.32	No	0.02	7	0.91	0.008	4.16
	Methodist Hospital, Philadelphia	5.6	0.0%	1.35	No	0.06	2	1.57	0.036	4.20
	Monongahela Valley Hospital, Monongahela	5.6	0.0%	1.26	No	0.00	6	0.72	0.007	5.47
	Montgomery Hospital, Norristown	6.4	0.0%	0.90	No	0.12	6	0.61	0.011	2.76
	Moses Taylor Hospital, Scranton	5.8	0.0%	1.05	No	0.04	3	0.73	0.023	5.07
	Nazareth Hospital, Philadelphia	6.2	0.0%	1.12	No	0.00	7	0.76	0.031	4.53
	Northeastern Hospital of Philadelphia	3.4	0.0%	1.49	No	0.02	4	0.71	0.030	4.06
	Northwest Medical Center, Franklin	4.6	0.0%	1.26	No	0.00	9	0.64	0.003	2.60
	Polyclinic Medical Center, Harrisburg	4.8	0.0%	1.30	No	0.20	8	0.66	0.015	2.27
	Presbyterian Medical Center of Philadelphia	6.3	0.0%	1.16	No	0.64	4	0.72	0.048	2.76
	Reading Hospital and Medical Center, Reading	6.8	0.0%	1.19	No	0.20	8	0.84	0.010	4.16
	Robert Packer Hospital, Sayre	7.1	0.0%	1.23	No	0.27	10	0.97	0.011	3.07

Natl. Rank	Hospital	U.S. News index	Reputational score	Gastro-enterology mortality rate	COTH member	Interns and residents to beds	Technology score (of 11)	R.N.'s to beds	Board-certified gastroenterologists to beds	Procedures to beds
	Sacred Heart Hospital, Allentown	6.8	0.0%	1.09	No	0.15	7	0.85	0.012	3.97
	St. Agnes Medical Center, Philadelphia	4.6	0.0%	1.11	No	0.13	4	0.58	0.034	3.03
	St. Francis Medical Center, Pittsburgh	7.1	0.0%	1.17	Yes	0.14	8	0.69	0.000	1.13
	St. Joseph Hospital, Reading	4.0	0.0%	1.67	No	0.11	7	0.77	0.016	3.75
	St. Luke's Hospital, Bethlehem	5.7	0.0%	1.26	No	0.14	7	0.85	0.007	3.74
	St. Vincent Health System, Erie	5.4	0.0%	1.20	No	0.08	5	1.11	0.007	3.23
	The Medical Center, Beaver	6.3	0.0%	1.14	No	0.08	8	0.80	0.009	3.91
	Washington Hospital, Washington	7.1	0.0%	1.18	No	0.12	8	0.78	0.023	5.30
	Wilkes-Barre General Hospital, Wilkes-Barre	4.2	0.0%	1.49	No	0.01	7	0.75	0.016	3.91
	Williamsport Hospital and Medical Center, Williamsport	4.0	0.0%	1.41	No	0.13	5	0.73	0.015	3.49

GERIATRICS

Natl. Rank	Hospital	U.S. News index	Reputational score	Hospital-wide mortality rate	COTH member	Service mix	Interns and residents to beds	Technology score (of 13)	R.N.'s to beds	Discharge planning (of 2)	Geriatric services (of 9)	Board-certified internists to beds
TIER ONE												
23	Hospital of the University of Pennsylvania, Philadelphia	30.3	2.1%	0.97	Yes	8	1.72	12	1.33	2	4	0.007
TIER TWO												
36	Albert Einstein Medical Center, Philadelphia	26.2	2.3%	1.07	Yes	8	0.75	12	0.89	2	8	0.098
81	Bryn Mawr Hospital, Bryn Mawr	22.2	0.0%	0.80	Yes	7	0.14	9	1.35	2	2	0.083
75	Mercy Hospital of Pittsburgh, Pittsburgh	22.4	0.0%	0.90	Yes	6	0.37	11	0.94	2	5	0.053
70	Penn State's Milton S. Hershey Medical Ctr., Hershey	22.6	0.0%	1.03	Yes	7	1.55	10	1.57	2	6	0.023
79	Temple University Hospital, Philadelphia	22.2	1.4%	1.05	Yes	4	1.25	12	1.15	2	1	0.055
34	Thomas Jefferson University Hospital, Philadelphia	26.6	0.5%	0.85	Yes	8	0.96	11	1.44	2	3	0.042
43	University of Pittsburgh-Presbyterian University Hospital	25.0	1.5%	1.10	Yes	5	1.48	10	2.10	2	1	0.291
82	Western Pennsylvania Hospital, Pittsburgh	22.1	0.0%	0.95	Yes	6	0.43	12	1.44	2	5	0.091
TIER THREE												
	Abington Memorial Hospital, Abington	19.8	0.0%	0.93	No	8	0.36	8	0.84	2	6	0.088
	Allegheny General Hospital, Pittsburgh	19.3	0.0%	1.04	Yes	9	0.52	11	1.36	2	1	0.025
	Chester County Hospital, Westchester	16.7	0.0%	0.91	No	4	0.00	10	0.69	2	2	0.074
	Conemaugh Memorial Hospital, Johnstown	19.8	0.0%	0.79	No	5	0.43	9	1.14	2	4	0.043
	Crozer-Chester Medical Center, Upland	15.4	0.0%	1.22	Yes	10	0.12	11	0.72	2	8	0.058
	Easton Hospital, Easton	13.9	0.0%	1.01	No	4	0.20	6	0.99	2	1	0.106
	Forbes Regional Hospital, Monroeville	16.5	0.0%	0.94	No	5	0.11	8	0.85	2	3	0.068
	Frankford Hospital, Philadelphia	15.0	0.0%	1.06	Yes	5	0.17	6	1.07	2	1	0.077
	Geisinger Medical Center, Danville	19.6	0.0%	1.06	Yes	7	0.68	10	1.23	2	5	0.140
	Graduate Hospital, Philadelphia	18.7	0.0%	1.04	Yes	6	0.74	12	1.07	2	1	0.109
	Hahnemann University Hospital, Philadelphia	16.2	0.0%	1.22	Yes	8	1.19	9	1.11	2	3	0.045
	Latrobe Area Hospital, Latrobe	16.8	0.0%	0.97	No	7	0.10	6	0.80	2	7	0.030
	Lee Hospital, Johnstown	14.4	0.0%	1.09	No	6	0.00	9	1.20	2	5	0.138
	Lehigh Valley Hospital, Allentown	18.5	0.5%	1.08	Yes	8	0.19	10	1.19	2	3	0.044
	McKeesport Hospital, McKeesport	14.1	0.0%	1.03	No	4	0.28	10	0.78	2	3	0.064
	Medical College Hospital, Philadelphia	18.1	0.0%	1.13	Yes	7	1.39	9	0.81	2	3	0.138
	Paoli Memorial Hospital, Paoli	17.7	0.0%	0.94	No	7	0.00	9	0.82	2	3	0.113
	Shadyside Hospital, Pittsburgh	17.8	0.0%	1.02	Yes	4	0.23	11	0.88	2	6	0.103
	University of Pittsburgh-Montefiore Hospital	16.5	0.0%	1.08	No	5	0.93	5	1.43	2	2	0.388
	Washington Hospital, Washington	14.2	0.0%	0.98	No	4	0.12	10	0.78	1	3	0.074
	Westmoreland Hospital, Greensburg	15.5	0.0%	1.01	No	7	0.00	10	1.09	2	2	0.022
	York Hospital, York	15.0	0.0%	1.13	Yes	6	0.33	9	0.92	2	4	0.063
TIER FOUR												
	Allegheny Valley Hospital, Natrona Heights	12.2	0.0%	1.04	No	4	0.00	11	0.85	1	2	0.061
	Altoona Hospital, Altoona	9.5	0.0%	1.36	No	7	0.12	8	1.15	2	6	0.069
	Chestnut Hill Hospital, Philadelphia	13.2	0.0%	1.03	No	3	0.26	5	0.99	2	2	0.121
	Delaware Valley Medical Center, Langhorne	11.3	0.0%	1.19	No	4	0.47	9	0.45	2	1	0.393

Natl. Rank	Hospital	U.S. News index	Reputational score	Hospital-wide mortality rate	COTH member	Service mix	Interns and residents to beds	Technology score (of 13)	R.N.'s to beds	Discharge planning (of 2)	Geriatric services (of 9)	Board-certified internists to beds
	Divine Providence Hospital, Williamsport	9.5	0.0%	1.11	No	4	0.00	8	0.85	1	1	0.017
	Dubois Regional Medical Center, Dubois	11.1	0.0%	1.13	No	6	0.00	9	0.77	2	2	0.014
	Germantown Hospital and Medical Center, Philadelphia	12.1	0.0%	1.24	Yes	6	0.21	8	0.99	2	2	0.097
	Good Samaritan Hospital, Lebanon	8.2	0.0%	1.21	No	5	0.06	3	0.72	2	3	0.021
	Hamot Medical Center, Erie	10.7	0.0%	1.29	Yes	7	0.10	8	0.95	1	5	0.016
	Harrisburg Hospital, Harrisburg	7.2	0.0%	1.34	No	5	0.17	7	0.96	2	1	0.065
	Lancaster General Hospital, Lancaster	11.6	0.0%	1.12	No	5	0.14	10	0.85	2	2	0.009
	Lankenau Hospital, Wynnewood	12.4	0.0%	1.18	No	6	0.47	10	1.21	2	1	0.072
	Lewistown Hospital, Lewistown	11.8	0.0%	1.07	No	7	0.00	9	0.68	1	1	0.070
	Lower Bucks Hospital, Bristol	8.8	0.0%	1.25	No	5	0.01	7	0.87	2	3	0.070
	Mercy Health Corporation, Bala Cynwyd	7.7	0.0%	1.47	Yes	6	0.32	9	0.54	2	1	0.051
	Mercy Hospital of Scranton, Scranton	8.8	0.0%	1.29	No	7	0.02	9	0.91	2	1	0.044
	Methodist Hospital, Philadelphia	11.4	0.0%	1.15	No	4	0.06	3	1.57	2	1	0.254
	Monongahela Valley Hospital, Monongahela	7.3	0.0%	1.27	No	3	0.00	9	0.72	2	3	0.032
	Montgomery Hospital, Norristown	12.2	0.0%	1.11	No	6	0.12	9	0.61	2	3	0.076
	Moses Taylor Hospital, Scranton	9.9	0.0%	1.11	No	3	0.04	3	0.73	2	4	0.056
	Nazareth Hospital, Philadelphia	11.3	0.0%	1.10	No	4	0.00	11	0.76	2	1	0.037
	Northeastern Hospital of Philadelphia	9.0	0.0%	1.16	No	4	0.02	4	0.71	2	3	0.046
	Northwest Medical Center, Franklin	12.9	0.0%	1.03	No	4	0.00	9	0.64	2	3	0.022
	Polyclinic Medical Center, Harrisburg	8.4	0.0%	1.35	No	4	0.20	10	0.66	2	8	0.041
	Presbyterian Medical Center of Philadelphia	13.3	0.0%	1.08	No	5	0.64	6	0.72	2	2	0.114
	Reading Hospital and Medical Center, Reading	9.0	0.0%	1.29	No	6	0.20	11	0.84	2	1	0.057
	Sacred Heart Hospital, Allentown	10.6	0.0%	1.20	No	4	0.15	10	0.85	2	1	0.231
	St. Agnes Medical Center, Philadelphia	9.0	0.0%	1.20	No	4	0.13	5	0.58	2	4	0.085
	St. Francis Medical Center, Pittsburgh	10.8	0.0%	1.33	Yes	5	0.14	11	0.69	2	4	0.130
	St. Joseph Hospital, Reading	8.7	0.0%	1.25	No	5	0.11	9	0.77	2	2	0.047
	St. Margaret Memorial Hospital, Pittsburgh	11.4	0.6%	1.11	No	3	0.27	5	0.64	1	4	0.109
	St. Vincent Health System, Erie	12.7	0.0%	1.14	No	6	0.08	8	1.11	2	6	0.026
	The Medical Center, Beaver	10.3	0.0%	1.24	No	5	0.08	11	0.80	2	6	0.040
	Wilkes-Barre General Hospital, Wilkes-Barre	6.8	0.0%	1.32	No	3	0.01	11	0.75	2	3	0.009
	Williamsport Hospital and Medical Center, Williamsport	10.6	0.0%	1.17	No	5	0.13	9	0.73	2	3	0.055

GYNECOLOGY

Natl. Rank	Hospital	U.S. News index	Reputational score	Hospital-wide mortality rate	Interns and residents to beds	Technology score (of 10)	R.N.'s to beds	Board-certified OB-GYNs to beds	Procedures to beds
	TIER ONE								
15	Hospital of the University of Pennsylvania, Philadelphia	39.7	4.5%	0.97	1.72	10	1.33	0.036	0.35
22	Thomas Jefferson University Hospital, Philadelphia	33.4	1.9%	0.85	0.96	9	1.44	0.102	0.41
	TIER TWO								
44	Penn State's Milton S. Hershey Medical Ctr., Hershey	27.4	1.1%	1.03	1.55	8	1.57	0.021	0.61
63	Temple University Hospital, Philadelphia	24.4	0.6%	1.05	1.25	9	1.15	0.069	0.24
	TIER THREE								
	Abington Memorial Hospital, Abington	18.8	0.0%	0.93	0.36	6	0.84	0.065	0.49
	Albert Einstein Medical Center, Philadelphia	18.7	0.0%	1.07	0.75	9	0.89	0.056	0.17
	Allegheny General Hospital, Pittsburgh	20.4	0.6%	1.04	0.52	8	1.36	0.020	0.18
98	Bryn Mawr Hospital, Bryn Mawr	21.3	0.0%	0.80	0.14	6	1.35	0.058	0.30
	Chester County Hospital, Westchester	16.7	0.0%	0.91	0.00	6	0.69	0.052	0.41
	Chestnut Hill Hospital, Philadelphia	15.1	0.0%	1.03	0.26	4	0.99	0.084	0.53
	Conemaugh Memorial Hospital, Johnstown	20.8	0.0%	0.79	0.43	6	1.14	0.020	0.31
	Forbes Regional Hospital, Monroeville	15.7	0.0%	0.94	0.11	5	0.85	0.025	0.33
	Frankford Hospital, Philadelphia	14.5	0.0%	1.06	0.17	5	1.07	0.058	0.33
	Geisinger Medical Center, Danville	18.9	0.4%	1.06	0.68	7	1.23	0.016	0.32
	Graduate Hospital, Philadelphia	17.9	0.0%	1.04	0.74	7	1.07	0.016	0.30
	Hahnemann University Hospital, Philadelphia	18.1	0.4%	1.22	1.19	7	1.11	0.054	0.18

Natl. Rank	Hospital	U.S. News index	Reputa- tional score	Hospital- wide mortality rate	Interns and residents to beds	Tech- nology score (of 10)	R.N.'s to beds	Board- certified OB-GYNs to beds	Procedures to beds
	Lankenau Hospital, Wynnewood	16.9	0.0%	1.18	0.47	9	1.21	0.072	0.62
	Lehigh Valley Hospital, Allentown	16.0	0.0%	1.08	0.19	8	1.19	0.028	0.41
	Medical College Hospital, Philadelphia	17.5	0.0%	1.13	1.39	6	0.81	0.042	0.26
	Mercy Hospital of Pittsburgh, Pittsburgh	19.9	0.0%	0.90	0.37	7	0.94	0.016	0.21
	Paoli Memorial Hospital, Paoli	15.7	0.0%	0.94	0.00	5	0.82	0.048	0.47
	Robert Packer Hospital, Sayre	15.4	0.0%	1.06	0.27	8	0.97	0.014	0.30
	Shadyside Hospital, Pittsburgh	15.3	0.0%	1.02	0.23	7	0.88	0.016	0.24
	Washington Hospital, Washington	14.7	0.0%	0.98	0.12	6	0.78	0.013	0.44
90	Western Pennsylvania Hospital, Pittsburgh	22.0	0.0%	0.95	0.43	8	1.44	0.045	0.36
	Westmoreland Hospital, Greensburg	15.7	0.0%	1.01	0.00	7	1.09	0.025	0.30
TIER FOUR									
	Allegheny Valley Hospital, Natrona Heights	13.5	0.0%	1.04	0.00	7	0.85	0.011	0.49
	Altoona Hospital, Altoona	6.6	0.0%	1.36	0.12	3	1.15	0.026	0.54
	Crozer-Chester Medical Center, Upland	11.3	0.0%	1.22	0.12	8	0.72	0.055	0.26
	Delaware County Memorial Hospital, Drexel Hill	14.0	0.0%	1.05	0.09	7	0.81	0.038	0.34
	Delaware Valley Medical Center, Langhorne	10.6	0.0%	1.19	0.47	5	0.45	0.080	0.16
	Divine Providence Hospital, Williamsport	11.8	0.0%	1.11	0.00	6	0.85	0.039	0.57
	Dubois Regional Medical Center, Dubois	11.7	0.0%	1.13	0.00	8	0.77	0.014	0.30
	Easton Hospital, Easton	13.9	0.0%	1.01	0.20	4	0.99	0.020	0.34
	Germantown Hospital and Medical Center, Philadelphia	10.4	0.0%	1.24	0.21	5	0.99	0.060	0.24
	Good Samaritan Hospital, Lebanon	7.3	0.0%	1.21	0.06	3	0.72	0.041	0.80
	Hamot Medical Center, Erie	8.6	0.0%	1.29	0.10	6	0.95	0.014	0.27
	Harrisburg Hospital, Harrisburg	7.8	0.0%	1.34	0.17	4	0.96	0.062	0.47
	Lancaster General Hospital, Lancaster	12.5	0.0%	1.12	0.14	7	0.85	0.025	0.36
	Latrobe Area Hospital, Latrobe	13.1	0.0%	0.97	0.10	3	0.80	0.027	0.31
	Lee Hospital, Johnstown	13.0	0.0%	1.09	0.00	5	1.20	0.038	0.33
	Lewistown Hospital, Lewistown	11.9	0.0%	1.07	0.00	7	0.68	0.009	0.54
	Lower Bucks Hospital, Bristol	8.6	0.0%	1.25	0.01	5	0.87	0.045	0.31
	McKeesport Hospital, McKeesport	13.8	0.0%	1.03	0.28	6	0.78	0.003	0.51
	Mercy Health Corporation, Bala Cynwyd	5.3	0.0%	1.47	0.32	6	0.54	0.019	0.33
	Mercy Hospital of Scranton, Scranton	8.1	0.0%	1.29	0.02	6	0.91	0.014	0.34
	Methodist Hospital, Philadelphia	13.6	0.0%	1.15	0.06	4	1.57	0.067	0.27
	Monongahela Valley Hospital, Monongahela	6.6	0.0%	1.27	0.00	5	0.72	0.011	0.35
	Montgomery Hospital, Norristown	10.7	0.0%	1.11	0.12	6	0.61	0.019	0.25
	Moses Taylor Hospital, Scranton	8.8	0.0%	1.11	0.04	3	0.73	0.019	0.17
	Nazareth Hospital, Philadelphia	12.3	0.0%	1.10	0.00	7	0.76	0.040	0.30
	Northeastern Hospital of Philadelphia	8.8	0.0%	1.16	0.02	4	0.71	0.046	0.24
	Northwest Medical Center, Franklin	12.8	0.0%	1.03	0.00	7	0.64	0.005	0.26
	Polyclinic Medical Center, Harrisburg	7.9	0.0%	1.35	0.20	7	0.66	0.029	0.18
	Presbyterian Medical Center of Philadelphia	12.9	0.0%	1.08	0.64	4	0.72	0.018	0.10
	Reading Hospital and Medical Center, Reading	10.5	0.0%	1.29	0.20	8	0.84	0.038	0.60
	Sacred Heart Hospital, Allentown	11.8	0.0%	1.20	0.15	7	0.85	0.057	0.43
	St. Agnes Medical Center, Philadelphia	7.4	0.0%	1.20	0.13	4	0.58	0.017	0.10
	St. Francis Medical Center, Pittsburgh	6.9	0.0%	1.33	0.14	6	0.69	0.007	0.10
	St. Joseph Hospital, Reading	8.8	0.0%	1.25	0.11	6	0.77	0.027	0.26
	St. Luke's Hospital, Bethlehem	10.1	0.0%	1.27	0.14	7	0.85	0.046	0.52
	St. Margaret Memorial Hospital, Pittsburgh	11.0	0.0%	1.11	0.27	4	0.64	0.052	0.27
	St. Vincent Health System, Erie	11.5	0.0%	1.14	0.08	5	1.11	0.026	0.31
	The Medical Center, Beaver	10.2	0.0%	1.24	0.08	8	0.80	0.021	0.42
	Wilkes-Barre General Hospital, Wilkes-Barre	6.6	0.0%	1.32	0.01	6	0.75	0.004	0.34
	Williamsport Hospital and Medical Center, Williamsport	8.8	0.0%	1.17	0.13	4	0.73	0.026	0.46
	York Hospital, York	13.9	0.0%	1.13	0.33	7	0.92	0.047	0.61

NEUROLOGY

Natl. Rank	Hospital	U.S. News index	Reputa-tional score	Neurology mortality rate	COTH member	Interns and residents to beds	Tech-nology score (of 9)	R.N.'s to beds	Board-certified neurologists to beds
	TIER ONE								
10	Hospital of the University of Pennsylvania, Philadelphia	36.1	9.2%	1.02	Yes	1.72	9	1.33	0.051
20	University of Pittsburgh-Presbyterian University Hospital	26.0	2.1%	1.05	Yes	1.48	7	2.10	0.066
	TIER TWO								
65	Bryn Mawr Hospital, Bryn Mawr	18.5	0.0%	0.75	Yes	0.14	5	1.35	0.017
64	Geisinger Medical Center, Danville	18.5	0.0%	0.82	Yes	0.68	6	1.23	0.014
56	Graduate Hospital, Philadelphia	19.1	0.0%	0.85	Yes	0.74	7	1.07	0.034
55	Medical College Hospital, Philadelphia	19.3	0.0%	0.86	Yes	1.39	5	0.81	0.026
34	Temple University Hospital, Philadelphia	22.9	0.0%	0.75	Yes	1.25	8	1.15	0.025
26	Thomas Jefferson University Hospital, Philadelphia	24.1	0.6%	0.59	Yes	0.96	8	1.44	0.031
87	University of Pittsburgh-Montefiore Hospital	17.9	0.4%	0.99	No	0.93	3	1.43	0.074
46	Western Pennsylvania Hospital, Pittsburgh	20.7	0.0%	0.65	Yes	0.43	7	1.44	0.024
	TIER THREE								
	Abington Memorial Hospital, Abington	11.4	0.0%	0.93	No	0.36	5	0.84	0.011
	Albert Einstein Medical Center, Philadelphia	16.9	0.0%	0.90	Yes	0.75	8	0.89	0.017
	Allegheny General Hospital, Pittsburgh	16.3	2.1%	1.15	Yes	0.52	7	1.36	0.012
	Conemaugh Memorial Hospital, Johnstown	14.3	0.0%	0.81	No	0.43	5	1.14	0.003
	Easton Hospital, Easton	13.7	0.0%	0.80	No	0.20	4	0.99	0.010
	Forbes Regional Hospital, Monroeville	14.2	0.0%	0.81	No	0.11	5	0.85	0.025
	Frankford Hospital, Philadelphia	11.9	0.0%	1.00	Yes	0.17	4	1.07	0.008
	Germantown Hospital and Medical Center, Philadelphia	12.0	0.0%	1.04	Yes	0.21	5	0.99	0.014
	Hahnemann University Hospital, Philadelphia	15.0	0.0%	1.09	Yes	1.19	6	1.11	0.014
	Lankenau Hospital, Wynnewood	11.9	0.0%	1.03	No	0.47	8	1.21	0.010
	Latrobe Area Hospital, Latrobe	12.9	0.0%	0.78	No	0.10	3	0.80	0.008
	Lehigh Valley Hospital, Allentown	11.8	0.0%	1.13	Yes	0.19	7	1.19	0.014
	Mercy Hospital of Pittsburgh, Pittsburgh	13.0	0.0%	0.99	Yes	0.37	6	0.94	0.006
	Penn State's Milton S. Hershey Medical Ctr., Hershey	16.0	0.0%	1.20	Yes	1.55	7	1.57	0.009
	Shadyside Hospital, Pittsburgh	15.9	0.0%	0.87	Yes	0.23	7	0.88	0.021
	Washington Hospital, Washington	13.1	0.0%	0.81	No	0.12	6	0.78	0.006
	TIER FOUR								
	Allegheny Valley Hospital, Natrona Heights	7.3	0.0%	1.16	No	0.00	7	0.85	0.007
	Altoona Hospital, Altoona	8.8	0.0%	1.02	No	0.12	3	1.15	0.003
	Chester County Hospital, Westchester	10.1	0.0%	0.93	No	0.00	6	0.69	0.009
	Chestnut Hill Hospital, Philadelphia	9.1	0.0%	1.11	No	0.26	4	0.99	0.021
	Crozer-Chester Medical Center, Upland	9.0	0.0%	1.28	Yes	0.12	8	0.72	0.013
	Delaware County Memorial Hospital, Drexel Hill	9.5	0.0%	1.04	No	0.09	6	0.81	0.019
	Delaware Valley Medical Center, Langhorne	8.6	0.0%	1.16	No	0.47	5	0.45	0.031
	Divine Providence Hospital, Williamsport	7.7	0.0%	1.09	No	0.00	6	0.85	0.006
	Dubois Regional Medical Center, Dubois	7.3	0.0%	1.12	No	0.00	7	0.77	0.005
	Good Samaritan Hospital, Lebanon	4.4	0.0%	1.29	No	0.06	3	0.72	0.005
	Hamot Medical Center, Erie	9.1	0.0%	1.17	Yes	0.10	5	0.95	0.002
	Harrisburg Hospital, Harrisburg	7.4	0.0%	1.12	No	0.17	3	0.96	0.007
	Lancaster General Hospital, Lancaster	8.5	0.0%	1.07	No	0.14	6	0.85	0.007
	Lee Hospital, Johnstown	5.8	0.0%	1.30	No	0.00	5	1.20	0.004
	Lewistown Hospital, Lewistown	8.5	0.0%	1.02	No	0.00	7	0.68	0.005
	Lower Bucks Hospital, Bristol	10.9	0.0%	0.95	No	0.01	5	0.87	0.025
	McKeesport Hospital, McKeesport	8.1	0.0%	1.10	No	0.28	6	0.78	0.003
	Mercy Health Corporation, Bala Cynwyd	9.0	0.0%	1.18	Yes	0.32	5	0.54	0.008
	Mercy Hospital of Scranton, Scranton	6.3	0.0%	1.24	No	0.02	6	0.91	0.008
	Methodist Hospital, Philadelphia	9.4	0.0%	1.14	No	0.06	2	1.57	0.027
	Monongahela Valley Hospital, Monongahela	4.6	0.0%	1.30	No	0.00	5	0.72	0.004
	Montgomery Hospital, Norristown	6.3	0.0%	1.24	No	0.12	5	0.61	0.019
	Moses Taylor Hospital, Scranton	7.3	0.0%	1.06	No	0.04	3	0.73	0.009
	Nazareth Hospital, Philadelphia	8.6	0.0%	1.03	No	0.00	6	0.76	0.009

Natl. Rank	Hospital	U.S. News index	Reputational score	Neurology mortality rate	COTH member	Interns and residents to beds	Technology score (of 9)	R.N.'s to beds	Board-certified neurologists to beds
	Northeastern Hospital of Philadelphia	5.9	0.0%	1.28	No	0.02	4	0.71	0.025
	Northwest Medical Center, Franklin	6.2	0.0%	1.17	No	0.00	7	0.64	0.003
	Paoli Memorial Hospital, Paoli	10.3	0.0%	0.98	No	0.00	5	0.82	0.024
	Polyclinic Medical Center, Harrisburg	6.1	0.0%	1.23	No	0.20	6	0.66	0.004
	Presbyterian Medical Center of Philadelphia	7.5	0.0%	1.27	No	0.64	4	0.72	0.018
	Reading Hospital and Medical Center, Reading	9.0	0.0%	1.05	No	0.20	7	0.84	0.002
	Robert Packer Hospital, Sayre	10.8	0.0%	1.01	No	0.27	8	0.97	0.008
	Sacred Heart Hospital, Allentown	5.9	0.0%	1.37	No	0.15	6	0.85	0.016
	St. Agnes Medical Center, Philadelphia	7.0	0.0%	1.21	No	0.13	4	0.58	0.030
	St. Joseph Hospital, Reading	6.5	0.0%	1.27	No	0.11	6	0.77	0.016
	St. Luke's Hospital, Bethlehem	8.0	0.0%	1.13	No	0.14	6	0.85	0.011
	St. Margaret Memorial Hospital, Pittsburgh	6.2	0.0%	1.18	No	0.27	4	0.64	0.004
	St. Vincent Health System, Erie	8.7	0.0%	1.04	No	0.08	4	1.11	0.005
	The Medical Center, Beaver	6.7	0.0%	1.22	No	0.08	7	0.80	0.009
	Westmoreland Hospital, Greensburg	8.7	0.0%	1.09	No	0.00	7	1.09	0.006
	Wilkes-Barre General Hospital, Wilkes-Barre	8.0	0.0%	1.06	No	0.01	6	0.75	0.007
	Williamsport Hospital and Medical Center, Williamsport	7.4	0.0%	1.07	No	0.13	4	0.73	0.004
	York Hospital, York	9.7	0.0%	1.20	Yes	0.33	6	0.92	0.002

ORTHOPEDICS

Natl. Rank	Hospital	U.S. News index	Reputational score	Orthopedics mortality rate	COTH member	Interns and residents to beds	Technology score (of 5)	R.N.'s to beds	Board-certified orthopedists to beds	Procedures to beds
TIER ONE										
11	Hospital of the University of Pennsylvania, Philadelphia	28.7	3.9%	0.61	Yes	1.72	5	1.33	0.036	1.65
17	Thomas Jefferson University Hospital, Philadelphia	22.9	2.5%	0.61	Yes	0.96	4	1.44	0.034	1.73
TIER TWO										
47	Allegheny General Hospital, Pittsburgh	16.7	1.4%	0.84	Yes	0.52	4	1.36	0.020	2.13
49	Penn State's Milton S. Hershey Medical Ctr., Hershey	16.6	0.5%	1.10	Yes	1.55	4	1.57	0.016	1.71
59	Temple University Hospital, Philadelphia	15.8	0.4%	0.89	Yes	1.25	4	1.15	0.030	0.91
26	University of Pittsburgh-Presbyterian University Hospital	19.9	2.8%	1.79	Yes	1.48	3	2.10	0.103	1.80
67	Western Pennsylvania Hospital, Pittsburgh	15.2	0.0%	0.70	Yes	0.43	4	1.44	0.012	1.66
TIER THREE										
	Albert Einstein Medical Center, Philadelphia	11.1	0.0%	1.12	Yes	0.75	4	0.89	0.028	2.08
	Allegheny Valley Hospital, Natrona Heights	10.0	0.0%	0.70	No	0.00	4	0.85	0.029	2.94
	Bryn Mawr Hospital, Bryn Mawr	13.0	0.0%	0.73	Yes	0.14	2	1.35	0.042	3.64
	Chester County Hospital, Westchester	8.6	0.0%	0.72	No	0.00	3	0.69	0.030	2.62
	Chestnut Hill Hospital, Philadelphia	10.9	0.0%	0.68	No	0.26	3	0.99	0.026	3.65
	Conemaugh Memorial Hospital, Johnstown	10.6	0.0%	0.75	No	0.43	3	1.14	0.020	2.28
	Crozer-Chester Medical Center, Upland	9.1	0.0%	1.01	Yes	0.12	4	0.72	0.020	1.35
	Divine Providence Hospital, Williamsport	8.3	0.0%	0.74	No	0.00	2	0.85	0.039	3.37
	Dubois Regional Medical Center, Dubois	9.8	0.0%	0.59	No	0.00	4	0.77	0.005	1.34
	Frankford Hospital, Philadelphia	8.5	0.0%	1.25	Yes	0.17	3	1.07	0.027	2.68
	Geisinger Medical Center, Danville	11.0	0.4%	1.32	Yes	0.68	3	1.23	0.012	2.54
	Germantown Hospital and Medical Center, Philadelphia	9.1	0.0%	0.99	Yes	0.21	2	0.99	0.019	2.14
	Graduate Hospital, Philadelphia	11.4	0.0%	1.20	Yes	0.74	4	1.07	0.094	1.57
	Hahnemann University Hospital, Philadelphia	11.3	0.0%	1.18	Yes	1.19	2	1.11	0.009	1.34
	Latrobe Area Hospital, Latrobe	9.1	0.0%	0.68	No	0.10	2	0.80	0.019	3.36
	Lehigh Valley Hospital, Allentown	9.8	0.0%	1.05	Yes	0.19	3	1.19	0.017	2.03
	Lower Bucks Hospital, Bristol	8.3	0.0%	0.81	No	0.01	4	0.87	0.029	2.06
	Medical College Hospital, Philadelphia	11.2	0.4%	1.52	Yes	1.39	3	0.81	0.023	1.00
	Mercy Hospital of Pittsburgh, Pittsburgh	10.0	0.0%	1.03	Yes	0.37	3	0.94	0.016	2.67
	Robert Packer Hospital, Sayre	8.2	0.0%	0.97	No	0.27	4	0.97	0.016	3.01
	Shadyside Hospital, Pittsburgh	10.6	0.0%	0.95	Yes	0.23	4	0.88	0.016	2.82
	St. Margaret Memorial Hospital, Pittsburgh	8.6	0.4%	0.98	No	0.27	3	0.64	0.067	6.88

Natl. Rank	Hospital	U.S. News index	Reputa-tional score	Orthopedics mortality rate	COTH member	Interns and residents to beds	Tech-nology score (of 5)	R.N.'s to beds	Board-certified orthopedists to beds	Pro-cedures to beds
	University of Pittsburgh-Montefiore Hospital	11.2	0.0%	0.99	No	0.93	3	1.43	0.077	3.13
TIER FOUR										
	Abington Memorial Hospital, Abington	6.8	0.0%	0.97	No	0.36	2	0.84	0.024	2.60
	Altoona Hospital, Altoona	2.6	0.0%	2.04	No	0.12	2	1.15	0.007	2.39
	Delaware County Memorial Hospital, Drexel Hill	6.4	0.0%	1.01	No	0.09	3	0.81	0.023	3.37
	Easton Hospital, Easton	6.8	0.0%	0.97	No	0.20	2	0.99	0.033	2.77
	Forbes Regional Hospital, Monroeville	6.7	0.0%	1.08	No	0.11	4	0.85	0.031	3.25
	Good Samaritan Hospital, Lebanon	7.7	0.0%	0.77	No	0.06	2	0.72	0.021	3.72
	Hamot Medical Center, Erie	5.8	0.0%	1.61	Yes	0.10	2	0.95	0.018	2.39
	Harrisburg Hospital, Harrisburg	3.8	0.0%	1.48	No	0.17	2	0.96	0.020	2.64
	Lancaster General Hospital, Lancaster	6.1	0.0%	1.09	No	0.14	3	0.85	0.022	3.62
	Lankenau Hospital, Wynnewood	7.2	0.0%	1.32	No	0.47	4	1.21	0.017	2.12
	Lee Hospital, Johnstown	4.8	0.0%	1.32	No	0.00	2	1.20	0.033	3.58
	Lewistown Hospital, Lewistown	3.6	0.0%	1.49	No	0.00	4	0.68	0.014	2.24
	McKeesport Hospital, McKeesport	5.4	0.0%	1.19	No	0.28	3	0.78	0.009	2.31
	Mercy Health Corporation, Bala Cynwyd	7.4	0.0%	1.20	Yes	0.32	3	0.54	0.013	1.41
	Mercy Hospital of Scranton, Scranton	2.8	0.0%	1.90	No	0.02	3	0.91	0.030	2.76
	Methodist Hospital, Philadelphia	5.3	0.0%	1.39	No	0.06	2	1.57	0.036	1.51
	Monongahela Valley Hospital, Monongahela	5.0	0.0%	1.01	No	0.00	2	0.72	0.014	3.10
	Montgomery Hospital, Norristown	6.0	0.0%	0.87	No	0.12	2	0.61	0.019	2.01
	Moses Taylor Hospital, Scranton	5.3	0.0%	1.01	No	0.04	2	0.73	0.019	3.28
	Nazareth Hospital, Philadelphia	4.3	0.0%	1.24	No	0.00	3	0.76	0.025	2.52
	Northeastern Hospital of Philadelphia	3.7	0.0%	1.32	No	0.02	3	0.71	0.020	1.80
	Northwest Medical Center, Franklin	5.6	0.0%	1.02	No	0.00	4	0.64	0.008	1.39
	Paoli Memorial Hospital, Paoli	6.3	0.0%	0.93	No	0.00	2	0.82	0.036	4.13
	Polyclinic Medical Center, Harrisburg	3.0	0.0%	1.67	No	0.20	3	0.66	0.019	1.83
	Reading Hospital and Medical Center, Reading	7.3	0.0%	1.08	No	0.20	4	0.84	0.023	4.76
	Sacred Heart Hospital, Allentown	3.9	0.0%	1.54	No	0.15	3	0.85	0.020	2.50
	Shriners Hospital for Crippled Children, Philadelphia	3.7	0.0%	1.24	No	0.08	0	0.46	0.037	10.11
	St. Agnes Medical Center, Philadelphia	5.3	0.0%	1.02	No	0.13	3	0.58	0.025	1.58
	St. Francis Medical Center, Pittsburgh	6.0	0.0%	1.43	Yes	0.14	3	0.69	0.004	0.75
	St. Joseph Hospital, Reading	2.0	0.0%	1.90	No	0.11	2	0.77	0.016	2.69
	St. Luke's Hospital, Bethlehem	4.1	0.0%	1.46	No	0.14	3	0.85	0.025	2.23
	St. Vincent Health System, Erie	5.1	0.0%	1.32	No	0.08	3	1.11	0.019	2.28
	The Medical Center, Beaver	6.0	0.0%	1.11	No	0.08	4	0.80	0.015	2.48
	Washington Hospital, Washington	4.4	0.0%	1.36	No	0.12	3	0.78	0.016	3.49
	Westmoreland Hospital, Greensburg	7.9	0.0%	0.91	No	0.00	4	1.09	0.014	2.53
	Wilkes-Barre General Hospital, Wilkes-Barre	3.8	0.0%	1.36	No	0.01	3	0.75	0.013	2.70
	Williamsport Hospital and Medical Center, Williamsport	7.6	0.0%	0.86	No	0.13	3	0.73	0.026	3.61
	York Hospital, York	7.7	0.0%	1.48	Yes	0.33	3	0.92	0.020	2.88

OTOLARYNGOLOGY

Natl. Rank	Hospital	U.S. News index	Reputa-tional score	Hospital-wide mortality rate	COTH member	Interns and residents to beds	Tech-nology score (of 9)	R.N.'s to beds	Board-certified internists to beds	Procedures to beds
TIER ONE										
8	University of Pittsburgh-Presbyterian University Hospital	47.0	8.5%	1.10	Yes	1.48	7	2.10	0.291	0.285
25	Hospital of the University of Pennsylvania, Philadelphia	23.7	2.2%	0.97	Yes	1.72	9	1.33	0.007	0.315
TIER TWO										
94	Geisinger Medical Center, Danville	14.0	0.5%	1.06	Yes	0.68	6	1.23	0.140	0.324
63	Hosp. of the Philadelphia College of Osteopathic Medicine	16.1	0.0%	1.08	No	2.33	6	1.54	0.053	0.468
	Medical College Hospital, Philadelphia	13.7	0.0%	1.13	Yes	1.39	5	0.81	0.138	0.214
60	Penn State's Milton S. Hershey Medical Ctr., Hershey	16.3	0.0%	1.03	Yes	1.55	7	1.57	0.023	0.312
87	Temple University Hospital, Philadelphia	14.4	0.0%	1.05	Yes	1.25	8	1.15	0.055	0.206
57	Thomas Jefferson University Hospital, Philadelphia	16.9	0.8%	0.85	Yes	0.96	8	1.44	0.042	0.359

Natl. Rank	Hospital	U.S. News index	Reputational score	Hospital-wide mortality rate	COTH member	Interns and residents to beds	Technology score (of 9)	R.N.'s to beds	Board-certified internists to beds	Procedures to beds
39	**University of Pittsburgh-Montefiore Hospital**	19.6	2.4%	1.09	No	0.93	2	1.43	0.388	1.069
	TIER THREE									
	Albert Einstein Medical Center, Philadelphia	11.9	0.0%	1.07	Yes	0.75	8	0.89	0.098	0.140
	Allegheny General Hospital, Pittsburgh	11.6	0.0%	1.04	Yes	0.52	7	1.36	0.025	0.212
	Bryn Mawr Hospital, Bryn Mawr	10.3	0.0%	0.80	Yes	0.14	5	1.35	0.083	0.346
	Conemaugh Memorial Hospital, Johnstown	7.3	0.0%	0.79	No	0.43	5	1.14	0.043	0.506
	Crozer-Chester Medical Center, Upland	8.5	0.0%	1.22	Yes	0.12	8	0.72	0.058	0.184
	Delaware Valley Medical Center, Langhorne	7.9	0.0%	1.19	No	0.47	5	0.45	0.393	0.362
	Episcopal Hospital, Philadelphia	7.4	0.0%	1.21	Yes	0.40	3	0.54	0.033	0.073
	Fox Chase Cancer Center, Philadelphia	7.8	0.0%	0.23	No	0.36	6	1.42	0.000	0.420
	Frankford Hospital, Philadelphia	8.6	0.0%	1.06	Yes	0.17	3	1.07	0.077	0.261
	Germantown Hospital and Medical Center, Philadelphia	9.2	0.0%	1.25	Yes	0.21	5	0.99	0.097	0.333
	Graduate Hospital, Philadelphia	12.3	0.0%	1.04	Yes	0.74	7	1.07	0.109	0.253
	Hahnemann University Hospital, Philadelphia	13.2	0.0%	1.22	Yes	1.19	6	1.11	0.045	0.194
	Hamot Medical Center, Erie	7.9	0.0%	1.28	Yes	0.10	5	0.95	0.016	0.204
	Lankenau Hospital, Wynnewood	8.3	0.0%	1.18	No	0.47	8	1.21	0.072	0.199
	Lehigh Valley Hospital, Allentown	9.9	0.0%	1.08	Yes	0.19	7	1.19	0.044	0.172
	Mercy Health Corporation, Bala Cynwyd	7.7	0.0%	1.47	Yes	0.32	5	0.54	0.051	0.238
	Mercy Hospital of Pittsburgh, Pittsburgh	9.8	0.0%	0.90	Yes	0.37	6	0.94	0.053	0.398
	Methodist Hospital, Philadelphia	7.5	0.0%	1.15	No	0.06	1	1.57	0.254	0.281
	Shadyside Hospital, Pittsburgh	9.7	0.0%	1.02	Yes	0.23	7	0.88	0.103	0.371
	St. Francis Medical Center, Pittsburgh	8.5	0.0%	1.33	Yes	0.14	6	0.69	0.130	0.102
	Western Pennsylvania Hospital, Pittsburgh	12.1	0.0%	0.95	Yes	0.43	7	1.44	0.091	0.217
	York Hospital, York	9.5	0.0%	1.13	Yes	0.33	6	0.92	0.063	0.237
	TIER FOUR									
	Abington Memorial Hospital, Abington	6.0	0.0%	0.93	No	0.36	4	0.84	0.088	0.207
	Allegheny Valley Hospital, Natrona Heights	5.2	0.0%	1.04	No	0.00	7	0.85	0.061	0.496
	Altoona Hospital, Altoona	5.3	0.0%	1.36	No	0.12	3	1.15	0.069	0.383
	Chester County Hospital, Westchester	4.6	0.0%	0.91	No	0.00	6	0.69	0.074	0.509
	Chestnut Hill Hospital, Philadelphia	5.7	0.0%	1.03	No	0.26	2	0.99	0.121	0.279
	Delaware County Memorial Hospital, Drexel Hill	5.3	0.0%	1.06	No	0.09	6	0.81	0.083	0.455
	Divine Providence Hospital, Williamsport	4.4	0.0%	1.11	No	0.00	6	0.85	0.017	0.311
	Dubois Regional Medical Center, Dubois	4.4	0.0%	1.13	No	0.00	7	0.77	0.014	0.414
	Easton Hospital, Easton	5.4	0.0%	1.01	No	0.20	2	0.99	0.106	0.262
	Forbes Regional Hospital, Monroeville	5.2	0.0%	0.94	No	0.11	5	0.85	0.068	0.584
	Good Samaritan Hospital, Lebanon	2.9	0.0%	1.21	No	0.06	1	0.72	0.021	0.675
	Harrisburg Hospital, Harrisburg	4.6	0.0%	1.34	No	0.17	2	0.96	0.065	0.209
	Lancaster General Hospital, Lancaster	4.9	0.0%	1.12	No	0.14	6	0.85	0.009	0.231
	Latrobe Area Hospital, Latrobe	3.5	0.0%	0.97	No	0.10	1	0.80	0.030	0.727
	Lee Hospital, Johnstown	6.3	0.0%	1.09	No	0.00	5	1.20	0.138	0.983
	Lewistown Hospital, Lewistown	4.4	0.0%	1.07	No	0.00	6	0.68	0.070	0.469
	Lower Bucks Hospital, Bristol	4.0	0.0%	1.24	No	0.01	3	0.87	0.070	0.243
	McKeesport Hospital, McKeesport	5.8	0.0%	1.03	No	0.28	6	0.78	0.064	0.343
	Mercy Hospital of Scranton, Scranton	4.8	0.0%	1.29	No	0.02	6	0.91	0.044	0.288
	Monongahela Valley Hospital, Monongahela	3.8	0.0%	1.27	No	0.00	5	0.72	0.032	0.646
	Montgomery Hospital, Norristown	4.4	0.0%	1.11	No	0.12	5	0.61	0.076	0.176
	Moses Taylor Hospital, Scranton	3.1	0.0%	1.11	No	0.04	1	0.73	0.056	0.316
	Nazareth Hospital, Philadelphia	4.3	0.0%	1.10	No	0.00	6	0.76	0.037	0.240
	Northeastern Hospital of Philadelphia	3.2	0.0%	1.16	No	0.02	2	0.71	0.046	0.670
	Northwest Medical Center, Franklin	4.2	0.0%	1.03	No	0.00	7	0.64	0.022	0.353
	Paoli Memorial Hospital, Paoli	5.0	0.0%	0.94	No	0.00	5	0.82	0.113	0.327
	Polyclinic Medical Center, Harrisburg	4.7	0.0%	1.35	No	0.20	6	0.66	0.041	0.212
	Presbyterian Medical Center of Philadelphia	6.3	0.0%	1.08	No	0.64	2	0.72	0.114	0.254
	Reading Hospital and Medical Center, Reading	5.7	0.0%	1.29	No	0.20	7	0.84	0.057	0.412
	Robert Packer Hospital, Sayre	6.5	0.0%	1.06	No	0.27	8	0.97	0.022	0.454
	Sacred Heart Hospital, Allentown	6.8	0.0%	1.20	No	0.15	6	0.85	0.231	0.611

Natl. Rank	Hospital	U.S. News index	Reputa-tional score	Hospital-wide mortality rate	COTH member	Interns and residents to beds	Tech-nology score (of 9)	R.N.'s to beds	Board-certified internists to beds	Procedures to beds
	St. Agnes Medical Center, Philadelphia	3.5	0.0%	1.20	No	0.13	2	0.58	0.085	0.271
	St. Joseph Hospital, Reading	4.8	0.0%	1.25	No	0.11	6	0.77	0.047	0.372
	St. Luke's Hospital, Bethlehem	5.2	0.0%	1.27	No	0.14	6	0.85	0.053	0.518
	St. Margaret Memorial Hospital, Pittsburgh	4.8	0.0%	1.11	No	0.27	3	0.64	0.109	0.341
	St. Vincent Health System, Erie	5.0	0.0%	1.14	No	0.08	4	1.11	0.026	0.311
	The Medical Center, Beaver	5.0	0.0%	1.24	No	0.08	7	0.80	0.040	0.277
	Thomas Jefferson University Hospital, Philadelphia	3.3	0.0%	1.29	No	0.01	2	0.55	0.140	0.170
	Washington Hospital, Washington	5.3	0.0%	0.98	No	0.12	6	0.78	0.074	0.297
	Westmoreland Hospital, Greensburg	5.3	0.0%	1.01	No	0.00	6	1.09	0.022	0.402
	Wilkes-Barre General Hospital, Wilkes-Barre	4.0	0.0%	1.32	No	0.01	6	0.75	0.009	0.510
	Williamsport Hospital and Medical Center, Williamsport	4.3	0.0%	1.17	No	0.13	4	0.73	0.055	0.326

RHEUMATOLOGY

Natl. Rank	Hospital	U.S. News index	Reputa-tional score	Hospital-wide mortality rate	COTH member	Interns and residents to beds	Tech-nology score (of 5)	R.N.'s to beds	Board-certified internists to beds
	TIER ONE								
10	University of Pittsburgh-Presbyterian University Hospital	35.8	7.2%	1.10	Yes	1.48	3	2.10	0.291
19	Hospital of the University of Pennsylvania, Philadelphia	25.6	3.2%	0.97	Yes	1.72	5	1.33	0.007
	TIER TWO								
72	Hosp. of the Philadelphia College of Osteopathic Medicine	16.5	0.0%	1.08	No	2.33	2	1.54	0.053
52	Penn State's Milton S. Hershey Medical Ctr., Hershey	17.7	0.0%	1.03	Yes	1.55	4	1.57	0.023
35	Thomas Jefferson University Hospital, Philadelphia	20.3	1.3%	0.85	Yes	0.96	4	1.44	0.042
	TIER THREE								
	Abington Memorial Hospital, Abington	10.0	0.0%	0.93	No	0.36	2	0.84	0.088
	Albert Einstein Medical Center, Philadelphia	13.5	0.0%	1.07	Yes	0.75	4	0.89	0.098
	Allegheny General Hospital, Pittsburgh	14.8	0.5%	1.04	Yes	0.52	4	1.36	0.025
	Bryn Mawr Hospital, Bryn Mawr	14.1	0.0%	0.80	Yes	0.14	2	1.35	0.083
	Chestnut Hill Hospital, Philadelphia	9.8	0.0%	1.03	No	0.26	3	0.99	0.121
	Conemaugh Memorial Hospital, Johnstown	12.2	0.0%	0.79	No	0.43	3	1.14	0.043
	Crozer-Chester Medical Center, Upland	9.7	0.0%	1.22	Yes	0.12	4	0.72	0.058
	Delaware Valley Medical Center, Langhorne	9.8	0.0%	1.19	No	0.47	3	0.45	0.393
	Forbes Regional Hospital, Monroeville	9.8	0.0%	0.94	No	0.11	4	0.85	0.068
	Frankford Hospital, Philadelphia	11.7	0.0%	1.06	Yes	0.17	3	1.07	0.077
95	Geisinger Medical Center, Danville	15.1	0.4%	1.06	Yes	0.68	3	1.23	0.140
	Germantown Hospital and Medical Center, Philadelphia	9.9	0.0%	1.25	Yes	0.21	2	0.99	0.097
	Graduate Hospital, Philadelphia	14.3	0.0%	1.04	Yes	0.74	4	1.07	0.109
	Hahnemann University Hospital, Philadelphia	13.2	0.0%	1.22	Yes	1.19	2	1.11	0.045
	Lankenau Hospital, Wynnewood	10.0	0.0%	1.18	No	0.47	4	1.21	0.072
	Lehigh Valley Hospital, Allentown	11.6	0.0%	1.08	Yes	0.19	3	1.19	0.044
100	Medical College Hospital, Philadelphia	14.8	0.0%	1.13	Yes	1.39	3	0.81	0.138
	Mercy Hospital of Pittsburgh, Pittsburgh	13.3	0.0%	0.90	Yes	0.37	3	0.94	0.053
	Methodist Hospital, Philadelphia	10.3	0.0%	1.15	No	0.06	2	1.57	0.254
	Paoli Memorial Hospital, Paoli	9.7	0.4%	0.94	No	0.00	2	0.82	0.113
	Presbyterian Medical Center of Philadelphia	10.4	0.3%	1.08	No	0.64	3	0.72	0.114
	Shadyside Hospital, Pittsburgh	12.3	0.0%	1.02	Yes	0.23	4	0.88	0.103
86	Temple University Hospital, Philadelphia	15.7	0.0%	1.05	Yes	1.25	4	1.15	0.055
	University of Pittsburgh-Montefiore Hospital	14.6	0.0%	1.09	No	0.93	3	1.43	0.388
97	Western Pennsylvania Hospital, Pittsburgh	15.0	0.0%	0.95	Yes	0.43	4	1.44	0.091
	Wills Eye Hospital, Philadelphia	10.7	0.0%	0.08	No	0.57	2	0.69	0.000
	York Hospital, York	11.1	0.0%	1.13	Yes	0.33	3	0.92	0.063
	TIER FOUR								
	Allegheny Valley Hospital, Natrona Heights	7.5	0.0%	1.04	No	0.00	4	0.85	0.061
	Altoona Hospital, Altoona	6.8	0.0%	1.36	No	0.12	2	1.15	0.069
	Chester County Hospital, Westchester	9.0	0.0%	0.91	No	0.00	3	0.69	0.074

Natl. Rank	Hospital	U.S. News index	Reputa-tional score	Hospital-wide mortality rate	COTH member	Interns and residents to beds	Tech-nology score (of 5)	R.N.'s to beds	Board-certified internists to beds
	Delaware County Memorial Hospital, Drexel Hill	7.3	0.0%	1.06	No	0.09	3	0.81	0.083
	Divine Providence Hospital, Williamsport	5.8	0.0%	1.11	No	0.00	2	0.85	0.017
	Dubois Regional Medical Center, Dubois	7.3	0.0%	1.13	No	0.00	4	0.77	0.014
	Easton Hospital, Easton	9.3	0.0%	1.01	No	0.20	2	0.99	0.106
	Episcopal Hospital, Philadelphia	9.1	0.0%	1.21	Yes	0.40	2	0.54	0.033
	Good Samaritan Hospital, Lebanon	5.9	0.0%	1.21	No	0.06	2	0.72	0.021
	Hamot Medical Center, Erie	7.7	0.0%	1.28	Yes	0.10	2	0.95	0.016
	Harrisburg Hospital, Harrisburg	6.5	0.0%	1.34	No	0.17	2	0.96	0.065
	Lancaster General Hospital, Lancaster	7.5	0.0%	1.12	No	0.14	3	0.85	0.009
	Latrobe Area Hospital, Latrobe	8.2	0.0%	0.97	No	0.10	2	0.80	0.030
	Lee Hospital, Johnstown	8.7	0.0%	1.09	No	0.00	2	1.20	0.138
	Lewistown Hospital, Lewistown	6.9	0.0%	1.07	No	0.00	4	0.68	0.070
	Lower Bucks Hospital, Bristol	7.2	0.0%	1.24	No	0.01	4	0.87	0.070
	McKeesport Hospital, McKeesport	8.9	0.0%	1.03	No	0.28	3	0.78	0.064
	Mercy Health Corporation, Bala Cynwyd	8.1	0.0%	1.47	Yes	0.32	3	0.54	0.051
	Mercy Hospital of Scranton, Scranton	6.5	0.0%	1.29	No	0.02	3	0.91	0.044
	Monongahela Valley Hospital, Monongahela	5.4	0.0%	1.27	No	0.00	2	0.72	0.032
	Montgomery Hospital, Norristown	6.9	0.0%	1.11	No	0.12	2	0.61	0.076
	Moses Taylor Hospital, Scranton	6.8	0.0%	1.11	No	0.04	2	0.73	0.056
	Nazareth Hospital, Philadelphia	7.2	0.0%	1.10	No	0.00	3	0.76	0.037
	Northeastern Hospital of Philadelphia	6.7	0.0%	1.16	No	0.02	3	0.71	0.046
	Northwest Medical Center, Franklin	7.8	0.0%	1.03	No	0.00	4	0.64	0.022
	Polyclinic Medical Center, Harrisburg	6.1	0.0%	1.35	No	0.20	3	0.66	0.041
	Reading Hospital and Medical Center, Reading	7.4	0.0%	1.29	No	0.20	4	0.84	0.057
	Robert Packer Hospital, Sayre	8.2	0.0%	1.06	No	0.27	4	0.97	0.022
	Sacred Heart Hospital, Allentown	8.6	0.0%	1.20	No	0.15	3	0.85	0.231
	St. Agnes Medical Center, Philadelphia	6.8	0.0%	1.20	No	0.13	3	0.58	0.085
	St. Francis Medical Center, Pittsburgh	9.2	0.0%	1.33	Yes	0.14	3	0.69	0.130
	St. Joseph Hospital, Reading	6.2	0.0%	1.25	No	0.11	2	0.77	0.047
	St. Luke's Hospital, Bethlehem	5.9	0.0%	1.27	No	0.14	3	0.85	0.053
	St. Margaret Memorial Hospital, Pittsburgh	8.8	0.7%	1.11	No	0.27	3	0.64	0.109
	St. Vincent Health System, Erie	8.0	0.0%	1.14	No	0.08	3	1.11	0.026
	The Medical Center, Beaver	7.0	0.0%	1.24	No	0.08	4	0.80	0.040
	Washington Hospital, Washington	7.9	0.0%	0.98	No	0.12	3	0.78	0.074
	Westmoreland Hospital, Greensburg	9.1	0.0%	1.01	No	0.00	4	1.09	0.022
	Wilkes-Barre General Hospital, Wilkes-Barre	5.6	0.0%	1.32	No	0.01	3	0.75	0.009
	Williamsport Hospital and Medical Center, Williamsport	7.2	0.0%	1.17	No	0.13	3	0.73	0.055

UROLOGY

Natl. Rank	Hospital	U.S. News index	Reputa-tional score	Urology mortality rate	COTH member	Interns and residents to beds	Tech-nology score (of 11)	R.N.'s to beds	Board-certified internists to beds	Procedures to beds
TIER ONE										
16	University of Pittsburgh-Presbyterian University Hospital	26.8	2.9%	0.73	Yes	1.48	8	2.10	0.291	2.86
17	Hospital of the University of Pennsylvania, Philadelphia	25.6	4.6%	0.87	Yes	1.72	11	1.33	0.007	2.56
TIER TWO										
90	Allegheny General Hospital, Pittsburgh	15.1	0.0%	0.85	Yes	0.52	9	1.36	0.025	1.35
64	Graduate Hospital, Philadelphia	16.9	0.0%	0.77	Yes	0.74	9	1.07	0.109	2.09
33	Penn State's Milton S. Hershey Medical Ctr., Hershey	19.8	0.6%	0.87	Yes	1.55	9	1.57	0.023	2.00
55	Temple University Hospital, Philadelphia	17.5	0.5%	0.88	Yes	1.25	9	1.15	0.055	1.22
26	Thomas Jefferson University Hospital, Philadelphia	21.3	1.8%	0.73	Yes	0.96	10	1.44	0.042	1.73
TIER THREE										
	Abington Memorial Hospital, Abington	8.7	0.0%	1.00	No	0.36	5	0.84	0.088	2.46
	Albert Einstein Medical Center, Philadelphia	12.4	0.5%	1.29	Yes	0.75	9	0.89	0.098	2.51
	Bryn Mawr Hospital, Bryn Mawr	11.8	0.0%	1.02	Yes	0.14	6	1.35	0.083	2.29

Natl. Rank	Hospital	U.S. News index	Reputational score	Urology mortality rate	COTH member	Interns and residents to beds	Technology score (of 11)	R.N.'s to beds	Board-certified internists to beds	Procedures to beds
	Conemaugh Memorial Hospital, Johnstown	11.1	0.0%	0.86	No	0.43	6	1.14	0.043	2.14
	Divine Providence Hospital, Williamsport	9.4	0.0%	0.83	No	0.00	7	0.85	0.017	2.33
	Dubois Regional Medical Center, Dubois	10.0	0.0%	0.79	No	0.00	8	0.77	0.014	2.16
	Easton Hospital, Easton	10.2	0.0%	0.88	No	0.20	4	0.99	0.106	4.39
	Frankford Hospital, Philadelphia	9.9	0.0%	1.16	Yes	0.17	5	1.07	0.077	2.46
	Geisinger Medical Center, Danville	12.2	0.0%	1.28	Yes	0.68	8	1.23	0.140	1.71
	Germantown Hospital and Medical Center, Philadelphia	9.3	0.0%	1.29	Yes	0.21	6	0.99	0.097	2.09
	Hahnemann University Hospital, Philadelphia	13.0	0.8%	1.41	Yes	1.19	7	1.11	0.045	1.27
	Lancaster General Hospital, Lancaster	8.7	0.0%	0.92	No	0.14	7	0.85	0.009	2.03
	Lehigh Valley Hospital, Allentown	10.8	0.0%	1.13	Yes	0.19	8	1.19	0.044	1.52
	Lewistown Hospital, Lewistown	10.8	0.0%	0.71	No	0.00	7	0.68	0.070	2.20
	Medical College Hospital, Philadelphia	12.0	0.0%	1.45	Yes	1.39	6	0.81	0.138	0.94
	Mercy Hospital of Pittsburgh, Pittsburgh	11.8	0.0%	0.98	Yes	0.37	7	0.94	0.053	1.74
	Paoli Memorial Hospital, Paoli	11.4	0.0%	0.61	No	0.00	6	0.82	0.113	2.95
	Shadyside Hospital, Pittsburgh	12.4	0.0%	0.92	Yes	0.23	8	0.88	0.103	1.68
	St. Francis Medical Center, Pittsburgh	9.7	0.0%	1.12	Yes	0.14	8	0.69	0.130	0.68
	Washington Hospital, Washington	9.3	0.0%	0.91	No	0.12	8	0.78	0.074	2.37
	Western Pennsylvania Hospital, Pittsburgh	13.5	0.0%	1.02	Yes	0.43	8	1.44	0.091	1.81
	York Hospital, York	9.4	0.0%	1.34	Yes	0.33	7	0.92	0.063	2.35
TIER FOUR										
	Allegheny Valley Hospital, Natrona Heights	7.9	0.0%	1.03	No	0.00	8	0.85	0.061	2.64
	Altoona Hospital, Altoona	4.0	0.0%	1.83	No	0.12	4	1.15	0.069	1.97
	Chester County Hospital, Westchester	6.7	0.0%	1.08	No	0.00	7	0.69	0.074	1.69
	Chestnut Hill Hospital, Philadelphia	4.9	0.0%	1.74	No	0.26	4	0.99	0.121	2.84
	Crozer-Chester Medical Center, Upland	7.1	0.0%	1.75	Yes	0.12	10	0.72	0.058	1.41
	Delaware County Memorial Hospital, Drexel Hill	7.1	0.0%	1.13	No	0.09	7	0.81	0.083	2.27
	Delaware Valley Medical Center, Langhorne	7.5	0.0%	1.13	No	0.47	6	0.45	0.393	1.70
	Forbes Regional Hospital, Monroeville	7.2	0.0%	1.14	No	0.11	6	0.85	0.068	3.53
	Good Samaritan Hospital, Lebanon	3.0	0.0%	1.65	No	0.06	3	0.72	0.021	3.13
	Hamot Medical Center, Erie	7.4	0.0%	1.43	Yes	0.10	6	0.95	0.016	1.26
	Harrisburg Hospital, Harrisburg	5.4	0.0%	1.35	No	0.17	4	0.96	0.065	1.68
	Lankenau Hospital, Wynnewood	7.2	0.0%	1.63	No	0.47	9	1.21	0.072	1.89
	Latrobe Area Hospital, Latrobe	7.5	0.0%	0.93	No	0.10	3	0.80	0.030	2.51
	Lee Hospital, Johnstown	7.9	0.0%	1.12	No	0.00	6	1.20	0.138	2.16
	Lower Bucks Hospital, Bristol	3.4	0.0%	1.73	No	0.01	5	0.87	0.070	1.71
	McKeesport Hospital, McKeesport	7.8	0.0%	1.11	No	0.28	7	0.78	0.064	2.59
	Mercy Health Corporation, Bala Cynwyd	6.4	0.0%	1.85	Yes	0.32	7	0.54	0.051	2.29
	Mercy Hospital of Scranton, Scranton	4.8	0.0%	1.49	No	0.02	7	0.91	0.044	1.65
	Methodist Hospital, Philadelphia	7.3	0.0%	1.28	No	0.06	2	1.57	0.254	2.71
	Monongahela Valley Hospital, Monongahela	5.5	0.0%	1.21	No	0.00	6	0.72	0.032	2.45
	Montgomery Hospital, Norristown	3.9	0.0%	1.58	No	0.12	6	0.61	0.076	1.58
	Moses Taylor Hospital, Scranton	3.6	0.0%	1.50	No	0.04	3	0.73	0.056	2.61
	Nazareth Hospital, Philadelphia	6.5	0.0%	1.10	No	0.00	7	0.76	0.037	1.90
	Northeastern Hospital of Philadelphia	4.1	0.0%	1.40	No	0.02	4	0.71	0.046	2.60
	Northwest Medical Center, Franklin	8.0	0.0%	0.93	No	0.00	9	0.64	0.022	1.25
	Polyclinic Medical Center, Harrisburg	4.1	0.0%	1.68	No	0.20	8	0.66	0.041	1.00
	Presbyterian Medical Center of Philadelphia	7.1	0.0%	1.26	No	0.64	4	0.72	0.114	1.52
	Reading Hospital and Medical Center, Reading	8.3	0.0%	1.03	No	0.20	8	0.84	0.057	1.89
	Robert Packer Hospital, Sayre	7.3	0.0%	1.31	No	0.27	10	0.97	0.022	1.90
	Sacred Heart Hospital, Allentown	3.7	0.0%	2.15	No	0.15	7	0.85	0.231	1.28
	St. Agnes Medical Center, Philadelphia	3.7	0.0%	1.52	No	0.13	4	0.58	0.085	2.08
	St. Joseph Hospital, Reading	4.9	0.0%	1.45	No	0.11	7	0.77	0.047	1.77
	St. Luke's Hospital, Bethlehem	4.5	0.0%	1.65	No	0.14	7	0.85	0.053	1.94
	St. Margaret Memorial Hospital, Pittsburgh	4.7	0.0%	1.55	No	0.27	5	0.64	0.109	2.30
	St. Vincent Health System, Erie	5.4	0.0%	1.35	No	0.08	5	1.11	0.026	1.51
	The Medical Center, Beaver	5.2	0.0%	1.43	No	0.08	8	0.80	0.040	2.03

AMERICA'S BEST HOSPITALS

Natl. Rank	Hospital	U.S. News index	Reputa- tional score	Urology mortality rate	COTH member	Interns and residents to beds	Tech- nology score (of 11)	R.N.'s to beds	Board- certified internists to beds	Procedures to beds
	University of Pittsburgh-Montefiore Hospital	8.5	0.0%	1.60	No	0.93	4	1.43	0.388	1.40
	Westmoreland Hospital, Greensburg	7.8	0.0%	1.04	No	0.00	7	1.09	0.022	2.29
	Wilkes-Barre General Hospital, Wilkes-Barre	5.2	0.0%	1.27	No	0.01	7	0.75	0.009	1.86
	Williamsport Hospital and Medical Center, Williamsport	5.2	0.0%	1.32	No	0.13	5	0.73	0.055	2.30

AIDS

Natl. Rank	Hospital	U.S. News index	Reputa- tional score	Hospital- wide mortality rate	COTH member	Interns and residents to beds	Tech- nology score (of 11)	Discharge planning (of 2)	R.N.'s to beds	Board- certified internists to beds
				TIER TWO						
85	Roger Williams Medical Center, Providence	25.3	0.0%	0.89	Yes	0.58	5	2	1.03	0.178
				TIER THREE						
	Rhode Island Hospital, Providence	24.4	0.0%	1.04	Yes	0.82	9	2	0.84	0.210
	Women and Infants Hospital of Rhode Island, Providence	20.5	0.0%	0.98	Yes	0.26	2	2	0.65	0.005
				TIER FOUR						
	Memorial Hospital of Rhode Island, Pawtucket	18.8	0.0%	1.15	Yes	0.48	4	1	0.71	0.075
	Miriam Hospital, Providence	19.6	0.0%	1.15	Yes	0.44	5	1	0.62	0.215

CANCER

Natl. Rank	Hospital	U.S. News index	Reputa- tional score	Cancer mortality rate	COTH member	Interns and residents to beds	Tech- nology score (of 12)	R.N.'s to beds	Board- certified oncologists to beds	Procedures to beds
				TIER THREE						
	Memorial Hospital of Rhode Island, Pawtucket	5.9	0.0%	1.12	Yes	0.48	2	0.71	0.020	2.35
	Miriam Hospital, Providence	5.8	0.0%	0.85	Yes	0.44	2	0.62	0.049	1.69
	Rhode Island Hospital, Providence	9.7	0.0%	0.83	Yes	0.82	9	0.84	0.035	2.04
	Roger Williams Medical Center, Providence	9.4	0.0%	0.59	Yes	0.58	6	1.03	0.040	4.22

CARDIOLOGY

Natl. Rank	Hospital	U.S. News index	Reputa- tional score	Cardiology mortality rate	COTH member	Interns and residents to beds	Tech- nology score (of 10)	R.N.'s to beds	Board- certified cardiologists to beds	Procedures to beds
				TIER TWO						
59	Roger Williams Medical Center, Providence	22.6	0.0%	0.74	Yes	0.58	4	1.03	0.063	10.10
				TIER THREE						
	Memorial Hospital of Rhode Island, Pawtucket	20.3	0.0%	0.88	Yes	0.48	3	0.71	0.037	7.76
	Miriam Hospital, Providence	17.8	0.0%	1.03	Yes	0.44	7	0.62	0.093	16.29
100	Rhode Island Hospital, Providence	20.7	0.0%	1.00	Yes	0.82	9	0.84	0.047	8.70

ENDOCRINOLOGY

Natl. Rank	Hospital	U.S. News index	Reputa- tional score	Endocrinology mortality rate	COTH member	Interns and residents to beds	Tech- nology score (of 11)	R.N.'s to beds	Board- certified internists to beds
				TIER TWO					
78	Rhode Island Hospital, Providence	15.1	0.5%	0.85	Yes	0.82	9	0.84	0.210
				TIER THREE					
	Memorial Hospital of Rhode Island, Pawtucket	9.5	0.0%	1.01	Yes	0.48	3	0.71	0.075
	Miriam Hospital, Providence	8.3	0.0%	1.35	Yes	0.44	2	0.62	0.215
100	Roger Williams Medical Center, Providence	13.6	0.0%	0.85	Yes	0.58	7	1.03	0.178

GASTROENTEROLOGY

Natl. Rank	Hospital	U.S. News index	Reputa-tional score	Gastro-enterology mortality rate	COTH member	Interns and residents to beds	Tech-nology score (of 11)	R.N.'s to beds	Board-certified gastro-enterologists to beds	Pro-cedures to beds
	TIER TWO									
68	Roger Williams Medical Center, Providence	13.5	0.0%	0.87	Yes	0.58	6	1.03	0.029	5.20
	TIER THREE									
	Memorial Hospital of Rhode Island, Pawtucket	7.3	0.0%	1.40	Yes	0.48	3	0.71	0.020	3.51
	Miriam Hospital, Providence	8.1	0.0%	1.33	Yes	0.44	2	0.62	0.045	5.36
86	Rhode Island Hospital, Providence	12.8	0.0%	0.92	Yes	0.82	8	0.84	0.033	2.93

GERIATRICS

Natl. Rank	Hospital	U.S. News index	Reputa-tional score	Hospital-wide mortality rate	COTH member	Service mix	Interns and residents to beds	Tech-nology score (of 13)	R.N.'s to beds	Discharge planning (of 2)	Geriatric services (of 9)	Board-certified internists to beds
	TIER TWO											
61	Roger Williams Medical Center, Providence	23.2	0.5%	0.89	Yes	4	0.58	8	1.03	2	3	0.178
	TIER THREE											
	Rhode Island Hospital, Providence	20.5	0.6%	1.04	Yes	6	0.82	11	0.84	2	2	0.210
	TIER FOUR											
	Memorial Hospital of Rhode Island, Pawtucket	10.7	0.0%	1.15	Yes	4	0.48	3	0.71	1	1	0.075
	Miriam Hospital, Providence	11.5	0.0%	1.15	Yes	4	0.44	4	0.62	1	1	0.215

GYNECOLOGY

Natl. Rank	Hospital	U.S. News index	Reputa-tional score	Hospital-wide mortality rate	Interns and residents to beds	Tech-nology score (of 10)	R.N.'s to beds	Board-certified OB-GYNs to beds	Procedures to beds
	TIER THREE								
	Rhode Island Hospital, Providence	18.4	0.0%	1.04	0.82	7	0.84	0.064	0.12
	Roger Williams Medical Center, Providence	19.9	0.0%	0.89	0.58	5	1.03	0.011	0.24
	TIER FOUR								
	Memorial Hospital of Rhode Island, Pawtucket	9.9	0.0%	1.15	0.48	3	0.71	0.024	0.33
	Miriam Hospital, Providence	9.9	0.0%	1.15	0.44	3	0.62	0.045	0.13

NEUROLOGY

Natl. Rank	Hospital	U.S. News index	Reputa-tional score	Neurology mortality rate	COTH member	Interns and residents to beds	Tech-nology score (of 9)	R.N.'s to beds	Board-certified neurologists to beds
	TIER TWO								
57	Roger Williams Medical Center, Providence	19.1	0.0%	0.66	Yes	0.58	5	1.03	0.017
	TIER THREE								
	Miriam Hospital, Providence	11.5	0.0%	1.01	Yes	0.44	2	0.62	0.016
	Rhode Island Hospital, Providence	13.9	0.0%	1.12	Yes	0.82	7	0.84	0.028
	TIER FOUR								
	Memorial Hospital of Rhode Island, Pawtucket	9.0	0.0%	1.18	Yes	0.48	3	0.71	0.003

ORTHOPEDICS

Natl. Rank	Hospital	U.S. News index	Reputational score	Orthopedics mortality rate	COTH member	Interns and residents to beds	Technology score (of 5)	R.N.'s to beds	Board-certified orthopedists to beds	Procedures to beds
	TIER THREE									
	Rhode Island Hospital, Providence	**11.9**	0.0%	1.06	Yes	0.82	4	0.84	0.057	2.38
	Roger Williams Medical Center, Providence	**13.0**	0.0%	0.85	Yes	0.58	3	1.03	0.069	3.36
	TIER FOUR									
	Memorial Hospital of Rhode Island, Pawtucket	**8.1**	0.0%	1.18	Yes	0.48	2	0.71	0.034	1.95
	Miriam Hospital, Providence	**7.0**	0.0%	1.43	Yes	0.44	2	0.62	0.053	3.14

OTOLARYNGOLOGY

Natl. Rank	Hospital	U.S. News index	Reputational score	Hospital-wide mortality rate	COTH member	Interns and residents to beds	Technology score (of 9)	R.N.'s to beds	Board-certified internists to beds	Procedures to beds
	TIER THREE									
	Memorial Hospital of Rhode Island, Pawtucket	**8.1**	0.0%	1.15	Yes	0.48	1	0.71	0.075	0.303
	Miriam Hospital, Providence	**8.9**	0.0%	1.15	Yes	0.44	1	0.62	0.215	0.470
	Rhode Island Hospital, Providence	**12.8**	0.0%	1.04	Yes	0.82	7	0.84	0.210	0.271
	Roger Williams Medical Center, Providence	**11.7**	0.0%	0.89	Yes	0.58	5	1.03	0.178	0.259

RHEUMATOLOGY

Natl. Rank	Hospital	U.S. News index	Reputational score	Hospital-wide mortality rate	COTH member	Interns and residents to beds	Technology score (of 5)	R.N.'s to beds	Board-certified internists to beds
	TIER THREE								
	Miriam Hospital, Providence	**10.2**	0.0%	1.15	Yes	0.44	2	0.62	0.215
	Rhode Island Hospital, Providence	**14.7**	0.0%	1.04	Yes	0.82	4	0.84	0.210
93	Roger Williams Medical Center, Providence	**15.2**	0.0%	0.89	Yes	0.58	3	1.03	0.178
	TIER FOUR								
	Memorial Hospital of Rhode Island, Pawtucket	**9.5**	0.0%	1.15	Yes	0.48	2	0.71	0.075

UROLOGY

Natl. Rank	Hospital	U.S. News index	Reputational score	Urology mortality rate	COTH member	Interns and residents to beds	Technology score (of 11)	R.N.'s to beds	Board-certified internists to beds	Procedures to beds
	TIER TWO									
67	Roger Williams Medical Center, Providence	**16.6**	0.0%	0.64	Yes	0.58	6	1.03	0.178	2.40
	TIER THREE									
	Memorial Hospital of Rhode Island, Pawtucket	**8.6**	0.0%	1.30	Yes	0.48	3	0.71	0.075	2.14
	Miriam Hospital, Providence	**10.6**	0.0%	1.01	Yes	0.44	2	0.62	0.215	2.89
	Rhode Island Hospital, Providence	**14.3**	0.0%	0.96	Yes	0.82	8	0.84	0.210	1.86

AIDS

Natl. Rank	Hospital	U.S. News index	Reputa- tional score	Hospital- wide mortality rate	COTH member	Interns and residents to beds	Tech- nology score (of 11)	Discharge planning (of 2)	R.N.'s to beds	Board- certified internists to beds
	TIER THREE									
	Medical University of South Carolina, Charleston	24.2	0.0%	1.07	Yes	1.42	6	2	1.39	0.022
	TIER FOUR									
	Aiken Regional Medical Centers, Aiken	15.2	0.0%	1.41	No	0.00	5	2	1.08	0.044
	Allen Bennett Memorial Hospital, Greer	11.9	0.0%	1.55	No	0.00	4	1	0.35	0.019
	Anderson Area Medical Center, Anderson	17.0	0.0%	1.23	No	0.11	7	2	0.59	0.037
	Baptist Medical Center-Columbia, Columbia	15.8	0.0%	1.44	No	0.00	7	2	0.90	0.135
	Charleston Memorial Hospital, Charleston	14.9	0.0%	1.22	No	0.26	3	1	0.45	0.000
	Greenville Memorial Hospital, Greenville	18.2	0.0%	1.32	Yes	0.33	7	1	0.92	0.081
	HCA Trident Regional Medical Center, Charleston	16.9	0.0%	1.27	No	0.00	7	2	0.89	0.032
	Hillcrest Hospital, Simpsonville	15.0	0.0%	1.26	No	0.00	4	1	0.82	0.018
	Lexington Medical Center, West Columbia	14.4	0.0%	1.57	No	0.00	7	2	0.88	0.034
	McLeod Regional Medical Center, Florence	15.5	0.0%	1.47	No	0.11	7	2	0.99	0.023
	Richland Memorial Hospital, Columbia	18.2	0.0%	1.70	Yes	0.59	8	2	1.64	0.089
	Roper Hospital, Charleston	16.1	0.0%	1.36	No	0.00	6	2	0.99	0.096
	Self Memorial Hospital, Greenwood	16.0	0.0%	1.30	No	0.11	6	2	0.69	0.015
	Spartanburg Regional Medical Center, Spartanburg	15.4	0.0%	1.52	No	0.19	7	2	1.05	0.023

CANCER

Natl. Rank	Hospital	U.S. News index	Reputa- tional score	Cancer mortality rate	COTH member	Interns and residents to beds	Tech- nology score (of 12)	R.N.'s to beds	Board- certified oncologists to beds	Procedures to beds
	TIER TWO									
55	Medical University of South Carolina, Charleston	12.7	0.0%	0.88	Yes	1.42	9	1.39	0.007	0.88
	TIER THREE									
	Greenville Memorial Hospital, Greenville	7.3	0.0%	1.20	Yes	0.33	8	0.92	0.014	1.43
86	Richland Memorial Hospital, Columbia	10.8	0.0%	1.45	Yes	0.59	10	1.64	0.012	2.20
	TIER FOUR									
	Aiken Regional Medical Centers, Aiken	3.8	0.0%	1.18	No	0.00	7	1.08	0.000	1.21
	Anderson Area Medical Center, Anderson	4.0	0.0%	1.02	No	0.11	10	0.59	0.009	2.05
	Baptist Medical Center-Columbia, Columbia	3.6	0.0%	1.47	No	0.00	8	0.90	0.000	2.03
	HCA Trident Regional Medical Center, Charleston	3.6	0.0%	1.20	No	0.00	8	0.89	0.006	1.05
	Lexington Medical Center, West Columbia	3.7	0.0%	1.27	No	0.00	8	0.88	0.010	1.75
	McLeod Regional Medical Center, Florence	4.3	0.0%	1.26	No	0.11	8	0.99	0.006	1.61
	Roper Hospital, Charleston	4.0	0.0%	1.39	No	0.00	8	0.99	0.016	2.06
	Self Memorial Hospital, Greenwood	3.2	0.0%	1.15	No	0.11	7	0.69	0.003	1.09
	Spartanburg Regional Medical Center, Spartanburg	4.9	0.0%	1.53	No	0.19	9	1.05	0.008	1.44

CARDIOLOGY

Natl. Rank	Hospital	U.S. News index	Reputa- tional score	Cardiology mortality rate	COTH member	Interns and residents to beds	Tech- nology score (of 10)	R.N.'s to beds	Board- certified cardiologists to beds	Procedures to beds
	TIER TWO									
76	Medical University of South Carolina, Charleston	21.5	0.0%	1.09	Yes	1.42	8	1.39	0.031	3.97
	TIER FOUR									
	Aiken Regional Medical Centers, Aiken	7.1	0.0%	1.42	No	0.00	7	1.08	0.011	6.95
	Anderson Area Medical Center, Anderson	7.4	0.0%	1.32	No	0.11	7	0.59	0.013	6.34
	Baptist Medical Center-Columbia, Columbia	9.4	0.0%	1.17	No	0.00	6	0.90	0.000	3.40
	Greenville Memorial Hospital, Greenville	12.4	0.0%	1.32	Yes	0.33	8	0.92	0.023	8.19
	HCA Trident Regional Medical Center, Charleston	7.8	0.0%	1.39	No	0.00	9	0.89	0.029	6.03

Natl. Rank	Hospital	U.S. News index	Reputa-tional score	Cardiology mortality rate	COTH member	Interns and residents to beds	Tech-nology score (of 10)	R.N.'s to beds	Board-certified cardiologists to beds	Procedures to beds
	Lexington Medical Center, West Columbia	6.6	0.0%	1.38	No	0.00	5	0.88	0.024	6.12
	McLeod Regional Medical Center, Florence	7.3	0.0%	1.50	No	0.11	9	0.99	0.026	8.95
	Richland Memorial Hospital, Columbia	12.0	0.0%	1.67	Yes	0.59	9	1.64	0.037	5.63
	Roper Hospital, Charleston	9.9	0.0%	1.27	No	0.00	8	0.99	0.049	6.98
	Self Memorial Hospital, Greenwood	8.9	0.0%	1.20	No	0.11	6	0.69	0.006	4.80
	Spartanburg Regional Medical Center, Spartanburg	9.0	0.0%	1.38	No	0.19	9	1.05	0.019	7.08

ENDOCRINOLOGY

Natl. Rank	Hospital	U.S. News index	Reputa-tional score	Endocrinology mortality rate	COTH member	Interns and residents to beds	Tech-nology score (of 11)	R.N.'s to beds	Board-certified internists to beds
	TIER TWO								
68	Medical University of South Carolina, Charleston	15.9	0.6%	1.08	Yes	1.42	10	1.39	0.022
	TIER THREE								
	Greenville Memorial Hospital, Greenville	8.7	0.0%	1.43	Yes	0.33	8	0.92	0.081
	Richland Memorial Hospital, Columbia	10.1	0.0%	2.07	Yes	0.59	8	1.64	0.089
	TIER FOUR								
	Aiken Regional Medical Centers, Aiken	4.5	0.0%	1.72	No	0.00	8	1.08	0.044
	Anderson Area Medical Center, Anderson	5.5	0.0%	1.22	No	0.11	10	0.59	0.037
	Baptist Medical Center-Columbia, Columbia	7.3	0.0%	1.06	No	0.00	9	0.90	0.135
	HCA Trident Regional Medical Center, Charleston	4.7	0.0%	1.48	No	0.00	9	0.89	0.032
	Lexington Medical Center, West Columbia	3.2	0.0%	2.18	No	0.00	9	0.88	0.034
	McLeod Regional Medical Center, Florence	5.2	0.0%	1.51	No	0.11	9	0.99	0.023
	Roper Hospital, Charleston	4.7	0.0%	1.79	No	0.00	9	0.99	0.096
	Self Memorial Hospital, Greenwood	5.4	0.0%	1.19	No	0.11	8	0.69	0.015
	Spartanburg Regional Medical Center, Spartanburg	6.0	0.0%	1.40	No	0.19	9	1.05	0.023

GASTROENTEROLOGY

Natl. Rank	Hospital	U.S. News index	Reputa-tional score	Gastro-enterology mortality rate	COTH member	Interns and residents to beds	Tech-nology score (of 11)	R.N.'s to beds	Board-certified gastro-enterologists to beds	Pro-cedures to beds
	TIER TWO									
49	Medical University of South Carolina, Charleston	15.2	0.9%	1.15	Yes	1.42	9	1.39	0.011	1.14
	TIER THREE									
	Greenville Memorial Hospital, Greenville	8.6	0.0%	1.23	Yes	0.33	7	0.92	0.018	2.55
	Richland Memorial Hospital, Columbia	10.6	0.5%	1.43	Yes	0.59	7	1.64	0.012	1.72
	TIER FOUR									
	Aiken Regional Medical Centers, Aiken	4.3	0.0%	1.66	No	0.00	7	1.08	0.005	3.74
	Anderson Area Medical Center, Anderson	5.0	0.0%	1.36	No	0.11	9	0.59	0.004	3.59
	Baptist Medical Center-Columbia, Columbia	4.6	0.0%	1.43	No	0.00	9	0.90	0.000	2.64
	HCA Trident Regional Medical Center, Charleston	5.3	0.0%	1.32	No	0.00	9	0.89	0.010	3.17
	Lexington Medical Center, West Columbia	4.6	0.0%	1.57	No	0.00	8	0.88	0.017	4.01
	McLeod Regional Medical Center, Florence	5.2	0.0%	1.35	No	0.11	9	0.99	0.011	2.19
	Roper Hospital, Charleston	6.0	0.0%	1.14	No	0.00	8	0.99	0.016	3.10
	Self Memorial Hospital, Greenwood	5.7	0.0%	1.04	No	0.11	7	0.69	0.006	2.55
	Spartanburg Regional Medical Center, Spartanburg	5.4	0.0%	1.59	No	0.19	9	1.05	0.006	3.10

GERIATRICS

Natl. Rank	Hospital	U.S. News index	Reputa- tional score	Hospital- wide mortality rate	COTH member	Service mix	Interns and residents to beds	Tech- nology score (of 13)	R.N.'s to beds	Discharge planning (of 2)	Geriatric services (of 9)	Board- certified internists to beds
	TIER THREE											
	Medical University of South Carolina, Charleston	**19.6**	0.0%	1.07	Yes	7	1.42	10	1.39	2	1	0.022
	TIER FOUR											
	Aiken Regional Medical Centers, Aiken	**5.6**	0.0%	1.41	No	3	0.00	9	1.08	2	2	0.044
	Anderson Area Medical Center, Anderson	**10.4**	0.0%	1.23	No	7	0.11	12	0.59	2	3	0.037
	Baptist Medical Center-Columbia, Columbia	**7.1**	0.0%	1.44	No	6	0.00	11	0.90	2	2	0.135
	Greenville Memorial Hospital, Greenville	**9.4**	0.0%	1.32	Yes	5	0.33	10	0.92	1	1	0.081
	HCA Trident Regional Medical Center, Charleston	**8.2**	0.0%	1.27	No	3	0.00	11	0.89	2	3	0.032
	Lexington Medical Center, West Columbia	**3.1**	0.0%	1.57	No	3	0.00	9	0.88	2	2	0.034
	McLeod Regional Medical Center, Florence	**6.3**	0.0%	1.47	No	5	0.11	11	0.99	2	3	0.023
	Richland Memorial Hospital, Columbia	**9.5**	0.0%	1.70	Yes	8	0.59	11	1.64	2	2	0.089
	Roper Hospital, Charleston	**7.0**	0.0%	1.36	No	3	0.00	10	0.99	2	3	0.096
	Self Memorial Hospital, Greenwood	**8.1**	0.0%	1.30	No	6	0.11	10	0.69	2	2	0.015
	Spartanburg Regional Medical Center, Spartanburg	**7.1**	0.0%	1.52	No	6	0.19	12	1.05	2	5	0.023

GYNECOLOGY

Natl. Rank	Hospital	U.S. News index	Reputa- tional score	Hospital- wide mortality rate	Interns and residents to beds	Tech- nology score (of 10)	R.N.'s to beds	Board- certified OB-GYNs to beds	Procedures to beds
	TIER TWO								
65	**Medical University of South Carolina, Charleston**	**24.2**	0.4%	1.07	1.42	9	1.39	0.024	0.37
	TIER FOUR								
	Aiken Regional Medical Centers, Aiken	**7.3**	0.0%	1.41	0.00	6	1.08	0.033	0.43
	Anderson Area Medical Center, Anderson	**9.7**	0.0%	1.23	0.11	8	0.59	0.026	0.45
	Baptist Medical Center-Columbia, Columbia	**8.2**	0.0%	1.44	0.00	8	0.90	0.061	0.65
	Greenville Memorial Hospital, Greenville	**10.2**	0.0%	1.32	0.33	7	0.92	0.040	0.53
	HCA Trident Regional Medical Center, Charleston	**9.4**	0.0%	1.27	0.00	7	0.89	0.032	0.30
	Lexington Medical Center, West Columbia	**5.2**	0.0%	1.57	0.00	7	0.88	0.037	0.42
	McLeod Regional Medical Center, Florence	**8.0**	0.0%	1.47	0.11	8	0.99	0.031	0.40
	Richland Memorial Hospital, Columbia	**10.7**	0.0%	1.70	0.59	8	1.64	0.046	0.60
	Roper Hospital, Charleston	**9.4**	0.0%	1.36	0.00	7	0.99	0.078	0.59
	Self Memorial Hospital, Greenwood	**8.2**	0.0%	1.30	0.11	7	0.69	0.024	0.43
	Spartanburg Regional Medical Center, Spartanburg	**8.1**	0.0%	1.52	0.19	8	1.05	0.034	0.30

NEUROLOGY

Natl. Rank	Hospital	U.S. News index	Reputa- tional score	Neurology mortality rate	COTH member	Interns and residents to beds	Tech- nology score (of 9)	R.N.'s to beds	Board- certified neurologists to beds
	TIER THREE								
	Medical University of South Carolina, Charleston	**16.2**	0.0%	1.17	Yes	1.42	8	1.39	0.016
	Richland Memorial Hospital, Columbia	**11.3**	0.0%	1.39	Yes	0.59	6	1.64	0.014
	TIER FOUR								
	Aiken Regional Medical Centers, Aiken	**6.4**	0.0%	1.25	No	0.00	6	1.08	0.005
	Anderson Area Medical Center, Anderson	**7.8**	0.0%	1.10	No	0.11	8	0.59	0.004
	Baptist Medical Center-Columbia, Columbia	**5.9**	0.0%	1.31	No	0.00	7	0.90	0.009
	Greenville Memorial Hospital, Greenville	**9.2**	0.3%	1.32	Yes	0.33	6	0.92	0.007
	Lexington Medical Center, West Columbia	**4.6**	0.0%	1.47	No	0.00	7	0.88	0.010
	McLeod Regional Medical Center, Florence	**8.6**	0.0%	1.12	No	0.11	7	0.99	0.009
	Roper Hospital, Charleston	**5.9**	0.0%	1.36	No	0.00	7	0.99	0.013
	Self Memorial Hospital, Greenwood	**3.6**	0.0%	1.48	No	0.11	6	0.69	0.003
	Spartanburg Regional Medical Center, Spartanburg	**4.9**	0.0%	1.54	No	0.19	7	1.05	0.006

ORTHOPEDICS

Natl. Rank	Hospital	U.S. News index	Reputational score	Orthopedics mortality rate	COTH member	Interns and residents to beds	Technology score (of 5)	R.N.'s to beds	Board-certified orthopedists to beds	Procedures to beds
	TIER TWO									
75	**Medical University of South Carolina, Charleston**	14.7	0.0%	1.06	Yes	1.42	4	1.39	0.013	0.78
	TIER THREE									
	Greenville Memorial Hospital, Greenville	8.6	0.5%	1.53	Yes	0.33	3	0.92	0.041	2.54
	Richland Memorial Hospital, Columbia	11.7	0.0%	1.33	Yes	0.59	4	1.64	0.037	2.34
	TIER FOUR									
	Aiken Regional Medical Centers, Aiken	3.8	0.0%	1.66	No	0.00	3	1.08	0.027	2.82
	Anderson Area Medical Center, Anderson	5.0	0.0%	1.19	No	0.11	4	0.59	0.015	2.19
	Baptist Medical Center-Columbia, Columbia	5.8	0.0%	1.17	No	0.00	4	0.90	0.044	2.30
	HCA Trident Regional Medical Center, Charleston	5.4	0.0%	1.20	No	0.00	4	0.89	0.019	2.06
	Lexington Medical Center, West Columbia	4.0	0.0%	1.58	No	0.00	4	0.88	0.034	2.30
	McLeod Regional Medical Center, Florence	5.1	0.0%	1.47	No	0.11	4	0.99	0.028	2.97
	Roper Hospital, Charleston	4.5	0.0%	1.37	No	0.00	3	0.99	0.044	2.40
	Self Memorial Hospital, Greenwood	4.0	0.0%	1.29	No	0.11	3	0.69	0.012	1.73
	Spartanburg Regional Medical Center, Spartanburg	6.5	0.0%	1.19	No	0.19	4	1.05	0.021	1.93

OTOLARYNGOLOGY

Natl. Rank	Hospital	U.S. News index	Reputational score	Hospital-wide mortality rate	COTH member	Interns and residents to beds	Technology score (of 9)	R.N.'s to beds	Board-certified internists to beds	Procedures to beds
	TIER TWO									
68	**Medical University of South Carolina, Charleston**	15.5	0.0%	1.07	Yes	1.42	8	1.39	0.022	0.154
	TIER THREE									
	Greenville Memorial Hospital, Greenville	9.8	0.0%	1.32	Yes	0.33	7	0.92	0.081	0.095
	Richland Memorial Hospital, Columbia	13.0	0.0%	1.70	Yes	0.59	7	1.64	0.089	0.128
	TIER FOUR									
	Aiken Regional Medical Centers, Aiken	5.2	0.0%	1.41	No	0.00	6	1.08	0.044	0.202
	Allen Bennett Memorial Hospital, Greer	1.3	0.0%	1.55	No	0.00	1	0.35	0.019	0.032
	Anderson Area Medical Center, Anderson	4.7	0.0%	1.23	No	0.11	8	0.59	0.037	0.277
	Baptist Medical Center-Columbia, Columbia	5.7	0.0%	1.44	No	0.00	7	0.90	0.135	0.161
	Charleston Memorial Hospital, Charleston	2.3	0.0%	1.22	No	0.26	0	0.45	0.000	0.033
	HCA Trident Regional Medical Center, Charleston	4.9	0.0%	1.27	No	0.00	7	0.89	0.032	0.190
	Hillcrest Hospital, Simpsonville	2.8	0.0%	1.26	No	0.00	1	0.82	0.018	0.054
	Lexington Medical Center, West Columbia	4.7	0.0%	1.57	No	0.00	7	0.88	0.034	0.176
	McLeod Regional Medical Center, Florence	5.4	0.0%	1.47	No	0.11	7	0.99	0.023	0.179
	Roper Hospital, Charleston	5.7	0.0%	1.36	No	0.00	7	0.99	0.096	0.260
	Self Memorial Hospital, Greenwood	4.2	0.0%	1.30	No	0.11	6	0.69	0.015	0.120
	Spartanburg Regional Medical Center, Spartanburg	5.9	0.0%	1.52	No	0.19	7	1.05	0.023	0.129

RHEUMATOLOGY

Natl. Rank	Hospital	U.S. News index	Reputational score	Hospital-wide mortality rate	COTH member	Interns and residents to beds	Technology score (of 5)	R.N.'s to beds	Board-certified internists to beds
	TIER TWO								
31	**Medical University of South Carolina, Charleston**	20.8	2.0%	1.07	Yes	1.42	4	1.39	0.022
	TIER THREE								
	Richland Memorial Hospital, Columbia	11.7	0.0%	1.70	Yes	0.59	4	1.64	0.089
	TIER FOUR								
	Aiken Regional Medical Centers, Aiken	6.2	0.0%	1.41	No	0.00	3	1.08	0.044
	Anderson Area Medical Center, Anderson	6.6	0.0%	1.23	No	0.11	4	0.59	0.037
	Baptist Medical Center-Columbia, Columbia	6.7	0.0%	1.44	No	0.00	4	0.90	0.135
	Greenville Memorial Hospital, Greenville	9.0	0.0%	1.32	Yes	0.33	3	0.92	0.081

Natl. Rank	Hospital	U.S. News index	Reputa- tional score	Hospital- wide mortality rate	COTH member	Interns and residents to beds	Tech- nology score (of 5)	R.N.'s to beds	Board- certified internists to beds
	HCA Trident Regional Medical Center, Charleston	6.8	0.0%	1.27	No	0.00	4	0.89	0.032
	Lexington Medical Center, West Columbia	5.4	0.0%	1.57	No	0.00	4	0.88	0.034
	McLeod Regional Medical Center, Florence	6.4	0.0%	1.47	No	0.11	4	0.99	0.023
	Roper Hospital, Charleston	6.6	0.0%	1.36	No	0.00	3	0.99	0.096
	Self Memorial Hospital, Greenwood	5.9	0.0%	1.30	No	0.11	3	0.69	0.015
	Spartanburg Regional Medical Center, Spartanburg	6.6	0.0%	1.52	No	0.19	4	1.05	0.023

UROLOGY

Natl. Rank	Hospital	U.S. News index	Reputa- tional score	Urology mortality rate	COTH member	Interns and residents to beds	Tech- nology score (of 11)	R.N.'s to beds	Board- certified internists to beds	Procedures to beds
	TIER TWO									
46	Medical University of South Carolina, Charleston	18.6	0.7%	0.89	Yes	1.42	9	1.39	0.022	1.39
	TIER THREE									
	Greenville Memorial Hospital, Greenville	9.5	0.0%	1.29	Yes	0.33	7	0.92	0.081	1.44
	TIER FOUR									
	Aiken Regional Medical Centers, Aiken	3.7	0.0%	2.01	No	0.00	7	1.08	0.044	2.37
	Allen Bennett Memorial Hospital, Greer	0.0	0.0%	2.08	No	0.00	2	0.35	0.019	1.62
	Anderson Area Medical Center, Anderson	5.1	0.0%	1.41	No	0.11	9	0.59	0.037	1.72
	Baptist Medical Center-Columbia, Columbia	5.3	0.0%	1.59	No	0.00	9	0.90	0.135	1.31
	HCA Trident Regional Medical Center, Charleston	4.0	0.0%	1.82	No	0.00	9	0.89	0.032	1.74
	Lexington Medical Center, West Columbia	3.6	0.0%	1.93	No	0.00	8	0.88	0.034	2.18
	McLeod Regional Medical Center, Florence	4.9	0.0%	1.67	No	0.11	9	0.99	0.023	1.57
	Richland Memorial Hospital, Columbia	8.4	0.0%	2.75	Yes	0.59	7	1.64	0.089	1.12
	Roper Hospital, Charleston	5.1	0.0%	1.65	No	0.00	8	0.99	0.096	2.25
	Self Memorial Hospital, Greenwood	3.9	0.0%	1.63	No	0.11	7	0.69	0.015	2.00
	Spartanburg Regional Medical Center, Spartanburg	4.7	0.7%	2.33	No	0.19	9	1.05	0.023	1.36

AIDS

Natl. Rank	Hospital	U.S. News index	Reputational score	Hospital-wide mortality rate	COTH member	Interns and residents to beds	Technology score (of 11)	Discharge planning (of 2)	R.N.'s to beds	Board-certified internists to beds
TIER THREE										
	Sioux Valley Hospital, Sioux Falls	20.4	0.0%	1.03	No	0.04	5	2	1.57	0.053
TIER FOUR										
	McKennan Hospital, Sioux Falls	17.1	0.0%	1.25	No	0.09	6	2	0.99	0.054
	Rapid City Regional Hospital, Rapid City	19.1	0.0%	1.06	No	0.00	8	2	0.45	0.032
	St. Luke's Midland Regional Medical Center, Aberdeen	18.4	0.0%	1.12	No	0.00	6	2	1.03	0.027

CANCER

Natl. Rank	Hospital	U.S. News index	Reputational score	Cancer mortality rate	COTH member	Interns and residents to beds	Technology score (of 12)	R.N.'s to beds	Board-certified oncologists to beds	Procedures to beds
TIER THREE										
	Sioux Valley Hospital, Sioux Falls	5.7	0.0%	0.71	No	0.04	5	1.57	0.013	2.46
TIER FOUR										
	McKennan Hospital, Sioux Falls	3.7	0.0%	1.35	No	0.09	6	0.99	0.010	1.87
	Rapid City Regional Hospital, Rapid City	3.4	0.0%	0.80	No	0.00	10	0.45	0.005	1.50
	St. Luke's Midland Regional Medical Center, Aberdeen	3.9	0.0%	1.10	No	0.00	7	1.03	0.004	1.66

CARDIOLOGY

Natl. Rank	Hospital	U.S. News index	Reputational score	Cardiology mortality rate	COTH member	Interns and residents to beds	Technology score (of 10)	R.N.'s to beds	Board-certified cardiologists to beds	Procedures to beds
TIER THREE										
	Sioux Valley Hospital, Sioux Falls	16.2	0.0%	1.03	No	0.04	8	1.57	0.044	9.15
TIER FOUR										
	McKennan Hospital, Sioux Falls	10.2	0.0%	1.27	No	0.09	8	0.99	0.049	6.34
	Rapid City Regional Hospital, Rapid City	8.7	0.0%	1.19	No	0.00	8	0.45	0.011	5.57
	St. Luke's Midland Regional Medical Center, Aberdeen	10.2	0.0%	1.12	No	0.00	4	1.03	0.000	4.75

ENDOCRINOLOGY

Natl. Rank	Hospital	U.S. News index	Reputational score	Endocrinology mortality rate	COTH member	Interns and residents to beds	Technology score (of 11)	R.N.'s to beds	Board-certified internists to beds
TIER THREE									
	Rapid City Regional Hospital, Rapid City	8.7	0.0%	0.70	No	0.00	9	0.45	0.032
	Sioux Valley Hospital, Sioux Falls	10.1	0.4%	0.83	No	0.04	5	1.57	0.053
	St. Luke's Midland Regional Medical Center, Aberdeen	8.8	0.0%	0.80	No	0.00	8	1.03	0.027
TIER FOUR									
	McKennan Hospital, Sioux Falls	5.1	0.0%	1.34	No	0.09	5	0.99	0.054

GASTROENTEROLOGY

Natl. Rank Hospital	U.S. News index	Reputa- tional score	Gastro- enterology mortality rate	COTH member	Interns and residents to beds	Tech- nology score (of 11)	R.N.'s to beds	Board- certified gastro- enterologists to beds	Pro- cedures to beds
TIER THREE									
Sioux Valley Hospital, Sioux Falls	7.7	0.0%	0.93	No	0.04	4	1.57	0.013	2.95
TIER FOUR									
McKennan Hospital, Sioux Falls	3.6	0.0%	1.38	No	0.09	4	0.99	0.015	2.24
Rapid City Regional Hospital, Rapid City	3.5	0.0%	1.42	No	0.00	9	0.45	0.008	2.55
St. Luke's Midland Regional Medical Center, Aberdeen	5.8	0.0%	1.31	No	0.00	8	1.03	0.000	4.00

GERIATRICS

Natl. Rank Hospital	U.S. News index	Reputa- tional score	Hospital- wide mortality rate	COTH member	Service mix	Interns and residents to beds	Tech- nology score (of 13)	R.N.'s to beds	Discharge planning (of 2)	Geriatric services (of 9)	Board- certified internists to beds
TIER THREE											
Sioux Valley Hospital, Sioux Falls	16.4	0.0%	1.03	No	8	0.04	7	1.57	2	4	0.053
TIER FOUR											
McKennan Hospital, Sioux Falls	10.4	0.0%	1.25	No	6	0.09	8	0.99	2	6	0.054
Rapid City Regional Hospital, Rapid City	13.7	0.0%	1.06	No	7	0.00	11	0.45	2	4	0.032
St. Luke's Midland Regional Medical Center, Aberdeen	12.2	0.0%	1.12	No	7	0.00	8	1.03	2	2	0.027

GYNECOLOGY

Natl. Rank Hospital	U.S. News index	Reputa- tional score	Hospital- wide mortality rate	Interns and residents to beds	Tech- nology score (of 10)	R.N.'s to beds	Board- certified OB-GYNs to beds	Procedures to beds
TIER THREE								
Sioux Valley Hospital, Sioux Falls	16.1	0.0%	1.03	0.04	5	1.57	0.032	0.55
TIER FOUR								
McKennan Hospital, Sioux Falls	8.9	0.0%	1.25	0.09	5	0.99	0.027	0.54
Rapid City Regional Hospital, Rapid City	12.1	0.0%	1.06	0.00	8	0.45	0.016	0.41
St. Luke's Midland Regional Medical Center, Aberdeen	11.7	0.0%	1.12	0.00	6	1.03	0.013	0.51

NEUROLOGY

Natl. Rank Hospital	U.S. News index	Reputa- tional score	Neurology mortality rate	COTH member	Interns and residents to beds	Tech- nology score (of 9)	R.N.'s to beds	Board- certified neurologists to beds
TIER THREE								
Sioux Valley Hospital, Sioux Falls	13.0	0.0%	0.87	No	0.04	4	1.57	0.008
TIER FOUR								
McKennan Hospital, Sioux Falls	7.0	0.0%	1.17	No	0.09	4	0.99	0.010
Rapid City Regional Hospital, Rapid City	9.5	0.0%	0.97	No	0.00	7	0.45	0.016

ORTHOPEDICS

Natl. Rank Hospital	U.S. News index	Reputa- tional score	Orthopedics mortality rate	COTH member	Interns and residents to beds	Tech- nology score (of 5)	R.N.'s to beds	Board- certified orthopedists to beds	Pro- cedures to beds
TIER THREE									
Sioux Valley Hospital, Sioux Falls	11.3	0.0%	0.73	No	0.04	3	1.57	0.032	4.29
TIER FOUR									
McKennan Hospital, Sioux Falls	5.6	0.0%	1.26	No	0.09	3	0.99	0.034	4.17
Rapid City Regional Hospital, Rapid City	6.2	0.0%	0.94	No	0.00	4	0.45	0.011	3.35
St. Luke's Midland Regional Medical Center, Aberdeen	7.9	0.0%	0.86	No	0.00	3	1.03	0.004	3.94

OTOLARYNGOLOGY

Natl. Rank	Hospital	U.S. News index	Reputa-tional score	Hospital-wide mortality rate	COTH member	Interns and residents to beds	Tech-nology score (of 9)	R.N.'s to beds	Board-certified internists to beds	Procedures to beds
	TIER FOUR									
	McKennan Hospital, Sioux Falls	**4.6**	0.0%	1.25	No	0.09	3	0.99	0.054	0.199
	Rapid City Regional Hospital, Rapid City	**3.6**	0.0%	1.06	No	0.00	7	0.45	0.032	0.183
	Sioux Valley Hospital, Sioux Falls	**6.3**	0.0%	1.03	No	0.04	3	1.57	0.053	0.250
	St. Luke's Midland Regional Medical Center, Aberdeen	**5.1**	0.0%	1.12	No	0.00	6	1.03	0.027	0.204

RHEUMATOLOGY

Natl. Rank	Hospital	U.S. News index	Reputa-tional score	Hospital-wide mortality rate	COTH member	Interns and residents to beds	Tech-nology score (of 5)	R.N.'s to beds	Board-certified internists to beds
	TIER THREE								
	Sioux Valley Hospital, Sioux Falls	**10.1**	0.0%	1.03	No	0.04	3	1.57	0.053
	TIER FOUR								
	McKennan Hospital, Sioux Falls	**7.2**	0.0%	1.25	No	0.09	3	0.99	0.054
	Rapid City Regional Hospital, Rapid City	**7.1**	0.0%	1.06	No	0.00	4	0.45	0.032
	St. Luke's Midland Regional Medical Center, Aberdeen	**7.7**	0.0%	1.12	No	0.00	3	1.03	0.027

UROLOGY

Natl. Rank	Hospital	U.S. News index	Reputa-tional score	Urology mortality rate	COTH member	Interns and residents to beds	Tech-nology score (of 11)	R.N.'s to beds	Board-certified internists to beds	Procedures to beds
	TIER THREE									
	Rapid City Regional Hospital, Rapid City	**9.7**	0.0%	0.77	No	0.00	9	0.45	0.032	1.97
	Sioux Valley Hospital, Sioux Falls	**10.8**	0.0%	0.82	No	0.04	4	1.57	0.053	1.86
	St. Luke's Midland Regional Medical Center, Aberdeen	**11.4**	0.0%	0.78	No	0.00	8	1.03	0.027	3.92
	TIER FOUR									
	McKennan Hospital, Sioux Falls	**3.4**	0.0%	1.73	No	0.09	4	0.99	0.054	1.06

AIDS

Natl. Rank	Hospital	U.S. News index	Reputa-tional score	Hospital-wide mortality rate	COTH member	Interns and residents to beds	Tech-nology score (of 11)	Discharge planning (of 2)	R.N.'s to beds	Board-certified internists to beds
	TIER TWO									
39	**Vanderbilt University Hospital and Clinic, Nashville**	28.5	1.5%	1.01	Yes	1.21	10	2	1.29	0.171
	TIER THREE									
	Baptist Hospital, Nashville	19.9	0.0%	1.05	No	0.04	6	2	1.17	0.077
	Erlanger Medical Center, Chattanooga	22.7	0.0%	0.98	No	0.33	8	2	1.40	0.077
	Fort Sanders-Parkwest Medical Center, Knoxville	20.5	0.0%	0.99	No	0.00	6	2	1.03	0.049
	Nashville Memorial Hospital, Madison	19.8	0.0%	1.00	No	0.00	6	2	0.73	0.032
	St. Thomas Hospital, Nashville	21.6	0.0%	0.92	No	0.07	5	2	1.01	0.077
	TIER FOUR									
	Baptist Hospital of East Tennessee, Knoxville	13.6	0.0%	1.62	No	0.00	5	2	0.93	0.067
	Baptist Memorial Hospital, Memphis	18.7	0.0%	1.29	Yes	0.10	7	2	0.80	0.103
	Blount Memorial Hospital, Maryville	18.5	0.0%	1.06	No	0.00	7	1	0.69	0.039
	Bristol Regional Medical Center, Bristol	16.4	0.0%	1.26	No	0.07	7	1	0.87	0.042
	Clarksville Memorial Hospital, Clarksville	19.2	0.0%	1.00	No	0.00	6	1	0.82	0.032
	Fort Sanders Regional Medical Center, Knoxville	16.2	0.0%	1.28	No	0.00	6	2	0.74	0.033
	HCA Indian Path Medical Center, Kingsport	17.7	0.0%	1.13	No	0.00	6	2	0.56	0.048
	HCA Southern Hills Medical Center, Nashville	18.7	0.0%	1.06	No	0.00	6	1	1.10	0.048
	Holston Valley Hospital and Medical Center, Kingsport	18.0	0.0%	1.20	No	0.08	8	2	0.76	0.055
	Hubbard Hospital Meharry Medical College, Nashville	15.1	0.0%	1.59	Yes	0.21	6	2	0.17	0.098
	Jackson-Madison County General Hospital, Jackson	14.6	0.0%	1.48	No	0.04	6	2	0.80	0.018
	Johnson City Medical Center Hospital, Johnson City	18.2	0.0%	1.24	No	0.11	8	2	1.17	0.029
	Maury Regional Hospital, Columbia	18.5	0.0%	1.07	No	0.00	6	2	0.63	0.025
	Memorial Hospital, Chattanooga	19.2	0.0%	1.05	No	0.00	5	2	0.98	0.107
	Methodist Hospitals of Memphis	16.3	0.0%	1.33	No	0.13	7	2	0.75	0.023
	Methodist Medical Center of Oak Ridge, Oak Ridge	15.2	0.0%	1.39	No	0.00	6	2	0.85	0.007
	Metro Nashville General Hospital	15.2	0.0%	1.66	No	0.44	5	2	1.44	0.095
	Regional Medical Center at Memphis	16.2	0.6%	1.86	Yes	0.32	6	2	1.18	0.092
	St. Francis Hospital, Memphis	14.7	0.0%	1.45	No	0.02	8	2	0.30	0.011
	St. Joseph Hospital and Health Centers, Memphis	15.2	0.0%	1.26	No	0.00	7	1	0.23	0.013
	St. Mary's Medical Center, Knoxville	17.1	0.0%	1.26	No	0.00	7	2	1.00	0.017
	University of Tennessee Medical Center, Memphis	16.8	0.0%	1.23	No	0.23	4	2	0.72	0.127
	University of Tennessee Memorial Hospital, Knoxville	19.4	0.0%	1.24	No	0.39	9	2	1.22	0.058

CANCER

Natl. Rank	Hospital	U.S. News index	Reputa-tional score	Cancer mortality rate	COTH member	Interns and residents to beds	Tech-nology score (of 12)	R.N.'s to beds	Board-certified oncologists to beds	Procedures to beds
	TIER TWO									
24	**Vanderbilt University Hospital and Clinic, Nashville**	15.6	1.9%	0.64	Yes	1.21	12	1.29	0.011	1.82
	TIER THREE									
	Baptist Memorial Hospital, Memphis	6.6	0.0%	1.03	Yes	0.10	9	0.80	0.000	1.59
	Erlanger Medical Center, Chattanooga	6.9	0.0%	0.95	No	0.33	10	1.40	0.007	1.36
	Johnson City Medical Center Hospital, Johnson City	5.5	0.0%	1.24	No	0.11	10	1.17	0.017	1.78
	University of Tennessee Memorial Hospital, Knoxville	7.1	0.0%	0.95	No	0.39	11	1.22	0.012	2.15
	TIER FOUR									
	Baptist Hospital of East Tennessee, Knoxville	3.3	0.0%	1.45	No	0.00	6	0.93	0.014	2.52
	Baptist Hospital, Nashville	5.0	0.0%	0.84	No	0.04	8	1.17	0.011	1.43
	Blount Memorial Hospital, Maryville	2.8	0.0%	1.10	No	0.00	6	0.69	0.020	1.82
	Bristol Regional Medical Center, Bristol	4.3	0.0%	1.26	No	0.07	9	0.87	0.006	2.42
	Clarksville Memorial Hospital, Clarksville	3.8	0.0%	1.07	No	0.00	8	0.82	0.011	2.31
	Fort Sanders Regional Medical Center, Knoxville	4.3	0.6%	1.23	No	0.00	8	0.74	0.023	2.12

Natl. Rank	Hospital	U.S. News index	Reputational score	Cancer mortality rate	COTH member	Interns and residents to beds	Technology score (of 12)	R.N.'s to beds	Board-certified oncologists to beds	Procedures to beds
	Fort Sanders-Parkwest Medical Center, Knoxville	3.3	0.0%	1.01	No	0.00	4	1.03	0.022	1.93
	HCA Indian Path Medical Center, Kingsport	2.0	0.0%	1.20	No	0.00	5	0.56	0.014	1.44
	HCA Southern Hills Medical Center, Nashville	4.0	0.0%	1.11	No	0.00	7	1.10	0.007	1.14
	Holston Valley Hospital and Medical Center, Kingsport	4.2	0.0%	1.32	No	0.08	10	0.76	0.010	2.09
	Jackson-Madison County General Hospital, Jackson	3.4	0.0%	1.12	No	0.04	7	0.80	0.005	2.10
	Maury Regional Hospital, Columbia	2.6	0.0%	1.49	No	0.00	7	0.63	0.007	1.80
	Memorial Hospital, Chattanooga	4.0	0.0%	0.83	No	0.00	6	0.98	0.009	2.68
	Methodist Hospitals of Memphis	4.4	0.0%	1.04	No	0.13	10	0.75	0.005	1.67
	Methodist Medical Center of Oak Ridge, Oak Ridge	2.7	0.0%	1.51	No	0.00	5	0.85	0.017	1.78
	Nashville Memorial Hospital, Madison	3.6	0.0%	0.91	No	0.00	8	0.73	0.010	1.77
	St. Francis Hospital, Memphis	2.2	0.0%	1.51	No	0.02	9	0.30	0.004	1.27
	St. Joseph Hospital and Health Centers, Memphis	1.7	0.0%	1.48	No	0.00	8	0.23	0.003	1.53
	St. Mary's Medical Center, Knoxville	5.0	0.6%	1.45	No	0.00	9	1.00	0.012	1.82
	St. Thomas Hospital, Nashville	4.7	0.5%	0.87	No	0.07	5	1.01	0.018	2.52
	University of Tennessee Medical Center, Memphis	3.3	0.0%	0.97	No	0.23	3	0.72	0.068	2.09

CARDIOLOGY

Natl. Rank	Hospital	U.S. News index	Reputational score	Cardiology mortality rate	COTH member	Interns and residents to beds	Technology score (of 10)	R.N.'s to beds	Board-certified cardiologists to beds	Procedures to beds
	TIER TWO									
58	Vanderbilt University Hospital and Clinic, Nashville	22.7	0.3%	1.02	Yes	1.21	9	1.29	0.030	3.40
	TIER THREE									
	Baptist Hospital, Nashville	14.8	0.3%	1.02	No	0.04	8	1.17	0.013	6.00
	Clarksville Memorial Hospital, Clarksville	15.4	0.0%	0.89	No	0.00	4	0.82	0.005	6.98
	Erlanger Medical Center, Chattanooga	17.4	0.0%	0.99	No	0.33	9	1.40	0.028	5.53
	St. Thomas Hospital, Nashville	20.1	1.9%	0.92	No	0.07	7	1.01	0.049	16.30
	TIER FOUR									
	Baptist Hospital of East Tennessee, Knoxville	5.7	0.0%	1.57	No	0.00	7	0.93	0.032	12.97
	Baptist Memorial Hospital, Memphis	12.3	1.8%	1.43	Yes	0.10	9	0.80	0.000	5.86
	Blount Memorial Hospital, Maryville	13.0	0.0%	1.02	No	0.00	7	0.69	0.020	10.35
	Bristol Regional Medical Center, Bristol	10.7	0.0%	1.20	No	0.07	9	0.87	0.009	9.57
	Fort Sanders Regional Medical Center, Knoxville	8.6	0.0%	1.28	No	0.00	8	0.74	0.036	5.94
	Fort Sanders-Parkwest Medical Center, Knoxville	11.3	0.0%	1.16	No	0.00	8	1.03	0.022	7.57
	HCA Indian Path Medical Center, Kingsport	8.2	0.0%	1.23	No	0.00	6	0.56	0.024	7.09
	HCA Southern Hills Medical Center, Nashville	13.4	0.0%	1.05	No	0.00	6	1.10	0.048	6.83
	Holston Valley Hospital and Medical Center, Kingsport	11.3	0.0%	1.17	No	0.08	9	0.76	0.023	10.62
	Jackson-Madison County General Hospital, Jackson	4.6	0.0%	1.63	No	0.04	8	0.80	0.014	6.84
	Johnson City Medical Center Hospital, Johnson City	8.8	0.0%	1.37	No	0.11	8	1.17	0.015	7.59
	Maury Regional Hospital, Columbia	11.2	0.0%	1.06	No	0.00	6	0.63	0.007	6.27
	Memorial Hospital, Chattanooga	10.3	0.0%	1.22	No	0.00	6	0.98	0.047	11.65
	Methodist Hospitals of Memphis	7.3	0.4%	1.48	No	0.13	9	0.75	0.014	8.01
	Methodist Medical Center of Oak Ridge, Oak Ridge	6.7	0.0%	1.47	No	0.00	9	0.85	0.017	7.91
	Nashville Memorial Hospital, Madison	13.5	0.0%	1.01	No	0.00	8	0.73	0.019	6.54
	St. Francis Hospital, Memphis	2.9	0.0%	1.63	No	0.02	8	0.30	0.010	4.68
	St. Joseph Hospital and Health Centers, Memphis	7.4	0.0%	1.24	No	0.00	8	0.23	0.008	5.80
	St. Mary's Medical Center, Knoxville	8.9	0.0%	1.33	No	0.00	9	1.00	0.015	8.35
	University of Tennessee Memorial Hospital, Knoxville	10.6	0.0%	1.38	No	0.39	9	1.22	0.045	6.58

ENDOCRINOLOGY

Natl. Rank	Hospital	U.S. News index	Reputa-tional score	Endocrinology mortality rate	COTH member	Interns and residents to beds	Tech-nology score (of 11)	R.N.'s to beds	Board-certified internists to beds
TIER ONE
14	Vanderbilt University Hospital and Clinic, Nashville	26.8	7.9%	0.93	Yes	1.21	11	1.29	0.171
TIER THREE
	Blount Memorial Hospital, Maryville	9.6	0.0%	0.64	No	0.00	7	0.69	0.039
	Clarksville Memorial Hospital, Clarksville	9.1	0.0%	0.73	No	0.00	8	0.82	0.032
	Erlanger Medical Center, Chattanooga	11.7	0.0%	0.79	No	0.33	10	1.40	0.077
	Fort Sanders-Parkwest Medical Center, Knoxville	9.6	0.0%	0.69	No	0.00	5	1.03	0.049
	St. Thomas Hospital, Nashville	8.4	0.0%	0.86	No	0.07	6	1.01	0.077
	University of Tennessee Medical Center, Memphis	10.4	0.0%	0.66	No	0.23	4	0.72	0.127
	University of Tennessee Memorial Hospital, Knoxville	8.6	0.0%	1.16	No	0.39	10	1.22	0.058
TIER FOUR
	Baptist Hospital of East Tennessee, Knoxville	4.9	0.0%	1.41	No	0.00	7	0.93	0.067
	Baptist Hospital, Nashville	6.3	0.0%	1.31	No	0.04	8	1.17	0.077
	Baptist Memorial Hospital, Memphis	7.6	0.0%	1.54	Yes	0.10	9	0.80	0.103
	Bristol Regional Medical Center, Bristol	6.4	0.0%	1.14	No	0.07	9	0.87	0.042
	Fort Sanders Regional Medical Center, Knoxville	3.9	0.0%	1.57	No	0.00	8	0.74	0.033
	HCA Indian Path Medical Center, Kingsport	3.4	0.0%	1.47	No	0.00	6	0.56	0.048
	Holston Valley Hospital and Medical Center, Kingsport	5.7	0.0%	1.29	No	0.08	10	0.76	0.055
	Hubbard Hospital Meharry Medical College, Nashville	6.0	0.0%	1.37	Yes	0.21	5	0.17	0.098
	Jackson-Madison County General Hospital, Jackson	4.6	0.0%	1.40	No	0.04	8	0.80	0.018
	Johnson City Medical Center Hospital, Johnson City	6.1	0.0%	1.47	No	0.11	10	1.17	0.029
	Maury Regional Hospital, Columbia	7.2	0.0%	0.84	No	0.00	8	0.63	0.025
	Memorial Hospital, Chattanooga	5.5	0.0%	1.37	No	0.00	7	0.98	0.107
	Methodist Hospitals of Memphis	4.6	0.0%	1.58	No	0.13	10	0.75	0.023
	Methodist Medical Center of Oak Ridge, Oak Ridge	6.4	0.0%	0.94	No	0.00	6	0.85	0.007
	Nashville Memorial Hospital, Madison	6.5	0.0%	1.01	No	0.00	9	0.73	0.032
	Regional Medical Center at Memphis	7.1	0.0%	2.86	Yes	0.32	8	1.18	0.092
	St. Francis Hospital, Memphis	4.4	0.0%	1.15	No	0.02	9	0.30	0.011
	St. Joseph Hospital and Health Centers, Memphis	3.0	0.0%	1.43	No	0.00	9	0.23	0.013
	St. Mary's Medical Center, Knoxville	6.7	0.0%	1.11	No	0.00	10	1.00	0.017

GASTROENTEROLOGY

Natl. Rank	Hospital	U.S. News index	Reputa-tional score	Gastro-enterology mortality rate	COTH member	Interns and residents to beds	Tech-nology score (of 11)	R.N.'s to beds	Board-certified gastro-enterologists to beds	Pro-cedures to beds
TIER TWO
33	Vanderbilt University Hospital and Clinic, Nashville	16.7	0.5%	0.77	Yes	1.21	10	1.29	0.019	1.54
TIER THREE
	Baptist Hospital, Nashville	8.2	0.0%	0.92	No	0.04	8	1.17	0.020	3.16
	Baptist Memorial Hospital, Memphis	8.6	0.5%	1.20	Yes	0.10	8	0.80	0.000	2.43
	Erlanger Medical Center, Chattanooga	9.5	0.0%	0.93	No	0.33	9	1.40	0.017	2.39
	Johnson City Medical Center Hospital, Johnson City	7.9	0.0%	1.04	No	0.11	9	1.17	0.010	3.21
	Memorial Hospital, Chattanooga	8.7	0.0%	0.87	No	0.00	6	0.98	0.038	5.17
	St. Thomas Hospital, Nashville	8.4	0.0%	0.80	No	0.07	5	1.01	0.018	3.72
TIER FOUR
	Baptist Hospital of East Tennessee, Knoxville	3.2	0.0%	1.74	No	0.00	6	0.93	0.017	3.15
	Blount Memorial Hospital, Maryville	6.7	0.0%	1.04	No	0.00	7	0.69	0.015	4.76
	Bristol Regional Medical Center, Bristol	5.6	0.0%	1.30	No	0.07	8	0.87	0.006	3.68
	Clarksville Memorial Hospital, Clarksville	5.4	0.0%	1.25	No	0.00	7	0.82	0.005	4.11
	Fort Sanders Regional Medical Center, Knoxville	6.4	0.0%	1.01	No	0.00	8	0.74	0.018	3.25
	Fort Sanders-Parkwest Medical Center, Knoxville	6.8	0.0%	1.05	No	0.00	6	1.03	0.019	4.31
	HCA Indian Path Medical Center, Kingsport	4.3	0.0%	1.47	No	0.00	7	0.56	0.038	4.52
	Holston Valley Hospital and Medical Center, Kingsport	5.5	0.0%	1.32	No	0.08	9	0.76	0.018	3.51

Natl. Rank	Hospital	U.S. News index	Reputa-tional score	Gastro-enterology mortality rate	COTH member	Interns and residents to beds	Tech-nology score (of 11)	R.N.'s to beds	Board-certified gastro-enterologists to beds	Pro-cedures to beds
	Jackson-Madison County General Hospital, Jackson	3.5	0.0%	1.66	No	0.04	8	0.80	0.008	2.66
	Maury Regional Hospital, Columbia	5.5	0.0%	1.07	No	0.00	7	0.63	0.011	3.42
	Methodist Hospitals of Memphis	5.3	0.0%	1.33	No	0.13	9	0.75	0.008	2.96
	Methodist Medical Center of Oak Ridge, Oak Ridge	4.2	0.0%	1.42	No	0.00	6	0.85	0.014	3.70
	Nashville Memorial Hospital, Madison	5.2	0.0%	1.18	No	0.00	8	0.73	0.006	3.03
	St. Francis Hospital, Memphis	2.2	0.0%	1.61	No	0.02	8	0.30	0.004	2.25
	St. Joseph Hospital and Health Centers, Memphis	3.1	0.0%	1.39	No	0.00	9	0.23	0.000	2.57
	St. Mary's Medical Center, Knoxville	7.3	0.0%	1.09	No	0.00	10	1.00	0.012	3.68
	University of Tennessee Memorial Hospital, Knoxville	6.6	0.0%	1.57	No	0.39	10	1.22	0.016	2.56

GERIATRICS

Natl. Rank	Hospital	U.S. News index	Reputa-tional score	Hospital-wide mortality rate	COTH member	Service mix	Interns and residents to beds	Tech-nology score (of 13)	R.N.'s to beds	Discharge planning (of 2)	Geriatric services (of 9)	Board-certified internists to beds
TIER TWO												
47	Vanderbilt University Hospital and Clinic, Nashville	24.4	0.3%	1.01	Yes	8	1.21	12	1.29	2	7	0.171
TIER THREE												
	Baptist Hospital, Nashville	14.4	0.0%	1.05	No	5	0.04	11	1.17	2	3	0.077
	Erlanger Medical Center, Chattanooga	16.6	0.0%	0.98	No	4	0.33	11	1.40	2	1	0.077
	Fort Sanders-Parkwest Medical Center, Knoxville	14.6	0.0%	0.99	No	4	0.00	6	1.03	2	4	0.049
	Nashville Memorial Hospital, Madison	13.9	0.0%	1.00	No	4	0.00	10	0.73	2	2	0.032
	St. Thomas Hospital, Nashville	17.0	0.0%	0.92	No	5	0.07	7	1.01	2	1	0.077
TIER FOUR												
	Baptist Hospital of East Tennessee, Knoxville	4.5	0.4%	1.62	No	5	0.00	9	0.93	2	1	0.067
	Baptist Memorial Hospital, Memphis	12.1	0.6%	1.29	Yes	4	0.10	12	0.80	2	2	0.103
	Blount Memorial Hospital, Maryville	12.0	0.0%	1.06	No	7	0.00	9	0.69	1	1	0.039
	Clarksville Memorial Hospital, Clarksville	13.5	0.0%	1.00	No	6	0.00	10	0.82	1	1	0.032
	Fort Sanders Regional Medical Center, Knoxville	8.4	0.0%	1.28	No	6	0.00	11	0.74	2	1	0.033
	HCA Indian Path Medical Center, Kingsport	9.8	0.0%	1.13	No	4	0.00	7	0.56	2	2	0.048
	Holston Valley Hospital and Medical Center, Kingsport	10.3	0.0%	1.20	No	5	0.08	11	0.76	2	3	0.055
	Jackson-Madison County General Hospital, Jackson	5.4	0.0%	1.48	No	5	0.04	10	0.80	2	3	0.018
	Johnson City Medical Center Hospital, Johnson City	10.1	0.0%	1.24	No	5	0.11	10	1.17	2	3	0.029
	Maury Regional Hospital, Columbia	12.3	0.0%	1.07	No	5	0.00	10	0.63	2	2	0.025
	Memorial Hospital, Chattanooga	13.1	0.0%	1.05	No	4	0.00	8	0.98	2	3	0.107
	Methodist Hospitals of Memphis	9.6	0.6%	1.33	No	4	0.13	12	0.75	2	5	0.023
	Methodist Medical Center of Oak Ridge, Oak Ridge	5.9	0.0%	1.39	No	5	0.00	8	0.85	2	2	0.007
	St. Francis Hospital, Memphis	6.0	0.0%	1.45	No	8	0.02	11	0.30	2	2	0.011
	St. Joseph Hospital and Health Centers, Memphis	6.0	0.0%	1.26	No	5	0.00	10	0.23	1	1	0.013
	St. Mary's Medical Center, Knoxville	10.0	0.0%	1.26	No	6	0.00	11	1.00	2	4	0.017
	University of Tennessee Memorial Hospital, Knoxville	12.0	0.0%	1.24	No	7	0.39	13	1.22	2	1	0.058

GYNECOLOGY

Natl. Rank	Hospital	U.S. News index	Reputa-tional score	Hospital-wide mortality rate	Interns and residents to beds	Tech-nology score (of 10)	R.N.'s to beds	Board-certified OB-GYNs to beds	Procedures to beds
TIER TWO									
32	Vanderbilt University Hospital and Clinic, Nashville	30.2	2.4%	1.01	1.21	10	1.29	0.024	0.39
TIER THREE									
	Baptist Hospital, Nashville	16.0	0.0%	1.05	0.04	7	1.17	0.069	0.85
	Clarksville Memorial Hospital, Clarksville	14.4	0.0%	1.00	0.00	6	0.82	0.037	0.46
97	Erlanger Medical Center, Chattanooga	21.3	0.0%	0.98	0.33	9	1.40	0.052	0.34
	Fort Sanders-Parkwest Medical Center, Knoxville	14.4	0.0%	0.99	0.00	5	1.03	0.015	0.70
	Memorial Hospital, Chattanooga	14.4	0.0%	1.05	0.00	5	0.98	0.107	1.02

Natl. Rank	Hospital	U.S. News index	Reputa-tional score	Hospital-wide mortality rate	Interns and residents to beds	Tech-nology score (of 10)	R.N.'s to beds	Board-certified OB-GYNs to beds	Procedures to beds
	Nashville Memorial Hospital, Madison	14.1	0.0%	1.00	0.00	7	0.73	0.013	0.26
	St. Thomas Hospital, Nashville	18.0	0.4%	0.92	0.07	5	1.01	0.023	0.33
	University of Tennessee Memorial Hospital, Knoxville	18.0	1.4%	1.24	0.39	9	1.22	0.031	0.51
TIER FOUR									
	Baptist Hospital of East Tennessee, Knoxville	3.6	0.0%	1.62	0.00	5	0.93	0.043	0.84
	Baptist Memorial Hospital, Memphis	12.6	1.4%	1.29	0.10	7	0.80	0.036	0.45
	Blount Memorial Hospital, Maryville	12.8	0.0%	1.06	0.00	7	0.69	0.030	0.40
	Bristol Regional Medical Center, Bristol	9.1	0.0%	1.26	0.07	7	0.87	0.009	0.40
	Fort Sanders Regional Medical Center, Knoxville	8.3	0.0%	1.28	0.00	6	0.74	0.053	0.50
	HCA Indian Path Medical Center, Kingsport	10.1	0.0%	1.13	0.00	5	0.56	0.067	0.51
	Holston Valley Hospital and Medical Center, Kingsport	12.1	0.0%	1.20	0.08	9	0.76	0.048	0.32
	Jackson-Madison County General Hospital, Jackson	5.6	0.0%	1.48	0.04	7	0.80	0.017	0.51
	Johnson City Medical Center Hospital, Johnson City	12.9	0.0%	1.24	0.11	9	1.17	0.027	0.42
	Maury Regional Hospital, Columbia	11.5	0.0%	1.07	0.00	6	0.63	0.025	0.26
	Methodist Hospitals of Memphis	8.6	0.0%	1.33	0.13	8	0.75	0.017	0.34
	Methodist Medical Center of Oak Ridge, Oak Ridge	5.4	0.0%	1.39	0.00	5	0.85	0.017	0.42
	St. Francis Hospital, Memphis	3.5	0.0%	1.45	0.02	7	0.30	0.005	0.33
	St. Mary's Medical Center, Knoxville	10.8	0.0%	1.26	0.00	8	1.00	0.034	0.57

NEUROLOGY

Natl. Rank	Hospital	U.S. News index	Reputa-tional score	Neurology mortality rate	COTH member	Interns and residents to beds	Tech-nology score (of 9)	R.N.'s to beds	Board-certified neurologists to beds
TIER TWO									
84	Vanderbilt University Hospital and Clinic, Nashville	17.9	0.6%	1.09	Yes	1.21	9	1.29	0.021
TIER THREE									
	Baptist Memorial Hospital, Memphis	11.0	0.3%	1.09	Yes	0.10	7	0.80	0.007
	Erlanger Medical Center, Chattanooga	13.3	0.0%	0.97	No	0.33	8	1.40	0.015
	Fort Sanders-Parkwest Medical Center, Knoxville	11.4	0.0%	0.91	No	0.00	5	1.03	0.015
	Memorial Hospital, Chattanooga	12.6	0.0%	0.85	No	0.00	5	0.98	0.016
	St. Thomas Hospital, Nashville	11.0	0.0%	0.93	No	0.07	5	1.01	0.012
TIER FOUR									
	Baptist Hospital of East Tennessee, Knoxville	6.4	0.0%	1.23	No	0.00	5	0.93	0.012
	Baptist Hospital, Nashville	8.3	0.0%	1.15	No	0.04	6	1.17	0.011
	Blount Memorial Hospital, Maryville	6.3	0.0%	1.19	No	0.00	7	0.69	0.005
	Bristol Regional Medical Center, Bristol	6.2	0.0%	1.31	No	0.07	7	0.87	0.012
	Clarksville Memorial Hospital, Clarksville	9.6	0.0%	0.96	No	0.00	6	0.82	0.005
	Fort Sanders Regional Medical Center, Knoxville	6.1	0.0%	1.21	No	0.00	6	0.74	0.008
	HCA Indian Path Medical Center, Kingsport	8.4	0.0%	1.01	No	0.00	5	0.56	0.014
	HCA Southern Hills Medical Center, Nashville	6.3	0.0%	1.33	No	0.00	6	1.10	0.014
	Holston Valley Hospital and Medical Center, Kingsport	8.5	0.0%	1.12	No	0.08	8	0.76	0.013
	Jackson-Madison County General Hospital, Jackson	4.6	0.0%	1.37	No	0.04	6	0.80	0.005
	Johnson City Medical Center Hospital, Johnson City	9.0	0.0%	1.15	No	0.11	8	1.17	0.010
	Methodist Hospitals of Memphis	7.6	0.0%	1.15	No	0.13	8	0.75	0.004
	Methodist Medical Center of Oak Ridge, Oak Ridge	6.4	0.0%	1.22	No	0.00	6	0.85	0.010
	Nashville Memorial Hospital, Madison	10.6	0.2%	0.93	No	0.00	7	0.73	0.006
	Regional Medical Center at Memphis	7.4	0.0%	1.72	Yes	0.32	6	1.18	0.019
	St. Francis Hospital, Memphis	4.1	0.0%	1.32	No	0.02	7	0.30	0.005
	St. Joseph Hospital and Health Centers, Memphis	4.3	0.0%	1.26	No	0.00	7	0.23	0.003
	St. Mary's Medical Center, Knoxville	10.2	0.0%	1.02	No	0.00	8	1.00	0.012
	University of Tennessee Memorial Hospital, Knoxville	9.5	0.0%	1.17	No	0.39	8	1.22	0.007

ORTHOPEDICS

Natl. Rank	Hospital	U.S. News index	Reputational score	Orthopedics mortality rate	COTH member	Interns and residents to beds	Technology score (of 5)	R.N.'s to beds	Board-certified orthopedists to beds	Procedures to beds
TIER ONE											
18	Vanderbilt University Hospital and Clinic, Nashville	21.6	2.3%	0.80	Yes	1.21	5	1.29	0.018	1.62
TIER THREE											
	Baptist Memorial Hospital, Memphis	10.5	0.9%	1.11	Yes	0.10	4	0.80	0.020	1.94
	Clarksville Memorial Hospital, Clarksville	9.0	0.0%	0.71	No	0.00	3	0.82	0.016	2.92
	Erlanger Medical Center, Chattanooga	10.7	0.0%	0.83	No	0.33	4	1.40	0.040	2.00
	Fort Sanders-Parkwest Medical Center, Knoxville	8.8	0.0%	0.83	No	0.00	4	1.03	0.060	2.41
	HCA Southern Hills Medical Center, Nashville	9.5	0.0%	0.80	No	0.00	4	1.10	0.041	3.55
	Johnson City Medical Center Hospital, Johnson City	8.8	0.0%	0.88	No	0.11	4	1.17	0.027	2.17
	Memorial Hospital, Chattanooga	9.8	0.0%	0.67	No	0.00	2	0.98	0.085	3.03
	Nashville Memorial Hospital, Madison	9.1	0.0%	0.69	No	0.00	3	0.73	0.022	3.25
TIER FOUR											
	Baptist Hospital of East Tennessee, Knoxville	1.9	0.0%	1.97	No	0.00	2	0.93	0.032	2.16
	Baptist Hospital, Nashville	7.8	0.0%	0.92	No	0.04	3	1.17	0.036	3.15
	Blount Memorial Hospital, Maryville	5.9	0.0%	1.05	No	0.00	4	0.69	0.020	2.66
	Bristol Regional Medical Center, Bristol	6.3	0.0%	1.09	No	0.07	4	0.87	0.021	2.34
	Fort Sanders Regional Medical Center, Knoxville	5.0	0.0%	1.16	No	0.00	3	0.74	0.043	3.48
	HCA Indian Path Medical Center, Kingsport	4.5	0.0%	1.22	No	0.00	4	0.56	0.034	2.08
	Holston Valley Hospital and Medical Center, Kingsport	6.3	0.0%	1.05	No	0.08	4	0.76	0.025	2.21
	Jackson-Madison County General Hospital, Jackson	3.9	0.0%	1.31	No	0.04	3	0.80	0.009	1.65
	Maury Regional Hospital, Columbia	8.1	0.0%	0.74	No	0.00	3	0.63	0.018	2.87
	Methodist Hospitals of Memphis	5.2	0.0%	1.23	No	0.13	4	0.75	0.013	1.86
	Methodist Medical Center of Oak Ridge, Oak Ridge	2.8	0.0%	2.12	No	0.00	4	0.85	0.021	2.99
	St. Francis Hospital, Memphis	2.6	0.0%	1.46	No	0.02	4	0.30	0.008	1.54
	St. Joseph Hospital and Health Centers, Memphis	2.7	0.0%	1.35	No	0.00	4	0.23	0.010	1.10
	St. Mary's Medical Center, Knoxville	6.0	0.0%	1.22	No	0.00	4	1.00	0.029	3.88
	St. Thomas Hospital, Nashville	7.4	0.0%	0.91	No	0.07	3	1.01	0.021	2.71
	University of Tennessee Memorial Hospital, Knoxville	7.8	0.0%	1.25	No	0.39	5	1.22	0.010	1.42

OTOLARYNGOLOGY

Natl. Rank	Hospital	U.S. News index	Reputational score	Hospital-wide mortality rate	COTH member	Interns and residents to beds	Technology score (of 9)	R.N.'s to beds	Board-certified internists to beds	Procedures to beds
TIER ONE											
14	Vanderbilt University Hospital and Clinic, Nashville	36.7	6.5%	1.02	Yes	1.21	9	1.29	0.171	0.463
TIER THREE											
	Baptist Hospital, Nashville	10.3	1.3%	1.05	No	0.04	6	1.17	0.077	0.322
	Baptist Memorial Hospital, Memphis	8.7	0.0%	1.29	Yes	0.10	7	0.80	0.103	0.158
	Erlanger Medical Center, Chattanooga	8.6	0.0%	0.98	No	0.33	8	1.40	0.077	0.217
	Metro Nashville General Hospital	7.2	0.0%	1.65	No	0.44	2	1.44	0.095	0.171
	Regional Medical Center at Memphis	10.2	0.0%	1.86	Yes	0.32	6	1.18	0.092	0.092
	University of Tennessee Memorial Hospital, Knoxville	7.9	0.0%	1.24	No	0.39	8	1.22	0.058	0.227
TIER FOUR											
	Baptist Hospital of East Tennessee, Knoxville	4.6	0.0%	1.62	No	0.00	5	0.93	0.067	0.281
	Blount Memorial Hospital, Maryville	3.9	0.0%	1.06	No	0.00	5	0.69	0.039	0.266
	Bristol Regional Medical Center, Bristol	5.2	0.0%	1.26	No	0.07	7	0.87	0.042	0.336
	Clarksville Memorial Hospital, Clarksville	4.5	0.0%	1.00	No	0.00	6	0.82	0.032	0.186
	Fort Sanders Regional Medical Center, Knoxville	4.1	0.0%	1.28	No	0.00	6	0.74	0.033	0.267
	Fort Sanders-Parkwest Medical Center, Knoxville	4.5	0.0%	0.99	No	0.00	3	1.03	0.049	0.180
	HCA Indian Path Medical Center, Kingsport	3.2	0.0%	1.13	No	0.00	4	0.56	0.048	0.192
	HCA Southern Hills Medical Center, Nashville	5.5	0.0%	1.06	No	0.00	6	1.10	0.048	0.301
	Holston Valley Hospital and Medical Center, Kingsport	5.3	0.0%	1.20	No	0.08	8	0.76	0.055	0.204
	Hubbard Hospital Meharry Medical College, Nashville	6.2	0.0%	1.59	Yes	0.21	4	0.17	0.098	0.070

Natl. Rank	Hospital	U.S. News index	Reputational score	Hospital-wide mortality rate	COTH member	Interns and residents to beds	Technology score (of 9)	R.N.'s to beds	Board-certified internists to beds	Procedures to beds
	Jackson-Madison County General Hospital, Jackson	4.2	0.0%	1.48	No	0.04	6	0.80	0.018	0.140
	Johnson City Medical Center Hospital, Johnson City	6.4	0.0%	1.24	No	0.11	8	1.17	0.029	0.236
	Maury Regional Hospital, Columbia	3.8	0.0%	1.07	No	0.00	6	0.63	0.025	0.167
	Memorial Hospital, Chattanooga	5.4	0.0%	1.05	No	0.00	5	0.98	0.107	0.372
	Methodist Hospitals of Memphis	5.1	0.0%	1.33	No	0.13	8	0.75	0.023	0.230
	Methodist Medical Center of Oak Ridge, Oak Ridge	3.6	0.0%	1.39	No	0.00	4	0.85	0.007	0.334
	Nashville Memorial Hospital, Madison	4.5	0.0%	1.00	No	0.00	7	0.73	0.032	0.239
	St. Francis Hospital, Memphis	2.9	0.0%	1.45	No	0.02	7	0.30	0.011	0.098
	St. Joseph Hospital and Health Centers, Memphis	2.7	0.0%	1.26	No	0.00	7	0.23	0.013	0.126
	St. Mary's Medical Center, Knoxville	5.4	0.0%	1.26	No	0.00	8	1.00	0.017	0.309
	St. Thomas Hospital, Nashville	5.3	0.0%	0.92	No	0.07	4	1.01	0.077	0.266
	University of Tennessee Medical Center, Memphis	6.9	0.7%	1.24	No	0.23	2	0.72	0.127	0.322

RHEUMATOLOGY

Natl. Rank	Hospital	U.S. News index	Reputational score	Hospital-wide mortality rate	COTH member	Interns and residents to beds	Technology score (of 5)	R.N.'s to beds	Board-certified internists to beds
TIER TWO									
37	Vanderbilt University Hospital and Clinic, Nashville	20.2	1.2%	1.02	Yes	1.21	5	1.29	0.171
TIER THREE									
	Baptist Hospital, Nashville	9.9	0.4%	1.05	No	0.04	3	1.17	0.077
	Baptist Memorial Hospital, Memphis	9.8	0.0%	1.29	Yes	0.10	4	0.80	0.103
	Erlanger Medical Center, Chattanooga	11.7	0.0%	0.98	No	0.33	4	1.40	0.077
	St. Thomas Hospital, Nashville	10.0	0.0%	0.92	No	0.07	3	1.01	0.077
	University of Tennessee Memorial Hospital, Knoxville	9.8	0.0%	1.24	No	0.39	5	1.22	0.058
TIER FOUR									
	Baptist Hospital of East Tennessee, Knoxville	4.7	0.0%	1.62	No	0.00	2	0.93	0.067
	Blount Memorial Hospital, Maryville	6.8	0.0%	1.06	No	0.00	4	0.69	0.039
	Bristol Regional Medical Center, Bristol	6.1	0.0%	1.26	No	0.07	4	0.87	0.042
	Clarksville Memorial Hospital, Clarksville	7.1	0.0%	1.00	No	0.00	3	0.82	0.032
	Fort Sanders Regional Medical Center, Knoxville	5.9	0.0%	1.28	No	0.00	3	0.74	0.033
	Fort Sanders-Parkwest Medical Center, Knoxville	9.4	0.0%	0.99	No	0.00	4	1.03	0.049
	HCA Indian Path Medical Center, Kingsport	7.0	0.0%	1.13	No	0.00	4	0.56	0.048
	HCA Southern Hills Medical Center, Nashville	7.9	0.0%	1.06	No	0.00	4	1.10	0.048
	Holston Valley Hospital and Medical Center, Kingsport	7.3	0.0%	1.20	No	0.08	4	0.76	0.055
	Jackson-Madison County General Hospital, Jackson	5.1	0.0%	1.48	No	0.04	3	0.80	0.018
	Johnson City Medical Center Hospital, Johnson City	8.1	0.0%	1.24	No	0.11	4	1.17	0.029
	Maury Regional Hospital, Columbia	7.0	0.0%	1.07	No	0.00	3	0.63	0.025
	Memorial Hospital, Chattanooga	8.2	0.0%	1.05	No	0.00	2	0.98	0.107
	Methodist Hospitals of Memphis	6.4	0.0%	1.33	No	0.13	4	0.75	0.023
	Methodist Medical Center of Oak Ridge, Oak Ridge	5.9	0.0%	1.39	No	0.00	4	0.85	0.007
	Nashville Memorial Hospital, Madison	7.9	0.0%	1.00	No	0.00	3	0.73	0.032
	St. Francis Hospital, Memphis	4.3	0.0%	1.45	No	0.02	4	0.30	0.011
	St. Joseph Hospital and Health Centers, Memphis	4.0	0.0%	1.26	No	0.00	4	0.23	0.013
	St. Mary's Medical Center, Knoxville	7.1	0.0%	1.26	No	0.00	4	1.00	0.017

UROLOGY

Natl. Rank	Hospital	U.S. News index	Reputa-tional score	Urology mortality rate	COTH member	Interns and residents to beds	Tech-nology score (of 11)	R.N.'s to beds	Board-certified internists to beds	Procedures to beds
	TIER TWO									
79	**Vanderbilt University Hospital and Clinic, Nashville**	**16.0**	1.7%	1.47	Yes	1.21	10	1.29	0.171	1.44
	TIER THREE									
	Baptist Memorial Hospital, Memphis	**10.0**	0.0%	1.10	Yes	0.10	8	0.80	0.103	1.04
	Clarksville Memorial Hospital, Clarksville	**9.4**	0.0%	0.84	No	0.00	7	0.82	0.032	2.69
	Erlanger Medical Center, Chattanooga	**9.9**	0.0%	1.10	No	0.33	9	1.40	0.077	1.53
	University of Tennessee Medical Center, Memphis	**12.7**	0.0%	0.66	No	0.23	3	0.72	0.127	7.62
	TIER FOUR									
	Baptist Hospital of East Tennessee, Knoxville	**1.9**	0.0%	2.64	No	0.00	6	0.93	0.067	1.66
	Baptist Hospital, Nashville	**6.6**	0.0%	1.45	No	0.04	8	1.17	0.077	3.24
	Blount Memorial Hospital, Maryville	**5.8**	0.0%	1.19	No	0.00	7	0.69	0.039	2.22
	Bristol Regional Medical Center, Bristol	**5.5**	0.0%	1.40	No	0.07	8	0.87	0.042	1.88
	Fort Sanders Regional Medical Center, Knoxville	**3.5**	0.0%	1.79	No	0.00	8	0.74	0.033	2.11
	Fort Sanders-Parkwest Medical Center, Knoxville	**6.8**	0.0%	1.14	No	0.00	6	1.03	0.049	2.18
	HCA Indian Path Medical Center, Kingsport	**6.7**	0.0%	1.02	No	0.00	7	0.56	0.048	1.92
	HCA Southern Hills Medical Center, Nashville	**6.8**	0.0%	1.19	No	0.00	7	1.10	0.048	1.83
	Holston Valley Hospital and Medical Center, Kingsport	**4.8**	0.0%	1.56	No	0.08	9	0.76	0.055	1.46
	Jackson-Madison County General Hospital, Jackson	**3.3**	0.0%	1.97	No	0.04	8	0.80	0.018	2.39
	Johnson City Medical Center Hospital, Johnson City	**5.6**	0.0%	1.66	No	0.11	9	1.17	0.029	1.90
	Maury Regional Hospital, Columbia	**3.3**	0.0%	1.70	No	0.00	7	0.63	0.025	2.53
	Memorial Hospital, Chattanooga	**7.1**	0.0%	1.17	No	0.00	6	0.98	0.107	2.98
	Methodist Hospitals of Memphis	**5.3**	0.0%	1.45	No	0.13	9	0.75	0.023	1.73
	Methodist Medical Center of Oak Ridge, Oak Ridge	**5.9**	0.0%	1.16	No	0.00	6	0.85	0.007	2.07
	Nashville Memorial Hospital, Madison	**6.3**	0.0%	1.13	No	0.00	8	0.73	0.032	1.36
	St. Francis Hospital, Memphis	**2.9**	0.0%	1.56	No	0.02	8	0.30	0.011	1.38
	St. Joseph Hospital and Health Centers, Memphis	**4.1**	0.0%	1.30	No	0.00	9	0.23	0.013	1.31
	St. Mary's Medical Center, Knoxville	**6.6**	0.0%	1.32	No	0.00	10	1.00	0.017	2.62
	St. Thomas Hospital, Nashville	**8.2**	0.0%	0.97	No	0.07	5	1.01	0.077	1.76
	University of Tennessee Memorial Hospital, Knoxville	**8.3**	0.0%	1.35	No	0.39	10	1.22	0.058	1.65

AIDS

Natl. Rank	Hospital	U.S. News index	Reputational score	Hospital-wide mortality rate	COTH member	Interns and residents to beds	Technology score (of 11)	Discharge planning (of 2)	R.N.'s to beds	Board-certified internists to beds
TIER TWO									
54	Baylor University Medical Center, Dallas	26.8	1.2%	0.89	Yes	0.29	6	2	1.38	0.093
41	University of Texas M.D. Anderson Cancer Ctr., Houston	28.2	0.4%	0.38	Yes	0.70	8	2	1.88	0.083
TIER THREE									
	Bexar County Hospital District, San Antonio	21.2	0.0%	1.25	Yes	1.12	8	2	0.83	0.028
	Citizens Medical Center, Victoria	20.3	0.0%	0.98	No	0.00	7	2	0.59	0.034
	Clear Lake Regional Medical Center, Webbster	20.0	0.0%	0.96	No	0.00	6	2	0.52	0.019
	East Texas Medical Center, Tyler	22.1	0.0%	0.89	No	0.00	6	2	0.85	0.059
	HCA Medical Center of Plano, Plano	21.0	0.0%	0.94	No	0.00	5	2	1.04	0.063
	HCA Medical Plaza Hospital, Fort Worth	20.7	0.0%	0.94	No	0.00	6	2	0.65	0.065
	HCA Spring Branch Medical Center, Houston	19.7	0.0%	1.00	No	0.00	6	2	0.80	0.006
	Harris Methodist Fort Worth	20.4	0.0%	1.03	No	0.01	6	2	1.29	0.082
	Harris Methodist-HEB, Bedford	21.4	0.0%	0.84	No	0.00	5	2	0.65	0.053
	Hermann Hospital, Houston	20.2	0.0%	1.26	Yes	0.48	6	2	1.42	0.062
	Medical City Dallas Hospital	21.5	0.0%	0.98	No	0.00	9	1	1.15	0.114
	Memorial City Medical Center, Houston	22.0	0.0%	0.86	No	0.00	7	2	0.55	0.046
	Methodist Hospital, Houston	20.3	0.4%	1.25	Yes	0.19	7	2	1.33	0.026
	Northeast Medical Center Hospital, Humble	20.7	0.0%	0.98	No	0.00	7	2	0.96	0.018
97	Parkland Memorial Hospital, Dallas	24.6	1.3%	1.22	Yes	1.35	10	2	0.93	0.039
	Presbyterian Hospital, Dallas	21.7	0.0%	0.89	No	0.19	5	1	1.03	0.065
	Sam Houston Memorial Hospital, Houston	19.9	0.0%	1.06	No	0.00	6	2	1.05	0.172
	San Antonio Regional Hospital	20.7	0.0%	0.98	No	0.04	6	1	0.91	0.271
	Santa Rosa Health Care Corp, San Antonio	21.2	0.0%	0.98	No	0.00	8	2	0.81	0.085
	Scott and White Memorial Hospital, Temple	24.0	0.0%	1.01	Yes	0.71	7	2	1.32	0.059
	Southwest Texas Methodist Hospital, San Antonio	19.9	0.0%	1.02	No	0.00	8	1	0.95	0.042
	St. Mary Hospital, Port Arthur	21.4	0.0%	0.85	No	0.05	5	2	0.68	0.019
	St. Paul Medical Center, Dallas	21.2	0.0%	1.13	Yes	0.25	7	2	1.17	0.077
	Tomball Regional Hospital, Tomball	20.6	0.0%	0.98	No	0.00	5	2	1.29	0.033
	University Medical Center, Lubbock	19.7	0.0%	1.26	Yes	0.43	8	2	0.75	0.043
	University of Texas Medical Branch Hospitals, Galveston	23.6	0.0%	1.16	Yes	1.09	10	2	1.19	0.068
TIER FOUR									
	AMI Brownsville Medical Center, Brownsville	17.0	0.0%	1.15	No	0.00	6	2	0.38	0.024
	All Saints Episcopal Hospital, Fort Worth	18.6	0.0%	1.08	No	0.00	6	2	0.85	0.013
	Amarillo Hospital District, Amarillo	18.1	0.0%	1.22	No	0.10	7	2	1.26	0.019
	Arlington Memorial Hospital, Arlington	16.6	0.0%	1.13	No	0.00	4	1	0.86	0.036
	Baptist Hospital of Southeast Texas, Beaumont	18.4	0.0%	1.09	No	0.00	7	2	0.53	0.019
	Baptist Medical Center, San Antonio	17.6	0.0%	1.24	No	0.00	6	2	0.79	0.260
	Bethania Regional Health Center, Wichita Falls	17.6	0.0%	1.11	No	0.03	5	2	0.61	0.030
	Good Shepherd Medical Center, Longview	16.8	0.0%	1.29	No	0.00	6	2	1.17	0.050
	HCA Rio Grande Regional Hospital, McAllen	17.8	0.0%	1.12	No	0.00	5	2	0.74	0.061
	HCA South Austin Medical Center, Austin	18.9	0.0%	1.00	No	0.00	4	1	0.88	0.122
	Harris County Hospital District, Houston	17.7	0.0%	1.56	Yes	0.46	10	1	0.75	0.163
	Hendrick Medical Center, Abilene	16.7	0.0%	1.30	No	0.00	6	2	0.98	0.105
	High Plains Baptist Health System, Amarillo	18.6	0.0%	1.11	No	0.02	5	2	1.11	0.088
	Hillcrest Baptist Medical Center, Waco	15.3	0.0%	1.44	No	0.06	7	2	0.80	0.016
	Houston Northwest Medical Center	18.2	0.0%	1.05	No	0.00	4	2	0.73	0.012
	Irving Healthcare System, Irving	18.6	0.0%	1.10	No	0.00	5	2	1.10	0.066
	John Peter Smith Hospital, Fort Worth	15.7	0.0%	1.71	No	0.79	6	2	1.47	0.010
	McAllen Medical Center, McAllen	18.3	0.0%	1.13	No	0.03	7	2	0.71	0.038
	Medical Center Hospital, Conroe	18.2	0.0%	1.18	No	0.00	6	2	1.37	0.018
	Medical Center Hospital, Odessa	16.7	0.0%	1.21	No	0.05	7	2	0.30	0.031
	Memorial Hospital System, Houston	18.8	0.0%	1.12	No	0.04	7	2	0.96	0.033

STATE RANKINGS ■ TEXAS

Natl. Rank	Hospital	U.S. News index	Reputa-tional score	Hospital-wide mortality rate	COTH member	Interns and residents to beds	Tech-nology score (of 11)	Discharge planning (of 2)	R.N.'s to beds	Board-certified internists to beds
	Memorial Hospital and Medical Center, Midland	16.5	0.0%	1.26	No	0.00	6	2	0.85	0.030
	Memorial Medical Center of East Texas, Lufkin	19.3	0.0%	1.05	No	0.00	7	2	0.66	0.026
	Memorial Medical Center, Corpus Christi	18.4	0.0%	1.24	No	0.21	9	2	0.85	0.057
	Methodist Hospital, Lubbock	19.5	0.0%	1.03	No	0.00	6	2	0.89	0.025
	Methodist Medical Center, Dallas	19.5	0.0%	1.22	Yes	0.19	7	2	0.90	0.046
	Mother Frances Hospital Regional Center, Tyler	18.5	0.0%	1.15	No	0.00	6	2	1.16	0.071
	Northeast Baptist Hospital, San Antonio	19.5	0.0%	1.24	No	0.01	6	2	1.11	0.602
	Osteopathic Medical Center of Texas, Fort Worth	19.6	0.0%	1.05	No	0.38	6	2	0.66	0.035
	Providence Memorial Hospital, El Paso	17.7	0.0%	1.18	No	0.00	7	2	0.67	0.071
	R.E. Thomason General Hospital, El Paso	15.1	0.0%	1.42	No	0.37	5	2	0.66	0.013
	RHD Memorial Medical Center, Dallas	18.7	0.0%	1.05	No	0.00	5	2	0.80	0.041
	San Jacinto Methodist Hospital, Baytown	15.6	0.0%	1.17	No	0.15	3	1	0.66	0.011
	Seton Medical Center, Austin	17.8	0.0%	1.14	No	0.00	6	2	0.71	0.050
	Shannon Medical Center, San Angelo	15.6	0.0%	1.35	No	0.00	6	2	0.77	0.031
	Sierra Medical Center, El Paso	16.1	0.0%	1.27	No	0.00	5	2	0.82	0.043
	Spohn Health System, Corpus Christi	18.3	0.0%	1.11	No	0.00	6	2	0.74	0.062
	St. Anthony's Hospital, Amarillo	19.6	0.0%	0.97	No	0.00	6	2	0.42	0.023
	St. David's Hospital, Austin	18.4	0.0%	1.13	No	0.00	5	2	0.76	0.242
	St. Elizabeth Hospital, Beaumont	17.0	0.0%	1.22	No	0.00	6	2	0.92	0.024
	St. Joseph Hospital and Health Center, Bryan	18.4	0.0%	1.06	No	0.00	6	1	0.85	0.052
	St. Joseph Hospital, Fort Worth	16.5	0.0%	1.24	No	0.00	6	2	0.68	0.035
	St. Joseph Hospital, Houston	19.3	0.0%	1.07	No	0.15	7	2	0.73	0.041
	St. Mary of the Plains Hospital, Lubbock	16.3	0.0%	1.24	No	0.02	5	2	0.74	0.042
	Texas Heart Institute-St. Luke's Episcopal, Houston	19.0	0.0%	1.31	Yes	0.26	6	2	1.36	0.045
	Texoma Medical Center, Denison	16.2	0.0%	1.29	No	0.00	6	2	0.80	0.016
	University of Texas Health Center, Tyler	15.4	0.0%	1.29	No	0.14	5	1	0.78	0.042
	Valley Baptist Medical Center, Harlingen	18.4	0.0%	1.16	No	0.00	8	2	0.87	0.021
	Wadley Regional Medical Center, Texarkana	17.1	0.0%	1.24	No	0.00	7	2	0.83	0.039
	Wichita General Hospital, Wichita Falls	15.0	0.0%	1.36	No	0.04	5	2	0.62	0.038

CANCER

Natl. Rank	Hospital	U.S. News index	Reputa-tional score	Cancer mortality rate	COTH member	Interns and residents to beds	Tech-nology score (of 12)	R.N.'s to beds	Board-certified oncologists to beds	Procedures to beds
	TIER ONE									
2	University of Texas M.D. Anderson Cancer Ctr., Houston	93.2	63.1%	0.27	Yes	0.70	11	1.88	0.010	7.18
	TIER TWO									
68	Parkland Memorial Hospital, Dallas	11.7	0.0%	0.69	Yes	1.35	10	0.93	0.010	0.36
75	University of Texas Medical Branch Hospitals, Galveston	11.3	0.0%	1.11	Yes	1.09	11	1.19	0.013	0.48
	TIER THREE									
	Amarillo Hospital District, Amarillo	5.9	0.0%	0.39	No	0.10	9	1.26	0.006	0.87
	Baylor University Medical Center, Dallas	9.7	0.4%	0.66	Yes	0.29	8	1.38	0.006	1.55
	Bexar County Hospital District, San Antonio	9.4	0.0%	1.05	Yes	1.12	7	0.83	0.015	0.32
	Harris County Hospital District, Houston	7.2	0.0%	0.97	Yes	0.46	8	0.75	0.000	0.19
	Hermann Hospital, Houston	9.1	0.0%	0.88	Yes	0.48	7	1.42	0.017	0.59
	Methodist Hospital, Houston	8.6	0.0%	1.18	Yes	0.19	10	1.33	0.008	1.35
	Methodist Medical Center, Dallas	7.1	0.0%	0.93	Yes	0.19	8	0.90	0.012	1.54
90	Scott and White Memorial Hospital, Temple	10.5	0.0%	0.54	Yes	0.71	8	1.32	0.021	1.72
	Southwest Texas Methodist Hospital, San Antonio	6.3	1.3%	1.11	No	0.00	10	0.95	0.020	1.88
	St. Paul Medical Center, Dallas	8.1	0.0%	0.82	Yes	0.25	8	1.17	0.016	0.88
	Texas Heart Institute-St. Luke's Episcopal, Houston	7.6	0.0%	1.18	Yes	0.26	6	1.36	0.009	0.83
	Zale Lipshy University Hospital, Dallas	5.4	0.0%	0.73	No	0.24	4	1.33	0.047	1.87
	TIER FOUR									
	All Saints Episcopal Hospital, Fort Worth	4.1	0.0%	0.80	No	0.00	7	0.85	0.020	3.00
	Arlington Memorial Hospital, Arlington	2.1	0.0%	1.35	No	0.00	3	0.86	0.008	1.59

Natl. Rank	Hospital	U.S. News index	Reputa- tional score	Cancer mortality rate	COTH member	Interns and residents to beds	Tech- nology score (of 12)	R.N.'s to beds	Board- certified oncologists to beds	Procedures to beds
	Baptist Hospital of Southeast Texas, Beaumont	2.6	0.0%	0.96	No	0.00	7	0.53	0.013	1.18
	Baptist Medical Center, San Antonio	3.6	0.0%	1.19	No	0.00	8	0.79	0.000	2.51
	Bethania Regional Health Center, Wichita Falls	2.6	0.0%	0.77	No	0.03	4	0.61	0.010	2.85
	Citizens Medical Center, Victoria	3.8	0.0%	0.54	No	0.00	8	0.59	0.004	2.64
	Clear Lake Regional Medical Center, Webbster	2.9	0.0%	0.87	No	0.00	8	0.52	0.009	1.22
	East Texas Medical Center, Tyler	3.5	0.0%	0.64	No	0.00	5	0.85	0.013	1.78
	Good Shepherd Medical Center, Longview	4.1	0.0%	1.47	No	0.00	7	1.17	0.007	2.00
	HCA Medical Center of Plano, Plano	3.7	0.0%	1.01	No	0.00	6	1.04	0.013	1.19
	HCA Medical Plaza Hospital, Fort Worth	3.0	0.0%	0.53	No	0.00	5	0.65	0.015	2.03
	HCA Rio Grande Regional Hospital, McAllen	2.3	0.0%	0.76	No	0.00	3	0.74	0.010	1.15
	HCA South Austin Medical Center, Austin	3.0	0.0%	0.77	No	0.00	4	0.88	0.014	1.31
	HCA Spring Branch Medical Center, Houston	2.4	0.0%	1.00	No	0.00	4	0.80	0.006	1.17
	Harris Methodist Fort Worth	4.6	0.0%	0.86	No	0.01	6	1.29	0.007	1.36
	Harris Methodist-HEB, Bedford	3.0	0.0%	0.71	No	0.00	6	0.65	0.009	1.08
	Hendrick Medical Center, Abilene	3.9	0.0%	1.14	No	0.00	7	0.98	0.007	2.76
	High Plains Baptist Health System, Amarillo	4.8	0.0%	0.54	No	0.02	6	1.11	0.015	2.54
	Hillcrest Baptist Medical Center, Waco	4.1	0.0%	1.10	No	0.06	9	0.80	0.009	2.13
	Houston Northwest Medical Center	2.7	0.0%	0.82	No	0.00	5	0.73	0.007	1.03
	Irving Healthcare System, Irving	4.0	0.0%	1.14	No	0.00	7	1.10	0.004	1.35
	McAllen Medical Center, McAllen	3.3	0.0%	0.56	No	0.03	6	0.71	0.007	0.62
	Medical Center Hospital, Conroe	5.0	0.0%	0.80	No	0.00	7	1.37	0.006	1.05
	Medical Center Hospital, Odessa	2.2	0.0%	1.14	No	0.05	8	0.30	0.010	1.08
	Medical City Dallas Hospital	5.2	0.0%	1.25	No	0.00	11	1.15	0.016	1.06
	Memorial City Medical Center, Houston	3.0	0.0%	0.88	No	0.00	8	0.55	0.019	1.05
	Memorial Hospital System, Houston	4.6	0.0%	0.77	No	0.04	8	0.96	0.009	1.87
	Memorial Hospital and Medical Center, Midland	3.0	0.0%	1.64	No	0.00	7	0.85	0.007	1.37
	Memorial Medical Center of East Texas, Lufkin	3.6	0.0%	0.61	No	0.00	8	0.66	0.004	0.88
	Methodist Hospital, Lubbock	3.8	0.0%	0.98	No	0.00	7	0.89	0.007	2.40
	Mother Frances Hospital Regional Center, Tyler	4.3	0.0%	1.23	No	0.00	7	1.16	0.026	1.85
	Northeast Baptist Hospital, San Antonio	4.3	0.0%	1.19	No	0.01	5	1.11	0.000	5.82
	Northeast Medical Center Hospital, Humble	3.9	0.0%	1.12	No	0.00	8	0.96	0.018	0.97
	Osteopathic Medical Center of Texas, Fort Worth	3.8	0.0%	0.75	No	0.38	5	0.66	0.013	0.77
	Presbyterian Hospital, Dallas	5.2	0.0%	0.75	No	0.19	8	1.03	0.009	1.48
	Providence Memorial Hospital, El Paso	2.9	0.0%	0.93	No	0.00	6	0.67	0.017	1.98
	RHD Memorial Medical Center, Dallas	3.3	0.0%	0.85	No	0.00	6	0.80	0.000	1.97
	San Antonio Regional Hospital	4.0	0.0%	0.89	No	0.04	7	0.91	0.013	1.61
	San Jacinto Methodist Hospital, Baytown	3.0	0.0%	0.52	No	0.15	4	0.66	0.008	0.65
	Santa Rosa Health Care Corp, San Antonio	4.1	0.0%	0.63	No	0.00	8	0.81	0.012	0.71
	Seton Medical Center, Austin	3.0	0.0%	1.31	No	0.00	7	0.71	0.006	2.32
	Shannon Medical Center, San Angelo	3.1	0.0%	0.89	No	0.00	6	0.77	0.009	1.46
	Sierra Medical Center, El Paso	2.3	0.0%	1.01	No	0.00	3	0.82	0.013	1.76
	Spohn Health System, Corpus Christi	3.4	0.0%	1.09	No	0.00	8	0.74	0.010	1.80
	St. Anthony's Hospital, Amarillo	2.8	0.0%	0.39	No	0.00	7	0.42	0.000	1.75
	St. David's Hospital, Austin	2.2	0.0%	1.16	No	0.00	4	0.76	0.017	1.31
	St. Elizabeth Hospital, Beaumont	4.3	0.4%	1.25	No	0.00	8	0.92	0.006	2.01
	St. Joseph Hospital and Health Center, Bryan	3.2	0.0%	0.71	No	0.00	5	0.85	0.005	1.18
	St. Joseph Hospital, Fort Worth	2.3	0.0%	0.84	No	0.00	4	0.68	0.018	1.08
	St. Joseph Hospital, Houston	3.8	0.0%	1.01	No	0.15	8	0.73	0.003	1.06
	St. Mary Hospital, Port Arthur	3.1	0.0%	0.77	No	0.05	6	0.68	0.009	1.07
	St. Mary of the Plains Hospital, Lubbock	3.1	0.0%	0.69	No	0.02	5	0.74	0.012	1.22
	Texoma Medical Center, Denison	3.7	0.0%	1.14	No	0.00	8	0.80	0.000	2.68
	University of Texas Health Center, Tyler	4.0	1.0%	0.87	No	0.14	3	0.78	0.012	1.54
	Valley Baptist Medical Center, Harlingen	4.6	0.0%	0.53	No	0.00	9	0.87	0.005	1.48
	Wadley Regional Medical Center, Texarkana	3.2	0.0%	1.57	No	0.00	8	0.83	0.003	1.24
	Wichita General Hospital, Wichita Falls	2.5	0.0%	1.52	No	0.04	6	0.62	0.008	2.21

CARDIOLOGY

STATE RANKINGS ■ TEXAS

Natl. Rank	Hospital	U.S. News index	Reputa-tional score	Cardiology mortality rate	COTH member	Interns and residents to beds	Tech-nology score (of 10)	R.N.'s to beds	Board-certified cardiologists to beds	Procedures to beds
	TIER ONE									
3	Texas Heart Institute-St. Luke's Episcopal, Houston	81.4	24.6%	1.52	Yes	0.26	9	1.36	0.064	10.00
17	Methodist Hospital, Houston	29.6	8.6%	1.13	Yes	0.19	9	1.33	0.058	5.03
	TIER TWO									
91	Parkland Memorial Hospital, Dallas	21.0	1.7%	1.15	Yes	1.35	9	0.93	0.020	1.41
	TIER THREE									
97	Baylor University Medical Center, Dallas	20.8	2.9%	1.12	Yes	0.29	8	1.38	0.019	6.06
	East Texas Medical Center, Tyler	15.7	0.0%	0.92	No	0.00	6	0.85	0.036	4.20
	HCA South Austin Medical Center, Austin	14.7	0.0%	0.99	No	0.00	7	0.88	0.050	7.64
	Harris Methodist-HEB, Bedford	13.6	0.0%	0.96	No	0.00	6	0.65	0.018	5.59
	Hermann Hospital, Houston	16.9	0.0%	1.19	Yes	0.48	8	1.42	0.073	3.90
	Medical City Dallas Hospital	18.5	0.0%	0.91	No	0.00	10	1.15	0.049	5.53
	Methodist Hospital, Lubbock	15.4	0.7%	1.00	No	0.00	8	0.89	0.020	10.14
	Northeast Medical Center Hospital, Humble	15.0	0.0%	0.97	No	0.00	6	0.96	0.041	7.57
	Osteopathic Medical Center of Texas, Fort Worth	14.7	0.0%	1.00	No	0.38	8	0.66	0.017	5.14
	Presbyterian Hospital, Dallas	15.8	0.0%	0.97	No	0.19	7	1.03	0.033	4.58
	Scott and White Memorial Hospital, Temple	16.2	0.0%	1.21	Yes	0.71	7	1.32	0.026	6.53
	St. Joseph Hospital and Health Center, Bryan	17.9	0.0%	0.82	No	0.00	9	0.85	0.021	8.89
	St. Mary Hospital, Port Arthur	14.0	0.0%	0.97	No	0.05	6	0.68	0.033	6.66
	St. Paul Medical Center, Dallas	13.8	0.0%	1.28	Yes	0.25	9	1.17	0.038	4.65
	University of Texas Medical Branch Hospitals, Galveston	17.2	0.0%	1.22	Yes	1.09	9	1.19	0.017	1.85
	TIER FOUR									
	AMI Brownsville Medical Center, Brownsville	9.4	0.0%	1.16	No	0.00	8	0.38	0.018	7.22
	All Saints Episcopal Hospital, Fort Worth	8.0	0.0%	1.37	No	0.00	9	0.85	0.026	7.58
	Amarillo Hospital District, Amarillo	11.7	0.0%	1.18	No	0.10	8	1.26	0.022	3.21
	Arlington Memorial Hospital, Arlington	10.1	0.0%	1.19	No	0.00	7	0.86	0.030	5.07
	Baptist Hospital of Southeast Texas, Beaumont	10.1	0.0%	1.14	No	0.00	7	0.53	0.042	4.90
	Baptist Medical Center, San Antonio	9.1	0.0%	1.24	No	0.00	8	0.79	0.000	12.58
	Bethania Regional Health Center, Wichita Falls	10.2	0.0%	1.19	No	0.03	8	0.61	0.030	11.23
	Citizens Medical Center, Victoria	10.9	0.0%	1.10	No	0.00	8	0.59	0.013	6.49
	Clear Lake Regional Medical Center, Webbster	10.5	0.0%	1.09	No	0.00	7	0.52	0.019	3.82
	Good Shepherd Medical Center, Longview	13.0	0.0%	1.09	No	0.00	8	1.17	0.014	9.16
	HCA Medical Center of Plano, Plano	11.9	0.0%	1.13	No	0.00	7	1.04	0.054	3.82
	HCA Medical Plaza Hospital, Fort Worth	11.5	0.0%	1.11	No	0.00	8	0.65	0.040	8.18
	HCA Rio Grande Regional Hospital, McAllen	9.6	0.0%	1.26	No	0.00	8	0.74	0.056	9.42
	HCA Spring Branch Medical Center, Houston	11.7	0.0%	1.09	No	0.00	7	0.80	0.032	3.82
	Harris County Hospital District, Houston	11.6	0.0%	1.36	Yes	0.46	10	0.75	0.000	1.20
	Harris Methodist Fort Worth	10.9	0.0%	1.25	No	0.01	9	1.29	0.028	5.79
	Hendrick Medical Center, Abilene	3.7	0.0%	1.77	No	0.00	7	0.98	0.026	5.13
	High Plains Baptist Health System, Amarillo	7.8	0.0%	1.46	No	0.02	8	1.11	0.040	7.87
	Hillcrest Baptist Medical Center, Waco	4.8	0.0%	1.51	No	0.06	5	0.80	0.012	4.89
	Houston Northwest Medical Center	5.3	0.0%	1.45	No	0.00	6	0.73	0.015	3.71
	Irving Healthcare System, Irving	11.6	0.0%	1.16	No	0.00	8	1.10	0.018	8.80
	McAllen Medical Center, McAllen	11.4	0.0%	1.13	No	0.03	8	0.71	0.041	8.57
	Medical Center Hospital, Conroe	12.9	0.0%	1.14	No	0.00	8	1.37	0.036	8.12
	Medical Center Hospital, Odessa	9.8	0.0%	1.14	No	0.05	9	0.30	0.007	6.55
	Memorial City Medical Center, Houston	9.0	0.0%	1.21	No	0.00	8	0.55	0.035	4.24
	Memorial Hospital System, Houston	11.5	0.0%	1.16	No	0.04	8	0.96	0.040	5.71
	Memorial Hospital and Medical Center, Midland	7.7	0.0%	1.32	No	0.00	7	0.85	0.017	5.51
	Memorial Medical Center of East Texas, Lufkin	9.0	0.0%	1.18	No	0.00	5	0.66	0.013	7.84
	Memorial Medical Center, Corpus Christi	11.3	0.0%	1.22	No	0.21	10	0.85	0.045	5.14
	Methodist Medical Center, Dallas	12.5	0.3%	1.31	Yes	0.19	9	0.90	0.020	5.52
	Mother Frances Hospital Regional Center, Tyler	13.1	0.0%	1.13	No	0.00	9	1.16	0.041	15.84
	Northeast Baptist Hospital, San Antonio	10.4	0.0%	1.24	No	0.01	9	1.11	0.000	29.16

Natl. Rank	Hospital	U.S. News index	Reputa-tional score	Cardiology mortality rate	COTH member	Interns and residents to beds	Tech-nology score (of 10)	R.N.'s to beds	Board-certified cardiologists to beds	Procedures to beds
	Providence Memorial Hospital, El Paso	10.2	0.0%	1.18	No	0.00	9	0.67	0.039	3.54
	RHD Memorial Medical Center, Dallas	11.3	0.0%	1.14	No	0.00	7	0.80	0.068	6.16
	San Antonio Regional Hospital	10.1	0.0%	1.25	No	0.04	7	0.91	0.102	7.18
	San Jacinto Methodist Hospital, Baytown	8.0	0.0%	1.20	No	0.15	3	0.66	0.008	3.38
	Santa Rosa Health Care Corp, San Antonio	10.2	0.0%	1.17	No	0.00	7	0.81	0.034	3.49
	Seton Medical Center, Austin	10.2	0.0%	1.19	No	0.00	8	0.71	0.038	7.77
	Shannon Medical Center, San Angelo	9.3	0.0%	1.26	No	0.00	8	0.77	0.031	8.68
	Sierra Medical Center, El Paso	8.3	0.0%	1.34	No	0.00	8	0.82	0.043	6.09
	Southwest Texas Methodist Hospital, San Antonio	11.9	0.0%	1.17	No	0.00	10	0.95	0.042	6.65
	Spohn Health System, Corpus Christi	11.1	0.0%	1.14	No	0.00	7	0.74	0.037	10.58
	St. Anthony's Hospital, Amarillo	3.3	0.0%	1.59	No	0.00	7	0.42	0.012	5.02
	St. David's Hospital, Austin	11.6	0.0%	1.10	No	0.00	7	0.76	0.040	6.09
	St. Elizabeth Hospital, Beaumont	8.8	0.0%	1.31	No	0.00	8	0.92	0.026	8.10
	St. Joseph Hospital, Fort Worth	7.9	0.0%	1.37	No	0.00	9	0.68	0.044	6.99
	St. Joseph Hospital, Houston	10.2	0.0%	1.19	No	0.15	9	0.73	0.008	3.87
	St. Mary of the Plains Hospital, Lubbock	7.4	0.0%	1.35	No	0.02	6	0.74	0.039	8.25
	Texoma Medical Center, Denison	9.8	0.0%	1.20	No	0.00	7	0.80	0.027	9.39
	Tomball Regional Hospital, Tomball	13.0	0.0%	1.11	No	0.00	7	1.29	0.022	11.47
	University of Texas Health Center, Tyler	5.6	0.0%	1.55	No	0.14	7	0.78	0.024	7.10
	Valley Baptist Medical Center, Harlingen	8.0	0.0%	1.36	No	0.00	9	0.87	0.010	8.05
	Wadley Regional Medical Center, Texarkana	5.8	0.0%	1.49	No	0.00	8	0.83	0.010	5.52
	Wichita General Hospital, Wichita Falls	9.0	0.0%	1.17	No	0.04	5	0.62	0.025	3.75

ENDOCRINOLOGY

Natl. Rank	Hospital	U.S. News index	Reputa-tional score	Endocrinology mortality rate	COTH member	Interns and residents to beds	Tech-nology score (of 11)	R.N.'s to beds	Board-certified internists to beds
	TIER ONE								
12	Parkland Memorial Hospital, Dallas	28.1	10.4%	1.00	Yes	1.35	10	0.93	0.039
24	University of Texas M.D. Anderson Cancer Ctr., Houston	21.7	2.2%	0.48	Yes	0.70	11	1.88	0.083
	TIER TWO								
47	Baylor University Medical Center, Dallas	17.7	1.9%	0.67	Yes	0.29	8	1.38	0.093
82	University of Texas Medical Branch Hospitals, Galveston	14.9	0.0%	0.92	Yes	1.09	10	1.19	0.068
	TIER THREE								
	Bexar County Hospital District, San Antonio	11.5	0.0%	1.18	Yes	1.12	7	0.83	0.028
	East Texas Medical Center, Tyler	8.2	0.0%	0.79	No	0.00	6	0.85	0.059
	Harris County Hospital District, Houston	8.4	0.0%	1.75	Yes	0.46	8	0.75	0.163
	Hermann Hospital, Houston	13.4	0.6%	0.93	Yes	0.48	6	1.42	0.062
	Houston Northwest Medical Center	9.1	0.0%	0.49	No	0.00	5	0.73	0.012
	Memorial City Medical Center, Houston	9.6	0.0%	0.28	No	0.00	9	0.55	0.046
	Methodist Hospital, Houston	8.5	0.4%	1.99	Yes	0.19	10	1.33	0.026
	Methodist Medical Center, Dallas	9.8	0.0%	1.06	Yes	0.19	9	0.90	0.046
	Northeast Baptist Hospital, San Antonio	9.0	0.0%	1.35	No	0.01	5	1.11	0.602
	Presbyterian Hospital, Dallas	8.2	0.0%	0.97	No	0.19	8	1.03	0.065
	San Antonio Regional Hospital	12.2	0.0%	0.56	No	0.04	8	0.91	0.271
	Scott and White Memorial Hospital, Temple	11.7	0.0%	1.23	Yes	0.71	8	1.32	0.059
	St. Anthony's Hospital, Amarillo	8.9	0.0%	0.53	No	0.00	8	0.42	0.023
	St. Paul Medical Center, Dallas	11.3	0.0%	1.01	Yes	0.25	9	1.17	0.077
	Texas Heart Institute-St. Luke's Episcopal, Houston	9.5	0.0%	1.34	Yes	0.26	7	1.36	0.045
	Wadley Regional Medical Center, Texarkana	10.4	0.0%	0.64	No	0.00	9	0.83	0.039
	TIER FOUR								
	AMI Brownsville Medical Center, Brownsville	2.1	0.0%	1.60	No	0.00	5	0.38	0.024
	All Saints Episcopal Hospital, Fort Worth	5.3	0.0%	1.16	No	0.00	7	0.85	0.013
	Amarillo Hospital District, Amarillo	4.3	0.0%	2.15	No	0.10	8	1.26	0.019
	Arlington Memorial Hospital, Arlington	5.5	0.0%	1.06	No	0.00	4	0.86	0.036

Natl. Rank	Hospital	U.S. News index	Reputa- tional score	Endocrinology mortality rate	COTH member	Interns and residents to beds	Tech- nology score (of 11)	R.N.'s to beds	Board- certified internists to beds
	Baptist Hospital of Southeast Texas, Beaumont	5.5	0.0%	0.97	No	0.00	6	0.53	0.019
	Baptist Medical Center, San Antonio	6.3	0.0%	1.35	No	0.00	8	0.79	0.260
	Bethania Regional Health Center, Wichita Falls	1.7	0.0%	2.07	No	0.03	4	0.61	0.030
	Citizens Medical Center, Victoria	7.0	0.0%	0.88	No	0.00	9	0.59	0.034
	Clear Lake Regional Medical Center, Webbster	6.8	0.0%	0.85	No	0.00	8	0.52	0.019
	Good Shepherd Medical Center, Longview	6.9	0.0%	1.12	No	0.00	8	1.17	0.050
	HCA Medical Plaza Hospital, Fort Worth	7.2	0.0%	0.84	No	0.00	6	0.65	0.065
	HCA Rio Grande Regional Hospital, McAllen	3.8	0.0%	1.41	No	0.00	4	0.74	0.061
	HCA South Austin Medical Center, Austin	7.7	0.0%	0.87	No	0.00	5	0.88	0.122
	HCA Spring Branch Medical Center, Houston	3.3	0.0%	1.63	No	0.00	6	0.80	0.006
	Harris Methodist Fort Worth	7.6	0.0%	1.03	No	0.01	6	1.29	0.082
	Hendrick Medical Center, Abilene	7.8	0.0%	0.95	No	0.00	8	0.98	0.105
	Hillcrest Baptist Medical Center, Waco	5.7	0.0%	1.23	No	0.06	10	0.80	0.016
	Irving Healthcare System, Irving	7.2	0.0%	1.06	No	0.00	8	1.10	0.066
	McAllen Medical Center, McAllen	4.4	0.0%	1.31	No	0.03	6	0.71	0.038
	Medical Center Hospital, Odessa	5.1	0.0%	1.06	No	0.05	9	0.30	0.031
	Medical City Dallas Hospital	7.7	0.0%	1.13	No	0.00	10	1.15	0.114
	Memorial Hospital System, Houston	6.6	0.0%	1.11	No	0.04	9	0.96	0.033
	Memorial Hospital and Medical Center, Midland	5.9	0.0%	1.11	No	0.00	8	0.85	0.030
	Memorial Medical Center of East Texas, Lufkin	5.6	0.0%	1.11	No	0.00	9	0.66	0.026
	Memorial Medical Center, Corpus Christi	7.3	0.0%	1.09	No	0.21	10	0.85	0.057
	Methodist Hospital, Lubbock	7.0	0.0%	0.96	No	0.00	8	0.89	0.025
	Mother Frances Hospital Regional Center, Tyler	6.4	0.0%	1.24	No	0.00	8	1.16	0.071
	Osteopathic Medical Center of Texas, Fort Worth	6.8	0.0%	1.00	No	0.38	5	0.66	0.035
	Providence Memorial Hospital, El Paso	5.6	0.0%	1.06	No	0.00	6	0.67	0.071
	Sam Houston Memorial Hospital, Houston	7.2	0.0%	1.06	No	0.00	5	1.05	0.172
	San Jacinto Methodist Hospital, Baytown	2.7	0.0%	1.87	No	0.15	5	0.66	0.011
	Santa Rosa Health Care Corp, San Antonio	5.4	0.0%	1.28	No	0.00	8	0.81	0.085
	Seton Medical Center, Austin	4.1	0.0%	1.44	No	0.00	7	0.71	0.050
	Shannon Medical Center, San Angelo	5.8	0.0%	1.06	No	0.00	7	0.77	0.031
	Sierra Medical Center, El Paso	3.9	0.0%	1.39	No	0.00	4	0.82	0.043
	Southwest Texas Methodist Hospital, San Antonio	6.0	0.0%	1.21	No	0.00	9	0.95	0.042
	Spohn Health System, Corpus Christi	5.8	0.0%	1.16	No	0.00	9	0.74	0.062
	St. David's Hospital, Austin	6.6	0.0%	1.11	No	0.00	5	0.76	0.242
	St. Elizabeth Hospital, Beaumont	6.5	0.0%	1.08	No	0.00	9	0.92	0.024
	St. Joseph Hospital and Health Center, Bryan	3.6	0.0%	1.78	No	0.00	7	0.85	0.052
	St. Joseph Hospital, Fort Worth	3.9	0.0%	1.32	No	0.00	5	0.68	0.035
	St. Joseph Hospital, Houston	4.8	0.0%	1.49	No	0.15	9	0.73	0.041
	St. Mary Hospital, Port Arthur	7.9	0.0%	0.77	No	0.05	6	0.68	0.019
	St. Mary of the Plains Hospital, Lubbock	5.1	0.0%	1.12	No	0.02	5	0.74	0.042
	Texoma Medical Center, Denison	4.2	0.0%	1.53	No	0.00	9	0.80	0.016
	Tomball Regional Hospital, Tomball	5.6	0.0%	1.31	No	0.00	5	1.29	0.033
	University of Texas Health Center, Tyler	4.3	0.0%	1.37	No	0.14	4	0.78	0.042
	Valley Baptist Medical Center, Harlingen	6.5	0.0%	1.04	No	0.00	9	0.87	0.021
	Wichita General Hospital, Wichita Falls	4.4	0.0%	1.32	No	0.04	7	0.62	0.038

GASTROENTEROLOGY

Natl. Rank	Hospital	U.S. News index	Reputational score	Gastro-enterology mortality rate	COTH member	Interns and residents to beds	Technology score (of 11)	R.N.'s to beds	Board-certified gastro-enterologists to beds	Pro-cedures to beds
TIER ONE										
15	**Baylor University Medical Center, Dallas**	**24.2**	7.6%	0.80	Yes	0.29	8	1.38	0.008	2.44
TIER TWO										
34	**University of Texas M.D. Anderson Cancer Ctr., Houston**	**16.5**	0.6%	0.26	Yes	0.70	10	1.88	0.012	1.66
TIER THREE										
	Bethania Regional Health Center, Wichita Falls	7.5	0.0%	0.83	No	0.03	4	0.61	0.020	5.00
	HCA Rio Grande Regional Hospital, McAllen	7.8	0.0%	0.66	No	0.00	5	0.74	0.015	4.25
	Hermann Hospital, Houston	8.3	0.4%	1.67	Yes	0.48	6	1.42	0.013	1.19
	Medical City Dallas Hospital	7.8	0.0%	0.92	No	0.00	10	1.15	0.014	1.82
	Methodist Hospital, Houston	9.2	0.4%	1.42	Yes	0.19	10	1.33	0.018	1.52
	Methodist Medical Center, Dallas	8.1	0.0%	1.31	Yes	0.19	8	0.90	0.012	2.71
	Mother Frances Hospital Regional Center, Tyler	8.6	0.0%	0.90	No	0.00	7	1.16	0.026	4.22
	Northeast Baptist Hospital, San Antonio	10.6	0.0%	1.82	No	0.01	6	1.11	0.000	15.74
	Presbyterian Hospital, Dallas	9.1	0.4%	0.81	No	0.19	7	1.03	0.008	2.05
	San Antonio Regional Hospital	8.5	0.0%	0.79	No	0.04	8	0.91	0.049	2.70
74	**Scott and White Memorial Hospital, Temple**	**13.2**	0.0%	0.99	Yes	0.71	8	1.32	0.021	3.43
	St. Paul Medical Center, Dallas	9.9	0.0%	1.05	Yes	0.25	8	1.17	0.007	2.07
	Texas Heart Institute-St. Luke's Episcopal, Houston	8.9	0.0%	1.21	Yes	0.26	6	1.36	0.018	2.09
TIER FOUR										
	AMI Brownsville Medical Center, Brownsville	1.9	0.0%	1.91	No	0.00	6	0.38	0.012	3.74
	All Saints Episcopal Hospital, Fort Worth	6.2	0.0%	1.06	No	0.00	6	0.85	0.013	4.12
	Amarillo Hospital District, Amarillo	6.5	0.0%	1.06	No	0.10	7	1.26	0.006	1.82
	Arlington Memorial Hospital, Arlington	3.0	0.0%	1.34	No	0.00	3	0.86	0.016	2.57
	Baptist Hospital of Southeast Texas, Beaumont	2.6	0.0%	1.43	No	0.00	6	0.53	0.016	2.13
	Baptist Medical Center, San Antonio	5.3	0.0%	1.82	No	0.00	8	0.79	0.000	6.79
	Citizens Medical Center, Victoria	5.0	0.0%	1.26	No	0.00	8	0.59	0.013	3.87
	Clear Lake Regional Medical Center, Webbster	6.0	0.0%	0.90	No	0.00	8	0.52	0.013	2.04
	East Texas Medical Center, Tyler	5.7	0.0%	1.13	No	0.00	7	0.85	0.026	3.40
	Good Shepherd Medical Center, Longview	5.2	0.0%	1.55	No	0.00	8	1.17	0.011	3.86
	HCA South Austin Medical Center, Austin	4.7	0.0%	1.34	No	0.00	5	0.88	0.036	4.30
	Harris Methodist Fort Worth	6.7	0.0%	0.95	No	0.01	5	1.29	0.018	2.30
	Harris Methodist-HEB, Bedford	6.7	0.0%	0.81	No	0.00	6	0.65	0.022	2.23
	Hendrick Medical Center, Abilene	5.1	0.0%	1.39	No	0.00	8	0.98	0.010	3.43
	High Plains Baptist Health System, Amarillo	6.9	0.0%	0.96	No	0.02	5	1.11	0.004	3.54
	Hillcrest Baptist Medical Center, Waco	4.7	0.0%	1.53	No	0.06	10	0.80	0.019	2.89
	Houston Northwest Medical Center	4.6	0.0%	1.01	No	0.00	5	0.73	0.010	1.75
	Irving Healthcare System, Irving	5.3	0.0%	1.25	No	0.00	7	1.10	0.018	2.83
	McAllen Medical Center, McAllen	6.4	0.0%	0.89	No	0.03	5	0.71	0.014	3.20
	Medical Center Hospital, Conroe	6.0	0.0%	1.29	No	0.00	7	1.37	0.018	3.17
	Medical Center Hospital, Odessa	4.4	0.0%	1.24	No	0.05	9	0.30	0.003	3.06
	Memorial City Medical Center, Houston	7.2	0.0%	0.73	No	0.00	9	0.55	0.028	1.86
	Memorial Hospital System, Houston	5.4	0.0%	1.22	No	0.04	8	0.96	0.016	2.47
	Memorial Hospital and Medical Center, Midland	4.3	0.0%	1.33	No	0.00	8	0.85	0.003	2.26
	Memorial Medical Center of East Texas, Lufkin	5.1	0.0%	1.26	No	0.00	8	0.66	0.009	3.79
	Memorial Medical Center, Corpus Christi	4.3	0.0%	1.58	No	0.21	9	0.85	0.012	1.97
	Methodist Hospital, Lubbock	6.2	0.0%	1.20	No	0.00	8	0.89	0.008	4.39
	Osteopathic Medical Center of Texas, Fort Worth	5.0	0.0%	1.22	No	0.38	5	0.66	0.009	2.50
	Providence Memorial Hospital, El Paso	3.5	0.0%	1.28	No	0.00	5	0.67	0.020	2.74
	San Jacinto Methodist Hospital, Baytown	2.7	0.0%	1.45	No	0.15	4	0.66	0.008	2.18
	Santa Rosa Health Care Corp, San Antonio	3.6	0.0%	1.33	No	0.00	7	0.81	0.015	1.59
	Seton Medical Center, Austin	5.1	0.0%	1.13	No	0.00	6	0.71	0.023	3.48
	Shannon Medical Center, San Angelo	4.6	0.0%	1.27	No	0.00	6	0.77	0.009	3.59
	Sierra Medical Center, El Paso	3.6	0.0%	1.35	No	0.00	4	0.82	0.020	3.28
	Southwest Texas Methodist Hospital, San Antonio	6.0	0.0%	1.13	No	0.00	8	0.95	0.024	2.97

Natl. Rank	Hospital	U.S. News index	Reputa-tional score	Gastro-enterology mortality rate	COTH member	Interns and residents to beds	Tech-nology score (of 11)	R.N.'s to beds	Board-certified gastro-enterologists to beds	Pro-cedures to beds
	Spohn Health System, Corpus Christi	6.8	0.0%	1.02	No	0.00	8	0.74	0.017	4.01
	St. Anthony's Hospital, Amarillo	6.8	0.0%	0.84	No	0.00	7	0.42	0.016	3.39
	St. David's Hospital, Austin	6.3	0.0%	0.88	No	0.00	5	0.76	0.020	2.70
	St. Elizabeth Hospital, Beaumont	6.0	0.0%	1.16	No	0.00	8	0.92	0.010	3.44
	St. Joseph Hospital and Health Center, Bryan	4.5	0.0%	1.34	No	0.00	6	0.85	0.015	3.66
	St. Joseph Hospital, Fort Worth	5.6	0.0%	0.95	No	0.00	5	0.68	0.018	2.92
	St. Joseph Hospital, Houston	5.6	0.0%	1.13	No	0.15	9	0.73	0.008	1.90
	St. Mary Hospital, Port Arthur	7.2	0.0%	0.65	No	0.05	5	0.68	0.009	3.18
	St. Mary of the Plains Hospital, Lubbock	3.7	0.0%	1.23	No	0.02	4	0.74	0.020	2.69
	Texoma Medical Center, Denison	4.4	0.0%	1.43	No	0.00	8	0.80	0.022	3.13
	Valley Baptist Medical Center, Harlingen	5.1	0.0%	1.25	No	0.00	8	0.87	0.008	2.97
	Wadley Regional Medical Center, Texarkana	3.8	0.0%	1.65	No	0.00	9	0.83	0.008	2.79
	Wichita General Hospital, Wichita Falls	1.7	0.0%	1.90	No	0.04	6	0.62	0.017	2.19

GERIATRICS

Natl. Rank	Hospital	U.S. News index	Reputa-tional score	Hospital-wide mortality rate	COTH member	Service mix	Interns and residents to beds	Tech-nology score (of 13)	R.N.'s to beds	Discharge planning (of 2)	Geriatric services (of 9)	Board-certified internists to beds
	TIER TWO											
42	Baylor University Medical Center, Dallas	25.6	0.6%	0.89	Yes	8	0.29	11	1.38	2	4	0.093
	TIER THREE											
	Citizens Medical Center, Victoria	15.1	0.0%	0.98	No	5	0.00	10	0.59	2	4	0.034
	Clear Lake Regional Medical Center, Webbster	14.5	0.0%	0.96	No	4	0.00	10	0.52	2	2	0.019
	East Texas Medical Center, Tyler	16.6	0.0%	0.89	No	3	0.00	7	0.85	2	2	0.059
	HCA Medical Plaza Hospital, Fort Worth	15.4	0.0%	0.94	No	4	0.00	8	0.65	2	3	0.065
	Harris Methodist Fort Worth	15.5	0.0%	1.03	No	7	0.01	9	1.29	2	2	0.082
	Harris Methodist-HEB, Bedford	17.6	0.0%	0.84	No	6	0.00	8	0.65	2	2	0.053
	Medical City Dallas Hospital	15.9	0.0%	0.98	No	5	0.00	13	1.15	1	3	0.114
	Memorial City Medical Center, Houston	16.7	0.0%	0.86	No	4	0.00	10	0.55	2	1	0.046
	Northeast Medical Center Hospital, Humble	15.1	0.0%	0.98	No	4	0.00	11	0.96	2	3	0.018
	Parkland Memorial Hospital, Dallas	17.4	0.6%	1.22	Yes	6	1.35	11	0.93	2	4	0.039
	Santa Rosa Health Care Corp, San Antonio	17.8	0.0%	0.98	No	9	0.00	9	0.81	2	6	0.085
99	Scott and White Memorial Hospital, Temple	20.6	0.0%	1.01	Yes	7	0.71	10	1.32	2	5	0.059
	St. Anthony's Hospital, Amarillo	14.5	0.0%	0.97	No	6	0.00	10	0.42	2	1	0.023
	St. Joseph Hospital, Houston	14.3	0.0%	1.07	No	7	0.15	11	0.73	2	4	0.041
	St. Mary Hospital, Port Arthur	16.6	0.0%	0.85	No	4	0.05	7	0.68	2	2	0.019
	St. Paul Medical Center, Dallas	16.5	0.0%	1.13	Yes	8	0.25	11	1.17	2	3	0.077
	University of Texas Medical Branch Hospitals, Galveston	19.4	0.0%	1.16	Yes	9	1.09	12	1.19	2	7	0.068
	TIER FOUR											
	AMI Brownsville Medical Center, Brownsville	8.6	0.0%	1.15	No	4	0.00	6	0.38	2	2	0.024
	All Saints Episcopal Hospital, Fort Worth	12.6	0.0%	1.08	No	6	0.00	10	0.85	2	2	0.013
	Amarillo Hospital District, Amarillo	9.8	0.0%	1.22	No	4	0.10	10	1.26	2	2	0.019
	Arlington Memorial Hospital, Arlington	8.2	0.0%	1.13	No	3	0.00	6	0.86	1	1	0.036
	Baptist Hospital of Southeast Texas, Beaumont	10.4	0.0%	1.09	No	4	0.00	7	0.53	2	2	0.019
	Baptist Medical Center, San Antonio	11.8	0.0%	1.24	No	7	0.00	11	0.79	2	5	0.260
	Bethania Regional Health Center, Wichita Falls	10.5	0.0%	1.11	No	4	0.03	7	0.61	2	3	0.030
	Good Shepherd Medical Center, Longview	8.2	0.0%	1.29	No	4	0.00	8	1.17	2	3	0.050
	HCA Rio Grande Regional Hospital, McAllen	10.5	0.0%	1.12	No	4	0.00	6	0.74	2	3	0.061
	HCA South Austin Medical Center, Austin	12.2	0.0%	1.00	No	3	0.00	7	0.88	1	1	0.122
	Hendrick Medical Center, Abilene	8.6	0.0%	1.30	No	5	0.00	9	0.98	2	3	0.105
	Hermann Hospital, Houston	12.5	0.0%	1.26	Yes	5	0.48	8	1.42	2	1	0.062
	High Plains Baptist Health System, Amarillo	10.8	0.0%	1.11	No	3	0.02	7	1.11	2	1	0.088
	Hillcrest Baptist Medical Center, Waco	6.7	0.0%	1.44	No	6	0.06	10	0.80	2	4	0.016
	Houston Northwest Medical Center	12.7	0.0%	1.05	No	6	0.00	7	0.73	2	2	0.012

Natl. Rank	Hospital	U.S. News index	Reputational score	Hospital-wide mortality rate	COTH member	Service mix	Interns and residents to beds	Technology score (of 13)	R.N.'s to beds	Discharge planning (of 2)	Geriatric services (of 9)	Board-certified internists to beds
	Irving Healthcare System, Irving	12.5	0.0%	1.10	No	4	0.00	9	1.10	2	4	0.066
	McAllen Medical Center, McAllen	10.0	0.0%	1.13	No	4	0.03	7	0.71	2	2	0.038
	Medical Center Hospital, Conroe	10.5	0.0%	1.18	No	3	0.00	10	1.37	2	3	0.018
	Medical Center Hospital, Odessa	8.5	0.0%	1.21	No	5	0.05	11	0.30	2	1	0.031
	Memorial Hospital System, Houston	12.4	0.0%	1.12	No	6	0.04	10	0.96	2	3	0.033
	Memorial Hospital and Medical Center, Midland	7.7	0.0%	1.26	No	3	0.00	9	0.85	2	3	0.030
	Memorial Medical Center of East Texas, Lufkin	13.5	0.0%	1.05	No	6	0.00	10	0.66	2	3	0.026
	Memorial Medical Center, Corpus Christi	10.2	0.0%	1.24	No	5	0.21	12	0.85	2	3	0.057
	Methodist Hospital, Houston	13.1	0.0%	1.25	Yes	7	0.19	12	1.33	2	1	0.026
	Methodist Hospital, Lubbock	13.4	0.0%	1.03	No	4	0.00	10	0.89	2	2	0.025
	Methodist Medical Center, Dallas	12.7	0.0%	1.22	Yes	6	0.19	11	0.90	2	2	0.046
	Mother Frances Hospital Regional Center, Tyler	11.2	0.0%	1.15	No	4	0.00	9	1.16	2	3	0.071
	Northeast Baptist Hospital, San Antonio	12.8	0.0%	1.24	No	5	0.01	8	1.11	2	5	0.602
	Osteopathic Medical Center of Texas, Fort Worth	12.8	0.0%	1.05	No	5	0.38	7	0.66	2	1	0.035
	Providence Memorial Hospital, El Paso	9.7	0.0%	1.18	No	5	0.00	8	0.67	2	2	0.071
	San Jacinto Methodist Hospital, Baytown	9.1	0.0%	1.17	No	7	0.15	6	0.66	1	2	0.011
	Seton Medical Center, Austin	10.9	0.0%	1.14	No	5	0.00	10	0.71	2	2	0.050
	Shannon Medical Center, San Angelo	6.1	0.0%	1.35	No	4	0.00	8	0.77	2	2	0.031
	Sierra Medical Center, El Paso	6.5	0.0%	1.27	No	3	0.00	6	0.82	2	1	0.043
	Southwest Texas Methodist Hospital, San Antonio	12.2	0.0%	1.02	No	3	0.00	11	0.95	1	1	0.042
	Spohn Health System, Corpus Christi	11.6	0.0%	1.11	No	5	0.00	10	0.74	2	2	0.062
	St. David's Hospital, Austin	12.1	0.0%	1.13	No	6	0.00	6	0.76	2	3	0.242
	St. Elizabeth Hospital, Beaumont	9.9	0.0%	1.22	No	5	0.00	10	0.92	2	4	0.024
	St. Joseph Hospital and Health Center, Bryan	11.3	0.0%	1.06	No	4	0.00	9	0.85	1	2	0.052
	St. Joseph Hospital, Fort Worth	8.0	0.0%	1.24	No	5	0.00	7	0.68	2	2	0.035
	St. Mary of the Plains Hospital, Lubbock	8.0	0.0%	1.24	No	4	0.02	7	0.74	2	3	0.042
	Texas Heart Institute-St. Luke's Episcopal, Houston	11.4	0.0%	1.31	Yes	6	0.26	9	1.36	2	1	0.045
	Texoma Medical Center, Denison	8.0	0.0%	1.29	No	5	0.00	9	0.80	2	3	0.016
	Valley Baptist Medical Center, Harlingen	11.4	0.0%	1.16	No	6	0.00	11	0.87	2	3	0.021
	Wadley Regional Medical Center, Texarkana	9.2	0.0%	1.24	No	5	0.00	10	0.83	2	3	0.039
	Wichita General Hospital, Wichita Falls	5.3	0.0%	1.36	No	3	0.04	9	0.62	2	1	0.038

GYNECOLOGY

Natl. Rank	Hospital	U.S. News index	Reputational score	Hospital-wide mortality rate	Interns and residents to beds	Technology score (of 10)	R.N.'s to beds	Board-certified OB-GYNs to beds	Procedures to beds
	TIER ONE								
3	University of Texas M.D. Anderson Cancer Ctr., Houston	85.9	22.5%	0.38	0.70	9	1.88	0.040	0.75
12	Parkland Memorial Hospital, Dallas	43.9	10.2%	1.22	1.35	9	0.93	0.024	0.11
27	Baylor University Medical Center, Dallas	32.0	4.0%	0.89	0.29	7	1.38	0.008	0.53
	TIER TWO								
73	Presbyterian Hospital, Dallas	23.4	0.9%	0.89	0.19	7	1.03	0.076	0.64
55	Scott and White Memorial Hospital, Temple	25.6	2.1%	1.01	0.71	7	1.32	0.039	0.64
	TIER THREE								
	East Texas Medical Center, Tyler	18.1	0.0%	0.89	0.00	6	0.85	0.043	0.52
	HCA Medical Plaza Hospital, Fort Worth	14.5	0.0%	0.94	0.00	5	0.65	0.035	0.35
	Harris Methodist Fort Worth	16.4	0.0%	1.03	0.01	6	1.29	0.067	0.82
	Harris Methodist-HEB, Bedford	16.7	0.0%	0.84	0.00	5	0.65	0.049	0.32
	Hermann Hospital, Houston	14.1	0.0%	1.26	0.48	6	1.42	0.067	0.15
	Medical City Dallas Hospital	20.0	0.0%	0.98	0.00	9	1.15	0.112	0.41
	Memorial City Medical Center, Houston	18.3	0.0%	0.86	0.00	8	0.55	0.046	0.25
	Methodist Hospital, Houston	14.6	0.5%	1.25	0.19	8	1.33	0.035	0.31
	Methodist Hospital, Lubbock	14.3	0.0%	1.03	0.00	7	0.89	0.023	0.55
	San Antonio Regional Hospital	15.0	0.0%	0.98	0.04	6	0.91	0.018	0.24
	Santa Rosa Health Care Corp, San Antonio	15.8	0.0%	0.98	0.00	7	0.81	0.045	0.24

Natl. Rank	Hospital	U.S. News index	Reputa-tional score	Hospital-wide mortality rate	Interns and residents to beds	Tech-nology score (of 10)	R.N.'s to beds	Board-certified OB-GYNs to beds	Procedures to beds
	Southwest Texas Methodist Hospital, San Antonio	17.1	0.0%	1.02	0.00	8	0.95	0.093	0.87
	St. Mary Hospital, Port Arthur	16.0	0.0%	0.85	0.05	4	0.68	0.033	0.34
	St. Paul Medical Center, Dallas	15.8	0.0%	1.13	0.25	8	1.17	0.061	0.39
	University of Texas Medical Branch Hospitals, Galveston	18.7	0.0%	1.16	1.09	9	1.19	0.024	0.13
TIER FOUR									
	All Saints Episcopal Hospital, Fort Worth	12.1	0.0%	1.08	0.00	6	0.85	0.029	0.60
	Amarillo Hospital District, Amarillo	12.4	0.0%	1.22	0.10	7	1.26	0.038	0.57
	Arlington Memorial Hospital, Arlington	10.1	0.0%	1.13	0.00	4	0.86	0.049	0.42
	Baptist Hospital of Southeast Texas, Beaumont	10.4	0.0%	1.09	0.00	6	0.53	0.023	0.16
	Baptist Medical Center, San Antonio	9.5	0.0%	1.24	0.00	6	0.79	0.069	0.80
	Bethania Regional Health Center, Wichita Falls	9.5	0.0%	1.11	0.03	4	0.61	0.045	0.55
	Citizens Medical Center, Victoria	14.0	0.0%	0.98	0.00	7	0.59	0.009	0.34
	Clear Lake Regional Medical Center, Webbster	13.7	0.0%	0.96	0.00	6	0.52	0.021	0.29
	Good Shepherd Medical Center, Longview	9.2	0.0%	1.29	0.00	6	1.17	0.018	0.47
	HCA Rio Grande Regional Hospital, McAllen	9.7	0.0%	1.12	0.00	4	0.74	0.040	0.58
	Harris County Hospital District, Houston	7.5	0.0%	1.56	0.46	7	0.75	0.068	0.09
	Hendrick Medical Center, Abilene	8.5	0.0%	1.30	0.00	6	0.98	0.033	0.44
	High Plains Baptist Health System, Amarillo	12.5	0.0%	1.11	0.02	5	1.11	0.048	0.68
	Hillcrest Baptist Medical Center, Waco	8.4	0.0%	1.44	0.06	9	0.80	0.044	0.71
	Houston Northwest Medical Center	10.2	0.0%	1.05	0.00	3	0.73	0.022	0.19
	Irving Healthcare System, Irving	13.7	0.0%	1.10	0.00	6	1.10	0.066	0.45
	McAllen Medical Center, McAllen	10.6	0.0%	1.13	0.03	6	0.71	0.031	0.44
	Medical Center Hospital, Conroe	13.3	0.0%	1.18	0.00	7	1.37	0.041	0.23
	Medical Center Hospital, Odessa	8.6	0.0%	1.21	0.05	8	0.30	0.027	0.25
	Memorial Hospital System, Houston	13.7	0.0%	1.12	0.04	8	0.96	0.045	0.30
	Memorial Hospital and Medical Center, Midland	8.6	0.0%	1.26	0.00	6	0.85	0.033	0.38
	Memorial Medical Center of East Texas, Lufkin	12.6	0.0%	1.05	0.00	7	0.66	0.013	0.39
	Memorial Medical Center, Corpus Christi	10.7	0.0%	1.24	0.21	7	0.85	0.040	0.25
	Methodist Medical Center, Dallas	12.4	0.0%	1.22	0.19	8	0.90	0.056	0.51
	Mother Frances Hospital Regional Center, Tyler	13.3	0.0%	1.15	0.00	7	1.16	0.052	0.94
	Northeast Baptist Hospital, San Antonio	11.0	0.0%	1.24	0.01	5	1.11	0.159	1.85
	Osteopathic Medical Center of Texas, Fort Worth	12.9	0.0%	1.05	0.38	5	0.66	0.022	0.35
	Providence Memorial Hospital, El Paso	10.4	0.0%	1.18	0.00	6	0.67	0.074	0.40
	San Jacinto Methodist Hospital, Baytown	7.5	0.0%	1.17	0.15	3	0.66	0.011	0.15
	Seton Medical Center, Austin	12.3	0.4%	1.14	0.00	6	0.71	0.065	0.68
	Shannon Medical Center, San Angelo	6.7	0.0%	1.35	0.00	6	0.77	0.026	0.34
	Sierra Medical Center, El Paso	8.6	0.0%	1.27	0.00	5	0.82	0.076	0.45
	Spohn Health System, Corpus Christi	12.7	0.0%	1.11	0.00	7	0.74	0.070	0.63
	St. Anthony's Hospital, Amarillo	12.6	0.0%	0.97	0.00	6	0.42	0.004	0.35
	St. David's Hospital, Austin	12.7	0.4%	1.13	0.00	5	0.76	0.106	0.82
	St. Elizabeth Hospital, Beaumont	11.0	0.0%	1.22	0.00	8	0.92	0.030	0.47
	St. Joseph Hospital and Health Center, Bryan	13.3	0.0%	1.06	0.00	6	0.85	0.052	0.44
	St. Joseph Hospital, Fort Worth	7.0	0.0%	1.24	0.00	5	0.68	0.009	0.11
	St. Joseph Hospital, Houston	14.0	0.0%	1.07	0.15	8	0.73	0.034	0.25
	St. Mary of the Plains Hospital, Lubbock	7.2	0.0%	1.24	0.02	4	0.74	0.037	0.41
	Texas Heart Institute-St. Luke's Episcopal, Houston	12.0	0.4%	1.31	0.26	5	1.36	0.052	0.25
	Texoma Medical Center, Denison	8.0	0.0%	1.29	0.00	7	0.80	0.005	0.24
	Valley Baptist Medical Center, Harlingen	11.8	0.0%	1.16	0.00	8	0.87	0.023	0.52
	Wadley Regional Medical Center, Texarkana	9.5	0.0%	1.24	0.00	7	0.83	0.028	0.42
	Wichita General Hospital, Wichita Falls	5.6	0.0%	1.36	0.04	5	0.62	0.038	0.80

NEUROLOGY

Natl. Rank	Hospital	U.S. News index	Reputa-tional score	Neurology mortality rate	COTH member	Interns and residents to beds	Tech-nology score (of 9)	R.N.'s to beds	Board-certified neurologists to beds
	TIER TWO								
63	Baylor University Medical Center, Dallas	18.6	2.6%	0.94	Yes	0.29	6	1.38	0.001
78	Scott and White Memorial Hospital, Temple	18.0	0.7%	0.90	Yes	0.71	6	1.32	0.013
	TIER THREE								
	Baptist Hospital of Southeast Texas, Beaumont	13.2	0.0%	0.58	No	0.00	5	0.53	0.010
	Citizens Medical Center, Victoria	14.1	0.0%	0.75	No	0.00	7	0.59	0.013
	East Texas Medical Center, Tyler	13.4	0.0%	0.80	No	0.00	6	0.85	0.013
	HCA Medical Plaza Hospital, Fort Worth	13.5	0.0%	0.67	No	0.00	5	0.65	0.010
	Harris Methodist-HEB, Bedford	13.4	0.0%	0.69	No	0.00	5	0.65	0.009
	Hermann Hospital, Houston	15.7	1.1%	1.18	Yes	0.48	5	1.42	0.040
	Irving Healthcare System, Irving	13.6	0.0%	0.84	No	0.00	6	1.10	0.018
	Memorial City Medical Center, Houston	14.0	0.0%	0.62	No	0.00	7	0.55	0.012
	Methodist Hospital, Houston	16.8	3.0%	1.25	Yes	0.19	8	1.33	0.029
	Methodist Hospital, Lubbock	12.9	0.0%	0.81	No	0.00	6	0.89	0.005
	Methodist Medical Center, Dallas	12.1	0.0%	1.04	Yes	0.19	7	0.90	0.010
	Northeast Medical Center Hospital, Humble	16.2	0.0%	0.59	No	0.00	7	0.96	0.030
	Parkland Memorial Hospital, Dallas	15.4	0.0%	1.13	Yes	1.35	8	0.93	0.018
	Presbyterian Hospital, Dallas	13.9	0.2%	0.84	No	0.19	6	1.03	0.011
	San Antonio Regional Hospital	15.3	0.0%	0.77	No	0.04	6	0.91	0.022
	San Jacinto Methodist Hospital, Baytown	13.3	0.0%	0.68	No	0.15	3	0.66	0.008
	Southwest Texas Methodist Hospital, San Antonio	14.1	0.0%	0.81	No	0.00	7	0.95	0.018
	St. Anthony's Hospital, Amarillo	12.9	0.0%	0.77	No	0.00	6	0.42	0.008
	St. David's Hospital, Austin	11.7	0.0%	0.93	No	0.00	4	0.76	0.040
	St. Joseph Hospital, Houston	12.2	0.0%	0.86	No	0.15	7	0.73	0.007
	St. Mary Hospital, Port Arthur	11.1	0.0%	0.84	No	0.05	4	0.68	0.005
	St. Paul Medical Center, Dallas	15.6	0.0%	0.89	Yes	0.25	7	1.17	0.012
	Texas Heart Institute-St. Luke's Episcopal, Houston	17.0	0.0%	0.85	Yes	0.26	5	1.36	0.022
	University of Texas Medical Branch Hospitals, Galveston	16.0	0.0%	1.04	Yes	1.09	8	1.19	0.011
	Valley Baptist Medical Center, Harlingen	13.6	0.0%	0.79	No	0.00	7	0.87	0.005
	TIER FOUR								
	All Saints Episcopal Hospital, Fort Worth	8.6	0.0%	1.01	No	0.00	5	0.85	0.007
	Amarillo Hospital District, Amarillo	5.6	0.0%	1.41	No	0.10	6	1.26	0.003
	Arlington Memorial Hospital, Arlington	9.5	0.0%	0.93	No	0.00	3	0.86	0.008
	Bethania Regional Health Center, Wichita Falls	7.6	0.0%	1.02	No	0.03	4	0.61	0.005
	Clear Lake Regional Medical Center, Webbster	8.3	0.0%	1.00	No	0.00	6	0.52	0.009
	Good Shepherd Medical Center, Longview	7.0	0.0%	1.23	No	0.00	6	1.17	0.007
	HCA Rio Grande Regional Hospital, McAllen	6.3	0.0%	1.16	No	0.00	4	0.74	0.010
	Harris County Hospital District, Houston	9.8	0.0%	1.31	Yes	0.46	6	0.75	0.022
	Hendrick Medical Center, Abilene	9.3	0.0%	1.05	No	0.00	6	0.98	0.016
	High Plains Baptist Health System, Amarillo	9.5	0.0%	0.99	No	0.02	4	1.11	0.007
	Hillcrest Baptist Medical Center, Waco	6.1	0.0%	1.31	No	0.06	8	0.80	0.009
	Houston Northwest Medical Center	7.6	0.0%	1.02	No	0.00	3	0.73	0.007
	McAllen Medical Center, McAllen	5.7	0.0%	1.22	No	0.03	5	0.71	0.007
	Medical City Dallas Hospital	9.7	0.0%	1.13	No	0.00	8	1.15	0.024
	Memorial Hospital System, Houston	9.4	0.0%	1.05	No	0.04	7	0.96	0.012
	Memorial Hospital and Medical Center, Midland	6.8	0.0%	1.17	No	0.00	6	0.85	0.007
	Memorial Medical Center of East Texas, Lufkin	8.7	0.0%	1.00	No	0.00	7	0.66	0.004
	Mother Frances Hospital Regional Center, Tyler	8.3	0.0%	1.16	No	0.00	6	1.16	0.015
	Osteopathic Medical Center of Texas, Fort Worth	7.8	0.0%	1.11	No	0.38	4	0.66	0.009
	Providence Memorial Hospital, El Paso	7.9	0.0%	1.06	No	0.00	5	0.67	0.015
	Santa Rosa Health Care Corp, San Antonio	10.6	0.0%	0.94	No	0.00	6	0.81	0.015
	Seton Medical Center, Austin	8.8	0.0%	1.03	No	0.00	5	0.71	0.019
	Shannon Medical Center, San Angelo	3.9	0.0%	1.40	No	0.00	5	0.77	0.004
	Sierra Medical Center, El Paso	7.9	0.0%	1.04	No	0.00	4	0.82	0.007

Natl. Rank	Hospital	U.S. News index	Reputational score	Neurology mortality rate	COTH member	Interns and residents to beds	Technology score (of 9)	R.N.'s to beds	Board-certified neurologists to beds
	Spohn Health System, Corpus Christi	9.7	0.0%	1.04	No	0.00	7	0.74	0.025
	St. Elizabeth Hospital, Beaumont	7.0	0.0%	1.19	No	0.00	7	0.92	0.006
	St. Joseph Hospital and Health Center, Bryan	8.0	0.0%	1.04	No	0.00	5	0.85	0.005
	St. Joseph Hospital, Fort Worth	9.3	0.0%	0.99	No	0.00	5	0.68	0.018
	St. Mary of the Plains Hospital, Lubbock	8.0	0.0%	1.02	No	0.02	3	0.74	0.010
	Texoma Medical Center, Denison	4.0	0.0%	1.47	No	0.00	7	0.80	0.005
	Wadley Regional Medical Center, Texarkana	8.8	0.0%	1.02	No	0.00	7	0.83	0.003
	Wichita General Hospital, Wichita Falls	9.5	0.0%	0.97	No	0.04	5	0.62	0.017

ORTHOPEDICS

Natl. Rank	Hospital	U.S. News index	Reputational score	Orthopedics mortality rate	COTH member	Interns and residents to beds	Technology score (of 5)	R.N.'s to beds	Board-certified orthopedists to beds	Procedures to beds
	TIER ONE									
14	University of Texas M.D. Anderson Cancer Ctr., Houston	24.4	2.9%	0.20	Yes	0.70	5	1.88	0.022	0.69
	TIER TWO									
61	Baylor University Medical Center, Dallas	15.7	0.5%	0.68	Yes	0.29	3	1.38	0.026	2.25
80	Parkland Memorial Hospital, Dallas	14.5	1.2%	1.25	Yes	1.35	4	0.93	0.008	0.40
	TIER THREE									
	Citizens Medical Center, Victoria	10.5	0.4%	0.53	No	0.00	4	0.59	0.026	2.01
	Clear Lake Regional Medical Center, Webbster	8.5	0.0%	0.66	No	0.00	3	0.52	0.013	1.28
	HCA Medical Plaza Hospital, Fort Worth	9.1	0.0%	0.71	No	0.00	4	0.65	0.020	2.42
	HCA Spring Branch Medical Center, Houston	10.0	0.0%	0.50	No	0.00	4	0.80	0.019	1.30
	Harris Methodist-HEB, Bedford	8.4	0.0%	0.47	No	0.00	2	0.65	0.022	1.72
	Hermann Hospital, Houston	10.8	0.0%	1.12	Yes	0.48	3	1.42	0.040	0.96
	High Plains Baptist Health System, Amarillo	8.2	0.0%	0.87	No	0.02	3	1.11	0.026	3.81
	Irving Healthcare System, Irving	10.4	0.0%	0.64	No	0.00	3	1.10	0.035	1.99
	Medical Center Hospital, Conroe	11.0	0.0%	0.32	No	0.00	3	1.37	0.018	1.96
	Medical City Dallas Hospital	11.7	0.0%	0.57	No	0.00	5	1.15	0.039	1.63
	Memorial City Medical Center, Houston	9.5	0.0%	0.16	No	0.00	4	0.55	0.014	2.45
	Memorial Medical Center of East Texas, Lufkin	9.6	0.0%	0.52	No	0.00	4	0.66	0.013	1.41
	Methodist Hospital, Houston	12.6	1.0%	1.12	Yes	0.19	4	1.33	0.042	2.62
	Methodist Medical Center, Dallas	10.4	0.0%	0.95	Yes	0.19	4	0.90	0.017	2.17
	Northeast Baptist Hospital, San Antonio	9.2	0.0%	1.07	No	0.01	4	1.11	0.109	10.35
	Osteopathic Medical Center of Texas, Fort Worth	9.4	0.0%	0.73	No	0.38	3	0.66	0.013	2.09
	Presbyterian Hospital, Dallas	9.4	0.0%	0.73	No	0.19	2	1.03	0.021	3.45
	San Antonio Regional Hospital	8.6	0.0%	0.80	No	0.04	3	0.91	0.102	2.42
	Santa Rosa Health Care Corp, San Antonio	9.3	0.0%	0.49	No	0.00	3	0.81	0.025	1.07
83	Scott and White Memorial Hospital, Temple	14.3	0.4%	0.89	Yes	0.71	3	1.32	0.016	3.03
	Southwest Texas Methodist Hospital, San Antonio	9.9	0.0%	0.79	No	0.00	5	0.95	0.078	2.74
	St. Joseph Hospital, Houston	9.2	0.0%	0.73	No	0.15	4	0.73	0.018	1.31
	St. Paul Medical Center, Dallas	9.9	0.0%	1.18	Yes	0.25	4	1.17	0.045	2.09
	Texas Heart Institute-St. Luke's Episcopal, Houston	10.9	0.0%	1.06	Yes	0.26	4	1.36	0.022	1.52
	University of Texas Medical Branch Hospitals, Galveston	11.9	0.4%	1.48	Yes	1.09	4	1.19	0.010	0.62
	TIER FOUR									
	All Saints Episcopal Hospital, Fort Worth	5.5	0.0%	1.27	No	0.00	4	0.85	0.039	3.98
	Amarillo Hospital District, Amarillo	3.4	0.0%	2.47	No	0.10	4	1.26	0.019	1.46
	Arlington Memorial Hospital, Arlington	3.4	0.0%	1.34	No	0.00	2	0.86	0.027	1.79
	Baptist Medical Center, San Antonio	5.9	0.0%	1.07	No	0.00	3	0.79	0.047	4.46
	Bethania Regional Health Center, Wichita Falls	4.1	0.0%	1.37	No	0.03	3	0.61	0.045	4.92
	East Texas Medical Center, Tyler	6.7	0.0%	1.04	No	0.00	4	0.85	0.033	3.96
	Good Shepherd Medical Center, Longview	6.5	0.0%	1.16	No	0.00	4	1.17	0.025	2.58
	HCA Medical Center of Plano, Plano	5.1	0.0%	1.28	No	0.00	3	1.04	0.081	1.90
	HCA Rio Grande Regional Hospital, McAllen	6.0	0.0%	0.95	No	0.00	3	0.74	0.030	2.05
	HCA South Austin Medical Center, Austin	5.2	0.0%	1.05	No	0.00	2	0.88	0.050	2.39

Natl. Rank	Hospital	U.S. News index	Reputa-tional score	Orthopedics mortality rate	COTH member	Interns and residents to beds	Tech-nology score (of 5)	R.N.'s to beds	Board-certified orthopedists to beds	Pro-cedures to beds
	Harris Methodist Fort Worth	8.1	0.0%	0.99	No	0.01	4	1.29	0.027	3.15
	Hendrick Medical Center, Abilene	7.7	0.0%	0.86	No	0.00	3	0.98	0.016	3.29
	Hillcrest Baptist Medical Center, Waco	5.0	0.0%	1.34	No	0.06	4	0.80	0.016	3.44
	Houston Northwest Medical Center	6.1	0.0%	0.85	No	0.00	2	0.73	0.015	1.54
	McAllen Medical Center, McAllen	3.7	0.0%	1.48	No	0.03	4	0.71	0.017	1.27
	Medical Center Hospital, Odessa	5.0	0.0%	1.01	No	0.05	4	0.30	0.003	1.78
	Memorial Hospital System, Houston	7.2	0.0%	0.97	No	0.04	4	0.96	0.025	1.93
	Memorial Hospital and Medical Center, Midland	3.7	0.0%	1.43	No	0.00	3	0.85	0.010	2.70
	Methodist Hospital, Lubbock	5.5	0.0%	1.16	No	0.00	3	0.89	0.027	4.22
	Mother Frances Hospital Regional Center, Tyler	5.4	0.0%	1.48	No	0.00	4	1.16	0.045	3.57
	Providence Memorial Hospital, El Paso	5.9	0.0%	1.03	No	0.00	4	0.67	0.047	1.78
	Seton Medical Center, Austin	5.2	0.0%	1.15	No	0.00	3	0.71	0.040	4.22
	Shannon Medical Center, San Angelo	5.3	0.0%	1.28	No	0.00	4	0.77	0.031	4.27
	Sierra Medical Center, El Paso	4.6	0.0%	1.31	No	0.00	3	0.82	0.063	3.29
	Spohn Health System, Corpus Christi	5.0	0.0%	1.18	No	0.00	3	0.74	0.047	3.57
	St. Anthony's Hospital, Amarillo	5.5	0.0%	0.99	No	0.00	3	0.42	0.027	4.88
	St. David's Hospital, Austin	4.3	0.0%	1.36	No	0.00	3	0.76	0.093	2.93
	St. Elizabeth Hospital, Beaumont	5.5	0.0%	1.10	No	0.00	3	0.92	0.020	2.48
	St. Joseph Hospital and Health Center, Bryan	6.1	0.0%	1.11	No	0.00	4	0.85	0.031	3.31
	St. Joseph Hospital, Fort Worth	5.9	0.0%	1.04	No	0.00	4	0.68	0.044	2.29
	St. Mary Hospital, Port Arthur	5.9	0.0%	0.86	No	0.05	2	0.68	0.019	1.41
	St. Mary of the Plains Hospital, Lubbock	5.0	0.0%	1.04	No	0.02	2	0.74	0.057	2.48
	Texoma Medical Center, Denison	3.9	0.0%	1.31	No	0.00	3	0.80	0.005	2.21
	Tomball Regional Hospital, Tomball	7.8	0.0%	0.95	No	0.00	3	1.29	0.033	3.20
	University Medical Center, Lubbock	7.9	0.0%	1.48	Yes	0.43	4	0.75	0.032	1.31
	Valley Baptist Medical Center, Harlingen	5.7	0.0%	1.18	No	0.00	4	0.87	0.013	3.30
	Wadley Regional Medical Center, Texarkana	4.5	0.0%	1.34	No	0.00	4	0.83	0.018	1.85
	Wichita General Hospital, Wichita Falls	5.8	0.0%	0.89	No	0.04	2	0.62	0.029	2.54

OTOLARYNGOLOGY

Natl. Rank	Hospital	U.S. News index	Reputa-tional score	Hospital-wide mortality rate	COTH member	Interns and residents to beds	Tech-nology score (of 9)	R.N.'s to beds	Board-certified internists to beds	Procedures to beds
TIER ONE										
9	University of Texas M.D. Anderson Cancer Ctr., Houston	42.7	8.6%	0.38	Yes	0.70	9	1.88	0.083	0.419
32	Parkland Memorial Hospital, Dallas	21.2	2.3%	1.22	Yes	1.35	8	0.93	0.039	0.050
TIER TWO										
51	Baylor University Medical Center, Dallas	18.1	2.2%	0.89	Yes	0.29	6	1.38	0.093	0.159
47	University of Texas Medical Branch Hospitals, Galveston	18.5	1.5%	1.16	Yes	1.09	8	1.19	0.068	0.072
TIER THREE										
	Bexar County Hospital District, San Antonio	11.6	0.0%	1.25	Yes	1.12	5	0.83	0.028	0.073
	Harris County Hospital District, Houston	10.1	0.0%	1.56	Yes	0.46	6	0.75	0.163	0.037
	Hermann Hospital, Houston	10.9	0.0%	1.26	Yes	0.48	4	1.42	0.062	0.099
	John Peter Smith Hospital, Fort Worth	8.2	0.0%	1.70	No	0.79	3	1.47	0.010	0.048
	Methodist Hospital, Houston	12.9	0.8%	1.25	Yes	0.19	8	1.33	0.026	0.173
	Methodist Medical Center, Dallas	8.9	0.0%	1.22	Yes	0.19	7	0.90	0.046	0.154
	Northeast Baptist Hospital, San Antonio	9.4	0.0%	1.24	No	0.01	3	1.11	0.602	0.881
	San Antonio Regional Hospital	7.0	0.0%	0.98	No	0.04	6	0.91	0.271	0.191
	Scott and White Memorial Hospital, Temple	12.2	0.0%	1.01	Yes	0.71	6	1.32	0.059	0.183
	St. Paul Medical Center, Dallas	10.3	0.0%	1.13	Yes	0.25	7	1.17	0.077	0.110
	Texas Heart Institute-St. Luke's Episcopal, Houston	11.6	0.5%	1.31	Yes	0.26	5	1.36	0.045	0.112
	University Medical Center, Lubbock	9.4	0.0%	1.26	Yes	0.43	7	0.75	0.043	0.103
	Zale Lipshy University Hospital, Dallas	9.1	0.0%	0.80	No	0.24	3	1.33	0.340	0.774
TIER FOUR										
	AMI Brownsville Medical Center, Brownsville	2.2	0.0%	1.15	No	0.00	3	0.38	0.024	0.107

Natl. Rank	Hospital	U.S. News index	Reputational score	Hospital-wide mortality rate	COTH member	Interns and residents to beds	Technology score (of 9)	R.N.'s to beds	Board-certified internists to beds	Procedures to beds
	All Saints Episcopal Hospital, Fort Worth	4.1	0.0%	1.08	No	0.00	5	0.85	0.013	0.290
	Amarillo Hospital District, Amarillo	6.0	0.0%	1.23	No	0.10	6	1.26	0.019	0.114
	Arlington Memorial Hospital, Arlington	3.5	0.0%	1.13	No	0.00	2	0.86	0.036	0.157
	Baptist Hospital of Southeast Texas, Beaumont	3.2	0.0%	1.09	No	0.00	5	0.53	0.019	0.168
	Baptist Medical Center, San Antonio	6.2	0.0%	1.24	No	0.00	6	0.79	0.260	0.380
	Bethania Regional Health Center, Wichita Falls	2.8	0.0%	1.11	No	0.03	2	0.61	0.030	0.228
	Citizens Medical Center, Victoria	4.1	0.0%	0.98	No	0.00	7	0.59	0.034	0.163
	Clear Lake Regional Medical Center, Webbster	3.5	0.0%	0.96	No	0.00	6	0.52	0.019	0.124
	East Texas Medical Center, Tyler	4.4	0.0%	0.89	No	0.00	4	0.85	0.059	0.119
	Good Shepherd Medical Center, Longview	5.6	0.0%	1.29	No	0.00	6	1.17	0.050	0.423
	HCA Medical Center of Plano, Plano	5.0	0.0%	0.94	No	0.00	4	1.04	0.063	0.081
	HCA Medical Plaza Hospital, Fort Worth	3.8	0.0%	0.94	No	0.00	4	0.65	0.065	0.100
	HCA Rio Grande Regional Hospital, McAllen	3.3	0.0%	1.12	No	0.00	2	0.74	0.061	0.207
	HCA South Austin Medical Center, Austin	4.7	0.0%	1.00	No	0.00	3	0.88	0.122	0.259
	HCA Spring Branch Medical Center, Houston	3.7	0.0%	1.00	No	0.00	4	0.80	0.006	0.071
	Harris Methodist Fort Worth	5.8	0.0%	1.03	No	0.01	4	1.29	0.082	0.102
	Harris Methodist-HEB, Bedford	4.1	0.0%	0.84	No	0.00	5	0.65	0.053	0.120
	Hendrick Medical Center, Abilene	5.5	0.0%	1.30	No	0.00	6	0.98	0.105	0.147
	High Plains Baptist Health System, Amarillo	5.6	0.0%	1.11	No	0.02	5	1.11	0.088	0.188
	Hillcrest Baptist Medical Center, Waco	4.9	0.0%	1.44	No	0.06	8	0.80	0.016	0.224
	Houston Northwest Medical Center	3.2	0.0%	1.05	No	0.00	3	0.73	0.012	0.111
	Irving Healthcare System, Irving	5.6	0.0%	1.10	No	0.00	6	1.10	0.066	0.168
	McAllen Medical Center, McAllen	3.7	0.0%	1.13	No	0.03	4	0.71	0.038	0.107
	Medical Center Hospital, Conroe	6.0	0.0%	1.18	No	0.00	6	1.37	0.018	0.166
	Medical Center Hospital, Odessa	3.3	0.0%	1.21	No	0.05	7	0.30	0.031	0.160
	Medical City Dallas Hospital	6.8	0.0%	0.98	No	0.00	8	1.15	0.114	0.138
	Memorial City Medical Center, Houston	4.2	0.0%	0.86	No	0.00	7	0.55	0.046	0.123
	Memorial Hospital System, Houston	5.3	0.0%	1.12	No	0.04	7	0.96	0.033	0.151
	Memorial Hospital and Medical Center, Midland	4.4	0.0%	1.26	No	0.00	6	0.85	0.030	0.145
	Memorial Medical Center of East Texas, Lufkin	4.2	0.0%	1.05	No	0.00	7	0.66	0.026	0.168
	Memorial Medical Center, Corpus Christi	6.0	0.0%	1.24	No	0.21	8	0.85	0.057	0.130
	Methodist Hospital, Lubbock	4.7	0.0%	1.03	No	0.00	6	0.89	0.025	0.321
	Mother Frances Hospital Regional Center, Tyler	5.8	0.0%	1.15	No	0.00	6	1.16	0.071	0.157
	Northeast Medical Center Hospital, Humble	5.2	0.0%	0.98	No	0.00	7	0.96	0.018	0.249
	Osteopathic Medical Center of Texas, Fort Worth	4.7	0.0%	1.05	No	0.38	3	0.66	0.035	0.100
	Presbyterian Hospital, Dallas	6.3	0.0%	0.89	No	0.19	6	1.03	0.065	0.074
	Providence Memorial Hospital, El Paso	3.7	0.0%	1.18	No	0.00	4	0.67	0.071	0.199
	R.E. Thomason General Hospital, El Paso	3.7	0.0%	1.42	No	0.37	1	0.66	0.013	0.020
	RHD Memorial Medical Center, Dallas	4.2	0.0%	1.05	No	0.00	5	0.80	0.041	0.088
	Sam Houston Memorial Hospital, Houston	5.5	0.0%	1.06	No	0.00	3	1.05	0.172	0.069
	San Jacinto Methodist Hospital, Baytown	3.5	0.0%	1.17	No	0.15	3	0.66	0.011	0.100
	Santa Rosa Health Care Corp, San Antonio	5.0	0.0%	0.98	No	0.00	6	0.81	0.085	0.098
	Seton Medical Center, Austin	4.0	0.0%	1.13	No	0.00	5	0.71	0.050	0.165
	Shannon Medical Center, San Angelo	3.9	0.0%	1.35	No	0.00	5	0.77	0.031	0.285
	Sierra Medical Center, El Paso	3.3	0.0%	1.27	No	0.00	2	0.82	0.043	0.214
	Southwest Texas Methodist Hospital, San Antonio	5.3	0.0%	1.02	No	0.00	7	0.95	0.042	0.364
	Spohn Health System, Corpus Christi	4.7	0.0%	1.11	No	0.00	7	0.74	0.062	0.192
	St. Anthony's Hospital, Amarillo	3.2	0.0%	0.97	No	0.00	6	0.42	0.023	0.124
	St. David's Hospital, Austin	5.2	0.0%	1.13	No	0.00	3	0.76	0.242	0.103
	St. Elizabeth Hospital, Beaumont	4.9	0.0%	1.22	No	0.00	7	0.92	0.024	0.237
	St. Joseph Hospital and Health Center, Bryan	4.5	0.0%	1.06	No	0.00	5	0.85	0.052	0.263
	St. Joseph Hospital, Fort Worth	3.1	0.0%	1.24	No	0.00	3	0.68	0.035	0.105
	St. Joseph Hospital, Houston	5.1	0.0%	1.07	No	0.15	7	0.73	0.041	0.093
	St. Mary Hospital, Port Arthur	4.0	0.0%	0.85	No	0.05	5	0.68	0.019	0.164
	St. Mary of the Plains Hospital, Lubbock	3.5	0.0%	1.24	No	0.02	3	0.74	0.042	0.192
	Texoma Medical Center, Denison	4.4	0.0%	1.29	No	0.00	7	0.80	0.016	0.143

Natl. Rank	Hospital	U.S. News index	Reputa-tional score	Hospital-wide mortality rate	COTH member	Interns and residents to beds	Tech-nology score (of 9)	R.N.'s to beds	Board-certified internists to beds	Procedures to beds
	Tomball Regional Hospital, Tomball	5.2	0.0%	0.98	No	0.00	3	1.29	0.033	0.473
	University of Texas Health Center, Tyler	3.7	0.0%	1.29	No	0.14	2	0.78	0.042	0.169
	Valley Baptist Medical Center, Harlingen	4.8	0.0%	1.16	No	0.00	7	0.87	0.021	0.156
	Wadley Regional Medical Center, Texarkana	4.8	0.0%	1.24	No	0.00	7	0.83	0.039	0.142
	Wichita General Hospital, Wichita Falls	3.6	0.0%	1.36	No	0.04	5	0.62	0.038	0.071

RHEUMATOLOGY

Natl. Rank	Hospital	U.S. News index	Reputa-tional score	Hospital-wide mortality rate	COTH member	Interns and residents to beds	Tech-nology score (of 5)	R.N.'s to beds	Board-certified internists to beds
TIER ONE									
21	Parkland Memorial Hospital, Dallas	24.7	4.8%	1.22	Yes	1.35	4	0.93	0.039
TIER TWO									
79	Baylor University Medical Center, Dallas	16.3	0.7%	0.89	Yes	0.29	3	1.38	0.093
34	University of Texas M.D. Anderson Cancer Ctr., Houston	20.3	0.7%	0.38	Yes	0.70	5	1.88	0.083
TIER THREE									
	East Texas Medical Center, Tyler	10.1	0.0%	0.89	No	0.00	4	0.85	0.059
	Harris Methodist Fort Worth	10.0	0.0%	1.03	No	0.01	4	1.29	0.082
	Hermann Hospital, Houston	12.1	0.0%	1.26	Yes	0.48	3	1.42	0.062
	Medical City Dallas Hospital	9.7	0.0%	0.98	No	0.00	5	1.15	0.114
	Methodist Hospital, Houston	11.1	0.0%	1.25	Yes	0.19	4	1.33	0.026
	Methodist Medical Center, Dallas	10.3	0.0%	1.22	Yes	0.19	4	0.90	0.046
	Northeast Baptist Hospital, San Antonio	11.8	0.0%	1.24	No	0.01	4	1.11	0.602
	Scott and White Memorial Hospital, Temple	14.3	0.0%	1.01	Yes	0.71	3	1.32	0.059
	St. Paul Medical Center, Dallas	12.1	0.0%	1.13	Yes	0.25	4	1.17	0.077
	Texas Heart Institute-St. Luke's Episcopal, Houston	11.2	0.0%	1.31	Yes	0.26	4	1.36	0.045
	University of Texas Medical Branch Hospitals, Galveston	14.5	0.0%	1.16	Yes	1.09	4	1.19	0.068
TIER FOUR									
	AMI Brownsville Medical Center, Brownsville	6.2	0.0%	1.15	No	0.00	4	0.38	0.024
	All Saints Episcopal Hospital, Fort Worth	7.8	0.0%	1.08	No	0.00	4	0.85	0.013
	Amarillo Hospital District, Amarillo	8.3	0.0%	1.23	No	0.10	4	1.26	0.019
	Arlington Memorial Hospital, Arlington	5.7	0.0%	1.13	No	0.00	2	0.86	0.036
	Baptist Hospital of Southeast Texas, Beaumont	6.5	0.0%	1.09	No	0.00	3	0.53	0.019
	Baptist Medical Center, San Antonio	7.9	0.0%	1.24	No	0.00	3	0.79	0.260
	Bethania Regional Health Center, Wichita Falls	6.7	0.0%	1.11	No	0.03	3	0.61	0.030
	Citizens Medical Center, Victoria	8.2	0.0%	0.98	No	0.00	4	0.59	0.034
	Clear Lake Regional Medical Center, Webbster	7.6	0.0%	0.96	No	0.00	3	0.52	0.019
	Good Shepherd Medical Center, Longview	7.6	0.0%	1.29	No	0.00	4	1.17	0.050
	HCA Medical Plaza Hospital, Fort Worth	9.0	0.0%	0.94	No	0.00	4	0.65	0.065
	HCA Rio Grande Regional Hospital, McAllen	7.2	0.0%	1.12	No	0.00	3	0.74	0.061
	HCA South Austin Medical Center, Austin	7.5	0.0%	1.00	No	0.00	2	0.88	0.122
	HCA Spring Branch Medical Center, Houston	8.4	0.0%	1.00	No	0.00	4	0.80	0.006
	Harris County Hospital District, Houston	9.4	0.0%	1.56	Yes	0.46	5	0.75	0.163
	Harris Methodist-HEB, Bedford	9.1	0.0%	0.84	No	0.00	2	0.65	0.053
	Hendrick Medical Center, Abilene	7.0	0.0%	1.30	No	0.00	3	0.98	0.105
	High Plains Baptist Health System, Amarillo	8.5	0.0%	1.11	No	0.02	3	1.11	0.088
	Hillcrest Baptist Medical Center, Waco	5.8	0.0%	1.44	No	0.06	4	0.80	0.016
	Houston Northwest Medical Center	6.9	0.0%	1.05	No	0.00	2	0.73	0.012
	Irving Healthcare System, Irving	8.3	0.0%	1.10	No	0.00	3	1.10	0.066
	McAllen Medical Center, McAllen	7.4	0.0%	1.13	No	0.03	4	0.71	0.038
	Medical Center Hospital, Conroe	8.1	0.0%	1.18	No	0.00	3	1.37	0.018
	Medical Center Hospital, Odessa	5.8	0.0%	1.21	No	0.05	4	0.30	0.031
	Memorial City Medical Center, Houston	9.5	0.0%	0.86	No	0.00	4	0.55	0.046
	Memorial Hospital System, Houston	8.1	0.0%	1.12	No	0.04	4	0.96	0.033
	Memorial Hospital and Medical Center, Midland	6.3	0.0%	1.26	No	0.00	3	0.85	0.030

Natl. Rank	Hospital	U.S. News index	Reputa-tional score	Hospital-wide mortality rate	COTH member	Interns and residents to beds	Tech-nology score (of 5)	R.N.'s to beds	Board-certified internists to beds
	Memorial Medical Center of East Texas, Lufkin	7.7	0.0%	1.05	No	0.00	4	0.66	0.026
	Memorial Medical Center, Corpus Christi	8.2	0.0%	1.24	No	0.21	5	0.85	0.057
	Methodist Hospital, Lubbock	8.0	0.0%	1.03	No	0.00	3	0.89	0.025
	Mother Frances Hospital Regional Center, Tyler	8.6	0.0%	1.15	No	0.00	4	1.16	0.071
	Northeast Medical Center Hospital, Humble	9.0	0.0%	0.98	No	0.00	4	0.96	0.018
	Osteopathic Medical Center of Texas, Fort Worth	8.5	0.0%	1.05	No	0.38	3	0.66	0.035
	Presbyterian Hospital, Dallas	9.2	0.0%	0.89	No	0.19	2	1.03	0.065
	Providence Memorial Hospital, El Paso	7.1	0.0%	1.18	No	0.00	4	0.67	0.071
	San Antonio Regional Hospital	9.4	0.0%	0.98	No	0.04	3	0.91	0.271
	San Jacinto Methodist Hospital, Baytown	4.8	0.0%	1.17	No	0.15	1	0.66	0.011
	Santa Rosa Health Care Corp, San Antonio	8.7	0.0%	0.98	No	0.00	3	0.81	0.085
	Seton Medical Center, Austin	6.9	0.0%	1.13	No	0.00	3	0.71	0.050
	Shannon Medical Center, San Angelo	6.1	0.0%	1.35	No	0.00	4	0.77	0.031
	Sierra Medical Center, El Paso	7.1	0.4%	1.27	No	0.00	3	0.82	0.043
	Southwest Texas Methodist Hospital, San Antonio	8.3	0.0%	1.02	No	0.00	5	0.95	0.042
	Spohn Health System, Corpus Christi	7.2	0.0%	1.11	No	0.00	3	0.74	0.062
	St. Anthony's Hospital, Amarillo	7.3	0.0%	0.97	No	0.00	3	0.42	0.023
	St. David's Hospital, Austin	8.5	0.0%	1.13	No	0.00	3	0.76	0.242
	St. Elizabeth Hospital, Beaumont	6.7	0.0%	1.22	No	0.00	3	0.92	0.024
	St. Joseph Hospital and Health Center, Bryan	7.3	0.0%	1.06	No	0.00	4	0.85	0.052
	St. Joseph Hospital, Fort Worth	6.5	0.0%	1.24	No	0.00	4	0.68	0.035
	St. Joseph Hospital, Houston	8.3	0.0%	1.07	No	0.15	4	0.73	0.041
	St. Mary Hospital, Port Arthur	9.0	0.0%	0.85	No	0.05	2	0.68	0.019
	St. Mary of the Plains Hospital, Lubbock	5.8	0.0%	1.24	No	0.02	2	0.74	0.042
	Texoma Medical Center, Denison	5.9	0.0%	1.29	No	0.00	3	0.80	0.016
	University of Texas Health Center, Tyler	5.4	0.0%	1.29	No	0.14	3	0.78	0.042
	Valley Baptist Medical Center, Harlingen	7.4	0.0%	1.16	No	0.00	4	0.87	0.021
	Wadley Regional Medical Center, Texarkana	6.9	0.0%	1.24	No	0.00	4	0.83	0.039
	Wichita General Hospital, Wichita Falls	4.9	0.0%	1.36	No	0.04	2	0.62	0.038

UROLOGY

Natl. Rank	Hospital	U.S. News index	Reputa-tional score	Urology mortality rate	COTH member	Interns and residents to beds	Tech-nology score (of 11)	R.N.'s to beds	Board-certified internists to beds	Procedures to beds
	TIER ONE									
9	University of Texas M.D. Anderson Cancer Ctr., Houston	37.7	13.7%	0.51	Yes	0.70	10	1.88	0.083	1.76
11	Baylor University Medical Center, Dallas	28.8	9.4%	0.72	Yes	0.29	8	1.38	0.093	1.44
	TIER TWO									
28	Parkland Memorial Hospital, Dallas	21.0	2.8%	0.81	Yes	1.35	9	0.93	0.039	0.71
68	Scott and White Memorial Hospital, Temple	16.6	0.8%	0.88	Yes	0.71	8	1.32	0.059	2.56
	TIER THREE									
	Amarillo Hospital District, Amarillo	11.9	0.0%	0.51	No	0.10	7	1.26	0.019	0.89
	Bexar County Hospital District, San Antonio	11.9	0.0%	1.15	Yes	1.12	6	0.83	0.028	0.52
	East Texas Medical Center, Tyler	9.5	0.0%	0.87	No	0.00	7	0.85	0.059	3.32
	Hermann Hospital, Houston	10.9	0.0%	1.29	Yes	0.48	6	1.42	0.062	1.32
	Medical City Dallas Hospital	12.8	0.0%	0.37	No	0.00	10	1.15	0.114	1.10
	Methodist Hospital, Houston	12.9	1.8%	1.29	Yes	0.19	10	1.33	0.026	1.31
	Methodist Hospital, Lubbock	11.5	0.0%	0.73	No	0.00	8	0.89	0.025	2.82
	Northeast Medical Center Hospital, Humble	11.4	0.0%	0.68	No	0.00	8	0.96	0.018	2.02
	Presbyterian Hospital, Dallas	8.7	0.0%	0.99	No	0.19	7	1.03	0.065	1.07
	San Antonio Regional Hospital	8.9	0.0%	1.07	No	0.04	8	0.91	0.271	3.77
	Southwest Texas Methodist Hospital, San Antonio	8.8	0.0%	0.92	No	0.00	8	0.95	0.042	1.68
	St. Anthony's Hospital, Amarillo	9.9	0.0%	0.72	No	0.00	7	0.42	0.023	2.35
	St. Mary Hospital, Port Arthur	10.3	0.0%	0.69	No	0.05	5	0.68	0.019	2.85
	St. Paul Medical Center, Dallas	8.7	0.0%	1.57	Yes	0.25	8	1.17	0.077	0.97

Natl. Rank Hospital	U.S. News index	Reputa- tional score	Urology mortality rate	COTH member	Interns and residents to beds	Tech- nology score (of 11)	R.N.'s to beds	Board- certified internists to beds	Procedures to beds
Texas Heart Institute-St. Luke's Episcopal, Houston	10.5	1.8%	1.73	Yes	0.26	6	1.36	0.045	1.72
University of Texas Medical Branch Hospitals, Galveston	12.7	0.0%	1.40	Yes	1.09	10	1.19	0.068	0.94
TIER FOUR									
AMI Brownsville Medical Center, Brownsville	4.9	0.0%	1.14	No	0.00	6	0.38	0.024	1.89
All Saints Episcopal Hospital, Fort Worth	7.8	0.0%	0.94	No	0.00	6	0.85	0.013	2.30
Arlington Memorial Hospital, Arlington	3.3	0.0%	1.50	No	0.00	3	0.86	0.036	1.50
Baptist Hospital of Southeast Texas, Beaumont	3.9	0.0%	1.34	No	0.00	6	0.53	0.019	1.39
Baptist Medical Center, San Antonio	5.8	0.0%	1.60	No	0.00	8	0.79	0.260	4.49
Bethania Regional Health Center, Wichita Falls	8.0	0.0%	0.86	No	0.03	4	0.61	0.030	2.76
Citizens Medical Center, Victoria	4.6	0.0%	1.39	No	0.00	8	0.59	0.034	1.92
Clear Lake Regional Medical Center, Webbster	6.6	0.0%	1.01	No	0.00	8	0.52	0.019	1.39
Good Shepherd Medical Center, Longview	6.8	0.0%	1.33	No	0.00	8	1.17	0.050	2.95
HCA Medical Plaza Hospital, Fort Worth	4.9	0.0%	1.33	No	0.00	6	0.65	0.065	2.44
HCA Rio Grande Regional Hospital, McAllen	5.9	0.0%	1.14	No	0.00	5	0.74	0.061	2.42
HCA South Austin Medical Center, Austin	7.4	0.0%	1.07	No	0.00	5	0.88	0.122	2.96
HCA Spring Branch Medical Center, Houston	7.3	0.0%	0.93	No	0.00	6	0.80	0.006	0.97
Harris County Hospital District, Houston	6.9	0.0%	2.12	Yes	0.46	7	0.75	0.163	0.37
Harris Methodist Fort Worth	6.2	0.0%	1.32	No	0.01	5	1.29	0.082	1.71
Hendrick Medical Center, Abilene	4.3	0.0%	1.87	No	0.00	8	0.98	0.105	1.93
High Plains Baptist Health System, Amarillo	6.5	0.0%	1.20	No	0.02	5	1.11	0.088	1.77
Hillcrest Baptist Medical Center, Waco	6.7	0.0%	1.25	No	0.06	10	0.80	0.016	2.60
Houston Northwest Medical Center	4.6	0.0%	1.25	No	0.00	5	0.73	0.012	1.49
Irving Healthcare System, Irving	7.4	0.0%	1.12	No	0.00	7	1.10	0.066	1.85
McAllen Medical Center, McAllen	6.8	0.0%	1.02	No	0.03	5	0.71	0.038	2.30
Medical Center Hospital, Conroe	3.4	0.0%	2.42	No	0.00	7	1.37	0.018	1.96
Medical Center Hospital, Odessa	3.6	0.0%	1.58	No	0.05	9	0.30	0.031	2.33
Memorial City Medical Center, Houston	7.5	0.0%	0.96	No	0.00	9	0.55	0.046	1.09
Memorial Hospital System, Houston	7.6	0.0%	1.06	No	0.04	8	0.96	0.033	1.61
Memorial Hospital and Medical Center, Midland	7.3	0.0%	1.05	No	0.00	8	0.85	0.030	1.66
Memorial Medical Center of East Texas, Lufkin	6.5	0.0%	1.10	No	0.00	8	0.66	0.026	2.16
Memorial Medical Center, Corpus Christi	3.6	0.0%	2.32	No	0.21	9	0.85	0.057	1.76
Methodist Medical Center, Dallas	7.8	0.8%	1.97	Yes	0.19	8	0.90	0.046	2.36
Mother Frances Hospital Regional Center, Tyler	5.6	0.0%	1.48	No	0.00	7	1.16	0.071	1.81
Northeast Baptist Hospital, San Antonio	7.9	0.0%	1.60	No	0.01	6	1.11	0.602	10.41
Osteopathic Medical Center of Texas, Fort Worth	5.2	0.0%	1.38	No	0.38	5	0.66	0.035	1.75
Providence Memorial Hospital, El Paso	4.4	0.0%	1.34	No	0.00	5	0.67	0.071	1.67
San Jacinto Methodist Hospital, Baytown	2.8	0.0%	1.67	No	0.15	4	0.66	0.011	1.63
Santa Rosa Health Care Corp, San Antonio	5.8	0.0%	1.24	No	0.00	7	0.81	0.085	1.08
Seton Medical Center, Austin	4.6	0.0%	1.37	No	0.00	6	0.71	0.050	1.94
Shannon Medical Center, San Angelo	2.4	0.0%	2.06	No	0.00	6	0.77	0.031	2.18
Sierra Medical Center, El Paso	3.7	0.0%	1.52	No	0.00	4	0.82	0.043	2.44
Spohn Health System, Corpus Christi	5.8	0.0%	1.32	No	0.00	8	0.74	0.062	2.83
St. David's Hospital, Austin	7.1	0.0%	1.08	No	0.00	5	0.76	0.242	2.36
St. Elizabeth Hospital, Beaumont	7.4	0.0%	1.08	No	0.00	8	0.92	0.024	2.26
St. Joseph Hospital and Health Center, Bryan	5.0	0.0%	1.34	No	0.00	6	0.85	0.052	1.72
St. Joseph Hospital, Fort Worth	2.2	0.0%	1.90	No	0.00	5	0.68	0.035	1.89
St. Joseph Hospital, Houston	6.6	0.0%	1.21	No	0.15	9	0.73	0.041	1.46
St. Mary of the Plains Hospital, Lubbock	2.4	0.0%	1.78	No	0.02	4	0.74	0.042	1.21
Texoma Medical Center, Denison	3.3	0.0%	1.90	No	0.00	8	0.80	0.016	2.15
Tomball Regional Hospital, Tomball	6.7	0.0%	1.23	No	0.00	4	1.29	0.033	3.69
Valley Baptist Medical Center, Harlingen	7.3	0.0%	1.05	No	0.00	8	0.87	0.021	1.85
Wadley Regional Medical Center, Texarkana	7.6	0.0%	1.05	No	0.00	9	0.83	0.039	1.88
Wichita General Hospital, Wichita Falls	4.5	0.0%	1.39	No	0.04	6	0.62	0.038	2.64

AIDS

Natl. Rank	Hospital	U.S. News index	Reputational score	Hospital-wide mortality rate	COTH member	Interns and residents to beds	Technology score (of 11)	Discharge planning (of 2)	R.N.'s to beds	Board-certified internists to beds
	TIER TWO									
52	University of Utah Hospitals and Clinics, Salt Lake City	26.8	0.0%	0.81	Yes	0.88	6	2	1.73	0.021
	TIER THREE									
	Cottonwood Hospital Medical Center, Murray	20.7	0.0%	0.99	No	0.00	6	2	0.99	0.109
	LDS Hospital, Salt Lake City	23.2	0.0%	0.81	No	0.13	7	2	1.04	0.077
	McKay-Dee Hospital Center, Ogden	21.2	0.0%	0.87	No	0.05	5	1	0.95	0.032
	TIER FOUR									
	St. Benedict's Hospital, Ogden	19.3	0.0%	1.03	No	0.00	6	2	0.74	0.042
	Utah Valley Regional Medical Center, Provo	18.8	0.0%	1.18	No	0.00	8	2	1.19	0.054

CANCER

Natl. Rank	Hospital	U.S. News index	Reputational score	Cancer mortality rate	COTH member	Interns and residents to beds	Technology score (of 12)	R.N.'s to beds	Board-certified oncologists to beds	Procedures to beds
	TIER TWO									
45	University of Utah Hospitals and Clinics, Salt Lake City	13.2	0.7%	0.68	Yes	0.88	9	1.73	0.028	0.95
	TIER THREE									
	LDS Hospital, Salt Lake City	5.7	0.0%	0.57	No	0.13	10	1.04	0.011	1.02
	TIER FOUR									
	Holy Cross Hospital, Salt Lake City	3.4	0.0%	0.84	No	0.10	5	0.89	0.005	1.15
	McKay-Dee Hospital Center, Ogden	2.9	0.0%	0.80	No	0.05	3	0.95	0.006	0.80
	St. Benedict's Hospital, Ogden	2.7	0.0%	1.49	No	0.00	7	0.74	0.008	0.70
	Utah Valley Regional Medical Center, Provo	4.8	0.0%	1.01	No	0.00	9	1.19	0.006	0.81

CARDIOLOGY

Natl. Rank	Hospital	U.S. News index	Reputational score	Cardiology mortality rate	COTH member	Interns and residents to beds	Technology score (of 10)	R.N.'s to beds	Board-certified cardiologists to beds	Procedures to beds
	TIER TWO									
63	LDS Hospital, Salt Lake City	22.1	1.8%	0.79	No	0.13	9	1.04	0.055	7.16
30	University of Utah Hospitals and Clinics, Salt Lake City	26.1	0.0%	0.54	Yes	0.88	7	1.73	0.075	2.84
	TIER THREE									
	McKay-Dee Hospital Center, Ogden	14.5	0.0%	0.99	No	0.05	8	0.95	0.020	4.27
	TIER FOUR									
	Holy Cross Hospital, Salt Lake City	12.3	0.0%	1.13	No	0.10	8	0.89	0.045	7.43
	Utah Valley Regional Medical Center, Provo	13.0	0.0%	1.10	No	0.00	9	1.19	0.020	5.69

ENDOCRINOLOGY

Natl. Rank	Hospital	U.S. News index	Reputational score	Endocrinology mortality rate	COTH member	Interns and residents to beds	Technology score (of 11)	R.N.'s to beds	Board-certified internists to beds
	TIER TWO								
61	University of Utah Hospitals and Clinics, Salt Lake City	16.2	0.0%	0.80	Yes	0.88	9	1.73	0.021
	TIER THREE								
	Holy Cross Hospital, Salt Lake City	9.5	0.0%	0.73	No	0.10	6	0.89	0.070
	LDS Hospital, Salt Lake City	8.4	0.0%	0.98	No	0.13	10	1.04	0.077

Natl. Rank	Hospital	U.S. News index	Reputational score	Endocrinology mortality rate	COTH member	Interns and residents to beds	Technology score (of 11)	R.N.'s to beds	Board-certified internists to beds
	McKay-Dee Hospital Center, Ogden	9.8	0.0%	0.31	No	0.05	4	0.95	0.032
	St. Benedict's Hospital, Ogden	9.9	0.0%	0.44	No	0.00	8	0.74	0.042
TIER FOUR									
	Utah Valley Regional Medical Center, Provo	5.7	0.0%	1.49	No	0.00	9	1.19	0.054

GASTROENTEROLOGY

Natl. Rank	Hospital	U.S. News index	Reputational score	Gastro-enterology mortality rate	COTH member	Interns and residents to beds	Technology score (of 11)	R.N.'s to beds	Board-certified gastro-enterologists to beds	Procedures to beds
TIER TWO										
61	University of Utah Hospitals and Clinics, Salt Lake City	14.1	0.0%	0.95	Yes	0.88	9	1.73	0.021	1.28
TIER THREE										
	LDS Hospital, Salt Lake City	9.5	0.0%	0.78	No	0.13	9	1.04	0.015	3.20
TIER FOUR										
	Holy Cross Hospital, Salt Lake City	6.7	0.0%	1.02	No	0.10	6	0.89	0.015	3.80
	McKay-Dee Hospital Center, Ogden	6.8	0.0%	0.76	No	0.05	4	0.95	0.009	1.99
	Utah Valley Regional Medical Center, Provo	5.2	0.0%	1.44	No	0.00	8	1.19	0.011	3.10

GERIATRICS

Natl. Rank	Hospital	U.S. News index	Reputational score	Hospital-wide mortality rate	COTH member	Service mix	Interns and residents to beds	Technology score (of 13)	R.N.'s to beds	Discharge planning (of 2)	Geriatric services (of 9)	Board-certified internists to beds
TIER TWO												
32	University of Utah Hospitals and Clinics, Salt Lake City	26.7	0.7%	0.81	Yes	6	0.88	10	1.73	2	5	0.021
TIER THREE												
	Holy Cross Hospital, Salt Lake City	13.9	0.0%	1.01	No	5	0.10	6	0.89	2	2	0.070
100	LDS Hospital, Salt Lake City	20.6	0.3%	0.81	No	6	0.13	12	1.04	2	3	0.077
	McKay-Dee Hospital Center, Ogden	17.4	0.0%	0.87	No	7	0.05	6	0.95	1	3	0.032
TIER FOUR												
	Utah Valley Regional Medical Center, Provo	12.1	0.0%	1.18	No	6	0.00	11	1.19	2	4	0.054

GYNECOLOGY

Natl. Rank	Hospital	U.S. News index	Reputational score	Hospital-wide mortality rate	Interns and residents to beds	Technology score (of 10)	R.N.'s to beds	Board-certified OB-GYNs to beds	Procedures to beds
TIER TWO									
74	LDS Hospital, Salt Lake City	23.4	0.4%	0.81	0.13	9	1.04	0.070	0.66
35	University of Utah Hospitals and Clinics, Salt Lake City	28.4	0.4%	0.81	0.88	8	1.73	0.044	0.35
TIER THREE									
	Holy Cross Hospital, Salt Lake City	16.0	0.0%	1.01	0.10	6	0.89	0.090	0.60
	McKay-Dee Hospital Center, Ogden	18.2	0.0%	0.87	0.05	5	0.95	0.049	0.51
	Utah Valley Regional Medical Center, Provo	14.5	0.4%	1.18	0.00	8	1.19	0.048	0.44

NEUROLOGY

Natl. Rank	Hospital	U.S. News index	Reputa-tional score	Neurology mortality rate	COTH member	Interns and residents to beds	Tech-nology score (of 9)	R.N.'s to beds	Board-certified neurologists to beds
TIER TWO									
47	University of Utah Hospitals and Clinics, Salt Lake City	20.7	0.6%	0.95	Yes	0.88	7	1.73	0.039
TIER FOUR									
	Holy Cross Hospital, Salt Lake City	10.8	0.0%	0.96	No	0.10	6	0.89	0.015
	LDS Hospital, Salt Lake City	9.9	0.0%	1.08	No	0.13	8	1.04	0.015
	Utah Valley Regional Medical Center, Provo	8.0	0.0%	1.23	No	0.00	7	1.19	0.017

ORTHOPEDICS

Natl. Rank	Hospital	U.S. News index	Reputa-tional score	Orthopedics mortality rate	COTH member	Interns and residents to beds	Tech-nology score (of 5)	R.N.'s to beds	Board-certified orthopedists to beds	Pro-cedures to beds
TIER TWO										
65	University of Utah Hospitals and Clinics, Salt Lake City	15.4	1.5%	1.32	Yes	0.88	3	1.73	0.021	2.35
TIER THREE										
	Holy Cross Hospital, Salt Lake City	10.8	0.0%	0.69	No	0.10	4	0.89	0.040	3.74
	LDS Hospital, Salt Lake City	10.7	0.0%	0.72	No	0.13	4	1.04	0.035	3.36
TIER FOUR										
	Cottonwood Hospital Medical Center, Murray	7.0	0.0%	1.19	No	0.00	4	0.99	0.156	4.18
	McKay-Dee Hospital Center, Ogden	6.9	0.0%	0.94	No	0.05	3	0.95	0.029	2.49
	St. Benedict's Hospital, Ogden	6.2	0.0%	0.91	No	0.00	3	0.74	0.021	1.67
	Utah Valley Regional Medical Center, Provo	5.3	0.0%	1.53	No	0.00	4	1.19	0.037	3.54

OTOLARYNGOLOGY

Natl. Rank	Hospital	U.S. News index	Reputa-tional score	Hospital-wide mortality rate	COTH member	Interns and residents to beds	Tech-nology score (of 9)	R.N.'s to beds	Board-certified internists to beds	Procedures to beds
TIER TWO										
88	University of Utah Hospitals and Clinics, Salt Lake City	14.3	0.0%	0.81	Yes	0.88	7	1.73	0.021	0.268
TIER FOUR										
	Cottonwood Hospital Medical Center, Murray	5.4	0.0%	0.99	No	0.00	5	0.99	0.109	0.184
	Holy Cross Hospital, Salt Lake City	4.9	0.0%	1.01	No	0.10	4	0.89	0.070	0.125
	LDS Hospital, Salt Lake City	6.9	0.0%	0.81	No	0.13	8	1.04	0.077	0.116
	McKay-Dee Hospital Center, Ogden	4.1	0.0%	0.87	No	0.05	2	0.95	0.032	0.187
	St. Benedict's Hospital, Ogden	4.3	0.0%	1.03	No	0.00	6	0.74	0.042	0.113
	Utah Valley Regional Medical Center, Provo	6.0	0.0%	1.18	No	0.00	7	1.19	0.054	0.130

RHEUMATOLOGY

Natl. Rank	Hospital	U.S. News index	Reputa-tional score	Hospital-wide mortality rate	COTH member	Interns and residents to beds	Tech-nology score (of 5)	R.N.'s to beds	Board-certified internists to beds
TIER TWO									
30	University of Utah Hospitals and Clinics, Salt Lake City	21.1	1.6%	0.81	Yes	0.88	3	1.73	0.021
TIER THREE									
	LDS Hospital, Salt Lake City	11.7	0.0%	0.81	No	0.13	4	1.04	0.077
TIER FOUR									
	Holy Cross Hospital, Salt Lake City	9.3	0.0%	1.01	No	0.10	4	0.89	0.070
	McKay-Dee Hospital Center, Ogden	9.0	0.0%	0.87	No	0.05	3	0.95	0.032
	Utah Valley Regional Medical Center, Provo	8.3	0.0%	1.18	No	0.00	4	1.19	0.054

UROLOGY

Natl. Rank	Hospital	U.S. News index	Reputa-tional score	Urology mortality rate	COTH member	Interns and residents to beds	Tech-nology score (of 11)	R.N.'s to beds	Board-certified internists to beds	Procedures to beds
TIER TWO										
47	**University of Utah Hospitals and Clinics, Salt Lake City**	**18.5**	1.4%	0.89	Yes	0.88	9	1.73	0.021	1.20
TIER THREE										
	Cottonwood Hospital Medical Center, Murray	8.6	0.0%	1.02	No	0.00	7	0.99	0.109	3.14
	LDS Hospital, Salt Lake City	12.2	0.6%	0.82	No	0.13	9	1.04	0.077	2.28
	McKay-Dee Hospital Center, Ogden	10.2	0.0%	0.66	No	0.05	4	0.95	0.032	0.83
	Utah Valley Regional Medical Center, Provo	9.8	0.0%	0.89	No	0.00	8	1.19	0.054	1.44
TIER FOUR										
	Holy Cross Hospital, Salt Lake City	6.8	0.0%	1.18	No	0.10	6	0.89	0.070	2.65

STATE RANKINGS ■ UTAH

AIDS

Natl. Rank	Hospital	U.S. News index	Reputa-tional score	Hospital-wide mortality rate	COTH member	Interns and residents to beds	Tech-nology score (of 11)	Discharge planning (of 2)	R.N.'s to beds	Board-certified internists to beds
	TIER THREE									
	Medical Center Hospital of Vermont, Burlington, Vt.	**21.2**	0.0%	1.23	Yes	0.79	7	2	0.78	0.241
	TIER FOUR									
	Fanny Allen Hospital, Colchester, Vt.	**16.6**	0.0%	1.15	No	0.07	4	2	0.42	0.060

CANCER

Natl. Rank	Hospital	U.S. News index	Reputa-tional score	Cancer mortality rate	COTH member	Interns and residents to beds	Tech-nology score (of 12)	R.N.'s to beds	Board-certified oncologists to beds	Procedures to beds
	TIER THREE									
	Medical Center Hospital of Vermont, Burlington, Vt.	**8.9**	0.0%	0.93	Yes	0.79	9	0.78	0.000	1.06
	TIER FOUR									
	Fanny Allen Hospital, Colchester, Vt.	**1.3**	0.0%	1.17	No	0.07	2	0.42	0.036	2.54

CARDIOLOGY

Natl. Rank	Hospital	U.S. News index	Reputa-tional score	Cardiology mortality rate	COTH member	Interns and residents to beds	Tech-nology score (of 10)	R.N.'s to beds	Board-certified cardiologists to beds	Procedures to beds
	TIER THREE									
	Medical Center Hospital of Vermont, Burlington, Vt.	**14.5**	0.0%	1.21	Yes	0.79	7	0.78	0.000	7.06

ENDOCRINOLOGY

Natl. Rank	Hospital	U.S. News index	Reputa-tional score	Endocrinology mortality rate	COTH member	Interns and residents to beds	Tech-nology score (of 11)	R.N.'s to beds	Board-certified internists to beds
	TIER THREE								
	Medical Center Hospital of Vermont, Burlington, Vt.	**13.2**	0.0%	1.03	Yes	0.79	10	0.78	0.241

GASTROENTEROLOGY

Natl. Rank	Hospital	U.S. News index	Reputa-tional score	Gastro-enterology mortality rate	COTH member	Interns and residents to beds	Tech-nology score (of 11)	R.N.'s to beds	Board-certified gastro-enterologists to beds	Pro-cedures to beds
	TIER THREE									
	Medical Center Hospital of Vermont, Burlington, Vt.	**11.6**	0.0%	0.99	Yes	0.79	9	0.78	0.000	2.01

GERIATRICS

Natl. Rank	Hospital	U.S. News index	Reputa-tional score	Hospital-wide mortality rate	COTH member	Service mix	Interns and residents to beds	Tech-nology score (of 13)	R.N.'s to beds	Discharge planning (of 2)	Geriatric services (of 9)	Board-certified internists to beds
	TIER THREE											
	Medical Center Hospital of Vermont, Burlington, Vt.	**14.0**	0.0%	1.23	Yes	5	0.79	10	0.78	2	2	0.241

GYNECOLOGY

Natl. Rank	Hospital	U.S. News index	Reputational score	Hospital-wide mortality rate	Interns and residents to beds	Technology score (of 10)	R.N.'s to beds	Board-certified OB-GYNs to beds	Procedures to beds
TIER FOUR									
	Medical Center Hospital of Vermont, Burlington, Vt.	14.0	0.0%	1.23	0.79	8	0.78	0.046	0.45

NEUROLOGY

Natl. Rank	Hospital	U.S. News index	Reputational score	Neurology mortality rate	COTH member	Interns and residents to beds	Technology score (of 9)	R.N.'s to beds	Board-certified neurologists to beds
TIER THREE									
	Medical Center Hospital of Vermont, Burlington, Vt.	12.5	0.8%	1.31	Yes	0.79	8	0.78	0.018

ORTHOPEDICS

Natl. Rank	Hospital	U.S. News index	Reputational score	Orthopedics mortality rate	COTH member	Interns and residents to beds	Technology score (of 5)	R.N.'s to beds	Board-certified orthopedists to beds	Procedures to beds
TIER THREE										
	Medical Center Hospital of Vermont, Burlington, Vt.	13.0	0.0%	0.86	Yes	0.79	4	0.78	0.038	1.95

OTOLARYNGOLOGY

Natl. Rank	Hospital	U.S. News index	Reputational score	Hospital-wide mortality rate	COTH member	Interns and residents to beds	Technology score (of 9)	R.N.'s to beds	Board-certified internists to beds	Procedures to beds
TIER THREE										
	Medical Center Hospital of Vermont, Burlington, Vt.	12.8	0.0%	1.23	Yes	0.79	8	0.78	0.241	0.157
TIER FOUR										
	Fanny Allen Hospital, Colchester, Vt.	2.3	0.0%	1.15	No	0.07	1	0.42	0.060	0.217

RHEUMATOLOGY

Natl. Rank	Hospital	U.S. News index	Reputational score	Hospital-wide mortality rate	COTH member	Interns and residents to beds	Technology score (of 5)	R.N.'s to beds	Board-certified internists to beds
TIER THREE									
	Medical Center Hospital of Vermont, Burlington, Vt.	13.3	0.0%	1.23	Yes	0.79	4	0.78	0.241

UROLOGY

Natl. Rank	Hospital	U.S. News index	Reputational score	Urology mortality rate	COTH member	Interns and residents to beds	Technology score (of 11)	R.N.'s to beds	Board-certified internists to beds	Procedures to beds
TIER THREE										
	Medical Center Hospital of Vermont, Burlington, Vt.	12.1	0.0%	1.20	Yes	0.79	9	0.78	0.241	1.10

AIDS

Natl. Rank	Hospital	U.S. News index	Reputa-tional score	Hospital-wide mortality rate	COTH member	Interns and residents to beds	Tech-nology score (of 11)	Discharge planning (of 2)	R.N.'s to beds	Board-certified internists to beds
	TIER TWO									
84	**Fairfax Hospital, Falls Church**	25.3	0.8%	0.97	Yes	0.15	8	2	1.34	0.122
90	**Medical College of Virginia Hospitals, Richmond**	25.0	0.9%	1.11	Yes	0.93	9	2	1.27	0.094
63	**University of Virginia Health Sciences Ctr., Charlottesville**	26.4	1.3%	1.21	Yes	1.41	9	2	1.92	0.101
	TIER THREE									
	Bon Secours-St. Mary's Hospital, Richmond	20.3	0.0%	1.03	No	0.02	7	2	0.87	0.116
	HCA Henrico Doctor's Hospital, Richmond	20.4	0.0%	1.07	No	0.00	8	2	1.35	0.014
	Sentara Norfolk General Hospital, Norfolk	19.8	0.0%	1.28	Yes	0.16	7	2	1.18	0.176
	Winchester Medical Center, Winchester	20.3	0.0%	0.97	No	0.00	5	2	0.90	0.060
	TIER FOUR									
	Alexandria Hospital, Alexandria	19.1	0.0%	1.03	No	0.00	5	2	0.67	0.116
	Arlington Hospital, Arlington	15.2	0.0%	1.41	No	0.06	6	2	0.71	0.049
	Bon Secours-Maryview Medical Center, Portsmouth	16.6	0.0%	1.24	No	0.02	7	2	0.50	0.040
	Community Hospital of Roanoke Valley, Roanoke	15.0	0.0%	1.47	No	0.08	5	2	1.14	0.032
	Danville Regional Medical Center, Danville	15.3	0.0%	1.36	No	0.00	6	2	0.71	0.021
	Fair Oaks Hospital, Fairfax	18.2	0.0%	1.11	No	0.01	5	2	0.78	0.103
	HCA Chippenham Medical Center, Richmond	19.3	0.0%	1.04	No	0.03	5	2	0.83	0.112
	HCA Lewis-Gale Hospital, Salem	16.1	0.0%	1.22	No	0.00	7	1	0.51	0.021
	Johnston-Willis Hospital, Richmond	18.5	0.0%	1.08	No	0.00	7	1	0.79	0.066
	Lynchburg General Hospital, Lynchburg	18.4	0.0%	1.08	No	0.02	6	2	0.51	0.074
	Mary Washington Hospital, Fredericksburg	14.7	0.0%	1.46	No	0.00	7	2	0.61	0.028
	Portsmouth General Hospital, Portsmouth	14.6	0.0%	1.42	No	0.04	5	2	0.58	0.098
	Richmond Memorial Hospital, Richmond	15.7	0.0%	1.30	No	0.00	5	2	0.72	0.068
	Riverside Regional Medical Center, Newport News	17.1	0.0%	1.30	No	0.28	6	2	0.91	0.085
	Roanoke Memorial Hospitals, Roanoke	17.3	0.0%	1.33	No	0.35	8	2	0.81	0.025
	Rockingham Memorial Hospital, Harrisonburg	16.9	0.0%	1.22	No	0.00	6	2	0.91	0.012
	Virginia Baptist Hospital, Lynchburg	16.3	0.0%	1.30	No	0.01	6	2	0.86	0.070
	Virginia Beach General Hospital, Virginia Beach	17.3	0.0%	1.12	No	0.01	7	1	0.53	0.021

CANCER

Natl. Rank	Hospital	U.S. News index	Reputa-tional score	Cancer mortality rate	COTH member	Interns and residents to beds	Tech-nology score (of 12)	R.N.'s to beds	Board-certified oncologists to beds	Procedures to beds
	TIER TWO									
65	**Medical College of Virginia Hospitals, Richmond**	12.0	0.5%	0.90	Yes	0.93	11	1.27	0.016	0.84
27	**University of Virginia Health Sciences Ctr., Charlottesville**	15.3	0.0%	0.58	Yes	1.41	11	1.92	0.012	1.86
	TIER THREE									
	Fairfax Hospital, Falls Church	8.8	0.0%	0.78	Yes	0.15	9	1.34	0.035	1.23
	Sentara Norfolk General Hospital, Norfolk	8.0	0.0%	1.31	Yes	0.16	10	1.18	0.011	1.31
	TIER FOUR									
	Alexandria Hospital, Alexandria	3.1	0.0%	0.90	No	0.00	7	0.67	0.022	1.11
	Arlington Hospital, Arlington	3.3	0.0%	1.08	No	0.06	7	0.71	0.013	1.61
	Bon Secours-Maryview Medical Center, Portsmouth	2.5	0.0%	1.24	No	0.02	8	0.50	0.003	1.12
	Bon Secours-St. Mary's Hospital, Richmond	4.3	0.0%	1.23	No	0.02	9	0.87	0.021	2.69
	Community Hospital of Roanoke Valley, Roanoke	3.2	0.0%	1.21	No	0.08	3	1.14	0.018	1.16
	Danville Regional Medical Center, Danville	2.2	0.0%	1.44	No	0.00	5	0.71	0.005	1.62
	Depaul Medical Center, Norfolk	5.0	0.0%	1.04	No	0.14	9	0.88	0.018	3.28
	HCA Chippenham Medical Center, Richmond	2.9	0.0%	0.72	No	0.03	4	0.83	0.007	0.90
	HCA Henrico Doctor's Hospital, Richmond	5.0	0.0%	1.23	No	0.00	8	1.35	0.019	1.58
	HCA Lewis-Gale Hospital, Salem	3.0	0.0%	1.18	No	0.00	9	0.51	0.012	1.68
	Johnston-Willis Hospital, Richmond	3.6	0.0%	1.05	No	0.00	8	0.79	0.004	2.01

Natl. Rank	Hospital	U.S. News index	Reputational score	Cancer mortality rate	COTH member	Interns and residents to beds	Technology score (of 12)	R.N.'s to beds	Board-certified oncologists to beds	Procedures to beds
	Lynchburg General Hospital, Lynchburg	1.9	0.0%	1.08	No	0.02	5	0.51	0.012	1.10
	Mary Washington Hospital, Fredericksburg	2.6	0.0%	1.81	No	0.00	8	0.61	0.006	1.54
	Richmond Memorial Hospital, Richmond	1.7	0.0%	1.05	No	0.00	2	0.72	0.013	1.48
	Riverside Regional Medical Center, Newport News	4.2	0.0%	1.51	No	0.28	7	0.91	0.012	1.47
	Roanoke Memorial Hospitals, Roanoke	5.1	0.0%	1.32	No	0.35	9	0.81	0.014	2.46
	Rockingham Memorial Hospital, Harrisonburg	3.4	0.0%	1.76	No	0.00	7	0.91	0.008	2.70
	Virginia Baptist Hospital, Lynchburg	3.5	0.0%	1.63	No	0.01	8	0.86	0.011	1.73
	Virginia Beach General Hospital, Virginia Beach	3.1	0.0%	1.36	No	0.01	9	0.53	0.025	1.84
	Winchester Medical Center, Winchester	2.9	0.0%	1.27	No	0.00	5	0.90	0.009	1.70

CARDIOLOGY

Natl. Rank	Hospital	U.S. News index	Reputational score	Cardiology mortality rate	COTH member	Interns and residents to beds	Technology score (of 10)	R.N.'s to beds	Board-certified cardiologists to beds	Procedures to beds
TIER TWO										
42	Fairfax Hospital, Falls Church	23.8	0.5%	0.88	Yes	0.15	9	1.34	0.099	8.00
51	University of Virginia Health Sciences Ctr., Charlottesville	23.0	1.1%	1.19	Yes	1.41	9	1.92	0.019	6.26
TIER THREE										
	Alexandria Hospital, Alexandria	15.3	0.0%	0.95	No	0.00	8	0.67	0.050	5.44
	Bon Secours-Maryview Medical Center, Portsmouth	14.0	0.0%	0.95	No	0.02	7	0.50	0.013	5.88
	Bon Secours-St. Mary's Hospital, Richmond	14.2	0.0%	1.04	No	0.02	8	0.87	0.077	6.78
	HCA Henrico Doctor's Hospital, Richmond	18.0	0.0%	0.96	No	0.00	9	1.35	0.106	10.73
	Johnston-Willis Hospital, Richmond	17.4	0.0%	0.88	No	0.00	7	0.79	0.052	5.24
	Lynchburg General Hospital, Lynchburg	15.4	0.0%	0.88	No	0.02	5	0.51	0.018	7.97
	Medical College of Virginia Hospitals, Richmond	18.9	0.0%	1.14	Yes	0.93	9	1.27	0.046	4.01
	Sentara Norfolk General Hospital, Norfolk	17.6	0.0%	1.08	Yes	0.16	9	1.18	0.062	8.38
	Winchester Medical Center, Winchester	17.4	0.0%	0.88	No	0.00	7	0.90	0.020	11.38
TIER FOUR										
	Arlington Hospital, Arlington	8.0	0.0%	1.36	No	0.06	8	0.71	0.054	5.44
	Community Hospital of Roanoke Valley, Roanoke	5.8	0.0%	1.54	No	0.08	5	1.14	0.021	5.45
	Danville Regional Medical Center, Danville	7.8	0.0%	1.28	No	0.00	6	0.71	0.011	8.28
	Depaul Medical Center, Norfolk	13.1	0.0%	1.07	No	0.14	7	0.88	0.036	6.84
	HCA Chippenham Medical Center, Richmond	13.4	0.0%	1.04	No	0.03	7	0.83	0.039	7.41
	HCA Lewis-Gale Hospital, Salem	8.4	0.0%	1.26	No	0.00	9	0.51	0.015	7.75
	Mary Washington Hospital, Fredericksburg	8.6	0.0%	1.25	No	0.00	8	0.61	0.019	8.17
	Portsmouth General Hospital, Portsmouth	4.8	0.0%	1.46	No	0.04	4	0.58	0.043	4.60
	Richmond Memorial Hospital, Richmond	10.3	0.0%	1.14	No	0.00	6	0.72	0.032	6.95
	Riverside Regional Medical Center, Newport News	13.0	0.0%	1.11	No	0.28	8	0.91	0.035	6.45
	Roanoke Memorial Hospitals, Roanoke	11.5	0.0%	1.23	No	0.35	9	0.81	0.032	11.06
	Rockingham Memorial Hospital, Harrisonburg	12.1	0.0%	1.05	No	0.00	5	0.91	0.016	8.88
	Virginia Baptist Hospital, Lynchburg	12.1	0.0%	1.08	No	0.01	8	0.86	0.017	4.97
	Virginia Beach General Hospital, Virginia Beach	12.2	0.0%	1.10	No	0.01	9	0.53	0.061	7.45

ENDOCRINOLOGY

Natl. Rank	Hospital	U.S. News index	Reputational score	Endocrinology mortality rate	COTH member	Interns and residents to beds	Technology score (of 11)	R.N.'s to beds	Board-certified internists to beds
TIER ONE									
15	University of Virginia Health Sciences Ctr., Charlottesville	26.3	6.0%	0.90	Yes	1.41	10	1.92	0.101
TIER THREE									
	Fairfax Hospital, Falls Church	11.5	0.0%	1.05	Yes	0.15	9	1.34	0.122
99	Medical College of Virginia Hospitals, Richmond	13.6	0.5%	1.23	Yes	0.93	10	1.27	0.094
	Sentara Norfolk General Hospital, Norfolk	10.1	0.0%	1.38	Yes	0.16	10	1.18	0.176
	Winchester Medical Center, Winchester	8.3	0.0%	0.82	No	0.00	7	0.90	0.060

Natl. Rank	Hospital	U.S. News index	Reputational score	Endocrinology mortality rate	COTH member	Interns and residents to beds	Technology score (of 11)	R.N.'s to beds	Board-certified internists to beds
	TIER FOUR								
	Alexandria Hospital, Alexandria	6.2	0.0%	1.05	No	0.00	7	0.67	0.116
	Arlington Hospital, Arlington	4.1	0.0%	1.57	No	0.06	8	0.71	0.049
	Bon Secours-Maryview Medical Center, Portsmouth	4.4	0.0%	1.30	No	0.02	9	0.50	0.040
	Bon Secours-St. Mary's Hospital, Richmond	7.2	0.0%	1.04	No	0.02	9	0.87	0.116
	Community Hospital of Roanoke Valley, Roanoke	5.6	0.0%	1.19	No	0.08	3	1.14	0.032
	Danville Regional Medical Center, Danville	3.0	0.0%	1.71	No	0.00	6	0.71	0.021
	Depaul Medical Center, Norfolk	6.7	0.0%	1.38	No	0.14	9	0.88	0.196
	Fair Oaks Hospital, Fairfax	2.7	0.0%	2.01	No	0.01	4	0.78	0.103
	HCA Chippenham Medical Center, Richmond	6.0	0.0%	1.09	No	0.03	5	0.83	0.112
	HCA Henrico Doctor's Hospital, Richmond	8.0	0.0%	0.98	No	0.00	8	1.35	0.014
	HCA Lewis-Gale Hospital, Salem	4.2	0.0%	1.36	No	0.00	10	0.51	0.021
	Johnston-Willis Hospital, Richmond	5.4	0.0%	1.29	No	0.00	9	0.79	0.066
	Lynchburg General Hospital, Lynchburg	6.0	0.0%	0.95	No	0.02	6	0.51	0.074
	Mary Washington Hospital, Fredericksburg	4.6	0.0%	1.28	No	0.00	9	0.61	0.028
	Portsmouth General Hospital, Portsmouth	3.3	0.0%	1.54	No	0.04	4	0.58	0.098
	Richmond Memorial Hospital, Richmond	3.2	0.0%	1.60	No	0.00	4	0.72	0.068
	Riverside Regional Medical Center, Newport News	6.8	0.0%	1.24	No	0.28	8	0.91	0.085
	Roanoke Memorial Hospitals, Roanoke	6.1	0.0%	1.33	No	0.35	9	0.81	0.025
	Rockingham Memorial Hospital, Harrisonburg	5.5	0.0%	1.20	No	0.00	8	0.91	0.012
	Virginia Baptist Hospital, Lynchburg	7.7	0.0%	0.91	No	0.01	8	0.86	0.070
	Virginia Beach General Hospital, Virginia Beach	4.4	0.0%	1.29	No	0.01	9	0.53	0.021

GASTROENTEROLOGY

Natl. Rank	Hospital	U.S. News index	Reputational score	Gastroenterology mortality rate	COTH member	Interns and residents to beds	Technology score (of 11)	R.N.'s to beds	Board-certified gastroenterologists to beds	Procedures to beds
	TIER TWO									
53	Medical College of Virginia Hospitals, Richmond	14.8	1.7%	1.11	Yes	0.93	10	1.27	0.018	1.10
22	University of Virginia Health Sciences Ctr., Charlottesville	19.0	1.2%	0.95	Yes	1.41	10	1.92	0.009	1.95
	TIER THREE									
	Depaul Medical Center, Norfolk	7.5	0.0%	1.01	No	0.14	8	0.88	0.036	3.73
	Fairfax Hospital, Falls Church	9.6	0.0%	1.18	Yes	0.15	8	1.34	0.046	2.56
	Johnston-Willis Hospital, Richmond	7.6	0.0%	0.92	No	0.00	9	0.79	0.015	3.56
	Sentara Norfolk General Hospital, Norfolk	7.7	0.0%	1.63	Yes	0.16	10	1.18	0.025	1.78
	TIER FOUR									
	Alexandria Hospital, Alexandria	3.8	0.0%	1.24	No	0.00	6	0.67	0.019	2.46
	Arlington Hospital, Arlington	3.8	0.0%	1.45	No	0.06	7	0.71	0.031	2.61
	Bon Secours-Maryview Medical Center, Portsmouth	3.3	0.0%	1.51	No	0.02	8	0.50	0.008	2.91
	Bon Secours-St. Mary's Hospital, Richmond	6.9	0.0%	1.05	No	0.02	9	0.87	0.039	3.39
	Community Hospital of Roanoke Valley, Roanoke	4.3	0.0%	1.55	No	0.08	4	1.14	0.009	4.01
	Danville Regional Medical Center, Danville	5.1	0.0%	1.14	No	0.00	6	0.71	0.008	3.62
	HCA Chippenham Medical Center, Richmond	4.5	0.0%	1.17	No	0.03	5	0.83	0.025	2.65
	HCA Henrico Doctor's Hospital, Richmond	7.2	0.0%	1.23	No	0.00	9	1.35	0.065	3.59
	HCA Lewis-Gale Hospital, Salem	4.5	0.0%	1.45	No	0.00	9	0.51	0.015	4.15
	Lynchburg General Hospital, Lynchburg	5.1	0.0%	1.07	No	0.02	6	0.51	0.009	3.66
	Mary Washington Hospital, Fredericksburg	5.0	0.0%	1.39	No	0.00	9	0.61	0.012	4.22
	Portsmouth General Hospital, Portsmouth	3.5	0.0%	1.22	No	0.04	4	0.58	0.027	2.88
	Richmond Memorial Hospital, Richmond	3.0	0.0%	1.54	No	0.00	4	0.72	0.016	3.80
	Riverside Regional Medical Center, Newport News	4.2	0.0%	1.68	No	0.28	7	0.91	0.014	2.59
	Roanoke Memorial Hospitals, Roanoke	5.4	0.0%	1.64	No	0.35	8	0.81	0.011	3.89
	Rockingham Memorial Hospital, Harrisonburg	6.0	0.0%	1.23	No	0.00	7	0.91	0.008	4.70

Natl. Rank	Hospital	U.S. News index	Reputa-tional score	Gastro-enterology mortality rate	COTH member	Interns and residents to beds	Tech-nology score (of 11)	R.N.'s to beds	Board-certified gastro-enterologists to beds	Pro-cedures to beds
	Virginia Baptist Hospital, Lynchburg	5.0	0.0%	1.19	No	0.01	7	0.86	0.008	2.76
	Virginia Beach General Hospital, Virginia Beach	4.3	0.0%	1.38	No	0.01	8	0.53	0.025	3.69
	Winchester Medical Center, Winchester	5.2	0.0%	1.27	No	0.00	6	0.90	0.009	4.07

GERIATRICS

Natl. Rank	Hospital	U.S. News index	Reputa-tional score	Hospital-wide mortality rate	COTH member	Service mix	Interns and residents to beds	Tech-nology score (of 13)	R.N.'s to beds	Discharge planning (of 2)	Geriatric services (of 9)	Board-certified internists to beds
	TIER TWO											
85	Medical College of Virginia Hospitals, Richmond	22.0	1.0%	1.11	Yes	9	0.93	12	1.27	2	2	0.094
	TIER THREE											
	Bon Secours-St. Mary's Hospital, Richmond	14.0	0.0%	1.03	No	5	0.02	10	0.87	2	1	0.116
	Depaul Medical Center, Norfolk	14.9	0.0%	1.05	No	4	0.14	12	0.88	2	4	0.196
	Fairfax Hospital, Falls Church	19.2	0.0%	0.97	Yes	5	0.15	11	1.34	2	1	0.122
	HCA Chippenham Medical Center, Richmond	13.9	0.0%	1.04	No	5	0.03	6	0.83	2	5	0.112
	HCA Henrico Doctor's Hospital, Richmond	14.0	0.0%	1.07	No	6	0.00	10	1.35	2	2	0.014
	Sentara Norfolk General Hospital, Norfolk	14.2	0.0%	1.28	Yes	9	0.16	12	1.18	2	2	0.176
97	University of Virginia Health Sciences Ctr., Charlottesville	20.6	0.0%	1.21	Yes	9	1.41	12	1.92	2	6	0.101
	Winchester Medical Center, Winchester	15.2	0.0%	0.97	No	5	0.00	9	0.90	2	1	0.060
	TIER FOUR											
	Alexandria Hospital, Alexandria	13.5	0.0%	1.03	No	4	0.00	10	0.67	2	3	0.116
	Arlington Hospital, Arlington	6.0	0.0%	1.41	No	4	0.06	10	0.71	2	3	0.049
	Bon Secours-Maryview Medical Center, Portsmouth	9.6	0.0%	1.24	No	7	0.02	11	0.50	2	3	0.040
	Community Hospital of Roanoke Valley, Roanoke	4.8	0.0%	1.47	No	5	0.08	5	1.14	2	1	0.032
	Danville Regional Medical Center, Danville	5.9	0.0%	1.36	No	5	0.00	8	0.71	2	1	0.021
	HCA Lewis-Gale Hospital, Salem	7.5	0.0%	1.22	No	5	0.00	11	0.51	1	1	0.021
	Johnston-Willis Hospital, Richmond	12.7	0.0%	1.08	No	7	0.00	11	0.79	1	3	0.066
	Lynchburg General Hospital, Lynchburg	11.2	0.0%	1.08	No	4	0.02	8	0.51	2	2	0.074
	Mary Washington Hospital, Fredericksburg	4.8	0.0%	1.46	No	4	0.00	11	0.61	2	2	0.028
	Richmond Memorial Hospital, Richmond	7.3	0.0%	1.30	No	5	0.00	5	0.72	2	4	0.068
	Riverside Regional Medical Center, Newport News	11.8	0.0%	1.30	No	8	0.28	10	0.91	2	8	0.085
	Roanoke Memorial Hospitals, Roanoke	10.6	0.0%	1.33	No	9	0.35	12	0.81	2	3	0.025
	Rockingham Memorial Hospital, Harrisonburg	9.3	0.0%	1.22	No	5	0.00	10	0.91	2	2	0.012
	Virginia Baptist Hospital, Lynchburg	9.8	0.0%	1.30	No	8	0.01	11	0.86	2	3	0.070

GYNECOLOGY

Natl. Rank	Hospital	U.S. News index	Reputa-tional score	Hospital-wide mortality rate	Interns and residents to beds	Tech-nology score (of 10)	R.N.'s to beds	Board-certified OB-GYNs to beds	Procedures to beds
	TIER TWO								
71	Medical College of Virginia Hospitals, Richmond	23.6	1.6%	1.11	0.93	9	1.27	0.020	0.27
38	University of Virginia Health Sciences Ctr., Charlottesville	28.1	2.2%	1.21	1.41	9	1.92	0.021	0.46
	TIER THREE								
	Alexandria Hospital, Alexandria	15.5	0.5%	1.03	0.00	6	0.67	0.146	0.33
	Bon Secours-St. Mary's Hospital, Richmond	16.4	0.0%	1.03	0.02	8	0.87	0.085	0.32
	Depaul Medical Center, Norfolk	15.5	0.0%	1.05	0.14	7	0.88	0.075	0.73
87	Fairfax Hospital, Falls Church	22.2	0.5%	0.97	0.15	8	1.34	0.143	0.41
	HCA Henrico Doctor's Hospital, Richmond	17.7	0.0%	1.07	0.00	8	1.35	0.093	0.50
	Sentara Norfolk General Hospital, Norfolk	15.4	0.6%	1.28	0.16	9	1.18	0.087	0.20
	Winchester Medical Center, Winchester	14.8	0.0%	0.97	0.00	5	0.90	0.034	0.44
	TIER FOUR								
	Arlington Hospital, Arlington	7.5	0.0%	1.41	0.06	7	0.71	0.069	0.32
	Bon Secours-Maryview Medical Center, Portsmouth	8.1	0.0%	1.24	0.02	7	0.50	0.028	0.18

Natl. Rank	Hospital	U.S. News index	Reputational score	Hospital-wide mortality rate	Interns and residents to beds	Technology score (of 10)	R.N.'s to beds	Board-certified OB-GYNs to beds	Procedures to beds
	Community Hospital of Roanoke Valley, Roanoke	6.1	0.0%	1.47	0.08	4	1.14	0.050	0.80
	Danville Regional Medical Center, Danville	5.3	0.0%	1.36	0.00	5	0.71	0.021	0.32
	HCA Chippenham Medical Center, Richmond	12.4	0.0%	1.04	0.03	5	0.83	0.023	0.31
	HCA Lewis-Gale Hospital, Salem	9.2	0.0%	1.22	0.00	8	0.51	0.027	0.41
	Johnston-Willis Hospital, Richmond	12.7	0.0%	1.08	0.00	7	0.79	0.030	0.25
	Lynchburg General Hospital, Lynchburg	10.1	0.0%	1.08	0.02	5	0.51	0.024	0.11
	Mary Washington Hospital, Fredericksburg	6.2	0.0%	1.46	0.00	8	0.61	0.043	0.27
	Richmond Memorial Hospital, Richmond	5.5	0.0%	1.30	0.00	3	0.72	0.045	0.26
	Riverside Regional Medical Center, Newport News	9.7	0.0%	1.30	0.28	6	0.91	0.045	0.38
	Rockingham Memorial Hospital, Harrisonburg	9.5	0.0%	1.22	0.00	6	0.91	0.031	0.56
	Virginia Baptist Hospital, Lynchburg	8.5	0.0%	1.30	0.01	7	0.86	0.023	0.44
	Virginia Beach General Hospital, Virginia Beach	12.7	0.0%	1.12	0.01	8	0.53	0.082	0.33

NEUROLOGY

Natl. Rank	Hospital	U.S. News index	Reputational score	Neurology mortality rate	COTH member	Interns and residents to beds	Technology score (of 9)	R.N.'s to beds	Board-certified neurologists to beds
TIER TWO									
88	Medical College of Virginia Hospitals, Richmond	17.8	0.5%	1.00	Yes	0.93	8	1.27	0.022
49	University of Virginia Health Sciences Ctr., Charlottesville	20.4	1.2%	1.10	Yes	1.41	8	1.92	0.018
TIER THREE									
	Alexandria Hospital, Alexandria	13.4	0.0%	0.83	No	0.00	5	0.67	0.033
	Bon Secours-St. Mary's Hospital, Richmond	15.2	0.0%	0.80	No	0.02	7	0.87	0.033
	Depaul Medical Center, Norfolk	11.7	0.0%	0.93	No	0.14	7	0.88	0.014
97	Fairfax Hospital, Falls Church	17.1	0.0%	0.90	Yes	0.15	7	1.34	0.035
	HCA Henrico Doctor's Hospital, Richmond	12.3	0.0%	0.93	No	0.00	7	1.35	0.014
TIER FOUR									
	Arlington Hospital, Arlington	5.8	0.0%	1.26	No	0.06	6	0.71	0.010
	Bon Secours-Maryview Medical Center, Portsmouth	5.4	0.0%	1.28	No	0.02	7	0.50	0.013
	Community Hospital of Roanoke Valley, Roanoke	3.7	0.0%	1.65	No	0.08	3	1.14	0.018
	Danville Regional Medical Center, Danville	3.7	0.0%	1.41	No	0.00	5	0.71	0.005
	HCA Chippenham Medical Center, Richmond	9.2	0.0%	0.97	No	0.03	4	0.83	0.009
	HCA Lewis-Gale Hospital, Salem	8.0	0.0%	1.06	No	0.00	8	0.51	0.009
	Johnston-Willis Hospital, Richmond	8.2	0.0%	1.14	No	0.00	7	0.79	0.022
	Lynchburg General Hospital, Lynchburg	6.3	0.0%	1.13	No	0.02	5	0.51	0.009
	Mary Washington Hospital, Fredericksburg	5.3	0.0%	1.29	No	0.00	7	0.61	0.009
	Richmond Memorial Hospital, Richmond	6.1	0.0%	1.18	No	0.00	4	0.72	0.013
	Riverside Regional Medical Center, Newport News	8.8	0.0%	1.13	No	0.28	6	0.91	0.014
	Roanoke Memorial Hospitals, Roanoke	6.3	0.0%	1.37	No	0.35	7	0.81	0.009
	Rockingham Memorial Hospital, Harrisonburg	3.4	0.0%	1.59	No	0.00	6	0.91	0.008
	Sentara Norfolk General Hospital, Norfolk	9.2	0.0%	1.43	Yes	0.16	8	1.18	0.017
	Virginia Beach General Hospital, Virginia Beach	7.7	0.0%	1.08	No	0.01	7	0.53	0.011
	Winchester Medical Center, Winchester	8.9	0.0%	1.03	No	0.00	5	0.90	0.014

ORTHOPEDICS

Natl. Rank	Hospital	U.S. News index	Reputational score	Orthopedics mortality rate	COTH member	Interns and residents to beds	Technology score (of 5)	R.N.'s to beds	Board-certified orthopedists to beds	Procedures to beds
TIER TWO										
76	Medical College of Virginia Hospitals, Richmond	14.7	0.0%	0.83	Yes	0.93	4	1.27	0.008	0.94
48	University of Virginia Health Sciences Ctr., Charlottesville	16.7	0.7%	1.24	Yes	1.41	4	1.92	0.007	1.75
TIER THREE										
	Depaul Medical Center, Norfolk	11.0	0.0%	0.66	No	0.14	4	0.88	0.039	2.25
	Fairfax Hospital, Falls Church	11.9	0.0%	0.91	Yes	0.15	4	1.34	0.055	1.77

Natl. Rank	Hospital	U.S. News index	Reputa-tional score	Orthopedics mortality rate	COTH member	Interns and residents to beds	Tech-nology score (of 5)	R.N.'s to beds	Board-certified orthopedists to beds	Pro-cedures to beds
	Sentara Norfolk General Hospital, Norfolk	9.4	0.0%	1.19	Yes	0.16	4	1.18	0.045	1.05
TIER FOUR										
	Alexandria Hospital, Alexandria	6.2	0.0%	0.89	No	0.00	3	0.67	0.025	1.48
	Arlington Hospital, Arlington	3.7	0.0%	1.41	No	0.06	3	0.71	0.046	1.99
	Bon Secours-Maryview Medical Center, Portsmouth	6.4	0.0%	0.91	No	0.02	4	0.50	0.033	1.59
	Bon Secours-St. Mary's Hospital, Richmond	6.6	0.0%	1.01	No	0.02	3	0.87	0.087	3.38
	Community Hospital of Roanoke Valley, Roanoke	2.4	0.0%	2.08	No	0.08	2	1.14	0.035	1.61
	Danville Regional Medical Center, Danville	3.2	0.0%	1.43	No	0.00	3	0.71	0.011	2.01
	Fair Oaks Hospital, Fairfax	7.7	0.0%	0.85	No	0.01	3	0.78	0.130	2.30
	HCA Chippenham Medical Center, Richmond	3.3	0.0%	1.55	No	0.03	3	0.83	0.021	2.04
	HCA Henrico Doctor's Hospital, Richmond	6.3	0.0%	1.35	No	0.00	4	1.35	0.035	3.48
	HCA Lewis-Gale Hospital, Salem	7.3	0.0%	0.85	No	0.00	4	0.51	0.027	3.76
	Johnston-Willis Hospital, Richmond	7.5	0.0%	0.88	No	0.00	4	0.79	0.033	2.71
	Lynchburg General Hospital, Lynchburg	6.8	0.0%	0.94	No	0.02	4	0.51	0.033	4.69
	Mary Washington Hospital, Fredericksburg	4.4	0.0%	1.25	No	0.00	4	0.61	0.025	1.89
	Richmond Memorial Hospital, Richmond	4.8	0.0%	1.01	No	0.00	2	0.72	0.032	1.85
	Riverside Regional Medical Center, Newport News	5.4	0.0%	1.28	No	0.28	3	0.91	0.026	2.34
	Roanoke Memorial Hospitals, Roanoke	6.8	0.0%	1.19	No	0.35	4	0.81	0.027	3.53
	Rockingham Memorial Hospital, Harrisonburg	5.0	0.0%	1.20	No	0.00	3	0.91	0.019	2.72
	Virginia Beach General Hospital, Virginia Beach	5.0	0.0%	1.15	No	0.01	4	0.53	0.046	2.67
	Winchester Medical Center, Winchester	7.0	0.0%	0.86	No	0.00	2	0.90	0.026	3.76

OTOLARYNGOLOGY

Natl. Rank	Hospital	U.S. News index	Reputa-tional score	Hospital-wide mortality rate	COTH member	Interns and residents to beds	Tech-nology score (of 9)	R.N.'s to beds	Board-certified internists to beds	Procedures to beds
TIER ONE										
12	University of Virginia Health Sciences Ctr., Charlottesville	38.1	6.4%	1.21	Yes	1.41	8	1.92	0.101	0.357
TIER TWO										
	Medical College of Virginia Hospitals, Richmond	13.7	0.0%	1.11	Yes	0.93	8	1.27	0.094	0.184
TIER THREE										
	Fairfax Hospital, Falls Church	11.0	0.0%	0.97	Yes	0.15	7	1.34	0.122	0.204
	Sentara Norfolk General Hospital, Norfolk	11.0	0.0%	1.28	Yes	0.16	8	1.18	0.176	0.175
TIER FOUR										
	Alexandria Hospital, Alexandria	4.5	0.0%	1.03	No	0.00	5	0.67	0.116	0.253
	Arlington Hospital, Arlington	4.3	0.0%	1.41	No	0.06	6	0.71	0.049	0.141
	Bon Secours-Maryview Medical Center, Portsmouth	3.8	0.0%	1.24	No	0.02	7	0.50	0.040	0.184
	Bon Secours-St. Mary's Hospital, Richmond	5.7	0.0%	1.03	No	0.02	7	0.87	0.116	0.347
	Community Hospital of Roanoke Valley, Roanoke	4.2	0.0%	1.47	No	0.08	1	1.14	0.032	0.271
	Danville Regional Medical Center, Danville	3.3	0.0%	1.36	No	0.00	4	0.71	0.021	0.265
	Depaul Medical Center, Norfolk	6.9	0.0%	1.05	No	0.14	7	0.88	0.196	0.246
	Fair Oaks Hospital, Fairfax	3.8	0.0%	1.11	No	0.01	2	0.78	0.103	0.240
	HCA Chippenham Medical Center, Richmond	4.5	0.0%	1.04	No	0.03	3	0.83	0.112	0.192
	HCA Henrico Doctor's Hospital, Richmond	6.0	0.0%	1.07	No	0.00	6	1.35	0.014	0.264
	HCA Lewis-Gale Hospital, Salem	3.9	0.0%	1.22	No	0.00	8	0.51	0.021	0.227
	Johnston-Willis Hospital, Richmond	5.0	0.0%	1.08	No	0.00	7	0.79	0.066	0.269
	Lynchburg General Hospital, Lynchburg	3.4	0.0%	1.08	No	0.02	4	0.51	0.074	0.223
	Mary Washington Hospital, Fredericksburg	3.9	0.0%	1.46	No	0.00	7	0.61	0.028	0.388
	Northern Virginia Doctors' Hospital, Arlington	3.4	0.0%	0.96	No	0.01	2	0.32	0.204	0.114
	Portsmouth General Hospital, Portsmouth	3.1	0.0%	1.42	No	0.04	2	0.58	0.098	0.179
	Richmond Memorial Hospital, Richmond	3.2	0.0%	1.30	No	0.00	2	0.72	0.068	0.181
	Riverside Regional Medical Center, Newport News	6.2	0.0%	1.30	No	0.28	6	0.91	0.085	0.243
	Roanoke Memorial Hospitals, Roanoke	5.9	0.0%	1.33	No	0.35	7	0.81	0.025	0.357
	Rockingham Memorial Hospital, Harrisonburg	4.5	0.0%	1.23	No	0.00	6	0.91	0.012	0.455

Natl. Rank	Hospital	U.S. News index	Reputational score	Hospital-wide mortality rate	COTH member	Interns and residents to beds	Technology score (of 9)	R.N.'s to beds	Board-certified internists to beds	Procedures to beds
	Virginia Baptist Hospital, Lynchburg	4.8	0.0%	1.31	No	0.01	6	0.86	0.070	0.161
	Virginia Beach General Hospital, Virginia Beach	3.8	0.0%	1.12	No	0.01	7	0.53	0.021	0.275
	Winchester Medical Center, Winchester	4.8	0.0%	0.97	No	0.00	5	0.90	0.060	0.255

RHEUMATOLOGY

Natl. Rank	Hospital	U.S. News index	Reputational score	Hospital-wide mortality rate	COTH member	Interns and residents to beds	Technology score (of 5)	R.N.'s to beds	Board-certified internists to beds
TIER TWO									
71	Medical College of Virginia Hospitals, Richmond	16.5	0.8%	1.11	Yes	0.93	4	1.27	0.094
41	University of Virginia Health Sciences Ctr., Charlottesville	19.1	0.7%	1.21	Yes	1.41	4	1.92	0.101
TIER THREE									
	Depaul Medical Center, Norfolk	10.0	0.0%	1.05	No	0.14	4	0.88	0.196
	Fairfax Hospital, Falls Church	13.9	0.0%	0.97	Yes	0.15	4	1.34	0.122
	HCA Henrico Doctor's Hospital, Richmond	10.1	0.4%	1.07	No	0.00	4	1.35	0.014
	Sentara Norfolk General Hospital, Norfolk	12.7	0.5%	1.28	Yes	0.16	4	1.18	0.176
TIER FOUR									
	Alexandria Hospital, Alexandria	8.1	0.0%	1.03	No	0.00	3	0.67	0.116
	Arlington Hospital, Arlington	5.5	0.0%	1.41	No	0.06	3	0.71	0.049
	Bon Secours-Maryview Medical Center, Portsmouth	6.1	0.0%	1.24	No	0.02	4	0.50	0.040
	Bon Secours-St. Mary's Hospital, Richmond	9.5	0.4%	1.03	No	0.02	3	0.87	0.116
	Community Hospital of Roanoke Valley, Roanoke	5.8	0.0%	1.47	No	0.08	2	1.14	0.032
	Danville Regional Medical Center, Danville	5.3	0.0%	1.36	No	0.00	3	0.71	0.021
	HCA Chippenham Medical Center, Richmond	8.5	0.0%	1.04	No	0.03	3	0.83	0.112
	HCA Lewis-Gale Hospital, Salem	5.1	0.0%	1.22	No	0.00	4	0.51	0.021
	Johnston-Willis Hospital, Richmond	7.1	0.0%	1.08	No	0.00	4	0.79	0.066
	Lynchburg General Hospital, Lynchburg	7.5	0.0%	1.08	No	0.02	4	0.51	0.074
	Mary Washington Hospital, Fredericksburg	5.1	0.0%	1.46	No	0.00	4	0.61	0.028
	Portsmouth General Hospital, Portsmouth	5.4	0.0%	1.42	No	0.04	3	0.58	0.098
	Richmond Memorial Hospital, Richmond	5.6	0.0%	1.30	No	0.00	2	0.72	0.068
	Riverside Regional Medical Center, Newport News	7.5	0.0%	1.30	No	0.28	3	0.91	0.085
	Roanoke Memorial Hospitals, Roanoke	7.4	0.0%	1.33	No	0.35	4	0.81	0.025
	Rockingham Memorial Hospital, Harrisonburg	6.5	0.0%	1.23	No	0.00	3	0.91	0.012
	Virginia Baptist Hospital, Lynchburg	6.4	0.0%	1.31	No	0.01	3	0.86	0.070
	Virginia Beach General Hospital, Virginia Beach	5.8	0.0%	1.12	No	0.01	4	0.53	0.021
	Winchester Medical Center, Winchester	8.4	0.0%	0.97	No	0.00	2	0.90	0.060

UROLOGY

Natl. Rank	Hospital	U.S. News index	Reputational score	Urology mortality rate	COTH member	Interns and residents to beds	Technology score (of 11)	R.N.'s to beds	Board-certified internists to beds	Procedures to beds
TIER TWO										
88	Medical College of Virginia Hospitals, Richmond	15.1	0.0%	1.01	Yes	0.93	10	1.27	0.094	1.08
34	University of Virginia Health Sciences Ctr., Charlottesville	19.7	3.0%	1.51	Yes	1.41	10	1.92	0.101	1.80
TIER THREE										
	Depaul Medical Center, Norfolk	9.9	0.0%	0.91	No	0.14	8	0.88	0.196	1.61
	Fairfax Hospital, Falls Church	12.9	0.0%	0.96	Yes	0.15	8	1.34	0.122	1.20
	Johnston-Willis Hospital, Richmond	10.4	0.0%	0.80	No	0.00	9	0.79	0.066	1.84
	Sentara Norfolk General Hospital, Norfolk	9.4	0.0%	1.60	Yes	0.16	10	1.18	0.176	1.32
TIER FOUR										
	Alexandria Hospital, Alexandria	5.6	0.0%	1.20	No	0.00	6	0.67	0.116	1.36
	Arlington Hospital, Arlington	4.8	0.0%	1.36	No	0.06	7	0.71	0.049	1.10
	Bon Secours-Maryview Medical Center, Portsmouth	4.0	0.0%	1.45	No	0.02	8	0.50	0.040	1.08
	Bon Secours-St. Mary's Hospital, Richmond	7.4	0.0%	1.18	No	0.02	9	0.87	0.116	2.36

Natl. Rank	Hospital	U.S. News index	Reputa- tional score	Urology mortality rate	COTH member	Interns and residents to beds	Tech- nology score (of 11)	R.N.'s to beds	Board- certified internists to beds	Procedures to beds
	Community Hospital of Roanoke Valley, Roanoke	7.4	0.0%	1.03	No	0.08	4	1.14	0.032	1.60
	Danville Regional Medical Center, Danville	3.3	0.0%	1.64	No	0.00	6	0.71	0.021	2.11
	HCA Chippenham Medical Center, Richmond	5.1	0.0%	1.35	No	0.03	5	0.83	0.112	1.43
	HCA Henrico Doctor's Hospital, Richmond	6.9	0.0%	1.31	No	0.00	9	1.35	0.014	1.51
	HCA Lewis-Gale Hospital, Salem	3.6	0.0%	1.62	No	0.00	9	0.51	0.021	1.83
	Lynchburg General Hospital, Lynchburg	3.3	0.0%	1.60	No	0.02	6	0.51	0.074	1.78
	Mary Washington Hospital, Fredericksburg	2.1	0.0%	2.44	No	0.00	9	0.61	0.028	2.14
	Northern Virginia Doctors' Hospital, Arlington	6.5	0.0%	0.93	No	0.01	3	0.32	0.204	1.46
	Portsmouth General Hospital, Portsmouth	3.1	0.0%	1.61	No	0.04	4	0.58	0.098	1.80
	Richmond Memorial Hospital, Richmond	1.5	0.0%	2.23	No	0.00	4	0.72	0.068	1.56
	Riverside Regional Medical Center, Newport News	6.2	0.0%	1.38	No	0.28	7	0.91	0.085	1.09
	Roanoke Memorial Hospitals, Roanoke	6.0	0.0%	1.45	No	0.35	8	0.81	0.025	1.88
	Rockingham Memorial Hospital, Harrisonburg	6.0	0.0%	1.24	No	0.00	7	0.91	0.012	2.51
	Virginia Baptist Hospital, Lynchburg	2.8	0.0%	2.06	No	0.01	7	0.86	0.070	0.85
	Virginia Beach General Hospital, Virginia Beach	4.0	0.0%	1.45	No	0.01	8	0.53	0.021	1.64
	Winchester Medical Center, Winchester	4.9	0.0%	1.42	No	0.00	6	0.90	0.060	2.19

AIDS

Natl. Rank	Hospital	U.S. News index	Reputa-tional score	Hospital-wide mortality rate	COTH member	Interns and residents to beds	Tech-nology score (of 11)	Discharge planning (of 2)	R.N.'s to beds	Board-certified internists to beds
TIER ONE										
10	University of Washington Medical Center, Seattle	35.6	4.3%	0.84	Yes	1.05	8	2	2.06	0.440
TIER TWO										
58	Harborview Medical Center, Seattle	26.5	2.8%	1.15	Yes	0.37	5	2	1.73	0.451
TIER THREE										
	Deaconess Rehabilitation Institute, Spokane	19.8	0.0%	0.85	No	0.06	2	1	0.71	0.046
	General Hospital Medical Center, Everett	21.9	0.0%	0.95	No	0.00	6	2	1.40	0.095
	Group Health Cooperative Hospital, Seattle	21.1	0.0%	1.02	No	0.04	8	2	1.34	0.022
	Overlake Hospital Medical Center, Bellevue	20.0	0.0%	0.96	No	0.00	6	2	0.43	0.051
	Providence Medical Center, Seattle	20.5	0.0%	1.01	No	0.22	6	2	0.96	0.067
	Sacred Heart Medical Center, Spokane	20.4	0.0%	0.93	No	0.12	6	1	0.62	0.058
	St. Mary Medical Center, Walla Walla	21.3	0.0%	0.72	No	0.00	6	1	0.56	0.125
	St. Peter Hospital, Olympia	21.0	0.0%	0.93	No	0.12	5	2	0.82	0.035
	Virginia Mason Medical Center, Seattle	20.8	0.0%	0.98	No	0.80	4	2	0.43	0.098
TIER FOUR										
	Affiliated Health Services, Mount Vernon	18.1	0.0%	1.07	No	0.00	7	1	0.56	0.045
	Kadlec Medical Center, Richland	18.4	0.0%	1.10	No	0.00	5	2	1.04	0.042
	Providence Hospital, Everett	18.1	0.0%	1.03	No	0.00	6	1	0.39	0.064
	Southwest Washington Medical Center, Vancouver	19.0	0.0%	1.05	No	0.00	6	2	0.70	0.042
	Swedish Medical Center, Seattle	18.9	0.0%	1.15	No	0.12	7	2	1.08	0.060
	Tacoma General Hospital, Tacoma	18.7	0.0%	1.16	No	0.06	6	2	0.80	0.255
	Valley Medical Center, Renton	17.4	0.0%	1.12	No	0.11	4	2	0.63	0.046
	Yakima Valley Memorial Hospital, Yakima	16.6	0.0%	1.19	No	0.00	6	1	0.68	0.084

CANCER

Natl. Rank	Hospital	U.S. News index	Reputa-tional score	Cancer mortality rate	COTH member	Interns and residents to beds	Tech-nology score (of 12)	R.N.'s to beds	Board-certified oncologists to beds	Procedures to beds
TIER ONE										
7	University of Washington Medical Center, Seattle	30.7	13.1%	0.58	Yes	1.05	9	2.06	0.039	2.11
TIER THREE										
	Group Health Cooperative Hospital, Seattle	6.1	0.0%	0.75	No	0.04	8	1.34	0.026	3.35
	Swedish Medical Center, Seattle	5.5	0.4%	1.42	No	0.12	9	1.08	0.034	1.98
TIER FOUR										
	Affiliated Health Services, Mount Vernon	3.0	0.0%	1.26	No	0.00	8	0.56	0.018	2.59
	Deaconess Medical Center, Spokane	2.0	0.0%	0.99	No	0.14	0	0.92	0.012	0.91
	Kadlec Medical Center, Richland	2.8	0.0%	1.39	No	0.00	4	1.04	0.007	1.35
	Overlake Hospital Medical Center, Bellevue	2.3	0.0%	1.16	No	0.00	7	0.43	0.017	1.62
	Providence Hospital, Everett	2.8	0.0%	0.86	No	0.00	8	0.39	0.021	1.69
	Providence Medical Center, Seattle	4.7	0.0%	0.91	No	0.22	7	0.96	0.013	1.71
	Sacred Heart Medical Center, Spokane	3.8	0.0%	0.83	No	0.12	8	0.62	0.016	1.51
	Southwest Washington Medical Center, Vancouver	3.0	0.0%	0.93	No	0.00	7	0.70	0.003	1.23
	St. Peter Hospital, Olympia	2.6	0.0%	1.08	No	0.12	3	0.82	0.004	1.89
	Tacoma General Hospital, Tacoma	3.2	0.0%	0.98	No	0.06	5	0.80	0.034	1.65
	Valley Medical Center, Renton	2.6	0.0%	1.13	No	0.11	5	0.63	0.008	1.71
	Virginia Mason Medical Center, Seattle	4.3	0.0%	0.95	No	0.80	2	0.43	0.029	4.43
	Yakima Valley Memorial Hospital, Yakima	2.9	0.0%	1.11	No	0.00	7	0.68	0.013	1.47

CARDIOLOGY

Natl. Rank	Hospital	U.S. News index	Reputa-tional score	Cardiology mortality rate	COTH member	Interns and residents to beds	Tech-nology score (of 10)	R.N.'s to beds	Board-certified cardiologists to beds	Procedures to beds
TIER TWO									
24	University of Washington Medical Center, Seattle	28.0	0.0%	0.75	Yes	1.05	8	2.06	0.132	4.35
TIER THREE									
	Affiliated Health Services, Mount Vernon	16.3	0.0%	0.85	No	0.00	7	0.56	0.018	7.19
	Deaconess Medical Center, Spokane	14.2	0.0%	0.94	No	0.14	0	0.92	0.034	7.88
	General Hospital Medical Center, Everett	16.5	0.0%	1.01	No	0.00	8	1.40	0.101	13.98
	Group Health Cooperative Hospital, Seattle	17.6	0.0%	0.91	No	0.04	6	1.34	0.026	13.98
	Overlake Hospital Medical Center, Bellevue	16.3	0.0%	0.89	No	0.00	7	0.43	0.068	8.52
	Providence Medical Center, Seattle	19.3	1.9%	0.97	No	0.22	8	0.96	0.032	10.51
	Sacred Heart Medical Center, Spokane	17.4	0.3%	0.89	No	0.12	6	0.62	0.051	9.71
	St. Peter Hospital, Olympia	17.4	0.0%	0.89	No	0.12	7	0.82	0.021	11.67
	Valley Medical Center, Renton	16.1	0.0%	0.89	No	0.11	6	0.63	0.017	7.21
	Virginia Mason Medical Center, Seattle	16.7	0.0%	0.92	No	0.80	2	0.43	0.049	10.88
TIER FOUR									
	Providence Hospital, Everett	8.3	0.0%	1.22	No	0.00	5	0.39	0.080	6.51
	Southwest Washington Medical Center, Vancouver	10.5	0.0%	1.11	No	0.00	6	0.70	0.016	6.73
	Swedish Medical Center, Seattle	12.5	0.0%	1.12	No	0.12	8	1.08	0.031	5.03
	Tacoma General Hospital, Tacoma	6.5	0.0%	1.51	No	0.06	8	0.80	0.048	7.47
	Yakima Valley Memorial Hospital, Yakima	8.0	0.0%	1.22	No	0.00	4	0.68	0.027	4.71

ENDOCRINOLOGY

Natl. Rank	Hospital	U.S. News index	Reputa-tional score	Endocrinology mortality rate	COTH member	Interns and residents to beds	Tech-nology score (of 11)	R.N.'s to beds	Board-certified internists to beds
TIER ONE								
10	University of Washington Medical Center, Seattle	34.2	11.3%	1.00	Yes	1.05	10	2.06	0.440
TIER TWO								
72	Harborview Medical Center, Seattle	15.6	0.0%	0.91	Yes	0.37	4	1.73	0.451
TIER THREE								
	Affiliated Health Services, Mount Vernon	9.6	0.0%	0.66	No	0.00	9	0.56	0.045
	General Hospital Medical Center, Everett	11.5	0.0%	0.64	No	0.00	5	1.40	0.095
	Overlake Hospital Medical Center, Bellevue	9.2	0.0%	0.65	No	0.00	8	0.43	0.051
	Southwest Washington Medical Center, Vancouver	9.8	0.0%	0.57	No	0.00	8	0.70	0.042
	St. Peter Hospital, Olympia	9.0	0.0%	0.70	No	0.12	4	0.82	0.035
	Tacoma General Hospital, Tacoma	11.4	0.0%	0.63	No	0.06	6	0.80	0.255
	Virginia Mason Medical Center, Seattle	9.2	0.0%	0.77	No	0.80	1	0.43	0.098
	Yakima Valley Memorial Hospital, Yakima	8.4	0.0%	0.78	No	0.00	8	0.68	0.084
TIER FOUR								
	Group Health Cooperative Hospital, Seattle	6.0	0.0%	1.49	No	0.04	9	1.34	0.022
	Providence Medical Center, Seattle	6.7	0.0%	1.21	No	0.22	8	0.96	0.067
	Sacred Heart Medical Center, Spokane	6.0	0.0%	1.02	No	0.12	6	0.62	0.058
	Swedish Medical Center, Seattle	7.4	0.0%	1.10	No	0.12	9	1.08	0.060
	Valley Medical Center, Renton	5.5	0.0%	1.10	No	0.11	6	0.63	0.046

GASTROENTEROLOGY

Natl. Rank	Hospital	U.S. News index	Reputa-tional score	Gastro-enterology mortality rate	COTH member	Interns and residents to beds	Tech-nology score (of 11)	R.N.'s to beds	Board-certified gastro-enterologists to beds	Pro-cedures to beds
	TIER THREE									
	General Hospital Medical Center, Everett	7.4	0.0%	1.01	No	0.00	6	1.40	0.045	3.20
	Group Health Cooperative Hospital, Seattle	9.7	0.0%	1.23	No	0.04	8	1.34	0.022	8.49
	Overlake Hospital Medical Center, Bellevue	7.6	0.0%	0.80	No	0.00	7	0.43	0.030	3.94
	Providence Medical Center, Seattle	9.2	0.0%	0.73	No	0.22	7	0.96	0.016	3.29
	St. Peter Hospital, Olympia	8.2	0.0%	0.69	No	0.12	4	0.82	0.014	4.41
92	Virginia Mason Medical Center, Seattle	12.3	2.0%	0.86	No	0.80	1	0.43	0.044	6.09
	TIER FOUR									
	Affiliated Health Services, Mount Vernon	7.2	0.0%	0.94	No	0.00	9	0.56	0.009	3.95
	Deaconess Medical Center, Spokane	3.5	0.0%	1.15	No	0.14	0	0.92	0.015	2.29
	Providence Hospital, Everett	5.9	0.0%	1.00	No	0.00	8	0.39	0.032	3.61
	Sacred Heart Medical Center, Spokane	6.1	0.0%	0.94	No	0.12	5	0.62	0.018	3.03
	Southwest Washington Medical Center, Vancouver	7.1	0.0%	0.91	No	0.00	7	0.70	0.006	3.89
	Swedish Medical Center, Seattle	5.4	0.0%	1.35	No	0.12	8	1.08	0.018	2.55
	Tacoma General Hospital, Tacoma	4.5	0.0%	1.27	No	0.06	5	0.80	0.024	3.40
	Valley Medical Center, Renton	6.0	0.0%	1.05	No	0.11	5	0.63	0.008	4.42
	Yakima Valley Memorial Hospital, Yakima	4.5	0.0%	1.26	No	0.00	7	0.68	0.009	3.16

GERIATRICS

Natl. Rank	Hospital	U.S. News index	Reputa-tional score	Hospital-wide mortality rate	COTH member	Service mix	Interns and residents to beds	Tech-nology score (of 13)	R.N.'s to beds	Discharge planning (of 2)	Geriatric services (of 9)	Board-certified internists to beds
	TIER ONE											
9	University of Washington Medical Center, Seattle	47.3	7.2%	0.84	Yes	7	1.05	10	2.06	2	4	0.440
	TIER TWO											
77	Harborview Medical Center, Seattle	22.3	1.7%	1.15	Yes	6	0.37	4	1.73	2	6	0.451
	TIER THREE											
	General Hospital Medical Center, Everett	15.8	0.0%	0.95	No	3	0.00	6	1.40	2	3	0.095
	Group Health Cooperative Hospital, Seattle	15.8	0.0%	1.02	No	6	0.04	9	1.34	2	5	0.022
	Overlake Hospital Medical Center, Bellevue	14.8	0.0%	0.96	No	3	0.00	9	0.43	2	6	0.051
	Providence Medical Center, Seattle	15.8	0.0%	1.01	No	6	0.22	10	0.96	2	3	0.067
	Sacred Heart Medical Center, Spokane	15.7	0.0%	0.93	No	6	0.12	9	0.62	1	2	0.058
	St. Peter Hospital, Olympia	16.4	0.0%	0.93	No	6	0.12	5	0.82	2	2	0.035
	Swedish Medical Center, Seattle	14.0	0.0%	1.15	No	9	0.12	11	1.08	2	4	0.060
	Virginia Mason Medical Center, Seattle	15.3	0.3%	0.98	No	4	0.80	1	0.43	2	3	0.098
	TIER FOUR											
	Affiliated Health Services, Mount Vernon	10.7	0.0%	1.07	No	4	0.00	10	0.56	1	2	0.045
	Providence Hospital, Everett	11.2	0.0%	1.03	No	4	0.00	9	0.39	1	2	0.064
	Southwest Washington Medical Center, Vancouver	13.6	0.0%	1.05	No	7	0.00	9	0.70	2	2	0.042
	Tacoma General Hospital, Tacoma	10.6	0.0%	1.16	No	3	0.06	7	0.80	2	3	0.255
	Valley Medical Center, Renton	10.8	0.0%	1.12	No	4	0.11	8	0.63	2	3	0.046
	Yakima Valley Memorial Hospital, Yakima	8.4	0.0%	1.19	No	5	0.00	9	0.68	1	1	0.084

GYNECOLOGY

Natl. Rank	Hospital	U.S. News index	Reputational score	Hospital-wide mortality rate	Interns and residents to beds	Technology score (of 10)	R.N.'s to beds	Board-certified OB-GYNs to beds	Procedures to beds
TIER ONE									
17	University of Washington Medical Center, Seattle	37.1	2.2%	0.84	1.05	9	2.06	0.093	0.59
TIER THREE									
	General Hospital Medical Center, Everett	19.3	0.0%	0.95	0.00	6	1.40	0.084	0.64
	Group Health Cooperative Hospital, Seattle	17.7	0.0%	1.02	0.04	7	1.34	0.074	1.13
	Harborview Medical Center, Seattle	14.7	0.0%	1.15	0.37	3	1.73	0.058	0.03
	Providence Medical Center, Seattle	15.1	0.0%	1.01	0.22	5	0.96	0.045	0.32
	Sacred Heart Medical Center, Spokane	16.3	0.0%	0.93	0.12	6	0.62	0.051	0.46
	St. Peter Hospital, Olympia	15.6	0.0%	0.93	0.12	4	0.82	0.039	0.65
TIER FOUR									
	Affiliated Health Services, Mount Vernon	11.9	0.0%	1.07	0.00	7	0.56	0.027	0.56
	Overlake Hospital Medical Center, Bellevue	13.8	0.0%	0.96	0.00	5	0.43	0.072	0.66
	Providence Hospital, Everett	12.9	0.0%	1.03	0.00	7	0.39	0.064	0.37
	Southwest Washington Medical Center, Vancouver	12.7	0.0%	1.05	0.00	6	0.70	0.048	0.70
	Tacoma General Hospital, Tacoma	11.3	0.0%	1.16	0.06	5	0.80	0.092	0.78
	Valley Medical Center, Renton	8.7	0.0%	1.12	0.11	3	0.63	0.029	0.55
	Virginia Mason Medical Center, Seattle	13.7	0.0%	0.98	0.80	0	0.43	0.088	0.88
	Yakima Valley Memorial Hospital, Yakima	10.3	0.0%	1.19	0.00	7	0.68	0.044	0.78

NEUROLOGY

Natl. Rank	Hospital	U.S. News index	Reputational score	Neurology mortality rate	COTH member	Interns and residents to beds	Technology score (of 9)	R.N.'s to beds	Board-certified neurologists to beds
TIER ONE									
17	University of Washington Medical Center, Seattle	27.0	2.6%	0.89	Yes	1.05	8	2.06	0.047
TIER THREE									
	General Hospital Medical Center, Everett	14.3	0.0%	0.89	No	0.00	5	1.40	0.039
TIER FOUR									
	Affiliated Health Services, Mount Vernon	5.3	0.0%	1.28	No	0.00	7	0.56	0.009
	Deaconess Medical Center, Spokane	8.3	0.0%	1.00	No	0.14	0	0.92	0.012
	Overlake Hospital Medical Center, Bellevue	7.1	0.0%	1.09	No	0.00	6	0.43	0.013
	Providence Hospital, Everett	7.1	0.0%	1.21	No	0.00	7	0.39	0.032
	Providence Medical Center, Seattle	9.4	0.0%	1.08	No	0.22	6	0.96	0.013
	Sacred Heart Medical Center, Spokane	8.1	0.0%	1.03	No	0.12	4	0.62	0.011
	Southwest Washington Medical Center, Vancouver	6.2	0.0%	1.18	No	0.00	6	0.70	0.006
	St. Peter Hospital, Olympia	9.6	0.0%	1.00	No	0.12	4	0.82	0.018
	Swedish Medical Center, Seattle	8.8	0.0%	1.17	No	0.12	7	1.08	0.017
	Tacoma General Hospital, Tacoma	6.5	0.0%	1.37	No	0.06	5	0.80	0.037
	Valley Medical Center, Renton	2.6	0.0%	1.57	No	0.11	4	0.63	0.008
	Virginia Mason Medical Center, Seattle	9.4	0.0%	1.05	No	0.80	0	0.43	0.029
	Yakima Valley Memorial Hospital, Yakima	2.9	0.0%	1.54	No	0.00	6	0.68	0.004

ORTHOPEDICS

Natl. Rank	Hospital	U.S. News index	Reputational score	Orthopedics mortality rate	COTH member	Interns and residents to beds	Technology score (of 5)	R.N.'s to beds	Board-certified orthopedists to beds	Procedures to beds
TIER ONE										
9	University of Washington Medical Center, Seattle	31.3	5.9%	0.72	Yes	1.05	4	2.06	0.070	1.54
21	Harborview Medical Center, Seattle	21.1	5.3%	1.24	Yes	0.37	2	1.73	0.049	1.21
TIER THREE										

Natl. Rank Hospital	U.S. News index	Reputa- tional score	Orthopedics mortality rate	COTH member	Interns and residents to beds	Tech- nology score (of 5)	R.N.'s to beds	Board- certified orthopedists to beds	Pro- cedures to beds
Group Health Cooperative Hospital, Seattle	10.3	0.0%	0.90	No	0.04	4	1.34	0.044	7.97
Swedish Medical Center, Seattle	9.4	0.8%	0.99	No	0.12	3	1.08	0.062	3.80
Virginia Mason Medical Center, Seattle	10.2	0.0%	0.56	No	0.80	0	0.43	0.044	5.19
TIER FOUR									
Affiliated Health Services, Mount Vernon	6.8	0.0%	0.92	No	0.00	4	0.56	0.041	3.07
General Hospital Medical Center, Everett	7.2	0.0%	1.19	No	0.00	4	1.40	0.056	2.70
Kadlec Medical Center, Richland	6.3	0.0%	1.06	No	0.00	3	1.04	0.042	3.01
Overlake Hospital Medical Center, Bellevue	8.0	0.0%	0.75	No	0.00	3	0.43	0.077	3.79
Providence Hospital, Everett	5.4	0.0%	0.94	No	0.00	3	0.39	0.059	2.55
Providence Medical Center, Seattle	6.1	0.0%	1.21	No	0.22	3	0.96	0.029	3.79
Sacred Heart Medical Center, Spokane	5.1	0.0%	1.03	No	0.12	2	0.62	0.042	2.86
Southwest Washington Medical Center, Vancouver	6.6	0.0%	0.92	No	0.00	3	0.70	0.032	3.78
St. Mary Medical Center, Walla Walla	5.3	0.0%	1.01	No	0.00	3	0.56	0.037	3.06
St. Peter Hospital, Olympia	6.3	0.0%	1.04	No	0.12	3	0.82	0.032	3.40
Tacoma General Hospital, Tacoma	5.1	0.0%	1.40	No	0.06	4	0.80	0.085	3.18
Valley Medical Center, Renton	2.9	0.0%	1.50	No	0.11	2	0.63	0.021	3.52
Yakima Valley Memorial Hospital, Yakima	5.9	0.0%	1.00	No	0.00	3	0.68	0.053	3.33

OTOLARYNGOLOGY

Natl. Rank Hospital	U.S. News index	Reputa- tional score	Hospital- wide mortality rate	COTH member	Interns and residents to beds	Tech- nology score (of 9)	R.N.'s to beds	Board- certified internists to beds	Procedures to beds
TIER ONE									
17 University of Washington Medical Center, Seattle	30.3	3.3%	0.84	Yes	1.05	8	2.06	0.440	0.225
TIER TWO									
89 Harborview Medical Center, Seattle	14.3	0.0%	1.15	Yes	0.37	2	1.73	0.451	0.095
TIER FOUR									
Affiliated Health Services, Mount Vernon	4.1	0.0%	1.07	No	0.00	7	0.56	0.045	0.153
Deaconess Medical Center, Spokane	4.1	0.0%	0.87	No	0.14	0	0.92	0.067	0.098
Deaconess Rehabilitation Institute, Spokane	3.0	0.0%	0.85	No	0.06	0	0.71	0.046	0.023
General Hospital Medical Center, Everett	6.1	0.0%	0.95	No	0.00	3	1.40	0.095	0.179
Group Health Cooperative Hospital, Seattle	6.5	0.0%	1.02	No	0.04	7	1.34	0.022	0.694
Kadlec Medical Center, Richland	4.6	0.0%	1.11	No	0.00	4	1.04	0.042	0.076
Overlake Hospital Medical Center, Bellevue	3.5	0.0%	0.96	No	0.00	6	0.43	0.051	0.174
Providence Hospital, Everett	3.7	0.0%	1.03	No	0.00	7	0.39	0.064	0.176
Providence Medical Center, Seattle	6.1	0.0%	1.01	No	0.22	6	0.96	0.067	0.192
Sacred Heart Medical Center, Spokane	4.4	0.0%	0.93	No	0.12	5	0.62	0.058	0.112
Southwest Washington Medical Center, Vancouver	4.2	0.0%	1.05	No	0.00	6	0.70	0.042	0.197
St. Mary Medical Center, Walla Walla	4.8	0.0%	0.72	No	0.00	6	0.56	0.125	0.213
St. Peter Hospital, Olympia	4.0	0.0%	0.93	No	0.12	2	0.82	0.035	0.240
Swedish Medical Center, Seattle	6.2	0.0%	1.15	No	0.12	7	1.08	0.060	0.238
Tacoma General Hospital, Tacoma	5.9	0.0%	1.16	No	0.06	4	0.80	0.255	0.119
Valley Medical Center, Renton	3.9	0.0%	1.12	No	0.11	4	0.63	0.046	0.218
Virginia Mason Medical Center, Seattle	5.7	0.0%	0.98	No	0.80	1	0.43	0.098	0.387
Yakima Valley Memorial Hospital, Yakima	4.4	0.0%	1.19	No	0.00	6	0.68	0.084	0.173

RHEUMATOLOGY

Natl. Rank	Hospital	U.S. News index	Reputa-tional score	Hospital-wide mortality rate	COTH member	Interns and residents to beds	Tech-nology score (of 5)	R.N.'s to beds	Board-certified internists to beds
	TIER ONE								
14	University of Washington Medical Center, Seattle	31.5	4.1%	0.84	Yes	1.05	4	2.06	0.440
	TIER THREE								
	General Hospital Medical Center, Everett	11.0	0.0%	0.95	No	0.00	4	1.40	0.095
	Group Health Cooperative Hospital, Seattle	9.8	0.0%	1.02	No	0.04	4	1.34	0.022
87	Harborview Medical Center, Seattle	15.6	0.0%	1.15	Yes	0.37	2	1.73	0.451
	Virginia Mason Medical Center, Seattle	11.4	1.1%	0.98	No	0.80	0	0.43	0.098
	TIER FOUR								
	Affiliated Health Services, Mount Vernon	6.4	0.0%	1.07	No	0.00	4	0.56	0.045
	Deaconess Medical Center, Spokane	7.1	0.0%	0.87	No	0.14	0	0.92	0.067
	Overlake Hospital Medical Center, Bellevue	7.6	0.0%	0.96	No	0.00	3	0.43	0.051
	Providence Hospital, Everett	5.9	0.0%	1.03	No	0.00	3	0.39	0.064
	Providence Medical Center, Seattle	9.4	0.0%	1.01	No	0.22	3	0.96	0.067
	Sacred Heart Medical Center, Spokane	7.4	0.0%	0.93	No	0.12	2	0.62	0.058
	Southwest Washington Medical Center, Vancouver	7.5	0.0%	1.05	No	0.00	3	0.70	0.042
	St. Peter Hospital, Olympia	9.3	0.0%	0.93	No	0.12	3	0.82	0.035
	Swedish Medical Center, Seattle	9.2	0.5%	1.15	No	0.12	3	1.08	0.060
	Tacoma General Hospital, Tacoma	9.1	0.0%	1.16	No	0.06	4	0.80	0.255
	Valley Medical Center, Renton	6.6	0.0%	1.12	No	0.11	2	0.63	0.046
	Yakima Valley Memorial Hospital, Yakima	5.7	0.0%	1.19	No	0.00	3	0.68	0.084

UROLOGY

Natl. Rank	Hospital	U.S. News index	Reputa-tional score	Urology mortality rate	COTH member	Interns and residents to beds	Tech-nology score (of 11)	R.N.'s to beds	Board-certified internists to beds	Procedures to beds
	TIER ONE									
15	University of Washington Medical Center, Seattle	26.9	4.9%	0.80	Yes	1.05	10	2.06	0.440	1.60
	TIER THREE									
	Deaconess Medical Center, Spokane	9.2	0.0%	0.78	No	0.14	0	0.92	0.067	2.16
	General Hospital Medical Center, Everett	9.6	0.0%	0.95	No	0.00	6	1.40	0.095	1.90
	Group Health Cooperative Hospital, Seattle	13.2	0.0%	0.63	No	0.04	8	1.34	0.022	4.22
	Providence Medical Center, Seattle	11.0	0.0%	0.80	No	0.22	7	0.96	0.067	1.62
	Sacred Heart Medical Center, Spokane	10.5	0.0%	0.72	No	0.12	5	0.62	0.058	2.36
	St. Peter Hospital, Olympia	10.6	0.0%	0.56	No	0.12	4	0.82	0.035	2.45
	Tacoma General Hospital, Tacoma	9.2	0.0%	0.86	No	0.06	5	0.80	0.255	1.31
	Valley Medical Center, Renton	10.3	0.0%	0.57	No	0.11	5	0.63	0.046	1.91
	Virginia Mason Medical Center, Seattle	11.9	1.2%	0.85	No	0.80	1	0.43	0.098	4.27
	TIER FOUR									
	Affiliated Health Services, Mount Vernon	2.3	0.0%	2.22	No	0.00	9	0.56	0.045	1.65
	Overlake Hospital Medical Center, Bellevue	5.8	0.0%	1.09	No	0.00	7	0.43	0.051	1.86
	Providence Hospital, Everett	7.6	0.0%	0.92	No	0.00	8	0.39	0.064	1.85
	Southwest Washington Medical Center, Vancouver	5.7	0.0%	1.20	No	0.00	7	0.70	0.042	1.85
	Swedish Medical Center, Seattle	6.8	0.0%	1.28	No	0.12	8	1.08	0.060	1.57
	Yakima Valley Memorial Hospital, Yakima	4.1	0.0%	1.61	No	0.00	7	0.68	0.084	2.36

AIDS

Natl. Rank Hospital	U.S. News index	Reputa-tional score	Hospital-wide mortality rate	COTH member	Interns and residents to beds	Tech-nology score (of 11)	Discharge planning (of 2)	R.N.'s to beds	Board-certified internists to beds
TIER THREE
Charleston Area Medical Center, Charleston, W.V.	**20.2**	0.0%	1.24	Yes	0.26	9	2	0.99	0.028
West Virginia University Hospitals, Morgantown	**22.3**	0.0%	1.23	Yes	1.15	7	2	1.51	0.034
TIER FOUR
Bluefield Regional Medical Center, Bluefield, W.V.	**15.1**	0.0%	1.26	No	0.00	5	1	0.65	0.011
Cabell Huntington Hospital, Huntington, W.V.	**14.8**	0.0%	1.58	No	0.08	7	2	1.07	0.034
Camden-Clark Memorial Hospital, Parkersburg, W.V.	**15.8**	0.0%	1.30	No	0.00	6	2	0.71	0.004
Monongalia General Hospital, Morgantown, W.V.	**16.3**	0.0%	1.28	No	0.01	5	2	0.88	0.083
Ohio Valley Medical Center, Wheeling, W.V.	**17.1**	0.0%	1.11	No	0.10	6	1	0.40	0.024
St. Mary's Hospital, Huntington, W.V.	**17.5**	0.0%	1.18	No	0.09	7	1	0.90	0.050
Thomas Memorial Hospital, South Charleston, W.V.	**16.1**	0.0%	1.14	No	0.00	5	1	0.37	0.013
United Hospital Center, Clarksburg, W.V.	**17.2**	0.0%	1.22	No	0.12	7	2	0.61	0.012
Wheeling Hospital, Wheeling, W.V.	**16.4**	0.0%	1.29	No	0.10	5	2	0.97	0.069

CANCER

Natl. Rank Hospital	U.S. News index	Reputa-tional score	Cancer mortality rate	COTH member	Interns and residents to beds	Tech-nology score (of 12)	R.N.'s to beds	Board-certified oncologists to beds	Procedures to beds
TIER TWO
60 West Virginia University Hospitals, Morgantown	**12.4**	0.0%	0.95	Yes	1.15	9	1.51	0.018	2.09
TIER THREE
Charleston Area Medical Center, Charleston, W.V.	**7.5**	0.0%	1.19	Yes	0.26	9	0.99	0.009	1.22
TIER FOUR
Bluefield Regional Medical Center, Bluefield, W.V.	**2.6**	0.0%	1.08	No	0.00	6	0.65	0.011	1.48
Cabell Huntington Hospital, Huntington, W.V.	**3.7**	0.0%	1.35	No	0.08	6	1.07	0.017	0.91
Camden-Clark Memorial Hospital, Parkersburg, W.V.	**3.4**	0.0%	1.15	No	0.00	8	0.71	0.000	2.63
Monongalia General Hospital, Morgantown, W.V.	**2.6**	0.0%	1.13	No	0.01	3	0.88	0.005	2.98
Ohio Valley Medical Center, Wheeling, W.V.	**2.9**	0.0%	1.17	No	0.10	9	0.40	0.010	0.91
St. Mary's Hospital, Huntington, W.V.	**4.0**	0.0%	1.27	No	0.09	8	0.90	0.011	1.76
Thomas Memorial Hospital, South Charleston, W.V.	**1.5**	0.0%	1.05	No	0.00	5	0.37	0.004	1.30
United Hospital Center, Clarksburg, W.V.	**3.8**	0.0%	0.78	No	0.12	8	0.61	0.006	1.68
Wheeling Hospital, Wheeling, W.V.	**4.3**	0.0%	1.01	No	0.10	7	0.97	0.014	2.41

CARDIOLOGY

Natl. Rank Hospital	U.S. News index	Reputa-tional score	Cardiology mortality rate	COTH member	Interns and residents to beds	Tech-nology score (of 10)	R.N.'s to beds	Board-certified cardiologists to beds	Procedures to beds
TIER THREE
Charleston Area Medical Center, Charleston, W.V.	**16.4**	0.0%	1.11	Yes	0.26	9	0.99	0.022	11.12
West Virginia University Hospitals, Morgantown	**17.2**	0.0%	1.30	Yes	1.15	8	1.51	0.015	7.60
TIER FOUR
Bluefield Regional Medical Center, Bluefield, W.V.	**12.2**	0.0%	1.02	No	0.00	5	0.65	0.023	8.07
Cabell Huntington Hospital, Huntington, W.V.	**6.0**	0.0%	1.49	No	0.08	4	1.07	0.030	6.36
Camden-Clark Memorial Hospital, Parkersburg, W.V.	**7.8**	0.0%	1.26	No	0.00	5	0.71	0.013	8.99
Monongalia General Hospital, Morgantown, W.V.	**8.5**	0.0%	1.31	No	0.01	8	0.88	0.000	15.01
Ohio Valley Medical Center, Wheeling, W.V.	**9.3**	0.0%	1.14	No	0.10	6	0.40	0.024	3.66
St. Mary's Hospital, Huntington, W.V.	**11.1**	0.0%	1.19	No	0.09	9	0.90	0.018	9.81
Thomas Memorial Hospital, South Charleston, W.V.	**8.4**	0.0%	1.14	No	0.00	4	0.37	0.009	7.71
United Hospital Center, Clarksburg, W.V.	**9.2**	0.0%	1.22	No	0.12	7	0.61	0.015	9.98
Wheeling Hospital, Wheeling, W.V.	**10.4**	0.0%	1.19	No	0.10	5	0.97	0.025	11.02

ENDOCRINOLOGY

Natl. Rank	Hospital	U.S. News index	Reputa-tional score	Endocrinology mortality rate	COTH member	Interns and residents to beds	Tech-nology score (of 11)	R.N.'s to beds	Board-certified internists to beds
	TIER TWO								
74	West Virginia University Hospitals, Morgantown	15.2	0.4%	1.04	Yes	1.15	9	1.51	0.034
	TIER THREE								
	Charleston Area Medical Center, Charleston, W.V.	11.0	0.0%	0.94	Yes	0.26	9	0.99	0.028
	TIER FOUR								
	Bluefield Regional Medical Center, Bluefield, W.V.	2.8	0.0%	1.75	No	0.00	7	0.65	0.011
	Cabell Huntington Hospital, Huntington, W.V.	4.4	0.0%	1.68	No	0.08	6	1.07	0.034
	Camden-Clark Memorial Hospital, Parkersburg, W.V.	3.5	0.0%	1.68	No	0.00	9	0.71	0.004
	Monongalia General Hospital, Morgantown, W.V.	2.8	0.0%	2.07	No	0.01	4	0.88	0.083
	Ohio Valley Medical Center, Wheeling, W.V.	7.6	0.0%	0.80	No	0.10	9	0.40	0.024
	St. Mary's Hospital, Huntington, W.V.	7.2	0.0%	1.03	No	0.09	9	0.90	0.050
	Thomas Memorial Hospital, South Charleston, W.V.	2.9	0.0%	1.39	No	0.00	6	0.37	0.013
	United Hospital Center, Clarksburg, W.V.	3.6	0.0%	1.72	No	0.12	9	0.61	0.012
	Wheeling Hospital, Wheeling, W.V.	4.6	0.0%	1.69	No	0.10	7	0.97	0.069

GASTROENTEROLOGY

Natl. Rank	Hospital	U.S. News index	Reputa-tional score	Gastro-enterology mortality rate	COTH member	Interns and residents to beds	Tech-nology score (of 11)	R.N.'s to beds	Board-certified gastro-enterologists to beds	Pro-cedures to beds
	TIER THREE									
	Charleston Area Medical Center, Charleston, W.V.	8.5	0.0%	1.43	Yes	0.26	9	0.99	0.009	2.91
90	West Virginia University Hospitals, Morgantown	12.5	0.0%	1.38	Yes	1.15	9	1.51	0.009	1.76
	TIER FOUR									
	Bluefield Regional Medical Center, Bluefield, W.V.	3.2	0.0%	1.62	No	0.00	6	0.65	0.011	3.80
	Cabell Huntington Hospital, Huntington, W.V.	2.9	0.0%	2.29	No	0.08	6	1.07	0.020	3.22
	Camden-Clark Memorial Hospital, Parkersburg, W.V.	5.6	0.0%	1.55	No	0.00	9	0.71	0.008	5.79
	Monongalia General Hospital, Morgantown, W.V.	4.6	0.0%	1.42	No	0.01	4	0.88	0.000	5.27
	Ohio Valley Medical Center, Wheeling, W.V.	3.2	0.0%	1.35	No	0.10	8	0.40	0.010	1.53
	St. Mary's Hospital, Huntington, W.V.	6.0	0.0%	1.27	No	0.09	9	0.90	0.005	3.48
	Thomas Memorial Hospital, South Charleston, W.V.	4.1	0.0%	1.28	No	0.00	6	0.37	0.009	4.56
	United Hospital Center, Clarksburg, W.V.	4.3	0.0%	1.65	No	0.12	8	0.61	0.000	4.39
	Wheeling Hospital, Wheeling, W.V.	6.5	0.0%	1.15	No	0.10	6	0.97	0.014	4.51

GERIATRICS

Natl. Rank	Hospital	U.S. News index	Reputa-tional score	Hospital-wide mortality rate	COTH member	Service mix	Interns and residents to beds	Tech-nology score (of 13)	R.N.'s to beds	Discharge planning (of 2)	Geriatric services (of 9)	Board-certified internists to beds
	TIER THREE											
	Charleston Area Medical Center, Charleston, W.V.	14.8	0.0%	1.24	Yes	9	0.26	11	0.99	2	6	0.028
	West Virginia University Hospitals, Morgantown	14.9	0.0%	1.23	Yes	4	1.15	10	1.51	2	2	0.034
	TIER FOUR											
	Bluefield Regional Medical Center, Bluefield, W.V.	5.8	0.0%	1.26	No	3	0.00	9	0.65	1	1	0.011
	Cabell Huntington Hospital, Huntington, W.V.	4.2	0.0%	1.58	No	6	0.08	6	1.07	2	2	0.034
	Camden-Clark Memorial Hospital, Parkersburg, W.V.	6.0	0.0%	1.30	No	2	0.00	9	0.71	2	2	0.004
	Monongalia General Hospital, Morgantown, W.V.	7.0	0.0%	1.28	No	3	0.01	6	0.88	2	2	0.083
	Ohio Valley Medical Center, Wheeling, W.V.	9.6	0.0%	1.11	No	3	0.10	11	0.40	1	3	0.024
	St. Mary's Hospital, Huntington, W.V.	9.7	0.0%	1.18	No	5	0.09	11	0.90	1	2	0.050
	Thomas Memorial Hospital, South Charleston, W.V.	8.5	0.0%	1.14	No	6	0.00	7	0.37	1	1	0.013
	United Hospital Center, Clarksburg, W.V.	8.2	0.0%	1.22	No	3	0.12	11	0.61	2	1	0.012
	Wheeling Hospital, Wheeling, W.V.	8.1	0.0%	1.29	No	5	0.10	8	0.97	2	1	0.069

GYNECOLOGY

Natl. Rank	Hospital	U.S. News index	Reputational score	Hospital-wide mortality rate	Interns and residents to beds	Technology score (of 10)	R.N.'s to beds	Board-certified OB-GYNs to beds	Procedures to beds
TIER THREE									
	West Virginia University Hospitals, Morgantown	18.4	0.0%	1.23	1.15	8	1.51	0.018	0.34
TIER FOUR									
	Bluefield Regional Medical Center, Bluefield, W.V.	6.6	0.0%	1.26	0.00	5	0.65	0.011	0.42
	Cabell Huntington Hospital, Huntington, W.V.	5.1	0.0%	1.58	0.08	5	1.07	0.047	0.54
	Camden-Clark Memorial Hospital, Parkersburg, W.V.	7.7	0.0%	1.30	0.00	7	0.71	0.017	0.72
	Charleston Area Medical Center, Charleston, W.V.	12.0	0.0%	1.24	0.26	8	0.99	0.026	0.32
	Monongalia General Hospital, Morgantown, W.V.	6.9	0.0%	1.28	0.01	4	0.88	0.024	0.82
	Ohio Valley Medical Center, Wheeling, W.V.	10.8	0.0%	1.11	0.10	7	0.40	0.029	0.19
	St. Mary's Hospital, Huntington, W.V.	10.9	0.0%	1.18	0.09	7	0.90	0.007	0.34
	Thomas Memorial Hospital, South Charleston, W.V.	7.8	0.0%	1.14	0.00	5	0.37	0.013	0.34
	United Hospital Center, Clarksburg, W.V.	9.0	0.0%	1.22	0.12	7	0.61	0.006	0.55
	Wheeling Hospital, Wheeling, W.V.	9.3	0.0%	1.29	0.10	6	0.97	0.043	0.78

NEUROLOGY

Natl. Rank	Hospital	U.S. News index	Reputational score	Neurology mortality rate	COTH member	Interns and residents to beds	Technology score (of 9)	R.N.'s to beds	Board-certified neurologists to beds
TIER THREE									
	Ohio Valley Medical Center, Wheeling, W.V.	13.4	0.0%	0.70	No	0.10	7	0.40	0.005
	West Virginia University Hospitals, Morgantown	16.9	0.2%	1.09	Yes	1.15	7	1.51	0.018
TIER FOUR									
	Bluefield Regional Medical Center, Bluefield, W.V.	6.7	0.0%	1.12	No	0.00	5	0.65	0.008
	Cabell Huntington Hospital, Huntington, W.V.	3.4	0.0%	1.59	No	0.08	4	1.07	0.007
	Camden-Clark Memorial Hospital, Parkersburg, W.V.	6.5	0.0%	1.19	No	0.00	7	0.71	0.008
	Charleston Area Medical Center, Charleston, W.V.	9.3	0.0%	1.28	Yes	0.26	7	0.99	0.006
	Monongalia General Hospital, Morgantown, W.V.	5.0	0.0%	1.28	No	0.01	4	0.88	0.005
	St. Mary's Hospital, Huntington, W.V.	7.5	0.0%	1.16	No	0.09	7	0.90	0.005
	Thomas Memorial Hospital, South Charleston, W.V.	10.4	0.0%	0.84	No	0.00	5	0.37	0.004
	United Hospital Center, Clarksburg, W.V.	6.6	0.0%	1.17	No	0.12	7	0.61	0.003
	Wheeling Hospital, Wheeling, W.V.	5.8	0.0%	1.33	No	0.10	5	0.97	0.011

ORTHOPEDICS

Natl. Rank	Hospital	U.S. News index	Reputational score	Orthopedics mortality rate	COTH member	Interns and residents to beds	Technology score (of 5)	R.N.'s to beds	Board-certified orthopedists to beds	Procedures to beds
TIER THREE										
	Charleston Area Medical Center, Charleston, W.V.	8.5	0.0%	1.35	Yes	0.26	4	0.99	0.017	2.05
92	West Virginia University Hospitals, Morgantown	13.5	0.6%	1.33	Yes	1.15	3	1.51	0.003	1.89
TIER FOUR										
	Bluefield Regional Medical Center, Bluefield, W.V.	2.1	0.0%	1.49	No	0.00	2	0.65	0.008	1.81
	Cabell Huntington Hospital, Huntington, W.V.	3.9	0.0%	1.63	No	0.08	3	1.07	0.034	1.80
	Camden-Clark Memorial Hospital, Parkersburg, W.V.	4.8	0.0%	1.15	No	0.00	3	0.71	0.017	3.24
	Monongalia General Hospital, Morgantown, W.V.	6.4	0.0%	1.03	No	0.01	3	0.88	0.029	4.26
	Ohio Valley Medical Center, Wheeling, W.V.	1.9	0.0%	1.63	No	0.10	3	0.40	0.014	1.12
	St. Mary's Hospital, Huntington, W.V.	5.7	0.0%	1.19	No	0.09	4	0.90	0.018	1.86
	Thomas Memorial Hospital, South Charleston, W.V.	3.7	0.0%	1.12	No	0.00	3	0.37	0.013	1.71
	United Hospital Center, Clarksburg, W.V.	5.2	0.0%	1.17	No	0.12	4	0.61	0.012	2.20
	Wheeling Hospital, Wheeling, W.V.	4.3	0.0%	1.35	No	0.10	2	0.97	0.022	3.46

OTOLARYNGOLOGY

Natl. Rank	Hospital	U.S. News index	Reputa- tional score	Hospital- wide mortality rate	COTH member	Interns and residents to beds	Tech- nology score (of 9)	R.N.'s to beds	Board- certified internists to beds	Procedures to beds
	TIER TWO									
62	**West Virginia University Hospitals, Morgantown**	**16.2**	0.5%	1.22	Yes	1.15	7	1.51	0.034	0.409
	TIER THREE									
	Charleston Area Medical Center, Charleston, W.V.	9.3	0.0%	1.24	Yes	0.26	7	0.99	0.028	0.236
	TIER FOUR									
	Bluefield Regional Medical Center, Bluefield, W.V.	3.4	0.0%	1.26	No	0.00	5	0.65	0.011	0.196
	Cabell Huntington Hospital, Huntington, W.V.	4.8	0.0%	1.59	No	0.08	4	1.07	0.034	0.255
	Camden-Clark Memorial Hospital, Parkersburg, W.V.	4.1	0.0%	1.30	No	0.00	7	0.71	0.004	0.450
	Monongalia General Hospital, Morgantown, W.V.	3.9	0.0%	1.28	No	0.01	2	0.88	0.083	0.366
	Ohio Valley Medical Center, Wheeling, W.V.	3.8	0.0%	1.11	No	0.10	7	0.40	0.024	0.074
	St. Mary's Hospital, Huntington, W.V.	5.5	0.0%	1.18	No	0.09	7	0.90	0.050	0.252
	Thomas Memorial Hospital, South Charleston, W.V.	2.3	0.0%	1.14	No	0.00	4	0.37	0.013	0.275
	United Hospital Center, Clarksburg, W.V.	4.3	0.0%	1.22	No	0.12	7	0.61	0.012	0.229
	Wheeling Hospital, Wheeling, W.V.	5.5	0.0%	1.29	No	0.10	6	0.97	0.069	0.290

RHEUMATOLOGY

Natl. Rank	Hospital	U.S. News index	Reputa- tional score	Hospital- wide mortality rate	COTH member	Interns and residents to beds	Tech- nology score (of 5)	R.N.'s to beds	Board- certified internists to beds
	TIER THREE								
	Charleston Area Medical Center, Charleston, W.V.	10.5	0.0%	1.24	Yes	0.26	4	0.99	0.028
	West Virginia University Hospitals, Morgantown	14.4	0.0%	1.22	Yes	1.15	3	1.51	0.034
	TIER FOUR								
	Bluefield Regional Medical Center, Bluefield, W.V.	4.2	0.0%	1.26	No	0.00	2	0.65	0.011
	Cabell Huntington Hospital, Huntington, W.V.	5.7	0.0%	1.59	No	0.08	3	1.07	0.034
	Camden-Clark Memorial Hospital, Parkersburg, W.V.	5.5	0.0%	1.30	No	0.00	3	0.71	0.004
	Monongalia General Hospital, Morgantown, W.V.	6.7	0.0%	1.28	No	0.01	3	0.88	0.083
	Ohio Valley Medical Center, Wheeling, W.V.	5.4	0.0%	1.11	No	0.10	3	0.40	0.024
	St. Mary's Hospital, Huntington, W.V.	6.8	0.0%	1.18	No	0.09	4	0.90	0.050
	Thomas Memorial Hospital, South Charleston, W.V.	4.7	0.0%	1.14	No	0.00	3	0.37	0.013
	United Hospital Center, Clarksburg, W.V.	6.6	0.0%	1.22	No	0.12	4	0.61	0.012
	Wheeling Hospital, Wheeling, W.V.	6.6	0.0%	1.29	No	0.10	2	0.97	0.069

UROLOGY

Natl. Rank	Hospital	U.S. News index	Reputa- tional score	Urology mortality rate	COTH member	Interns and residents to beds	Tech- nology score (of 11)	R.N.'s to beds	Board- certified internists to beds	Procedures to beds
	TIER THREE									
	Charleston Area Medical Center, Charleston, W.V.	9.7	0.0%	1.30	Yes	0.26	9	0.99	0.028	1.82
	Monongalia General Hospital, Morgantown, W.V.	10.0	0.0%	0.78	No	0.01	4	0.88	0.083	2.31
98	West Virginia University Hospitals, Morgantown	14.6	0.0%	1.22	Yes	1.15	9	1.51	0.034	2.11
	TIER FOUR									
	Bluefield Regional Medical Center, Bluefield, W.V.	5.3	0.0%	1.17	No	0.00	6	0.65	0.011	1.82
	Cabell Huntington Hospital, Huntington, W.V.	4.7	0.0%	1.64	No	0.08	6	1.07	0.034	2.42
	Camden-Clark Memorial Hospital, Parkersburg, W.V.	3.8	0.0%	1.78	No	0.00	9	0.71	0.004	2.82
	Ohio Valley Medical Center, Wheeling, W.V.	4.2	0.0%	1.35	No	0.10	8	0.40	0.024	0.75
	St. Mary's Hospital, Huntington, W.V.	5.4	0.0%	1.56	No	0.09	9	0.90	0.050	2.20
	Thomas Memorial Hospital, South Charleston, W.V.	3.8	0.0%	1.33	No	0.00	6	0.37	0.013	2.40
	United Hospital Center, Clarksburg, W.V.	5.3	0.0%	1.30	No	0.12	8	0.61	0.012	1.88
	Wheeling Hospital, Wheeling, W.V.	5.3	0.0%	1.47	No	0.10	6	0.97	0.069	2.32

AIDS

Natl. Rank	Hospital	U.S. News index	Reputational score	Hospital-wide mortality rate	COTH member	Interns and residents to beds	Technology score (of 11)	Discharge planning (of 2)	R.N.'s to beds	Board-certified internists to beds
	TIER TWO									
45	**University of Wisconsin Hospital and Clinics, Madison**	27.7	0.4%	0.95	Yes	1.30	10	2	1.24	0.037
	TIER THREE									
	Froedtert Memorial Lutheran Hospital, Milwaukee	22.1	0.0%	1.03	Yes	0.49	3	2	1.13	0.199
	Luther Hospital, Eau Claire, Wis.	20.6	0.0%	0.99	No	0.03	7	2	0.87	0.054
	Lutheran Hospital-La Crosse, La Crosse, Wis.	22.2	0.0%	0.95	No	0.12	9	2	0.93	0.026
	Mercy Hospital of Janesville, Janesville, Wis.	20.5	0.0%	0.99	No	0.03	7	2	0.74	0.085
	Mercy Medical Center, Oshkosh, Wis.	20.0	0.0%	0.99	No	0.00	6	2	0.68	0.055
	Meriter Hospital, Madison, Wis.	21.2	0.0%	0.91	No	0.10	5	2	0.62	0.079
	Milwaukee County Medical Complex	19.7	0.0%	1.28	Yes	0.43	8	2	0.81	0.081
	Sacred Heart Hospital, Eau Claire, Wis.	20.7	0.0%	0.94	No	0.02	7	2	0.39	0.042
	Sinai Samaritan Medical Center, Milwaukee	23.9	0.0%	1.00	Yes	0.66	7	2	0.86	0.170
	St. Elizabeth Hospital, Appleton, Wis.	20.5	0.0%	0.93	No	0.03	6	2	0.32	0.053
	St. Francis Medical Center, La Crosse, Wis.	21.1	0.0%	0.88	No	0.11	4	2	0.50	0.051
	St. Luke's Medical Center, Milwaukee	21.1	0.0%	1.07	Yes	0.20	8	1	0.76	0.125
	St. Mary's Hospital Medical Center, Madison, Wis.	20.5	0.0%	0.94	No	0.09	5	2	0.64	0.064
	Wausau Hospital, Wausau, Wis.	22.8	0.0%	0.83	No	0.06	7	2	0.98	0.034
	TIER FOUR									
	Appleton Medical Center, Appleton, Wis.	19.2	0.0%	0.99	No	0.05	4	2	0.55	0.095
	Columbia Hospital, Milwaukee	18.6	0.0%	1.12	No	0.06	7	2	0.68	0.093
	St. Agnes Hospital, Fond du Lac, Wis.	17.5	0.0%	1.22	No	0.00	8	2	0.70	0.026
	St. Catherine's Hospital, Kenosha, Wis.	18.7	0.0%	1.00	No	0.07	5	2	0.26	0.038
	St. Francis Hospital, Milwaukee	16.6	0.0%	1.28	No	0.00	6	2	0.62	0.158
	St. Joseph's Hospital, Marshfield, Wis.	17.2	0.0%	1.14	No	0.05	5	2	0.46	0.059
	St. Joseph's Hospital, Milwaukee	17.1	0.0%	1.26	No	0.14	7	2	0.71	0.075
	St. Mary's Hospital, Milwaukee	15.9	0.0%	1.31	No	0.11	6	1	1.09	0.027
	St. Michael Hospital, Milwaukee	17.6	0.0%	1.10	No	0.08	5	2	0.42	0.048
	St. Vincent Hospital, Green Bay, Wis.	18.7	0.0%	1.05	No	0.00	6	1	0.89	0.076
	Waukesha Memorial Hospital, Waukesha, Wis.	18.8	0.0%	1.08	No	0.04	7	2	0.53	0.047
	West Allis Memorial Hospital, West Allis, Wis.	19.1	0.0%	1.02	No	0.03	7	1	0.56	0.085

CANCER

Natl. Rank	Hospital	U.S. News index	Reputational score	Cancer mortality rate	COTH member	Interns and residents to beds	Technology score (of 12)	R.N.'s to beds	Board-certified oncologists to beds	Procedures to beds
	TIER TWO									
22	**University of Wisconsin Hospital and Clinics, Madison**	15.8	2.0%	0.62	Yes	1.30	11	1.24	0.039	2.14
	TIER THREE									
	Froedtert Memorial Lutheran Hospital, Milwaukee	7.8	0.5%	0.60	Yes	0.49	1	1.13	0.028	0.95
	Lutheran Hospital-La Crosse, La Crosse, Wis.	5.5	0.0%	0.68	No	0.12	10	0.93	0.014	1.67
	Milwaukee County Medical Complex	8.0	0.0%	0.77	Yes	0.43	8	0.81	0.041	1.15
	Sinai Samaritan Medical Center, Milwaukee	8.3	0.0%	0.91	Yes	0.66	7	0.86	0.028	1.14
	St. Luke's Medical Center, Milwaukee	7.2	0.0%	0.96	Yes	0.20	9	0.76	0.009	2.60
	TIER FOUR									
	Appleton Medical Center, Appleton, Wis.	1.4	0.0%	1.03	No	0.05	1	0.55	0.013	2.83
	Columbia Hospital, Milwaukee	3.1	0.0%	1.25	No	0.06	7	0.68	0.017	1.98
	Luther Hospital, Eau Claire, Wis.	4.3	0.0%	0.71	No	0.03	8	0.87	0.010	1.52
	Mercy Hospital of Janesville, Janesville, Wis.	3.8	0.0%	0.91	No	0.03	9	0.74	0.000	1.12
	Mercy Medical Center, Oshkosh, Wis.	2.8	0.0%	0.89	No	0.00	6	0.68	0.000	1.39
	Meriter Hospital, Madison, Wis.	2.8	0.0%	0.63	No	0.10	4	0.62	0.011	1.05
	Sacred Heart Hospital, Eau Claire, Wis.	2.8	0.0%	0.71	No	0.02	8	0.39	0.007	0.85

Natl. Rank	Hospital	U.S. News index	Reputational score	Cancer mortality rate	COTH member	Interns and residents to beds	Technology score (of 12)	R.N.'s to beds	Board-certified oncologists to beds	Procedures to beds
	St. Agnes Hospital, Fond du Lac, Wis.	3.0	0.0%	1.40	No	0.00	8	0.70	0.009	1.44
	St. Catherine's Hospital, Kenosha, Wis.	1.7	0.0%	0.83	No	0.07	5	0.26	0.005	1.46
	St. Elizabeth Hospital, Appleton, Wis.	2.1	0.0%	0.93	No	0.03	7	0.32	0.007	1.25
	St. Francis Hospital, Milwaukee	1.2	0.0%	1.94	No	0.00	3	0.62	0.011	1.41
	St. Francis Medical Center, La Crosse, Wis.	2.4	0.0%	0.56	No	0.11	4	0.50	0.000	1.05
	St. Joseph's Hospital, Marshfield, Wis.	3.0	0.0%	0.91	No	0.05	7	0.46	0.025	2.84
	St. Joseph's Hospital, Milwaukee	3.4	0.0%	2.04	No	0.14	8	0.71	0.013	2.00
	St. Mary's Hospital Medical Center, Madison, Wis.	3.0	0.0%	0.76	No	0.09	5	0.64	0.012	1.62
	St. Mary's Hospital, Milwaukee	3.9	0.0%	2.17	No	0.11	7	1.09	0.006	1.36
	St. Michael Hospital, Milwaukee	1.8	0.0%	0.71	No	0.08	3	0.42	0.018	1.32
	St. Vincent Hospital, Green Bay, Wis.	3.5	0.0%	1.10	No	0.00	6	0.89	0.015	2.61
	Waukesha Memorial Hospital, Waukesha, Wis.	2.7	0.0%	1.45	No	0.04	8	0.53	0.010	1.57
	Wausau Hospital, Wausau, Wis.	5.0	0.0%	0.65	No	0.06	8	0.98	0.008	2.05
	West Allis Memorial Hospital, West Allis, Wis.	3.2	0.0%	1.19	No	0.03	8	0.56	0.017	2.79

CARDIOLOGY

Natl. Rank	Hospital	U.S. News index	Reputational score	Cardiology mortality rate	COTH member	Interns and residents to beds	Technology score (of 10)	R.N.'s to beds	Board-certified cardiologists to beds	Procedures to beds
TIER TWO										
46	Sinai Samaritan Medical Center, Milwaukee	23.6	0.0%	0.77	Yes	0.66	8	0.86	0.097	9.01
72	University of Wisconsin Hospital and Clinics, Madison	21.7	0.0%	1.04	Yes	1.30	9	1.24	0.018	4.11
TIER THREE										
	Appleton Medical Center, Appleton, Wis.	15.4	0.4%	0.97	No	0.05	6	0.55	0.063	12.10
	Columbia Hospital, Milwaukee	16.4	0.0%	0.92	No	0.06	8	0.68	0.048	5.52
	Luther Hospital, Eau Claire, Wis.	14.9	0.0%	0.95	No	0.03	6	0.87	0.020	7.50
	St. Catherine's Hospital, Kenosha, Wis.	15.0	0.0%	0.84	No	0.07	5	0.26	0.016	6.99
	St. Elizabeth Hospital, Appleton, Wis.	13.7	0.0%	0.95	No	0.03	7	0.32	0.039	3.34
	St. Francis Medical Center, La Crosse, Wis.	15.2	0.0%	0.79	No	0.11	4	0.50	0.004	4.78
99	St. Luke's Medical Center, Milwaukee	20.7	1.7%	1.02	Yes	0.20	9	0.76	0.076	18.93
	St. Mary's Hospital Medical Center, Madison, Wis.	14.0	0.0%	0.98	No	0.09	7	0.64	0.020	8.20
	St. Vincent Hospital, Green Bay, Wis.	14.5	0.0%	0.96	No	0.00	6	0.89	0.021	4.54
	Waukesha Memorial Hospital, Waukesha, Wis.	17.1	0.0%	0.81	No	0.04	8	0.53	0.037	8.27
	Wausau Hospital, Wausau, Wis.	18.4	0.0%	0.80	No	0.06	8	0.98	0.034	8.39
	West Allis Memorial Hospital, West Allis, Wis.	13.6	0.0%	0.97	No	0.03	6	0.56	0.021	8.06
TIER FOUR										
	Lutheran Hospital-La Crosse, La Crosse, Wis.	13.4	0.0%	1.08	No	0.12	9	0.93	0.011	10.01
	Mercy Hospital of Janesville, Janesville, Wis.	12.0	0.0%	1.04	No	0.03	6	0.74	0.009	5.44
	Mercy Medical Center, Oshkosh, Wis.	12.2	0.0%	1.06	No	0.00	8	0.68	0.017	6.23
	Meriter Hospital, Madison, Wis.	13.4	0.0%	0.98	No	0.10	6	0.62	0.014	6.06
	Milwaukee County Medical Complex	12.4	0.5%	1.42	Yes	0.43	9	0.81	0.051	4.21
	Sacred Heart Hospital, Eau Claire, Wis.	13.2	0.0%	0.93	No	0.02	5	0.39	0.010	3.93
	St. Agnes Hospital, Fond du Lac, Wis.	9.8	0.0%	1.12	No	0.00	5	0.70	0.013	5.17
	St. Francis Hospital, Milwaukee	10.9	0.0%	1.13	No	0.00	8	0.62	0.036	6.50
	St. Joseph's Hospital, Marshfield, Wis.	10.2	0.6%	1.17	No	0.05	6	0.46	0.027	8.46
	St. Joseph's Hospital, Milwaukee	12.2	0.0%	1.10	No	0.14	7	0.71	0.039	8.89
	St. Mary's Hospital, Milwaukee	9.6	1.2%	1.48	No	0.11	8	1.09	0.045	7.16
	St. Michael Hospital, Milwaukee	11.9	0.0%	1.06	No	0.08	8	0.42	0.026	7.89

ENDOCRINOLOGY

Natl. Rank	Hospital	U.S. News index	Reputa-tional score	Endocrinology mortality rate	COTH member	Interns and residents to beds	Tech-nology score (of 11)	R.N.'s to beds	Board-certified internists to beds
	TIER TWO								
39	**University of Wisconsin Hospital and Clinics, Madison**	18.6	0.0%	0.61	Yes	1.30	11	1.24	0.037
	TIER THREE								
	Froedtert Memorial Lutheran Hospital, Milwaukee	10.7	0.0%	1.06	Yes	0.49	0	1.13	0.199
	Mercy Hospital of Janesville, Janesville, Wis.	10.7	0.0%	0.61	No	0.03	10	0.74	0.085
96	**Milwaukee County Medical Complex**	13.6	0.0%	0.72	Yes	0.43	9	0.81	0.081
	Sinai Samaritan Medical Center, Milwaukee	12.1	0.0%	1.04	Yes	0.66	8	0.86	0.170
	St. Agnes Hospital, Fond du Lac, Wis.	9.0	0.0%	0.72	No	0.00	9	0.70	0.026
	St. Francis Medical Center, La Crosse, Wis.	9.1	0.0%	0.33	No	0.11	5	0.50	0.051
	St. Luke's Medical Center, Milwaukee	9.2	0.0%	1.25	Yes	0.20	10	0.76	0.125
	Wausau Hospital, Wausau, Wis.	10.0	0.0%	0.72	No	0.06	9	0.98	0.034
	TIER FOUR								
	Columbia Hospital, Milwaukee	4.5	0.0%	1.50	No	0.06	8	0.68	0.093
	Lutheran Hospital-La Crosse, La Crosse, Wis.	7.8	0.0%	0.98	No	0.12	10	0.93	0.026
	Mercy Medical Center, Oshkosh, Wis.	4.5	0.0%	1.31	No	0.00	7	0.68	0.055
	Meriter Hospital, Madison, Wis.	5.1	0.0%	1.08	No	0.10	3	0.62	0.079
	St. Catherine's Hospital, Kenosha, Wis.	7.1	0.0%	0.76	No	0.07	6	0.26	0.038
	St. Francis Hospital, Milwaukee	6.2	0.0%	1.01	No	0.00	5	0.62	0.158
	St. Joseph's Hospital, Marshfield, Wis.	5.7	0.0%	0.98	No	0.05	6	0.46	0.059
	St. Joseph's Hospital, Milwaukee	6.1	0.0%	1.15	No	0.14	8	0.71	0.075
	St. Mary's Hospital Medical Center, Madison, Wis.	6.4	0.0%	0.91	No	0.09	4	0.64	0.064
	St. Mary's Hospital, Milwaukee	7.9	0.0%	0.96	No	0.11	8	1.09	0.027
	St. Michael Hospital, Milwaukee	4.9	0.0%	1.02	No	0.08	4	0.42	0.048
	St. Vincent Hospital, Green Bay, Wis.	6.8	0.0%	1.03	No	0.00	8	0.89	0.076
	Waukesha Memorial Hospital, Waukesha, Wis.	5.4	0.0%	1.13	No	0.04	9	0.53	0.047
	West Allis Memorial Hospital, West Allis, Wis.	5.1	0.0%	1.25	No	0.03	9	0.56	0.085

GASTROENTEROLOGY

Natl. Rank	Hospital	U.S. News index	Reputa-tional score	Gastro-enterology mortality rate	COTH member	Interns and residents to beds	Tech-nology score (of 11)	R.N.'s to beds	Board-certified gastro-enterologists to beds	Pro-cedures to beds
	TIER TWO									
25	**University of Wisconsin Hospital and Clinics, Madison**	18.3	2.0%	0.97	Yes	1.30	11	1.24	0.014	2.03
	TIER THREE									
	Froedtert Memorial Lutheran Hospital, Milwaukee	9.7	0.0%	0.90	Yes	0.49	0	1.13	0.028	2.39
	Luther Hospital, Eau Claire, Wis.	7.5	0.0%	0.90	No	0.03	8	0.87	0.015	2.92
	Lutheran Hospital-La Crosse, La Crosse, Wis.	9.8	0.0%	0.83	No	0.12	10	0.93	0.006	4.07
	Mercy Hospital of Janesville, Janesville, Wis.	7.8	0.0%	0.88	No	0.03	9	0.74	0.005	3.31
	Sinai Samaritan Medical Center, Milwaukee	10.5	0.0%	1.08	Yes	0.66	7	0.86	0.028	2.56
	St. Luke's Medical Center, Milwaukee	10.8	0.4%	1.06	Yes	0.20	10	0.76	0.024	3.63
	Wausau Hospital, Wausau, Wis.	9.4	0.0%	0.82	No	0.06	9	0.98	0.004	3.80
	TIER FOUR									
	Appleton Medical Center, Appleton, Wis.	5.7	0.0%	0.95	No	0.05	3	0.55	0.013	4.34
	Columbia Hospital, Milwaukee	6.8	0.0%	0.95	No	0.06	7	0.68	0.020	3.62
	Mercy Medical Center, Oshkosh, Wis.	6.2	0.0%	1.05	No	0.00	8	0.68	0.004	3.72
	Meriter Hospital, Madison, Wis.	6.3	0.0%	0.73	No	0.10	3	0.62	0.011	2.66
	Sacred Heart Hospital, Eau Claire, Wis.	4.5	0.0%	1.14	No	0.02	9	0.39	0.010	2.07
	St. Agnes Hospital, Fond du Lac, Wis.	5.5	0.0%	1.14	No	0.00	8	0.70	0.000	3.36
	St. Catherine's Hospital, Kenosha, Wis.	6.5	0.0%	0.75	No	0.07	6	0.26	0.011	3.11
	St. Elizabeth Hospital, Appleton, Wis.	4.8	0.0%	1.01	No	0.03	8	0.32	0.007	2.00
	St. Francis Hospital, Milwaukee	4.0	0.0%	1.31	No	0.00	5	0.62	0.014	4.02
	St. Francis Medical Center, La Crosse, Wis.	6.0	0.0%	0.89	No	0.11	4	0.50	0.008	3.33
	St. Joseph's Hospital, Marshfield, Wis.	4.1	0.0%	1.16	No	0.05	5	0.46	0.017	3.18

Natl. Rank	Hospital	U.S. News index	Reputa-tional score	Gastro-enterology mortality rate	COTH member	Interns and residents to beds	Tech-nology score (of 11)	R.N.'s to beds	Board-certified gastro-enterologists to beds	Pro-cedures to beds
	St. Joseph's Hospital, Milwaukee	5.2	0.0%	1.30	No	0.14	8	0.71	0.012	3.34
	St. Mary's Hospital Medical Center, Madison, Wis.	6.9	0.0%	0.73	No	0.09	3	0.64	0.009	3.69
	St. Mary's Hospital, Milwaukee	3.3	0.0%	1.87	No	0.11	7	1.09	0.012	2.04
	St. Michael Hospital, Milwaukee	5.0	0.0%	1.10	No	0.08	4	0.42	0.031	4.53
	St. Vincent Hospital, Green Bay, Wis.	6.0	0.0%	1.08	No	0.00	7	0.89	0.015	3.35
	Waukesha Memorial Hospital, Waukesha, Wis.	5.7	0.0%	1.09	No	0.04	9	0.53	0.010	3.05
	West Allis Memorial Hospital, West Allis, Wis.	6.6	0.0%	1.09	No	0.03	8	0.56	0.025	4.98

GERIATRICS

Natl. Rank	Hospital	U.S. News index	Reputa-tional score	Hospital-wide mortality rate	COTH member	Service mix	Interns and residents to beds	Tech-nology score (of 13)	R.N.'s to beds	Discharge planning (of 2)	Geriatric services (of 9)	Board-certified internists to beds
TIER ONE												
19	University of Wisconsin Hospital and Clinics, Madison	31.6	2.7%	0.95	Yes	9	1.30	11	1.24	2	5	0.037
TIER TWO												
83	Sinai Samaritan Medical Center, Milwaukee	22.1	0.0%	1.00	Yes	8	0.66	10	0.86	2	9	0.170
TIER THREE												
	Appleton Medical Center, Appleton, Wis.	14.2	0.0%	0.99	No	4	0.05	4	0.55	2	7	0.095
	Froedtert Memorial Lutheran Hospital, Milwaukee	17.2	0.0%	1.03	Yes	4	0.49	1	1.13	2	6	0.199
	Luther Hospital, Eau Claire, Wis.	16.0	0.3%	0.99	No	5	0.03	10	0.87	2	3	0.054
	Lutheran Hospital-La Crosse, La Crosse, Wis.	18.7	0.0%	0.95	No	10	0.12	11	0.93	2	2	0.026
	Mercy Hospital of Janesville, Janesville, Wis.	15.8	0.0%	0.99	No	5	0.03	10	0.74	2	6	0.085
	Mercy Medical Center, Oshkosh, Wis.	15.4	0.0%	0.99	No	7	0.00	7	0.68	2	4	0.055
	Meriter Hospital, Madison, Wis.	16.8	0.0%	0.91	No	6	0.10	5	0.62	2	6	0.079
	Sacred Heart Hospital, Eau Claire, Wis.	16.8	0.0%	0.94	No	6	0.02	9	0.39	2	6	0.042
	St. Elizabeth Hospital, Appleton, Wis.	15.9	0.0%	0.93	No	5	0.03	9	0.32	2	3	0.053
	St. Francis Medical Center, La Crosse, Wis.	17.5	0.0%	0.88	No	6	0.11	6	0.50	2	3	0.051
	St. Luke's Medical Center, Milwaukee	17.1	0.5%	1.07	Yes	6	0.20	12	0.76	1	5	0.125
	St. Mary's Hospital Medical Center, Madison, Wis.	16.4	0.0%	0.94	No	4	0.09	7	0.64	2	7	0.064
	Wausau Hospital, Wausau, Wis.	17.9	0.0%	0.83	No	4	0.06	10	0.98	2	2	0.034
TIER FOUR												
	Columbia Hospital, Milwaukee	13.4	0.0%	1.12	No	7	0.06	10	0.68	2	6	0.093
	Milwaukee County Medical Complex	11.9	0.0%	1.28	Yes	6	0.43	11	0.81	2	1	0.081
	St. Agnes Hospital, Fond du Lac, Wis.	10.6	0.0%	1.22	No	8	0.00	9	0.70	2	4	0.026
	St. Catherine's Hospital, Kenosha, Wis.	13.6	0.0%	1.00	No	5	0.07	7	0.26	2	5	0.038
	St. Francis Hospital, Milwaukee	7.8	0.0%	1.28	No	4	0.00	6	0.62	2	4	0.158
	St. Joseph's Hospital, Marshfield, Wis.	11.4	0.0%	1.14	No	6	0.05	7	0.46	2	6	0.059
	St. Joseph's Hospital, Milwaukee	10.3	0.0%	1.26	No	6	0.14	10	0.71	2	6	0.075
	St. Mary's Hospital, Milwaukee	7.1	0.0%	1.31	No	4	0.11	10	1.09	1	3	0.027
	St. Michael Hospital, Milwaukee	11.3	0.0%	1.10	No	5	0.08	6	0.42	2	5	0.048
	St. Vincent Hospital, Green Bay, Wis.	12.2	0.0%	1.05	No	5	0.00	9	0.89	1	2	0.076
	Waukesha Memorial Hospital, Waukesha, Wis.	12.4	0.0%	1.08	No	5	0.04	9	0.53	2	4	0.047
	West Allis Memorial Hospital, West Allis, Wis.	12.5	0.0%	1.02	No	4	0.03	9	0.56	1	4	0.085

GYNECOLOGY

Natl. Rank	Hospital	U.S. News index	Reputa-tional score	Hospital-wide mortality rate	Interns and residents to beds	Tech-nology score (of 10)	R.N.'s to beds	Board-certified OB-GYNs to beds	Pro-cedures to beds
TIER TWO									
41	University of Wisconsin Hospital and Clinics, Madison	27.6	0.9%	0.95	1.30	9	1.24	0.027	0.31
TIER THREE									
	Luther Hospital, Eau Claire, Wis.	16.9	0.0%	0.99	0.03	8	0.87	0.064	0.38
	Lutheran Hospital-La Crosse, La Crosse, Wis.	18.8	0.0%	0.95	0.12	9	0.93	0.031	0.52

Natl. Rank	Hospital	U.S. News index	Reputa-tional score	Hospital-wide mortality rate	Interns and residents to beds	Tech-nology score (of 10)	R.N.'s to beds	Board-certified OB-GYNs to beds	Procedures to beds
	Mercy Hospital of Janesville, Janesville, Wis.	15.5	0.0%	0.99	0.03	8	0.74	0.028	0.42
	Meriter Hospital, Madison, Wis.	15.3	0.0%	0.91	0.10	4	0.62	0.043	0.44
	Sacred Heart Hospital, Eau Claire, Wis.	14.5	0.0%	0.94	0.02	7	0.39	0.016	0.23
	Sinai Samaritan Medical Center, Milwaukee	19.8	0.0%	1.00	0.66	7	0.86	0.100	0.44
	St. Elizabeth Hospital, Appleton, Wis.	14.4	0.0%	0.93	0.03	6	0.32	0.036	0.32
	St. Francis Medical Center, La Crosse, Wis.	14.9	0.0%	0.88	0.11	4	0.50	0.008	0.29
	St. Vincent Hospital, Green Bay, Wis.	14.2	0.0%	1.05	0.00	7	0.89	0.044	0.44
	Wausau Hospital, Wausau, Wis.	19.3	0.0%	0.83	0.06	7	0.98	0.026	0.40
	West Allis Memorial Hospital, West Allis, Wis.	14.8	0.0%	1.02	0.03	7	0.56	0.093	0.80
TIER FOUR									
	Appleton Medical Center, Appleton, Wis.	12.5	0.0%	0.99	0.05	3	0.55	0.082	0.58
	Columbia Hospital, Milwaukee	11.4	0.0%	1.12	0.06	6	0.68	0.056	0.34
	Mercy Medical Center, Oshkosh, Wis.	13.5	0.0%	0.99	0.00	6	0.68	0.013	0.48
	Milwaukee County Medical Complex	12.1	0.0%	1.28	0.43	8	0.81	0.057	0.21
	St. Agnes Hospital, Fond du Lac, Wis.	9.2	0.0%	1.22	0.00	7	0.70	0.022	0.53
	St. Catherine's Hospital, Kenosha, Wis.	11.5	0.0%	1.00	0.07	5	0.26	0.043	0.28
	St. Francis Hospital, Milwaukee	8.1	0.0%	1.28	0.00	6	0.62	0.065	0.43
	St. Joseph's Hospital, Marshfield, Wis.	9.4	0.4%	1.14	0.05	5	0.46	0.019	0.49
	St. Joseph's Hospital, Milwaukee	9.4	0.0%	1.26	0.14	7	0.71	0.040	0.47
	St. Luke's Medical Center, Milwaukee	13.3	0.0%	1.07	0.20	7	0.76	0.020	0.34
	St. Mary's Hospital Medical Center, Madison, Wis.	14.0	0.0%	0.94	0.09	4	0.64	0.032	0.45
	St. Mary's Hospital, Milwaukee	10.3	0.0%	1.31	0.11	7	1.09	0.048	0.73
	St. Michael Hospital, Milwaukee	9.6	0.0%	1.10	0.08	4	0.42	0.066	0.43
	Waukesha Memorial Hospital, Waukesha, Wis.	12.9	0.0%	1.08	0.04	8	0.53	0.043	0.24

NEUROLOGY

Natl. Rank	Hospital	U.S. News index	Reputa-tional score	Neurology mortality rate	COTH member	Interns and residents to beds	Tech-nology score (of 9)	R.N.'s to beds	Board-certified neurologists to beds
TIER TWO									
74	University of Wisconsin Hospital and Clinics, Madison	18.3	1.7%	1.29	Yes	1.30	9	1.24	0.033
TIER THREE									
	Froedtert Memorial Lutheran Hospital, Milwaukee	14.0	0.0%	1.04	Yes	0.49	0	1.13	0.049
	Lutheran Hospital-La Crosse, La Crosse, Wis.	11.3	0.0%	0.97	No	0.12	8	0.93	0.014
	Sinai Samaritan Medical Center, Milwaukee	11.1	0.0%	1.24	Yes	0.66	6	0.86	0.017
	St. Elizabeth Hospital, Appleton, Wis.	13.3	0.0%	0.71	No	0.03	6	0.32	0.014
	St. Francis Medical Center, La Crosse, Wis.	11.2	0.0%	0.82	No	0.11	3	0.50	0.008
	Wausau Hospital, Wausau, Wis.	15.2	0.0%	0.74	No	0.06	7	0.98	0.011
TIER FOUR									
	Appleton Medical Center, Appleton, Wis.	3.2	0.0%	1.48	No	0.05	3	0.55	0.019
	Columbia Hospital, Milwaukee	8.1	0.0%	1.16	No	0.06	6	0.68	0.028
	Mercy Hospital of Janesville, Janesville, Wis.	6.9	0.0%	1.27	No	0.03	8	0.74	0.019
	Mercy Medical Center, Oshkosh, Wis.	8.8	0.0%	1.02	No	0.00	6	0.68	0.013
	Meriter Hospital, Madison, Wis.	6.7	0.0%	1.11	No	0.10	3	0.62	0.011
	Sacred Heart Hospital, Eau Claire, Wis.	10.4	0.0%	0.90	No	0.02	7	0.39	0.013
	St. Catherine's Hospital, Kenosha, Wis.	2.7	0.0%	1.41	No	0.07	5	0.26	0.005
	St. Francis Hospital, Milwaukee	4.4	0.0%	1.40	No	0.00	5	0.62	0.018
	St. Joseph's Hospital, Marshfield, Wis.	8.0	0.5%	1.11	No	0.05	5	0.46	0.021
	St. Joseph's Hospital, Milwaukee	5.8	0.0%	1.30	No	0.14	6	0.71	0.012
	St. Luke's Medical Center, Milwaukee	9.8	0.0%	1.19	Yes	0.20	8	0.76	0.007
	St. Mary's Hospital Medical Center, Madison, Wis.	6.6	0.0%	1.12	No	0.09	3	0.64	0.012
	St. Mary's Hospital, Milwaukee	9.9	0.0%	1.02	No	0.11	6	1.09	0.009
	St. Michael Hospital, Milwaukee	9.6	0.0%	0.95	No	0.08	4	0.42	0.022

Natl. Rank	Hospital	U.S. News index	Reputa-tional score	Neurology mortality rate	COTH member	Interns and residents to beds	Tech-nology score (of 9)	R.N.'s to beds	Board-certified neurologists to beds
	St. Vincent Hospital, Green Bay, Wis.	7.6	0.0%	1.14	No	0.00	6	0.89	0.012
	Waukesha Memorial Hospital, Waukesha, Wis.	7.7	0.0%	1.09	No	0.04	8	0.53	0.007
	West Allis Memorial Hospital, West Allis, Wis.	9.8	0.0%	0.94	No	0.03	7	0.56	0.008

ORTHOPEDICS

Natl. Rank	Hospital	U.S. News index	Reputa-tional score	Orthopedics mortality rate	COTH member	Interns and residents to beds	Tech-nology score (of 5)	R.N.'s to beds	Board-certified orthopedists to beds	Pro-cedures to beds
	TIER ONE									
20	University of Wisconsin Hospital and Clinics, Madison	21.1	1.0%	0.57	Yes	1.30	5	1.24	0.014	1.66
	TIER THREE									
	Luther Hospital, Eau Claire, Wis.	10.8	0.0%	0.45	No	0.03	4	0.87	0.059	2.77
	Mercy Medical Center, Oshkosh, Wis.	8.9	0.0%	0.74	No	0.00	4	0.68	0.021	3.15
	Meriter Hospital, Madison, Wis.	8.9	0.0%	0.65	No	0.10	2	0.62	0.023	2.73
	Milwaukee County Medical Complex	11.4	0.5%	1.02	Yes	0.43	4	0.81	0.027	1.30
	Sinai Samaritan Medical Center, Milwaukee	11.4	0.0%	0.91	Yes	0.66	3	0.86	0.021	1.57
	St. Elizabeth Hospital, Appleton, Wis.	8.5	0.0%	0.66	No	0.03	3	0.32	0.039	2.52
	St. Luke's Medical Center, Milwaukee	10.4	0.0%	0.93	Yes	0.20	4	0.76	0.024	2.69
	St. Mary's Hospital Medical Center, Madison, Wis.	9.1	0.0%	0.43	No	0.09	2	0.64	0.020	3.78
	St. Vincent Hospital, Green Bay, Wis.	9.6	0.0%	0.72	No	0.00	3	0.89	0.038	4.80
	Wausau Hospital, Wausau, Wis.	9.1	0.0%	0.84	No	0.06	4	0.98	0.030	4.23
	TIER FOUR									
	Appleton Medical Center, Appleton, Wis.	5.0	0.0%	1.03	No	0.05	2	0.55	0.070	3.42
	Columbia Hospital, Milwaukee	6.7	0.0%	0.96	No	0.06	3	0.68	0.039	5.01
	Lutheran Hospital-La Crosse, La Crosse, Wis.	6.2	0.0%	1.20	No	0.12	4	0.93	0.011	3.59
	Mercy Hospital of Janesville, Janesville, Wis.	7.9	0.0%	0.87	No	0.03	4	0.74	0.047	3.50
	Sacred Heart Hospital, Eau Claire, Wis.	6.1	0.0%	0.95	No	0.02	4	0.39	0.039	3.24
	St. Agnes Hospital, Fond du Lac, Wis.	4.6	0.0%	1.28	No	0.00	4	0.70	0.013	2.77
	St. Catherine's Hospital, Kenosha, Wis.	6.0	0.0%	0.82	No	0.07	3	0.26	0.022	1.68
	St. Francis Hospital, Milwaukee	4.8	0.0%	1.39	No	0.00	4	0.62	0.097	4.08
	St. Francis Medical Center, La Crosse, Wis.	4.7	0.0%	1.00	No	0.11	2	0.50	0.008	2.23
	St. Joseph's Hospital, Marshfield, Wis.	1.7	0.0%	1.42	No	0.05	1	0.46	0.011	2.99
	St. Joseph's Hospital, Milwaukee	3.3	0.0%	1.58	No	0.14	3	0.71	0.017	2.50
	St. Mary's Hospital, Milwaukee	3.1	0.0%	1.90	No	0.11	3	1.09	0.012	1.28
	St. Michael Hospital, Milwaukee	4.6	0.0%	1.14	No	0.08	3	0.42	0.057	3.08
	Waukesha Memorial Hospital, Waukesha, Wis.	5.6	0.0%	1.04	No	0.04	4	0.53	0.030	2.17
	West Allis Memorial Hospital, West Allis, Wis.	7.2	0.0%	0.94	No	0.03	4	0.56	0.072	4.49

OTOLARYNGOLOGY

Natl. Rank	Hospital	U.S. News index	Reputa-tional score	Hospital-wide mortality rate	COTH member	Interns and residents to beds	Tech-nology score (of 9)	R.N.'s to beds	Board-certified internists to beds	Procedures to beds
	TIER TWO									
74	University of Wisconsin Hospital and Clinics, Madison	15.0	0.0%	0.95	Yes	1.30	9	1.24	0.037	0.302
	TIER THREE									
	Froedtert Memorial Lutheran Hospital, Milwaukee	10.4	0.0%	1.03	Yes	0.49	0	1.13	0.199	0.813
	Milwaukee County Medical Complex	9.9	0.0%	1.28	Yes	0.43	7	0.81	0.081	0.068
	Sinai Samaritan Medical Center, Milwaukee	11.6	0.0%	1.00	Yes	0.66	6	0.86	0.170	0.239
	St. Luke's Medical Center, Milwaukee	9.6	0.0%	1.07	Yes	0.20	8	0.76	0.125	0.400
	TIER FOUR									
	Appleton Medical Center, Appleton, Wis.	3.1	0.0%	0.99	No	0.05	1	0.55	0.095	0.272
	Columbia Hospital, Milwaukee	4.8	0.0%	1.12	No	0.06	6	0.68	0.093	0.239
	Luther Hospital, Eau Claire, Wis.	5.3	0.0%	1.00	No	0.03	7	0.87	0.054	0.233
	Lutheran Hospital-La Crosse, La Crosse, Wis.	5.9	0.0%	0.95	No	0.12	8	0.93	0.026	0.328

Natl. Rank	Hospital	U.S. News index	Reputational score	Hospital-wide mortality rate	COTH member	Interns and residents to beds	Technology score (of 9)	R.N.'s to beds	Board-certified internists to beds	Procedures to beds
	Mercy Hospital of Janesville, Janesville, Wis.	5.4	0.0%	0.99	No	0.03	8	0.74	0.085	0.316
	Mercy Medical Center, Oshkosh, Wis.	4.0	0.0%	0.99	No	0.00	5	0.68	0.055	0.258
	Meriter Hospital, Madison, Wis.	3.4	0.0%	0.91	No	0.10	1	0.62	0.079	0.365
	Sacred Heart Hospital, Eau Claire, Wis.	3.7	0.0%	0.94	No	0.02	7	0.39	0.042	0.219
	St. Agnes Hospital, Fond du Lac, Wis.	4.2	0.0%	1.22	No	0.00	7	0.70	0.026	0.183
	St. Catherine's Hospital, Kenosha, Wis.	2.6	0.0%	1.00	No	0.07	4	0.26	0.038	0.158
	St. Elizabeth Hospital, Appleton, Wis.	3.3	0.0%	0.93	No	0.03	6	0.32	0.053	0.135
	St. Francis Hospital, Milwaukee	4.0	0.0%	1.27	No	0.00	3	0.62	0.158	0.280
	St. Francis Medical Center, La Crosse, Wis.	3.4	0.0%	0.88	No	0.11	3	0.50	0.051	0.248
	St. Joseph's Hospital, Marshfield, Wis.	3.5	0.0%	1.14	No	0.05	5	0.46	0.059	0.389
	St. Joseph's Hospital, Milwaukee	4.9	0.0%	1.26	No	0.14	6	0.71	0.075	0.262
	St. Mary's Hospital Medical Center, Madison, Wis.	3.6	0.0%	0.94	No	0.09	2	0.64	0.064	0.478
	St. Mary's Hospital, Milwaukee	5.5	0.0%	1.31	No	0.11	6	1.09	0.027	0.184
	St. Michael Hospital, Milwaukee	2.6	0.0%	1.10	No	0.08	2	0.42	0.048	0.414
	St. Vincent Hospital, Green Bay, Wis.	5.1	0.0%	1.05	No	0.00	6	0.89	0.076	0.302
	Waukesha Memorial Hospital, Waukesha, Wis.	4.2	0.0%	1.08	No	0.04	7	0.53	0.047	0.336
	Wausau Hospital, Wausau, Wis.	5.8	0.0%	0.83	No	0.06	7	0.98	0.034	0.294
	West Allis Memorial Hospital, West Allis, Wis.	4.6	0.0%	1.02	No	0.03	7	0.56	0.085	0.534

RHEUMATOLOGY

Natl. Rank	Hospital	U.S. News index	Reputational score	Hospital-wide mortality rate	COTH member	Interns and residents to beds	Technology score (of 5)	R.N.'s to beds	Board-certified internists to beds
TIER TWO									
61	University of Wisconsin Hospital and Clinics, Madison	17.3	0.0%	0.95	Yes	1.30	5	1.24	0.037
TIER THREE									
	Froedtert Memorial Lutheran Hospital, Milwaukee	12.6	0.0%	1.03	Yes	0.49	0	1.13	0.199
	Lutheran Hospital-La Crosse, La Crosse, Wis.	9.7	0.0%	0.95	No	0.12	4	0.93	0.026
	Milwaukee County Medical Complex	12.5	0.8%	1.28	Yes	0.43	4	0.81	0.081
	Sinai Samaritan Medical Center, Milwaukee	13.9	0.0%	1.00	Yes	0.66	3	0.86	0.170
	St. Luke's Medical Center, Milwaukee	11.9	0.6%	1.07	Yes	0.20	4	0.76	0.125
	Wausau Hospital, Wausau, Wis.	11.0	0.0%	0.83	No	0.06	4	0.98	0.034
TIER FOUR									
	Appleton Medical Center, Appleton, Wis.	7.7	0.0%	0.99	No	0.05	2	0.55	0.095
	Columbia Hospital, Milwaukee	8.5	0.5%	1.12	No	0.06	3	0.68	0.093
	Luther Hospital, Eau Claire, Wis.	9.0	0.0%	1.00	No	0.03	4	0.87	0.054
	Mercy Hospital of Janesville, Janesville, Wis.	8.9	0.0%	0.99	No	0.03	4	0.74	0.085
	Mercy Medical Center, Oshkosh, Wis.	8.5	0.0%	0.99	No	0.00	4	0.68	0.055
	Meriter Hospital, Madison, Wis.	8.7	0.0%	0.91	No	0.10	2	0.62	0.079
	Sacred Heart Hospital, Eau Claire, Wis.	8.2	0.0%	0.94	No	0.02	4	0.39	0.042
	St. Agnes Hospital, Fond du Lac, Wis.	6.6	0.0%	1.22	No	0.00	4	0.70	0.026
	St. Catherine's Hospital, Kenosha, Wis.	6.9	0.0%	1.00	No	0.07	3	0.26	0.038
	St. Elizabeth Hospital, Appleton, Wis.	7.8	0.0%	0.93	No	0.03	3	0.32	0.053
	St. Francis Hospital, Milwaukee	7.0	0.0%	1.27	No	0.00	4	0.62	0.158
	St. Francis Medical Center, La Crosse, Wis.	8.6	0.0%	0.88	No	0.11	2	0.50	0.051
	St. Joseph's Hospital, Marshfield, Wis.	5.5	0.0%	1.14	No	0.05	1	0.46	0.059
	St. Joseph's Hospital, Milwaukee	6.7	0.0%	1.26	No	0.14	3	0.71	0.075
	St. Mary's Hospital Medical Center, Madison, Wis.	8.3	0.0%	0.94	No	0.09	2	0.64	0.064
	St. Mary's Hospital, Milwaukee	5.9	0.0%	1.31	No	0.11	3	1.09	0.027
	St. Michael Hospital, Milwaukee	6.6	0.0%	1.10	No	0.08	3	0.42	0.048
	St. Vincent Hospital, Green Bay, Wis.	7.2	0.0%	1.05	No	0.00	3	0.89	0.076
	Waukesha Memorial Hospital, Waukesha, Wis.	7.4	0.0%	1.08	No	0.04	4	0.53	0.047
	West Allis Memorial Hospital, West Allis, Wis.	7.2	0.0%	1.02	No	0.03	4	0.56	0.085

UROLOGY

Natl. Rank	Hospital	U.S. News index	Reputa- tional score	Urology mortality rate	COTH member	Interns and residents to beds	Tech- nology score (of 11)	R.N.'s to beds	Board- certified internists to beds	Procedures to beds
	TIER TWO									
85	St. Luke's Medical Center, Milwaukee	15.3	0.0%	0.70	Yes	0.20	10	0.76	0.125	1.76
30	University of Wisconsin Hospital and Clinics, Madison	20.8	0.5%	0.55	Yes	1.30	11	1.24	0.037	2.85
	TIER THREE									
	Froedtert Memorial Lutheran Hospital, Milwaukee	14.0	0.0%	0.83	Yes	0.49	0	1.13	0.199	4.26
	Lutheran Hospital-La Crosse, La Crosse, Wis.	12.3	0.0%	0.68	No	0.12	10	0.93	0.026	1.95
	Meriter Hospital, Madison, Wis.	9.8	0.0%	0.34	No	0.10	3	0.62	0.079	1.58
	Sacred Heart Hospital, Eau Claire, Wis.	8.6	0.0%	0.84	No	0.02	9	0.39	0.042	1.34
	Sinai Samaritan Medical Center, Milwaukee	10.1	0.0%	1.48	Yes	0.66	7	0.86	0.170	1.49
	St. Elizabeth Hospital, Appleton, Wis.	9.8	0.0%	0.64	No	0.03	8	0.32	0.053	0.91
	Wausau Hospital, Wausau, Wis.	11.9	0.0%	0.45	No	0.06	9	0.98	0.034	1.76
	TIER FOUR									
	Appleton Medical Center, Appleton, Wis.	8.1	0.0%	0.84	No	0.05	3	0.55	0.095	2.23
	Columbia Hospital, Milwaukee	4.9	0.0%	1.41	No	0.06	7	0.68	0.093	1.48
	Luther Hospital, Eau Claire, Wis.	6.5	0.0%	1.19	No	0.03	8	0.87	0.054	1.46
	Mercy Hospital of Janesville, Janesville, Wis.	6.1	0.0%	1.30	No	0.03	9	0.74	0.085	1.86
	Mercy Medical Center, Oshkosh, Wis.	3.9	0.0%	1.66	No	0.00	8	0.68	0.055	1.96
	St. Agnes Hospital, Fond du Lac, Wis.	5.4	0.0%	1.24	No	0.00	8	0.70	0.026	1.27
	St. Francis Hospital, Milwaukee	3.0	0.0%	1.87	No	0.00	5	0.62	0.158	2.00
	St. Francis Medical Center, La Crosse, Wis.	3.3	0.0%	1.44	No	0.11	4	0.50	0.051	1.13
	St. Joseph's Hospital, Marshfield, Wis.	5.7	0.0%	1.08	No	0.05	5	0.46	0.059	1.72
	St. Joseph's Hospital, Milwaukee	5.9	0.0%	1.32	No	0.14	8	0.71	0.075	1.82
	St. Mary's Hospital Medical Center, Madison, Wis.	4.1	0.0%	1.35	No	0.09	3	0.64	0.064	2.06
	St. Mary's Hospital, Milwaukee	6.7	0.0%	1.21	No	0.11	7	1.09	0.027	1.16
	St. Michael Hospital, Milwaukee	4.1	0.0%	1.31	No	0.08	4	0.42	0.048	2.81
	St. Vincent Hospital, Green Bay, Wis.	4.6	0.0%	1.60	No	0.00	7	0.89	0.076	2.16
	Waukesha Memorial Hospital, Waukesha, Wis.	5.0	0.0%	1.33	No	0.04	9	0.53	0.047	1.23
	West Allis Memorial Hospital, West Allis, Wis.	8.5	0.0%	0.92	No	0.03	8	0.56	0.085	2.57

AIDS

Natl. Rank	Hospital	U.S. News index	Reputa-tional score	Hospital-wide mortality rate	COTH member	Interns and residents to beds	Tech-nology score (of 11)	Discharge planning (of 2)	R.N.'s to beds	Board-certified internists to beds
		TIER FOUR								
	De Paul Hospital, Cheyenne, Wyo.	16.1	0.0%	1.22	No	0.05	5	1	0.77	0.105
	Wyoming Medical Center, Casper	18.5	0.0%	1.14	No	0.08	6	2	1.08	0.040

CANCER

Natl. Rank	Hospital	U.S. News index	Reputa-tional score	Cancer mortality rate	COTH member	Interns and residents to beds	Tech-nology score (of 12)	R.N.'s to beds	Board-certified oncologists to beds	Procedures to beds
		TIER FOUR								
	Wyoming Medical Center, Casper	4.1	0.0%	1.10	No	0.08	7	1.08	0.000	1.08

CARDIOLOGY

Natl. Rank	Hospital	U.S. News index	Reputa-tional score	Cardiology mortality rate	COTH member	Interns and residents to beds	Tech-nology score (of 10)	R.N.'s to beds	Board-certified cardiologists to beds	Procedures to beds
		TIER FOUR								
	Wyoming Medical Center, Casper	9.5	0.0%	1.25	No	0.08	7	1.08	0.004	5.06

ENDOCRINOLOGY

Natl. Rank	Hospital	U.S. News index	Reputa-tional score	Endocrinology mortality rate	COTH member	Interns and residents to beds	Tech-nology score (of 11)	R.N.'s to beds	Board-certified internists to beds
		TIER FOUR							
	Wyoming Medical Center, Casper	7.8	0.0%	0.97	No	0.08	8	1.08	0.040

GASTROENTEROLOGY

Natl. Rank	Hospital	U.S. News index	Reputa-tional score	Gastro-enterology mortality rate	COTH member	Interns and residents to beds	Tech-nology score (of 11)	R.N.'s to beds	Board-certified gastro-enterologists to beds	Pro-cedures to beds
		TIER FOUR								
	Memorial Hospital of Laramie County, Cheyenne, Wyo.	2.4	0.0%	1.36	No	0.04	0	0.59	0.000	4.12
	Wyoming Medical Center, Casper	4.5	0.0%	1.47	No	0.08	7	1.08	0.000	2.55

GERIATRICS

Natl. Rank	Hospital	U.S. News index	Reputa-tional score	Hospital-wide mortality rate	COTH member	Service mix	Interns and residents to beds	Tech-nology score (of 13)	R.N.'s to beds	Discharge planning (of 2)	Geriatric services (of 9)	Board-certified internists to beds
		TIER FOUR										
	Wyoming Medical Center, Casper	11.4	0.0%	1.14	No	5	0.08	9	1.08	2	2	0.040

GYNECOLOGY

Natl. Rank	Hospital	U.S. News index	Reputa-tional score	Hospital-wide mortality rate	Interns and residents to beds	Tech-nology score (of 10)	R.N.'s to beds	Board-certified OB-GYNs to beds	Procedures to beds
		TIER FOUR							
	Wyoming Medical Center, Casper	11.9	0.0%	1.14	0.08	6	1.08	0.018	0.44

ORTHOPEDICS

Natl. Rank	Hospital	U.S. News index	Reputa-tional score	Orthopedics mortality rate	COTH member	Interns and residents to beds	Tech-nology score (of 5)	R.N.'s to beds	Board-certified orthopedists to beds	Pro-cedures to beds
	TIER THREE									
	Wyoming Medical Center, Casper	**8.9**	0.0%	0.79	No	0.08	3	1.08	0.018	2.72

OTOLARYNGOLOGY

Natl. Rank	Hospital	U.S. News index	Reputa-tional score	Hospital-wide mortality rate	COTH member	Interns and residents to beds	Tech-nology score (of 9)	R.N.'s to beds	Board-certified internists to beds	Procedures to beds
	TIER FOUR									
	De Paul Hospital, Cheyenne, Wyo.	**4.2**	0.0%	1.22	No	0.05	3	0.77	0.105	0.173
	Memorial Hospital of Laramie County, Cheyenne, Wyo.	**2.1**	0.0%	1.31	No	0.04	0	0.59	0.030	0.459
	Wyoming Medical Center, Casper	**5.6**	0.0%	1.15	No	0.08	6	1.08	0.040	0.218

RHEUMATOLOGY

Natl. Rank	Hospital	U.S. News index	Reputa-tional score	Hospital-wide mortality rate	COTH member	Interns and residents to beds	Tech-nology score (of 5)	R.N.'s to beds	Board-certified internists to beds
	TIER FOUR								
	Wyoming Medical Center, Casper	**8.0**	0.0%	1.15	No	0.08	3	1.08	0.040

UROLOGY

Natl. Rank	Hospital	U.S. News index	Reputa-tional score	Urology mortality rate	COTH member	Interns and residents to beds	Tech-nology score (of 11)	R.N.'s to beds	Board-certified internists to beds	Procedures to beds
	TIER FOUR									
	Wyoming Medical Center, Casper	**7.5**	0.0%	1.08	No	0.08	7	1.08	0.040	1.16

Boston

AIDS

Natl. Rank	Hospital
TIER ONE	
3	Massachusetts General Hospital, Boston
12	Beth Israel Hospital, Boston
13	New England Deaconess Hospital, Boston
21	Boston City Hospital
26	Brigham and Women's Hospital, Boston
TIER TWO	
49	Boston University Medical Center-University Hospital
31	New England Medical Center, Boston
57	University of Massachusetts Medical Center, Worcester
TIER THREE	
	Brockton Hospital, Brockton, Mass.
	Carney Hospital, Boston
	Faulkner Hospital, Boston
	Lahey Clinic Hospital, Burlington, Mass.
	Medical Center of Central Massachusetts, Worcester
	Metrowest Medical Center, Framingham, Mass.
	Mount Auburn Hospital, Cambridge, Mass.
	New England Baptist Hospital, Boston
	Newton-Wellesley Hospital, Newton, Mass.
100	St. Elizabeth's Hospital of Boston
	St. Vincent Hospital, Worcester, Mass.
	Walthamweston Hospital and Medical Center, Waltham, Mass.
TIER FOUR	
	Atlanticare Medical Center, Lynn, Mass.
	Burbank Hospital, Fitchburg, Mass.
	Cambridge Hospital, Cambridge, Mass.
	Cardinal Cushing General Hospital, Brockton, Mass.
	Elliot Hospital, Manchester, N.H.
	Holy Family Hospital and Medical Center, Methuen, Mass.
	Jewish Memorial Hospital, Boston
	Malden Hospital, Malden, Mass.
	North Shore Medical Center, Salem, Mass.
	St. Joseph Hospital and Trauma Center, Nashua, N.H.

CANCER

Natl. Rank	Hospital
TIER ONE	
3	Dana-Farber Cancer Institute, Boston
12	Massachusetts General Hospital, Boston
TIER TWO	
67	Beth Israel Hospital, Boston
32	Brigham and Women's Hospital, Boston
53	New England Deaconess Hospital, Boston
48	New England Medical Center, Boston
59	University of Massachusetts Medical Center, Worcester
TIER THREE	
	Boston City Hospital
99	Boston University Medical Center-University Hospital
	Faulkner Hospital, Boston
	Lahey Clinic Hospital, Burlington, Mass.

Natl. Rank	Hospital
	Mount Auburn Hospital, Cambridge, Mass.
	St. Elizabeth's Hospital of Boston
	St. Vincent Hospital, Worcester, Mass.
TIER FOUR	
	Atlanticare Medical Center, Lynn, Mass.
	Brockton Hospital, Brockton, Mass.
	Burbank Hospital, Fitchburg, Mass.
	Cardinal Cushing General Hospital, Brockton, Mass.
	Carney Hospital, Boston
	Elliot Hospital, Manchester, N.H.
	Holy Family Hospital and Medical Center, Methuen, Mass.
	Lawrence Memorial Hospital of Medford, Medford, Mass.
	Malden Hospital, Malden, Mass.
	Medical Center of Central Massachusetts, Worcester
	Metrowest Medical Center, Framingham, Mass.
	New England Baptist Hospital, Boston
	Newton-Wellesley Hospital, Newton, Mass.
	North Shore Medical Center, Salem, Mass.
	St. Joseph Hospital and Trauma Center, Nashua, N.H.
	Walthamweston Hospital and Medical Center, Waltham, Mass.

CARDIOLOGY

Natl. Rank	Hospital
TIER ONE	
4	Massachusetts General Hospital, Boston
6	Brigham and Women's Hospital, Boston
14	Beth Israel Hospital, Boston
TIER TWO	
85	Boston University Medical Center-University Hospital
27	New England Medical Center, Boston
94	University of Massachusetts Medical Center, Worcester
TIER THREE	
	Brockton Hospital, Brockton, Mass.
	Carney Hospital, Boston
	Faulkner Hospital, Boston
	Lahey Clinic Hospital, Burlington, Mass.
	Lawrence Memorial Hospital of Medford, Medford, Mass.
	Medical Center of Central Massachusetts, Worcester
	Metrowest Medical Center, Framingham, Mass.
	Mount Auburn Hospital, Cambridge, Mass.
	New England Baptist Hospital, Boston
	New England Deaconess Hospital, Boston
	Newton-Wellesley Hospital, Newton, Mass.
	North Shore Medical Center, Salem, Mass.
	St. Elizabeth's Hospital of Boston
	Walthamweston Hospital and Medical Center, Waltham, Mass.
TIER FOUR	
	Atlanticare Medical Center, Lynn, Mass.
	Burbank Hospital, Fitchburg, Mass.
	Cambridge Hospital, Cambridge, Mass.
	Cardinal Cushing General Hospital, Brockton, Mass.
	Elliot Hospital, Manchester, N.H.
	Holy Family Hospital and Medical Center, Methuen, Mass.
	Malden Hospital, Malden, Mass.
	St. Joseph Hospital and Trauma Center, Nashua, N.H.
	St. Vincent Hospital, Worcester, Mass.

ENDOCRINOLOGY

Natl. Rank	Hospital
TIER ONE	
2	Massachusetts General Hospital, Boston
9	New England Deaconess Hospital, Boston
11	Brigham and Women's Hospital, Boston
16	Beth Israel Hospital, Boston
TIER TWO	
31	Boston City Hospital
43	Boston University Medical Center-University Hospital
42	New England Medical Center, Boston
66	St. Elizabeth's Hospital of Boston
37	University of Massachusetts Medical Center, Worcester
TIER THREE	
	Carney Hospital, Boston
	Faulkner Hospital, Boston
	Lahey Clinic Hospital, Burlington, Mass.
	Mount Auburn Hospital, Cambridge, Mass.
	Newton-Wellesley Hospital, Newton, Mass.
	St. Vincent Hospital, Worcester, Mass.
TIER FOUR	
	Atlanticare Medical Center, Lynn, Mass.
	Brockton Hospital, Brockton, Mass.
	Burbank Hospital, Fitchburg, Mass.
	Cardinal Cushing General Hospital, Brockton, Mass.
	Elliot Hospital, Manchester, N.H.
	Holy Family Hospital and Medical Center, Methuen, Mass.
	Lawrence Memorial Hospital of Medford, Medford, Mass.
	Malden Hospital, Malden, Mass.
	Medical Center of Central Massachusetts, Worcester
	Metrowest Medical Center, Framingham, Mass.
	North Shore Medical Center, Salem, Mass.
	Walthamweston Hospital and Medical Center, Waltham, Mass.

GASTROENTEROLOGY

Natl. Rank	Hospital
TIER ONE	
3	Massachusetts General Hospital, Boston
10	Brigham and Women's Hospital, Boston
12	Beth Israel Hospital, Boston
TIER TWO	
51	Boston University Medical Center-University Hospital
43	Lahey Clinic Hospital, Burlington, Mass.
31	New England Deaconess Hospital, Boston
37	New England Medical Center, Boston
72	St. Elizabeth's Hospital of Boston
48	University of Massachusetts Medical Center, Worcester
TIER THREE	
	Faulkner Hospital, Boston
	Medical Center of Central Massachusetts, Worcester
	Mount Auburn Hospital, Cambridge, Mass.
	St. Vincent Hospital, Worcester, Mass.
TIER FOUR	
	Atlanticare Medical Center, Lynn, Mass.
	Brockton Hospital, Brockton, Mass.

Natl. Rank	Hospital
	Burbank Hospital, Fitchburg, Mass.
	Cardinal Cushing General Hospital, Brockton, Mass.
	Carney Hospital, Boston
	Elliot Hospital, Manchester, N.H.
	Holy Family Hospital and Medical Center, Methuen, Mass.
	Lawrence Memorial Hospital of Medford, Medford, Mass.
	Malden Hospital, Malden, Mass.
	Metrowest Medical Center, Framingham, Mass.
	New England Baptist Hospital, Boston
	Newton-Wellesley Hospital, Newton, Mass.
	North Shore Medical Center, Salem, Mass.
	St. Joseph Hospital and Trauma Center, Nashua, N.H.
	Walthamweston Hospital and Medical Center, Waltham, Mass.

GERIATRICS

Natl. Rank	Hospital
TIER ONE	
2	Massachusetts General Hospital, Boston
5	Beth Israel Hospital, Boston
10	Brigham and Women's Hospital, Boston
TIER TWO	
28	Boston University Medical Center-University Hospital
53	New England Deaconess Hospital, Boston
37	New England Medical Center, Boston
72	St. Elizabeth's Hospital of Boston
58	University of Massachusetts Medical Center, Worcester
TIER THREE	
	Carney Hospital, Boston
	Faulkner Hospital, Boston
	Lahey Clinic Hospital, Burlington, Mass.
	Medical Center of Central Massachusetts, Worcester
	Metrowest Medical Center, Framingham, Mass.
	Mount Auburn Hospital, Cambridge, Mass.
	New England Baptist Hospital, Boston
	Newton-Wellesley Hospital, Newton, Mass.
	St. Vincent Hospital, Worcester, Mass.
	Walthamweston Hospital and Medical Center, Waltham, Mass.
TIER FOUR	
	Atlanticare Medical Center, Lynn, Mass.
	Brockton Hospital, Brockton, Mass.
	Burbank Hospital, Fitchburg, Mass.
	Cardinal Cushing General Hospital, Brockton, Mass.
	Elliot Hospital, Manchester, N.H.
	Holy Family Hospital and Medical Center, Methuen, Mass.
	Lawrence Memorial Hospital of Medford, Medford, Mass.
	Malden Hospital, Malden, Mass.
	North Shore Medical Center, Salem, Mass.
	St. Joseph Hospital and Trauma Center, Nashua, N.H.

GYNECOLOGY

Natl. Rank	Hospital
TIER ONE	
4	Brigham and Women's Hospital, Boston
5	Massachusetts General Hospital, Boston

Natl. Rank	Hospital
19	Beth Israel Hospital, Boston
TIER TWO	
75	Boston University Medical Center-University Hospital
80	New England Deaconess Hospital, Boston
76	University of Massachusetts Medical Center, Worcester
TIER THREE	
	Brockton Hospital, Brockton, Mass.
	Carney Hospital, Boston
	Faulkner Hospital, Boston
	Lahey Clinic Hospital, Burlington, Mass.
	Medical Center of Central Massachusetts, Worcester
	Metrowest Medical Center, Framingham, Mass.
	Mount Auburn Hospital, Cambridge, Mass.
	Newton-Wellesley Hospital, Newton, Mass.
	St. Elizabeth's Hospital of Boston
	Walthamweston Hospital and Medical Center, Waltham, Mass.
TIER FOUR	
	Atlanticare Medical Center, Lynn, Mass.
	Burbank Hospital, Fitchburg, Mass.
	Cardinal Cushing General Hospital, Brockton, Mass.
	Elliot Hospital, Manchester, N.H.
	Holy Family Hospital and Medical Center, Methuen, Mass.
	Lawrence Memorial Hospital of Medford, Medford, Mass.
	Malden Hospital, Malden, Mass.
	North Shore Medical Center, Salem, Mass.
	St. Vincent Hospital, Worcester, Mass.

NEUROLOGY

Natl. Rank	Hospital
TIER ONE	
4	Massachusetts General Hospital, Boston
12	Brigham and Women's Hospital, Boston
18	Beth Israel Hospital, Boston
TIER TWO	
32	Boston University Medical Center-University Hospital
39	New England Deaconess Hospital, Boston
50	New England Medical Center, Boston
86	St. Elizabeth's Hospital of Boston
59	University of Massachusetts Medical Center, Worcester
TIER THREE	
	Faulkner Hospital, Boston
	Lahey Clinic Hospital, Burlington, Mass.
	Medical Center of Central Massachusetts, Worcester
	Mount Auburn Hospital, Cambridge, Mass.
	Newton-Wellesley Hospital, Newton, Mass.
	St. Vincent Hospital, Worcester, Mass.
	Walthamweston Hospital and Medical Center, Waltham, Mass.
TIER FOUR	
	Atlanticare Medical Center, Lynn, Mass.
	Brockton Hospital, Brockton, Mass.
	Burbank Hospital, Fitchburg, Mass.
	Cardinal Cushing General Hospital, Brockton, Mass.
	Carney Hospital, Boston
	Elliot Hospital, Manchester, N.H.
	Holy Family Hospital and Medical Center, Methuen, Mass.
	Lawrence Memorial Hospital of Medford, Medford, Mass.

Natl. Rank	Hospital
	Metrowest Medical Center, Framingham, Mass.
	North Shore Medical Center, Salem, Mass.

ORTHOPEDICS

Natl. Rank	Hospital
TIER ONE	
3	Massachusetts General Hospital, Boston
15	Brigham and Women's Hospital, Boston
TIER TWO	
35	Beth Israel Hospital, Boston
52	Boston University Medical Center-University Hospital
56	New England Medical Center, Boston
42	University of Massachusetts Medical Center, Worcester
TIER THREE	
	Brockton Hospital, Brockton, Mass.
	Carney Hospital, Boston
	Faulkner Hospital, Boston
	Lahey Clinic Hospital, Burlington, Mass.
	Mount Auburn Hospital, Cambridge, Mass.
	New England Baptist Hospital, Boston
98	New England Deaconess Hospital, Boston
	St. Elizabeth's Hospital of Boston
	St. Vincent Hospital, Worcester, Mass.
TIER FOUR	
	Atlanticare Medical Center, Lynn, Mass.
	Burbank Hospital, Fitchburg, Mass.
	Cardinal Cushing General Hospital, Brockton, Mass.
	Elliot Hospital, Manchester, N.H.
	Holy Family Hospital and Medical Center, Methuen, Mass.
	Lawrence Memorial Hospital of Medford, Medford, Mass.
	Malden Hospital, Malden, Mass.
	Medical Center of Central Massachusetts, Worcester
	Metrowest Medical Center, Framingham, Mass.
	Newton-Wellesley Hospital, Newton, Mass.
	North Shore Medical Center, Salem, Mass.
	St. Joseph Hospital and Trauma Center, Nashua, N.H.
	Walthamweston Hospital and Medical Center, Waltham, Mass.

OTOLARYNGOLOGY

Natl. Rank	Hospital
TIER ONE	
2	Massachusetts Eye and Ear Infirmary, Boston
35	Beth Israel Hospital, Boston
TIER TWO	
59	Boston City Hospital
100	Boston University Medical Center-University Hospital
48	Brigham and Women's Hospital, Boston
72	Lahey Clinic Hospital, Burlington, Mass.
80	New England Deaconess Hospital, Boston
46	New England Medical Center, Boston
	University of Massachusetts Medical Center, Worcester
TIER THREE	
	Carney Hospital, Boston
	Dana-Farber Cancer Institute, Boston

Natl. Rank	Hospital
	Faulkner Hospital, Boston
	Medical Center of Central Massachusetts, Worcester
	Mount Auburn Hospital, Cambridge, Mass.
	St. Elizabeth's Hospital of Boston
	St. Vincent Hospital, Worcester, Mass.
TIER FOUR	
	Atlanticare Medical Center, Lynn, Mass.
	Brockton Hospital, Brockton, Mass.
	Burbank Hospital, Fitchburg, Mass.
	Cambridge Hospital, Cambridge, Mass.
	Cardinal Cushing General Hospital, Brockton, Mass.
	Elliot Hospital, Manchester, N.H.
	Holy Family Hospital and Medical Center, Methuen, Mass.
	Jewish Memorial Hospital, Boston
	Lawrence Memorial Hospital of Medford, Medford, Mass.
	Lemuel Shattuck Hospital, Boston
	Malden Hospital, Malden, Mass.
	Metrowest Medical Center, Framingham, Mass.
	New England Baptist Hospital, Boston
	Newton-Wellesley Hospital, Newton, Mass.
	North Shore Medical Center, Salem, Mass.
	St. Joseph Hospital and Trauma Center, Nashua, N.H.
	Walthamweston Hospital and Medical Center, Waltham, Mass.

RHEUMATOLOGY

Natl. Rank	Hospital
TIER ONE	
3	Brigham and Women's Hospital, Boston
12	Massachusetts General Hospital, Boston
16	Beth Israel Hospital, Boston
TIER TWO	
57	Boston University Medical Center-University Hospital
65	New England Deaconess Hospital, Boston
40	New England Medical Center, Boston
51	University of Massachusetts Medical Center, Worcester
TIER THREE	
	Carney Hospital, Boston
	Faulkner Hospital, Boston
	Lahey Clinic Hospital, Burlington, Mass.
	Medical Center of Central Massachusetts, Worcester
	Mount Auburn Hospital, Cambridge, Mass.
	St. Elizabeth's Hospital of Boston
	St. Vincent Hospital, Worcester, Mass.
TIER FOUR	
	Atlanticare Medical Center, Lynn, Mass.
	Brockton Hospital, Brockton, Mass.
	Burbank Hospital, Fitchburg, Mass.
	Cardinal Cushing General Hospital, Brockton, Mass.
	Elliot Hospital, Manchester, N.H.
	Holy Family Hospital and Medical Center, Methuen, Mass.
	Lawrence Memorial Hospital of Medford, Medford, Mass.
	Malden Hospital, Malden, Mass.
	Metrowest Medical Center, Framingham, Mass.
	New England Baptist Hospital, Boston
	Newton-Wellesley Hospital, Newton, Mass.
	North Shore Medical Center, Salem, Mass.

Natl. Rank	Hospital
	St. Joseph Hospital and Trauma Center, Nashua, N.H.
	Walthamweston Hospital and Medical Center, Waltham, Mass.

UROLOGY

Natl. Rank	Hospital
TIER ONE	
7	Massachusetts General Hospital, Boston
22	Brigham and Women's Hospital, Boston
TIER TWO	
39	Beth Israel Hospital, Boston
57	Boston City Hospital
61	Boston University Medical Center-University Hospital
27	Lahey Clinic Hospital, Burlington, Mass.
31	New England Deaconess Hospital, Boston
42	New England Medical Center, Boston
78	St. Elizabeth's Hospital of Boston
36	University of Massachusetts Medical Center, Worcester
TIER THREE	
	Faulkner Hospital, Boston
	Metrowest Medical Center, Framingham, Mass.
	Mount Auburn Hospital, Cambridge, Mass.
	New England Baptist Hospital, Boston
	Newton-Wellesley Hospital, Newton, Mass.
	St. Vincent Hospital, Worcester, Mass.
	Walthamweston Hospital and Medical Center, Waltham, Mass.
TIER FOUR	
	Atlanticare Medical Center, Lynn, Mass.
	Brockton Hospital, Brockton, Mass.
	Burbank Hospital, Fitchburg, Mass.
	Cardinal Cushing General Hospital, Brockton, Mass.
	Carney Hospital, Boston
	Elliot Hospital, Manchester, N.H.
	Holy Family Hospital and Medical Center, Methuen, Mass.
	Lawrence Memorial Hospital of Medford, Medford, Mass.
	Malden Hospital, Malden, Mass.
	Medical Center of Central Massachusetts, Worcester
	North Shore Medical Center, Salem, Mass.

Chicago

AIDS

CANCER

Natl. Rank	Hospital
	St. Margaret Mercy Health Centers, Hammond, Ind.
	St. Mary of Nazareth Hospital Center, Chicago
	St. Mary's Hospital of Kankakee, Kankakee, Ill.
	Swedish Covenant Hospital, Chicago
	West Suburban Hospital Medical Center, Oak Park, Ill.

CARDIOLOGY

Natl. Rank	Hospital
TIER ONE	
16	University of Chicago Hospitals
TIER TWO	
36	Cook County Hospital, Chicago
53	Evanston Hospital, Evanston, Ill.
44	F.G. McGaw Hospital at Loyola University, Maywood, Ill.
71	Michael Reese Hospital and Medical Center, Chicago
65	Northwestern Memorial Hospital, Chicago
34	Rush-Presbyterian-St. Luke's Medical Center, Chicago
67	University of Illinois Hospital and Clinics, Chicago
TIER THREE	
	Alexian Brothers Medical Center, Elk Grove Village, Ill.
	Columbus Hospital, Chicago
	Edgewater Medical Center, Chicago
	Elmhurst Memorial Hospital, Elmhurst, Ill.
	Good Samaritan Hospital, Downers Grove, Ill.
	Gottlieb Memorial Hospital, Melrose Park, Ill.
	Grant Hospital of Chicago
	Hinsdale Hospital, Hinsdale, Ill.
	Holy Family Hospital, Des Plaines, Ill.
	Illinois Masonic Medical Center, Chicago
	La Grange Memorial Health System, La Grange, Ill.
	Louis A. Weiss Memorial Hospital, Chicago
	Lutheran General Healthsystem, Park Ridge, Ill.
98	MacNeal Hospital, Berwyn, Ill.
	Mercy Hospital and Medical Center, Chicago
	Methodist Hospitals, Gary, Ind.
	Northwest Community Hospital, Arlington Heights, Ill.
	Rush North Shore Medical Center, Skokie, Ill.
	St. Catherine's Hospital, Kenosha, Wis.
	St. Francis Hospital, Evanston, Ill.
	St. James Hospital and Health Center, Chicago Heights, Ill.
	Swedish Covenant Hospital, Chicago
	West Suburban Hospital Medical Center, Oak Park, Ill.
TIER FOUR	
	Central Du Page Hospital, Winfield, Ill.
	Christ Hospital and Medical Center, Oak Lawn, Ill.
	Copley Memorial Hospital, Aurora, Ill.
	Ingalls Memorial Hospital, Harvey, Ill.
	Lakeshore Health System, East Chicago, Ind.
	Little Company of Mary Hospital, Evergreen Park, Ill.
	Mercy Center for Health Care Services, Aurora, Ill.
	Oak Park Hospital, Oak Park, Ill.
	Porter Memorial Hospital, Valparaiso, Ind.
	Ravenswood Hospital Medical Center, Chicago
	Resurrection Medical Center, Chicago
	Riverside Medical Center, Kankakee, Ill.
	Sherman Hospital, Elgin, Ill.

Natl. Rank	Hospital
	St. Anthony Medical Center, Crown Point, Ind.
	St. Joseph Hospital and Health Care Center, Chicago
	St. Joseph Medical Center, Joliet, Ill.
	St. Margaret Mercy Health Centers, Hammond, Ind.
	St. Mary of Nazareth Hospital Center, Chicago
	St. Mary's Hospital of Kankakee, Kankakee, Ill.

ENDOCRINOLOGY

Natl. Rank	Hospital
TIER ONE	
7	University of Chicago Hospitals
26	University of Illinois Hospital and Clinics, Chicago
TIER TWO	
55	Cook County Hospital, Chicago
76	Evanston Hospital, Evanston, Ill.
33	F.G. McGaw Hospital at Loyola University, Maywood, Ill.
65	Northwestern Memorial Hospital, Chicago
41	Rush-Presbyterian-St. Luke's Medical Center, Chicago
TIER THREE	
	Alexian Brothers Medical Center, Elk Grove Village, Ill.
	Central Du Page Hospital, Winfield, Ill.
	Columbus Hospital, Chicago
	Edgewater Medical Center, Chicago
	Good Samaritan Hospital, Downers Grove, Ill.
	Grant Hospital of Chicago
	Illinois Masonic Medical Center, Chicago
	Louis A. Weiss Memorial Hospital, Chicago
	Lutheran General Healthsystem, Park Ridge, Ill.
	MacNeal Hospital, Berwyn, Ill.
	Mercy Hospital and Medical Center, Chicago
91	Michael Reese Hospital and Medical Center, Chicago
	Rush North Shore Medical Center, Skokie, Ill.
	St. Francis Hospital, Evanston, Ill.
	St. James Hospital and Health Center, Chicago Heights, Ill.
	St. Joseph Hospital and Health Care Center, Chicago
TIER FOUR	
	Christ Hospital and Medical Center, Oak Lawn, Ill.
	Elmhurst Memorial Hospital, Elmhurst, Ill.
	Gottlieb Memorial Hospital, Melrose Park, Ill.
	Hinsdale Hospital, Hinsdale, Ill.
	Holy Family Hospital, Des Plaines, Ill.
	Ingalls Memorial Hospital, Harvey, Ill.
	La Grange Memorial Health System, La Grange, Ill.
	Lakeshore Health System, East Chicago, Ind.
	Little Company of Mary Hospital, Evergreen Park, Ill.
	Mercy Center for Health Care Services, Aurora, Ill.
	Methodist Hospitals, Gary, Ind.
	Mount Sinai Hospital Medical Center, Chicago
	Northwest Community Hospital, Arlington Heights, Ill.
	Oak Park Hospital, Oak Park, Ill.
	Porter Memorial Hospital, Valparaiso, Ind.
	Ravenswood Hospital Medical Center, Chicago
	Resurrection Medical Center, Chicago
	Riverside Medical Center, Kankakee, Ill.
	Sherman Hospital, Elgin, Ill.
	St. Anthony Medical Center, Crown Point, Ind.

METRO RANKINGS

Natl. Rank — Hospital

Natl. Rank	Hospital
	St. Catherine's Hospital, Kenosha, Wis.
	St. Joseph Medical Center, Joliet, Ill.
	St. Margaret Mercy Health Centers, Hammond, Ind.
	St. Mary of Nazareth Hospital Center, Chicago
	St. Mary's Hospital of Kankakee, Kankakee, Ill.
	Swedish Covenant Hospital, Chicago
	West Suburban Hospital Medical Center, Oak Park, Ill.

GASTROENTEROLOGY

Natl. Rank — Hospital

Natl. Rank	Hospital
TIER ONE	
9	University of Chicago Hospitals
TIER TWO	
66	Cook County Hospital, Chicago
45	F.G. McGaw Hospital at Loyola University, Maywood, Ill.
57	Northwestern Memorial Hospital, Chicago
23	Rush-Presbyterian-St. Luke's Medical Center, Chicago
TIER THREE	
	Columbus Hospital, Chicago
	Edgewater Medical Center, Chicago
	Elmhurst Memorial Hospital, Elmhurst, Ill.
78	Evanston Hospital, Evanston, Ill.
	Hinsdale Hospital, Hinsdale, Ill.
	Holy Family Hospital, Des Plaines, Ill.
	Illinois Masonic Medical Center, Chicago
	Louis A. Weiss Memorial Hospital, Chicago
83	Lutheran General Healthsystem, Park Ridge, Ill.
	MacNeal Hospital, Berwyn, Ill.
	Mercy Hospital and Medical Center, Chicago
	Michael Reese Hospital and Medical Center, Chicago
	St. Francis Hospital, Evanston, Ill.
	West Suburban Hospital Medical Center, Oak Park, Ill.
TIER FOUR	
	Alexian Brothers Medical Center, Elk Grove Village, Ill.
	Central Du Page Hospital, Winfield, Ill.
	Christ Hospital and Medical Center, Oak Lawn, Ill.
	Copley Memorial Hospital, Aurora, Ill.
	Good Samaritan Hospital, Downers Grove, Ill.
	Gottlieb Memorial Hospital, Melrose Park, Ill.
	Grant Hospital of Chicago
	Ingalls Memorial Hospital, Harvey, Ill.
	La Grange Memorial Health System, La Grange, Ill.
	Lakeshore Health System, East Chicago, Ind.
	Little Company of Mary Hospital, Evergreen Park, Ill.
	Mercy Center for Health Care Services, Aurora, Ill.
	Northwest Community Hospital, Arlington Heights, Ill.
	Oak Park Hospital, Oak Park, Ill.
	Porter Memorial Hospital, Valparaiso, Ind.
	Ravenswood Hospital Medical Center, Chicago
	Resurrection Medical Center, Chicago
	Riverside Medical Center, Kankakee, Ill.
	Rush North Shore Medical Center, Skokie, Ill.
	Sherman Hospital, Elgin, Ill.
	St. Anthony Medical Center, Crown Point, Ind.
	St. Catherine's Hospital, Kenosha, Wis.
	St. James Hospital and Health Center, Chicago Heights, Ill.

Natl. Rank — Hospital

Natl. Rank	Hospital
	St. Joseph Hospital and Health Care Center, Chicago
	St. Joseph Medical Center, Joliet, Ill.
	St. Margaret Mercy Health Centers, Hammond, Ind.
	St. Mary of Nazareth Hospital Center, Chicago
	St. Mary's Hospital of Kankakee, Kankakee, Ill.
	Swedish Covenant Hospital, Chicago

GERIATRICS

Natl. Rank — Hospital

Natl. Rank	Hospital
TIER ONE	
11	University of Chicago Hospitals
16	Rush-Presbyterian-St. Luke's Medical Center, Chicago
TIER TWO	
49	Cook County Hospital, Chicago
46	Evanston Hospital, Evanston, Ill.
55	F.G. McGaw Hospital at Loyola University, Maywood, Ill.
80	Lutheran General Healthsystem, Park Ridge, Ill.
90	Michael Reese Hospital and Medical Center, Chicago
33	Northwestern Memorial Hospital, Chicago
29	University of Illinois Hospital and Clinics, Chicago
TIER THREE	
	Alexian Brothers Medical Center, Elk Grove Village, Ill.
	Columbus Hospital, Chicago
	Edgewater Medical Center, Chicago
	Elmhurst Memorial Hospital, Elmhurst, Ill.
	Good Samaritan Hospital, Downers Grove, Ill.
	Gottlieb Memorial Hospital, Melrose Park, Ill.
	Grant Hospital of Chicago
	Hinsdale Hospital, Hinsdale, Ill.
	Holy Family Hospital, Des Plaines, Ill.
	Illinois Masonic Medical Center, Chicago
	Ingalls Memorial Hospital, Harvey, Ill.
	La Grange Memorial Health System, La Grange, Ill.
	Little Company of Mary Hospital, Evergreen Park, Ill.
	Louis A. Weiss Memorial Hospital, Chicago
	MacNeal Hospital, Berwyn, Ill.
	Mercy Hospital and Medical Center, Chicago
	Northwest Community Hospital, Arlington Heights, Ill.
	Ravenswood Hospital Medical Center, Chicago
	Rush North Shore Medical Center, Skokie, Ill.
	St. Francis Hospital, Evanston, Ill.
	St. James Hospital and Health Center, Chicago Heights, Ill.
	St. Joseph Hospital and Health Care Center, Chicago
	Swedish Covenant Hospital, Chicago
	West Suburban Hospital Medical Center, Oak Park, Ill.
TIER FOUR	
	Central Du Page Hospital, Winfield, Ill.
	Christ Hospital and Medical Center, Oak Lawn, Ill.
	Copley Memorial Hospital, Aurora, Ill.
	Lakeshore Health System, East Chicago, Ind.
	Mercy Center for Health Care Services, Aurora, Ill.
	Methodist Hospitals, Gary, Ind.
	Resurrection Medical Center, Chicago
	Riverside Medical Center, Kankakee, Ill.
	Sherman Hospital, Elgin, Ill.
	St. Catherine's Hospital, Kenosha, Wis.

METRO RANKINGS ■ CHICAGO

	St. Joseph Medical Center, Joliet, Ill.
	St. Margaret Mercy Health Centers, Hammond, Ind.
	St. Mary of Nazareth Hospital Center, Chicago
	St. Mary's Hospital of Kankakee, Kankakee, Ill.

GYNECOLOGY

	TIER ONE
9	University of Chicago Hospitals
25	Northwestern Memorial Hospital, Chicago
28	Rush-Presbyterian-St. Luke's Medical Center, Chicago
30	University of Illinois Hospital and Clinics, Chicago
	TIER TWO
46	Cook County Hospital, Chicago
67	Evanston Hospital, Evanston, Ill.
47	F.G. McGaw Hospital at Loyola University, Maywood, Ill.
	TIER THREE
	Alexian Brothers Medical Center, Elk Grove Village, Ill.
	Columbus Hospital, Chicago
	Edgewater Medical Center, Chicago
	Elmhurst Memorial Hospital, Elmhurst, Ill.
	Good Samaritan Hospital, Downers Grove, Ill.
	Gottlieb Memorial Hospital, Melrose Park, Ill.
	Grant Hospital of Chicago
	Hinsdale Hospital, Hinsdale, Ill.
	Holy Family Hospital, Des Plaines, Ill.
	Illinois Masonic Medical Center, Chicago
	Ingalls Memorial Hospital, Harvey, Ill.
	Louis A. Weiss Memorial Hospital, Chicago
	Lutheran General Healthsystem, Park Ridge, Ill.
	MacNeal Hospital, Berwyn, Ill.
	Mercy Hospital and Medical Center, Chicago
93	Michael Reese Hospital and Medical Center, Chicago
	Northwest Community Hospital, Arlington Heights, Ill.
	Oak Park Hospital, Oak Park, Ill.
	Rush North Shore Medical Center, Skokie, Ill.
	Sherman Hospital, Elgin, Ill.
	St. Francis Hospital, Evanston, Ill.
	St. James Hospital and Health Center, Chicago Heights, Ill.
	St. Joseph Hospital and Health Care Center, Chicago
	West Suburban Hospital Medical Center, Oak Park, Ill.
	TIER FOUR
	Central Du Page Hospital, Winfield, Ill.
	Christ Hospital and Medical Center, Oak Lawn, Ill.
	Copley Memorial Hospital, Aurora, Ill.
	La Grange Memorial Health System, La Grange, Ill.
	Lakeshore Health System, East Chicago, Ind.
	Little Company of Mary Hospital, Evergreen Park, Ill.
	Mercy Center for Health Care Services, Aurora, Ill.
	Methodist Hospitals, Gary, Ind.
	Porter Memorial Hospital, Valparaiso, Ind.
	Ravenswood Hospital Medical Center, Chicago
	Resurrection Medical Center, Chicago
	Riverside Medical Center, Kankakee, Ill.
	St. Anthony Medical Center, Crown Point, Ind.
	St. Catherine's Hospital, Kenosha, Wis.

	St. Joseph Medical Center, Joliet, Ill.
	St. Margaret Mercy Health Centers, Hammond, Ind.
	St. Mary of Nazareth Hospital Center, Chicago
	St. Mary's Hospital of Kankakee, Kankakee, Ill.
	Swedish Covenant Hospital, Chicago

NEUROLOGY

	TIER ONE
14	University of Illinois Hospital and Clinics, Chicago
16	University of Chicago Hospitals
19	Rush-Presbyterian-St. Luke's Medical Center, Chicago
	TIER TWO
68	Evanston Hospital, Evanston, Ill.
72	Lutheran General Healthsystem, Park Ridge, Ill.
41	Northwestern Memorial Hospital, Chicago
	TIER THREE
	Alexian Brothers Medical Center, Elk Grove Village, Ill.
	Columbus Hospital, Chicago
	Edgewater Medical Center, Chicago
90	F.G. McGaw Hospital at Loyola University, Maywood, Ill.
	Good Samaritan Hospital, Downers Grove, Ill.
	Gottlieb Memorial Hospital, Melrose Park, Ill.
	Grant Hospital of Chicago
	Hinsdale Hospital, Hinsdale, Ill.
	Holy Family Hospital, Des Plaines, Ill.
	Illinois Masonic Medical Center, Chicago
	Ingalls Memorial Hospital, Harvey, Ill.
	La Grange Memorial Health System, La Grange, Ill.
	Little Company of Mary Hospital, Evergreen Park, Ill.
	Louis A. Weiss Memorial Hospital, Chicago
	MacNeal Hospital, Berwyn, Ill.
89	Mercy Hospital and Medical Center, Chicago
	Methodist Hospitals, Gary, Ind.
98	Michael Reese Hospital and Medical Center, Chicago
	Mount Sinai Hospital Medical Center, Chicago
	Oak Park Hospital, Oak Park, Ill.
	Rush North Shore Medical Center, Skokie, Ill.
	St. James Hospital and Health Center, Chicago Heights, Ill.
	St. Joseph Hospital and Health Care Center, Chicago
	St. Mary of Nazareth Hospital Center, Chicago
	TIER FOUR
	Central Du Page Hospital, Winfield, Ill.
	Christ Hospital and Medical Center, Oak Lawn, Ill.
	Elmhurst Memorial Hospital, Elmhurst, Ill.
	Lakeshore Health System, East Chicago, Ind.
	Northwest Community Hospital, Arlington Heights, Ill.
	Ravenswood Hospital Medical Center, Chicago
	Resurrection Medical Center, Chicago
	Riverside Medical Center, Kankakee, Ill.
	Sherman Hospital, Elgin, Ill.
	St. Anthony Medical Center, Crown Point, Ind.
	St. Catherine's Hospital, Kenosha, Wis.
	St. Francis Hospital, Evanston, Ill.
	St. Joseph Medical Center, Joliet, Ill.
	St. Margaret Mercy Health Centers, Hammond, Ind.

| St. Mary's Hospital of Kankakee, Kankakee, Ill. |
| Swedish Covenant Hospital, Chicago |
| West Suburban Hospital Medical Center, Oak Park, Ill. |

ORTHOPEDICS

Natl.
Rank   Hospital

TIER ONE	
19	University of Chicago Hospitals
TIER TWO	
31	F.G. McGaw Hospital at Loyola University, Maywood, Ill.
24	Rush-Presbyterian-St. Luke's Medical Center, Chicago
TIER THREE	
	Alexian Brothers Medical Center, Elk Grove Village, Ill.
	Evanston Hospital, Evanston, Ill.
	Good Samaritan Hospital, Downers Grove, Ill.
	Grant Hospital of Chicago
	Holy Family Hospital, Des Plaines, Ill.
	Illinois Masonic Medical Center, Chicago
	Lakeshore Health System, East Chicago, Ind.
	Louis A. Weiss Memorial Hospital, Chicago
	Lutheran General Healthsystem, Park Ridge, Ill.
	MacNeal Hospital, Berwyn, Ill.
	Mercy Hospital and Medical Center, Chicago
	Michael Reese Hospital and Medical Center, Chicago
	Northwest Community Hospital, Arlington Heights, Ill.
	Northwestern Memorial Hospital, Chicago
	Rush North Shore Medical Center, Skokie, Ill.
	St. Joseph Hospital and Health Care Center, Chicago
TIER FOUR	
	Central Du Page Hospital, Winfield, Ill.
	Christ Hospital and Medical Center, Oak Lawn, Ill.
	Columbus Hospital, Chicago
	Copley Memorial Hospital, Aurora, Ill.
	Elmhurst Memorial Hospital, Elmhurst, Ill.
	Gottlieb Memorial Hospital, Melrose Park, Ill.
	Hinsdale Hospital, Hinsdale, Ill.
	Ingalls Memorial Hospital, Harvey, Ill.
	La Grange Memorial Health System, La Grange, Ill.
	Little Company of Mary Hospital, Evergreen Park, Ill.
	Mercy Center for Health Care Services, Aurora, Ill.
	Oak Park Hospital, Oak Park, Ill.
	Porter Memorial Hospital, Valparaiso, Ind.
	Resurrection Medical Center, Chicago
	Riverside Medical Center, Kankakee, Ill.
	Sherman Hospital, Elgin, Ill.
	St. Anthony Medical Center, Crown Point, Ind.
	St. Catherine's Hospital, Kenosha, Wis.
	St. Francis Hospital, Evanston, Ill.
	St. James Hospital and Health Center, Chicago Heights, Ill.
	St. Joseph Medical Center, Joliet, Ill.
	St. Margaret Mercy Health Centers, Hammond, Ind.
	St. Mary's Hospital of Kankakee, Kankakee, Ill.
	Swedish Covenant Hospital, Chicago
	West Suburban Hospital Medical Center, Oak Park, Ill.

OTOLARYNGOLOGY

Natl.
Rank   Hospital

TIER ONE	
23	University of Illinois Hospital and Clinics, Chicago
28	Northwestern Memorial Hospital, Chicago
31	University of Chicago Hospitals
33	F.G. McGaw Hospital at Loyola University, Maywood, Ill.
TIER TWO	
71	Cook County Hospital, Chicago
67	Rush-Presbyterian-St. Luke's Medical Center, Chicago
TIER THREE	
	Columbus Hospital, Chicago
	Evanston Hospital, Evanston, Ill.
	Illinois Masonic Medical Center, Chicago
	Lutheran General Healthsystem, Park Ridge, Ill.
	MacNeal Hospital, Berwyn, Ill.
	Mercy Hospital and Medical Center, Chicago
	Michael Reese Hospital and Medical Center, Chicago
	Mount Sinai Hospital Medical Center, Chicago
TIER FOUR	
	Alexian Brothers Medical Center, Elk Grove Village, Ill.
	Central Du Page Hospital, Winfield, Ill.
	Christ Hospital and Medical Center, Oak Lawn, Ill.
	Copley Memorial Hospital, Aurora, Ill.
	Edgewater Medical Center, Chicago
	Elmhurst Memorial Hospital, Elmhurst, Ill.
	Good Samaritan Hospital, Downers Grove, Ill.
	Gottlieb Memorial Hospital, Melrose Park, Ill.
	Grant Hospital of Chicago
	Hinsdale Hospital, Hinsdale, Ill.
	Holy Family Hospital, Des Plaines, Ill.
	Ingalls Memorial Hospital, Harvey, Ill.
	La Grange Memorial Health System, La Grange, Ill.
	Lakeshore Health System, East Chicago, Ind.
	Little Company of Mary Hospital, Evergreen Park, Ill.
	Louis A. Weiss Memorial Hospital, Chicago
	Mercy Center for Health Care Services, Aurora, Ill.
	Methodist Hospitals, Gary, Ind.
	Northwest Community Hospital, Arlington Heights, Ill.
	Oak Forest Hospital of Cook County, Oak Forest, Ill.
	Oak Park Hospital, Oak Park, Ill.
	Porter Memorial Hospital, Valparaiso, Ind.
	Ravenswood Hospital Medical Center, Chicago
	Resurrection Medical Center, Chicago
	Riverside Medical Center, Kankakee, Ill.
	Rush North Shore Medical Center, Skokie, Ill.
	Sherman Hospital, Elgin, Ill.
	St. Anthony Medical Center, Crown Point, Ind.
	St. Catherine's Hospital, Kenosha, Wis.
	St. Francis Hospital, Evanston, Ill.
	St. James Hospital and Health Center, Chicago Heights, Ill.
	St. Joseph Hospital and Health Care Center, Chicago
	St. Joseph Medical Center, Joliet, Ill.
	St. Margaret Mercy Health Centers, Hammond, Ind.
	St. Mary of Nazareth Hospital Center, Chicago

	St. Mary's Hospital of Kankakee, Kankakee, Ill.
	Swedish Covenant Hospital, Chicago
	West Suburban Hospital Medical Center, Oak Park, Ill.

	St. Mary of Nazareth Hospital Center, Chicago
	St. Mary's Hospital of Kankakee, Kankakee, Ill.
	Swedish Covenant Hospital, Chicago
	West Suburban Hospital Medical Center, Oak Park, Ill.

RHEUMATOLOGY

Natl. Rank	Hospital
TIER ONE	
20	University of Chicago Hospitals
TIER TWO	
56	Cook County Hospital, Chicago
64	F.G. McGaw Hospital at Loyola University, Maywood, Ill.
82	Northwestern Memorial Hospital, Chicago
32	Rush-Presbyterian-St. Luke's Medical Center, Chicago
28	University of Illinois Hospital and Clinics, Chicago
TIER THREE	
	Alexian Brothers Medical Center, Elk Grove Village, Ill.
	Columbus Hospital, Chicago
	Elmhurst Memorial Hospital, Elmhurst, Ill.
89	Evanston Hospital, Evanston, Ill.
	Grant Hospital of Chicago
	Hinsdale Hospital, Hinsdale, Ill.
	Holy Family Hospital, Des Plaines, Ill.
	Illinois Masonic Medical Center, Chicago
	Louis A. Weiss Memorial Hospital, Chicago
85	Lutheran General Healthsystem, Park Ridge, Ill.
	MacNeal Hospital, Berwyn, Ill.
	Mercy Hospital and Medical Center, Chicago
	Michael Reese Hospital and Medical Center, Chicago
	Rush North Shore Medical Center, Skokie, Ill.
TIER FOUR	
	Central Du Page Hospital, Winfield, Ill.
	Christ Hospital and Medical Center, Oak Lawn, Ill.
	Copley Memorial Hospital, Aurora, Ill.
	Edgewater Medical Center, Chicago
	Good Samaritan Hospital, Downers Grove, Ill.
	Gottlieb Memorial Hospital, Melrose Park, Ill.
	Ingalls Memorial Hospital, Harvey, Ill.
	La Grange Memorial Health System, La Grange, Ill.
	Lakeshore Health System, East Chicago, Ind.
	Little Company of Mary Hospital, Evergreen Park, Ill.
	Mercy Center for Health Care Services, Aurora, Ill.
	Methodist Hospitals, Gary, Ind.
	Northwest Community Hospital, Arlington Heights, Ill.
	Oak Park Hospital, Oak Park, Ill.
	Porter Memorial Hospital, Valparaiso, Ind.
	Ravenswood Hospital Medical Center, Chicago
	Resurrection Medical Center, Chicago
	Riverside Medical Center, Kankakee, Ill.
	Sherman Hospital, Elgin, Ill.
	St. Anthony Medical Center, Crown Point, Ind.
	St. Catherine's Hospital, Kenosha, Wis.
	St. Francis Hospital, Evanston, Ill.
	St. James Hospital and Health Center, Chicago Heights, Ill.
	St. Joseph Hospital and Health Care Center, Chicago
	St. Joseph Medical Center, Joliet, Ill.
	St. Margaret Mercy Health Centers, Hammond, Ind.

UROLOGY

Natl. Rank	Hospital
TIER TWO	
44	Cook County Hospital, Chicago
65	F.G. McGaw Hospital at Loyola University, Maywood, Ill.
52	Northwestern Memorial Hospital, Chicago
43	Rush-Presbyterian-St. Luke's Medical Center, Chicago
32	University of Chicago Hospitals
62	University of Illinois Hospital and Clinics, Chicago
TIER THREE	
	Columbus Hospital, Chicago
	Edgewater Medical Center, Chicago
	Elmhurst Memorial Hospital, Elmhurst, Ill.
	Evanston Hospital, Evanston, Ill.
	Grant Hospital of Chicago
	Holy Family Hospital, Des Plaines, Ill.
	Illinois Masonic Medical Center, Chicago
	Little Company of Mary Hospital, Evergreen Park, Ill.
	Louis A. Weiss Memorial Hospital, Chicago
	Lutheran General Healthsystem, Park Ridge, Ill.
	Mercy Hospital and Medical Center, Chicago
97	Michael Reese Hospital and Medical Center, Chicago
	Mount Sinai Hospital Medical Center, Chicago
	Rush North Shore Medical Center, Skokie, Ill.
	Sherman Hospital, Elgin, Ill.
	St. James Hospital and Health Center, Chicago Heights, Ill.
TIER FOUR	
	Alexian Brothers Medical Center, Elk Grove Village, Ill.
	Central Du Page Hospital, Winfield, Ill.
	Christ Hospital and Medical Center, Oak Lawn, Ill.
	Copley Memorial Hospital, Aurora, Ill.
	Good Samaritan Hospital, Downers Grove, Ill.
	Gottlieb Memorial Hospital, Melrose Park, Ill.
	Hinsdale Hospital, Hinsdale, Ill.
	Ingalls Memorial Hospital, Harvey, Ill.
	La Grange Memorial Health System, La Grange, Ill.
	Lakeshore Health System, East Chicago, Ind.
	MacNeal Hospital, Berwyn, Ill.
	Methodist Hospitals, Gary, Ind.
	Northwest Community Hospital, Arlington Heights, Ill.
	Oak Park Hospital, Oak Park, Ill.
	Porter Memorial Hospital, Valparaiso, Ind.
	Ravenswood Hospital Medical Center, Chicago
	Resurrection Medical Center, Chicago
	Riverside Medical Center, Kankakee, Ill.
	St. Anthony Medical Center, Crown Point, Ind.
	St. Francis Hospital, Evanston, Ill.
	St. Joseph Hospital and Health Care Center, Chicago
	St. Joseph Medical Center, Joliet, Ill.
	St. Margaret Mercy Health Centers, Hammond, Ind.
	St. Mary of Nazareth Hospital Center, Chicago

| St. Mary's Hospital of Kankakee, Kankakee, Ill. |
| Swedish Covenant Hospital, Chicago |
| West Suburban Hospital Medical Center, Oak Park, Ill. |

Dallas-Fort Worth

AIDS

Natl. Rank	Hospital
TIER TWO	
54	Baylor University Medical Center, Dallas
TIER THREE	
	HCA Medical Center of Plano, Plano, Texas
	HCA Medical Plaza Hospital, Fort Worth
	Harris Methodist Fort Worth
	Harris Methodist-HEB, Bedford, Texas
	Medical City Dallas Hospital
97	Parkland Memorial Hospital, Dallas
	Presbyterian Hospital, Dallas
	St. Paul Medical Center, Dallas
TIER FOUR	
	All Saints Episcopal Hospital, Fort Worth
	Arlington Memorial Hospital, Arlington, Texas
	Irving Healthcare System, Irving, Texas
	John Peter Smith Hospital, Fort Worth
	Methodist Medical Center, Dallas
	Osteopathic Medical Center of Texas, Fort Worth
	RHD Memorial Medical Center, Dallas
	St. Joseph Hospital, Fort Worth

CANCER

Natl. Rank	Hospital
TIER TWO	
68	Parkland Memorial Hospital, Dallas
TIER THREE	
	Baylor University Medical Center, Dallas
	Methodist Medical Center, Dallas
	St. Paul Medical Center, Dallas
	Zale Lipshy University Hospital, Dallas
TIER FOUR	
	All Saints Episcopal Hospital, Fort Worth
	Arlington Memorial Hospital, Arlington, Texas
	HCA Medical Center of Plano, Plano, Texas
	HCA Medical Plaza Hospital, Fort Worth
	Harris Methodist Fort Worth
	Harris Methodist-HEB, Bedford, Texas
	Irving Healthcare System, Irving, Texas
	Medical City Dallas Hospital
	Osteopathic Medical Center of Texas, Fort Worth
	Presbyterian Hospital, Dallas
	RHD Memorial Medical Center, Dallas
	St. Joseph Hospital, Fort Worth

CARDIOLOGY

Natl. Rank	Hospital
TIER TWO	
91	Parkland Memorial Hospital, Dallas
TIER THREE	
97	Baylor University Medical Center, Dallas
	Harris Methodist-HEB, Bedford, Texas
	Medical City Dallas Hospital
	Osteopathic Medical Center of Texas, Fort Worth
	Presbyterian Hospital, Dallas
	St. Paul Medical Center, Dallas
TIER FOUR	
	All Saints Episcopal Hospital, Fort Worth
	Arlington Memorial Hospital, Arlington, Texas
	HCA Medical Center of Plano, Plano, Texas
	HCA Medical Plaza Hospital, Fort Worth
	Harris Methodist Fort Worth
	Irving Healthcare System, Irving, Texas
	Methodist Medical Center, Dallas
	RHD Memorial Medical Center, Dallas
	St. Joseph Hospital, Fort Worth

ENDOCRINOLOGY

Natl. Rank	Hospital
TIER ONE	
12	Parkland Memorial Hospital, Dallas
TIER TWO	
47	Baylor University Medical Center, Dallas
TIER THREE	
	Methodist Medical Center, Dallas
	Presbyterian Hospital, Dallas
	St. Paul Medical Center, Dallas
TIER FOUR	
	All Saints Episcopal Hospital, Fort Worth
	Arlington Memorial Hospital, Arlington, Texas
	HCA Medical Plaza Hospital, Fort Worth
	Harris Methodist Fort Worth
	Irving Healthcare System, Irving, Texas
	Medical City Dallas Hospital
	Osteopathic Medical Center of Texas, Fort Worth
	St. Joseph Hospital, Fort Worth

GASTROENTEROLOGY

Natl. Rank	Hospital
TIER ONE	
15	Baylor University Medical Center, Dallas
TIER THREE	
	Medical City Dallas Hospital
	Methodist Medical Center, Dallas
	Presbyterian Hospital, Dallas
	St. Paul Medical Center, Dallas

METRO RANKINGS ■ DALLAS

TIER FOUR
All Saints Episcopal Hospital, Fort Worth
Arlington Memorial Hospital, Arlington, Texas
Harris Methodist Fort Worth
Harris Methodist-HEB, Bedford, Texas
Irving Healthcare System, Irving, Texas
Osteopathic Medical Center of Texas, Fort Worth
St. Joseph Hospital, Fort Worth

GERIATRICS

Natl.
Rank   Hospital

Rank	TIER TWO
42	Baylor University Medical Center, Dallas
	TIER THREE
	HCA Medical Plaza Hospital, Fort Worth
	Harris Methodist Fort Worth
	Harris Methodist-HEB, Bedford, Texas
	Medical City Dallas Hospital
	Parkland Memorial Hospital, Dallas
	St. Paul Medical Center, Dallas
	TIER FOUR
	All Saints Episcopal Hospital, Fort Worth
	Arlington Memorial Hospital, Arlington, Texas
	Irving Healthcare System, Irving, Texas
	Methodist Medical Center, Dallas
	Osteopathic Medical Center of Texas, Fort Worth
	St. Joseph Hospital, Fort Worth

GYNECOLOGY

Natl.
Rank   Hospital

Rank	TIER ONE
12	Parkland Memorial Hospital, Dallas
27	Baylor University Medical Center, Dallas
	TIER TWO
73	Presbyterian Hospital, Dallas
	TIER THREE
	HCA Medical Plaza Hospital, Fort Worth
	Harris Methodist Fort Worth
	Harris Methodist-HEB, Bedford, Texas
	Medical City Dallas Hospital
	St. Paul Medical Center, Dallas
	TIER FOUR
	All Saints Episcopal Hospital, Fort Worth
	Arlington Memorial Hospital, Arlington, Texas
	Irving Healthcare System, Irving, Texas
	Methodist Medical Center, Dallas
	Osteopathic Medical Center of Texas, Fort Worth
	St. Joseph Hospital, Fort Worth

NEUROLOGY

Natl.
Rank   Hospital

Rank	TIER TWO
63	Baylor University Medical Center, Dallas
	TIER THREE
	HCA Medical Plaza Hospital, Fort Worth
	Harris Methodist-HEB, Bedford, Texas
	Irving Healthcare System, Irving, Texas
	Methodist Medical Center, Dallas
	Parkland Memorial Hospital, Dallas
	Presbyterian Hospital, Dallas
	St. Paul Medical Center, Dallas
	TIER FOUR
	All Saints Episcopal Hospital, Fort Worth
	Arlington Memorial Hospital, Arlington, Texas
	Medical City Dallas Hospital
	Osteopathic Medical Center of Texas, Fort Worth
	St. Joseph Hospital, Fort Worth

ORTHOPEDICS

Natl.
Rank   Hospital

Rank	TIER TWO
61	Baylor University Medical Center, Dallas
80	Parkland Memorial Hospital, Dallas
	TIER THREE
	HCA Medical Plaza Hospital, Fort Worth
	Harris Methodist-HEB, Bedford, Texas
	Irving Healthcare System, Irving, Texas
	Medical City Dallas Hospital
	Methodist Medical Center, Dallas
	Osteopathic Medical Center of Texas, Fort Worth
	Presbyterian Hospital, Dallas
	St. Paul Medical Center, Dallas
	TIER FOUR
	All Saints Episcopal Hospital, Fort Worth
	Arlington Memorial Hospital, Arlington, Texas
	HCA Medical Center of Plano, Plano, Texas
	Harris Methodist Fort Worth
	St. Joseph Hospital, Fort Worth

OTOLARYNGOLOGY

Natl.
Rank   Hospital

Rank	TIER ONE
32	Parkland Memorial Hospital, Dallas
	TIER TWO
51	Baylor University Medical Center, Dallas
	TIER THREE
	John Peter Smith Hospital, Fort Worth
	Methodist Medical Center, Dallas
	St. Paul Medical Center, Dallas
	Zale Lipshy University Hospital, Dallas

TIER FOUR
All Saints Episcopal Hospital, Fort Worth
Arlington Memorial Hospital, Arlington, Texas
HCA Medical Center of Plano, Plano, Texas
HCA Medical Plaza Hospital, Fort Worth
Harris Methodist Fort Worth
Harris Methodist-HEB, Bedford, Texas
Irving Healthcare System, Irving, Texas
Medical City Dallas Hospital
Osteopathic Medical Center of Texas, Fort Worth
Presbyterian Hospital, Dallas
RHD Memorial Medical Center, Dallas
St. Joseph Hospital, Fort Worth

RHEUMATOLOGY

Natl.
Rank   Hospital

	TIER ONE
21	Parkland Memorial Hospital, Dallas
	TIER TWO
79	Baylor University Medical Center, Dallas
	TIER THREE
	Harris Methodist Fort Worth
	Medical City Dallas Hospital
	Methodist Medical Center, Dallas
	St. Paul Medical Center, Dallas
	TIER FOUR
	All Saints Episcopal Hospital, Fort Worth
	Arlington Memorial Hospital, Arlington, Texas
	HCA Medical Plaza Hospital, Fort Worth
	Harris Methodist-HEB, Bedford, Texas
	Irving Healthcare System, Irving, Texas
	Osteopathic Medical Center of Texas, Fort Worth
	Presbyterian Hospital, Dallas
	St. Joseph Hospital, Fort Worth

UROLOGY

Natl.
Rank   Hospital

	TIER ONE
11	Baylor University Medical Center, Dallas
	TIER TWO
28	Parkland Memorial Hospital, Dallas
	TIER THREE
	Medical City Dallas Hospital
	Presbyterian Hospital, Dallas
	St. Paul Medical Center, Dallas
	TIER FOUR
	All Saints Episcopal Hospital, Fort Worth
	Arlington Memorial Hospital, Arlington, Texas
	HCA Medical Plaza Hospital, Fort Worth
	Harris Methodist Fort Worth
	Irving Healthcare System, Irving, Texas

Methodist Medical Center, Dallas
Osteopathic Medical Center of Texas, Fort Worth
St. Joseph Hospital, Fort Worth

Detroit

AIDS

Natl.
Rank   Hospital

	TIER ONE
24	Henry Ford Hospital, Detroit
	TIER TWO
37	University of Michigan Medical Center, Ann Arbor
	TIER THREE
	Bon Secours Hospital, Grosse Pointe, Mich.
	Catherine McAuley Health System, Ann Arbor, Mich.
	Detroit Riverview Hospital
96	Harper Hospital, Detroit
	Macomb Hospital Center, Warren, Mich.
	Mercy Hospital, Port Huron, Mich.
	North Oakland Medical Center, Pontiac, Mich.
	Providence Hospital, Southfield, Mich.
	Sinai Hospital, Detroit
	St. John Hospital and Medical Center, Detroit
	St. Joseph Mercy Hospital, Pontiac, Mich.
	William Beaumont Hospital, Royal Oak, Mich.
	TIER FOUR
	Detroit Receiving Hospital
	Genesys Regional Medical Center-St. Joseph, Flint, Mich.
	Grace Hospital, Detroit
	Hurley Medical Center, Flint, Mich.
	Hutzel Hospital, Detroit
	McLaren Regional Medical Center, Flint, Mich.
	Oakwood Hospital, Dearborn, Mich.
	St. Mary Hospital, Livonia, Mich.

CANCER

Natl.
Rank   Hospital

	TIER TWO
35	Henry Ford Hospital, Detroit
40	University of Michigan Medical Center, Ann Arbor
	TIER THREE
	Catherine McAuley Health System, Ann Arbor, Mich.
	Grace Hospital, Detroit
	Harper Hospital, Detroit
	Hurley Medical Center, Flint, Mich.
	Hutzel Hospital, Detroit
	Oakwood Hospital, Dearborn, Mich.
	Providence Hospital, Southfield, Mich.
	Sinai Hospital, Detroit
	St. John Hospital and Medical Center, Detroit
88	William Beaumont Hospital, Royal Oak, Mich.

TIER FOUR
Bon Secours Hospital, Grosse Pointe, Mich.
Genesys Regional Medical Center-St. Joseph, Flint, Mich.
Macomb Hospital Center, Warren, Mich.
McLaren Regional Medical Center, Flint, Mich.
Mercy Hospital, Port Huron, Mich.
North Oakland Medical Center, Pontiac, Mich.
St. Joseph Mercy Hospital, Pontiac, Mich.
St. Mary Hospital, Livonia, Mich.

CARDIOLOGY

Rank	TIER TWO
31	Henry Ford Hospital, Detroit
32	University of Michigan Medical Center, Ann Arbor
48	William Beaumont Hospital, Royal Oak, Mich.
	TIER THREE
	Bon Secours Hospital, Grosse Pointe, Mich.
	Catherine McAuley Health System, Ann Arbor, Mich.
	Grace Hospital, Detroit
	Harper Hospital, Detroit
	Mercy Hospital, Port Huron, Mich.
	North Oakland Medical Center, Pontiac, Mich.
	Providence Hospital, Southfield, Mich.
	Sinai Hospital, Detroit
	St. John Hospital and Medical Center, Detroit
	St. Joseph Mercy Hospital, Pontiac, Mich.
	St. Mary Hospital, Livonia, Mich.
	TIER FOUR
	Detroit Riverview Hospital
	Genesys Regional Medical Center-St. Joseph, Flint, Mich.
	Hurley Medical Center, Flint, Mich.
	Macomb Hospital Center, Warren, Mich.
	McLaren Regional Medical Center, Flint, Mich.
	Oakwood Hospital, Dearborn, Mich.

ENDOCRINOLOGY

Rank	TIER ONE
8	University of Michigan Medical Center, Ann Arbor
	TIER TWO
51	Henry Ford Hospital, Detroit
	TIER THREE
	Catherine McAuley Health System, Ann Arbor, Mich.
	Detroit Receiving Hospital
	Grace Hospital, Detroit
	Harper Hospital, Detroit
	Oakwood Hospital, Dearborn, Mich.
	Sinai Hospital, Detroit
	St. John Hospital and Medical Center, Detroit
	William Beaumont Hospital, Royal Oak, Mich.
	TIER FOUR
	Bon Secours Hospital, Grosse Pointe, Mich.
	Detroit Riverview Hospital

Genesys Regional Medical Center-St. Joseph, Flint, Mich.
Hurley Medical Center, Flint, Mich.
Macomb Hospital Center, Warren, Mich.
McLaren Regional Medical Center, Flint, Mich.
North Oakland Medical Center, Pontiac, Mich.
Providence Hospital, Southfield, Mich.
St. Joseph Mercy Hospital, Pontiac, Mich.
St. Mary Hospital, Livonia, Mich.

GASTROENTEROLOGY

Rank	TIER ONE
14	University of Michigan Medical Center, Ann Arbor
	TIER TWO
32	Henry Ford Hospital, Detroit
36	William Beaumont Hospital, Royal Oak, Mich.
	TIER THREE
	Bon Secours Hospital, Grosse Pointe, Mich.
	Catherine McAuley Health System, Ann Arbor, Mich.
	Grace Hospital, Detroit
97	Harper Hospital, Detroit
	Hurley Medical Center, Flint, Mich.
	Oakwood Hospital, Dearborn, Mich.
	Providence Hospital, Southfield, Mich.
	Sinai Hospital, Detroit
	St. John Hospital and Medical Center, Detroit
	St. Joseph Mercy Hospital, Pontiac, Mich.
	TIER FOUR
	Genesys Regional Medical Center-St. Joseph, Flint, Mich.
	Macomb Hospital Center, Warren, Mich.
	McLaren Regional Medical Center, Flint, Mich.
	Mercy Hospital, Port Huron, Mich.
	North Oakland Medical Center, Pontiac, Mich.
	St. Mary Hospital, Livonia, Mich.

GERIATRICS

Rank	TIER ONE
8	University of Michigan Medical Center, Ann Arbor
	TIER TWO
38	Henry Ford Hospital, Detroit
62	William Beaumont Hospital, Royal Oak, Mich.
	TIER THREE
	Bon Secours Hospital, Grosse Pointe, Mich.
	Catherine McAuley Health System, Ann Arbor, Mich.
	Detroit Riverview Hospital
	Harper Hospital, Detroit
	Macomb Hospital Center, Warren, Mich.
	Mercy Hospital, Port Huron, Mich.
	North Oakland Medical Center, Pontiac, Mich.
	Oakwood Hospital, Dearborn, Mich.
	Providence Hospital, Southfield, Mich.
	St. John Hospital and Medical Center, Detroit
	St. Joseph Mercy Hospital, Pontiac, Mich.

	TIER FOUR
	Detroit Receiving Hospital
	Genesys Regional Medical Center-St. Joseph, Flint, Mich.
	Grace Hospital, Detroit
	Hurley Medical Center, Flint, Mich.
	McLaren Regional Medical Center, Flint, Mich.
	Sinai Hospital, Detroit
	St. Mary Hospital, Livonia, Mich.

GYNECOLOGY

	TIER TWO
49	Henry Ford Hospital, Detroit
40	University of Michigan Medical Center, Ann Arbor
	TIER THREE
	Bon Secours Hospital, Grosse Pointe, Mich.
	Catherine McAuley Health System, Ann Arbor, Mich.
	Detroit Riverview Hospital
	Harper Hospital, Detroit
	Macomb Hospital Center, Warren, Mich.
	North Oakland Medical Center, Pontiac, Mich.
	Providence Hospital, Southfield, Mich.
	Sinai Hospital, Detroit
	St. John Hospital and Medical Center, Detroit
	St. Joseph Mercy Hospital, Pontiac, Mich.
88	William Beaumont Hospital, Royal Oak, Mich.
	TIER FOUR
	Detroit Receiving Hospital
	Genesys Regional Medical Center-St. Joseph, Flint, Mich.
	Grace Hospital, Detroit
	Hurley Medical Center, Flint, Mich.
	McLaren Regional Medical Center, Flint, Mich.
	Oakwood Hospital, Dearborn, Mich.
	St. Mary Hospital, Livonia, Mich.

NEUROLOGY

	TIER ONE
24	University of Michigan Medical Center, Ann Arbor
	TIER TWO
42	Harper Hospital, Detroit
45	Henry Ford Hospital, Detroit
61	William Beaumont Hospital, Royal Oak, Mich.
	TIER THREE
	Bon Secours Hospital, Grosse Pointe, Mich.
	Catherine McAuley Health System, Ann Arbor, Mich.
	Detroit Receiving Hospital
	Grace Hospital, Detroit
	Hurley Medical Center, Flint, Mich.
	Providence Hospital, Southfield, Mich.
	Sinai Hospital, Detroit
	St. John Hospital and Medical Center, Detroit

	TIER FOUR
	Genesys Regional Medical Center-St. Joseph, Flint, Mich.
	Macomb Hospital Center, Warren, Mich.
	McLaren Regional Medical Center, Flint, Mich.
	Mercy Hospital, Port Huron, Mich.
	North Oakland Medical Center, Pontiac, Mich.
	Oakwood Hospital, Dearborn, Mich.
	St. Joseph Mercy Hospital, Pontiac, Mich.
	St. Mary Hospital, Livonia, Mich.

ORTHOPEDICS

	TIER ONE
13	University of Michigan Medical Center, Ann Arbor
	TIER TWO
30	Henry Ford Hospital, Detroit
	TIER THREE
94	Catherine McAuley Health System, Ann Arbor, Mich.
	Detroit Receiving Hospital
	Grace Hospital, Detroit
	Oakwood Hospital, Dearborn, Mich.
	Providence Hospital, Southfield, Mich.
	Sinai Hospital, Detroit
	St. John Hospital and Medical Center, Detroit
	St. Joseph Mercy Hospital, Pontiac, Mich.
	William Beaumont Hospital, Royal Oak, Mich.
	TIER FOUR
	Bon Secours Hospital, Grosse Pointe, Mich.
	Genesys Regional Medical Center-St. Joseph, Flint, Mich.
	Hutzel Hospital, Detroit
	Macomb Hospital Center, Warren, Mich.
	McLaren Regional Medical Center, Flint, Mich.
	Mercy Hospital, Port Huron, Mich.
	North Oakland Medical Center, Pontiac, Mich.
	St. Mary Hospital, Livonia, Mich.

OTOLARYNGOLOGY

	TIER ONE
4	University of Michigan Medical Center, Ann Arbor
34	Henry Ford Hospital, Detroit
	TIER THREE
	Catherine McAuley Health System, Ann Arbor, Mich.
	Detroit Receiving Hospital
	Grace Hospital, Detroit
	Harper Hospital, Detroit
	Hurley Medical Center, Flint, Mich.
	Hutzel Hospital, Detroit
	Oakwood Hospital, Dearborn, Mich.
	Providence Hospital, Southfield, Mich.
	Sinai Hospital, Detroit
	St. John Hospital and Medical Center, Detroit
	William Beaumont Hospital, Royal Oak, Mich.

TIER FOUR
Bon Secours Hospital, Grosse Pointe, Mich.
Chelsea Community Hospital, Chelsea, Mich.
Detroit Riverview Hospital
Genesys Regional Medical Center-St. Joseph, Flint, Mich.
Macomb Hospital Center, Warren, Mich.
McLaren Regional Medical Center, Flint, Mich.
Mercy Hospital, Port Huron, Mich.
North Oakland Medical Center, Pontiac, Mich.
St. Joseph Mercy Hospital, Pontiac, Mich.
St. Mary Hospital, Livonia, Mich.

RHEUMATOLOGY

Natl. Rank	**TIER ONE**
13	University of Michigan Medical Center, Ann Arbor
	TIER TWO
27	Henry Ford Hospital, Detroit
76	William Beaumont Hospital, Royal Oak, Mich.
	TIER THREE
	Bon Secours Hospital, Grosse Pointe, Mich.
	Catherine McAuley Health System, Ann Arbor, Mich.
	Detroit Receiving Hospital
	Grace Hospital, Detroit
	Harper Hospital, Detroit
	Hurley Medical Center, Flint, Mich.
	North Oakland Medical Center, Pontiac, Mich.
	Oakwood Hospital, Dearborn, Mich.
	Providence Hospital, Southfield, Mich.
	Sinai Hospital, Detroit
	St. John Hospital and Medical Center, Detroit
	St. Joseph Mercy Hospital, Pontiac, Mich.
	TIER FOUR
	Detroit Riverview Hospital
	Genesys Regional Medical Center-St. Joseph, Flint, Mich.
	Macomb Hospital Center, Warren, Mich.
	McLaren Regional Medical Center, Flint, Mich.
	Mercy Hospital, Port Huron, Mich.
	St. Mary Hospital, Livonia, Mich.

UROLOGY

Natl. Rank	**TIER ONE**
24	University of Michigan Medical Center, Ann Arbor
	TIER TWO
70	Harper Hospital, Detroit
45	Henry Ford Hospital, Detroit
50	William Beaumont Hospital, Royal Oak, Mich.
	TIER THREE
	Catherine McAuley Health System, Ann Arbor, Mich.
	Detroit Receiving Hospital
	Detroit Riverview Hospital
	Grace Hospital, Detroit

Hospital
Hurley Medical Center, Flint, Mich.
Providence Hospital, Southfield, Mich.
Sinai Hospital, Detroit
St. John Hospital and Medical Center, Detroit
St. Joseph Mercy Hospital, Pontiac, Mich.
TIER FOUR
Bon Secours Hospital, Grosse Pointe, Mich.
Genesys Regional Medical Center-St. Joseph, Flint, Mich.
Macomb Hospital Center, Warren, Mich.
McLaren Regional Medical Center, Flint, Mich.
Oakwood Hospital, Dearborn, Mich.
St. Mary Hospital, Livonia, Mich.

Houston

AIDS

Natl. Rank	**TIER TWO**
41	University of Texas, M.D. Anderson Cancer Ctr., Houston
	TIER THREE
	Clear Lake Regional Medical Center, Webster, Texas
	HCA Spring Branch Medical Center, Houston
	Hermann Hospital, Houston
	Memorial City Medical Center, Houston
	Methodist Hospital, Houston
	Northeast Medical Center Hospital, Humble, Texas
	Sam Houston Memorial Hospital, Houston
	Tomball Regional Hospital, Tomball, Texas
	University of Texas Medical Branch Hospitals, Galveston
	TIER FOUR
	Harris County Hospital District, Houston
	Houston Northwest Medical Center
	Medical Center Hospital, Conroe, Texas
	Memorial Hospital System, Houston
	San Jacinto Methodist Hospital, Baytown, Texas
	St. Joseph Hospital, Houston
	Texas Heart Institute-St. Luke's Episcopal, Houston

CANCER

Natl. Rank	**TIER ONE**
2	University of Texas, M.D. Anderson Cancer Ctr., Houston
	TIER TWO
75	University of Texas Medical Branch Hospitals, Galveston
	TIER THREE
	Harris County Hospital District, Houston
	Hermann Hospital, Houston
	Methodist Hospital, Houston
	Texas Heart Institute-St. Luke's Episcopal, Houston
	TIER FOUR
	Clear Lake Regional Medical Center, Webster, Texas

METRO RANKINGS ■ HOUSTON

Natl.
Rank Hospital

	HCA Spring Branch Medical Center, Houston
	Houston Northwest Medical Center
	Medical Center Hospital, Conroe, Texas
	Memorial City Medical Center, Houston
	Memorial Hospital System, Houston
	Northeast Medical Center Hospital, Humble, Texas
	San Jacinto Methodist Hospital, Baytown, Texas
	St. Joseph Hospital, Houston

CARDIOLOGY

Natl.
Rank Hospital

	TIER ONE
3	Texas Heart Institute-St. Luke's Episcopal, Houston
17	Methodist Hospital, Houston
	TIER THREE
	Hermann Hospital, Houston
	Northeast Medical Center Hospital, Humble, Texas
	University of Texas Medical Branch Hospitals, Galveston
	TIER FOUR
	Clear Lake Regional Medical Center, Webster, Texas
	HCA Spring Branch Medical Center, Houston
	Harris County Hospital District, Houston
	Houston Northwest Medical Center
	Medical Center Hospital, Conroe, Texas
	Memorial City Medical Center, Houston
	Memorial Hospital System, Houston
	San Jacinto Methodist Hospital, Baytown, Texas
	St. Joseph Hospital, Houston
	Tomball Regional Hospital, Tomball, Texas

ENDOCRINOLOGY

Natl.
Rank Hospital

	TIER ONE
24	University of Texas, M.D. Anderson Cancer Ctr., Houston
	TIER TWO
82	University of Texas Medical Branch Hospitals, Galveston
	TIER THREE
	Harris County Hospital District, Houston
	Hermann Hospital, Houston
	Houston Northwest Medical Center
	Memorial City Medical Center, Houston
	Methodist Hospital, Houston
	Texas Heart Institute-St. Luke's Episcopal, Houston
	TIER FOUR
	Clear Lake Regional Medical Center, Webster, Texas
	HCA Spring Branch Medical Center, Houston
	Memorial Hospital System, Houston
	Sam Houston Memorial Hospital, Houston
	San Jacinto Methodist Hospital, Baytown, Texas
	St. Joseph Hospital, Houston
	Tomball Regional Hospital, Tomball, Texas

GASTROENTEROLOGY

Natl.
Rank Hospital

	TIER TWO
34	University of Texas, M.D. Anderson Cancer Ctr., Houston
	TIER THREE
	Hermann Hospital, Houston
	Methodist Hospital, Houston
	Texas Heart Institute-St. Luke's Episcopal, Houston
	TIER FOUR
	Clear Lake Regional Medical Center, Webster, Texas
	Houston Northwest Medical Center
	Medical Center Hospital, Conroe, Texas
	Memorial City Medical Center, Houston
	Memorial Hospital System, Houston
	San Jacinto Methodist Hospital, Baytown, Texas
	St. Joseph Hospital, Houston

GERIATRICS

Natl.
Rank Hospital

	TIER THREE
	Clear Lake Regional Medical Center, Webster, Texas
	Memorial City Medical Center, Houston
	Northeast Medical Center Hospital, Humble, Texas
	St. Joseph Hospital, Houston
	University of Texas Medical Branch Hospitals, Galveston
	TIER FOUR
	Hermann Hospital, Houston
	Houston Northwest Medical Center
	Medical Center Hospital, Conroe, Texas
	Memorial Hospital System, Houston
	Methodist Hospital, Houston
	San Jacinto Methodist Hospital, Baytown, Texas
	Texas Heart Institute-St. Luke's Episcopal, Houston

GYNECOLOGY

Natl.
Rank Hospital

	TIER ONE
3	University of Texas, M.D. Anderson Cancer Ctr., Houston
	TIER THREE
	Hermann Hospital, Houston
	Memorial City Medical Center, Houston
	Methodist Hospital, Houston
	University of Texas Medical Branch Hospitals, Galveston
	TIER FOUR
	Clear Lake Regional Medical Center, Webster, Texas
	Harris County Hospital District, Houston
	Houston Northwest Medical Center
	Medical Center Hospital, Conroe, Texas
	Memorial Hospital System, Houston
	San Jacinto Methodist Hospital, Baytown, Texas
	St. Joseph Hospital, Houston
	Texas Heart Institute-St. Luke's Episcopal, Houston

NEUROLOGY

TIER THREE
Hermann Hospital, Houston
Memorial City Medical Center, Houston
Methodist Hospital, Houston
Northeast Medical Center Hospital, Humble, Texas
San Jacinto Methodist Hospital, Baytown, Texas
St. Joseph Hospital, Houston
Texas Heart Institute-St. Luke's Episcopal, Houston
University of Texas Medical Branch Hospitals, Galveston

TIER FOUR
Clear Lake Regional Medical Center, Webster, Texas
Harris County Hospital District, Houston
Houston Northwest Medical Center
Memorial Hospital System, Houston

ORTHOPEDICS

Natl.
Rank   Hospital

	TIER ONE
14	University of Texas, M.D. Anderson Cancer Ctr., Houston

TIER THREE
Clear Lake Regional Medical Center, Webster, Texas
HCA Spring Branch Medical Center, Houston
Hermann Hospital, Houston
Medical Center Hospital, Conroe, Texas
Memorial City Medical Center, Houston
Methodist Hospital, Houston
St. Joseph Hospital, Houston
Texas Heart Institute-St. Luke's Episcopal, Houston
University of Texas Medical Branch Hospitals, Galveston

TIER FOUR
Houston Northwest Medical Center
Memorial Hospital System, Houston
Tomball Regional Hospital, Tomball, Texas

OTOLARYNGOLOGY

Natl.
Rank   Hospital

	TIER ONE
9	University of Texas, M.D. Anderson Cancer Ctr., Houston

	TIER TWO
47	University of Texas Medical Branch Hospitals, Galveston

TIER THREE
Harris County Hospital District, Houston
Hermann Hospital, Houston
Methodist Hospital, Houston
Texas Heart Institute-St. Luke's Episcopal, Houston

TIER FOUR
Clear Lake Regional Medical Center, Webster, Texas
HCA Spring Branch Medical Center, Houston
Houston Northwest Medical Center
Medical Center Hospital, Conroe, Texas

Memorial City Medical Center, Houston
Memorial Hospital System, Houston
Northeast Medical Center Hospital, Humble, Texas
Sam Houston Memorial Hospital, Houston
San Jacinto Methodist Hospital, Baytown, Texas
St. Joseph Hospital, Houston
Tomball Regional Hospital, Tomball, Texas

RHEUMATOLOGY

Natl.
Rank   Hospital

	TIER TWO
34	University of Texas, M.D. Anderson Cancer Ctr., Houston

TIER THREE
Hermann Hospital, Houston
Methodist Hospital, Houston
Texas Heart Institute-St. Luke's Episcopal, Houston
University of Texas Medical Branch Hospitals, Galveston

TIER FOUR
Clear Lake Regional Medical Center, Webster, Texas
HCA Spring Branch Medical Center, Houston
Harris County Hospital District, Houston
Houston Northwest Medical Center
Medical Center Hospital, Conroe, Texas
Memorial City Medical Center, Houston
Memorial Hospital System, Houston
Northeast Medical Center Hospital, Humble, Texas
San Jacinto Methodist Hospital, Baytown, Texas
St. Joseph Hospital, Houston

UROLOGY

Natl.
Rank   Hospital

	TIER ONE
9	University of Texas, M.D. Anderson Cancer Ctr., Houston

TIER THREE
Hermann Hospital, Houston
Methodist Hospital, Houston
Northeast Medical Center Hospital, Humble, Texas
Texas Heart Institute-St. Luke's Episcopal, Houston
University of Texas Medical Branch Hospitals, Galveston

TIER FOUR
Clear Lake Regional Medical Center, Webster, Texas
HCA Spring Branch Medical Center, Houston
Harris County Hospital District, Houston
Houston Northwest Medical Center
Medical Center Hospital, Conroe, Texas
Memorial City Medical Center, Houston
Memorial Hospital System, Houston
San Jacinto Methodist Hospital, Baytown, Texas
St. Joseph Hospital, Houston
Tomball Regional Hospital, Tomball, Texas

METRO RANKINGS ■ HOUSTON

Los Angeles

AIDS

	TIER ONE
5	UCLA Medical Center, Los Angeles
	TIER TWO
78	Cedars-Sinai Medical Center, Los Angeles
74	Kaiser Foundation Hospital, Los Angeles
36	Los Angeles County-Harbor-UCLA Medical Center
28	Los Angeles County-USC Medical Center
	TIER THREE
	Beverly Hospital, Montebello, Calif.
	Centinela Hospital Medical Center, Inglewood, Calif.
	Century City Hospital, Los Angeles
	Desert Hospital, Palm Springs, Calif.
	Downey Community Hospital, Downey, Calif.
	Eisenhower Memorial Hospital, Rancho Mirage, Calif.
	Encino-Tarzana Regional Medical Center, Tarzana, Calif.
	Fountain Valley Regional Hospital Med. Ctr., Fountain Valley, Calif.
	Garfield Medical Center, Monterey Park, Calif.
	Glendale Adventist Medical Center, Glendale, Calif.
	Hoag Memorial Hospital Presbyterian, Newport Beach, Calif.
	Hospital of the Good Samaritan, Los Angeles
	Huntington Memorial Hospital, Pasadena, Calif.
	Kaiser Foundation Hospital, Fontana, Calif.
	Kaiser Foundation Hospital, West Los Angeles
	Kaiser Foundation Hospital, Panorama City, Calif.
	Kaiser Foundation Hospital, Woodland Hills, Calif.
	L.A. County-Rancho Los Amigos Med. Ctr., Downey, Calif.
	Long Beach Community Hospital, Long Beach, Calif.
	Long Beach Memorial Medical Center, Long Beach, Calif.
	Los Angeles County-King-Drew Medical Center
	Methodist Hospital of Southern California, Arcadia, Calif.
	Northridge Hospital Medical Center, Northridge, Calif.
	Olive View Medical Center, Sylmar, Calif.
	Presbyterian Intercommunity Hospital, Whittier, Calif.
	Queen of Angels-Hollywood Center, Hollywood, Calif.
	Saddleback Memorial Medical Center, Laguna Hills, Calif.
	San Pedro Peninsula Hospital, San Pedro, Calif.
	Santa Monica Hospital Medical Center, Santa Monica, Calif.
	South Coast Medical Center, South Laguna, Calif.
	St. John's Hospital and Health Center, Santa Monica, Calif.
	St. Joseph Hospital, Orange, Calif.
	St. Joseph Medical Center, Burbank, Calif.
	St. Mary Medical Center, Long Beach, Calif.
	St. Vincent Medical Center, Los Angeles
	Torrance Memorial Medical Center, Torrance, Calif.
	University of California, Irvine Medical Center, Orange
	White Memorial Medical Center, Los Angeles
	TIER FOUR
	Antelope Valley Hospital Medical Center, Lancaster, Calif.
	California Medical Center, Los Angeles
	Community Memorial Hospital, Ventura, Calif.
	Glendale Memorial Hospital and Health Center, Glendale, Calif.
	Hemet Valley Medical Center, Hemet, Calif.
	Loma Linda Community Hospital, Loma Linda, Calif.

	Martin Luther Hospital, Anaheim, Calif.
	Riverside General Hospital-Medical Center, Riverside, Calif.
	San Bernardino County Medical Center, San Bernardino, Calif.
	San Gabriel Valley Medical Center, San Gabriel, Calif.
	St. Bernardine Medical Center, San Bernardino, Calif.
	St. Francis Medical Center, Lynwood, Calif.
	St. Jude Medical Center, Fullerton, Calif.
	USC Kenneth Norris Cancer Hospital, Los Angeles
	Western Medical Center, Santa Ana, Calif.

CANCER

	TIER ONE
13	UCLA Medical Center, Los Angeles
	TIER TWO
54	Loma Linda University Medical Center, Loma Linda, Calif.
63	Los Angeles County-USC Medical Center
37	USC Kenneth Norris Cancer Hospital, Los Angeles
	TIER THREE
	Cedars-Sinai Medical Center, Los Angeles
	City of Hope National Medical Center, Duarte, Calif.
	Hoag Memorial Hospital Presbyterian, Newport Beach, Calif.
	Hospital of the Good Samaritan, Los Angeles
	Huntington Memorial Hospital, Pasadena, Calif.
	Kaiser Foundation Hospital, Los Angeles
	Kaiser Foundation Hospital, Woodland Hills, Calif.
	Long Beach Memorial Medical Center, Long Beach, Calif.
	Pomona Valley Hospital Medical Center, Pomona, Calif.
	University of California, Irvine Medical Center, Orange
	TIER FOUR
	Antelope Valley Hospital Medical Center, Lancaster, Calif.
	Beverly Hospital, Montebello, Calif.
	California Medical Center, Los Angeles
	Centinela Hospital Medical Center, Inglewood, Calif.
	Community Memorial Hospital, Ventura, Calif.
	Daniel Freeman Memorial Hospital, Inglewood, Calif.
	Desert Hospital, Palm Springs, Calif.
	Downey Community Hospital, Downey, Calif.
	Eisenhower Memorial Hospital, Rancho Mirage, Calif.
	Encino-Tarzana Regional Medical Center, Tarzana, Calif.
	Fountain Valley Regional Hospital Med. Ctr., Fountain Valley, Calif.
	Garfield Medical Center, Monterey Park, Calif.
	Glendale Adventist Medical Center, Glendale, Calif.
	Glendale Memorial Hospital and Health Center, Glendale, Calif.
	Hemet Valley Medical Center, Hemet, Calif.
	Inter-Community Medical Center, Covina, Calif.
	Kaiser Foundation Hospital, Fontana, Calif.
	Kaiser Foundation Hospital, West Los Angeles
	Kaiser Foundation Hospital, Panorama City, Calif.
	Little Company of Mary Hospital, Torrance, Calif.
	Long Beach Community Hospital, Long Beach, Calif.
	Methodist Hospital of Southern California, Arcadia, Calif.
	Northridge Hospital Medical Center, Northridge, Calif.
	Presbyterian Intercommunity Hospital, Whittier, Calif.
	Queen of Angels-Hollywood Center, Hollywood, Calif.
	Saddleback Memorial Medical Center, Laguna Hills, Calif.

| San Antonio Community Hospital, Upland, Calif. |
| San Gabriel Valley Medical Center, San Gabriel, Calif. |
| San Pedro Peninsula Hospital, San Pedro, Calif. |
| Santa Monica Hospital Medical Center, Santa Monica, Calif. |
| St. Bernardine Medical Center, San Bernardino, Calif. |
| St. Francis Medical Center, Lynwood, Calif. |
| St. John's Hospital and Health Center, Santa Monica, Calif. |
| St. Joseph Hospital, Orange, Calif. |
| St. Joseph Medical Center, Burbank, Calif. |
| St. Jude Medical Center, Fullerton, Calif. |
| St. Mary Medical Center, Long Beach, Calif. |
| St. Vincent Medical Center, Los Angeles |
| Torrance Memorial Medical Center, Torrance, Calif. |
| Western Medical Center, Santa Ana, Calif. |
| White Memorial Medical Center, Los Angeles |

CARDIOLOGY

	TIER ONE
12	UCLA Medical Center, Los Angeles
18	Cedars-Sinai Medical Center, Los Angeles
	TIER TWO
77	Kaiser Foundation Hospital, Los Angeles
83	Loma Linda University Medical Center, Loma Linda, Calif.
	TIER THREE
	Beverly Hospital, Montebello, Calif.
	Community Memorial Hospital, Ventura, Calif.
	Desert Hospital, Palm Springs, Calif.
	Downey Community Hospital, Downey, Calif.
	Eisenhower Memorial Hospital, Rancho Mirage, Calif.
	Encino-Tarzana Regional Medical Center, Tarzana, Calif.
	Hemet Valley Medical Center, Hemet, Calif.
	Hospital of the Good Samaritan, Los Angeles
	Huntington Memorial Hospital, Pasadena, Calif.
	Kaiser Foundation Hospital, Fontana, Calif.
	Kaiser Foundation Hospital, West Los Angeles
	Kaiser Foundation Hospital, Panorama City, Calif.
	Kaiser Foundation Hospital, Woodland Hills, Calif.
	Little Company of Mary Hospital, Torrance, Calif.
	Long Beach Community Hospital, Long Beach, Calif.
	Long Beach Memorial Medical Center, Long Beach, Calif.
	Methodist Hospital of Southern California, Arcadia, Calif.
	Northridge Hospital Medical Center, Northridge, Calif.
	Presbyterian Intercommunity Hospital, Whittier, Calif.
	Saddleback Memorial Medical Center, Laguna Hills, Calif.
	Santa Monica Hospital Medical Center, Santa Monica, Calif.
	St. John's Hospital and Health Center, Santa Monica, Calif.
	St. Joseph Medical Center, Burbank, Calif.
	St. Mary Medical Center, Long Beach, Calif.
	St. Vincent Medical Center, Los Angeles
	Torrance Memorial Medical Center, Torrance, Calif.
	Western Medical Center, Santa Ana, Calif.
	White Memorial Medical Center, Los Angeles
	TIER FOUR
	Antelope Valley Hospital Medical Center, Lancaster, Calif.

| California Medical Center, Los Angeles |
| Centinela Hospital Medical Center, Inglewood, Calif. |
| Daniel Freeman Memorial Hospital, Inglewood, Calif. |
| Garfield Medical Center, Monterey Park, Calif. |
| Glendale Adventist Medical Center, Glendale, Calif. |
| Glendale Memorial Hospital and Health Center, Glendale, Calif. |
| Hoag Memorial Hospital Presbyterian, Newport Beach, Calif. |
| Inter-Community Medical Center, Covina, Calif. |
| Pomona Valley Hospital Medical Center, Pomona, Calif. |
| Queen of Angels-Hollywood Center, Hollywood, Calif. |
| San Antonio Community Hospital, Upland, Calif. |
| San Gabriel Valley Medical Center, San Gabriel, Calif. |
| San Pedro Peninsula Hospital, San Pedro, Calif. |
| St. Bernardine Medical Center, San Bernardino, Calif. |
| St. Francis Medical Center, Lynwood, Calif. |
| St. Joseph Hospital, Orange, Calif. |
| St. Jude Medical Center, Fullerton, Calif. |

ENDOCRINOLOGY

	TIER ONE
6	UCLA Medical Center, Los Angeles
	TIER TWO
81	Kaiser Foundation Hospital, Los Angeles
36	Loma Linda University Medical Center, Loma Linda, Calif.
30	Los Angeles County-USC Medical Center
	TIER THREE
	Beverly Hospital, Montebello, Calif.
	Cedars-Sinai Medical Center, Los Angeles
	Community Memorial Hospital, Ventura, Calif.
	Desert Hospital, Palm Springs, Calif.
	Eisenhower Memorial Hospital, Rancho Mirage, Calif.
	Encino-Tarzana Regional Medical Center, Tarzana, Calif.
	Garfield Medical Center, Monterey Park, Calif.
	Glendale Memorial Hospital and Health Center, Glendale, Calif.
	Hoag Memorial Hospital Presbyterian, Newport Beach, Calif.
	Inter-Community Medical Center, Covina, Calif.
	Kaiser Foundation Hospital, Fontana, Calif.
	Kaiser Foundation Hospital, West Los Angeles
	Kaiser Foundation Hospital, Panorama City, Calif.
	Little Company of Mary Hospital, Torrance, Calif.
	Long Beach Community Hospital, Long Beach, Calif.
	Long Beach Memorial Medical Center, Long Beach, Calif.
	Northridge Hospital Medical Center, Northridge, Calif.
	Pomona Valley Hospital Medical Center, Pomona, Calif.
	San Antonio Community Hospital, Upland, Calif.
	Santa Monica Hospital Medical Center, Santa Monica, Calif.
	St. John's Hospital and Health Center, Santa Monica, Calif.
	St. Joseph Hospital, Orange, Calif.
	St. Jude Medical Center, Fullerton, Calif.
	St. Mary Medical Center, Long Beach, Calif.
	St. Vincent Medical Center, Los Angeles
	Torrance Memorial Medical Center, Torrance, Calif.
	White Memorial Medical Center, Los Angeles
	TIER FOUR
	Antelope Valley Hospital Medical Center, Lancaster, Calif.

METRO RANKINGS ■ LOS ANGELES

California Medical Center, Los Angeles

Centinela Hospital Medical Center, Inglewood, Calif.

Daniel Freeman Memorial Hospital, Inglewood, Calif.

Downey Community Hospital, Downey, Calif.

Glendale Adventist Medical Center, Glendale, Calif.

Hemet Valley Medical Center, Hemet, Calif.

Hospital of the Good Samaritan, Los Angeles

Huntington Memorial Hospital, Pasadena, Calif.

Methodist Hospital of Southern California, Arcadia, Calif.

Presbyterian Intercommunity Hospital, Whittier, Calif.

Queen of Angels-Hollywood Center, Hollywood, Calif.

Saddleback Memorial Medical Center, Laguna Hills, Calif.

San Gabriel Valley Medical Center, San Gabriel, Calif.

San Pedro Peninsula Hospital, San Pedro, Calif.

St. Bernardine Medical Center, San Bernardino, Calif.

St. Francis Medical Center, Lynwood, Calif.

St. Joseph Medical Center, Burbank, Calif.

GASTROENTEROLOGY

	TIER ONE
5	UCLA Medical Center, Los Angeles
	TIER TWO
24	Cedars-Sinai Medical Center, Los Angeles
	TIER THREE
	Eisenhower Memorial Hospital, Rancho Mirage, Calif.
	Glendale Adventist Medical Center, Glendale, Calif.
	Hoag Memorial Hospital Presbyterian, Newport Beach, Calif.
	Hospital of the Good Samaritan, Los Angeles
	Kaiser Foundation Hospital, Fontana, Calif.
	Kaiser Foundation Hospital, Los Angeles
96	Kaiser Foundation Hospital, Woodland Hills, Calif.
77	Loma Linda University Medical Center, Loma Linda, Calif.
	Long Beach Memorial Medical Center, Long Beach, Calif.
	Methodist Hospital of Southern California, Arcadia, Calif.
	Presbyterian Intercommunity Hospital, Whittier, Calif.
	Saddleback Memorial Medical Center, Laguna Hills, Calif.
	Santa Monica Hospital Medical Center, Santa Monica, Calif.
	St. Francis Medical Center, Lynwood, Calif.
	St. John's Hospital and Health Center, Santa Monica, Calif.
	St. Joseph Medical Center, Burbank, Calif.
	St. Jude Medical Center, Fullerton, Calif.
	TIER FOUR
	Antelope Valley Hospital Medical Center, Lancaster, Calif.
	Beverly Hospital, Montebello, Calif.
	California Medical Center, Los Angeles
	Centinela Hospital Medical Center, Inglewood, Calif.
	Community Memorial Hospital, Ventura, Calif.
	Daniel Freeman Memorial Hospital, Inglewood, Calif.
	Desert Hospital, Palm Springs, Calif.
	Downey Community Hospital, Downey, Calif.
	Encino-Tarzana Regional Medical Center, Tarzana, Calif.
	Glendale Memorial Hospital and Health Center, Glendale, Calif.
	Hemet Valley Medical Center, Hemet, Calif.
	Huntington Memorial Hospital, Pasadena, Calif.
	Inter-Community Medical Center, Covina, Calif.

Kaiser Foundation Hospital, West Los Angeles

Kaiser Foundation Hospital, Panorama City, Calif.

Little Company of Mary Hospital, Torrance, Calif.

Long Beach Community Hospital, Long Beach, Calif.

Northridge Hospital Medical Center, Northridge, Calif.

Pomona Valley Hospital Medical Center, Pomona, Calif.

Queen of Angels-Hollywood Center, Hollywood, Calif.

San Antonio Community Hospital, Upland, Calif.

San Gabriel Valley Medical Center, San Gabriel, Calif.

St. Bernardine Medical Center, San Bernardino, Calif.

St. Joseph Hospital, Orange, Calif.

St. Mary Medical Center, Long Beach, Calif.

St. Vincent Medical Center, Los Angeles

Torrance Memorial Medical Center, Torrance, Calif.

GERIATRICS

	TIER ONE
1	UCLA Medical Center, Los Angeles
	TIER TWO
68	Kaiser Foundation Hospital, Los Angeles
	TIER THREE
	Beverly Hospital, Montebello, Calif.
	Cedars-Sinai Medical Center, Los Angeles
	Centinela Hospital Medical Center, Inglewood, Calif.
	Desert Hospital, Palm Springs, Calif.
	Downey Community Hospital, Downey, Calif.
	Eisenhower Memorial Hospital, Rancho Mirage, Calif.
	Encino-Tarzana Regional Medical Center, Tarzana, Calif.
	Garfield Medical Center, Monterey Park, Calif.
	Glendale Adventist Medical Center, Glendale, Calif.
	Hoag Memorial Hospital Presbyterian, Newport Beach, Calif.
	Huntington Memorial Hospital, Pasadena, Calif.
	Kaiser Foundation Hospital, Fontana, Calif.
	Kaiser Foundation Hospital, West Los Angeles
	Kaiser Foundation Hospital, Panorama City, Calif.
	Little Company of Mary Hospital, Torrance, Calif.
96	Loma Linda University Medical Center, Loma Linda, Calif.
	Long Beach Community Hospital, Long Beach, Calif.
	Long Beach Memorial Medical Center, Long Beach, Calif.
	Methodist Hospital of Southern California, Arcadia, Calif.
	Northridge Hospital Medical Center, Northridge, Calif.
	Presbyterian Intercommunity Hospital, Whittier, Calif.
	Queen of Angels-Hollywood Center, Hollywood, Calif.
	Saddleback Memorial Medical Center, Laguna Hills, Calif.
	San Antonio Community Hospital, Upland, Calif.
	San Pedro Peninsula Hospital, San Pedro, Calif.
	Santa Monica Hospital Medical Center, Santa Monica, Calif.
	St. Joseph Hospital, Orange, Calif.
	St. Joseph Medical Center, Burbank, Calif.
	St. Jude Medical Center, Fullerton, Calif.
	St. Mary Medical Center, Long Beach, Calif.
	St. Vincent Medical Center, Los Angeles
	Torrance Memorial Medical Center, Torrance, Calif.
	White Memorial Medical Center, Los Angeles

	TIER FOUR
	Antelope Valley Hospital Medical Center, Lancaster, Calif.
	California Medical Center, Los Angeles
	Community Memorial Hospital, Ventura, Calif.
	Glendale Memorial Hospital and Health Center, Glendale, Calif.
	Hemet Valley Medical Center, Hemet, Calif.
	Hospital of the Good Samaritan, Los Angeles
	Pomona Valley Hospital Medical Center, Pomona, Calif.
	San Gabriel Valley Medical Center, San Gabriel, Calif.
	St. Bernardine Medical Center, San Bernardino, Calif.
	St. Francis Medical Center, Lynwood, Calif.

GYNECOLOGY

	TIER ONE
6	Los Angeles County-USC Medical Center
10	UCLA Medical Center, Los Angeles
	TIER TWO
39	Cedars-Sinai Medical Center, Los Angeles
54	Kaiser Foundation Hospital, Los Angeles
79	Kaiser Foundation Hospital, Woodland Hills, Calif.
77	Santa Monica Hospital Medical Center, Santa Monica, Calif.
	TIER THREE
	Beverly Hospital, Montebello, Calif.
	Centinela Hospital Medical Center, Inglewood, Calif.
	Desert Hospital, Palm Springs, Calif.
	Downey Community Hospital, Downey, Calif.
	Eisenhower Memorial Hospital, Rancho Mirage, Calif.
95	Hoag Memorial Hospital Presbyterian, Newport Beach, Calif.
	Kaiser Foundation Hospital, Fontana, Calif.
	Kaiser Foundation Hospital, West Los Angeles
	Kaiser Foundation Hospital, Panorama City, Calif.
	Long Beach Community Hospital, Long Beach, Calif.
	Long Beach Memorial Medical Center, Long Beach, Calif.
	Methodist Hospital of Southern California, Arcadia, Calif.
	Northridge Hospital Medical Center, Northridge, Calif.
	Pomona Valley Hospital Medical Center, Pomona, Calif.
	Presbyterian Intercommunity Hospital, Whittier, Calif.
	Queen of Angels-Hollywood Center, Hollywood, Calif.
	Saddleback Memorial Medical Center, Laguna Hills, Calif.
	San Antonio Community Hospital, Upland, Calif.
	St. Francis Medical Center, Lynwood, Calif.
	St. John's Hospital and Health Center, Santa Monica, Calif.
	St. Joseph Hospital, Orange, Calif.
	St. Joseph Medical Center, Burbank, Calif.
	St. Jude Medical Center, Fullerton, Calif.
	St. Mary Medical Center, Long Beach, Calif.
	St. Vincent Medical Center, Los Angeles
	Torrance Memorial Medical Center, Torrance, Calif.
	White Memorial Medical Center, Los Angeles
	TIER FOUR
	Antelope Valley Hospital Medical Center, Lancaster, Calif.
	California Medical Center, Los Angeles
	Community Memorial Hospital, Ventura, Calif.
	Glendale Memorial Hospital and Health Center, Glendale, Calif.
	Hemet Valley Medical Center, Hemet, Calif.

	Huntington Memorial Hospital, Pasadena, Calif.
	Inter-Community Medical Center, Covina, Calif.
	San Gabriel Valley Medical Center, San Gabriel, Calif.
	St. Bernardine Medical Center, San Bernardino, Calif.

NEUROLOGY

	TIER ONE
6	UCLA Medical Center, Los Angeles
	TIER TWO
70	Kaiser Foundation Hospital, Los Angeles
36	Loma Linda University Medical Center, Loma Linda, Calif.
	TIER THREE
	Cedars-Sinai Medical Center, Los Angeles
	Centinela Hospital Medical Center, Inglewood, Calif.
	Desert Hospital, Palm Springs, Calif.
	Eisenhower Memorial Hospital, Rancho Mirage, Calif.
	Glendale Adventist Medical Center, Glendale, Calif.
	Glendale Memorial Hospital and Health Center, Glendale, Calif.
	Hemet Valley Medical Center, Hemet, Calif.
	Hoag Memorial Hospital Presbyterian, Newport Beach, Calif.
	Hospital of the Good Samaritan, Los Angeles
	Huntington Memorial Hospital, Pasadena, Calif.
	Kaiser Foundation Hospital, Fontana, Calif.
	Kaiser Foundation Hospital, West Los Angeles
	Kaiser Foundation Hospital, Woodland Hills, Calif.
	Little Company of Mary Hospital, Torrance, Calif.
	Long Beach Community Hospital, Long Beach, Calif.
	Long Beach Memorial Medical Center, Long Beach, Calif.
	Methodist Hospital of Southern California, Arcadia, Calif.
	Northridge Hospital Medical Center, Northridge, Calif.
	Pomona Valley Hospital Medical Center, Pomona, Calif.
	Queen of Angels-Hollywood Center, Hollywood, Calif.
	Saddleback Memorial Medical Center, Laguna Hills, Calif.
	San Antonio Community Hospital, Upland, Calif.
	Santa Monica Hospital Medical Center, Santa Monica, Calif.
	St. Francis Medical Center, Lynwood, Calif.
	St. John's Hospital and Health Center, Santa Monica, Calif.
	St. Joseph Hospital, Orange, Calif.
	St. Joseph Medical Center, Burbank, Calif.
	St. Jude Medical Center, Fullerton, Calif.
	St. Mary Medical Center, Long Beach, Calif.
	St. Vincent Medical Center, Los Angeles
	Torrance Memorial Medical Center, Torrance, Calif.
	TIER FOUR
	Antelope Valley Hospital Medical Center, Lancaster, Calif.
	Beverly Hospital, Montebello, Calif.
	California Medical Center, Los Angeles
	Community Memorial Hospital, Ventura, Calif.
	Daniel Freeman Memorial Hospital, Inglewood, Calif.
	Downey Community Hospital, Downey, Calif.
	Inter-Community Medical Center, Covina, Calif.
	Kaiser Foundation Hospital, Panorama City, Calif.
	Presbyterian Intercommunity Hospital, Whittier, Calif.
	San Gabriel Valley Medical Center, San Gabriel, Calif.
	St. Bernardine Medical Center, San Bernardino, Calif.

ORTHOPEDICS

Natl. Rank	Hospital
TIER ONE	
6	UCLA Medical Center, Los Angeles
TIER TWO	
57	Loma Linda University Medical Center, Loma Linda, Calif.
TIER THREE	
97	Cedars-Sinai Medical Center, Los Angeles
	Century City Hospital, Los Angeles
	Community Memorial Hospital, Ventura, Calif.
	Desert Hospital, Palm Springs, Calif.
	Downey Community Hospital, Downey, Calif.
	Eisenhower Memorial Hospital, Rancho Mirage, Calif.
	Encino-Tarzana Regional Medical Center, Tarzana, Calif.
	Hoag Memorial Hospital Presbyterian, Newport Beach, Calif.
	Hospital of the Good Samaritan, Los Angeles
	Kaiser Foundation Hospital, Fontana, Calif.
100	Kaiser Foundation Hospital, Los Angeles
	Kaiser Foundation Hospital, West Los Angeles
	Kaiser Foundation Hospital, Woodland Hills, Calif.
	Long Beach Community Hospital, Long Beach, Calif.
	Long Beach Memorial Medical Center, Long Beach, Calif.
	Methodist Hospital of Southern California, Arcadia, Calif.
	Pomona Valley Hospital Medical Center, Pomona, Calif.
	San Antonio Community Hospital, Upland, Calif.
	Santa Monica Hospital Medical Center, Santa Monica, Calif.
	St. John's Hospital and Health Center, Santa Monica, Calif.
	St. Joseph Medical Center, Burbank, Calif.
	St. Jude Medical Center, Fullerton, Calif.
	St. Mary Medical Center, Long Beach, Calif.
TIER FOUR	
	Antelope Valley Hospital Medical Center, Lancaster, Calif.
	Beverly Hospital, Montebello, Calif.
	Centinela Hospital Medical Center, Inglewood, Calif.
	Fountain Valley Regional Hospital Med. Ctr., Fountain Valley, Calif.
	Glendale Adventist Medical Center, Glendale, Calif.
	Glendale Memorial Hospital and Health Center, Glendale, Calif.
	Hemet Valley Medical Center, Hemet, Calif.
	Huntington Memorial Hospital, Pasadena, Calif.
	Inter-Community Medical Center, Covina, Calif.
	Kaiser Foundation Hospital, Panorama City, Calif.
	Little Company of Mary Hospital, Torrance, Calif.
	Northridge Hospital Medical Center, Northridge, Calif.
	Orthopaedic Hospital, Los Angeles
	Presbyterian Intercommunity Hospital, Whittier, Calif.
	Queen of Angels-Hollywood Center, Hollywood, Calif.
	Saddleback Memorial Medical Center, Laguna Hills, Calif.
	San Gabriel Valley Medical Center, San Gabriel, Calif.
	San Pedro Peninsula Hospital, San Pedro, Calif.
	St. Bernardine Medical Center, San Bernardino, Calif.
	St. Francis Medical Center, Lynwood, Calif.
	St. Joseph Hospital, Orange, Calif.
	St. Vincent Medical Center, Los Angeles
	Torrance Memorial Medical Center, Torrance, Calif.

OTOLARYNGOLOGY

Natl. Rank	Hospital
TIER ONE	
5	UCLA Medical Center, Los Angeles
20	Los Angeles County-USC Medical Center
TIER TWO	
58	Loma Linda University Medical Center, Loma Linda, Calif.
76	Los Angeles County-King-Drew Medical Center
TIER THREE	
	Cedars-Sinai Medical Center, Los Angeles
	Hospital of the Good Samaritan, Los Angeles
	Huntington Memorial Hospital, Pasadena, Calif.
	Kaiser Foundation Hospital, Los Angeles
	Kaiser Foundation Hospital, Woodland Hills, Calif.
	Long Beach Memorial Medical Center, Long Beach, Calif.
	Los Angeles County-Harbor-UCLA Medical Center
	Northridge Hospital Medical Center, Northridge, Calif.
	Olive View Medical Center, Sylmar, Calif.
	San Bernardino County Medical Center, San Bernardino, Calif.
	Santa Monica Hospital Medical Center, Santa Monica, Calif.
	St. Vincent Medical Center, Los Angeles
	Torrance Memorial Medical Center, Torrance, Calif.
	USC Kenneth Norris Cancer Hospital, Los Angeles
	University of California, Irvine Medical Center, Orange
TIER FOUR	
	Antelope Valley Hospital Medical Center, Lancaster, Calif.
	Beverly Hospital, Montebello, Calif.
	California Medical Center, Los Angeles
	Centinela Hospital Medical Center, Inglewood, Calif.
	Century City Hospital, Los Angeles
	City of Hope National Medical Center, Duarte, Calif.
	Community Memorial Hospital, Ventura, Calif.
	Daniel Freeman Memorial Hospital, Inglewood, Calif.
	Desert Hospital, Palm Springs, Calif.
	Downey Community Hospital, Downey, Calif.
	Eisenhower Memorial Hospital, Rancho Mirage, Calif.
	Encino-Tarzana Regional Medical Center, Tarzana, Calif.
	Fountain Valley Regional Hospital Med. Ctr., Fountain Valley, Calif.
	Garfield Medical Center, Monterey Park, Calif.
	Glendale Adventist Medical Center, Glendale, Calif.
	Glendale Memorial Hospital and Health Center, Glendale, Calif.
	Hemet Valley Medical Center, Hemet, Calif.
	Hoag Memorial Hospital Presbyterian, Newport Beach, Calif.
	Inter-Community Medical Center, Covina, Calif.
	Kaiser Foundation Hospital, Fontana, Calif.
	Kaiser Foundation Hospital, West Los Angeles
	Kaiser Foundation Hospital, Panorama City, Calif.
	L.A. County-Rancho Los Amigos Med. Ctr., Downey, Calif.
	Little Company of Mary Hospital, Torrance, Calif.
	Loma Linda Community Hospital, Loma Linda, Calif.
	Long Beach Community Hospital, Long Beach, Calif.
	Martin Luther Hospital, Anaheim, Calif.
	Methodist Hospital of Southern California, Arcadia, Calif.
	Pomona Valley Hospital Medical Center, Pomona, Calif.
	Presbyterian Intercommunity Hospital, Whittier, Calif.
	Queen of Angels-Hollywood Center, Hollywood, Calif.
	Riverside General Hospital-Medical Center, Riverside, Calif.

	Saddleback Memorial Medical Center, Laguna Hills, Calif.
	San Antonio Community Hospital, Upland, Calif.
	San Gabriel Valley Medical Center, San Gabriel, Calif.
	San Pedro Peninsula Hospital, San Pedro, Calif.
	South Coast Medical Center, South Laguna, Calif.
	St. Bernardine Medical Center, San Bernardino, Calif.
	St. Francis Medical Center, Lynwood, Calif.
	St. John's Hospital and Health Center, Santa Monica, Calif.
	St. Joseph Hospital, Orange, Calif.
	St. Joseph Medical Center, Burbank, Calif.
	St. Jude Medical Center, Fullerton, Calif.
	St. Mary Medical Center, Long Beach, Calif.
	Western Medical Center, Santa Ana, Calif.
	White Memorial Medical Center, Los Angeles

RHEUMATOLOGY

	TIER ONE
4	UCLA Medical Center, Los Angeles
	TIER TWO
74	Loma Linda University Medical Center, Loma Linda, Calif.
	TIER THREE
	Cedars-Sinai Medical Center, Los Angeles
	Desert Hospital, Palm Springs, Calif.
	Encino-Tarzana Regional Medical Center, Tarzana, Calif.
	Garfield Medical Center, Monterey Park, Calif.
	Hoag Memorial Hospital Presbyterian, Newport Beach, Calif.
	Hospital of the Good Samaritan, Los Angeles
	Huntington Memorial Hospital, Pasadena, Calif.
	Kaiser Foundation Hospital, Fontana, Calif.
	Kaiser Foundation Hospital, Los Angeles
	Kaiser Foundation Hospital, West Los Angeles
	Kaiser Foundation Hospital, Panorama City, Calif.
	Kaiser Foundation Hospital, Woodland Hills, Calif.
	Long Beach Memorial Medical Center, Long Beach, Calif.
	Northridge Hospital Medical Center, Northridge, Calif.
	Queen of Angels-Hollywood Center, Hollywood, Calif.
	Saddleback Memorial Medical Center, Laguna Hills, Calif.
	San Antonio Community Hospital, Upland, Calif.
	Santa Monica Hospital Medical Center, Santa Monica, Calif.
	St. John's Hospital and Health Center, Santa Monica, Calif.
	St. Joseph Medical Center, Burbank, Calif.
	St. Mary Medical Center, Long Beach, Calif.
	St. Vincent Medical Center, Los Angeles
	Torrance Memorial Medical Center, Torrance, Calif.
	White Memorial Medical Center, Los Angeles
	TIER FOUR
	Antelope Valley Hospital Medical Center, Lancaster, Calif.
	Beverly Hospital, Montebello, Calif.
	California Medical Center, Los Angeles
	Centinela Hospital Medical Center, Inglewood, Calif.
	Community Memorial Hospital, Ventura, Calif.
	Daniel Freeman Memorial Hospital, Inglewood, Calif.
	Downey Community Hospital, Downey, Calif.
	Eisenhower Memorial Hospital, Rancho Mirage, Calif.
	Glendale Adventist Medical Center, Glendale, Calif.

	Glendale Memorial Hospital and Health Center, Glendale, Calif.
	Hemet Valley Medical Center, Hemet, Calif.
	Inter-Community Medical Center, Covina, Calif.
	Little Company of Mary Hospital, Torrance, Calif.
	Long Beach Community Hospital, Long Beach, Calif.
	Methodist Hospital of Southern California, Arcadia, Calif.
	Pomona Valley Hospital Medical Center, Pomona, Calif.
	Presbyterian Intercommunity Hospital, Whittier, Calif.
	San Gabriel Valley Medical Center, San Gabriel, Calif.
	San Pedro Peninsula Hospital, San Pedro, Calif.
	St. Bernardine Medical Center, San Bernardino, Calif.
	St. Francis Medical Center, Lynwood, Calif.
	St. Joseph Hospital, Orange, Calif.
	St. Jude Medical Center, Fullerton, Calif.

UROLOGY

	TIER ONE
4	UCLA Medical Center, Los Angeles
	TIER TWO
29	Loma Linda University Medical Center, Loma Linda, Calif.
66	USC Kenneth Norris Cancer Hospital, Los Angeles
	TIER THREE
	Cedars-Sinai Medical Center, Los Angeles
	Daniel Freeman Memorial Hospital, Inglewood, Calif.
	Desert Hospital, Palm Springs, Calif.
	Downey Community Hospital, Downey, Calif.
	Eisenhower Memorial Hospital, Rancho Mirage, Calif.
	Encino-Tarzana Regional Medical Center, Tarzana, Calif.
	Garfield Medical Center, Monterey Park, Calif.
	Glendale Adventist Medical Center, Glendale, Calif.
	Glendale Memorial Hospital and Health Center, Glendale, Calif.
	Hoag Memorial Hospital Presbyterian, Newport Beach, Calif.
	Kaiser Foundation Hospital, Fontana, Calif.
	Kaiser Foundation Hospital, Los Angeles
	Kaiser Foundation Hospital, West Los Angeles
	Kaiser Foundation Hospital, Woodland Hills, Calif.
	Little Company of Mary Hospital, Torrance, Calif.
	Long Beach Community Hospital, Long Beach, Calif.
	Long Beach Memorial Medical Center, Long Beach, Calif.
	Methodist Hospital of Southern California, Arcadia, Calif.
	Pomona Valley Hospital Medical Center, Pomona, Calif.
	Presbyterian Intercommunity Hospital, Whittier, Calif.
	Queen of Angels-Hollywood Center, Hollywood, Calif.
	Saddleback Memorial Medical Center, Laguna Hills, Calif.
	San Antonio Community Hospital, Upland, Calif.
	Santa Monica Hospital Medical Center, Santa Monica, Calif.
	St. John's Hospital and Health Center, Santa Monica, Calif.
	St. Joseph Hospital, Orange, Calif.
	St. Mary Medical Center, Long Beach, Calif.
	White Memorial Medical Center, Los Angeles
	TIER FOUR
	Antelope Valley Hospital Medical Center, Lancaster, Calif.
	Beverly Hospital, Montebello, Calif.
	California Medical Center, Los Angeles
	Centinela Hospital Medical Center, Inglewood, Calif.

	Hospital
	Community Memorial Hospital, Ventura, Calif.
	Hemet Valley Medical Center, Hemet, Calif.
	Hospital of the Good Samaritan, Los Angeles
	Huntington Memorial Hospital, Pasadena, Calif.
	Inter-Community Medical Center, Covina, Calif.
	Kaiser Foundation Hospital, Panorama City, Calif.
	Northridge Hospital Medical Center, Northridge, Calif.
	San Gabriel Valley Medical Center, San Gabriel, Calif.
	San Pedro Peninsula Hospital, San Pedro, Calif.
	St. Bernardine Medical Center, San Bernardino, Calif.
	St. Francis Medical Center, Lynwood, Calif.
	St. Joseph Medical Center, Burbank, Calif.
	St. Jude Medical Center, Fullerton, Calif.
	St. Vincent Medical Center, Los Angeles
	Torrance Memorial Medical Center, Torrance, Calif.
	Western Medical Center, Santa Ana, Calif.

New York

AIDS

Natl. Rank	Hospital
TIER ONE	
7	Memorial Sloan-Kettering Cancer Center, New York
8	New York University Medical Center
9	New York Hospital-Cornell Medical Center
16	Columbia-Presbyterian Medical Center, New York
19	Mount Sinai Medical Center, New York
23	Montefiore Medical Center, Bronx, N.Y.
TIER TWO	
65	Beth Israel Medical Center, New York
88	Methodist Hospital, Brooklyn, N.Y.
80	North Shore University Hospital, Manhasset, N.Y.
73	St. Vincent's Hospital and Medical Center, New York
38	Yale-New Haven Hospital, New Haven, Conn.
TIER THREE	
	Bellevue Hospital Center, New York
	Bronx-Lebanon Hospital Center, Bronx, N.Y.
	Brooklyn Hospital Center, Brooklyn, N.Y.
	Cabrini Medical Center, New York
	Danbury Hospital, Danbury, Conn.
	Greenwich Hospital, Greenwich, Conn.
	Hackensack Medical Center, Hackensack, N.J.
	Hospital of St. Raphael, New Haven, Conn.
	Lenox Hill Hospital, New York
	Lincoln Medical and Mental Health Center, Bronx, N.Y.
	Long Island College Hospital, Brooklyn, N.Y.
	Long Island Jewish Medical Center, New York
	Maimonides Medical Center, Brooklyn, N.Y.
	Medical Center at Princeton, Princeton, N.J.
	Northern Westchester Hospital Center, Mount Kisco, N.Y.
	Overlook Hospital, Summit, N.J.
	Robert Wood Johnson University Hospital, New Brunswick, N.J.
	St. Barnabas Medical Center, Livingston, N.J.

	Hospital
	St. Luke's-Roosevelt Hospital Center, New York
	St. Mary's Hospital, Waterbury, Conn.
	Stamford Hospital, Stamford, Conn.
	University Hospital, Newark, N.J.
	University Hospital, Stony Brook, N.Y.
	Winthrop-University Hospital, Mineola, N.Y.
TIER FOUR	
	Bayley Seton Hospital, Staten Island, N.Y.
	Bergen Pines County Hospital, Paramus, N.J.
	Bridgeport Hospital, Bridgeport, Conn.
	Bronx Municipal Hospital Center, Bronx, N.Y.
	Brookdale Hospital Medical Center, Brooklyn, N.Y.
	Catholic Medical Center, Jamaica, N.Y.
	Central General Hospital, Plainview, N.Y.
	Christ Hospital, Jersey City, N.J.
	Community Medical Center, Toms River, N.J.
	Coney Island Hospital, Brooklyn, N.Y.
	Elizabeth General Medical Center, Elizabeth, N.J.
	Elmhurst Hospital Center, Elmhurst, N.Y.
	Englewood Hospital, Englewood, N.J.
	Flushing Hospital Medical Center, Flushing, N.Y.
	Franklin Hospital Medical Center, Valley Stream, N.Y.
	Goldwater Memorial Hospital, New York
	Good Samaritan Hospital, Suffern, N.Y.
	Good Samaritan Hospital, West Islip, N.Y.
	Griffin Hospital, Derby, Conn.
	Harlem Hospital Center, New York
	Helene Fuld Medical Center, Trenton, N.J.
	Hunterdon Medical Center, Flemington, N.J.
	Huntington Hospital, Huntington, N.Y.
	Interfaith Medical Center, Brooklyn, N.Y.
	JFK Medical Center, Edison, N.J.
	Jamaica Hospital, Jamaica, N.Y.
	Jersey City Medical Center, Jersey City, N.J.
	Jersey Shore Medical Center, Neptune, N.J.
	John T. Mather Memorial Hospital, Port Jefferson, N.Y.
	Kings County Hospital Center, Brooklyn, N.Y.
	Kingsboro Psychiatric Center, Brooklyn, N.Y.
	Kingsbrook Jewish Medical Center, Brooklyn, N.Y.
	La Guardia Hospital, Flushing, N.Y.
	Lutheran Medical Center, Brooklyn, N.Y.
	Mercer Medical Center, Trenton, N.J.
	Mercy Medical Center, Rockville Centre, N.Y.
	Metropolitan Hospital Center, New York
	Monmouth Medical Center, Long Branch, N.J.
	Morristown Memorial Hospital, Morristown, N.J.
	Mount Vernon Hospital, Mount Vernon, N.Y.
	Mountainside Hospital, Montclair, N.J.
	Muhlenberg Regional Medical Center, Plainfield, N.J.
	Nassau County Medical Center, East Meadow, N.Y.
	New Rochelle Hospital Medical Center, New Rochelle, N.Y.
	New York Downtown Hospital
	New York Hospital Medical Center, Flushing
	North Central Bronx Hospital, Bronx, N.Y.
	North General Hospital, New York
	North Shore University Hospital-Glen Cove, Glen Cove, N.Y.
	Norwalk Hospital, Norwalk, Conn.
	Nyack Hospital, Nyack, N.Y.

	Hospital
	Our Lady of Mercy Medical Center, Bronx, N.Y.
	Queens Hospital Center, Jamaica, N.Y.
	Raritan Bay Medical Center, Perth Amboy, N.J.
	Riverview Medical Center, Red Bank, N.J.
	Somerset Medical Center, Somerville, N.J.
	South Nassau Community Hospital, Oceanside, N.Y.
	Southampton Hospital, Southampton, N.Y.
	Southside Hospital, Bay Shore, N.Y.
	St. Charles Hospital and Rehabilitation Center, Port Jefferson, N.Y.
	St. Elizabeth Hospital, Elizabeth, N.J.
	St. Francis Medical Center, Trenton, N.J.
	St. John's Episcopal Hospital, Smithtown, N.Y.
	St. Joseph's Hospital and Medical Center, Paterson, N.J.
	St. Joseph's Medical Center, Yonkers, N.Y.
	St. Michael's Medical Center, Newark, N.J.
	St. Peter's Medical Center, New Brunswick, N.J.
	St. Vincent's Medical Center, Staten Island, N.Y.
	Staten Island University Hospital, Staten Island, N.Y.
	United Hospital Medical Center, Newark, N.J.
	University Hospital of Brooklyn-SUNY Center, Brooklyn
	Valley Hospital, Ridgewood, N.J.
	Vassar Brothers Hospital, Poughkeepsie, N.Y.
	Warren Hospital, Phillipsburg, N.J.
	Waterbury Hospital, Waterbury, Conn.
	Westchester County Medical Center, Valhalla, N.Y.

CANCER

Natl. Rank	Hospital
TIER ONE	
1	Memorial Sloan-Kettering Cancer Center, New York
TIER TWO	
76	Columbia-Presbyterian Medical Center, New York
69	Long Island Jewish Medical Center, New York
73	Montefiore Medical Center, Bronx, N.Y.
29	Mount Sinai Medical Center, New York
64	New York University Medical Center
78	University Hospital, Stony Brook, N.Y.
36	Yale-New Haven Hospital, New Haven, Conn.
TIER THREE	
	Bellevue Hospital Center, New York
	Beth Israel Medical Center, New York
	Bridgeport Hospital, Bridgeport, Conn.
	Bronx Municipal Hospital Center, Bronx, N.Y.
	Brookdale Hospital Medical Center, Brooklyn, N.Y.
	Brooklyn Hospital Center, Brooklyn, N.Y.
	Cabrini Medical Center, New York
	Catholic Medical Center, Jamaica, N.Y.
	Danbury Hospital, Danbury, Conn.
	Flushing Hospital Medical Center, Flushing, N.Y.
	Greenwich Hospital, Greenwich, Conn.
	Hackensack Medical Center, Hackensack, N.J.
	Harlem Hospital Center, New York
	Hospital of St. Raphael, New Haven, Conn.
	Jersey Shore Medical Center, Neptune, N.J.
	Kings County Hospital Center, Brooklyn, N.Y.
	Lenox Hill Hospital, New York

	Hospital
	Lincoln Medical and Mental Health Center, Bronx, N.Y.
	Long Island College Hospital, Brooklyn, N.Y.
	Maimonides Medical Center, Brooklyn, N.Y.
	Methodist Hospital, Brooklyn, N.Y.
	Monmouth Medical Center, Long Branch, N.J.
	Morristown Memorial Hospital, Morristown, N.J.
	New York Downtown Hospital
	New York Hospital Medical Center, Flushing
83	New York Hospital-Cornell Medical Center
	Newark Beth Israel Medical Center, Newark, N.J.
95	North Shore University Hospital, Manhasset, N.Y.
	Our Lady of Mercy Medical Center, Bronx, N.Y.
	Overlook Hospital, Summit, N.J.
	Robert Wood Johnson University Hospital, New Brunswick, N.J.
	St. Barnabas Medical Center, Livingston, N.J.
	St. Joseph's Hospital and Medical Center, Paterson, N.J.
	St. Luke's-Roosevelt Hospital Center, New York
	St. Mary's Hospital, Waterbury, Conn.
	St. Michael's Medical Center, Newark, N.J.
	St. Vincent's Hospital and Medical Center, New York
	Stamford Hospital, Stamford, Conn.
	University Hospital of Brooklyn-SUNY Center, Brooklyn
84	University Hospital, Newark, N.J.
91	Westchester County Medical Center, Valhalla, N.Y.
	Winthrop-University Hospital, Mineola, N.Y.
TIER FOUR	
	Bayley Seton Hospital, Staten Island, N.Y.
	Central General Hospital, Plainview, N.Y.
	Christ Hospital, Jersey City, N.J.
	Community Medical Center, Toms River, N.J.
	Coney Island Hospital, Brooklyn, N.Y.
	Elizabeth General Medical Center, Elizabeth, N.J.
	Englewood Hospital, Englewood, N.J.
	Franklin Hospital Medical Center, Valley Stream, N.Y.
	Good Samaritan Hospital, Suffern, N.Y.
	Good Samaritan Hospital, West Islip, N.Y.
	Griffin Hospital, Derby, Conn.
	Helene Fuld Medical Center, Trenton, N.J.
	Hospital Center at Orange, Orange, N.J.
	Hunterdon Medical Center, Flemington, N.J.
	Huntington Hospital, Huntington, N.Y.
	Interfaith Medical Center, Brooklyn, N.Y.
	JFK Medical Center, Edison, N.J.
	Jamaica Hospital, Jamaica, N.Y.
	John T. Mather Memorial Hospital, Port Jefferson, N.Y.
	Kingsboro Psychiatric Center, Brooklyn, N.Y.
	Kingsbrook Jewish Medical Center, Brooklyn, N.Y.
	La Guardia Hospital, Flushing, N.Y.
	Lutheran Medical Center, Brooklyn, N.Y.
	Medical Center at Princeton, Princeton, N.J.
	Mercer Medical Center, Trenton, N.J.
	Mercy Medical Center, Rockville Centre, N.Y.
	Mount Vernon Hospital, Mount Vernon, N.Y.
	Mountainside Hospital, Montclair, N.J.
	Muhlenberg Regional Medical Center, Plainfield, N.J.
	New Rochelle Hospital Medical Center, New Rochelle, N.Y.
	North Shore University Hospital-Glen Cove, Glen Cove, N.Y.
	Northern Westchester Hospital Center, Mount Kisco, N.Y.

Natl. Rank	Hospital
	Norwalk Hospital, Norwalk, Conn.
	Nyack Hospital, Nyack, N.Y.
	Raritan Bay Medical Center, Perth Amboy, N.J.
	Riverview Medical Center, Red Bank, N.J.
	Somerset Medical Center, Somerville, N.J.
	South Nassau Community Hospital, Oceanside, N.Y.
	Southampton Hospital, Southampton, N.Y.
	Southside Hospital, Bay Shore, N.Y.
	St. Barnabas Hospital, Bronx, N.Y.
	St. Charles Hospital and Rehabilitation Center, Port Jefferson, N.Y.
	St. Elizabeth Hospital, Elizabeth, N.J.
	St. Francis Medical Center, Trenton, N.J.
	St. John's Episcopal Hospital, Far Rockaway, N.Y.
	St. Joseph's Medical Center, Yonkers, N.Y.
	St. Peter's Medical Center, New Brunswick, N.J.
	St. Vincent's Medical Center, Bridgeport, Conn.
	St. Vincent's Medical Center, Staten Island, N.Y.
	Staten Island University Hospital, Staten Island, N.Y.
	United Hospital Medical Center, Newark, N.J.
	Valley Hospital, Ridgewood, N.J.
	Vassar Brothers Hospital, Poughkeepsie, N.Y.
	Warren Hospital, Phillipsburg, N.J.
	Waterbury Hospital, Waterbury, Conn.

CARDIOLOGY

Natl. Rank	Hospital
TIER ONE	
11	Columbia-Presbyterian Medical Center, New York
19	Mount Sinai Medical Center, New York
23	New York Hospital-Cornell Medical Center
TIER TWO	
70	Beth Israel Medical Center, New York
64	Hackensack Medical Center, Hackensack, N.J.
28	New York University Medical Center
49	Yale-New Haven Hospital, New Haven, Conn.
TIER THREE	
	Bronx Municipal Hospital Center, Bronx, N.Y.
	Bronx-Lebanon Hospital Center, Bronx, N.Y.
	Brooklyn Hospital Center, Brooklyn, N.Y.
	Cabrini Medical Center, New York
	Danbury Hospital, Danbury, Conn.
	Englewood Hospital, Englewood, N.J.
	Greenwich Hospital, Greenwich, Conn.
	Griffin Hospital, Derby, Conn.
	Helene Fuld Medical Center, Trenton, N.J.
	Hospital of St. Raphael, New Haven, Conn.
	Hunterdon Medical Center, Flemington, N.J.
	Huntington Hospital, Huntington, N.Y.
	Lenox Hill Hospital, New York
	Lincoln Medical and Mental Health Center, Bronx, N.Y.
	Long Island College Hospital, Brooklyn, N.Y.
	Long Island Jewish Medical Center, New York
	Maimonides Medical Center, Brooklyn, N.Y.
	Medical Center at Princeton, Princeton, N.J.
	Mercy Medical Center, Rockville Centre, N.Y.
	Methodist Hospital, Brooklyn, N.Y.

Natl. Rank	Hospital
	Monmouth Medical Center, Long Branch, N.J.
	Montefiore Medical Center, Bronx, N.Y.
	Morristown Memorial Hospital, Morristown, N.J.
	Mount Vernon Hospital, Mount Vernon, N.Y.
	North Shore University Hospital, Manhasset, N.Y.
	Northern Westchester Hospital Center, Mount Kisco, N.Y.
	Overlook Hospital, Summit, N.J.
	Robert Wood Johnson University Hospital, New Brunswick, N.J.
	St. Barnabas Medical Center, Livingston, N.J.
	St. Elizabeth Hospital, Elizabeth, N.J.
	St. Francis Medical Center, Trenton, N.J.
	St. Luke's-Roosevelt Hospital Center, New York
	St. Mary's Hospital, Waterbury, Conn.
	St. Peter's Medical Center, New Brunswick, N.J.
	St. Vincent's Hospital and Medical Center, New York
	Stamford Hospital, Stamford, Conn.
	University Hospital of Brooklyn-SUNY Center, Brooklyn
	University Hospital, Stony Brook, N.Y.
	Westchester County Medical Center, Valhalla, N.Y.
	Winthrop-University Hospital, Mineola, N.Y.
TIER FOUR	
	Bayley Seton Hospital, Staten Island, N.Y.
	Bellevue Hospital Center, New York
	Bridgeport Hospital, Bridgeport, Conn.
	Brookdale Hospital Medical Center, Brooklyn, N.Y.
	Catholic Medical Center, Jamaica, N.Y.
	Central General Hospital, Plainview, N.Y.
	Christ Hospital, Jersey City, N.J.
	Community Medical Center, Toms River, N.J.
	Coney Island Hospital, Brooklyn, N.Y.
	Elizabeth General Medical Center, Elizabeth, N.J.
	Elmhurst Hospital Center, Elmhurst, N.Y.
	Flushing Hospital Medical Center, Flushing, N.Y.
	Franklin Hospital Medical Center, Valley Stream, N.Y.
	Good Samaritan Hospital, Suffern, N.Y.
	Good Samaritan Hospital, West Islip, N.Y.
	Harlem Hospital Center, New York
	Hospital Center at Orange, Orange, N.J.
	JFK Medical Center, Edison, N.J.
	Jamaica Hospital, Jamaica, N.Y.
	Jersey Shore Medical Center, Neptune, N.J.
	John T. Mather Memorial Hospital, Port Jefferson, N.Y.
	Kingsbrook Jewish Medical Center, Brooklyn, N.Y.
	La Guardia Hospital, Flushing, N.Y.
	Lutheran Medical Center, Brooklyn, N.Y.
	Mercer Medical Center, Trenton, N.J.
	Mountainside Hospital, Montclair, N.J.
	Muhlenberg Regional Medical Center, Plainfield, N.J.
	Nassau County Medical Center, East Meadow, N.Y.
	New Rochelle Hospital Medical Center, New Rochelle, N.Y.
	New York Downtown Hospital
	New York Hospital Medical Center, Flushing
	Newark Beth Israel Medical Center, Newark, N.J.
	North Shore University Hospital-Glen Cove, Glen Cove, N.Y.
	Norwalk Hospital, Norwalk, Conn.
	Nyack Hospital, Nyack, N.Y.
	Our Lady of Mercy Medical Center, Bronx, N.Y.
	Queens Hospital Center, Jamaica, N.Y.

Natl. Rank	Hospital
	Raritan Bay Medical Center, Perth Amboy, N.J.
	Riverview Medical Center, Red Bank, N.J.
	Somerset Medical Center, Somerville, N.J.
	South Nassau Community Hospital, Oceanside, N.Y.
	Southampton Hospital, Southampton, N.Y.
	Southside Hospital, Bay Shore, N.Y.
	St. Barnabas Hospital, Bronx, N.Y.
	St. Charles Hospital and Rehabilitation Center, Port Jefferson, N.Y.
	St. John's Episcopal Hospital, Far Rockaway, N.Y.
	St. John's Episcopal Hospital, Smithtown, N.Y.
	St. Joseph's Hospital and Medical Center, Paterson, N.J.
	St. Joseph's Medical Center, Yonkers, N.Y.
	St. Michael's Medical Center, Newark, N.J.
	St. Vincent's Medical Center, Bridgeport, Conn.
	St. Vincent's Medical Center, Staten Island, N.Y.
	Staten Island University Hospital, Staten Island, N.Y.
	University Hospital, Newark, N.J.
	Valley Hospital, Ridgewood, N.J.
	Vassar Brothers Hospital, Poughkeepsie, N.Y.
	Warren Hospital, Phillipsburg, N.J.
	Waterbury Hospital, Waterbury, Conn.

ENDOCRINOLOGY

Natl. Rank	Hospital
TIER ONE	
21	Columbia-Presbyterian Medical Center, New York
TIER TWO	
48	Mount Sinai Medical Center, New York
52	New York Hospital-Cornell Medical Center
53	New York University Medical Center
54	Yale-New Haven Hospital, New Haven, Conn.
TIER THREE	
	Beth Israel Medical Center, New York
	Bronx Municipal Hospital Center, Bronx, N.Y.
	Bronx-Lebanon Hospital Center, Bronx, N.Y.
	Brooklyn Hospital Center, Brooklyn, N.Y.
	Cabrini Medical Center, New York
	Hackensack Medical Center, Hackensack, N.J.
	Hospital of St. Raphael, New Haven, Conn.
	Lenox Hill Hospital, New York
	Lincoln Medical and Mental Health Center, Bronx, N.Y.
	Long Island College Hospital, Brooklyn, N.Y.
	Long Island Jewish Medical Center, New York
	Maimonides Medical Center, Brooklyn, N.Y.
	Memorial Sloan-Kettering Cancer Center, New York
	Methodist Hospital, Brooklyn, N.Y.
	Metropolitan Hospital Center, New York
	Montefiore Medical Center, Bronx, N.Y.
	Morristown Memorial Hospital, Morristown, N.J.
	Nassau County Medical Center, East Meadow, N.Y.
	Newark Beth Israel Medical Center, Newark, N.J.
	North Shore University Hospital, Manhasset, N.Y.
	Northern Westchester Hospital Center, Mount Kisco, N.Y.
	Overlook Hospital, Summit, N.J.
	Robert Wood Johnson University Hospital, New Brunswick, N.J.
	St. Luke's-Roosevelt Hospital Center, New York

Natl. Rank	Hospital
	St. Mary's Hospital, Waterbury, Conn.
	St. Vincent's Hospital and Medical Center, New York
	Stamford Hospital, Stamford, Conn.
	University Hospital, Stony Brook, N.Y.
	Waterbury Hospital, Waterbury, Conn.
	Westchester County Medical Center, Valhalla, N.Y.
TIER FOUR	
	Bayley Seton Hospital, Staten Island, N.Y.
	Bergen Pines County Hospital, Paramus, N.J.
	Bridgeport Hospital, Bridgeport, Conn.
	Brookdale Hospital Medical Center, Brooklyn, N.Y.
	Catholic Medical Center, Jamaica, N.Y.
	Central General Hospital, Plainview, N.Y.
	Christ Hospital, Jersey City, N.J.
	Community Medical Center, Toms River, N.J.
	Coney Island Hospital, Brooklyn, N.Y.
	Elizabeth General Medical Center, Elizabeth, N.J.
	Englewood Hospital, Englewood, N.J.
	Flushing Hospital Medical Center, Flushing, N.Y.
	Franklin Hospital Medical Center, Valley Stream, N.Y.
	Good Samaritan Hospital, Suffern, N.Y.
	Good Samaritan Hospital, West Islip, N.Y.
	Greenwich Hospital, Greenwich, Conn.
	Griffin Hospital, Derby, Conn.
	Harlem Hospital Center, New York
	Helene Fuld Medical Center, Trenton, N.J.
	Hospital Center at Orange, Orange, N.J.
	Huntington Hospital, Huntington, N.Y.
	Interfaith Medical Center, Brooklyn, N.Y.
	JFK Medical Center, Edison, N.J.
	Jamaica Hospital, Jamaica, N.Y.
	Jersey Shore Medical Center, Neptune, N.J.
	John T. Mather Memorial Hospital, Port Jefferson, N.Y.
	Kingsbrook Jewish Medical Center, Brooklyn, N.Y.
	La Guardia Hospital, Flushing, N.Y.
	Lutheran Medical Center, Brooklyn, N.Y.
	Medical Center at Princeton, Princeton, N.J.
	Mercer Medical Center, Trenton, N.J.
	Mercy Medical Center, Rockville Centre, N.Y.
	Monmouth Medical Center, Long Branch, N.J.
	Mount Vernon Hospital, Mount Vernon, N.Y.
	Mountainside Hospital, Montclair, N.J.
	Muhlenberg Regional Medical Center, Plainfield, N.J.
	New Rochelle Hospital Medical Center, New Rochelle, N.Y.
	New York Downtown Hospital
	New York Hospital Medical Center, Flushing
	North Shore University Hospital-Glen Cove, Glen Cove, N.Y.
	Norwalk Hospital, Norwalk, Conn.
	Nyack Hospital, Nyack, N.Y.
	Our Lady of Mercy Medical Center, Bronx, N.Y.
	Queens Hospital Center, Jamaica, N.Y.
	Raritan Bay Medical Center, Perth Amboy, N.J.
	Riverview Medical Center, Red Bank, N.J.
	Somerset Medical Center, Somerville, N.J.
	South Nassau Community Hospital, Oceanside, N.Y.
	Southampton Hospital, Southampton, N.Y.
	Southside Hospital, Bay Shore, N.Y.
	St. Barnabas Hospital, Bronx, N.Y.

St. Barnabas Medical Center, Livingston, N.J.

St. Charles Hospital and Rehabilitation Center, Port Jefferson, N.Y.

St. Elizabeth Hospital, Elizabeth, N.J.

St. Francis Medical Center, Trenton, N.J.

St. John's Episcopal Hospital, Far Rockaway, N.Y.

St. John's Episcopal Hospital, Smithtown, N.Y.

St. Joseph's Hospital and Medical Center, Paterson, N.J.

St. Joseph's Medical Center, Yonkers, N.Y.

St. Michael's Medical Center, Newark, N.J.

St. Peter's Medical Center, New Brunswick, N.J.

St. Vincent's Medical Center, Bridgeport, Conn.

St. Vincent's Medical Center, Staten Island, N.Y.

Staten Island University Hospital, Staten Island, N.Y.

United Hospital Medical Center, Newark, N.J.

Valley Hospital, Ridgewood, N.J.

Vassar Brothers Hospital, Poughkeepsie, N.Y.

Warren Hospital, Phillipsburg, N.J.

Winthrop-University Hospital, Mineola, N.Y.

GASTROENTEROLOGY

Natl.
Rank   Hospital

Natl. Rank	Hospital
TIER ONE	
7	Mount Sinai Medical Center, New York
16	Yale-New Haven Hospital, New Haven, Conn.
20	Memorial Sloan-Kettering Cancer Center, New York
TIER TWO	
67	Beth Israel Medical Center, New York
50	Columbia-Presbyterian Medical Center, New York
60	Hospital of St. Raphael, New Haven, Conn.
54	Montefiore Medical Center, Bronx, N.Y.
41	New York Hospital-Cornell Medical Center
30	New York University Medical Center
TIER THREE	
	Bridgeport Hospital, Bridgeport, Conn.
	Bronx Municipal Hospital Center, Bronx, N.Y.
	Bronx-Lebanon Hospital Center, Bronx, N.Y.
	Brooklyn Hospital Center, Brooklyn, N.Y.
	Cabrini Medical Center, New York
	Community Medical Center, Toms River, N.J.
	Greenwich Hospital, Greenwich, Conn.
87	Hackensack Medical Center, Hackensack, N.J.
	Huntington Hospital, Huntington, N.Y.
	Lenox Hill Hospital, New York
100	Long Island College Hospital, Brooklyn, N.Y.
81	Long Island Jewish Medical Center, New York
	Maimonides Medical Center, Brooklyn, N.Y.
	Medical Center at Princeton, Princeton, N.J.
	Methodist Hospital, Brooklyn, N.Y.
	Monmouth Medical Center, Long Branch, N.J.
93	North Shore University Hospital, Manhasset, N.Y.
	Northern Westchester Hospital Center, Mount Kisco, N.Y.
	Norwalk Hospital, Norwalk, Conn.
	Our Lady of Mercy Medical Center, Bronx, N.Y.
	Overlook Hospital, Summit, N.J.
	Robert Wood Johnson University Hospital, New Brunswick, N.J.
	St. Barnabas Medical Center, Livingston, N.J.

Natl. Rank	Hospital
	St. Joseph's Hospital and Medical Center, Paterson, N.J.
	St. Joseph's Medical Center, Yonkers, N.Y.
	St. Luke's-Roosevelt Hospital Center, New York
	St. Mary's Hospital, Waterbury, Conn.
	St. Vincent's Hospital and Medical Center, New York
	Stamford Hospital, Stamford, Conn.
95	University Hospital, Stony Brook, N.Y.
	Valley Hospital, Ridgewood, N.J.
	Westchester County Medical Center, Valhalla, N.Y.
	Winthrop-University Hospital, Mineola, N.Y.
TIER FOUR	
	Brookdale Hospital Medical Center, Brooklyn, N.Y.
	Catholic Medical Center, Jamaica, N.Y.
	Central General Hospital, Plainview, N.Y.
	Christ Hospital, Jersey City, N.J.
	Danbury Hospital, Danbury, Conn.
	Elizabeth General Medical Center, Elizabeth, N.J.
	Englewood Hospital, Englewood, N.J.
	Flushing Hospital Medical Center, Flushing, N.Y.
	Franklin Hospital Medical Center, Valley Stream, N.Y.
	Good Samaritan Hospital, Suffern, N.Y.
	Good Samaritan Hospital, West Islip, N.Y.
	Griffin Hospital, Derby, Conn.
	Helene Fuld Medical Center, Trenton, N.J.
	Hospital Center at Orange, Orange, N.J.
	Hunterdon Medical Center, Flemington, N.J.
	JFK Medical Center, Edison, N.J.
	Jamaica Hospital, Jamaica, N.Y.
	Jersey Shore Medical Center, Neptune, N.J.
	John T. Mather Memorial Hospital, Port Jefferson, N.Y.
	Kingsbrook Jewish Medical Center, Brooklyn, N.Y.
	La Guardia Hospital, Flushing, N.Y.
	Lutheran Medical Center, Brooklyn, N.Y.
	Mercer Medical Center, Trenton, N.J.
	Mercy Medical Center, Rockville Centre, N.Y.
	Morristown Memorial Hospital, Morristown, N.J.
	Mount Vernon Hospital, Mount Vernon, N.Y.
	Mountainside Hospital, Montclair, N.J.
	Muhlenberg Regional Medical Center, Plainfield, N.J.
	New Rochelle Hospital Medical Center, New Rochelle, N.Y.
	New York Downtown Hospital
	New York Hospital Medical Center, Flushing
	Newark Beth Israel Medical Center, Newark, N.J.
	North Shore University Hospital-Glen Cove, Glen Cove, N.Y.
	Nyack Hospital, Nyack, N.Y.
	Raritan Bay Medical Center, Perth Amboy, N.J.
	Riverview Medical Center, Red Bank, N.J.
	Somerset Medical Center, Somerville, N.J.
	South Nassau Community Hospital, Oceanside, N.Y.
	Southampton Hospital, Southampton, N.Y.
	Southside Hospital, Bay Shore, N.Y.
	St. Barnabas Hospital, Bronx, N.Y.
	St. Charles Hospital and Rehabilitation Center, Port Jefferson, N.Y.
	St. Elizabeth Hospital, Elizabeth, N.J.
	St. Francis Medical Center, Trenton, N.J.
	St. John's Episcopal Hospital, Far Rockaway, N.Y.
	St. John's Episcopal Hospital, Smithtown, N.Y.
	St. Peter's Medical Center, New Brunswick, N.J.

	St. Vincent's Medical Center, Bridgeport, Conn.
	St. Vincent's Medical Center, Staten Island, N.Y.
	Staten Island University Hospital, Staten Island, N.Y.
	Vassar Brothers Hospital, Poughkeepsie, N.Y.
	Warren Hospital, Phillipsburg, N.J.
	Waterbury Hospital, Waterbury, Conn.

GERIATRICS

Natl.
Rank Hospital

	TIER ONE
3	Mount Sinai Medical Center, New York
15	New York University Medical Center
20	Yale-New Haven Hospital, New Haven, Conn.
25	New York Hospital-Cornell Medical Center
	TIER TWO
26	Columbia-Presbyterian Medical Center, New York
88	Hospital of St. Raphael, New Haven, Conn.
31	Montefiore Medical Center, Bronx, N.Y.
	TIER THREE
	Bellevue Hospital Center, New York
	Beth Israel Medical Center, New York
	Greenwich Hospital, Greenwich, Conn.
98	Hackensack Medical Center, Hackensack, N.J.
	Hunterdon Medical Center, Flemington, N.J.
	Long Island College Hospital, Brooklyn, N.Y.
93	Long Island Jewish Medical Center, New York
	Maimonides Medical Center, Brooklyn, N.Y.
	Medical Center at Princeton, Princeton, N.J.
92	Methodist Hospital, Brooklyn, N.Y.
	North Shore University Hospital, Manhasset, N.Y.
	Northern Westchester Hospital Center, Mount Kisco, N.Y.
	Overlook Hospital, Summit, N.J.
	St. Mary's Hospital, Waterbury, Conn.
	St. Vincent's Hospital and Medical Center, New York
	Stamford Hospital, Stamford, Conn.
	University Hospital, Stony Brook, N.Y.
	Winthrop-University Hospital, Mineola, N.Y.
	TIER FOUR
	Bridgeport Hospital, Bridgeport, Conn.
	Bronx Municipal Hospital Center, Bronx, N.Y.
	Bronx-Lebanon Hospital Center, Bronx, N.Y.
	Brookdale Hospital Medical Center, Brooklyn, N.Y.
	Brooklyn Hospital Center, Brooklyn, N.Y.
	Cabrini Medical Center, New York
	Catholic Medical Center, Jamaica, N.Y.
	Central General Hospital, Plainview, N.Y.
	Christ Hospital, Jersey City, N.J.
	Community Medical Center, Toms River, N.J.
	Coney Island Hospital, Brooklyn, N.Y.
	Elizabeth General Medical Center, Elizabeth, N.J.
	Flushing Hospital Medical Center, Flushing, N.Y.
	Franklin Hospital Medical Center, Valley Stream, N.Y.
	Good Samaritan Hospital, Suffern, N.Y.
	Good Samaritan Hospital, West Islip, N.Y.
	Griffin Hospital, Derby, Conn.
	Harlem Hospital Center, New York

	Helene Fuld Medical Center, Trenton, N.J.
	JFK Medical Center, Edison, N.J.
	Jamaica Hospital, Jamaica, N.Y.
	Jersey Shore Medical Center, Neptune, N.J.
	John T. Mather Memorial Hospital, Port Jefferson, N.Y.
	Kingsboro Psychiatric Center, Brooklyn, N.Y.
	Kingsbrook Jewish Medical Center, Brooklyn, N.Y.
	La Guardia Hospital, Flushing, N.Y.
	Lenox Hill Hospital, New York
	Lutheran Medical Center, Brooklyn, N.Y.
	Mercer Medical Center, Trenton, N.J.
	Mercy Medical Center, Rockville Centre, N.Y.
	Monmouth Medical Center, Long Branch, N.J.
	Morristown Memorial Hospital, Morristown, N.J.
	Mount Vernon Hospital, Mount Vernon, N.Y.
	Mountainside Hospital, Montclair, N.J.
	Muhlenberg Regional Medical Center, Plainfield, N.J.
	Nassau County Medical Center, East Meadow, N.Y.
	New Rochelle Hospital Medical Center, New Rochelle, N.Y.
	New York Downtown Hospital
	New York Hospital Medical Center, Flushing
	North Shore University Hospital-Glen Cove, Glen Cove, N.Y.
	Norwalk Hospital, Norwalk, Conn.
	Our Lady of Mercy Medical Center, Bronx, N.Y.
	Raritan Bay Medical Center, Perth Amboy, N.J.
	Riverview Medical Center, Red Bank, N.J.
	Robert Wood Johnson University Hospital, New Brunswick, N.J.
	Somerset Medical Center, Somerville, N.J.
	South Nassau Community Hospital, Oceanside, N.Y.
	Southside Hospital, Bay Shore, N.Y.
	St. Barnabas Medical Center, Livingston, N.J.
	St. Charles Hospital and Rehabilitation Center, Port Jefferson, N.Y.
	St. Elizabeth Hospital, Elizabeth, N.J.
	St. Francis Medical Center, Trenton, N.J.
	St. John's Episcopal Hospital, Smithtown, N.Y.
	St. Joseph's Hospital and Medical Center, Paterson, N.J.
	St. Joseph's Medical Center, Yonkers, N.Y.
	St. Luke's-Roosevelt Hospital Center, New York
	St. Michael's Medical Center, Newark, N.J.
	St. Peter's Medical Center, New Brunswick, N.J.
	St. Vincent's Medical Center, Staten Island, N.Y.
	Staten Island University Hospital, Staten Island, N.Y.
	University Hospital of Brooklyn-SUNY Center, Brooklyn
	Valley Hospital, Ridgewood, N.J.
	Vassar Brothers Hospital, Poughkeepsie, N.Y.
	Warren Hospital, Phillipsburg, N.J.
	Waterbury Hospital, Waterbury, Conn.
	Westchester County Medical Center, Valhalla, N.Y.

GYNECOLOGY

Natl.
Rank Hospital

	TIER ONE
11	Memorial Sloan-Kettering Cancer Center, New York
16	Yale-New Haven Hospital, New Haven, Conn.
29	New York Hospital-Cornell Medical Center
31	New York University Medical Center

TIER TWO	
33	Columbia-Presbyterian Medical Center, New York
36	Mount Sinai Medical Center, New York

TIER THREE
Beth Israel Medical Center, New York
Greenwich Hospital, Greenwich, Conn.
Hackensack Medical Center, Hackensack, N.J.
Hospital of St. Raphael, New Haven, Conn.
Lenox Hill Hospital, New York
Long Island College Hospital, Brooklyn, N.Y.
Long Island Jewish Medical Center, New York
Medical Center at Princeton, Princeton, N.J.
Methodist Hospital, Brooklyn, N.Y.
Montefiore Medical Center, Bronx, N.Y.
North Shore University Hospital, Manhasset, N.Y.
Northern Westchester Hospital Center, Mount Kisco, N.Y.
Overlook Hospital, Summit, N.J.
St. Barnabas Medical Center, Livingston, N.J.
St. Elizabeth Hospital, Elizabeth, N.J.
St. Vincent's Hospital and Medical Center, New York
Stamford Hospital, Stamford, Conn.
University Hospital, Stony Brook, N.Y.

TIER FOUR
Bellevue Hospital Center, New York
Bridgeport Hospital, Bridgeport, Conn.
Bronx Municipal Hospital Center, Bronx, N.Y.
Bronx-Lebanon Hospital Center, Bronx, N.Y.
Brookdale Hospital Medical Center, Brooklyn, N.Y.
Brooklyn Hospital Center, Brooklyn, N.Y.
Cabrini Medical Center, New York
Catholic Medical Center, Jamaica, N.Y.
Central General Hospital, Plainview, N.Y.
Christ Hospital, Jersey City, N.J.
Community Medical Center, Toms River, N.J.
Coney Island Hospital, Brooklyn, N.Y.
Elizabeth General Medical Center, Elizabeth, N.J.
Englewood Hospital, Englewood, N.J.
Flushing Hospital Medical Center, Flushing, N.Y.
Franklin Hospital Medical Center, Valley Stream, N.Y.
Good Samaritan Hospital, Suffern, N.Y.
Good Samaritan Hospital, West Islip, N.Y.
Griffin Hospital, Derby, Conn.
Helene Fuld Medical Center, Trenton, N.J.
Hunterdon Medical Center, Flemington, N.J.
Huntington Hospital, Huntington, N.Y.
JFK Medical Center, Edison, N.J.
Jamaica Hospital, Jamaica, N.Y.
Jersey Shore Medical Center, Neptune, N.J.
John T. Mather Memorial Hospital, Port Jefferson, N.Y.
Kingsbrook Jewish Medical Center, Brooklyn, N.Y.
La Guardia Hospital, Flushing, N.Y.
Lutheran Medical Center, Brooklyn, N.Y.
Maimonides Medical Center, Brooklyn, N.Y.
Mercer Medical Center, Trenton, N.J.
Mercy Medical Center, Rockville Centre, N.Y.
Monmouth Medical Center, Long Branch, N.J.
Morristown Memorial Hospital, Morristown, N.J.
Muhlenberg Regional Medical Center, Plainfield, N.J.

Nassau County Medical Center, East Meadow, N.Y.
New Rochelle Hospital Medical Center, New Rochelle, N.Y.
New York Downtown Hospital
New York Hospital Medical Center, Flushing
North Shore University Hospital-Glen Cove, Glen Cove, N.Y.
Norwalk Hospital, Norwalk, Conn.
Our Lady of Mercy Medical Center, Bronx, N.Y.
Raritan Bay Medical Center, Perth Amboy, N.J.
Riverview Medical Center, Red Bank, N.J.
Robert Wood Johnson University Hospital, New Brunswick, N.J.
Somerset Medical Center, Somerville, N.J.
South Nassau Community Hospital, Oceanside, N.Y.
Southside Hospital, Bay Shore, N.Y.
St. Charles Hospital and Rehabilitation Center, Port Jefferson, N.Y.
St. Francis Medical Center, Trenton, N.J.
St. John's Episcopal Hospital, Smithtown, N.Y.
St. Joseph's Hospital and Medical Center, Paterson, N.J.
St. Joseph's Medical Center, Yonkers, N.Y.
St. Luke's-Roosevelt Hospital Center, New York
St. Mary's Hospital, Waterbury, Conn.
St. Michael's Medical Center, Newark, N.J.
St. Peter's Medical Center, New Brunswick, N.J.
St. Vincent's Medical Center, Staten Island, N.Y.
Staten Island University Hospital, Staten Island, N.Y.
Valley Hospital, Ridgewood, N.J.
Vassar Brothers Hospital, Poughkeepsie, N.Y.
Warren Hospital, Phillipsburg, N.J.
Waterbury Hospital, Waterbury, Conn.
Westchester County Medical Center, Valhalla, N.Y.
Winthrop-University Hospital, Mineola, N.Y.

NEUROLOGY

TIER ONE	
5	Columbia-Presbyterian Medical Center, New York
8	New York Hospital-Cornell Medical Center
13	New York University Medical Center
22	Mount Sinai Medical Center, New York

TIER TWO	
75	Montefiore Medical Center, Bronx, N.Y.
80	North Shore University Hospital, Manhasset, N.Y.
62	Yale-New Haven Hospital, New Haven, Conn.

TIER THREE
Beth Israel Medical Center, New York
Bronx-Lebanon Hospital Center, Bronx, N.Y.
Cabrini Medical Center, New York
Greenwich Hospital, Greenwich, Conn.
Hackensack Medical Center, Hackensack, N.J.
Hospital of St. Raphael, New Haven, Conn.
JFK Medical Center, Edison, N.J.
Lenox Hill Hospital, New York
Long Island College Hospital, Brooklyn, N.Y.
Long Island Jewish Medical Center, New York
Maimonides Medical Center, Brooklyn, N.Y.
Memorial Sloan-Kettering Cancer Center, New York
Northern Westchester Hospital Center, Mount Kisco, N.Y.

99	Robert Wood Johnson University Hospital, New Brunswick, N.J.
	St. Luke's-Roosevelt Hospital Center, New York
	St. Mary's Hospital, Waterbury, Conn.
	St. Vincent's Hospital and Medical Center, New York
	United Hospital Medical Center, Newark, N.J.
	University Hospital, Newark, N.J.
	University Hospital, Stony Brook, N.Y.
	Valley Hospital, Ridgewood, N.J.
	Winthrop-University Hospital, Mineola, N.Y.

TIER FOUR

	Bridgeport Hospital, Bridgeport, Conn.
	Bronx Municipal Hospital Center, Bronx, N.Y.
	Brookdale Hospital Medical Center, Brooklyn, N.Y.
	Brooklyn Hospital Center, Brooklyn, N.Y.
	Central General Hospital, Plainview, N.Y.
	Christ Hospital, Jersey City, N.J.
	Community Medical Center, Toms River, N.J.
	Coney Island Hospital, Brooklyn, N.Y.
	Elizabeth General Medical Center, Elizabeth, N.J.
	Englewood Hospital, Englewood, N.J.
	Flushing Hospital Medical Center, Flushing, N.Y.
	Franklin Hospital Medical Center, Valley Stream, N.Y.
	Good Samaritan Hospital, Suffern, N.Y.
	Good Samaritan Hospital, West Islip, N.Y.
	Harlem Hospital Center, New York
	Helene Fuld Medical Center, Trenton, N.J.
	Hospital Center at Orange, Orange, N.J.
	Huntington Hospital, Huntington, N.Y.
	Jamaica Hospital, Jamaica, N.Y.
	Jersey Shore Medical Center, Neptune, N.J.
	John T. Mather Memorial Hospital, Port Jefferson, N.Y.
	Kings County Hospital Center, Brooklyn, N.Y.
	Kingsbrook Jewish Medical Center, Brooklyn, N.Y.
	La Guardia Hospital, Flushing, N.Y.
	Medical Center at Princeton, Princeton, N.J.
	Mercer Medical Center, Trenton, N.J.
	Mercy Medical Center, Rockville Centre, N.Y.
	Monmouth Medical Center, Long Branch, N.J.
	Morristown Memorial Hospital, Morristown, N.J.
	Mount Vernon Hospital, Mount Vernon, N.Y.
	Mountainside Hospital, Montclair, N.J.
	Muhlenberg Regional Medical Center, Plainfield, N.J.
	Nassau County Medical Center, East Meadow, N.Y.
	New Rochelle Hospital Medical Center, New Rochelle, N.Y.
	New York Downtown Hospital
	New York Hospital Medical Center, Flushing
	Newark Beth Israel Medical Center, Newark, N.J.
	North Shore University Hospital-Glen Cove, Glen Cove, N.Y.
	Norwalk Hospital, Norwalk, Conn.
	Nyack Hospital, Nyack, N.Y.
	Our Lady of Mercy Medical Center, Bronx, N.Y.
	Overlook Hospital, Summit, N.J.
	Raritan Bay Medical Center, Perth Amboy, N.J.
	Riverview Medical Center, Red Bank, N.J.
	Somerset Medical Center, Somerville, N.J.
	South Nassau Community Hospital, Oceanside, N.Y.
	Southside Hospital, Bay Shore, N.Y.
	St. Barnabas Hospital, Bronx, N.Y.

	St. Barnabas Medical Center, Livingston, N.J.
	St. Charles Hospital and Rehabilitation Center, Port Jefferson, N.Y.
	St. Elizabeth Hospital, Elizabeth, N.J.
	St. Francis Medical Center, Trenton, N.J.
	St. John's Episcopal Hospital, Far Rockaway, N.Y.
	St. John's Episcopal Hospital, Smithtown, N.Y.
	St. Joseph's Hospital and Medical Center, Paterson, N.J.
	St. Joseph's Medical Center, Yonkers, N.Y.
	St. Peter's Medical Center, New Brunswick, N.J.
	St. Vincent's Medical Center, Bridgeport, Conn.
	St. Vincent's Medical Center, Staten Island, N.Y.
	Stamford Hospital, Stamford, Conn.
	Staten Island University Hospital, Staten Island, N.Y.
	Vassar Brothers Hospital, Poughkeepsie, N.Y.
	Warren Hospital, Phillipsburg, N.J.
	Waterbury Hospital, Waterbury, Conn.
	Westchester County Medical Center, Valhalla, N.Y.

ORTHOPEDICS

TIER ONE

| 2 | Hospital for Special Surgery, New York |
| 8 | Hospital for Joint Diseases-Orthopedic Institute, New York |

TIER TWO

43	Columbia-Presbyterian Medical Center, New York
68	Mount Sinai Medical Center, New York
27	New York University Medical Center
77	North Shore University Hospital, Manhasset, N.Y.
60	Yale-New Haven Hospital, New Haven, Conn.

TIER THREE

	Beth Israel Medical Center, New York
	Brooklyn Hospital Center, Brooklyn, N.Y.
	Danbury Hospital, Danbury, Conn.
	Greenwich Hospital, Greenwich, Conn.
89	Hackensack Medical Center, Hackensack, N.J.
	Hospital of St. Raphael, New Haven, Conn.
	Lenox Hill Hospital, New York
	Long Island College Hospital, Brooklyn, N.Y.
91	Long Island Jewish Medical Center, New York
	Maimonides Medical Center, Brooklyn, N.Y.
81	Memorial Sloan-Kettering Cancer Center, New York
	Montefiore Medical Center, Bronx, N.Y.
	Overlook Hospital, Summit, N.J.
	Robert Wood Johnson University Hospital, New Brunswick, N.J.
	St. Barnabas Medical Center, Livingston, N.J.
	St. Luke's-Roosevelt Hospital Center, New York
	St. Vincent's Hospital and Medical Center, New York
	University Hospital, Stony Brook, N.Y.
	Westchester County Medical Center, Valhalla, N.Y.
	Winthrop-University Hospital, Mineola, N.Y.

TIER FOUR

	Bridgeport Hospital, Bridgeport, Conn.
	Brookdale Hospital Medical Center, Brooklyn, N.Y.
	Cabrini Medical Center, New York
	Central General Hospital, Plainview, N.Y.
	Christ Hospital, Jersey City, N.J.

	Hospital
	Community Medical Center, Toms River, N.J.
	Coney Island Hospital, Brooklyn, N.Y.
	Elizabeth General Medical Center, Elizabeth, N.J.
	Englewood Hospital, Englewood, N.J.
	Flushing Hospital Medical Center, Flushing, N.Y.
	Franklin Hospital Medical Center, Valley Stream, N.Y.
	Good Samaritan Hospital, Suffern, N.Y.
	Good Samaritan Hospital, West Islip, N.Y.
	Griffin Hospital, Derby, Conn.
	Helene Fuld Medical Center, Trenton, N.J.
	Hunterdon Medical Center, Flemington, N.J.
	Huntington Hospital, Huntington, N.Y.
	JFK Medical Center, Edison, N.J.
	Jamaica Hospital, Jamaica, N.Y.
	Jersey Shore Medical Center, Neptune, N.J.
	John T. Mather Memorial Hospital, Port Jefferson, N.Y.
	Kingsbrook Jewish Medical Center, Brooklyn, N.Y.
	La Guardia Hospital, Flushing, N.Y.
	Lutheran Medical Center, Brooklyn, N.Y.
	Medical Center at Princeton, Princeton, N.J.
	Mercer Medical Center, Trenton, N.J.
	Mercy Medical Center, Rockville Centre, N.Y.
	Monmouth Medical Center, Long Branch, N.J.
	Morristown Memorial Hospital, Morristown, N.J.
	Mountainside Hospital, Montclair, N.J.
	Muhlenberg Regional Medical Center, Plainfield, N.J.
	New Rochelle Hospital Medical Center, New Rochelle, N.Y.
	New York Hospital Medical Center, Flushing
	North Shore University Hospital-Glen Cove, Glen Cove, N.Y.
	Northern Westchester Hospital Center, Mount Kisco, N.Y.
	Norwalk Hospital, Norwalk, Conn.
	Nyack Hospital, Nyack, N.Y.
	Our Lady of Mercy Medical Center, Bronx, N.Y.
	Raritan Bay Medical Center, Perth Amboy, N.J.
	Riverview Medical Center, Red Bank, N.J.
	Somerset Medical Center, Somerville, N.J.
	South Nassau Community Hospital, Oceanside, N.Y.
	Southampton Hospital, Southampton, N.Y.
	Southside Hospital, Bay Shore, N.Y.
	St. Charles Hospital and Rehabilitation Center, Port Jefferson, N.Y.
	St. Elizabeth Hospital, Elizabeth, N.J.
	St. Francis Medical Center, Trenton, N.J.
	St. John's Episcopal Hospital, Smithtown, N.Y.
	St. Joseph's Hospital and Medical Center, Paterson, N.J.
	St. Joseph's Medical Center, Yonkers, N.Y.
	St. Mary's Hospital, Waterbury, Conn.
	St. Peter's Medical Center, New Brunswick, N.J.
	St. Vincent's Medical Center, Staten Island, N.Y.
	Stamford Hospital, Stamford, Conn.
	Staten Island University Hospital, Staten Island, N.Y.
	Valley Hospital, Ridgewood, N.J.
	Vassar Brothers Hospital, Poughkeepsie, N.Y.
	Warren Hospital, Phillipsburg, N.J.
	Waterbury Hospital, Waterbury, Conn.

OTOLARYNGOLOGY

Natl. Rank	Hospital
TIER ONE	
13	Mount Sinai Medical Center, New York
15	New York University Medical Center
21	Manhattan Eye, Ear and Throat Hospital, New York
TIER TWO	
38	Columbia-Presbyterian Medical Center, New York
97	Hackensack Medical Center, Hackensack, N.J.
86	Long Island Jewish Medical Center, New York
61	Memorial Sloan-Kettering Cancer Center, New York
65	Montefiore Medical Center, Bronx, N.Y.
50	New York Eye and Ear Infirmary
70	New York Hospital-Cornell Medical Center
95	North Shore University Hospital, Manhasset, N.Y.
55	St. Vincent's Hospital and Medical Center, New York
69	University Hospital, Newark, N.J.
93	University Hospital, Stony Brook, N.Y.
40	Yale-New Haven Hospital, New Haven, Conn.
TIER THREE	
	Bellevue Hospital Center, New York
	Beth Israel Medical Center, New York
	Bridgeport Hospital, Bridgeport, Conn.
	Bronx Municipal Hospital Center, Bronx, N.Y.
	Bronx-Lebanon Hospital Center, Bronx, N.Y.
	Brookdale Hospital Medical Center, Brooklyn, N.Y.
	Brooklyn Hospital Center, Brooklyn, N.Y.
	Cabrini Medical Center, New York
	Catholic Medical Center, Jamaica, N.Y.
	Danbury Hospital, Danbury, Conn.
	Elmhurst Hospital Center, Elmhurst, N.Y.
	Flushing Hospital Medical Center, Flushing, N.Y.
	Greenwich Hospital, Greenwich, Conn.
	Harlem Hospital Center, New York
	Hospital for Joint Diseases-Orthopedic Institute, New York
	Hospital for Special Surgery, New York
	Hospital of St. Raphael, New Haven, Conn.
	Jersey Shore Medical Center, Neptune, N.J.
	Kings County Hospital Center, Brooklyn, N.Y.
	Lenox Hill Hospital, New York
	Lincoln Medical and Mental Health Center, Bronx, N.Y.
	Long Island College Hospital, Brooklyn, N.Y.
	Maimonides Medical Center, Brooklyn, N.Y.
	Methodist Hospital, Brooklyn, N.Y.
	Metropolitan Hospital Center, New York
	Monmouth Medical Center, Long Branch, N.J.
	Morristown Memorial Hospital, Morristown, N.J.
	Nassau County Medical Center, East Meadow, N.Y.
	New York Hospital Medical Center, Flushing
	Newark Beth Israel Medical Center, Newark, N.J.
	North Shore University Hospital-Glen Cove, Glen Cove, N.Y.
	Northern Westchester Hospital Center, Mount Kisco, N.Y.
	Norwalk Hospital, Norwalk, Conn.
	Our Lady of Mercy Medical Center, Bronx, N.Y.
	Overlook Hospital, Summit, N.J.
	Robert Wood Johnson University Hospital, New Brunswick, N.J.
	St. Barnabas Medical Center, Livingston, N.J.

St. Joseph's Hospital and Medical Center, Paterson, N.J.

St. Luke's-Roosevelt Hospital Center, New York

St. Mary's Hospital, Waterbury, Conn.

St. Michael's Medical Center, Newark, N.J.

Stamford Hospital, Stamford, Conn.

United Hospital Medical Center, Newark, N.J.

University Hospital of Brooklyn-SUNY Center, Brooklyn

Westchester County Medical Center, Valhalla, N.Y.

Winthrop-University Hospital, Mineola, N.Y.

TIER FOUR

Bayley Seton Hospital, Staten Island, N.Y.

Bergen Pines County Hospital, Paramus, N.J.

Central General Hospital, Plainview, N.Y.

Christ Hospital, Jersey City, N.J.

Community Medical Center, Toms River, N.J.

Coney Island Hospital, Brooklyn, N.Y.

Elizabeth General Medical Center, Elizabeth, N.J.

Englewood Hospital, Englewood, N.J.

Franklin Hospital Medical Center, Valley Stream, N.Y.

Goldwater Memorial Hospital, New York

Good Samaritan Hospital, Suffern, N.Y.

Good Samaritan Hospital, West Islip, N.Y.

Griffin Hospital, Derby, Conn.

Helene Fuld Medical Center, Trenton, N.J.

Hospital Center at Orange, Orange, N.J.

Hunterdon Medical Center, Flemington, N.J.

Huntington Hospital, Huntington, N.Y.

Interfaith Medical Center, Brooklyn, N.Y.

JFK Medical Center, Edison, N.J.

Jamaica Hospital, Jamaica, N.Y.

Jersey City Medical Center, Jersey City, N.J.

John T. Mather Memorial Hospital, Port Jefferson, N.Y.

Kingsbrook Jewish Medical Center, Brooklyn, N.Y.

La Guardia Hospital, Flushing, N.Y.

Lutheran Medical Center, Brooklyn, N.Y.

Medical Center at Princeton, Princeton, N.J.

Mercer Medical Center, Trenton, N.J.

Mercy Medical Center, Rockville Centre, N.Y.

Mount Vernon Hospital, Mount Vernon, N.Y.

Mountainside Hospital, Montclair, N.J.

Muhlenberg Regional Medical Center, Plainfield, N.J.

New Rochelle Hospital Medical Center, New Rochelle, N.Y.

New York Downtown Hospital

North Central Bronx Hospital, Bronx, N.Y.

North General Hospital, New York

Nyack Hospital, Nyack, N.Y.

Queens Hospital Center, Jamaica, N.Y.

Raritan Bay Medical Center, Perth Amboy, N.J.

Riverview Medical Center, Red Bank, N.J.

Somerset Medical Center, Somerville, N.J.

South Nassau Community Hospital, Oceanside, N.Y.

Southampton Hospital, Southampton, N.Y.

Southside Hospital, Bay Shore, N.Y.

St. Barnabas Hospital, Bronx, N.Y.

St. Charles Hospital and Rehabilitation Center, Port Jefferson, N.Y.

St. Elizabeth Hospital, Elizabeth, N.J.

St. Francis Medical Center, Trenton, N.J.

St. John's Episcopal Hospital, Far Rockaway, N.Y.

St. John's Episcopal Hospital, Smithtown, N.Y.

St. Joseph's Medical Center, Yonkers, N.Y.

St. Peter's Medical Center, New Brunswick, N.J.

St. Vincent's Medical Center, Bridgeport, Conn.

St. Vincent's Medical Center, Staten Island, N.Y.

Staten Island University Hospital, Staten Island, N.Y.

Valley Hospital, Ridgewood, N.J.

Vassar Brothers Hospital, Poughkeepsie, N.Y.

Warren Hospital, Phillipsburg, N.J.

Waterbury Hospital, Waterbury, Conn.

RHEUMATOLOGY

Natl. Rank	Hospital
TIER ONE	
5	Hospital for Special Surgery, New York
9	New York University Medical Center
17	Yale-New Haven Hospital, New Haven, Conn.
22	Hospital for Joint Diseases-Orthopedic Institute, New York
25	Mount Sinai Medical Center, New York
TIER TWO	
67	Columbia-Presbyterian Medical Center, New York
68	Long Island Jewish Medical Center, New York
75	Memorial Sloan-Kettering Cancer Center, New York
80	Montefiore Medical Center, Bronx, N.Y.
63	New York Hospital-Cornell Medical Center
TIER THREE	
	Bellevue Hospital Center, New York
91	Beth Israel Medical Center, New York
	Bridgeport Hospital, Bridgeport, Conn.
	Bronx Municipal Hospital Center, Bronx, N.Y.
	Bronx-Lebanon Hospital Center, Bronx, N.Y.
	Brooklyn Hospital Center, Brooklyn, N.Y.
	Cabrini Medical Center, New York
	Danbury Hospital, Danbury, Conn.
	Greenwich Hospital, Greenwich, Conn.
94	Hackensack Medical Center, Hackensack, N.J.
	Hospital of St. Raphael, New Haven, Conn.
	Lenox Hill Hospital, New York
	Long Island College Hospital, Brooklyn, N.Y.
	Maimonides Medical Center, Brooklyn, N.Y.
	Methodist Hospital, Brooklyn, N.Y.
	Nassau County Medical Center, East Meadow, N.Y.
	New York Eye and Ear Infirmary
92	North Shore University Hospital, Manhasset, N.Y.
	Northern Westchester Hospital Center, Mount Kisco, N.Y.
	Overlook Hospital, Summit, N.J.
	Robert Wood Johnson University Hospital, New Brunswick, N.J.
	St. Barnabas Medical Center, Livingston, N.J.
	St. Luke's-Roosevelt Hospital Center, New York
	St. Mary's Hospital, Waterbury, Conn.
	St. Vincent's Hospital and Medical Center, New York
	Stamford Hospital, Stamford, Conn.
	University Hospital of Brooklyn-SUNY Center, Brooklyn
	University Hospital, Stony Brook, N.Y.
	Westchester County Medical Center, Valhalla, N.Y.
	Winthrop-University Hospital, Mineola, N.Y.

TIER FOUR

	Brookdale Hospital Medical Center, Brooklyn, N.Y.
	Catholic Medical Center, Jamaica, N.Y.
	Central General Hospital, Plainview, N.Y.
	Christ Hospital, Jersey City, N.J.
	Community Medical Center, Toms River, N.J.
	Coney Island Hospital, Brooklyn, N.Y.
	Elizabeth General Medical Center, Elizabeth, N.J.
	Englewood Hospital, Englewood, N.J.
	Flushing Hospital Medical Center, Flushing, N.Y.
	Franklin Hospital Medical Center, Valley Stream, N.Y.
	Good Samaritan Hospital, Suffern, N.Y.
	Good Samaritan Hospital, West Islip, N.Y.
	Griffin Hospital, Derby, Conn.
	Harlem Hospital Center, New York
	Helene Fuld Medical Center, Trenton, N.J.
	Hospital Center at Orange, Orange, N.J.
	Hunterdon Medical Center, Flemington, N.J.
	Huntington Hospital, Huntington, N.Y.
	JFK Medical Center, Edison, N.J.
	Jamaica Hospital, Jamaica, N.Y.
	Jersey Shore Medical Center, Neptune, N.J.
	John T. Mather Memorial Hospital, Port Jefferson, N.Y.
	Kingsbrook Jewish Medical Center, Brooklyn, N.Y.
	La Guardia Hospital, Flushing, N.Y.
	Lutheran Medical Center, Brooklyn, N.Y.
	Medical Center at Princeton, Princeton, N.J.
	Mercer Medical Center, Trenton, N.J.
	Mercy Medical Center, Rockville Centre, N.Y.
	Monmouth Medical Center, Long Branch, N.J.
	Morristown Memorial Hospital, Morristown, N.J.
	Mount Vernon Hospital, Mount Vernon, N.Y.
	Mountainside Hospital, Montclair, N.J.
	Muhlenberg Regional Medical Center, Plainfield, N.J.
	New Rochelle Hospital Medical Center, New Rochelle, N.Y.
	New York Downtown Hospital
	New York Hospital Medical Center, Flushing
	Newark Beth Israel Medical Center, Newark, N.J.
	North Shore University Hospital-Glen Cove, Glen Cove, N.Y.
	Norwalk Hospital, Norwalk, Conn.
	Nyack Hospital, Nyack, N.Y.
	Our Lady of Mercy Medical Center, Bronx, N.Y.
	Raritan Bay Medical Center, Perth Amboy, N.J.
	Riverview Medical Center, Red Bank, N.J.
	Somerset Medical Center, Somerville, N.J.
	South Nassau Community Hospital, Oceanside, N.Y.
	Southampton Hospital, Southampton, N.Y.
	Southside Hospital, Bay Shore, N.Y.
	St. Barnabas Hospital, Bronx, N.Y.
	St. Charles Hospital and Rehabilitation Center, Port Jefferson, N.Y.
	St. Elizabeth Hospital, Elizabeth, N.J.
	St. Francis Medical Center, Trenton, N.J.
	St. John's Episcopal Hospital, Far Rockaway, N.Y.
	St. John's Episcopal Hospital, Smithtown, N.Y.
	St. Joseph's Hospital and Medical Center, Paterson, N.J.
	St. Joseph's Medical Center, Yonkers, N.Y.
	St. Michael's Medical Center, Newark, N.J.
	St. Peter's Medical Center, New Brunswick, N.J.

	St. Vincent's Medical Center, Bridgeport, Conn.
	St. Vincent's Medical Center, Staten Island, N.Y.
	Staten Island University Hospital, Staten Island, N.Y.
	Valley Hospital, Ridgewood, N.J.
	Vassar Brothers Hospital, Poughkeepsie, N.Y.
	Warren Hospital, Phillipsburg, N.J.
	Waterbury Hospital, Waterbury, Conn.

UROLOGY

TIER ONE

Natl. Rank	Hospital
10	Memorial Sloan-Kettering Cancer Center, New York
12	New York Hospital-Cornell Medical Center
20	Columbia-Presbyterian Medical Center, New York

TIER TWO

Natl. Rank	Hospital
80	Mount Sinai Medical Center, New York
49	New York University Medical Center
89	Stamford Hospital, Stamford, Conn.
41	Yale-New Haven Hospital, New Haven, Conn.

TIER THREE

Natl. Rank	Hospital
	Bellevue Hospital Center, New York
	Beth Israel Medical Center, New York
	Bridgeport Hospital, Bridgeport, Conn.
	Brooklyn Hospital Center, Brooklyn, N.Y.
	Cabrini Medical Center, New York
	Greenwich Hospital, Greenwich, Conn.
	Hackensack Medical Center, Hackensack, N.J.
	Hospital of St. Raphael, New Haven, Conn.
	Hunterdon Medical Center, Flemington, N.J.
	Huntington Hospital, Huntington, N.Y.
	Lenox Hill Hospital, New York
	Lincoln Medical and Mental Health Center, Bronx, N.Y.
	Long Island College Hospital, Brooklyn, N.Y.
	Long Island Jewish Medical Center, New York
	Maimonides Medical Center, Brooklyn, N.Y.
	Methodist Hospital, Brooklyn, N.Y.
	Metropolitan Hospital Center, New York
	Montefiore Medical Center, Bronx, N.Y.
	Nassau County Medical Center, East Meadow, N.Y.
	North Shore University Hospital, Manhasset, N.Y.
	Overlook Hospital, Summit, N.J.
	Robert Wood Johnson University Hospital, New Brunswick, N.J.
	St. Luke's-Roosevelt Hospital Center, New York
	St. Mary's Hospital, Waterbury, Conn.
	St. Vincent's Hospital and Medical Center, New York
	University Hospital of Brooklyn-SUNY Center, Brooklyn
92	University Hospital, Stony Brook, N.Y.
	Westchester County Medical Center, Valhalla, N.Y.

TIER FOUR

	Bergen Pines County Hospital, Paramus, N.J.
	Bronx Municipal Hospital Center, Bronx, N.Y.
	Bronx-Lebanon Hospital Center, Bronx, N.Y.
	Brookdale Hospital Medical Center, Brooklyn, N.Y.
	Catholic Medical Center, Jamaica, N.Y.

Central General Hospital, Plainview, N.Y.

Christ Hospital, Jersey City, N.J.

Community Medical Center, Toms River, N.J.

Coney Island Hospital, Brooklyn, N.Y.

Elizabeth General Medical Center, Elizabeth, N.J.

Englewood Hospital, Englewood, N.J.

Flushing Hospital Medical Center, Flushing, N.Y.

Franklin Hospital Medical Center, Valley Stream, N.Y.

Good Samaritan Hospital, Suffern, N.Y.

Good Samaritan Hospital, West Islip, N.Y.

Griffin Hospital, Derby, Conn.

Helene Fuld Medical Center, Trenton, N.J.

Hospital Center at Orange, Orange, N.J.

JFK Medical Center, Edison, N.J.

Jamaica Hospital, Jamaica, N.Y.

Jersey Shore Medical Center, Neptune, N.J.

John T. Mather Memorial Hospital, Port Jefferson, N.Y.

Kingsbrook Jewish Medical Center, Brooklyn, N.Y.

La Guardia Hospital, Flushing, N.Y.

Lutheran Medical Center, Brooklyn, N.Y.

Medical Center at Princeton, Princeton, N.J.

Mercer Medical Center, Trenton, N.J.

Mercy Medical Center, Rockville Centre, N.Y.

Monmouth Medical Center, Long Branch, N.J.

Morristown Memorial Hospital, Morristown, N.J.

Mount Vernon Hospital, Mount Vernon, N.Y.

Mountainside Hospital, Montclair, N.J.

Muhlenberg Regional Medical Center, Plainfield, N.J.

New Rochelle Hospital Medical Center, New Rochelle, N.Y.

New York Downtown Hospital

New York Hospital Medical Center, Flushing

Newark Beth Israel Medical Center, Newark, N.J.

North Shore University Hospital-Glen Cove, Glen Cove, N.Y.

Northern Westchester Hospital Center, Mount Kisco, N.Y.

Norwalk Hospital, Norwalk, Conn.

Nyack Hospital, Nyack, N.Y.

Our Lady of Mercy Medical Center, Bronx, N.Y.

Raritan Bay Medical Center, Perth Amboy, N.J.

Riverview Medical Center, Red Bank, N.J.

Somerset Medical Center, Somerville, N.J.

South Nassau Community Hospital, Oceanside, N.Y.

Southside Hospital, Bay Shore, N.Y.

St. Barnabas Hospital, Bronx, N.Y.

St. Barnabas Medical Center, Livingston, N.J.

St. Charles Hospital and Rehabilitation Center, Port Jefferson, N.Y.

St. Elizabeth Hospital, Elizabeth, N.J.

St. Francis Medical Center, Trenton, N.J.

St. John's Episcopal Hospital, Far Rockaway, N.Y.

St. John's Episcopal Hospital, Smithtown, N.Y.

St. Joseph's Hospital and Medical Center, Paterson, N.J.

St. Joseph's Medical Center, Yonkers, N.Y.

St. Michael's Medical Center, Newark, N.J.

St. Peter's Medical Center, New Brunswick, N.J.

St. Vincent's Medical Center, Bridgeport, Conn.

St. Vincent's Medical Center, Staten Island, N.Y.

Staten Island University Hospital, Staten Island, N.Y.

Valley Hospital, Ridgewood, N.J.

Vassar Brothers Hospital, Poughkeepsie, N.Y.

Warren Hospital, Phillipsburg, N.J.

Waterbury Hospital, Waterbury, Conn.

Winthrop-University Hospital, Mineola, N.Y.

Philadelphia

AIDS

	TIER ONE
27	Hospital of the University of Pennsylvania, Philadelphia
	TIER TWO
83	Graduate Hospital, Philadelphia
91	Temple University Hospital, Philadelphia
40	Thomas Jefferson University Hospital, Philadelphia
	TIER THREE
	Abington Memorial Hospital, Abington, Pa.
	Albert Einstein Medical Center, Philadelphia
	Atlantic City Medical Center, Atlantic City, N.J.
	Bryn Mawr Hospital, Bryn Mawr, Pa.
	Chester County Hospital, Westchester, Pa.
	Chestnut Hill Hospital, Philadelphia
	Cooper Hospital-University Medical Center, Camden, N.J.
	Frankford Hospital, Philadelphia
	Hahnemann University Hospital, Philadelphia
	Medical Center of Delaware, Wilmington
	Medical College Hospital, Philadelphia
	Paoli Memorial Hospital, Paoli, Pa.
	Presbyterian Medical Center of Philadelphia
	TIER FOUR
	Crozer-Chester Medical Center, Upland, Pa.
	Delaware County Memorial Hospital, Drexel Hill, Pa.
	Delaware Valley Medical Center, Langhorne, Pa.
	Episcopal Hospital, Philadelphia
	Germantown Hospital and Medical Center, Philadelphia
	Kennedy Memorial Hospital–University Med. Ctr., Cherry Hill, N.J.
	Lankenau Hospital, Wynnewood, Pa.
	Lower Bucks Hospital, Bristol, Pa.
	Memorial Hospital of Burlington County, Mount Holly, N.J.
	Mercy Health Corporation, Bala Cynwyd, Pa.
	Methodist Hospital, Philadelphia
	Montgomery Hospital, Norristown, Pa.
	Nazareth Hospital, Philadelphia
	Northeastern Hospital of Philadelphia
	Our Lady of Lourdes Medical Center, Camden, N.J.
	St. Agnes Medical Center, Philadelphia
	St. Francis Hospital, Wilmington, Del.
	Thomas Jefferson University Hospital, Philadelphia
	West Jersey Hospital-Voorhees, Voorhees, N.J.

CANCER

TIER ONE	
14	Hospital of the University of Pennsylvania, Philadelphia

TIER TWO	
19	Fox Chase Cancer Center, Philadelphia
62	Temple University Hospital, Philadelphia
66	Thomas Jefferson University Hospital, Philadelphia

TIER THREE	
96	Albert Einstein Medical Center, Philadelphia
	Bryn Mawr Hospital, Bryn Mawr, Pa.
	Cooper Hospital-University Medical Center, Camden, N.J.
	Crozer-Chester Medical Center, Upland, Pa.
	Frankford Hospital, Philadelphia
	Germantown Hospital and Medical Center, Philadelphia
	Graduate Hospital, Philadelphia
85	Hahnemann University Hospital, Philadelphia
	Lankenau Hospital, Wynnewood, Pa.
	Medical Center of Delaware, Wilmington
98	Medical College Hospital, Philadelphia
	Mercy Health Corporation, Bala Cynwyd, Pa.

TIER FOUR	
	Abington Memorial Hospital, Abington, Pa.
	Atlantic City Medical Center, Atlantic City, N.J.
	Chester County Hospital, Westchester, Pa.
	Chestnut Hill Hospital, Philadelphia
	Delaware County Memorial Hospital, Drexel Hill, Pa.
	Delaware Valley Medical Center, Langhorne, Pa.
	Kennedy Memorial Hospital–University Med. Ctr., Cherry Hill, N.J.
	Lower Bucks Hospital, Bristol, Pa.
	Memorial Hospital of Burlington County, Mount Holly, N.J.
	Methodist Hospital, Philadelphia
	Montgomery Hospital, Norristown, Pa.
	Nazareth Hospital, Philadelphia
	Northeastern Hospital of Philadelphia
	Our Lady of Lourdes Medical Center, Camden, N.J.
	Paoli Memorial Hospital, Paoli, Pa.
	Presbyterian Medical Center of Philadelphia
	St. Agnes Medical Center, Philadelphia
	St. Francis Hospital, Wilmington, Del.
	Underwood-Memorial Hospital, Woodbury, N.J.
	West Jersey Hospital-Voorhees, Voorhees, N.J.

CARDIOLOGY

TIER ONE	
22	Hospital of the University of Pennsylvania, Philadelphia

TIER TWO	
79	Albert Einstein Medical Center, Philadelphia
61	Bryn Mawr Hospital, Bryn Mawr, Pa.
92	Graduate Hospital, Philadelphia
47	Temple University Hospital, Philadelphia
33	Thomas Jefferson University Hospital, Philadelphia

TIER THREE	
	Abington Memorial Hospital, Abington, Pa.

	Atlantic City Medical Center, Atlantic City, N.J.
	Chester County Hospital, Westchester, Pa.
	Chestnut Hill Hospital, Philadelphia
	Crozer-Chester Medical Center, Upland, Pa.
	Deborah Heart and Lung Center, Browns Mills, N.J.
	Delaware County Memorial Hospital, Drexel Hill, Pa.
	Frankford Hospital, Philadelphia
	Hahnemann University Hospital, Philadelphia
	Lankenau Hospital, Wynnewood, Pa.
	Medical Center of Delaware, Wilmington
	Medical College Hospital, Philadelphia
	Methodist Hospital, Philadelphia
	Montgomery Hospital, Norristown, Pa.
	Nazareth Hospital, Philadelphia
	Northeastern Hospital of Philadelphia
	Paoli Memorial Hospital, Paoli, Pa.
	Presbyterian Medical Center of Philadelphia
	St. Agnes Medical Center, Philadelphia
	Underwood-Memorial Hospital, Woodbury, N.J.

TIER FOUR	
	Cooper Hospital-University Medical Center, Camden, N.J.
	Delaware Valley Medical Center, Langhorne, Pa.
	Episcopal Hospital, Philadelphia
	Germantown Hospital and Medical Center, Philadelphia
	Kennedy Memorial Hospital–University Med. Ctr., Cherry Hill, N.J.
	Lower Bucks Hospital, Bristol, Pa.
	Memorial Hospital of Burlington County, Mount Holly, N.J.
	Mercy Health Corporation, Bala Cynwyd, Pa.
	Our Lady of Lourdes Medical Center, Camden, N.J.
	St. Francis Hospital, Wilmington, Del.
	West Jersey Hospital-Voorhees, Voorhees, N.J.

ENDOCRINOLOGY

TIER ONE	
23	Hospital of the University of Pennsylvania, Philadelphia

TIER TWO	
84	Bryn Mawr Hospital, Bryn Mawr, Pa.
70	Temple University Hospital, Philadelphia
50	Thomas Jefferson University Hospital, Philadelphia

TIER THREE	
	Abington Memorial Hospital, Abington, Pa.
	Albert Einstein Medical Center, Philadelphia
	Atlantic City Medical Center, Atlantic City, N.J.
	Chester County Hospital, Westchester, Pa.
	Cooper Hospital-University Medical Center, Camden, N.J.
	Crozer-Chester Medical Center, Upland, Pa.
	Frankford Hospital, Philadelphia
	Graduate Hospital, Philadelphia
88	Hahnemann University Hospital, Philadelphia
	Medical Center of Delaware, Wilmington
	Medical College Hospital, Philadelphia
	Methodist Hospital, Philadelphia
	Montgomery Hospital, Norristown, Pa.

TIER FOUR	
	Chestnut Hill Hospital, Philadelphia

Natl. Rank	Hospital
	Delaware County Memorial Hospital, Drexel Hill, Pa.
	Delaware Valley Medical Center, Langhorne, Pa.
	Episcopal Hospital, Philadelphia
	Germantown Hospital and Medical Center, Philadelphia
	Kennedy Memorial Hospital–University Med. Ctr., Cherry Hill, N.J.
	Lankenau Hospital, Wynnewood, Pa.
	Lower Bucks Hospital, Bristol, Pa.
	Memorial Hospital of Burlington County, Mount Holly, N.J.
	Mercy Health Corporation, Bala Cynwyd, Pa.
	Nazareth Hospital, Philadelphia
	Northeastern Hospital of Philadelphia
	Our Lady of Lourdes Medical Center, Camden, N.J.
	Paoli Memorial Hospital, Paoli, Pa.
	Presbyterian Medical Center of Philadelphia
	St. Agnes Medical Center, Philadelphia
	St. Francis Hospital, Wilmington, Del.
	Underwood-Memorial Hospital, Woodbury, N.J.
	West Jersey Hospital-Voorhees, Voorhees, N.J.

GASTROENTEROLOGY

Natl. Rank	Hospital
TIER ONE	
13	Hospital of the University of Pennsylvania, Philadelphia
TIER TWO	
71	Graduate Hospital, Philadelphia
73	Temple University Hospital, Philadelphia
35	Thomas Jefferson University Hospital, Philadelphia
TIER THREE	
	Abington Memorial Hospital, Abington, Pa.
	Albert Einstein Medical Center, Philadelphia
	Bryn Mawr Hospital, Bryn Mawr, Pa.
	Chester County Hospital, Westchester, Pa.
	Chestnut Hill Hospital, Philadelphia
	Cooper Hospital-University Medical Center, Camden, N.J.
	Crozer-Chester Medical Center, Upland, Pa.
	Frankford Hospital, Philadelphia
	Hahnemann University Hospital, Philadelphia
	Lankenau Hospital, Wynnewood, Pa.
	Medical Center of Delaware, Wilmington
	Medical College Hospital, Philadelphia
	Paoli Memorial Hospital, Paoli, Pa.
89	West Jersey Hospital-Voorhees, Voorhees, N.J.
TIER FOUR	
	Atlantic City Medical Center, Atlantic City, N.J.
	Delaware County Memorial Hospital, Drexel Hill, Pa.
	Germantown Hospital and Medical Center, Philadelphia
	Kennedy Memorial Hospital–University Med. Ctr., Cherry Hill, N.J.
	Lower Bucks Hospital, Bristol, Pa.
	Memorial Hospital of Burlington County, Mount Holly, N.J.
	Mercy Health Corporation, Bala Cynwyd, Pa.
	Methodist Hospital, Philadelphia
	Montgomery Hospital, Norristown, Pa.
	Nazareth Hospital, Philadelphia
	Northeastern Hospital of Philadelphia
	Our Lady of Lourdes Medical Center, Camden, N.J.
	Presbyterian Medical Center of Philadelphia

Natl. Rank	Hospital
	St. Agnes Medical Center, Philadelphia
	St. Francis Hospital, Wilmington, Del.
	Underwood-Memorial Hospital, Woodbury, N.J.

GERIATRICS

Natl. Rank	Hospital
TIER ONE	
23	Hospital of the University of Pennsylvania, Philadelphia
TIER TWO	
36	Albert Einstein Medical Center, Philadelphia
81	Bryn Mawr Hospital, Bryn Mawr, Pa.
79	Temple University Hospital, Philadelphia
34	Thomas Jefferson University Hospital, Philadelphia
TIER THREE	
	Abington Memorial Hospital, Abington, Pa.
	Atlantic City Medical Center, Atlantic City, N.J.
	Chester County Hospital, Westchester, Pa.
	Crozer-Chester Medical Center, Upland, Pa.
	Frankford Hospital, Philadelphia
	Graduate Hospital, Philadelphia
	Hahnemann University Hospital, Philadelphia
	Medical Center of Delaware, Wilmington
	Medical College Hospital, Philadelphia
	Paoli Memorial Hospital, Paoli, Pa.
TIER FOUR	
	Chestnut Hill Hospital, Philadelphia
	Cooper Hospital-University Medical Center, Camden, N.J.
	Delaware Valley Medical Center, Langhorne, Pa.
	Germantown Hospital and Medical Center, Philadelphia
	Kennedy Memorial Hospital–University Med. Ctr., Cherry Hill, N.J.
	Lankenau Hospital, Wynnewood, Pa.
	Lower Bucks Hospital, Bristol, Pa.
	Memorial Hospital of Burlington County, Mount Holly, N.J.
	Mercy Health Corporation, Bala Cynwyd, Pa.
	Methodist Hospital, Philadelphia
	Montgomery Hospital, Norristown, Pa.
	Nazareth Hospital, Philadelphia
	Northeastern Hospital of Philadelphia
	Our Lady of Lourdes Medical Center, Camden, N.J.
	Presbyterian Medical Center of Philadelphia
	St. Agnes Medical Center, Philadelphia
	St. Francis Hospital, Wilmington, Del.
	Underwood-Memorial Hospital, Woodbury, N.J.
	West Jersey Hospital-Voorhees, Voorhees, N.J.

GYNECOLOGY

Natl. Rank	Hospital
TIER ONE	
15	Hospital of the University of Pennsylvania, Philadelphia
22	Thomas Jefferson University Hospital, Philadelphia
TIER TWO	
63	Temple University Hospital, Philadelphia
TIER THREE	
	Abington Memorial Hospital, Abington, Pa.

METRO RANKINGS ■ PHILADELPHIA

Natl. Rank	Hospital
	Albert Einstein Medical Center, Philadelphia
	Atlantic City Medical Center, Atlantic City, N.J.
98	Bryn Mawr Hospital, Bryn Mawr, Pa.
	Chester County Hospital, Westchester, Pa.
	Chestnut Hill Hospital, Philadelphia
	Frankford Hospital, Philadelphia
	Graduate Hospital, Philadelphia
	Hahnemann University Hospital, Philadelphia
	Lankenau Hospital, Wynnewood, Pa.
	Medical Center of Delaware, Wilmington
	Medical College Hospital, Philadelphia
	Paoli Memorial Hospital, Paoli, Pa.

TIER FOUR

Natl. Rank	Hospital
	Cooper Hospital-University Medical Center, Camden, N.J.
	Crozer-Chester Medical Center, Upland, Pa.
	Delaware County Memorial Hospital, Drexel Hill, Pa.
	Delaware Valley Medical Center, Langhorne, Pa.
	Germantown Hospital and Medical Center, Philadelphia
	Kennedy Memorial Hospital–University Med. Ctr., Cherry Hill, N.J.
	Lower Bucks Hospital, Bristol, Pa.
	Memorial Hospital of Burlington County, Mount Holly, N.J.
	Mercy Health Corporation, Bala Cynwyd, Pa.
	Methodist Hospital, Philadelphia
	Montgomery Hospital, Norristown, Pa.
	Nazareth Hospital, Philadelphia
	Northeastern Hospital of Philadelphia
	Our Lady of Lourdes Medical Center, Camden, N.J.
	Presbyterian Medical Center of Philadelphia
	St. Agnes Medical Center, Philadelphia
	St. Francis Hospital, Wilmington, Del.
	Underwood-Memorial Hospital, Woodbury, N.J.
	West Jersey Hospital-Voorhees, Voorhees, N.J.

NEUROLOGY

Natl. Rank	Hospital

TIER ONE
Natl. Rank	Hospital
10	Hospital of the University of Pennsylvania, Philadelphia

TIER TWO
Natl. Rank	Hospital
65	Bryn Mawr Hospital, Bryn Mawr, Pa.
56	Graduate Hospital, Philadelphia
55	Medical College Hospital, Philadelphia
34	Temple University Hospital, Philadelphia
26	Thomas Jefferson University Hospital, Philadelphia

TIER THREE
Natl. Rank	Hospital
	Abington Memorial Hospital, Abington, Pa.
	Albert Einstein Medical Center, Philadelphia
	Frankford Hospital, Philadelphia
	Germantown Hospital and Medical Center, Philadelphia
	Hahnemann University Hospital, Philadelphia
	Lankenau Hospital, Wynnewood, Pa.
	Medical Center of Delaware, Wilmington
	West Jersey Hospital-Voorhees, Voorhees, N.J.

TIER FOUR
Natl. Rank	Hospital
	Atlantic City Medical Center, Atlantic City, N.J.
	Chester County Hospital, Westchester, Pa.
	Chestnut Hill Hospital, Philadelphia

Natl. Rank	Hospital
	Cooper Hospital-University Medical Center, Camden, N.J.
	Crozer-Chester Medical Center, Upland, Pa.
	Delaware County Memorial Hospital, Drexel Hill, Pa.
	Delaware Valley Medical Center, Langhorne, Pa.
	Kennedy Memorial Hospital–University Med. Ctr., Cherry Hill, N.J.
	Lower Bucks Hospital, Bristol, Pa.
	Memorial Hospital of Burlington County, Mount Holly, N.J.
	Mercy Health Corporation, Bala Cynwyd, Pa.
	Methodist Hospital, Philadelphia
	Montgomery Hospital, Norristown, Pa.
	Nazareth Hospital, Philadelphia
	Northeastern Hospital of Philadelphia
	Our Lady of Lourdes Medical Center, Camden, N.J.
	Paoli Memorial Hospital, Paoli, Pa.
	Presbyterian Medical Center of Philadelphia
	St. Agnes Medical Center, Philadelphia
	St. Francis Hospital, Wilmington, Del.
	Underwood-Memorial Hospital, Woodbury, N.J.

ORTHOPEDICS

Natl. Rank	Hospital

TIER ONE
Natl. Rank	Hospital
11	Hospital of the University of Pennsylvania, Philadelphia
17	Thomas Jefferson University Hospital, Philadelphia

TIER TWO
Natl. Rank	Hospital
59	Temple University Hospital, Philadelphia

TIER THREE
Natl. Rank	Hospital
	Albert Einstein Medical Center, Philadelphia
	Bryn Mawr Hospital, Bryn Mawr, Pa.
	Chester County Hospital, Westchester, Pa.
	Chestnut Hill Hospital, Philadelphia
	Cooper Hospital-University Medical Center, Camden, N.J.
	Crozer-Chester Medical Center, Upland, Pa.
	Frankford Hospital, Philadelphia
	Germantown Hospital and Medical Center, Philadelphia
	Graduate Hospital, Philadelphia
	Hahnemann University Hospital, Philadelphia
	Lower Bucks Hospital, Bristol, Pa.
	Medical Center of Delaware, Wilmington
	Medical College Hospital, Philadelphia
	West Jersey Hospital-Voorhees, Voorhees, N.J.

TIER FOUR
Natl. Rank	Hospital
	Abington Memorial Hospital, Abington, Pa.
	Atlantic City Medical Center, Atlantic City, N.J.
	Delaware County Memorial Hospital, Drexel Hill, Pa.
	Kennedy Memorial Hospital–University Med. Ctr., Cherry Hill, N.J.
	Lankenau Hospital, Wynnewood, Pa.
	Memorial Hospital of Burlington County, Mount Holly, N.J.
	Mercy Health Corporation, Bala Cynwyd, Pa.
	Methodist Hospital, Philadelphia
	Montgomery Hospital, Norristown, Pa.
	Nazareth Hospital, Philadelphia
	Northeastern Hospital of Philadelphia
	Our Lady of Lourdes Medical Center, Camden, N.J.
	Paoli Memorial Hospital, Paoli, Pa.
	Shriners Hospital for Crippled Children, Philadelphia

	St. Agnes Medical Center, Philadelphia
	St. Francis Hospital, Wilmington, Del.
	Underwood-Memorial Hospital, Woodbury, N.J.

OTOLARYNGOLOGY

Natl.
Rank   Hospital

Natl. Rank	Hospital
TIER ONE	
25	Hospital of the University of Pennsylvania, Philadelphia
TIER TWO	
63	Hospital of the Philadelphia College of Osteopathic Medicine
	Medical College Hospital, Philadelphia
87	Temple University Hospital, Philadelphia
57	Thomas Jefferson University Hospital, Philadelphia
TIER THREE	
	Albert Einstein Medical Center, Philadelphia
	Bryn Mawr Hospital, Bryn Mawr, Pa.
	Cooper Hospital-University Medical Center, Camden, N.J.
	Crozer-Chester Medical Center, Upland, Pa.
	Delaware Valley Medical Center, Langhorne, Pa.
	Episcopal Hospital, Philadelphia
	Fox Chase Cancer Center, Philadelphia
	Frankford Hospital, Philadelphia
	Germantown Hospital and Medical Center, Philadelphia
	Graduate Hospital, Philadelphia
	Hahnemann University Hospital, Philadelphia
	Lankenau Hospital, Wynnewood, Pa.
	Medical Center of Delaware, Wilmington
	Mercy Health Corporation, Bala Cynwyd, Pa.
	Methodist Hospital, Philadelphia
TIER FOUR	
	Abington Memorial Hospital, Abington, Pa.
	Atlantic City Medical Center, Atlantic City, N.J.
	Chester County Hospital, Westchester, Pa.
	Chestnut Hill Hospital, Philadelphia
	Deborah Heart and Lung Center, Browns Mills, N.J.
	Delaware County Memorial Hospital, Drexel Hill, Pa.
	Kennedy Memorial Hospital–University Med. Ctr., Cherry Hill, N.J.
	Lower Bucks Hospital, Bristol, Pa.
	Memorial Hospital of Burlington County, Mount Holly, N.J.
	Montgomery Hospital, Norristown, Pa.
	Nazareth Hospital, Philadelphia
	Northeastern Hospital of Philadelphia
	Our Lady of Lourdes Medical Center, Camden, N.J.
	Paoli Memorial Hospital, Paoli, Pa.
	Presbyterian Medical Center of Philadelphia
	St. Agnes Medical Center, Philadelphia
	St. Francis Hospital, Wilmington, Del.
	Thomas Jefferson University Hospital, Philadelphia
	Underwood-Memorial Hospital, Woodbury, N.J.
	West Jersey Hospital-Voorhees, Voorhees, N.J.

RHEUMATOLOGY

Natl.
Rank   Hospital

Natl. Rank	Hospital
TIER ONE	
19	Hospital of the University of Pennsylvania, Philadelphia
TIER TWO	
72	Hospital of the Philadelphia College of Osteopathic Medicine
35	Thomas Jefferson University Hospital, Philadelphia
TIER THREE	
	Abington Memorial Hospital, Abington, Pa.
	Albert Einstein Medical Center, Philadelphia
	Bryn Mawr Hospital, Bryn Mawr, Pa.
	Chestnut Hill Hospital, Philadelphia
	Cooper Hospital-University Medical Center, Camden, N.J.
	Crozer-Chester Medical Center, Upland, Pa.
	Deborah Heart and Lung Center, Browns Mills, N.J.
	Delaware Valley Medical Center, Langhorne, Pa.
	Frankford Hospital, Philadelphia
	Germantown Hospital and Medical Center, Philadelphia
	Graduate Hospital, Philadelphia
	Hahnemann University Hospital, Philadelphia
	Lankenau Hospital, Wynnewood, Pa.
	Medical Center of Delaware, Wilmington
100	Medical College Hospital, Philadelphia
	Methodist Hospital, Philadelphia
	Paoli Memorial Hospital, Paoli, Pa.
	Presbyterian Medical Center of Philadelphia
86	Temple University Hospital, Philadelphia
	Wills Eye Hospital, Philadelphia
TIER FOUR	
	Atlantic City Medical Center, Atlantic City, N.J.
	Chester County Hospital, Westchester, Pa.
	Delaware County Memorial Hospital, Drexel Hill, Pa.
	Episcopal Hospital, Philadelphia
	Kennedy Memorial Hospital–University Med. Ctr., Cherry Hill, N.J.
	Lower Bucks Hospital, Bristol, Pa.
	Memorial Hospital of Burlington County, Mount Holly, N.J.
	Mercy Health Corporation, Bala Cynwyd, Pa.
	Montgomery Hospital, Norristown, Pa.
	Nazareth Hospital, Philadelphia
	Northeastern Hospital of Philadelphia
	Our Lady of Lourdes Medical Center, Camden, N.J.
	St. Agnes Medical Center, Philadelphia
	St. Francis Hospital, Wilmington, Del.
	Underwood-Memorial Hospital, Woodbury, N.J.
	West Jersey Hospital-Voorhees, Voorhees, N.J.

UROLOGY

Natl.
Rank   Hospital

Natl. Rank	Hospital
TIER ONE	
17	Hospital of the University of Pennsylvania, Philadelphia
TIER TWO	
64	Graduate Hospital, Philadelphia
55	Temple University Hospital, Philadelphia
26	Thomas Jefferson University Hospital, Philadelphia

TIER THREE	
Abington Memorial Hospital, Abington, Pa.	
Albert Einstein Medical Center, Philadelphia	
Bryn Mawr Hospital, Bryn Mawr, Pa.	
Frankford Hospital, Philadelphia	
Germantown Hospital and Medical Center, Philadelphia	
Hahnemann University Hospital, Philadelphia	
Medical Center of Delaware, Wilmington	
Medical College Hospital, Philadelphia	
Paoli Memorial Hospital, Paoli, Pa.	
TIER FOUR	
Atlantic City Medical Center, Atlantic City, N.J.	
Chester County Hospital, Westchester, Pa.	
Chestnut Hill Hospital, Philadelphia	
Cooper Hospital-University Medical Center, Camden, N.J.	
Crozer-Chester Medical Center, Upland, Pa.	
Delaware County Memorial Hospital, Drexel Hill, Pa.	
Delaware Valley Medical Center, Langhorne, Pa.	
Kennedy Memorial Hospital–University Med. Ctr., Cherry Hill, N.J.	
Lankenau Hospital, Wynnewood, Pa.	
Lower Bucks Hospital, Bristol, Pa.	
Memorial Hospital of Burlington County, Mount Holly, N.J.	
Mercy Health Corporation, Bala Cynwyd, Pa.	
Methodist Hospital, Philadelphia	
Montgomery Hospital, Norristown, Pa.	
Nazareth Hospital, Philadelphia	
Northeastern Hospital of Philadelphia	
Our Lady of Lourdes Medical Center, Camden, N.J.	
Presbyterian Medical Center of Philadelphia	
St. Agnes Medical Center, Philadelphia	
St. Francis Hospital, Wilmington, Del.	
Underwood-Memorial Hospital, Woodbury, N.J.	
West Jersey Hospital-Voorhees, Voorhees, N.J.	

San Francisco

AIDS

TIER ONE	
1	San Francisco General Hospital Medical Center
4	University of California, San Francisco Medical Center
11	Stanford University Hospital, Stanford, Calif.
TIER THREE	
Alta Bates Medical Center, Berkeley, Calif.	
Davies Medical Center, San Francisco	
Highland General Hospital, Oakland, Calif.	
Kaiser Foundation Hospital, Oakland, Calif.	
Kaiser Foundation Hospital, Redwood City, Calif.	
Kaiser Foundation Hospital, San Francisco	
Kaiser Foundation Hospital, Santa Clara, Calif.	
Mills-Peninsula Hospitals, Burlingame, Calif.	
O'Connor Hospital, San Jose, Calif.	
Queen of the Valley Hospital, Napa, Calif.	

Santa Clara Veterans Affairs Medical Center, San Jose, Calif.	
Sequoia Hospital District, Redwood City, Calif.	
Seton Medical Center, Daly City, Calif.	
St. Mary's Hospital and Medical Center, San Francisco	
Washington Hospital, Fremont, Calif.	
TIER FOUR	
Brookside Hospital, San Pablo, Calif.	
Community Hospital, Santa Rosa, Calif.	
Good Samaritan Hospital, San Jose, Calif.	
John Muir Medical Center, Walnut Creek, Calif.	
Kaiser Foundation Hospital, Walnut Creek, Calif.	
Marin General Hospital, Greenbrae, Calif.	
Merrithew Memorial Hospital, Martinez, Calif.	
Northbay Medical Center, Fairfield, Calif.	
San Jose Medical Center, San Jose, Calif.	
Santa Rosa Memorial Hospital, Santa Rosa, Calif.	
St. Francis Memorial Hospital, San Francisco	

CANCER

TIER ONE	
6	Stanford University Hospital, Stanford, Calif.
11	University of California, San Francisco Medical Center
TIER THREE	
California Pacific Medical Center, San Francisco	
Kaiser Foundation Hospital, Santa Clara, Calif.	
St. Mary's Hospital and Medical Center, San Francisco	
TIER FOUR	
Alta Bates Medical Center, Berkeley, Calif.	
Brookside Hospital, San Pablo, Calif.	
Good Samaritan Hospital, San Jose, Calif.	
John Muir Medical Center, Walnut Creek, Calif.	
Kaiser Foundation Hospital, Oakland, Calif.	
Kaiser Foundation Hospital, Redwood City, Calif.	
Kaiser Foundation Hospital, San Francisco	
Kaiser Foundation Hospital, Walnut Creek, Calif.	
Marin General Hospital, Greenbrae, Calif.	
Mills-Peninsula Hospitals, Burlingame, Calif.	
Mount Diablo Medical Center, Concord, Calif.	
Mount Zion Medical Center, San Francisco	
O'Connor Hospital, San Jose, Calif.	
Queen of the Valley Hospital, Napa, Calif.	
San Jose Medical Center, San Jose, Calif.	
Santa Rosa Memorial Hospital, Santa Rosa, Calif.	
Sequoia Hospital District, Redwood City, Calif.	
St. Francis Memorial Hospital, San Francisco	
Washington Hospital, Fremont, Calif.	

CARDIOLOGY

ENDOCRINOLOGY

GASTROENTEROLOGY

GERIATRICS

TIER FOUR
Brookside Hospital, San Pablo, Calif.
Good Samaritan Hospital, San Jose, Calif.
John Muir Medical Center, Walnut Creek, Calif.
Kaiser Foundation Hospital, Walnut Creek, Calif.
Marin General Hospital, Greenbrae, Calif.
Mount Diablo Medical Center, Concord, Calif.
San Jose Medical Center, San Jose, Calif.
Santa Rosa Memorial Hospital, Santa Rosa, Calif.
St. Francis Memorial Hospital, San Francisco

GYNECOLOGY

Natl. Rank	TIER ONE
13	Stanford University Hospital, Stanford, Calif.
14	University of California, San Francisco Medical Center
	TIER TWO
56	California Pacific Medical Center, San Francisco
	TIER THREE
	Alta Bates Medical Center, Berkeley, Calif.
	Kaiser Foundation Hospital, San Francisco
	Kaiser Foundation Hospital, Santa Clara, Calif.
	O'Connor Hospital, San Jose, Calif.
	Queen of the Valley Hospital, Napa, Calif.
	Sequoia Hospital District, Redwood City, Calif.
	Washington Hospital, Fremont, Calif.
	TIER FOUR
	Brookside Hospital, San Pablo, Calif.
	Good Samaritan Hospital, San Jose, Calif.
	John Muir Medical Center, Walnut Creek, Calif.
	Kaiser Foundation Hospital, Oakland, Calif.
	Kaiser Foundation Hospital, Walnut Creek, Calif.
	Marin General Hospital, Greenbrae, Calif.
	Mount Diablo Medical Center, Concord, Calif.
	San Jose Medical Center, San Jose, Calif.
	Santa Rosa Memorial Hospital, Santa Rosa, Calif.
	St. Francis Memorial Hospital, San Francisco
	St. Mary's Hospital and Medical Center, San Francisco

NEUROLOGY

Natl. Rank	TIER ONE
3	University of California, San Francisco Medical Center
15	Stanford University Hospital, Stanford, Calif.
	TIER TWO
54	California Pacific Medical Center, San Francisco
	TIER THREE
	Good Samaritan Hospital, San Jose, Calif.
	Kaiser Foundation Hospital, Oakland, Calif.
	Kaiser Foundation Hospital, Redwood City, Calif.
	Kaiser Foundation Hospital, San Francisco
	Queen of the Valley Hospital, Napa, Calif.
93	San Francisco General Hospital Medical Center

Sequoia Hospital District, Redwood City, Calif.
St. Mary's Hospital and Medical Center, San Francisco
Washington Hospital, Fremont, Calif.
TIER FOUR
Alta Bates Medical Center, Berkeley, Calif.
Brookside Hospital, San Pablo, Calif.
John Muir Medical Center, Walnut Creek, Calif.
Kaiser Foundation Hospital, Santa Clara, Calif.
Marin General Hospital, Greenbrae, Calif.
Mills-Peninsula Hospitals, Burlingame, Calif.
Mount Diablo Medical Center, Concord, Calif.
Mount Zion Medical Center, San Francisco
O'Connor Hospital, San Jose, Calif.
San Jose Medical Center, San Jose, Calif.
Santa Rosa Memorial Hospital, Santa Rosa, Calif.
St. Francis Memorial Hospital, San Francisco

ORTHOPEDICS

Natl. Rank	TIER ONE
12	Stanford University Hospital, Stanford, Calif.
	TIER TWO
55	University of California, San Francisco Medical Center
	TIER THREE
	Alta Bates Medical Center, Berkeley, Calif.
	California Pacific Medical Center, San Francisco
	Kaiser Foundation Hospital, Oakland, Calif.
	Kaiser Foundation Hospital, Santa Clara, Calif.
	Mills-Peninsula Hospitals, Burlingame, Calif.
	Mount Diablo Medical Center, Concord, Calif.
	St. Mary's Hospital and Medical Center, San Francisco
	TIER FOUR
	Brookside Hospital, San Pablo, Calif.
	Good Samaritan Hospital, San Jose, Calif.
	John Muir Medical Center, Walnut Creek, Calif.
	Kaiser Foundation Hospital, Redwood City, Calif.
	Kaiser Foundation Hospital, San Francisco
	Kaiser Foundation Hospital, Walnut Creek, Calif.
	Marin General Hospital, Greenbrae, Calif.
	O'Connor Hospital, San Jose, Calif.
	Queen of the Valley Hospital, Napa, Calif.
	San Jose Medical Center, San Jose, Calif.
	Santa Rosa Memorial Hospital, Santa Rosa, Calif.
	Sequoia Hospital District, Redwood City, Calif.
	St. Francis Memorial Hospital, San Francisco
	Washington Hospital, Fremont, Calif.

OTOLARYNGOLOGY

TIER ONE	
11	Stanford University Hospital, Stanford, Calif.
16	University of California, San Francisco Medical Center

TIER THREE
California Pacific Medical Center, San Francisco
Good Samaritan Hospital, San Jose, Calif.
Kaiser Foundation Hospital, Santa Clara, Calif.
San Francisco General Hospital Medical Center
Santa Clara Veterans Affairs Medical Center, San Jose, Calif.
St. Mary's Hospital and Medical Center, San Francisco

TIER FOUR
Alta Bates Medical Center, Berkeley, Calif.
Brookside Hospital, San Pablo, Calif.
Community Hospital, Santa Rosa, Calif.
Davies Medical Center, San Francisco
Highland General Hospital, Oakland, Calif.
John Muir Medical Center, Walnut Creek, Calif.
Kaiser Foundation Hospital, Oakland, Calif.
Kaiser Foundation Hospital, Redwood City, Calif.
Kaiser Foundation Hospital, San Francisco
Kaiser Foundation Hospital, Walnut Creek, Calif.
Marin General Hospital, Greenbrae, Calif.
Merrithew Memorial Hospital, Martinez, Calif.
Mills-Peninsula Hospitals, Burlingame, Calif.
Mount Diablo Medical Center, Concord, Calif.
Mount Zion Medical Center, San Francisco
Northbay Medical Center, Fairfield, Calif.
O'Connor Hospital, San Jose, Calif.
Queen of the Valley Hospital, Napa, Calif.
San Jose Medical Center, San Jose, Calif.
Santa Rosa Memorial Hospital, Santa Rosa, Calif.
Sequoia Hospital District, Redwood City, Calif.
Seton Medical Center, Daly City, Calif.
St. Francis Memorial Hospital, San Francisco
Washington Hospital, Fremont, Calif.

RHEUMATOLOGY

TIER ONE	
11	Stanford University Hospital, Stanford, Calif.
15	University of California, San Francisco Medical Center

TIER TWO	
81	California Pacific Medical Center, San Francisco

TIER THREE
Kaiser Foundation Hospital, Redwood City, Calif.
Kaiser Foundation Hospital, San Francisco
Kaiser Foundation Hospital, Santa Clara, Calif.
Queen of the Valley Hospital, Napa, Calif.
St. Mary's Hospital and Medical Center, San Francisco
Washington Hospital, Fremont, Calif.

TIER FOUR
Alta Bates Medical Center, Berkeley, Calif.
Brookside Hospital, San Pablo, Calif.

Good Samaritan Hospital, San Jose, Calif.
John Muir Medical Center, Walnut Creek, Calif.
Kaiser Foundation Hospital, Oakland, Calif.
Kaiser Foundation Hospital, Walnut Creek, Calif.
Marin General Hospital, Greenbrae, Calif.
Mills-Peninsula Hospitals, Burlingame, Calif.
Mount Diablo Medical Center, Concord, Calif.
Mount Zion Medical Center, San Francisco
O'Connor Hospital, San Jose, Calif.
San Jose Medical Center, San Jose, Calif.
Santa Rosa Memorial Hospital, Santa Rosa, Calif.
Sequoia Hospital District, Redwood City, Calif.
St. Francis Memorial Hospital, San Francisco

UROLOGY

TIER ONE	
5	Stanford University Hospital, Stanford, Calif.
13	University of California, San Francisco Medical Center

TIER TWO	
63	California Pacific Medical Center, San Francisco

TIER THREE
Alta Bates Medical Center, Berkeley, Calif.
Kaiser Foundation Hospital, San Francisco
Kaiser Foundation Hospital, Santa Clara, Calif.
Queen of the Valley Hospital, Napa, Calif.
Santa Clara Veterans Affairs Medical Center, San Jose, Calif.
Sequoia Hospital District, Redwood City, Calif.
St. Francis Memorial Hospital, San Francisco
St. Mary's Hospital and Medical Center, San Francisco
Washington Hospital, Fremont, Calif.

TIER FOUR
Brookside Hospital, San Pablo, Calif.
Good Samaritan Hospital, San Jose, Calif.
John Muir Medical Center, Walnut Creek, Calif.
Kaiser Foundation Hospital, Oakland, Calif.
Kaiser Foundation Hospital, Redwood City, Calif.
Kaiser Foundation Hospital, Walnut Creek, Calif.
Marin General Hospital, Greenbrae, Calif.
Mills-Peninsula Hospitals, Burlingame, Calif.
Mount Diablo Medical Center, Concord, Calif.
Mount Zion Medical Center, San Francisco
O'Connor Hospital, San Jose, Calif.
San Jose Medical Center, San Jose, Calif.
Santa Rosa Memorial Hospital, Santa Rosa, Calif.

Washington, D.C.–Baltimore

AIDS

CANCER

CARDIOLOGY

TIER FOUR
Arlington Hospital, Arlington, Va.
Francis Scott Key Medical Center, Baltimore
Greater Southeast Community Hospital, Washington, D.C.
Howard County General Hospital, Columbia, Md.
Mary Washington Hospital, Fredericksburg, Va.
Prince George's Hospital Center, Cheverly, Md.
Providence Hospital, Washington, D.C.
Sibley Memorial Hospital, Washington, D.C.
St. Agnes Hospital, Baltimore

ENDOCRINOLOGY

Natl.
Rank   Hospital

Rank	TIER ONE
4	Johns Hopkins Hospital, Baltimore

Rank	TIER TWO
67	George Washington University Hospital, Washington, D.C.
69	Georgetown University Hospital, Washington, D.C.
57	University of Maryland Medical System, Baltimore

Rank	TIER THREE
	Anne Arundel Medical Center, Annapolis, Md.
	Fairfax Hospital, Falls Church, Va.
	Franklin Square Hospital Center, Baltimore
	Greater Baltimore Medical Center
	Harbor Hospital Center, Baltimore
	Holy Cross Hospital, Silver Spring, Md.
98	Howard University Hospital, Washington, D.C.
	Sinai Hospital of Baltimore, Baltimore

TIER FOUR
Alexandria Hospital, Alexandria, Va.
Arlington Hospital, Arlington, Va.
District of Columbia General Hospital, Washington, D.C.
Fair Oaks Hospital, Fairfax, Va.
Francis Scott Key Medical Center, Baltimore
Good Samaritan Hospital, Baltimore
Greater Southeast Community Hospital, Washington, D.C.
Howard County General Hospital, Columbia, Md.
Mary Washington Hospital, Fredericksburg, Va.
Maryland General Hospital, Baltimore
Mercy Medical Center, Baltimore
Northwest Hospital Center, Randallstown, Md.
Prince George's Hospital Center, Cheverly, Md.
Providence Hospital, Washington, D.C.
Sibley Memorial Hospital, Washington, D.C.
St. Agnes Hospital, Baltimore
Suburban Hospital, Bethesda, Md.
Union Memorial Hospital, Baltimore
Washington Adventist Hospital, Takoma Park, Md.
Washington County Hospital Assn., Hagerstown, Md.
Washington Hospital Center, Washington, D.C.

GASTROENTEROLOGY

Natl.
Rank   Hospital

Rank	TIER ONE
2	Johns Hopkins Hospital, Baltimore
19	Georgetown University Hospital, Washington, D.C.

Rank	TIER TWO
69	Sinai Hospital of Baltimore, Baltimore
38	University of Maryland Medical System, Baltimore

Rank	TIER THREE
	Anne Arundel Medical Center, Annapolis, Md.
	Fairfax Hospital, Falls Church, Va.
	Francis Scott Key Medical Center, Baltimore
	Franklin Square Hospital Center, Baltimore
75	George Washington University Hospital, Washington, D.C.
	Greater Baltimore Medical Center
	Holy Cross Hospital, Silver Spring, Md.
	Maryland General Hospital, Baltimore
	Mercy Medical Center, Baltimore
	Northwest Hospital Center, Randallstown, Md.
	Washington County Hospital Assn., Hagerstown, Md.

TIER FOUR
Alexandria Hospital, Alexandria, Va.
Arlington Hospital, Arlington, Va.
Good Samaritan Hospital, Baltimore
Greater Southeast Community Hospital, Washington, D.C.
Harbor Hospital Center, Baltimore
Howard County General Hospital, Columbia, Md.
Mary Washington Hospital, Fredericksburg, Va.
Prince George's Hospital Center, Cheverly, Md.
Providence Hospital, Washington, D.C.
Sibley Memorial Hospital, Washington, D.C.
St. Agnes Hospital, Baltimore
Suburban Hospital, Bethesda, Md.
Union Memorial Hospital, Baltimore
Washington Adventist Hospital, Takoma Park, Md.
Washington Hospital Center, Washington, D.C.

GERIATRICS

Natl.
Rank   Hospital

Rank	TIER ONE
6	Johns Hopkins Hospital, Baltimore

Rank	TIER TWO
66	Francis Scott Key Medical Center, Baltimore
44	Georgetown University Hospital, Washington, D.C.
59	Greater Baltimore Medical Center
73	Sinai Hospital of Baltimore, Baltimore
48	University of Maryland Medical System, Baltimore

TIER THREE
Anne Arundel Medical Center, Annapolis, Md.
Fairfax Hospital, Falls Church, Va.
Franklin Square Hospital Center, Baltimore
George Washington University Hospital, Washington, D.C.
Harbor Hospital Center, Baltimore
Holy Cross Hospital, Silver Spring, Md.
Howard University Hospital, Washington, D.C.

	Mercy Medical Center, Baltimore
	Suburban Hospital, Bethesda, Md.
	Union Memorial Hospital, Baltimore
	Washington County Hospital Assn., Hagerstown, Md.
TIER FOUR	
	Alexandria Hospital, Alexandria, Va.
	Arlington Hospital, Arlington, Va.
	Good Samaritan Hospital, Baltimore
	Greater Southeast Community Hospital, Washington, D.C.
	Howard County General Hospital, Columbia, Md.
	Mary Washington Hospital, Fredericksburg, Va.
	Maryland General Hospital, Baltimore
	Northwest Hospital Center, Randallstown, Md.
	Prince George's Hospital Center, Cheverly, Md.
	Providence Hospital, Washington, D.C.
	Sibley Memorial Hospital, Washington, D.C.
	Spring Grove Hospital Center, Catonsville, Md.
	St. Agnes Hospital, Baltimore
	Washington Adventist Hospital, Takoma Park, Md.
	Washington Hospital Center, Washington, D.C.

GYNECOLOGY

TIER ONE	
1	Johns Hopkins Hospital, Baltimore
TIER TWO	
34	Georgetown University Hospital, Washington, D.C.
82	Sinai Hospital of Baltimore, Baltimore
51	University of Maryland Medical System, Baltimore
TIER THREE	
	Alexandria Hospital, Alexandria, Va.
100	Anne Arundel Medical Center, Annapolis, Md.
87	Fairfax Hospital, Falls Church, Va.
92	George Washington University Hospital, Washington, D.C.
89	Greater Baltimore Medical Center
	Harbor Hospital Center, Baltimore
	Holy Cross Hospital, Silver Spring, Md.
	Howard University Hospital, Washington, D.C.
	Mercy Medical Center, Baltimore
	Northwest Hospital Center, Randallstown, Md.
	St. Agnes Hospital, Baltimore
	Washington Adventist Hospital, Takoma Park, Md.
	Washington County Hospital Assn., Hagerstown, Md.
TIER FOUR	
	Arlington Hospital, Arlington, Va.
	Francis Scott Key Medical Center, Baltimore
	Franklin Square Hospital Center, Baltimore
	Good Samaritan Hospital, Baltimore
	Greater Southeast Community Hospital, Washington, D.C.
	Mary Washington Hospital, Fredericksburg, Va.
	Maryland General Hospital, Baltimore
	Prince George's Hospital Center, Cheverly, Md.
	Providence Hospital, Washington, D.C.
	Sibley Memorial Hospital, Washington, D.C.

	Suburban Hospital, Bethesda, Md.
	Union Memorial Hospital, Baltimore
	Washington Hospital Center, Washington, D.C.

NEUROLOGY

TIER ONE	
2	Johns Hopkins Hospital, Baltimore
25	Georgetown University Hospital, Washington, D.C.
TIER TWO	
37	George Washington University Hospital, Washington, D.C.
67	Greater Baltimore Medical Center
40	University of Maryland Medical System, Baltimore
TIER THREE	
	Alexandria Hospital, Alexandria, Va.
	Anne Arundel Medical Center, Annapolis, Md.
97	Fairfax Hospital, Falls Church, Va.
	Franklin Square Hospital Center, Baltimore
	Harbor Hospital Center, Baltimore
	Holy Cross Hospital, Silver Spring, Md.
	Howard County General Hospital, Columbia, Md.
	Howard University Hospital, Washington, D.C.
	Maryland General Hospital, Baltimore
	Mercy Medical Center, Baltimore
	Northwest Hospital Center, Randallstown, Md.
	Sinai Hospital of Baltimore, Baltimore
	St. Agnes Hospital, Baltimore
	Washington Adventist Hospital, Takoma Park, Md.
TIER FOUR	
	Arlington Hospital, Arlington, Va.
	Francis Scott Key Medical Center, Baltimore
	Good Samaritan Hospital, Baltimore
	Greater Southeast Community Hospital, Washington, D.C.
	Mary Washington Hospital, Fredericksburg, Va.
	Prince George's Hospital Center, Cheverly, Md.
	Providence Hospital, Washington, D.C.
	Sibley Memorial Hospital, Washington, D.C.
	Suburban Hospital, Bethesda, Md.
	Union Memorial Hospital, Baltimore
	Washington County Hospital Assn., Hagerstown, Md.
	Washington Hospital Center, Washington, D.C.

ORTHOPEDICS

TIER ONE	
4	Johns Hopkins Hospital, Baltimore
TIER TWO	
39	Georgetown University Hospital, Washington, D.C.
71	Sinai Hospital of Baltimore, Baltimore
69	University of Maryland Medical System, Baltimore
TIER THREE	
	Anne Arundel Medical Center, Annapolis, Md.
	Fairfax Hospital, Falls Church, Va.
	Francis Scott Key Medical Center, Baltimore

Natl. Rank	Hospital
	George Washington University Hospital, Washington, D.C.
	Good Samaritan Hospital, Baltimore
	Greater Baltimore Medical Center
	Harbor Hospital Center, Baltimore
	Holy Cross Hospital, Silver Spring, Md.
	Mercy Medical Center, Baltimore
	Northwest Hospital Center, Randallstown, Md.
	St. Agnes Hospital, Baltimore
	Washington County Hospital Assn., Hagerstown, Md.
TIER FOUR	
	Alexandria Hospital, Alexandria, Va.
	Arlington Hospital, Arlington, Va.
	Fair Oaks Hospital, Fairfax, Va.
	Franklin Square Hospital Center, Baltimore
	Greater Southeast Community Hospital, Washington, D.C.
	Howard County General Hospital, Columbia, Md.
	Mary Washington Hospital, Fredericksburg, Va.
	Prince George's Hospital Center, Cheverly, Md.
	Providence Hospital, Washington, D.C.
	Sibley Memorial Hospital, Washington, D.C.
	Suburban Hospital, Bethesda, Md.
	Union Memorial Hospital, Baltimore
	Washington Adventist Hospital, Takoma Park, Md.
	Washington Hospital Center, Washington, D.C.

OTOLARYNGOLOGY

Natl. Rank	Hospital
TIER ONE	
1	Johns Hopkins Hospital, Baltimore
TIER TWO	
43	George Washington University Hospital, Washington, D.C.
73	Georgetown University Hospital, Washington, D.C.
96	Howard University Hospital, Washington, D.C.
37	University of Maryland Medical System, Baltimore
TIER THREE	
	District of Columbia General Hospital, Washington, D.C.
	Fairfax Hospital, Falls Church, Va.
	Francis Scott Key Medical Center, Baltimore
	Franklin Square Hospital Center, Baltimore
	Greater Baltimore Medical Center
	Holy Cross Hospital, Silver Spring, Md.
	Sinai Hospital of Baltimore, Baltimore
	Washington Hospital Center, Washington, D.C.
TIER FOUR	
	Alexandria Hospital, Alexandria, Va.
	Anne Arundel Medical Center, Annapolis, Md.
	Arlington Hospital, Arlington, Va.
	Deaton Hospital and Medical Center, Baltimore
	Fair Oaks Hospital, Fairfax, Va.
	Good Samaritan Hospital, Baltimore
	Greater Southeast Community Hospital, Washington, D.C.
	Harbor Hospital Center, Baltimore
	Howard County General Hospital, Columbia, Md.
	Mary Washington Hospital, Fredericksburg, Va.
	Maryland General Hospital, Baltimore
	Mercy Medical Center, Baltimore

Natl. Rank	Hospital
	Northern Virginia Doctors' Hospital, Arlington, Va.
	Northwest Hospital Center, Randallstown, Md.
	Prince George's Hospital Center, Cheverly, Md.
	Providence Hospital, Washington, D.C.
	Sibley Memorial Hospital, Washington, D.C.
	St. Agnes Hospital, Baltimore
	Suburban Hospital, Bethesda, Md.
	Union Memorial Hospital, Baltimore
	Washington Adventist Hospital, Takoma Park, Md.
	Washington County Hospital Assn., Hagerstown, Md.

RHEUMATOLOGY

Natl. Rank	Hospital
TIER ONE	
2	Johns Hopkins Hospital, Baltimore
TIER TWO	
36	George Washington University Hospital, Washington, D.C.
47	Georgetown University Hospital, Washington, D.C.
45	University of Maryland Medical System, Baltimore
TIER THREE	
	Anne Arundel Medical Center, Annapolis, Md.
	Fairfax Hospital, Falls Church, Va.
	Francis Scott Key Medical Center, Baltimore
	Franklin Square Hospital Center, Baltimore
	Good Samaritan Hospital, Baltimore
	Greater Baltimore Medical Center
	Harbor Hospital Center, Baltimore
	Holy Cross Hospital, Silver Spring, Md.
	Howard University Hospital, Washington, D.C.
	Mercy Medical Center, Baltimore
96	Sinai Hospital of Baltimore, Baltimore
	Washington Hospital Center, Washington, D.C.
TIER FOUR	
	Alexandria Hospital, Alexandria, Va.
	Arlington Hospital, Arlington, Va.
	Greater Southeast Community Hospital, Washington, D.C.
	Howard County General Hospital, Columbia, Md.
	Mary Washington Hospital, Fredericksburg, Va.
	Maryland General Hospital, Baltimore
	Northwest Hospital Center, Randallstown, Md.
	Prince George's Hospital Center, Cheverly, Md.
	Providence Hospital, Washington, D.C.
	Sibley Memorial Hospital, Washington, D.C.
	St. Agnes Hospital, Baltimore
	Suburban Hospital, Bethesda, Md.
	Union Memorial Hospital, Baltimore
	Washington Adventist Hospital, Takoma Park, Md.
	Washington County Hospital Assn., Hagerstown, Md.

METRO RANKINGS ■ WASHINGTON, D.C.

UROLOGY

Natl.
Rank   Hospital

TIER ONE	
1	Johns Hopkins Hospital, Baltimore
TIER TWO	
75	Howard University Hospital, Washington, D.C.
59	University of Maryland Medical System, Baltimore
TIER THREE	
	Anne Arundel Medical Center, Annapolis, Md.
	Fairfax Hospital, Falls Church, Va.
	Francis Scott Key Medical Center, Baltimore
	Franklin Square Hospital Center, Baltimore
95	George Washington University Hospital, Washington, D.C.
	Georgetown University Hospital, Washington, D.C.
	Greater Baltimore Medical Center
	Harbor Hospital Center, Baltimore
	Maryland General Hospital, Baltimore
	Mercy Medical Center, Baltimore
	Sinai Hospital of Baltimore, Baltimore
	Washington Hospital Center, Washington, D.C.
TIER FOUR	
	Alexandria Hospital, Alexandria, Va.
	Arlington Hospital, Arlington, Va.
	Good Samaritan Hospital, Baltimore
	Greater Southeast Community Hospital, Washington, D.C.
	Holy Cross Hospital, Silver Spring, Md.
	Howard County General Hospital, Columbia, Md.
	Mary Washington Hospital, Fredericksburg, Va.
	Northern Virginia Doctors' Hospital, Arlington, Va.
	Northwest Hospital Center, Randallstown, Md.
	Prince George's Hospital Center, Cheverly, Md.
	Providence Hospital, Washington, D.C.
	Sibley Memorial Hospital, Washington, D.C.
	St. Agnes Hospital, Baltimore
	Suburban Hospital, Bethesda, Md.
	Union Memorial Hospital, Baltimore
	Washington Adventist Hospital, Takoma Park, Md.
	Washington County Hospital Assn., Hagerstown, Md.

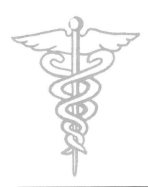

Subject Index

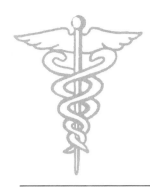

Hospital Index

SPECIAL INTRODUCTORY OFFER

☐ **YES,** send me 30 weeks of *U.S. News* and my FREE *Family Health Almanac* for only $15 — all at a savings of 83% off the cover price.

_____
Name

_____
Address

_____
City   State   Zip

☐ Payment Enclosed   ☐ Bill Me

Clip & mail to:
U.S. News Subscription Dept.
P.O. Box 55929
Boulder, CO 80322-5929

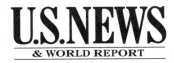

U.S.NEWS
& WORLD REPORT

59BR

FREE HEATH ALMANAC
with your subscription

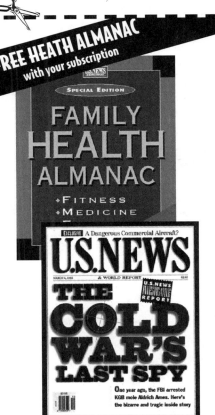

SPECIAL EDITION

FAMILY HEALTH ALMANAC
+FITNESS
+MEDICINE

EXCLUSIVE A Dangerous Commercial Aircraft?

U.S.NEWS
& WORLD REPORT

MARCH 6, 1995

THE COLD WAR'S LAST SPY

One year ago, the FBI arrested KGB mole Aldrich Ames. Here's the bizarre and tragic inside story

SAVE 83%*

on *U.S. News* and get the *Family Health Almanac* absolutely FREE.

The *Family Health Almanac* is a practical guide to everyday nutrition, fitness and medicine. Discover the latest finds in medicine, including new warnings about prescription drugs and the latest treatments for cancer and heart disease. PLUS, you get family medical record worksheets, a fitness planner and delicious low-fat recipes.

Subscribe now to *U.S.News* and get great savings -- 83% off the cover price. You'll also get intelligent news coverage and exclusive *News You Can Use*® about your health, home, career, education and personal finances.

*OFF THE COVER PRICE

Price offer and free gift subject to availability

Getting The Most From *U.S. News* Is As Easy As:

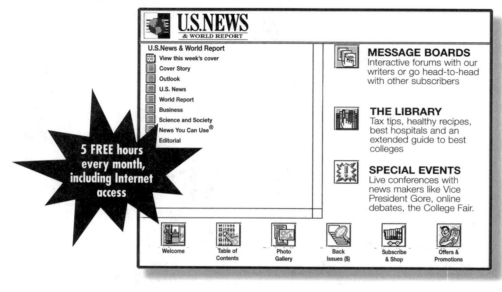

5 FREE hours every month, including Internet access

MESSAGE BOARDS
Interactive forums with our writers or go head-to-head with other subscribers

THE LIBRARY
Tax tips, healthy recipes, best hospitals and an extended guide to best colleges

SPECIAL EVENTS
Live conferences with news makers like Vice President Gore, online debates, the College Fair.

CompuServe®

U.S.NEWS ONLINE

1. To order simply complete and mail the card below or call 1-800-487-6227 and ask for the *U.S. News* representative. If you're wired, go to http://www.compuserve.com.

YOUR FIRST MONTH OF MEMBERSHIP IS FREE!

2. Next, you'll get everything you'll need to get started with U.S. News Online. You'll connect with the *U.S. News* forums, with writers, a library of useful information, access to *U.S. News* back issues, maps, photos and more! Plus, access to 3,000 services and the Internet.

3. Your first month of membership is FREE and you'll get ten hours to explore the service. Then, for just $9.95 a month you'll receive:
- 5 FREE hours. Additional hours only $2.95 each.
- Ask about our Super Value Plan.
